Th... te D... or R... n Ra... ers

A ... de
to O ... rders
from ... zation
for Rare Disorders, Inc.

Disorder Descriptions

Books, Newsletters, Journals

Grey House Publishing

LAKEVILLE, CT 06039

Publisher/Editor : Leslie E. Mackenzie

National Organization for
Rare Disorders, Inc. (NORD)
Editors : Joy E. Bartnett
Debra L. Madden
Robert P. Tomaino

Grey House Publishing

Published by Grey House Publishing, Inc.
Pocket Knife Square
Lakeville, CT 06039
860 • 435 • 0868
FAX 860 • 435 • 0867

Library of Congress Cataloging in Publication Data Available

ISBN 0-939300-98-2

1998/99

The Complete Directory for People with Rare Disorders

TABLE OF CONTENTS

Introduction to The National Organization for Rare Disorders Mission Statement

The National Organization for Rare Disorders, Inc. (NORD) is the unique federation of voluntary health organizations dedicated to helping people with rare "orphan" diseases and assisting the organizations that serve them. NORD is committed to the identification, treatment, and cure of rare disorders through programs of education, advocacy, research, and service.

What is a Rare or "Orphan" Disorder?

An "orphan disease" is any disorder that affects fewer than 200,000 people in the United States. There are more than 5,000 rare disorders that, taken together, affect approximately 20 million Americans. One in every 12 people in the United States has a rare disease.

A Message from NORD's President, Abbey S. Meyers

Fifteen years ago, a small group of dedicated individuals who were devoted to finding treatments and cures for rare "orphan diseases" decided to create the National Organization for Rare Disorders (NORD). They saw needs that were not being met by any other government or private agencies. They knew that the most pressing need was for medical information that had always been impossible to locate and difficult to understand for most families. They knew that they would have to put their individual differences aside to work for the common good, because together they could accomplish so much more than they would ever do alone.

So many people with disabilities rely on NORD's assistance, leadership, and multitude of services. Fifteen years later, we can be proud of NORD's accomplishments...the millions of people we have helped and the lives we have touched...simply because the vision remains in our hearts. We know that *The Complete Directory for People with Rare Disorders* will continue to help us make a difference.

What is NORD?

NORD is the only organization of its kind: a federation of more than 140 not-for-profit health organizations serving people with rare disorders. Each year, hundreds of thousands of affected individuals and their families--as well as support groups, health care and human service professionals, and advocates for people with disabilities--rely on NORD's assistance, leadership, and multitude of services.

NORD's Programs and Services

<u>*Information and Referral Services*</u>

NORD's primary goal is to educate the public as well as the medical community by serving as an international clearinghouse for information on rare "orphan" diseases. NORD provides information about orphan diseases as well as referrals to additional sources of information, assistance, and services to affected individuals, family members, medical professionals, researchers, educators, social workers, medical libraries, corporations, and the general public. For these purposes, NORD offers the following:

- ➢NORD's Rare Disease Database (RDB) provides information in understandable, lay terminology on over 1,100 rare disorders.
- ➢NORD's Abstract Database provides concise overviews of certain rare disorders. These abstracts are published on NORD's website at <http://www.nord-rdb.com/~orphan>.
- ➢NORD's Organizational Database (ODB), created in part with the National Institutes of Health (NIH), contains information on approximately 1,600 disease-specific and umbrella organizations, support groups, agencies, clearinghouses, registries, and other organizations that serve the needs of individuals with rare disorders or disabilities.
- ➢NORD's Orphan Drug Designation Database (ODD) provides information on drugs that have received FDA orphan drug designations including their trade and generic names, the disorder the drug has been designated for, the pharmaceutical company sponsor, etc.

➢ Special Rare Disease Publications for Physicians including the *Physicians' Guide to Rare Diseases*, a printed version of the RDB written in medical terminology for physicians and other health care professionals that is produced in association with Dowden Publishing Company.

NORD's Family Networking Program
NORD's Family Networking Program puts individuals and/or family members that are affected by the same rare disorders in touch with one another. In addition to promoting mutual support and the exchange of information, networking promotes the formation of new voluntary agencies for specific diseases.

NORD's Medication Assistance Programs
During NORD's 15 years of service, it has been dedicated to creating new innovative services to help fulfill the diverse needs of the medically disenfranchised. For example, NORD's Medication Assistance Programs provide certain prescription pharmaceuticals to needy patients who cannot afford to purchase them. In general, these are life-sustaining drugs for chronic conditions that must be used for the remainder of a patient's life. In addition, NORD runs early access programs for certain investigational drugs that are on the FDA Express Approval Track as well as limited and/or emergency access programs for certain vital medications that are in limited supply.

Research
There continues to be a serious shortage of funding for clinical research on orphan diseases. NORD attempts to fill this void by funding seed grants for new treatments for rare disorders, advocating for increased government research funds, and referring affected individuals to clinical trials and genetic investigations. NORD's funding and advocacy have enabled researchers to develop breakthrough treatments that have dramatically improved the length and quality of life for thousands of children and adults with rare disorders.

Patient Services
NORD's Patient Services Department counsels and advises affected individuals and family members who need assistance in accessing benefits and services in their local communities.

Advocacy
NORD continues to play a vital, prominent role in Washington, D.C. advocating for public policy issues on behalf of families with rare diseases, particularly when government programs and policies do not adequately address their needs.

Development and Fundraising
As a private charity that receives no government funding, NORD relies on the generosity of individual donors to fulfill its vitally important mission. Individuals can support NORD by becoming a member...playing an essential role in enabling the organization to continue its essential work for all individuals with rare disorders.

NORD Field Services and Chapter Development
NORD provides technical assistance to support groups and voluntary health agencies, helping them avoid duplication and maximize effectiveness. NORD's Field Services also helps develop local chapters that serve as regional support systems for individuals and family members affected by rare disorders. Run by local NORD members, these chapters offer a forum for increased understanding, more personalized, individualized, support and information exchange, and local networking.

How Congress Works: A Guide for Rare Disorder Advocates
Prepared by Michael S. Langan, NORD's Vice President of Public Policy

Introduction

Our representative system of government places a special responsibility on each of us to make ourselves heard in Washington. In fact, no more important source of information is available to members of Congress than the people who live and work in their State or district. As a constituent, you represent more than an abstract theme or a statistic. You offer personal experiences that make you uniquely qualified to talk about the issues that matter most to you--issues such as health care reform, Medicaid, rare disease research, and orphan drug development.

The more effectively you communicate with your elected officials, the more effective the representative system of government becomes. But to be effective requires more than a willingness to get involved. It requires a good understanding of how the policy-making process works and who the key players are. But most importantly, it requires that you know when your contact with lawmakers can have the greatest impact on the decision-making process. Because no matter how compelling your message is, it will count for little if decisions have already been made.

This guide will outline a common-sense approach to understanding the legislative decision-making process. While I'll offer some general tips on getting your point across to members of Congress, my primary goal is to give you - the rare disease advocate - basic information about the legislative process, how it works, and when you can have the greatest impact on the decisions that affect the lives of children and adults with orphan diseases.

The Legislative Process

To the average person, the process of getting a bill through Congress appears highly complex and technical. Actually, the process itself is fairly simple. What can be confusing to the lay person is (1) the volume of legislation pending before Congress and (2) the system Congress has for distributing its work. It is true that a great deal of legislation is handled by Congress each year. But only a handful of bills are of particular interest to the orphan disease community. So long as you keep your sights on the legislation dealing only with orphan disease-related issues, you should have no trouble following the progress of those bills. And once you familiarize yourself with the key committees responsible for handling rare disease-related issues, following the progress of legislation will become much easier.

The key to deciphering the legislative process is in understanding that legislation is grouped into three main categories. Authorizing legislation is a bill that creates a new federal program or extends the life of an existing program. Authorizing bills usually set a ceiling on the maximum amount of funds that can be spent by a program for a period of 3 to 5 years. An authorizing bill only establishes a framework for a federal program--it does not provide funds to operate the program. This year, Congress is scheduled to review at least 2 orphan disease-related authorizing laws: the National Institutes of Health authorization that funds medical research and a number of amendments to the Food, Drug and Cosmetic Act, under the name of "FDA reform."

An appropriations bill allocates funding for specific federal programs. Unlike authorizing legislation which remains in effect for 3 or more years, an appropriations bill must be enacted into law every year. A good example is the health appropriations bill that provides funding for research into rare disorders.

The third type of bill is entitlement legislation. This is a measure that guarantees a certain level of benefits to persons who meet eligibility requirements set by law. The Medicare and Medicaid programs are examples of existing entitlement programs. An example of entitlement legislation that the National Organization for Rare Disorders (NORD) is currently tracking is the effort in Congress to shift primary responsibility for Medicaid to the states.

Laying the Groundwork: The Role of Individual Members of Congress

Generally speaking, the earlier you get involved, the better your chances of having an impact on decision-making. The further along a bill advances in the legislative process, the more difficult it becomes to change or modify. This is especially true now that Congress often groups several issues into one bill.

The first formal step in the legislative process occurs when a bill is introduced by one or more members of Congress. But from an advocate's perspective, the work begins much earlier than that. For example, once NORD has identified an issue or a problem that merits special attention--like the need for coordination of rare disease research--our Washington office will select one or two members of Congress whose philosophy and voting record indicate that they would be willing to play a leadership role in supporting the issue. After extensive discussions with the senator or representative and their staff, formal legislation is prepared for introduction. Bills introduced in the House are assigned an "H.R." number (e.g., H.R.2027) and bills introduced in the Senate are given an "S." number.

Of course, having legislation introduced and getting it enacted into law are two different things. In order to prevent a bill from languishing in someone's files requires that we demonstrate broad support for the issue. In order to do that, NORD member organizations, and individual members, must contact their own senators and representatives and ask them to cosponsor the bill. The way that is done is by having the lawmaker's staff contact the original sponsor and ask to have his or her name listed as supporting the bill.

The Importance of the Committee System

Congressional committees are the "workhorses" of Congress. As the number of issues brought before Congress grows, lawmakers increasingly rely on the committee system to sift through the facts and determine how issues should be resolved.

Currently, there are 17 standing committees in the Senate and 19 in the House of Representatives. Both chambers also maintain certain select committees. Generally, standing committees have the power to generate legislation in their particular areas of jurisdiction, like tax-writing or appropriations. Select committees, like the Senate Special Committee on Aging, are primarily advisory in nature.

Most committees have delegated specific issues under their jurisdiction to subcommittees, whose job it is to analyze each issue and eventually make a recommendation to their parent committee, or full committee as it is sometimes called. Here again, it is vitally important that contact be made with the subcommittees as early in the process as possible.

In their earliest stages of review, subcommittees welcome input from interested organizations and individuals. At this point, letters and personal visits with members of the subcommittee and their staff can have a tremendous effect on the panel's recommendations. In many instances, a subcommittee will hold public hearings, either in Washington, D.C. or some other region of the country, where NORD member organizations may ask to present their positions. If your senator or representative is not on the subcommittee, does that mean you have no influence over the outcome?

It is true that members of a subcommittee are regarded as "specialists" by their colleagues and therefore can wield considerable power in deciding whether or not a bill will be advanced through the legislative process. However, your own senators or representatives, whether or not they are on the subcommittee, can often be effective intermediaries, depending on their personal or political relationships with the subcommittee members.

Floor Action

Once legislation has been approved by a committee, it becomes eligible for debate on the House and Senate floors, where it may be passed, defeated, or amended significantly.

When orphan disease-related legislation is about to be debated, NORD notifies member organizations of the need for communications with senators or representatives. Since floor debates are often scheduled on short notice, patient advocates are encouraged to prepare their messages (e.g., letters, telephone calls, etc.) well in advance. However, keep in mind that timing is extremely critical. Any communications about legislation that is coming up for floor debate should arrive as close to the time of voting as possible.

Conference Action

If the House and Senate pass different versions of the same bill, a handful of members from each chamber will be named to a conference committee where they will attempt to work out a compromise. Representation on the conference committee will usually consist of selected members of the House and Senate subcommittees that originally developed the legislation. In some instances, conference committees may only need to resolve a few issues. In the case of appropriations bills, there may be more than one hundred different items to be resolved. Orphan disease patient advocates whose senators or representatives happen to be on a conference committee can play a crucial role in the deliberations. Usually, NORD will contact selected member organizations and ask them to target their communications on members of the conference committee. But here again, the timing of your communications is very important because most conference committees meet for only one or two days. The end product of the meetings is a conference report containing the compromise bill and usually a section-by-section explanation of the compromise that was agreed on. Once the conference report is agreed to by both the House and Senate, the measure is sent to the President for approval (or veto).

The Importance of Staff Contacts

Lastly, while senators and representatives are the ultimate decision-makers, it is important to recognize that staff can have significant influence over the course and content of legislation. Rare disease advocates are urged to maintain ongoing contacts with these individuals, especially subcommittee staff and the lawmakers' own legislative aides. When the time comes to contact a lawmaker about specific orphan disease-related legislation, your staff contact should also be notified. This is one way of insuring that our issues are not lost or overlooked among the stack of legislation that is discussed every day. Also, keep in mind that every senator and representative maintains an office(s) in his or her home state. These district offices offer an excellent opportunity to build relationships with key staff, channel the latest rare disorder-related information back to senators and representatives, and generally get your message across to the legislator.

Glossary of Congressional Terms

The following is a listing of terms commonly used in connection with the legislative process.

➢ Act - The term for legislation that has been passed by Congress and signed into law by the President.
➢ Amendment - The proposal of a member of Congress to alter the wording of a bill being considered by a subcommittee, committee, or on the House or Senate floor. Amendments can also be offered to add or delete entire sections of a bill.
➢ Appropriation - Legislation that directs the spending of funds from the federal treasury for a specific purpose, e.g., funding for rare disorder research. By custom, an appropriations bill originates in the House, where it is assigned an H.R. number (e.g., H.R.2027) until it becomes law or is vetoed by the President. Typically, each appropriations bill includes funding for several hundred federal programs.
➢ Authorization - A law creating a new federal program or extending the life of an existing program. An authorization establishes the framework for operating a federal program, and usually sets the maximum amount of funds that can be given to a program for a period of 3 to 5 years. Under the rules of Congress, an authorization must be enacted into law before appropriations can be made to the program.
➢ Bill - A proposed law introduced by a member(s) of Congress.
➢ Budget - The document the President sends to Congress each year outlining federal expenditures and revenues for the upcoming fiscal year. The President's budget is usually submitted to Congress in late January or early February.

- Budget Resolution - Legislation passed by Congress each year which sets overall limits on spending and revenues. Congressional committees use the budget resolution as a guide for allocating funds to specific federal programs. The budget resolution does not require the President's approval.
- Conference - A meeting between House and Senate members to reconcile differences between bills passed by their respective chambers of Congress. Once a compromise has been ironed out a conference report is issued and voted on by the full House and Senate. The measure is then sent to the President for approval.
- Continuing Resolution - An emergency appropriations bill providing funding for federal agencies whose regular appropriations bills have not been passed before the end of the fiscal year.
- Entitlement - A federal program that guarantees a certain level of benefits to persons who meet requirements set by law, such as Social Security and unemployment benefits. Congress and the President generally have very little discretion over spending by these programs.
- Fiscal Year - For the federal government, the fiscal year runs from October 1 through September 30.
- Hearings - Committee meetings where testimony is taken from witnesses representing government agencies, private sector organizations, and the general public. Most congressional hearings are open to the public. Hearings may be held in Washington, D.C. or in local communities.
- Mark-Up - A subcommittee or committee meeting for the purpose of writing legislation. Once completed, the measure is ready for debate on the floor of the House or Senate.
- Public Law - A bill after it has been passed by the House and Senate and subsequently approved by the President.
- Reconciliation Bill - Legislation that contains changes (usually spending cuts) to existing laws so as to conform--or reconcile--with policies adopted in the budget resolution.
- Rescission - The act of canceling appropriations already enacted into law.
- Standing Committee - A committee that is permanently established by House and Senate rules. Standing committees are empowered to prepare and review legislation. (As opposed to select committees, which serve only to advise Congress on a limited range of issues.)
- Veto - The President's formal disapproval of legislation passed by Congress. When Congress is in session, the President must veto a bill within 10 days after receiving it from Congress, otherwise it becomes law without his approval. A bill can become law after a Presidential veto if two-thirds of Congress vote to override the veto.

1 **5 OXOPROLINURIA**

5-Oxoprolinuria is a metabolic disorder caused by an inborn error of glutathione metabolism. It is characterized by excretion of massive amounts of 5-oxoproline (pyroglutamic acid) in the urine, and abnormally high levels of this acid in the blood and cerebrospinal fluid. The disorder is caused by a deficiency of the enzyme glutathione synthetase. Functioning of the central nervous system is impaired. High acidity levels in the blood and body tissues (metabolic acidosis) usually occur.

In addition to The National Organization for Rare Disorders (NORD) listed in Section III, the following organizations in Section II (Disease Specific) and in Section III (Umbrella) and Section IV (Government Agencies) can provide more information:

Metabolic Information Network, *III*
NIH/National Institute of Neurological Disorders and Stroke, *IV*
Research Trust for Metabolic Diseases in Children, *III*
The Arc (a national organization on mental retardation), *III*

2 **ACTH DEFICIENCY**

ACTH Deficiency is characterized by adrenal insufficiency symptoms such as weight loss, lack of appetite (anorexia), weakness, nausea, vomiting, and low blood pressure (hypotension). The pituitary hormone called "adrenocorticotropic hormone" (ACTH) is decreased or absent, and other cortisol and other steroid hormone levels in the blood are abnormally low.

In addition to The National Organization for Rare Disorders (NORD) listed in Section III, the following organizations in Section II (Disease Specific) and in Section III (Umbrella) and Section IV (Government Agencies) can provide more information:

Brain and Pituitary Foundation of America, *III*
NIH/National Institute of Diabetes, Digestive and Kidney Diseases, *IV*
National Adrenal Diseases Foundation, *III*

3 **AIDS (ACQUIRED IMMUNE DEFICIENCY SYNDROME)**

AIDS is an infectious disorder that suppresses the normal function of the immune system. It is caused by the human immunodeficiency virus (HIV), which destroys the body's ability to fight infections. Specific cells of the immune system that are responsible for the proper response to infections (T cells) are destroyed by this virus. Characteristically a person infected with HIV initially experiences no symptoms for a long period of time. This may be followed by the development of persistent generalized swelling of the lymph nodes (AIDS-related lymphadenopathy). Eventually most patients infected with HIV experience a syndrome of symptoms that includes excessive fatigue, weight loss, and/or skin rashes.

The later stages of HIV infection are characterized by the progressive depression of T cells and infections that can even occur during a course of antibiotic therapy for another infection (superinfections). People with AIDS are particularly vulnerable to "opportunistic infections" from bacteria that other people normally fight off. Pneumocystis carinii, which causes severe inflammation of the lungs (pneumonia), is a common infection that effects people with AIDS. Cancers (malignant neoplasms), and a wide variety of neurological abnormalities, most notably the AIDS dementia complex, may also be present. These neurological symptoms appear to be a direct result of HIV infection of the nervous system.

In addition to The National Organization for Rare Disorders (NORD) listed in Section III, the following organizations in Section II (Disease Specific) and in Section III (Umbrella) and Section IV (Government Agencies) can provide more information:

AmFAR—American Foundation for AIDS Research, *II*
American Social Health Association, *III*
CDC Business Responds to AIDS and Labor Responds to AIDS, *II*
Centers for Disease Control and Prevention, *IV*
HIV/AIDS Treatment Information Service, *IV*
NIH/National Institute of Allergy and Infectious Diseases, *IV*
Sexuality Information and Education Council of the U.S., *III*

4 **AIDS DYSMORPHIC SYNDROME**

AIDS Dysmorphic Syndrome is an inborn infectious disorder affecting children. The AIDS virus (HIV virus) is transmitted to a fetus during pregnancy by an infected woman who may or may not have any symptoms of AIDS. AIDS Dysmorphic Syndrome is characterized by the development of abnormal facial and skull features. In addition, children with this disorder usually experience delays in physical and mental development. The virus is thought to act directly on the central nervous system. The basic characteristic of AIDS (Acquired Immune Deficiency Syndrome) is a severely impaired immune system. Children with AIDS Dysmorphic Syndrome are extremely susceptible to infections by bacteria and viruses, especially a form of pneumonia caused by the Pneumocystis carinii bacterium. However, treatment with intravenous gamma globulin (IGIV) and the drug azidothymidine (AZT) may be beneficial to children with Dysmorphic AIDS.

In addition to The National Organization for Rare Disorders (NORD) listed in Section III, the following organizations in Section II (Disease Specific) and in Section III (Umbrella) and Section IV (Government Agencies) can provide more information:
AmFAR—American Foundation for AIDS Research, *II*
Centers for Disease Control and Prevention, *IV*
NIH/National Institute of Allergy and Infectious Diseases, *IV*
The Arc (a national organization on mental retardation), *III*

5 APECED SYNDROME

APECED Syndrome is a very rare genetic syndrome involving the autoimmune system. It is a combination of several distinct disorders. APECED stands for Autoimmune Polyendocrinopathy (APE), Candidiasis (C) and Ectodermal Dysplasia (ED). Major symptoms may include low calcium and phosphate levels in the blood (hypoparathyroidism), lack of tooth enamel (enamel dystrophy), loss of hair (alopecia) and absence of pigment in areas of the skin (vitiligo). An eye disorder, corneal dystrophy (keratopathy), may also occur. There may be failure of sexual development, yeast infections of the mouth and nails (candidiasis), and the inability to properly absorb nutrients from food (malabsorption). Patients may develop liver disease or insulin- dependent diabetes as well as any combination of the various disorders.

In addition to The National Organization for Rare Disorders (NORD) listed in Section III, the following organizations in Section II (Disease Specific) and in Section III (Umbrella) and Section IV (Government Agencies) can provide more information:
American Lung Association, *III*
NIH/National Digestive Diseases Information Clearinghouse, *IV*
National Adrenal Diseases Foundation, *III*
National Foundation for Ectodermal Dysplasias, *II*

6 AARSKOG SYNDROME

Aarskog Syndrome is an extremely rare genetic disorder marked by distinctive structural abnormalities. Major symptoms may include stunted growth, broad facial features, short broad hands and feet, genital abnormalities, and mild mental retardation.

In addition to The National Organization for Rare Disorders (NORD) listed in Section III, the following organizations in Section II (Disease Specific) and in Section III (Umbrella) and Section IV (Government Agencies) can provide more information:
Aarskog Syndrome Parents Support Group, *II*
NIH/National Institute of Child Health and Human Development, *IV*

7 AASE SYNDROME

Aase Syndrome is a rare congenital disorder characterized by low levels of red blood cells (hypoplastic anemia) accompanied by the presence of an extra bone and joint in the thumb (triphalangeal thumb). Other abnormalities may also occur.

In addition to The National Organization for Rare Disorders (NORD) listed in Section III, the following organizations in Section II (Disease Specific) and in Section III (Umbrella) and Section IV (Government Agencies) can provide more information:
March of Dimes Birth Defects Foundation, *III*
NIH/National Heart, Lung and Blood Institute, *IV*
NIH/National Institute of Child Health and Human Development, *IV*

8 ABLEPHARON MACROSTOMIA SYNDROME

Ablepharon-Macrostomia Syndrome (AMS) is an extremely rare inherited disorder characterized by various physical abnormalities affecting the head and facial (craniofacial) area, the skin, the fingers, and the genitals. In addition, affected individuals may have malformations of the nipples and the abdominal wall. Infants and children with AMS may also experience delays in language development and, in some cases, mental retardation.

In infants with Ablepharon-Macrostomia Syndrome, characteristic craniofacial features may include absence or severe underdevelopment of the upper and lower eyelids (ablepharon or microblepharon) as well as absence of eyelashes and eyebrows; an unusually wide, "fish-like" mouth (macrostomia); and/or incompletely developed (rudimentary), low-set ears (pinnae). Abnormalities of the eyes may occur due to or in association with ablepharon or microblepharon. Individuals with AMS may also have additional characteristic features including abnormally sparse, thin hair; coarse, dry, unusually thickened skin with excess (redundant) folds;

webbed fingers with limited extension; and/or malformations of the external genitals. In some cases, additional features associated with AMS may include absent or abnormally small (hypoplastic) nipples and/or protrusion of portions of the large intestine through an abnormal opening in the abdominal wall (abdominal or ventral hernia). Although the exact cause of Ablepharon-Macrostomia Syndrome is not fully understood, some cases suggest that the disorder may be inherited as an autosomal recessive genetic trait.

In addition to The National Organization for Rare Disorders (NORD) listed in Section III, the following organizations in Section II (Disease Specific) and in Section III (Umbrella) and Section IV (Government Agencies) can provide more information:
Ambiguous Genitalia Support Network, *III*
Children's Craniofacial Association, *III*
FACES: The National Craniofacial Association, *III*
Forward Face, Inc., *III*
NIH/National Eye Institute, *IV*
NIH/National Institute of Arthritis and Musculoskeletal and Skin Diseases, *IV*
NIH/National Institute of Child Health and Human Development, *IV*

9 **ACANTHOCHEILONEMIASIS**

Acanthocheilonemiasis is a rare tropical infectious disease caused by a parasite known as Acanthocheilonema perstans, which belongs to a group of parasitic diseases known as filarial diseases (nematode). This parasite is found, for the most part, in Africa. Symptoms of infection may include red, itchy skin (pruritis), abdominal and chest pain, muscular pain (myalgia), and areas of localized swelling (edema). In addition, the liver and spleen may become abnormally enlarged (hepatosplenomegaly). Laboratory testing may also reveal abnormally elevated levels of certain specialized white blood cells (eosinophilia). The parasite is transmitted through the bite of small flies (A. coliroides).

In addition to The National Organization for Rare Disorders (NORD) listed in Section III, the following organizations in Section II (Disease Specific) and in Section III (Umbrella) and Section IV (Government Agencies) can provide more information:
Centers for Disease Control and Prevention, *IV*
NIH/National Institute of Allergy and Infectious Diseases, *IV*
World Health Organization (WHO) Regional Office for the Americas (AMRO), *III*

10 **ACANTHOCYTOSIS**

Acanthocytosis is a digestive disorder that is characterized by the absence of very low density lipoproteins (VLDL) and chylamicrons in the plasma, and fat malabsorption resulting in excessive fats excretion (steatorrhea). Other symptoms include abnormal red blood cells (acanthocytes), a vision disorder (retinitis pigmentosa), and impaired muscle coordination (ataxia).

In addition to The National Organization for Rare Disorders (NORD) listed in Section III, the following organizations in Section II (Disease Specific) and in Section III (Umbrella) and Section IV (Government Agencies) can provide more information:
Foundation Fighting Blindness, *III*
Metabolic Information Network, *III*
NIH/National Institute of Diabetes, Digestive and Kidney Diseases, *IV*
National Tay-Sachs and Allied Diseases Association, Inc., *III*
Research Trust for Metabolic Diseases in Children, *III*
Retinitis Pigmentosa International, *II*

11 **ACANTHOSIS NIGRICANS**

Acanthosis Nigricans is a rare skin disorder characterized by skin lesions that become thick (hyperkeratotic) and have a brownish-gray color (hyperpigmentation). Four types of Acanthosis Nigricans are recognized. Miescher Syndrome is an inherited benign form of Acanthosis Nigricans. Gougerot-Carteaud Syndrome is a benign, possibly inherited form of the disease that usually occurs in young adult females. Pseudoacanthosis Nigricans is a benign juvenile form that is associated with obesity and/or endocrine disorders. An adult form of Acanthosis Nigricans, known as Malignant Acanthosis, is frequently associated with cancer in another part of the body.

In addition to The National Organization for Rare Disorders (NORD) listed in Section III, the following organizations in Section II (Disease Specific) and in Section III (Umbrella) and Section IV (Government Agencies) can provide more information:
March of Dimes Birth Defects Foundation, *III*
NIH/National Institute of Arthritis and Musculoskeletal and Skin Diseases, *IV*

12 **ACHALASIA**

Achalasia is a rare disorder of the esophagus characterized by the abnormal enlargement of the esophagus, impairment of the ability of the esophagus to push food down toward the stomach (peristalsis), and the failure of the ring-shaped muscle (sphincter) at the bottom of the esophagus to relax.

In addition to The National Organization for Rare Disorders (NORD) listed in Section III, the following organizations in Section II (Disease Specific) and in Section III (Umbrella) and Section IV (Government Agencies) can provide more information:
March of Dimes Birth Defects Foundation, *III*
NIH/National Digestive Diseases Information Clearinghouse, *IV*

13 **ACHARD THIERS SYNDROME**
Achard-Thiers Syndrome is a rare disorder that affects postmenopausal women and is characterized by diabetes and the development of secondary male sexual traits (virilization). Symptoms develop due to the overproduction of male hormones (androgens) and other adrenocortical hormones (i.e., 11-oxysteroid) by the adrenal glands. If Achard-Thiers Syndrome is not treated, complications may occur including abnormally high blood pressure and heart disease.

In addition to The National Organization for Rare Disorders (NORD) listed in Section III, the following organizations in Section II (Disease Specific) and in Section III (Umbrella) and Section IV (Government Agencies) can provide more information:
NIH/National Institute of Diabetes, Digestive and Kidney Diseases, *IV*
National Adrenal Diseases Foundation, *III*

14 **ACHONDROGENESIS**
Achondrogenesis is a very rare disorder that is inherited as an autosomal recessive genetic trait. Major symptoms include extreme short limbed dwarfism, lack of development of ribs and other major bone formation. The head may be either soft or enlarged depending on the type of Achondrogenesis involved. The disorder is often fatal either in utero (in the womb) or shortly after birth.

In addition to The National Organization for Rare Disorders (NORD) listed in Section III, the following organizations in Section II (Disease Specific) and in Section III (Umbrella) and Section IV (Government Agencies) can provide more information:
Human Growth Foundation, *III*
Little People of America, *III*
Little People's Research Fund, Inc., *III*
MAGIC Foundation for Children's Growth, *III*
NIH/National Institute of Child Health and Human Development, *IV*
Short Stature Foundation, *III*

15 **ACHONDROPLASIA**
Achondroplasia is a rare genetic disorder characterized by an unusually large head (macrocephaly) with a prominent forehead (frontal bossing) and flat (depressed) nasal bridge; short upper arms and legs (rhizomelic dwarfism); unusually prominent abdomen and buttocks; and short hands with fingers that assume a "trident" or three-pronged position during extension. An autosomal dominant genetic trait, Achondroplasia occurs as a result of a fresh (new) spontaneous change (mutation) in genetic material in about 90 percent of cases. In Achondroplasia, affected individuals have impaired ability to form bone from cartilage (endochondral bone formation).

In addition to The National Organization for Rare Disorders (NORD) listed in Section III, the following organizations in Section II (Disease Specific) and in Section III (Umbrella) and Section IV (Government Agencies) can provide more information:
Alliance of Genetic Support Groups, *III*
Human Growth Foundation, *III*
Little People of America, *III*
Little People's Research Fund, Inc., *III*
MAGIC Foundation for Children's Growth, *III*
March of Dimes Birth Defects Foundation, *III*
NIH/National Arthritis and Musculoskeletal and Skin Diseases Information Clearinghouse, *IV*
Short Stature Foundation, *III*

16 **ACIDEMIA, ISOVALERIC**
Isovaleric Acidemia is a hereditary metabolic disorder. It is characterized by a deficiency of the enzyme isovaleryl CoA dehydrogenase. The disorder occurs in both an acute and a chronic intermittent form. In the acute form of Isovaleric Acidemia, vomiting, refusal to eat, and listlessness usually occur. With treatment and low protein diet, the disorder becomes chronically intermittent, and a nearly normal life is possible.

In addition to The National Organization for Rare Disorders (NORD) listed in Section III, the following organizations in Section II (Disease Specific) and in Section III (Umbrella) and Section IV (Government Agencies) can provide more information:
Association for Neuro-Metabolic Disorders, *III*
Metabolic Information Network, *III*
NIH/National Digestive Diseases Information Clearinghouse, *IV*
Organic Acidemia Association, *III*
Research Trust for Metabolic Diseases in Children, *III*
The Arc (a national organization on mental retardation), *III*

17 **ACIDEMIA, METHYLMALONIC**
Methylmalonic Acidemias are one type of organic acidemia. All known organic acidemias are inherited as autosomal recessive traits. They are caused by an enzymatic defect in the

metabolism of one amino acid. This results in an abnormally high level of acid in the blood and body tissues and concomitant metabolic acidosis. Acutely, drowsiness, coma, and seizures may occur. Mental retardation is a long-term consequence. The disorders may be caused either by a deficiency of the enzyme methylmalonyl CoA mutase, methylmalonyl racemase, or of adenosylcobalamin synthetic enzymes. Excretion of methylmalonate, a product of amino acid metabolism, in the urine is abnormally high.

In addition to The National Organization for Rare Disorders (NORD) listed in Section III, the following organizations in Section II (Disease Specific) and in Section III (Umbrella) and Section IV (Government Agencies) can provide more information:

Association for Neuro-Metabolic Disorders, *III*
Metabolic Information Network, *III*
NIH/National Digestive Diseases Information Clearinghouse, *IV*
Organic Acidemia Association, *III*
Research Trust for Metabolic Diseases in Children, *III*
Taking Action Against Language Disorders for Kids, Inc., *III*
The Arc (a national organization on mental retardation), *III*

18 ACIDEMIA, PROPIONIC

Propionic Acidemia is a very rare genetic form of Ketotic Hyperglycinemia. The disorder is due to deficiency of the enzyme propionyl CoA carboxylase, one of the enzymes necessary in the process of breaking down amino acids.

In addition to The National Organization for Rare Disorders (NORD) listed in Section III, the following organizations in Section II (Disease Specific) and in Section III (Umbrella) and Section IV (Government Agencies) can provide more information:

Metabolic Information Network, *III*
NIH/National Digestive Diseases Information Clearinghouse, *IV*
Organic Acidemia Association, *III*
Research Trust for Metabolic Diseases in Children, *III*
The Arc (a national organization on mental retardation), *III*

19 ACNE ROSACEA

Acne Rosacea is a skin disorder limited to the nose, cheeks, chin, and forehead, typically beginning during adulthood. The facial skin becomes oily, reddened and bumpy. Small red blood vessels are visible. In extreme cases, the nose may appear very red and bulbous.

In addition to The National Organization for Rare Disorders (NORD) listed in Section III, the following organizations in Section II (Disease Specific) and in Section III (Umbrella) and Section IV (Government Agencies) can provide more information:

NIH/National Arthritis and Musculoskeletal and Skin Diseases Information Clearinghouse, *IV*
National Rosacea Society, *II*

20 ACOUSTIC NEUROMA

Acoustic Neuroma is a benign (noncancerous) tumor of the 8th cranial nerve. This nerve lies within the ear (auditory) canal, and is associated with hearing loss and sending balance information from the inner ear to the brain.

In addition to The National Organization for Rare Disorders (NORD) listed in Section III, the following organizations in Section II (Disease Specific) and in Section III (Umbrella) and Section IV (Government Agencies) can provide more information:

Acoustic Neuroma Association, *II*
Acoustic Neuroma Association of Canada, *II*
Alexander Graham Bell Association for the Deaf, Inc., *III*
American Tinnitus Association, *II*
Better Hearing Institute, *III*
Deafness Research Foundation, *III*
NIH/National Institute on Deafness and Other Communication Disorders (Balance), *IV*
National Neurofibromatosis Foundation, Inc., *II*

21 ACROCALLOSAL SYNDROME, SCHINZEL TYPE

Schinzel Acrocallosal Syndrome is a very rare disorder inherited as an autosomal recessive genetic trait. This disorder is characterized by craniofacial abnormalities, absence or underdevelopment of the mass of white matter that unites the two halves of the brain (corpus callosum), additional fingers and/or toes (polydactyly), loss of muscle tone (hypotonia), and mental retardation.

In addition to The National Organization for Rare Disorders (NORD) listed in Section III, the following organizations in Section II (Disease Specific) and in Section III (Umbrella) and Section IV (Government Agencies) can provide more information:

Epilepsy Foundation of America, *III*
Guardians of Hydrocephalus Research Foundation, *II*
Hydrocephalus Association, *II*
NIH/National Institute of Child Health and Human Development, *IV*
National Hydrocephalus Foundation, *II*

22 ACRODERMATITIS ENTEROPATHICA

Acrodermatitis Enteropathica occurs in two forms: an inborn (congenital) form and an acquired form. The inborn form of AE is a rare genetic disorder characterized by intestinal abnormalities. Skin inflammation with pimples (pustular dermatitis) occurs around the mouth and/or anus, the nails (paronychial), and eyes. In the acute phase, irritability and emotional disturbances are evident due to wasting (atrophy) of the brain cortex.

Similar symptoms can be caused by special intravenous nutritional programs, for patients who cannot eat, which are almost always devoid of zinc. This is sometimes referred to as an acquired form of AE.

In addition to The National Organization for Rare Disorders (NORD) listed in Section III, the following organizations in Section II (Disease Specific) and in Section III (Umbrella) and Section IV (Government Agencies) can provide more information:
American Autoimmune Related Diseases Association, Inc., *III*
Metabolic Information Network, *III*
NIH/National Digestive Diseases Information Clearinghouse, *IV*
Research Trust for Metabolic Diseases in Children, *III*

23 ACRODYSOSTOSIS

Acrodysostosis is an extremely rare disorder characterized by abnormally short and malformed bones of the hands and feet (peripheral dysostosis), underdevelopment of the nose (nasal hypoplasia), and mental retardation. Other findings may include progressive growth delays, short stature, and/or unusual head and facial (craniofacial) features. Affected infants may exhibit premature maturation of bones of the hands and feet, malformation and shortening of the forearm bones (radius and ulna) near the wrist, and/or abnormally short fingers and toes (brachydactyly). Characteristic facial features may include a flattened, underdeveloped (hypoplastic) "pug" nose, an underdeveloped upper jaw bone (maxilliary hypoplasia), widely spaced eyes (ocular hypertelorism), and/or an extra fold of skin on either side of the nose that may cover the eyes' inner corners (epicanthal folds). In most cases, Acrodysostosis is thought to occur randomly, for no apparent reason (sporadic).

Some researchers believe that, in some cases, Acrodysostosis may be a form of Albright Hereditary Osteodystrophy (pseudohypoparathyroidism) in which normal calcium levels are present in the body (normocalcemic).

In addition to The National Organization for Rare Disorders (NORD) listed in Section III, the following organizations in Section II (Disease Specific) and in Section III (Umbrella) and Section IV (Government Agencies) can provide more information:
Little People of America, *III*
MAGIC Foundation for Children's Growth, *III*
NIH/National Institute of Child Health and Human Development, *IV*
Short Stature Foundation, *III*

24 ACROMEGALY

Acromegaly is a rare, slowly progressive chronic disorder characterized by an excess of growth hormone. Symptoms include abnormal enlargement in bones of the arms, legs, and head. The bones in the jaws and in the front of the skull are typically the most affected. Acromegaly may also cause thickening of the soft tissues of the body, particularly the heart and accelerated growth leading to tall stature.

In addition to The National Organization for Rare Disorders (NORD) listed in Section III, the following organizations in Section II (Disease Specific) and in Section III (Umbrella) and Section IV (Government Agencies) can provide more information:
Brain and Pituitary Foundation of America, *III*
NIH/National Arthritis and Musculoskeletal and Skin Diseases Information Clearinghouse, *IV*

25 ACROMESOMELIC DYSPLASIA

Acromesomelic Dysplasia is an extremely rare inherited progressive disorder characterized by premature fusion of the regions (metaphyses) where the shafts (diaphyses) of certain long bones (i.e., bones of the arms and legs) meet their growing ends (epiphyses). As a result, affected individuals exhibit unusually short forearms, abnormal shortening of bones of the lower (distal) legs, and short stature (short-limbed dwarfism), findings that typically become apparent during the first years of life. Abnormal cartilage and bone development may also affect other bones of the body, particularly those of the hands and feet (i.e., metacarpals, phalanges, metatarsals). Although the hands and feet may appear abnormally short and broad at birth, abnormalities of bone development in these areas are also progressive. As a result, bones of the hands and feet may appear increasingly shorter and wider during the first years of life. The fingernails and toenails may also appear unusually short and wide.

Affected individuals may also have additional

abnormalities resulting from abnormal cartilage and bone development including limited extension of the elbows and arms and/or progressive abnormal curvature of the spine (low thoracic kyphosis and/or lumbar hyperlordosis). Many individuals with Acromesomelic Dysplasia also have additional characteristic abnormalities including a relatively enlarged head (macrocephaly), slightly flattened midface, and/or small, pug nose. Acromesomelic Dysplasia is inherited as an autosomal recessive genetic trait.

In addition to The National Organization for Rare Disorders (NORD) listed in Section III, the following organizations in Section II (Disease Specific) and in Section III (Umbrella) and Section IV (Government Agencies) can provide more information:
Little People of America, *III*
MAGIC Foundation for Children's Growth, *III*
NIH/National Arthritis and Musculoskeletal and Skin Diseases Information Clearinghouse, *IV*
NIH/National Institute of Child Health and Human Development, *IV*
Short Stature Foundation, *III*

26 ACROMICRIC DYSPLASIA

Acromicric Dysplasia is an extremely rare inherited disorder characterized by abnormally short hands and feet, growth retardation and delayed bone maturation leading to short stature, and mild facial abnormalities. Most cases have occurred randomly for no apparent reason (sporadically). However, autosomal dominant inheritance has not been ruled out.

In addition to The National Organization for Rare Disorders (NORD) listed in Section III, the following organizations in Section II (Disease Specific) and in Section III (Umbrella) and Section IV (Government Agencies) can provide more information:
Human Growth Foundation, *III*
Little People of America, *III*
MAGIC Foundation for Children's Growth, *III*
NIH/National Institute of Child Health and Human Development, *IV*
Short Stature Foundation, *III*

27 ADAMS OLIVER SYNDROME

Adams-Oliver Syndrome is an extremely rare inherited disorder characterized by defects of the scalp and abnormalities of the fingers, toes, arms, and/or legs. The physical abnormalities associated with this disorder vary greatly among affected individuals. Some cases may be very mild while others may be severe. In infants with Adams-Oliver Syndrome, scalp defects are present at birth (congenital) and may include one or multiple hairless scarred areas (lesions) that may have abnormally wide (dilated) blood vessels directly under the affected skin. In severe cases, an underlying defect of the bones of the skull may also be present. In addition, infants with this disorder typically have malformations of the hands, arms, feet, and/or legs. These range from abnormally short (hypoplastic) fingers and toes to absent hands and/or lower legs. In some cases, additional abnormalities may also be present. Some cases of Adams-Oliver Syndrome occur randomly for unknown reasons (sporadically). Other cases are thought to be inherited as an autosomal dominant genetic trait.

In addition to The National Organization for Rare Disorders (NORD) listed in Section III, the following organizations in Section II (Disease Specific) and in Section III (Umbrella) and Section IV (Government Agencies) can provide more information:
Adams Oliver Syndrome Support Group, *II*
CHERUB—Association of Families and Friends of Children with Limb Disorders, *III*
NIH/National Arthritis and Musculoskeletal and Skin Diseases Information Clearinghouse, *IV*
NIH/National Institute of Child Health and Human Development, *IV*
Superkids, Inc. (newsletter for families and friends of children with limb differences), *III*

28 ADDISON'S DISEASE

Addison's Disease is a rare disorder characterized by chronic, usually progressive, insufficient functioning of the outer layer of the adrenal glands (adrenal cortex). Deficiencies of cortisol and aldosterone (hormones manufactured in the adrenals) result in low levels of sodium and chloride in the blood and body tissues, and high levels of potassium (electrolyte imbalance) in the body. Increased excretion of water and low blood pressure (hypotension) can lead to dehydration (extremely low levels of water in the body). Major symptoms of Addison's Disease include fatigue, gastrointestinal discomfort, and changes in skin color (pigmentation).

In addition to The National Organization for Rare Disorders (NORD) listed in Section III, the following organizations in Section II (Disease Specific) and in Section III (Umbrella) and Section IV (Government Agencies) can provide more information:
American Autoimmune Related Diseases Association, Inc., *III*
NIH/National Digestive Diseases Information Clearinghouse, *IV*
NIH/National Institute of Child Health and Human

Development, *IV*
National Adrenal Diseases Foundation, *III*

29 ADIE SYNDROME

Adie Syndrome is a rare neurological disorder affecting the pupil of the eye. In most patients with Adie Syndrome, the pupil is dilated (larger than normal) and slow to react to light on nearby objects. In some patients, however, the pupil may be constricted (smaller than normal) rather than dilated. Absent or poor reflexes are also associated with this disorder. Adie Syndrome is not progressive, life threatening, nor does it cause disability.

In addition to The National Organization for Rare Disorders (NORD) listed in Section III, the following organizations in Section II (Disease Specific) and in Section III (Umbrella) and Section IV (Government Agencies) can provide more information:
NIH/National Eye Institute, *IV*
NIH/National Institute of Neurological Disorders and Stroke, *IV*

30 ADRENAL HYPERPLASIA, CONGENITAL (GENERAL)

Congenital Adrenal Hyperplasia refers to a group of disorders that result from the impaired ability of the adrenal glands to produce hormones known as corticosteriods. Glucocorticoids and mineralocorticoids are the two corticosteriod hormones that are active in the body. Low levels of glucocorticoids, especially the hormone cortisol, can result in metabolic problems. Low levels of circulating cortisol cause the anterior pituitary gland to produce abnormally high amounts of adrenocorticotropin hormone (ACTH). Deficiencies of mineralocorticoids, especially the hormone aldosterone, cause sodium and water imbalance in the body; in some cases, this can be life-threatening.

The various forms of Congenital Adrenal Hyperplasia represent enzyme deficiencies at different stages of hormone production. These include 3-Beta Hydroxy-Steroid Dehydrogenase (HSD) Deficiency, 17-Hydroxylase Deficiency, 21-Hydroxylase Deficiency, 17-20 Desmolase Deficiency, 11-Beta Hydroxylase Deficiency, and 17-Alpha Hydroxylase.

One rare form of Congenital Adrenal Hyperplasia can result from the overgrowth of fatty-like cells in the adrenal glands (congenital lipoid hyperplasia). This is also known as male pseudohermaphroditism or 20-22 Desmolase Deficiency.

In addition to The National Organization for Rare Disorders (NORD) listed in Section III, the following organizations in Section II (Disease Specific) and in Section III (Umbrella) and Section IV (Government Agencies) can provide more information:
Ambiguous Genitalia Support Network, *III*
MAGIC Foundation for Children's Growth, *III*
March of Dimes Birth Defects Foundation, *III*
Metabolic Information Network, *III*
NIH/National Institute of Child Health and Human Development, *IV*
National Adrenal Diseases Foundation, *III*
Research Trust for Metabolic Diseases in Children, *III*

31 ADRENOLEUKODYSTROPHY

Adrenoleukodystrophy is a rare inherited metabolic disorder characterized by the loss of the fatty covering (myelin sheath) on nerve fibers within the brain (cerebral demyelination) and the progressive degeneration of the adrenal gland (adrenal atrophy). Adrenoleukodystrophy that is inherited as an X-linked genetic trait may begin in childhood or adulthood. However, Adrenoleukodystrophy that is inherited as an autosomal recessive genetic trait typically begins during infancy (neonatal period).

In addition to The National Organization for Rare Disorders (NORD) listed in Section III, the following organizations in Section II (Disease Specific) and in Section III (Umbrella) and Section IV (Government Agencies) can provide more information:
Alliance of Genetic Support Groups, *III*
Association for Neuro-Metabolic Disorders, *III*
Attia Research Trust Into ALD, *II*
March of Dimes Birth Defects Foundation, *III*
Metabolic Information Network, *III*
NIH/National Institute of Neurological Disorders and Stroke, *IV*
Research Trust for Metabolic Diseases in Children, *III*
The Arc (a national organization on mental retardation), *III*
United Leukodystrophy Foundation, *III*

32 AFIBRINOGENEMIA, CONGENITAL

Congenital Afibrinogenemia is a rare disorder in which the patient is born with little or no fibrinogen. Fibrinogen is a protein necessary in the blood clotting process. As a result, the blood does not coagulate causing the patient to bleed uncontrollably. Many patients may experience severe hemorrhaging during childhood while others may have very little trouble with bleeding. Congenital Afibrinogenemia is thought to be inherited as an autosomal recessive genetic trait.

In addition to The National Organization for Rare Disorders (NORD) listed in Section III, the following organizations in Section II (Disease Specific) and in Section III (Umbrella) and Section IV (Government Agencies) can provide more information:
NIH/National Heart, Lung and Blood Institute Information Center, *IV*
National Hemophilia Foundation, *II*

33 AGAMMAGLOBULINEMIAS, PRIMARY

Primary Agammaglobulinemias are a group of inherited immune deficiencies characterized by insufficient antibodies. Antibodies are composed of certain proteins (immunoglobulins) that are essential to the immune system. They are produced by specialized cells (i.e., B lymphocytes) that circulate in the lymphatic fluid and blood. Antibodies fight off bacteria, viruses, and other foreign substances that threaten the body. Agammaglobulinemias are also characterized by the abnormal function of specialized white blood cells called B lymphocytes. The B lymphocytes are supposed to search out and identify bacteria, viruses, or other foreign substances in the body. T lymphocytes, also known as the "killer cells," assist B lymphocytes to respond to infection and other antigens. However, in some forms of Primary Agammaglobulinemias, neither the B nor the T lymphocytes function normally.

There are three types of Primary Agammaglobulinemias: X-linked Agammaglobulinemia (XLA), X-linked Agammaglobulinemia with growth hormone deficiency, and autosomal recessive Agammaglobulinemia. All of these disorders are characterized by a weakened immune system that must be enhanced by gammaglobulin in order to fight infections.

In addition to The National Organization for Rare Disorders (NORD) listed in Section III, the following organizations in Section II (Disease Specific) and in Section III (Umbrella) and Section IV (Government Agencies) can provide more information:
Alliance of Genetic Support Groups, *III*
Centers for Disease Control and Prevention, *IV*
Immune Deficiency Foundation, *III*
International Patient Organization for Primary Immunodeficiencies, *III*
Jeffrey Modell Foundation, *III*
March of Dimes Birth Defects Foundation, *III*
NIH/National Institute of Allergy and Infectious Diseases, *IV*

34 AGENESIS OF CORPUS CALLOSUM

Agenesis of Corpus Callosum (ACC) is a rare disorder that is present at birth (congenital). It is characterized by a partial or complete absence (agenesis) of an area of the brain that connects the two cerebral hemispheres. This part of the brain is normally composed of transverse fibers. Agenesis of Corpus Callosum is usually inherited as either an autosomal recessive trait or an X-linked dominant trait. It can also be caused by an infection during the twelfth to the twenty-second week of pregnancy (intrauterine) leading to developmental disturbance of the fetal brain. In some cases mental retardation may result, but in other cases, no evident symptoms may appear and intelligence may not be impaired.

ACC is diagnosed in approximately ninety percent of patients during the first two years of life. An epileptic seizure is usually the initial symptom indicating that a child should be tested for a brain dysfunction. The disorder can also be without apparent symptoms in the mildest cases for many years. A normal lifespan may be expected for patients with ACC.

In addition to The National Organization for Rare Disorders (NORD) listed in Section III, the following organizations in Section II (Disease Specific) and in Section III (Umbrella) and Section IV (Government Agencies) can provide more information:
Agenesis of Corpus Callosum (ACC) Network, *II*
Brain and Pituitary Foundation of America, *III*
Guardians of Hydrocephalus Research Foundation, *II*
Hydrocephalus Association, *II*
NIH/National Institute of Neurological Disorders and Stroke, *IV*
National Hydrocephalus Foundation, *II*
The Arc (a national organization on mental retardation), *III*

35 AGNOSIA, PRIMARY VISUAL

Primary Visual Agnosia is a rare neurological disorder characterized by the total or partial loss of the ability to recognize and identify familiar objects and/or people by sight. This occurs without loss of the ability to actually see the object or person. The symptoms of Visual Agnosia occur as a result of damage to certain areas of the brain (primary) or in association with other disorders (secondary).

In addition to The National Organization for Rare Disorders (NORD) listed in Section III, the following organizations in Section II (Disease Specific) and in Section III (Umbrella) and Section IV (Government Agencies) can provide more information:

NIH/National Institute of Neurological Disorders and Stroke, *IV*
National Head Injury Foundation, Inc. (and Family Helpline), *III*

36 AGRANULOCYTOSIS, ACQUIRED

Acquired Agranulocytosis is a rare drug-induced blood disorder that is characterized by a severe reduction in the number of white blood cells (granulocytes) in the circulating blood. There are three types of granulocytes, namely basophils, eosinophils, and neutrophils. Acquired Agranulocytosis may be caused by a variety of drugs, including chemotherapeutic agents, used for cancer treatment, or antipsychotic medications (e.g., clozapine). The symptoms of Agranulocytosis develop because of impairment in the production of granulocytes in the bone marrow. People with Acquired Agranulocytosis are susceptible to a variety of bacterial infections that may cause flu-like symptoms. Painful ulcers in mucous membranes that line the mouth and/or the gastrointestinal tract may also develop.

In addition to The National Organization for Rare Disorders (NORD) listed in Section III, the following organizations in Section II (Disease Specific) and in Section III (Umbrella) and Section IV (Government Agencies) can provide more information:
NIH/National Heart, Lung and Blood Institute Information Center, *IV*

37 AHUMADA DEL CASTILLO SYNDROME

Ahumada Del Castillo is a rare endocrine disorder affecting adult females and is characterized by impairment in the function of the pituitary and hypothalamus glands. Symptoms may include the production of breast milk (lactation) not associated with nursing and the absence of menstrual periods (amenorrhea) due to the lack of monthly ovulation (anovulation). The exact cause of Ahumada Del Castillo is not known although some research suggests that small tumors in the pituitary and/or hypothalamus gland may be responsible for some cases of this disorder.

In addition to The National Organization for Rare Disorders (NORD) listed in Section III, the following organizations in Section II (Disease Specific) and in Section III (Umbrella) and Section IV (Government Agencies) can provide more information:
NIH/National Institute of Child Health and Human Development, *IV*
National Women's Health Network, *III*
National Women's Health Resource Center, *III*

38 AICARDI SYNDROME

Aicardi Syndrome is an extremely rare congenital disorder in which the structure linking the two cerebral hemispheres of the brain (corpus callosum) fails to develop. The absence of the corpus callosum is associated with frequent seizures, marked abnormalities of the retina and choroid (the thin membrane that covers the retina) of the eyes, and/or mental retardation.

In addition to The National Organization for Rare Disorders (NORD) listed in Section III, the following organizations in Section II (Disease Specific) and in Section III (Umbrella) and Section IV (Government Agencies) can provide more information:
Aicardi Syndrome Awareness and Support Group, *II*
Aicardi Syndrome Newsletter, Inc., *II*
Alliance of Genetic Support Groups, *III*
Blind Children's Fund, *III*
March of Dimes Birth Defects Foundation, *III*
NIH/National Institute of Neurological Disorders and Stroke, *IV*
National Association for Visually Handicapped, *III*
The Arc (a national organization on mental retardation), *III*

39 ALAGILLE SYNDROME

Alagille Syndrome is a genetic liver disorder usually present at birth. It is characterized by insufficient passage of bile due to a lower than normal number of bile ducts inside the liver. In some cases, the child may be born with no bile ducts. Major symptoms include prolonged yellow skin discoloration (jaundice), eye and heart structure anomalies, abnormally shaped vertebrae of the spine, compression of nerve space inside the lower spine, an absence of deep tendon reflexes, mental deficiency, facial abnormalities, and shortened fingers.

In addition to The National Organization for Rare Disorders (NORD) listed in Section III, the following organizations in Section II (Disease Specific) and in Section III (Umbrella) and Section IV (Government Agencies) can provide more information:
Alagille Syndrome Alliance, *II*
American Liver Foundation, *III*
Children's Liver Alliance, *III*
Digestive Disease National Coalition, *III*
NIH/National Digestive Diseases Information Clearinghouse, *IV*
The Arc (a national organization on mental retardation), *III*
United Liver Association, *III*

40 ALBINISM

Albinism is a group of rare inherited disorders characterized by the absence at birth of color (pigmentation) in the skin, hair, and eyes. Albinism is also associated with certain syndromes that produce defects in the eyes (ocular abnormalities). The syndromes of this disorder are categorized as Tyrosinase-Negative Oculocutaneous Albinism, Tyrosinase- Positive Oculocutaneous Albinism (Albinoidism), and Ocular Albinism.

In addition to The National Organization for Rare Disorders (NORD) listed in Section III, the following organizations in Section II (Disease Specific) and in Section III (Umbrella) and Section IV (Government Agencies) can provide more information:

Albino Fellowship, *II*
Alliance of Genetic Support Groups, *III*
March of Dimes Birth Defects Foundation, *III*
NIH/National Institute of Child Health and Human Development, *IV*
National Organization for Albinism and Hypopigmentation, *III*

41 **ALEXANDER'S DISEASE**

Alexander's Disease is an extremely rare, progressive, metabolic, neurological disorder that is frequently inherited. It is one of a group of diseases known as the leukodystrophies. Alexander's Disease is characterized by loss of the fatty layers that cover nerves (demyelination), and the formation of abnormal bodies (Rosenthal fibers) in supporting cells (astrocytes) of the brain. These Rosenthal fibers most frequently form on the surface of the brain and around the blood vessels within the brain. The symptoms of Alexander's Disease usually begin during infancy and are associated with mental and physical retardation. Juvenile (occuring later than infancy) and adult-onset Alexander's Disease are recognized forms of this disorder but occur very infrequently.

In addition to The National Organization for Rare Disorders (NORD) listed in Section III, the following organizations in Section II (Disease Specific) and in Section III (Umbrella) and Section IV (Government Agencies) can provide more information:

Alliance of Genetic Support Groups, *III*
Association for Neuro-Metabolic Disorders, *III*
Children's Brain Diseases Foundation, *II*
March of Dimes Birth Defects Foundation, *III*
Metabolic Information Network, *III*
NIH/National Institute of Neurological Disorders and Stroke, *IV*
The Arc (a national organization on mental retardation), *III*
United Leukodystrophy Foundation, *III*

42 **ALKAPTONURIA**

Alkaptonuria is a very rare hereditary disorder that is characterized by the excretion of large volumes of dark colored urine. The darkened urine is the result of the exposure to the air (spontaneous oxidation) of homogentisic acid that accumulates in the urine. Homogentisic acid also accumulates in the body tissues. In normal functioning, the amino acid tyrosine is metabolized into homogentisic acid, and further into maleylacetoacetic acid. In alkaptonuria, this metabolic pathway is not completed because of a deficiency of the enzyme homogentisic acid oxidase; therefore, the further metabolism of homogentisic acid is prevented. Excess accumulation of this acid leads to the severe degeneration of the cartilage of the spine and other major joints, and ultimately to osteoarthritis.

In addition to The National Organization for Rare Disorders (NORD) listed in Section III, the following organizations in Section II (Disease Specific) and in Section III (Umbrella) and Section IV (Government Agencies) can provide more information:

Alliance of Genetic Support Groups, *III*
March of Dimes Birth Defects Foundation, *III*
Metabolic Information Network, *III*
NIH/National Arthritis and Musculoskeletal and Skin Diseases Information Clearinghouse, *IV*
Research Trust for Metabolic Diseases in Children, *III*

43 **ALLAN HERNDON SYNDROME**

Allan-Herndon Syndrome is an extremely rare inherited disorder characterized by severe mental retardation; an inability to form words and speak clearly (dysarthria); diminished muscle tone (hypotonia); slow involuntary purposeless movements (athetoid movements) of the arms, hands, legs, and feet (extremities); impaired ability to coordinate voluntary movements (ataxia); and/or lack of control of voluntary movements of the legs (spastic paraplegia), resulting in "jerky" (athetoid) movements. In most cases, affected infants appear normal until approximately six months of age, when it becomes apparent that they have unusually weak neck muscles resulting in an inability to control head movements. In some cases, affected individuals may be unable to talk and/or walk. Other characteristic abnormalities may include underdevelopment (hypoplasia) and/or wasting away (atrophy) of various muscles; fixation of several joints in a permanently flexed position (joint contractures); and/or unusual head and facial (craniofacial) features. Allan-Herndon Syndrome is thought to be inherited as an X-linked recessive genetic trait.

In addition to The National Organization for Rare Disorders (NORD) listed in Section III, the following organizations in Section II (Disease Specific) and in Section III (Umbrella) and Section IV (Government Agencies) can provide more information:

NIH/National Institute of Child Health and Human Development, *IV*
NIH/National Institute on Deafness and Other Communication Disorders Information Clearinghouse, *IV*
WE MOVE, *III*

44 ALOPECIA AREATA

Alopecia Areata is a progressive condition characterized by loss of hair. The cause is unknown, and unpredictable hair loss is the only noticeable symptom. Regrowth of hair may or may not occur. Some cases may be associated with endocrine abnormalities, infection of the scalp, or an autoimmune reaction. Hair loss is usually confined to the head and face, although the entire body may be involved.

In addition to The National Organization for Rare Disorders (NORD) listed in Section III, the following organizations in Section II (Disease Specific) and in Section III (Umbrella) and Section IV (Government Agencies) can provide more information:

NIH/National Arthritis and Musculoskeletal and Skin Diseases Information Clearinghouse, *IV*
NIH/National Cancer Institute, *IV*
National Alopecia Areata Foundation, *II*

45 ALPERS DISEASE

Alpers Disease is a progressive neurologic (brain) disorder that occurs early in life. Symptoms include increased muscle tone with exaggerated reflexes (spasticity), seizures, loss of cognitive ability (dementia) and, in many cases, liver disease.

In addition to The National Organization for Rare Disorders (NORD) listed in Section III, the following organizations in Section II (Disease Specific) and in Section III (Umbrella) and Section IV (Government Agencies) can provide more information:

Association for Neuro-Metabolic Disorders, *III*
Epilepsy Foundation of America, *III*
NIH/National Institute of Neurological Disorders and Stroke, *IV*
National Association for Visually Handicapped, *III*
THRESHOLD (for uncontrolled seizure disorders), *III*
United Mitochondrial Disease Foundation, *III*

46 ALPHA-1-ANTITRYPSIN DEFICIENCY

Alpha-1-Antitrypsin Deficiency is a rare hereditary metabolic disease characterized by low levels of the enzyme Alpha-1-Antitrypsin. A deficiency of this enzyme allows substances that break down protein (proteolytic enzymes) to attack various tissues of the body. This results in destructive changes in the lungs (emphysema) and may also affect the liver and joints. Alpha-1-Antitrypsin is ordinarily released by specialized, granular white blood cells (neutrophils) in response to infection or inflammation. A deficiency of Alpha-1-Antitrypsin results in uncontrolled rapid breakdown of proteins (protease activity), especially in the foundation membranes (basilar) of the lungs.

In addition to The National Organization for Rare Disorders (NORD) listed in Section III, the following organizations in Section II (Disease Specific) and in Section III (Umbrella) and Section IV (Government Agencies) can provide more information:

Alliance of Genetic Support Groups, *III*
Alpha-1-Antitrypsin Deficiency National Association, *II*
American Liver Foundation, *III*
American Lung Association, *III*
Children's Liver Alliance, *III*
Children's Liver Disease Foundation, *III*
March of Dimes Birth Defects Foundation, *III*
Metabolic Information Network, *III*
NIH/National Heart, Lung and Blood Institute Information Center, *IV*

47 ALPORT SYNDROME

Alport Syndrome is a group of hereditary kidney disorders characterized by progressive deterioration of the glomerular basement membranes (GBMs), which are microscopic parts of the kidney. This deterioration may lead to chronic renal (kidney) failure causing excess waste products in the blood (uremia). Eventually severe renal failure (end-stage renal disease or ESRD) may develop. Uremia and kidney failure may cause heart and bone problems. Some types of Alport Syndrome also affect vision and hearing.

In addition to The National Organization for Rare Disorders (NORD) listed in Section III, the following organizations in Section II (Disease Specific) and in Section III (Umbrella) and Section IV (Government Agencies) can provide more information:

Alport Syndrome—Hereditary Nephritis Study, *II*
American Foundation for Urologic Disease, *III*
American Kidney Fund, Inc., *III*
Hereditary Nephritis Foundation, *III*
NIH/National Kidney and Urologic Diseases

Information Clearinghouse, *IV*
National Kidney Foundation, *III*

48 ALSTROM SYNDROME

Alstrom Syndrome is a rare disorder inherited as an autosomal recessive genetic trait. Characteristic features of this disorder include progressive loss of vision and hearing beginning in early childhood, diabetes mellitus, and obesity. Degeneration of the retina of the eye (retinitis pigmentosa) may be apparent in the first year of life. Other symptoms may include progressive kidney disease (chronic nephropathy), which may lead to serious complications. Intelligence is not affected.

In addition to The National Organization for Rare Disorders (NORD) listed in Section III, the following organizations in Section II (Disease Specific) and in Section III (Umbrella) and Section IV (Government Agencies) can provide more information:

American Society for Deaf Children, *III*
Better Hearing Institute, *III*
Blind Children's Center, *III*
Blind Children's Fund, *III*
Foundation Fighting Blindness, *III*
International Alstrom's Syndrome Newsletter, *II*
Juvenile Diabetes Foundation International, *II*
Little People of America, *III*
NIH/National Eye Institute, *IV*
NIH/National Institute on Deafness and Other Communication Disorders (Balance), *IV*
National Association for Parents of the Visually Impaired, *III*
National Association for Visually Handicapped, *III*
National Information Center on Deafness, *III*
Retinitis Pigmentosa International, *II*

49 ALTERNATING HEMIPLEGIA OF CHILDHOOD

Alternating Hemiplegia of Childhood (AHC) is a rare neurological disorder characterized by frequent, temporary episodes of paralysis on one side of the body (hemiplegia). Symptoms usually begin before the age of 18 months. This syndrome may be characterized by temporary (transient) hemiplegia of varying degrees; temporary paralysis of the muscles that control eye movement (transient ocular palsies); sudden, involuntary movements of limbs and facial muscles (choreoathetosis); and/or excessive sweating with changes in skin color and body temperature (autonomic nervous system dysfunction). Mental capacity may be affected. The exact cause of AHC is unknown. Some cases of AHC may be inherited as an autosomal dominant genetic trait.

In addition to The National Organization for Rare Disorders (NORD) listed in Section III, the following organizations in Section II (Disease Specific) and in Section III (Umbrella) and Section IV (Government Agencies) can provide more information:

International Foundation for Alternating Hemiplegia of Childhood, *II*
NIH/National Institute of Neurological Disorders and Stroke, *IV*

50 ALVEOLITIS, EXTRINSIC ALLERGIC

Extrinsic Allergic Alveolitis is a lung disorder resulting from repeated inhalation of organic dust, usually in a specific occupational setting. In the acute form, respiratory symptoms and fever begin several hours after exposure to the dust. The chronic form is characterized by gradual changes in the lung tissue associated with several years of exposure to the irritant.

In addition to The National Organization for Rare Disorders (NORD) listed in Section III, the following organizations in Section II (Disease Specific) and in Section III (Umbrella) and Section IV (Government Agencies) can provide more information:

American Lung Association, *III*
NIH/National Institute of Allergy and Infectious Diseases, *IV*
NIH/National Institute of Environmental Health Sciences Clearinghouse, *IV*

51 ALVEOLITIS, FIBROSING

Fibrosing Alveolitis is an inflammatory lung disorder characterized by abnormal formation of fibrous tissue between tiny air sacs (alveoli) or ducts in the lungs. Coughing and rapid, shallow breathing occur with moderate exercise. The skin may appear slightly bluish (cyanotic) due to lack of circulating oxygen. Complications such as infection, emphysema or heart problems may develop.

In addition to The National Organization for Rare Disorders (NORD) listed in Section III, the following organizations in Section II (Disease Specific) and in Section III (Umbrella) and Section IV (Government Agencies) can provide more information:

American Autoimmune Related Diseases Association, Inc., *III*
American Lung Association, *III*
NIH/National Heart, Lung and Blood Institute, *IV*

52 ALZHEIMER'S DISEASE

Alzheimer's Disease is a progressive condition of the brain affecting memory, thought and language. The degenerative changes of Alzheimer's Disease lead to patches or plaques in the brain and the entanglement of nerve fibers (neurofibrillary tangles). Memory loss and behavioral changes occur as a result of these changes in brain tissue.

In addition to The National Organization for Rare Disorders (NORD) listed in Section III, the following organizations in Section II (Disease Specific) and in Section III (Umbrella) and Section IV (Government Agencies) can provide more information:
Alliance of Genetic Support Groups, *III*
Alzheimer's Association, *II*
Alzheimer's Disease Education and Referral Center, *II*
March of Dimes Birth Defects Foundation, *III*
NIH/National Institute of Neurological Disorders and Stroke, *IV*
NIH/National Institute on Aging, *IV*

53 **AMELOBLASTOMA**

Ameloblastoma is a very rare disorder of the jaw and sinuses. Major symptoms may include cysts or tumors in the dental area. They may also occur in the sinuses, nose and/or eye sockets. In some cases, the ameloblastoma may become malignant and spread to other areas of the body.

In addition to The National Organization for Rare Disorders (NORD) listed in Section III, the following organizations in Section II (Disease Specific) and in Section III (Umbrella) and Section IV (Government Agencies) can provide more information:
American Cancer Society, Inc., *III*
NIH/National Oral Health Information Clearinghouse, *IV*

54 **AMELOGENESIS IMPERFECTA**

Amelogenesis Imperfecta is a rare inherited disorder characterized by brown discoloration of the teeth, resulting from a lack calcium (hypocalcification) or underdevelopment (hypoplasia) of the hard outer covering of teeth (enamel). The disorder is divided into numerous forms based on the severity of the enamel defect (e.g., complete absence [agenesis], underdevelopment, etc.). Individuals with Amelogenesis Imperfecta may be prone to early tooth loss and/or disease of the structures that surround and support the teeth (periodontal disease). Amelogenesis Imperfecta may be inherited as an X-linked, autosomal dominant, or autosomal recessive genetic trait, depending on the form present.

In addition to The National Organization for Rare Disorders (NORD) listed in Section III, the following organizations in Section II (Disease Specific) and in Section III (Umbrella) and Section IV (Government Agencies) can provide more information:
NIH/National Oral Health Information Clearinghouse, *IV*
National Foundation for Ectodermal Dysplasias, *II*

55 **AMENORRHEA, PRIMARY**

Primary Amenorrhea is a rare gynecological disorder characterized by the absence of menstrual flow (menses) in a female age 18 or older. The beginning of regular menstruation (menarche) usually begins within two years after the onset of puberty. Absence of menses by age 18 or older constitutes Primary Amenorrhea.

In addition to The National Organization for Rare Disorders (NORD) listed in Section III, the following organizations in Section II (Disease Specific) and in Section III (Umbrella) and Section IV (Government Agencies) can provide more information:
American Autoimmune Related Diseases Association, Inc., *III*
NIH/National Institute of Child Health and Human Development, *IV*
National Adrenal Diseases Foundation, *III*
National Women's Health Network, *III*

56 **AMNIOTIC BANDS**

Amniotic Bands is a rare condition that occurs when the level of amniotic fluid is insufficient during pregnancy. The severity of the resulting disorder is associated with the stage of fetal development at the time the amniotic fluid decrease begins in the uterus. Major symptoms may include abnormalities of the feet, spine, lungs and face.

In addition to The National Organization for Rare Disorders (NORD) listed in Section III, the following organizations in Section II (Disease Specific) and in Section III (Umbrella) and Section IV (Government Agencies) can provide more information:
CHERUB—Association of Families and Friends of Children with Limb Disorders, *III*
NIH/National Institute of Child Health and Human Development, *IV*

57 **AMYLOIDOSIS**

Amyloidosis is the term applied to a group of metabolic disorders in which amyloid (a fibrous protein) accumulates in tissues of the body. The excessive accumulation of amyloid causes the affected organ to malfunction. The accumulation may be localized, general, or systemic. There are various systems used to classify the different forms of the disorder. The most widely used classification system is based on the chemical properties of the fiber-like structures within amyloid (fibrils).

The most common form of Amyloidosis is AL

or light-chain-related (Primary Amyloidosis). This form of the disease may occur independently of other disease, or in the presence of multiple tumors arising from the bone marrow (myeloma). This form of the disorder generally effects the tongue, thyroid gland, intestinal tract, liver and spleen. Cardiac involvement may result in congestive heart failure.

AA Amyloidosis, or Secondary Amyloidosis, is most often discovered during the course of a chronic inflammatory disease, such as rheumatoid arthritis, chronic infections or familial Mediterranean fever. AA Amyloidosis commonly impairs the proper functioning of the kidneys, liver and spleen. The adrenal glands, lymph nodes, and vascular system may be affected as well. The skin inflammation that occurs with recurrent injections that are given to treat some inflammatory diseases seems to induce AA Amyloidosis. Malfunctioning of the kidneys, as in nephrotic syndrome and kidney (renal) failure, causes the most fatalities in AA Amyloidosis. This type of Amyloidosis is reported in approximately one percent of cases of chronic inflammatory diseases in the United States.

Amyloidosis of Aging commonly affects the heart. Sometimes this form of Amyloidosis also affects the pancreas and brain.

Hemodialysis-Associated Amyloidosis is seen in patients who have experienced long-term hemodialysis (a procedure in which impurities or wastes are removed from the blood due to the malfunctioning of the kidneys).

Familial Amyloidosis is found in a series of genetically transmitted diseases that typically affect the kidney, heart, skin and other areas of the body.

In addition to The National Organization for Rare Disorders (NORD) listed in Section III, the following organizations in Section II (Disease Specific) and in Section III (Umbrella) and Section IV (Government Agencies) can provide more information:

Alliance of Genetic Support Groups, *III*
Association for Neuro-Metabolic Disorders, *III*
March of Dimes Birth Defects Foundation, *III*
Metabolic Information Network, *III*
NIH/National Arthritis and Musculoskeletal and Skin Diseases Information Clearinghouse, *IV*

58 AMYOTROPHIC LATERAL SCLEROSIS

Amyotrophic Lateral Sclerosis (ALS) is a disease that causes progressive degeneration and eventual loss of function of both upper and lower motor neurons resulting in progressive skeletal muscular wasting and weakness.

There are a number of different forms of Amyotrophic Lateral Sclerosis and other motor neuron diseases with similar symptoms. These include: Slow Motor Neuron Disease, Focal Motor Neuron Disease, Spinal Muscular Atrophy (Kugelberg-Welander Disease and Juvenile Spinal Muscular Atrophy), Progressive Bulbar Palsy, Benign Focal Amyotrophy, Primary Lateral Sclerosis, Infantile Spinal Muscular Atrophy (Werdnig-Hoffmann Disease), Wohlfart- Kugelberg-Welander Disease, and Floppy Infant Syndrome.

In addition to The National Organization for Rare Disorders (NORD) listed in Section III, the following organizations in Section II (Disease Specific) and in Section III (Umbrella) and Section IV (Government Agencies) can provide more information:

Amyotrophic Lateral Sclerosis Association, *II*
Amyotrophic Lateral Sclerosis Society of Canada, *II*
Families of Spinal Muscular Atrophy, *III*
International Alliance of ALS/MND Associations, *III*
Les Turner Amyotrophic Lateral Sclerosis Foundation, Ltd., *II*
Muscular Dystrophy Association, *III*
NIH/National Institute of Neurological Disorders and Stroke, *IV*

59 ANAPHYLAXIS

Anaphylaxis is an abnormally severe reaction to a substance that a person is allergic to. Major symptoms may include severe itching, hives, flushing, swelling, vomiting, diarrhea, difficulty breathing and unconsciousness.

In addition to The National Organization for Rare Disorders (NORD) listed in Section III, the following organizations in Section II (Disease Specific) and in Section III (Umbrella) and Section IV (Government Agencies) can provide more information:

Asthma and Allergy Foundation of America, Inc., *III*
NIH/National Institute of Allergy and Infectious Diseases, *IV*

60 ANDERSEN DISEASE

Andersen Disease is a glycogen storage disease inherited through recessive genes. Symptoms of this disorder are caused by a lack of a brancher enzyme. Alpha-1,4-glucan 6-glucasyltransferase is abnormal in the liver, skin, fibroblasts, and other tissue. The lack of this enzyme causes an abnormality in the structure of the main carbohydrate storage material (glycogen). Andersen Disease is characterized by scarring of the liver (cirrhosis) that may lead to liver failure.

In addition to The National Organization for Rare Disorders (NORD) listed in Section III, the following organizations in Section II (Disease Specific) and in Section III (Umbrella) and Section IV (Government Agencies) can provide more information:
Association for Glycogen Storage Disease, *III*
Metabolic Information Network, *III*
NIH/National Institute of Diabetes, Digestive and Kidney Diseases, *IV*
Research Trust for Metabolic Diseases in Children, *III*

61 ANEMIA, APLASTIC

Aplastic Anemia is a rare blood disorder characterized by decreased function of the bone marrow that results in abnormally low levels of all the cellular elements of the blood (pancytopenia). In some cases, the disorder may affect primarily single cell lines (i.e., red blood cells, white cells, or platelets). The initial symptoms may include increasing weakness, fatigue, recurrent or persistent infections, and/or lethargy. In about 50 percent of cases, the exact cause is not known. In some cases, certain toxic agents (e.g., inorganic arsenic) or drugs (e.g., phenylbutazone, choramphenicol, etc.) may cause Aplastic Anemia.

In addition to The National Organization for Rare Disorders (NORD) listed in Section III, the following organizations in Section II (Disease Specific) and in Section III (Umbrella) and Section IV (Government Agencies) can provide more information:
Aplastic Anemia Association of Canada, *II*
Aplastic Anemia Foundation of America, Inc., *II*
MPD (Myeloproliferative Disease) Research Center, Inc., *III*
NIH/Hematology Branch, National Heart, Lung and Blood Institute (NHLBI), *IV*
NIH/National Heart, Lung and Blood Institute, *IV*

62 ANEMIA, BLACKFAN DIAMOND

Blackfan-Diamond Anemia is a rare blood disorder of unknown cause characterized by deficiency of red blood cells at birth (congenital hypoplastic anemia) and various other symptoms and findings including slow growth, abnormal weakness and fatigue, paleness of the skin, characteristic facial abnormalities, protruding shoulder blades (scapulae), webbing or abnormal shortening of the neck due to fusion of certain bones in the spine (cervical vertebrae), hand deformities, congenital heart defects, and/or other abnormalities. The symptoms and physical findings associated with Blackfan-Diamond Anemia vary greatly from case to case. A consistent "pattern" of symptoms and physical findings has not been identified. Blackfan-Diamond Anemia may be inherited as either an autosomal dominant or recessive genetic trait.

In addition to The National Organization for Rare Disorders (NORD) listed in Section III, the following organizations in Section II (Disease Specific) and in Section III (Umbrella) and Section IV (Government Agencies) can provide more information:
Alliance of Genetic Support Groups, *III*
Aplastic Anemia Foundation of America, Inc., *II*
Diamond Blackfan Anemia Registry, *II*
NIH/National Heart, Lung and Blood Institute, *IV*

63 ANEMIA, FANCONI'S

Fanconi's Anemia is an inherited condition that leads to a deficiency of certain blood cells that are produced by the bone marrow. This disorder occurs mainly in children and is characterized by abnormalities of the heart, kidneys, and skeleton. Skin color (pigmentation) changes may also occur.

In both types of Fanconi's Anemia (Type I and Type II) the symptoms are the same. Although the location of the defective gene that causes Fanconi's Anemia is unknown, it is thought that the gene that causes each type of Fanconi's Anemia is at a different location on the chromosome.

In addition to The National Organization for Rare Disorders (NORD) listed in Section III, the following organizations in Section II (Disease Specific) and in Section III (Umbrella) and Section IV (Government Agencies) can provide more information:
Alliance of Genetic Support Groups, *III*
Aplastic Anemia Foundation of America, Inc., *II*
Canadian Fanconi Anemia Research Fund, *II*
Fanconi Anemia Research Fund, Inc., *II*
March of Dimes Birth Defects Foundation, *III*
NIH/Hematology Branch, National Heart, Lung and Blood Institute (NHLBI), *IV*
NIH/National Heart, Lung and Blood Institute, *IV*

64 ANEMIA, HEMOLYTIC, ACQUIRED AUTOIMMUNE

Acquired Autoimmune Hemolytic Anemia is a rare autoimmune disorder characterized by the premature destruction of red blood cells. Autoimmune diseases occur when the body's natural defenses against invading organisms (e.g., lymphocytes, antibodies) destroy healthy tissue for unknown reasons. Normally, the red blood cells have a life span of approximately 120 days before they are removed by the spleen. In an individual affected with Acquired Autoimmune Hemolytic Anemia, the red blood cells are destroyed prematurely and bone marrow production of new cells can no longer compensate for their loss. The severity of this type of anemia is determined by the time the red blood cell is allowed to survive in an affected person, and by the capacity of the bone marrow to continue red cell production.

Acquired Autoimmune Hemolytic Anemia is a disorder that occurs in individuals who previously had a normal red blood cell system. The disorder commonly occurs as the result of, or in conjunction with some other medical condition. It less commonly occurs alone without a precipitating factor.

In addition to The National Organization for Rare Disorders (NORD) listed in Section III, the following organizations in Section II (Disease Specific) and in Section III (Umbrella) and Section IV (Government Agencies) can provide more information:

American Autoimmune Related Diseases Association, Inc., *III*

NIH/National Heart, Lung and Blood Institute Information Center, *IV*

65 ANEMIA, HEMOLYTIC, COLD ANTIBODY

Cold Antibody Hemolytic Anemia is a rare autoimmune disorder characterized by the premature destruction of red blood cells by the body's natural defenses against invading organisms (antibodies). Normally, the red blood cells have a life span of approximately 120 days before they are removed by the spleen. In individuals with Cold Antibody Hemolytic Anemia, the red blood cells are destroyed prematurely and bone marrow production of new cells can no longer compensate for their loss. The severity of the anemia is determined by the length of time that the red blood cells survive and by the capacity of the bone marrow to continue new red blood cell production.

Immune Hemolytic Anemias may be subdivided by the temperatures at which the antibodies destroy red blood cells. As its name implies, Cold Antibody Hemolytic Anemia occurs at temperatures of approximately 0 to 10 degrees centigrade (while Warm Antibody Hemolytic Anemia, for example, occurs at temperatures of 37 degrees or higher).

In most cases, Cold Antibody Hemolytic Anemia is a primary disorder that typically becomes apparent from approximately 50 to 60 years of age. Symptoms and findings associated with the disorder may include fatigue; low levels of circulating red blood cells (anemia); persistent yellowing of the skin, mucous membranes, and whites of the eyes (jaundice); and/or sweating and coldness of the fingers and/or toes (digits) and uneven bluish or reddish discoloration of the skin of the digits, ankles, and wrists (acrocyanosis or Raynauds sign).

Cold Antibody Hemolytic Anemia may also occur due to or in association with a number of different underlying disorders such as certain infectious diseases (e.g., mycoplasma infection, mumps, cytomegalovirus, infectious mononucleosis), immunoproliferative diseases (e.g., non-Hodgkins lymphoma, chronic lymphocytic leukemia), or connective tissue disorders (e.g., systemic lupus erythematosus). Although Cold Antibody Hemolytic Anemia is known to be an autoimmune disorder, its exact underlying cause is not fully understood.

In addition to The National Organization for Rare Disorders (NORD) listed in Section III, the following organizations in Section II (Disease Specific) and in Section III (Umbrella) and Section IV (Government Agencies) can provide more information:

American Autoimmune Related Diseases Association, Inc., *III*

NIH/National Heart, Lung and Blood Institute Information Center, *IV*

66 ANEMIA, HEMOLYTIC, WARM ANTIBODY

Warm Antibody Hemolytic Anemia is an autoimmune disorder characterized by the premature destruction of red blood cells by the body's natural defenses against invading organisms (antibodies). Normally, the red blood cells have a life span of approximately 120 days before they are removed by the spleen. In an individual affected with Warm Antibody Hemolytic Anemia, the red blood cells are destroyed prematurely and bone marrow production of new cells can no longer compensate for their loss. The severity of the anemia is determined by the time the red blood cells are allowed to survive and by the capacity of the bone marrow to continue new red blood cell production.

Immune Hemolytic Anemias are subdivided by the optimal temperature at which the antibodies destroy red blood cells. As their names imply, Warm Antibody Hemolytic Anemia occurs at temperatures of 37 degrees centigrade or higher while Cold Antibody Hemolytic Anemia usually occurs at approximately 0 to 10 degrees.

In addition to The National Organization for Rare Disorders (NORD) listed in Section III, the following organizations in Section II (Disease Specific) and in Section III (Umbrella) and Section IV (Government Agencies) can provide more information:
American Autoimmune Related Diseases Association, Inc., *III*
NIH/National Heart, Lung and Blood Institute, *IV*

67 **ANEMIA, HEREDITARY NONSPHEROCYTIC HEMOLYTIC**

Hereditary Nonspherocytic Hemolytic Anemia is a term used to describe a group of rare genetic blood disorders characterized by defective red blood cells (erythrocytes) that are not abnormally "sphere-shaped" (spherocytes). These disorders are thought to be caused by defects in the membranes of red blood cells, abnormal metabolism of a chemical contained in hemoglobin (porphyrin), and deficiencies in certain enzymes such as glucose-6-phosphate dehydrogenase (G6PD) or pyruvate kinase. There are approximately 16 red blood cell enzyme abnormalities that may cause Hereditary Nonspherocytic Hemolytic Anemia.

Glucose-6-Phosphate Dehydrogenase Deficiency is one of the most common inherited enzyme abnormalities in humans. There are close to 300 different varieties of enzymatic disorders that have been classified into 5 main groups according to their relationship to red blood cells and the premature destruction of red blood cells (hemolysis). Generally people with Hereditary Nonspherocytic Hemolytic Anemia who also have a glucose-6-phosphate dehydrogenase deficiency have inherited an uncommon variant of this enzyme deficiency characterized by decreased enzyme activity, extremely abnormal kinetics, and reduced heat stability. These factors could account for the defective function of glucose-6-phosphate dehydrogenase.

In addition to The National Organization for Rare Disorders (NORD) listed in Section III, the following organizations in Section II (Disease Specific) and in Section III (Umbrella) and Section IV (Government Agencies) can provide more information:
March of Dimes Birth Defects Foundation, *III*
NIH/National Heart, Lung and Blood Institute, *IV*

68 **ANEMIA, HEREDITARY SPHEROCYTIC HEMOLYTIC**

Hereditary Spherocytic Hemolytic Anemia is a rare blood disorder characterized by defects within red blood cells (intracorpuscular) that result in a shortened survival time for these cells. Red blood cells (erythrocytes) normally circulate for a few months and when they die off are replaced by new erythrocytes. However, in Hereditary Spherocytic Hemolytic Anemia, the cells die prematurely. They also have low amounts of fats (lipid) in the cell membranes and an abnormally small amount of surface area. The red blood cells are sphere shaped (spherocytic) making it difficult for them to pass through the spleen, resulting in the early destruction of these cells (hemolysis). The sphere shape of the red blood cells is the hallmark of Hereditary Spherocytic Hemolytic Anemia, and this abnormality may be identified under a microscope. Hereditary Spherocytic Hemolytic Anemia is caused by an inherited metabolic defect.

In addition to The National Organization for Rare Disorders (NORD) listed in Section III, the following organizations in Section II (Disease Specific) and in Section III (Umbrella) and Section IV (Government Agencies) can provide more information:
March of Dimes Birth Defects Foundation, *III*
NIH/National Heart, Lung and Blood Institute, *IV*

69 **ANEMIA, MEGALOBLASTIC**

Megaloblastic Anemia is a rare blood disorder characterized by the presence of large, abnormal, immature red blood cells (megaloblasts). Decreased numbers and immaturity of white blood cells (leukocytes) and blood platelets (thrombocytes) may also occur. This disorder may be caused by a deficiency or defective absorption of vitamin B12 or folic acid. Certain antitumor or immunosuppressive drugs may also cause Megaloblastic Anemia.

In addition to The National Organization for Rare Disorders (NORD) listed in Section III, the following organizations in Section II (Disease Specific) and in Section III (Umbrella) and Section IV (Government Agencies) can provide more information:
NIH/National Heart, Lung and Blood Institute, *IV*

70 **ANEMIA, PERNICIOUS**

Pernicious Anemia is a rare blood disorder characterized by the inability of the body to properly utilize vitamin B12 (a cobalamin), which is essential for the development of red blood cells. The symptoms of Pernicious Anemia may include weakness, fatigue, an upset stomach, an abnormally rapid heartbeat (tachycardia), and/or chest pains. Recurring episodes of anemia (megaloblastic) and an abnormal yellow coloration of the skin (jaundice) are also common. Pernicious Anemia is thought to be an autoimmune disorder, and certain people may have a genetic predisposition to this disorder.

The three recognized forms of Pernicious Anemia include: Congenital Pernicious Anemia, Juvenile Pernicious Anemia, and Adult Onset Pernicious Anemia. The subdivisions are based on the age at onset and the precise nature of the defect causing impaired B12 utilization (e.g., absence of intrinsic factor).

In addition to The National Organization for Rare Disorders (NORD) listed in Section III, the following organizations in Section II (Disease Specific) and in Section III (Umbrella) and Section IV (Government Agencies) can provide more information:

American Autoimmune Related Diseases Association, Inc., *III*
March of Dimes Birth Defects Foundation, *III*
NIH/National Heart, Lung and Blood Institute, *IV*
The Arc (a national organization on mental retardation), *III*

71 **ANEMIA, SIDEROBLASTIC**

Sideroblastic Anemias are a group of blood disorders characterized by an impaired ability of the bone marrow to produce normal red blood cells. The iron inside red blood cells is inadequately used to make hemoglobin, despite adequate or increased amounts of iron. Abnormal red blood cells called sideroblasts are found in the blood of people with these types of anemia.

In addition to The National Organization for Rare Disorders (NORD) listed in Section III, the following organizations in Section II (Disease Specific) and in Section III (Umbrella) and Section IV (Government Agencies) can provide more information:

Leukemia Society of America, Inc., *II*
NIH/National Heart, Lung and Blood Institute Information Center, *IV*

72 **ANENCEPHALY**

Anencephaly is characterized by the absence of the two hemispheres of the brain. The absent brain tissue is sometimes replaced by abnormal cystic nerve tissue, which may be either exposed or covered with skin. Additionally, varying portions of the brainstem and spinal cord may be missing or malformed.

In addition to The National Organization for Rare Disorders (NORD) listed in Section III, the following organizations in Section II (Disease Specific) and in Section III (Umbrella) and Section IV (Government Agencies) can provide more information:

Anencephaly Support Foundation, *II*
Association of Birth Defect Children, Inc., *III*
Fighters for Encephaly Support Group, *III*
NIH/National Institute of Child Health and Human Development, *IV*
NIH/National Institute of Neurological Disorders and Stroke, *IV*

73 **ANGELMAN SYNDROME**

Angelman Syndrome is an extremely rare disorder characterized by congenital mental retardation, the absence of speech, unprovoked laughter, unusual facial features, and muscular abnormalities. Children with this disorder smile often and easily and may have episodes of excessive laughter. This syndrome was first described as the Happy Puppet Syndrome; however, this term is now obsolete.

In addition to The National Organization for Rare Disorders (NORD) listed in Section III, the following organizations in Section II (Disease Specific) and in Section III (Umbrella) and Section IV (Government Agencies) can provide more information:

Alliance of Genetic Support Groups, *III*
Angelman Syndrome Foundation, Inc., *II*
Angelman Syndrome Support Group, *II*
Canadian Angelman Syndrome Society, *II*
NIH/National Institute of Child Health and Human Development, *IV*
NIH/National Institute of Neurological Disorders and Stroke, *IV*
The Arc (a national organization on mental retardation), *III*

74 **ANGIOEDEMA, HEREDITARY**

Hereditary Angioedema is a rare inherited vascular disorder characterized by an excessive accumulation of body fluids that results in areas of obstruction in lymphatic vessels or veins. The blockage of the normal flow of blood or lymphatic fluid results in temporary swelling of the skin and mucous membranes. Symptoms develop due to deficiency or improper functioning of certain proteins that help to maintain the normal flow of fluids through very small blood vessels (capillaries). In some cases fluid may accumulate in other internal organs. The severity of the disease varies greatly among affected individuals.

There are two recognized forms of this disorder. The most common is Hereditary Angioedema Type I, which is the result of abnormally low levels of certain complex proteins in the blood (C1 esterase inhibitors) known as complements. They help to regulate various body functions (e.g., flow of body fluids in and out of cells). Hereditary Angioedema Type II, a rarer form of the disorder, occurs as the result of the production of abnormal complement proteins.

In addition to The National Organization for Rare Disorders (NORD) listed in Section III, the following organizations in Section II (Disease Specific) and in Section III (Umbrella) and Section IV (Government Agencies) can provide more information:
March of Dimes Birth Defects Foundation, *III*
NIH/National Heart, Lung and Blood Institute, *IV*

75 ANIRIDIA

Aniridia is a rare genetic vision disorder characterized by lack of normal development of the eye's iris. The iris is the circular colored membrane in the middle of the eyeball. It is perforated in the center by an opening known as the pupil, which regulates the amount of light that enters the eye. Aniridia is characterized by partial or complete absence of the iris. Four forms of Aniridia have been identified to date. Each can be distinguished by accompanying symptoms. Some cases are thought to occur sporadically, although a chromosome defect is the cause of most forms of this disorder.

In addition to The National Organization for Rare Disorders (NORD) listed in Section III, the following organizations in Section II (Disease Specific) and in Section III (Umbrella) and Section IV (Government Agencies) can provide more information:
Blind Children's Fund, *III*
NIH/National Eye Institute, *IV*
National Association for Parents of the Visually Impaired, *III*
National Association for Visually Handicapped, *III*
The Arc (a national organization on mental retardation), *III*
Vision Foundation, Inc., *III*

76 ANIRIDIA CEREBELLAR ATAXIA MENTAL DEFICIENCY

Aniridia-Cerebellar Ataxia-Mental Deficiency, also known as Gillespie Syndrome, is an extremely rare inherited disorder that is characterized by partial absence (aplasia) of the colored portion (iris) of the eye (Partial Aniridia), impaired coordination of voluntary movements due to underdevelopment (hypoplasia) of the brain's cerebellum (cerebellar ataxia), and mental retardation. Many affected individuals also exhibit a delay in the acquisition of skills requiring coordination of muscular and mental activity (psychomotor retardation). Aniridia-Cerebellar Ataxia-Mental Deficiency is believed to be inherited as an autosomal recessive genetic trait.

In addition to The National Organization for Rare Disorders (NORD) listed in Section III, the following organizations in Section II (Disease Specific) and in Section III (Umbrella) and Section IV (Government Agencies) can provide more information:
Glaucoma Research Foundation, *II*
NIH/National Eye Institute, *IV*
NIH/National Institute of Neurological Disorders and Stroke, *IV*
National Association for Parents of the Visually Impaired, *III*
National Association for Visually Handicapped, *III*
National Ataxia Foundation, *III*
National Eye Research Foundation, *III*
Vision Foundation, Inc., *III*

77 ANKYLOSING SPONDYLITIS

Ankylosing Spondylitis is a form of arthritis characterized by inflammation and eventual immobility of the spine (ankylosis), pelvis (sacroiliac), and other joints near the spine (paraspinal). Symptoms include varying degrees of back pain and abnormal postures. Other complications that may occur include inflammation of the iris of the eyes (iritis), difficulty breathing, and/or abnormal reflexes. The exact cause of Ankylosing Spondylitis is not known, although some people may have a genetic predisposition to this disorder.

In addition to The National Organization for Rare Disorders (NORD) listed in Section III, the following organizations in Section II (Disease Specific) and in Section III (Umbrella) and Section IV (Government Agencies) can provide more information:
American Juvenile Arthritis Organization, *II*
Arthritis Foundation, *III*
March of Dimes Birth Defects Foundation, *III*
NIH/National Arthritis and Musculoskeletal and Skin Diseases Information Clearinghouse, *IV*

78 ANODONTIA

Anodontia is a genetic disorder characterized by partial or complete absence of the primary or permanent teeth. It is associated with a group of non-progressive skin and nerve syndromes called the Ectodermal Dysplasias. Anodontia is usually part of a syndrome and seldom occurs as an isolated entity.

In addition to The National Organization for Rare Disorders (NORD) listed in Section III, the following organizations in Section II (Disease Specific) and in Section III (Umbrella) and Section IV (Government Agencies) can provide more information:

NIH/National Oral Health Information Clearinghouse, *IV*
National Foundation for Ectodermal Dysplasias, *II*

79 ANOREXIA NERVOSA

Anorexia Nervosa is an illness of self-starvation resulting in marked weight loss and characterized by a disturbed sense of body image and anxiety about weight gain. Females with this disorder may also experience absence of menstrual periods.

In addition to The National Organization for Rare Disorders (NORD) listed in Section III, the following organizations in Section II (Disease Specific) and in Section III (Umbrella) and Section IV (Government Agencies) can provide more information:

American Anorexia and Bulimia Association, Inc., *III*
Anorexia Nervosa & Related Eating Disorders, Inc., *III*
Depression and Related Affective Disorders Association, *III*
Eating Disorders Awareness and Prevention, Inc., *III*
NIH/National Institute of Mental Health, *IV*
National Alliance for the Mentally Ill, *III*
National Association of Anorexia Nervosa and Associated Disorders, Inc., *III*
National Eating Disorders Organization, *III*
National Mental Health Association, *III*
National Mental Health Consumer Self-Help Clearinghouse, *III*

80 ANTIPHOSPHOLIPID SYNDROME

Antiphospholipid Syndrome (APLS) is a very rare blood disorder characterized by recurring blood clots that usually appear before 45 years of age. It may also be associated with repeated spontaneous abortions for no apparent reason in young women. There may be a family history of blood clotting disorders in some cases.

In addition to The National Organization for Rare Disorders (NORD) listed in Section III, the following organizations in Section II (Disease Specific) and in Section III (Umbrella) and Section IV (Government Agencies) can provide more information:

American Autoimmune Related Diseases Association, Inc., *III*
Lupus Foundation of America, Inc., *II*
NIH/National Heart, Lung and Blood Institute Information Center, *IV*
National Stroke Association, *II*

81 ANTISOCIAL PERSONALITY DISORDER

Antisocial Personality Disorder is a mental illness that usually becomes apparent before the age of fifteen. Major symptoms may include antisocial behavior in which there is little concern for the rights of others. Excessive drinking, fighting and irresponsibility may also occur.

In addition to The National Organization for Rare Disorders (NORD) listed in Section III, the following organizations in Section II (Disease Specific) and in Section III (Umbrella) and Section IV (Government Agencies) can provide more information:

NIH/National Institute of Mental Health, *IV*
National Alliance for the Mentally Ill, *III*
National Mental Health Association, *III*
National Mental Health Consumer Self-Help Clearinghouse, *III*

82 ANTITHROMBIN III DEFICIENCY

Antithrombin III (AT III) Deficiency is a blood disorder characterized by the tendency to form clots in the arteries and/or veins (thrombosis). An inherited tendency to thrombosis is known as thrombophilia. Antithrombin III is a substance in the blood that limits the blood's ability to clot (coagulation). In people with Congenital Antithrombin III Deficiency, there is usually a reduced amount of this substance in the blood due to a genetic abnormality. Antithrombin III Deficiency may also be acquired; in such cases, the disorder may be reversible with treatment.

In addition to The National Organization for Rare Disorders (NORD) listed in Section III, the following organizations in Section II (Disease Specific) and in Section III (Umbrella) and Section IV (Government Agencies) can provide more information:

American Liver Foundation, *III*
March of Dimes Birth Defects Foundation, *III*
NIH/National Heart, Lung and Blood Institute, *IV*
United Liver Association, *III*

83 ANTLEY BIXLER SYNDROME

Antley-Bixler Syndrome is a very rare disorder characterized by inappropriate knitting together of bones in the body (skeletal fusions), especially the bones of the skull, hips, and arms. Children with this disorder have unusual facial features including a large prominent forehead and a flat nasal bridge. The exact cause of Antley-Bixler Syndrome is not fully understood although some studies suggest that it may be inherited as an autosomal recessive genetic trait.

In addition to The National Organization for Rare Disorders (NORD) listed in Section III, the following organizations in Section II (Disease Specific) and in Section III (Umbrella) and Section IV (Government Agencies) can provide more information:
Children's Craniofacial Association, *III*
FACES: The National Craniofacial Association, *III*
NIH/National Institute of Child Health and Human Development, *IV*

84 APERT SYNDROME

Apert Syndrome is a rare inherited disorder characterized by premature closure of the bones of the skull (craniosynostosis) causing the head to appear long and pointed at the top (acrocephaly). Other features of this disorder include fusion or webbing (syndactyly) of the fingers and/or toes and unusual facial features such as widely spaced, protruding eyes and dental crowding. Apert Syndrome may be inherited as an autosomal dominant genetic trait, or it may occur for no apparent reason (sporadic).

In addition to The National Organization for Rare Disorders (NORD) listed in Section III, the following organizations in Section II (Disease Specific) and in Section III (Umbrella) and Section IV (Government Agencies) can provide more information:
AboutFace U.S.A., *III*
Alliance of Genetic Support Groups, *III*
American Heart Association, *III*
Apert Support and Information Network, *II*
Apert Syndrome Pen Pals, *II*
Apert Syndrome Support Group, *II*
Children's Craniofacial Association, *III*
Congenital Heart Anomalies, Support, Education, & Resources, *III*
Craniofacial Support Group, *III*
Danish Apert Syndrome Association (Danmarks Apertforening), *II*
FACES: The National Craniofacial Association, *III*
Forward Face, Inc., *III*
Let's Face It, Inc., *III*
NIH/National Institute of Child Health and Human Development, *IV*
National Foundation for Facial Reconstruction, *III*
The Arc (a national organization on mental retardation), *III*

85 APLASIA CUTIS CONGENITA

Aplasia Cutis Congenita is a rare disorder that may be inherited as an autosomal dominant or autosomal recessive genetic trait. Individuals are born with the absence of certain layer(s) of skin on the scalp, trunk, and/or arms and legs. The affected area typically is covered with a thin, transparent membrane. The skull and/or underlying areas may be visible and be abnormally developed. Aplasia Cutis Congenita may be a primary disorder or it may occur in association with other underlying disorders.

In addition to The National Organization for Rare Disorders (NORD) listed in Section III, the following organizations in Section II (Disease Specific) and in Section III (Umbrella) and Section IV (Government Agencies) can provide more information:
NIH/National Arthritis and Musculoskeletal and Skin Diseases Information Clearinghouse, *IV*

86 APNEA, INFANTILE

Apnea is a term used to describe the temporary absence of spontaneous breathing. Infantile apnea occurs in children under the age of one year. Apnea may occur because of neurological impairment of the respiratory rhythm or obstruction of air flow through the air passages. The symptoms of infantile apnea include the stoppage of breathing during sleep, an abnormal bluish discoloration to the skin (cyanosis) and sometimes an unusually slow heartbeat (bradycardia). Infantile apnea may be related to some cases of sudden infant death syndrome. Episodes of apnea may decrease with age. However, several forms of adult sleep apnea also exist.

In addition to The National Organization for Rare Disorders (NORD) listed in Section III, the following organizations in Section II (Disease Specific) and in Section III (Umbrella) and Section IV (Government Agencies) can provide more information:
American Sleep Apnea Association, *II*
Center for Research in Sleep Disorders, *III*
NIH/National Institute of Child Health and Human Development, *IV*
NIH/National Institute of Neurological Disorders and Stroke, *IV*
Sudden Infant Death Syndrome Alliance, Inc., *II*

87 APNEA, SLEEP

Sleep apnea is a sleep disorder characterized by temporary, recurrent interruptions of breathing (respiration) during sleep. Symptoms of this disorder include periodic wakefulness during the night, excessive sleepiness during the day, and loud snoring during sleep. People with this disorder are frequently overweight. Diagnosis and treatment of sleep apnea can avoid serious medical problems that may arise as a consequence of oxygen deprivation in untreated patients.

Sleep apnea occurs in several forms. In some apneas, breathing (respiratory) drive is normal while in others it is abnormal. The rate of respiration is regulated by group of nerve cells in the brain that control the rhythm of breathing in response to changing oxygen levels in the blood (respiratory drive). Obstructive sleep apnea (upper airway apnea), is the most common form of sleep apnea. It results from the blockage of the respiratory passages during sleep. Affected individuals may struggle to breathe and experience increased respiratory effort. Respiratory drive is normal in people with this form of sleep apnea but the blockage prevents them from breathing normally. Obstructive apnea is more likely than central apnea to be associated with snorting and arousal from sleep.

In the rarer central sleep apnea, the brain does not send adequate signals to the diaphragm and lungs during sleep, resulting in low respiratory drive. In this form of sleep apnea, breathing stops and does not resume until the oxygen-deprived brain finally sends impulses to the diaphragm and lungs, and breathing resumes. In infants, central sleep apnea is defined as lasting 20 seconds or more.

In some cases, sleep apnea is referred to as "Pickwickian Syndrome." In these cases, obstructive apnea is combined with obesity and a short neck. Infantile sleep apnea affects children and its cause is unknown.

In addition to The National Organization for Rare Disorders (NORD) listed in Section III, the following organizations in Section II (Disease Specific) and in Section III (Umbrella) and Section IV (Government Agencies) can provide more information:

American Sleep Apnea Association, *II*
Center for Research in Sleep Disorders, *III*
NIH/National Institute of Neurological Disorders and Stroke, *IV*
Narcolepsy Network, Inc., *II*
Narcolepsy and Cataplexy Foundation of America, *III*

88 APRAXIA

Apraxia is a disorder of brain function characterized by the inability to perform learned movements on command, even though the command is understood and there is a willingness to perform the movement. The affected individual has the physical ability to move, but cannot. Apraxia is believed to be caused by a lesion in the neural pathways of the brain that contain the learned patterns cf movement. It is often a symptom of neurological, metabolic, or other disorders that can involve the brain.

In addition to The National Organization for Rare Disorders (NORD) listed in Section III, the following organizations in Section II (Disease Specific) and in Section III (Umbrella) and Section IV (Government Agencies) can provide more information:

NIH/National Institute of Neurological Disorders and Stroke, *IV*
National Aphasia Association, *II*

89 APRAXIA, OCULAR MOTOR, COGAN TYPE

Cogan Type Ocular Motor Apraxia is a rare inherited eye disorder that is present at birth (congenital). The disorder is characterized by a defect in side-to-side (horizontal) eye movements, both voluntary and responsive. When affected infants rotate their heads to look at an object to the side, their eyes will "lag" and then move in the opposite direction. In order to compensate for this, the infants will sharply jerk their heads past the desired object in an effort to bring the eyes to a position where they can view the object. As affected children reach school age, the disorder may also be associated with poor reading skills and clumsiness. Symptoms of this disorder usually improve throughout the first and second decades of life. Cogan Type Ocular Motor Apraxia is thought to be inherited as an autosomal recessive genetic trait.

In addition to The National Organization for Rare Disorders (NORD) listed in Section III, the following organizations in Section II (Disease Specific) and in Section III (Umbrella) and Section IV (Government Agencies) can provide more information:

NIH/National Eye Institute, *IV*
NIH/National Institute of Child Health and Human Development, *IV*
National Eye Research Foundation, *III*

90 ARACHNOID CYSTS

Arachnoid Cysts are fluid-filled sacs that occur on the arachnoid membrane that covers the brain and the spinal cord. There are three membranes covering these components of the central nervous system: dura mater, arachnoid, and pia mater. Arachnoid cysts appear on the arachnoid membrane, and they may also expand into the space between the pia mater and arachnoid membranes (subarachnoid space). While Arachnoid Cysts in general are not rare, they are extremely rare in some locations. Arachnoid Cysts do not usually appear within the two hemispheres of the brain (cerebrum) or within the cavities (ventricles) of the brain.

In addition to The National Organization for Rare Disorders (NORD) listed in Section III, the following organizations in Section II (Disease Specific) and in Section III (Umbrella) and Section IV (Government Agencies) can provide more information:
Brain and Pituitary Foundation of America, *III*
NIH/National Institute of Neurological Disorders and Stroke, *IV*

91 **ARACHNOIDITIS**

Arachnoiditis is a progressive inflammatory disorder affecting the middle membrane surrounding the spinal cord and brain (arachnoid membrane). Either the spinal cord or the brain may be involved; in some cases, both are affected. This disorder can also be associated with Meningitis. The condition may be caused by foreign solutions such as anesthesia drugs or testing dyes injected into the spine or arachnoid membrane.

In addition to The National Organization for Rare Disorders (NORD) listed in Section III, the following organizations in Section II (Disease Specific) and in Section III (Umbrella) and Section IV (Government Agencies) can provide more information:
Arachnoiditis Information and Support Network, *II*
Canadian Syringomyelia Network, *II*
NIH/National Institute of Neurological Disorders and Stroke, *IV*
National Spinal Cord Injury Association, *III*
National Spinal Cord Injury Hotline, *III*
Spinal Cord Society, *III*

92 **ARGINASE DEFICIENCY**

Arginase Deficiency is one of several hereditary urea cycle disorders. These disorders are caused by a deficiency of one of the enzymes needed for the incorporation of ammonia into urea, which is normally excreted in the urine. These deficiencies cause an excess of ammonia in the blood and body tissues. Affected infants may exhibit mental retardation, seizures, and spasticity. Arginase Deficiency is inherited as an autosomal recessive genetic trait.

In addition to The National Organization for Rare Disorders (NORD) listed in Section III, the following organizations in Section II (Disease Specific) and in Section III (Umbrella) and Section IV (Government Agencies) can provide more information:
Association for Neuro-Metabolic Disorders, *III*
Metabolic Information Network, *III*
NIH/National Digestive Diseases Information Clearinghouse, *IV*
National Urea Cycle Disorders Foundation, *III*
Research Trust for Metabolic Diseases in Children, *III*
The Arc (a national organization on mental retardation), *III*

93 **ARGININO SUCCINIC ACIDURIA**

Arginino Succinic Aciduria is one of several hereditary urea cycle disorders. These disorders are caused by a deficiency of one of the enzymes needed for the breakdown of ammonia into urea, which is normally excreted in the urine. The deficiencies cause an excess of ammonia in the blood and body tissues.

In Arginino Succinic Aciduria, the deficient enzyme is argininosuccinase. If left untreated, the disorder manifests itself by an elevated level of toxic ammonia in the blood (hyperammonemia). This imbalance may lead to brain damage and eventually to coma.

In addition to The National Organization for Rare Disorders (NORD) listed in Section III, the following organizations in Section II (Disease Specific) and in Section III (Umbrella) and Section IV (Government Agencies) can provide more information:
American Kidney Fund, Inc., *III*
Metabolic Information Network, *III*
NIH/National Digestive Diseases Information Clearinghouse, *IV*
National Kidney Foundation, *III*
National Urea Cycle Disorders Foundation, *III*
Research Trust for Metabolic Diseases in Children, *III*

94 **ARNOLD CHIARI SYNDROME**

Arnold-Chiari Syndrome is a rare malformation of the brain that is present at birth. Abnormalities at the base of the brain may include the displacement of the lower portion of the brain (cerebellum) and/or brain stem through the opening in the back of the skull (foramen magnum). Portions of the brain typically reach the spinal canal (upper cervical area). A developmental defect of the central nervous system may occur in some infants with Arnold-Chiari Syndrome. A sac (myelomeningocele or herniated pouch) may bulge through an abnormal opening in the spinal column and may contain portions of the spinal cord, spinal membranes, and/or cerebrospinal fluid. Some infants may also have abnormal accumulations of cerebrospinal fluid in the skull (hydrocephalus). Other malformations of the brain and spinal cord (i.e., spina bifida) may also occur.

Recently the term Arnold-Chiari Syndrome has been limited to congenital malformations of the cerebellum and brain stem that displace these parts of the brain into the spinal canal. Chiari Type I is used to describe individuals who have an extension of the brain into the spinal canal without a myelomeningocele. Chiari Type II describes this brain malformation along with myelomeningocele.

In addition to The National Organization for Rare Disorders (NORD) listed in Section III, the following organizations in Section II (Disease Specific) and in Section III (Umbrella) and Section IV (Government Agencies) can provide more information:
Canadian Syringomyelia Network, *II*
Hydrocephalus Association, *II*
Hydrocephalus Research Foundation, Inc., *II*
Hydrocephalus Support Group, Inc., *II*
March of Dimes Birth Defects Foundation, *III*
NIH/National Institute of Neurological Disorders and Stroke, *IV*

95 ARTERIOVENOUS MALFORMATION

Arteriovenous Malformation (AVM) is an inborn disorder affecting the central nervous system that occurs in two main types: i.e., in the spine or the brain (cranial). Blood vessels in these areas of the central nervous system are enlarged and tortuous. Arteries and veins may connect directly rather than being connected by fine capillaries. The malformation may be small and localized or may involve a large area (e.g., half the spinal cord). It may, like a mass lesion, compress or even replace normal tissue, or it may rupture, causing local or generalized bleeding. The most common location in the spinal cord is on the back of the cord at the level of the chest. An angioma visible on the skin may sometimes overlie the spinal AVM.

In addition to The National Organization for Rare Disorders (NORD) listed in Section III, the following organizations in Section II (Disease Specific) and in Section III (Umbrella) and Section IV (Government Agencies) can provide more information:
NIH/National Institute of Neurological Disorders and Stroke, *IV*
National Vascular Malformations Foundation, Inc., *III*

96 ARTERITIS, GIANT CELL

Giant cell arteritis is a chronic inflammatory disease characterized by the progressive inflammation of many arteries of the body (panarteritis). Granular material and abnormally large cells (giant cells) accumulate in the elastic lining of the arteries. Chronic inflammation is sometimes confined to the different branches of the heart's main artery (aorta) and any large arteries can become inflamed. However, the temporal arteries of the head are most frequently affected (temporal arteritis). In rare cases, veins may also be affected by giant cell arteritis.

The symptoms of giant cell arteritis may include stiffness, muscle pain, fever, and/or headaches. The exact cause of this disease is not fully understood, although it is thought to be an autoimmune disease that occurs when the body's own immune system attacks healthy tissue.

In addition to The National Organization for Rare Disorders (NORD) listed in Section III, the following organizations in Section II (Disease Specific) and in Section III (Umbrella) and Section IV (Government Agencies) can provide more information:
American Autoimmune Related Diseases Association, Inc., *III*
NIH/National Heart, Lung and Blood Institute Information Center, *IV*

97 ARTERITIS, TAKAYASU

Takayasu arteritis is a rare disorder characterized by inflammation of the large elastic arteries. The main artery of the heart (aorta) and the pulmonary (lung) artery are affected. This disorder causes progressive inflammation of many arteries in the body (polyarteritis), resulting in the reduction of blood flow. Arteries in the head and arms may be affected, and this can result in the loss of the major pulse points in the body. Some people with takayasu arteritis have irregular narrowing of portions of the large arteries (segmental stenosis) and abnormal backward flow of blood from the aorta into the left ventricle of the heart (aortic regurgitation).

In addition to The National Organization for Rare Disorders (NORD) listed in Section III, the following organizations in Section II (Disease Specific) and in Section III (Umbrella) and Section IV (Government Agencies) can provide more information:
American Autoimmune Related Diseases Association, Inc., *III*
NIH/National Heart, Lung and Blood Institute Information Center, *IV*

98 ARTHRITIS, INFECTIOUS

Infectious Arthritis occurs as a result of infection of tissues of a joint by bacteria, viruses or fungi. Although the symptoms of Infectious Arthritis depend upon which agent has caused the infection, associated symptoms often include fever, chills, general weakness, and headaches, followed by inflammation and painful swelling of one or more joints of the body.

In addition to The National Organization for Rare Disorders (NORD) listed in Section III, the following organizations in Section II (Disease Specific) and in Section III (Umbrella) and Section IV (Government Agencies) can provide more information:
Arthritis Foundation, *III*
Arthritis Society, *II*
Centers for Disease Control and Prevention, *IV*
NIH/National Institute of Arthritis and Musculoskeletal and Skin Diseases, *IV*

99 ARTHRITIS, JUVENILE

Juvenile Arthritis is a relatively rare disorder. However, it is the most common pediatric rheumatic disease and is responsible for the largest percentage of childhood disability. Major symptoms may include swollen and painful joints, fever, skin rash, swollen lymph glands and enlarged spleen and liver. There may also be associated blood disorders and a feeling of fatigue. The symptoms may be mild or severe.

In addition to The National Organization for Rare Disorders (NORD) listed in Section III, the following organizations in Section II (Disease Specific) and in Section III (Umbrella) and Section IV (Government Agencies) can provide more information:
American Juvenile Arthritis Organization, *II*
Arthritis Society, *II*
Juvenile Diabetes Foundation International, *II*
NIH/National Arthritis and Musculoskeletal and Skin Diseases Information Clearinghouse, *IV*

100 ARTHRITIS, PSORIATIC

Psoriatic Arthritis is a rheumatoid-like arthritic condition that is associated with psoriasis of the skin or nails and a negative rheumatoid arthritis (RA) serology laboratory test. The disorder is more common in females than males.

In addition to The National Organization for Rare Disorders (NORD) listed in Section III, the following organizations in Section II (Disease Specific) and in Section III (Umbrella) and Section IV (Government Agencies) can provide more information:
Arthritis Foundation, *III*
Arthritis Society, *II*
NIH/National Arthritis and Musculoskeletal and Skin Diseases Information Clearinghouse, *IV*
National Psoriasis Foundation, *II*
Psoriatic Arthropathy Alliance, *II*

101 ARTHROGRYPOSIS MULTIPLEX CONGENITA

Arthrogryposis Multiplex Congenita, a rare disorder that is present at birth (congenital), is characterized by reduced mobility of many joints of the body. Impairment of mobility is due to the overgrowth (proliferation) of fibrous tissue in the joints (fibrous ankylosis). There are many different types of Arthrogryposis Multiplex Congenita and the symptoms vary widely among affected individuals. In the most common form of Arthrogryposis Multiplex Congenita, the range of motion of the joints in the arms and legs (limbs) is limited or fixed. Other findings may include inward rotation of the shoulders, abnormal extension of the elbows, and bending of the wrists and fingers. In addition, the hips may be dislocated and the heels of the feet may be inwardly bent from the midline of the leg while the feet are inwardly bent at the ankle (clubfoot). The cause of Arthrogryposis Multiplex Congenita (AMC) is unknown. Most types of Arthrogryposis Multiplex Congenita are not inherited; however, a rare autosomal recessive form of the disease has been reported in one large inbred Arabic kindred in Israel.

In addition to The National Organization for Rare Disorders (NORD) listed in Section III, the following organizations in Section II (Disease Specific) and in Section III (Umbrella) and Section IV (Government Agencies) can provide more information:
Alliance of Genetic Support Groups, *III*
Arthrogryposis Group, *II*
Human Growth Foundation, *III*
MAGIC Foundation for Children's Growth, *III*
NIH/National Arthritis and Musculoskeletal and Skin Diseases Information Clearinghouse, *IV*
Short Stature Foundation, *III*

102 ASHERMAN'S SYNDROME

Asherman's Syndrome is a gynecological disorder in which affected females experience a gradual decrease in menstrual flow, increased cramping and abdominal pain, eventual cessation of menstrual cycles (amenorrhea), and infertility. In females with the disorder, such symptoms and findings occur due to inflammation of the lining of the uterus (endometritis) and the development of bands of scar tissue abnormally joining portions of the uterus (intrauterine adhesions and synechiae). Endometrial scarring and intrauterine adhesions may occur due to surgical scraping or cleaning of tissue from the uterine wall (dilatation and curettage [D and C]), infections of the endometrium (e.g., tuberculosis), or other factors.

In addition to The National Organization for Rare Disorders (NORD) listed in Section III, the following organizations in Section II (Disease Specific) and in

Section III (Umbrella) and Section IV (Government Agencies) can provide more information:
NIH/National Institute of Child Health and Human Development, *IV*
National Women's Health Network, *III*

103 ASPARTYLGLYCOSAMINURIA

Aspartylglycosaminuria is a very rare genetic disorder that is found most commonly in persons of Finnish decent. However, it is also found in other populations around the world. It is a lysosomal storage disease that becomes apparent after the infant is a few months old. Major symptoms may include coarse facial features, spine and eye deformities, behavior problems and mental retardation. The disorder is caused by an glycoprotein enzyme deficiency.

In addition to The National Organization for Rare Disorders (NORD) listed in Section III, the following organizations in Section II (Disease Specific) and in Section III (Umbrella) and Section IV (Government Agencies) can provide more information:
Association for Neuro-Metabolic Disorders, *III*
NIH/National Institute of Child Health & Human Development (Preg & Perinat), *IV*
NIH/National Institute of Diabetes, Digestive & Kidney Diseases, *IV*
National MPS (Mucopolysaccharidoses/Mucolipidoses) Society, Inc., *III*
Research Trust for Metabolic Diseases in Children, *III*

104 ASPERGER'S SYNDROME

Asperger's Syndrome is a neuropsychiatric disorder. The inability to understand other's feelings, single-mindedness, lack of verbal skills, social withdrawal and over-sensitivity are characteristic of this syndrome. Many scientists believe that Asperger's Syndrome is a sub-type of autism that is differentiated by a later onset (i.e., it is usually not recognized before 30 months of age) and speech is not delayed as it usually is in children with autism.

In addition to The National Organization for Rare Disorders (NORD) listed in Section III, the following organizations in Section II (Disease Specific) and in Section III (Umbrella) and Section IV (Government Agencies) can provide more information:
NIH/National Institute of Neurological Disorders and Stroke, *IV*
National Autistic Society, *II*

105 ASPERGILLOSIS

Aspergillosis is a term used to describe a group of pulmonary infections caused by inhaling the fungus Aspergillus. Most people who are exposed to this common fungus are not affected by it, but those with an impaired immune system, or an abnormal immune response, can become ill.

In addition to The National Organization for Rare Disorders (NORD) listed in Section III, the following organizations in Section II (Disease Specific) and in Section III (Umbrella) and Section IV (Government Agencies) can provide more information:
Centers for Disease Control and Prevention, *IV*
NIH/National Institute of Allergy and Infectious Diseases, *IV*

106 ASTROCYTOMA, BENIGN

Benign astrocytomas are abnormal growths or tumors that occur in the brain and spinal cord. They are composed of star-shaped neurological cells called astrocytes. Astrocytomas may be benign (noncancerous) or malignant (cancerous), and either type can be disabling. The bones of the skull prevent the brain from expanding outward as the tumor grows and takes up space. Consequently, healthy brain tissue is compressed, causing symptoms controlled by the area of the brain that is compressed. Because of the pressure either type of astrocytoma (benign or malignant) exerts upon the brain and the resulting symptoms, the distinction between benign (noncancerous) and malignant (cancerous) tumors of the brain is less critical than for tumors occurring elsewhere in the body.

Benign astrocytomas are usually more slow growing than the malignant forms. Astrocytomas can occur anywhere in the brain or spinal cord, with the subcortical (beneath the brain covering) white matter (fibrous tissue) of the brain hemispheres being the most common location in adults. The brainstem, cerebellum, and optic nerve are the most common locations of benign astrocytomas in children.

In addition to The National Organization for Rare Disorders (NORD) listed in Section III, the following organizations in Section II (Disease Specific) and in Section III (Umbrella) and Section IV (Government Agencies) can provide more information:
American Brain Tumor Association, *III*
Brain Tumor Society, *III*
Candlelighters Childhood Cancer Foundation, *III*
National Brain Tumor Foundation, *III*

107 ASTROCYTOMA, MALIGNANT

Malignant Astrocytoma is an infiltrating, primary brain tumor, with tentacles that may invade surrounding tissue. This provides a butterfly-like distribution pattern through the white matter of the cerebral hemispheres. The tumor may invade a membrane covering the brain (the dura), or spread via the spinal fluid through the ventricles of the brain. Spread of the tumor (metastasis) outside the brain and spinal cord is rare.

In addition to The National Organization for Rare Disorders (NORD) listed in Section III, the following organizations in Section II (Disease Specific) and in Section III (Umbrella) and Section IV (Government Agencies) can provide more information:

American Brain Tumor Association, *III*
American Cancer Society, Inc., *III*
Brain Tumor Society, *III*
Brain and Pituitary Foundation of America, *III*
Candlelighters Childhood Cancer Foundation, *III*
NIH/National Institute of Neurological Disorders and Stroke, *IV*
National Brain Tumor Foundation, *III*

108 ATAXIA TELANGIECTASIA

Ataxia Telangiectasia, also known as Louis Bar Syndrome, is an inherited progressive form of cerebellar ataxia that usually begins during infancy. It involves progressive loss of coordination of the limbs, head, and eyes and decreased immune responses against infections. During the course of the disorder, dilated blood vessels (telangiectasias) appear in the eyes and skin. Individuals with this form of ataxia are more susceptible to sinus and lung infections and may also develop tumors (neoplasia). Ataxia Telangiectasia may be misdiagnosed as Friedreich's Ataxia until telangiectasias appear. (Friedreich's Ataxia is a hereditary neuromuscular syndrome characterized by slow degenerative changes of the spinal cord and the brain.)

In addition to The National Organization for Rare Disorders (NORD) listed in Section III, the following organizations in Section II (Disease Specific) and in Section III (Umbrella) and Section IV (Government Agencies) can provide more information:

Alliance of Genetic Support Groups, *III*
American Cancer Society, Inc., *III*
Ataxia-Telangiectasia Children's Project, *II*
Juvenile Diabetes Foundation International, *II*
NIH/National Institute of Neurological Disorders and Stroke, *IV*
NIH/Patient Referral Services Unit, *IV*
National Ataxia Foundation, *III*
WE MOVE, *III*

109 ATAXIA, FRIEDREICH'S

Friedreich's Ataxia is a progressive, hereditary neuromuscular syndrome that generally becomes apparent in childhood or adolescence. Slow deterioration (degenerative changes) of the spinal chord and brain occur. These degenerative changes affect speech and movement (motor coordination) producing numbness or weakness of the arms and legs, curvature of the spine (secondary lateral scoliosis), and lower limb paralysis. Although the disorder is progressive and treatment is symptomatic, unexplained sudden (spontaneous) remissions of 5 to 10 years in duration have been reported.

In addition to The National Organization for Rare Disorders (NORD) listed in Section III, the following organizations in Section II (Disease Specific) and in Section III (Umbrella) and Section IV (Government Agencies) can provide more information:

Alliance of Genetic Support Groups, *III*
Juvenile Diabetes Foundation International, *II*
March of Dimes Birth Defects Foundation, *III*
Muscular Dystrophy Association, *III*
NIH/National Institute of Neurological Disorders and Stroke, *IV*
National Ataxia Foundation, *III*
National Scoliosis Foundation, *II*
WE MOVE, *III*

110 ATAXIA, HEREDITARY

Hereditary Ataxia is a group of rare genetic neuromuscular disorders. It is characterized by degenerative changes in the brain and spinal cord. It can affect a person anytime between infancy through adulthood. Major symptoms include lack of coordination of the muscles used for voluntary movement.

In addition to The National Organization for Rare Disorders (NORD) listed in Section III, the following organizations in Section II (Disease Specific) and in Section III (Umbrella) and Section IV (Government Agencies) can provide more information:

NIH/National Institute of Neurological Disorders and Stroke, *IV*
National Ataxia Foundation, *III*
WE MOVE, *III*

111 ATAXIA, MARIE'S

Marie's Ataxia is an inherited disorder of impaired muscle coordination usually beginning during young adulthood or middle age. This hereditary form of ataxia is characterized by unsteady walking. Nerve degeneration and muscle atrophy in the legs, head and neck area and arms may occur. Cases that begin later in life may be mild with symptoms that can often be treated successfully.

In addition to The National Organization for Rare Disorders (NORD) listed in Section III, the following

organizations in Section II (Disease Specific) and in Section III (Umbrella) and Section IV (Government Agencies) can provide more information:
Muscular Dystrophy Association, *III*
NIH/National Institute of Neurological Disorders and Stroke, *IV*
National Ataxia Foundation, *III*
WE MOVE, *III*

112 ATRIAL SEPTAL DEFECTS

Atrial septal defects are a group of rare heart defects that are present at birth (congenital). The normal heart has four chambers with two upper chambers known as atria. They are separated from each other by a fibrous partition known as the atrial septum. The two lower chambers are known as ventricles and are separated from each other by the ventricular septum. Valves connect the atria (left and right) to their respective ventricles. A small opening between the two atria (foramen ovale) is present at birth. Shortly after birth, the atrial septum gradually closes and covers this opening. In infants with atrial septal defects, the atrial septum may not close properly or may be malformed during fetal development. In this disorder, the opening between the atria persists long after it should be closed, resulting in an increase in the workload on the right side of the heart and excessive blood flow to the lungs.

Initially the symptoms associated with atrial septal defects may be absent or so mild that they may go unnoticed. Frequently this disorder is not recognized until school age or even adulthood. In adults with undetected atrial septal defects, various respiratory problems and/or heart failure may develop.

There are several forms of atrial septal defects, including ostium primum atrial defects, ostium secundum defects, and coronary sinus venosus (sinus venous defect). Most cases of atrial septal defects occur for no apparent reason (sporadic). Other cases are thought to be inherited as autosomal recessive or dominant genetic traits. Atrial septal defects may also occur in association with other disorders such as Down Syndrome or Ellis van-Creveld Syndrome.

In addition to The National Organization for Rare Disorders (NORD) listed in Section III, the following organizations in Section II (Disease Specific) and in Section III (Umbrella) and Section IV (Government Agencies) can provide more information:
American Heart Association, *III*
American Lung Association, *III*
Congenital Heart Anomalies, Support, Education, & Resources, *III*
March of Dimes Birth Defects Foundation, *III*
NIH/National Heart, Lung and Blood Institute Information Center, *IV*

113 ATRIOVENTRICULAR SEPTAL DEFECT

Atrioventricular septal defect is a rare heart defect that is present at birth (congenital). The normal heart has four chambers. Two chambers are called atria which are separated from each other by a partition called the atrial septum. The other two chambers, known as ventricles, are also separated by a septum. Valves connect the atria (left and right) to their respective ventricles. Infants with atrioventricular septal defect have improperly developed septa and valves (atrial and ventricular septa and atrioventricular valves).

There are three forms of atrioventricular septal defect: incomplete mild ASD (atrial septal defect primum), a transitional form (atrial septal defect and small ventricular septal defect), or a more severe or complete form (large atrial and ventricular defects). The symptoms of atrioventricular septal defect vary greatly and depend on the severity of the malformations (e.g., valve leakage between ventricles and ventricular size). About half the cases of atrioventricular septal defect occur in children with Down Syndrome.

In addition to The National Organization for Rare Disorders (NORD) listed in Section III, the following organizations in Section II (Disease Specific) and in Section III (Umbrella) and Section IV (Government Agencies) can provide more information:
American Heart Association, *III*
American Lung Association, *III*
Congenital Heart Anomalies, Support, Education, & Resources, *III*
NIH/National Heart, Lung and Blood Institute Information Center, *IV*

114 ATTENTION DEFICIT HYPERACTIVITY DISORDER

Attention Deficit Hyperactivity Disorder is a behavioral disorder of childhood characterized by short attention span, excessive impulsiveness, and inappropriate hyperactivity.

In addition to The National Organization for Rare Disorders (NORD) listed in Section III, the following organizations in Section II (Disease Specific) and in Section III (Umbrella) and Section IV (Government

Agencies) can provide more information:
ADHD Challenge, Inc., *II*
Children and Adults with Attention Deficit Disorder, *II*
Learning Disabilities Association of America, *III*
NIH/National Institute of Mental Health, *IV*
NIH/National Institute of Neurological Disorders and Stroke, *IV*
National Alliance for the Mentally Ill, *III*
National Attention Deficit Disorder Association, *II*
National Center for Learning Disabilities, *III*
National Mental Health Association, *III*
National Mental Health Consumer Self-Help Clearinghouse, *III*
The Arc (a national organization on mental retardation), *III*

115 AUTISM

Autism is a lifelong, nonprogressive neurologic disorder typically appearing before the age of thirty months. It is characterized by language and communication deficits, withdrawal from social contacts and extreme reactions to changes in the immediate environment. About seventy-five percent of autistic children have low scores on standardized intelligence tests. The outlook for independent living may be improved with intensive training. The life span is normal.

In addition to The National Organization for Rare Disorders (NORD) listed in Section III, the following organizations in Section II (Disease Specific) and in Section III (Umbrella) and Section IV (Government Agencies) can provide more information:
Alliance of Genetic Support Groups, *III*
Autism Network International, *II*
Autism Network for Hearing and Visually Impaired Persons, *II*
Autism Society of America, *II*
C.A.N.D.L.E., *III*
Federation of Families for Children's Mental Health, *III*
MAAP Services, Inc., *II*
March of Dimes Birth Defects Foundation, *III*
NIH/National Institute of Child Health and Human Development, *IV*
NIH/National Institute of Mental Health, *IV*
NIH/National Institute of Neurological Disorders and Stroke, *IV*
NIH/National Institute on Deafness and Other Communication Disorders Information Clearinghouse, *IV*
NIH/National Society for Children and Adults with Autism, *IV*
National Alliance for the Mentally Ill, *III*
National Autistic Society, *II*
National Mental Health Association, *III*
National Mental Health Consumer Self-Help Clearinghouse, *III*

116 BABESIOSIS

Babesiosis is a rare infectious disease in humans. It normally infects animals. Babesiosis is caused by a single-celled organism (protozoa) known as Babesia microti. The symptoms of the disease are similar to those of malaria. A severe form of Babesiosis, which can be life-threatening if untreated, can occur in people who have had their spleen removed (splenectomized) or have an impaired immune system.

In addition to The National Organization for Rare Disorders (NORD) listed in Section III, the following organizations in Section II (Disease Specific) and in Section III (Umbrella) and Section IV (Government Agencies) can provide more information:
Centers for Disease Control and Prevention, *IV*
NIH/National Institute of Allergy and Infectious Diseases, *IV*
World Health Organization (WHO) Regional Office for the Americas (AMRO), *III*

117 BALANTIDIASIS

Balantidiasis is a rare intestinal infection caused by the bacteria Balantidium coli, a single celled parasite (ciliate protozoan) that frequently infects pigs. B. coli rarely infects humans. When infected, people may have no symptoms or mild diarrhea and abdominal discomfort. Others may experience symptoms associated with acute inflammation of the intestines. Symptoms of Balantidiasis may be similar to those of other infections that cause intestinal inflammation (i.e., amoebic dysentery).

In addition to The National Organization for Rare Disorders (NORD) listed in Section III, the following organizations in Section II (Disease Specific) and in Section III (Umbrella) and Section IV (Government Agencies) can provide more information:
Centers for Disease Control and Prevention, *IV*
NIH/National Institute of Allergy and Infectious Diseases, *IV*
World Health Organization (WHO) Regional Office for the Americas (AMRO), *III*

118 BALLER GEROLD SYNDROME

Baller-Gerold Syndrome is a very rare disorder that is thought to be inherited as an autosomal recessive trait. Major features of this disorder are premature fusion or closure of the fibrous or "soft" parts of the skull causing an upward growth of the head (craniosynostosis), a deformity of the large bone of the forearm (ulnar) causing the bone to be short and curved, and a missing or underdeveloped short bone of the forearm (radius).

In addition to The National Organization for Rare Disorders (NORD) listed in Section III, the following organizations in Section II (Disease Specific) and in Section III (Umbrella) and Section IV (Government Agencies) can provide more information:
AboutFace U.S.A., *III*
Children's Craniofacial Association, *III*
FACES: The National Craniofacial Association, *III*
Forward Face, Inc., *III*
Let's Face It, Inc., *III*
NIH/National Institute of Child Health and Human Development, *IV*

119 BALO DISEASE

Balo Disease is a rare neurological disorder characterized by the rapid, progressive loss of the fatty covering (myelin sheath) around nerve fibers in the brain (demyelination). This disease typically affects children, although some cases have been reported in adults. Symptoms include gradual paralysis, involuntary muscle spasms, and other neurological problems. The symptoms of Balo Disease vary according to the areas of the brain that are affected. Damage to the brain (demyelinating lesions) may be localized to any part of the brain (i.e., cerebrum, cerebellum, or brain stem). Lesions consist of irregular patches of demyelination in a series of widening concentric circles. The symptoms of Balo Disease, which can be life-threatening, progress rapidly over several weeks, or more slowly over 2 to 3 years.

In addition to The National Organization for Rare Disorders (NORD) listed in Section III, the following organizations in Section II (Disease Specific) and in Section III (Umbrella) and Section IV (Government Agencies) can provide more information:
American Autoimmune Related Diseases Association, Inc., *III*
NIH/National Institute of Neurological Disorders and Stroke, *IV*
United Leukodystrophy Foundation, *III*

120 BANTI'S SYNDROME

Banti's Syndrome is a disorder of the spleen, the large, gland-like organ in the upper left side of the abdomen that produces red blood cells before birth and in newborns, removes and destroys aged red blood cells, and plays a role in fighting infection. Bantis Syndrome is characterized by abnormal enlargement of the spleen (splenomegaly) due to obstruction of and abnormally increased blood pressure (hypertension) within certain veins of the liver (e.g., hepatic or portal veins) or the spleen (splenic veins). Symptoms may include abnormal accumulation of fluid in the abdominal cavity (ascites); weakness; fatigue; abnormally low levels of circulating red blood cells (anemia), white blood cells (leukopenia), and/or platelets (thrombocytopenia); and/or episodes of bleeding (hemorrhage) from the gastrointestinal tract. Bantis Syndrome may be due to a number of different factors causing obstruction of portal, hepatic, or splenic veins including congenital abnormalities of such veins, blood clots, or various underlying disorders causing inflammation and obstruction of veins (vascular obstruction) of the liver.

In addition to The National Organization for Rare Disorders (NORD) listed in Section III, the following organizations in Section II (Disease Specific) and in Section III (Umbrella) and Section IV (Government Agencies) can provide more information:
American Liver Foundation, *III*
NIH/National Digestive Diseases Information Clearinghouse, *IV*
United Liver Association, *III*

121 BARDET BIEDL SYNDROME

Bardet-Biedl Syndrome is a rare disorder inherited as an autosomal recessive genetic trait. Major symptoms of this disorder may include mental retardation, obesity, delayed sexual development or underdeveloped reproductive organs, degeneration of the retinas of the eyes, kidney abnormalities and/or abnormal fingers and/or toes. Confusion exists in the medical literature regarding the difference between Bardet-Biedl Syndrome and Laurence-Moon Syndrome. Some researchers still believe that Bardet-Biedl Syndrome is a subdivision of Laurence-Moon-Biedl Syndrome.

In addition to The National Organization for Rare Disorders (NORD) listed in Section III, the following organizations in Section II (Disease Specific) and in Section III (Umbrella) and Section IV (Government Agencies) can provide more information:
American Council of the Blind, Inc., *III*
American Foundation for the Blind, *III*
American Printing House for the Blind, *III*
Blind Children's Fund, *III*
Foundation Fighting Blindness, *III*
Laurence Moon Bardet Biedl Syndrome, *II*
NIH/National Institute of Child Health and Human Development, *IV*
National Association for Parents of the Visually Impaired, *III*
National Association for Visually Handicapped, *III*
Prevent Blindness America, *III*
Retinitis Pigmentosa International, *II*
Vision Foundation, Inc., *III*

122 **BARRETT ESOPHAGUS**

Barrett Esophagus is a rare disorder characterized by chronic inflammation and ulceration of the esophagus. Symptoms develop due to the reflux of stomach acid (peptic) into the esophagus and may include episodes of heartburn and recurring pain behind the breastbone (sternum). Late symptoms may also include a narrowing (stricture) of the esophagus and difficulty swallowing.

In addition to The National Organization for Rare Disorders (NORD) listed in Section III, the following organizations in Section II (Disease Specific) and in Section III (Umbrella) and Section IV (Government Agencies) can provide more information:
Digestive Disease National Coalition, *III*
NIH/National Digestive Diseases Information Clearinghouse, *IV*

123 **BARTONELLOSIS**

Bartonellosis is a rare infectious disease characterized by anemia, an abnormally high fever, and chronic skin rashes that may be accompanied by pain. The disease is found only in South America. Sandflies that bite during the night transmit the bacteria (Bartonella bacilliformis) to humans. Treatment with antibiotics cures this disease. However, if left untreated, the symptoms can be life-threatening.

In addition to The National Organization for Rare Disorders (NORD) listed in Section III, the following organizations in Section II (Disease Specific) and in Section III (Umbrella) and Section IV (Government Agencies) can provide more information:
Centers for Disease Control and Prevention, *IV*
NIH/National Institute of Allergy and Infectious Diseases, *IV*
World Health Organization (WHO) Regional Office for the Americas (AMRO), *III*

124 **BARTTER'S SYNDROME**

Bartter's Syndrome, also known as is hypokalemic alkalosis with hypercalciuria, is a rare inherited disorder characterized by growth deficiency, potentially resulting in short stature; muscle weakness; cramps; and/or loss of potassium from the kidneys (renal potassium wasting). In some cases, affected individuals may exhibit mental retardation. Individuals with Bartter's Syndrome have a disturbance in their acid-base ratio (i.e., an accumulation of base or loss of acid) associated with a loss of potassium (hypokalemic alkalosis). Low amounts of potassium may result from overproduction of a certain hormone (aldosterone) that is essential in controlling blood pressure and regulating sodium and potassium levels (hyperaldosteronism). The exact cause of Bartter's Syndrome is not known; in some cases, it may be inherited as an autosomal recessive genetic trait.

In addition to The National Organization for Rare Disorders (NORD) listed in Section III, the following organizations in Section II (Disease Specific) and in Section III (Umbrella) and Section IV (Government Agencies) can provide more information:
American Kidney Fund, Inc., *III*
Metabolic Information Network, *III*
NIH/National Institute of Diabetes, Digestive and Kidney Diseases, *IV*
National Kidney Foundation, *III*
The Arc (a national organization on mental retardation), *III*

125 **BATTEN DISEASE**

Batten Disease is the juvenile form of a group of progressive neurological diseases known as neuronal ceroid lipofuscinoses (NCL). It is characterized by accumulation of a fatty substance (lipopigment) in the brain as well as in tissue that does not contain nerve cells. This lipopigment storage disorder is inherited, and is marked by rapidly progressive vision failure (optic atrophy), and neurological disturbances, which may begin before eight years of age. Occurring mostly in families of Northern European Scandinavian ancestry, the disorder affects the brain and may cause both deterioration of intellect and neurological functions.

In addition to The National Organization for Rare Disorders (NORD) listed in Section III, the following organizations in Section II (Disease Specific) and in Section III (Umbrella) and Section IV (Government Agencies) can provide more information:
Alliance of Genetic Support Groups, *III*
Batten Disease Support and Research Association, *II*
Children's Brain Diseases Foundation, *II*
Metabolic Information Network, *III*
NIH/National Institute of Neurological Disorders and Stroke, *IV*
National Pediatric Myoclonus Center, *II*
National Tay-Sachs and Allied Diseases Association, Inc., *III*
Research Trust for Metabolic Diseases in Children, *III*

126 **BEALS SYNDROME**

Beals Syndrome is a rare genetic connective tissue disorder inherited as an autosomal dominant trait. The major features of this disorder are long, thin, spiderlike fingers and toes; congenital contractures of the fingers, hips, elbows, knees and ankles; and unusual ears that appear crumpled.

In addition to The National Organization for Rare Disorders (NORD) listed in Section III, the following organizations in Section II (Disease Specific) and in Section III (Umbrella) and Section IV (Government Agencies) can provide more information:
British Coalition of Heritable Disorders of Connective Tissue, *III*

127 BECKWITH WIEDEMANN SYNDROME

Beckwith-Wiedemann Syndrome is a rare congenital disorder characterized by an abnormally enlarged tongue (macroglossia), an opening in the abdominal wall through which the organs of the abdomen may protrude (omphalocele), excessive size and height (macrosomia), and unusual ear creases.

In addition to The National Organization for Rare Disorders (NORD) listed in Section III, the following organizations in Section II (Disease Specific) and in Section III (Umbrella) and Section IV (Government Agencies) can provide more information:
Alliance of Genetic Support Groups, *III*
Beckwith Wiedemann Support Network, *II*
Candlelighters Childhood Cancer Foundation, *III*
March of Dimes Birth Defects Foundation, *III*
NIH/National Cancer Institute, *IV*
NIH/National Institute of Child Health and Human Development, *IV*
Neuroblastoma Children's Cancer Society, *II*
The Arc (a national organization on mental retardation), *III*

128 BEHCET'S SYNDROME

Behcet's Syndrome is a rare chronic relapsing inflammatory disorder characterized by inflammation of the eyes and ulcers of the mouth and genitals. The cause is unknown. Symptoms include areas of abnormal skin changes (ulcers or lesions) of the mouth and genitals that tend to recur spontaneously. Other systems of the body may also be effected including the joints, blood vessels, central nervous system, and/or digestive tract.

In addition to The National Organization for Rare Disorders (NORD) listed in Section III, the following organizations in Section II (Disease Specific) and in Section III (Umbrella) and Section IV (Government Agencies) can provide more information:
American Behcet's Disease Association, *II*
Arthritis Foundation, *III*
NIH/National Arthritis and Musculoskeletal and Skin Diseases Information Clearinghouse, *IV*
NIH/National Eye Institute, *IV*
NIH/National Institute of Neurological Disorders and Stroke, *IV*
National Association for Visually Handicapped, *III*

129 BEJEL

Bejel is an infectious disease that is rare in the United States but common in certain parts of the world. It is characterized by lesions of the skin and bones. The infection is very similar to syphilis but is not sexually transmitted. The organism that causes Bejel is from the same group of bacteria that causes syphilis (Treponema). Also known as endemic syphilis, the symptoms of Bejel occur in gradual stages, the late stage being the most severe.

In addition to The National Organization for Rare Disorders (NORD) listed in Section III, the following organizations in Section II (Disease Specific) and in Section III (Umbrella) and Section IV (Government Agencies) can provide more information:
Centers for Disease Control and Prevention, *IV*
NIH/National Institute of Allergy and Infectious Diseases, *IV*
World Health Organization (WHO) Regional Office for the Americas (AMRO), *III*

130 BELL'S PALSY

Bell's Palsy is a nonprogressive neurological disorder of one of the facial nerves (7th cranial nerve). This disorder is characterized by the sudden onset of facial paralysis, which may be preceded by a slight fever, pain behind the ear on the affected side, a stiff neck, and weakness and/or stiffness on one side of the face. Paralysis results from decreased blood supply (ischemia) and/or compression of the 7th cranial nerve. The exact cause of Bell's Palsy is not known. Viral (e.g., herpes zoster virus) and immune disorders are frequently implicated as a cause for this disorder. There may also be an inherited tendency toward developing Bell's Palsy.

In addition to The National Organization for Rare Disorders (NORD) listed in Section III, the following organizations in Section II (Disease Specific) and in Section III (Umbrella) and Section IV (Government Agencies) can provide more information:
Bell's Palsy Web Site and Online Support Group, *II*
NIH/National Institute of Neurological Disorders and Stroke, *IV*

131 BENIGN ESSENTIAL TREMOR

Benign Essential Tremor is a prevalent neurological disorder characterized by rapid tremors primarily of the hands and head. This disorder may be slowly progressive and eventually affect other parts of the body. Benign Essential Tremor is most commonly inherited but it may occur sporadically.

In addition to The National Organization for Rare Disorders (NORD) listed in Section III, the following

organizations in Section II (Disease Specific) and in Section III (Umbrella) and Section IV (Government Agencies) can provide more information:
International Tremor Foundation, *III*
March of Dimes Birth Defects Foundation, *III*
NIH/National Institute of Neurological Disorders and Stroke, *IV*

132 BERNARD SOULIER SYNDROME

Bernard-Soulier Syndrome is a rare inherited disorder of blood clotting (coagulation) characterized by unusually large and irregularly shaped platelets in the blood that do not clump together normally. Affected individuals tend to bleed excessively and bruise easily. Most cases of Bernard-Soulier Disease are inherited as an autosomal recessive genetic trait.

In addition to The National Organization for Rare Disorders (NORD) listed in Section III, the following organizations in Section II (Disease Specific) and in Section III (Umbrella) and Section IV (Government Agencies) can provide more information:
NIH/National Heart, Lung and Blood Institute Information Center, *IV*

133 BERYLLIOSIS

Berylliosis is a metal poisoning or allergic disorder caused by exposure to beryllium dust or fumes, usually in occupational settings. Symptoms may affect the lungs, skin, eyes, blood or various other organs of the body. Symptoms can be chronic or acute and may begin after short- or long-term exposure. Some cases may be delayed as long as twenty years after initial exposure to beryllium, which is a metal that is primarily used in the aerospace and nuclear power industry.

In addition to The National Organization for Rare Disorders (NORD) listed in Section III, the following organizations in Section II (Disease Specific) and in Section III (Umbrella) and Section IV (Government Agencies) can provide more information:
American Lung Association, *III*
Centers for Disease Control and Prevention, *IV*
NIH/National Institute of Allergy and Infectious Diseases, *IV*
NIH/National Institute of Environmental Health Sciences Clearinghouse, *IV*

134 BILIARY ATRESIA, EXTRAHEPATIC

Extrahepatic Biliary Atresia is a rare gastrointestinal disorder characterized by the absence of the normal opening of the bile duct into the liver (porta hepatis). This results in the obstruction of the bile duct from outside the liver (extrahepatic), and bile that is produced in the liver is not able reach the small intestine. A less common form of Extrahepatic Biliary Atresia occurs when the blockage of the bile duct occurs in an area that is closer to the small intestine (Distal Biliary Atresia).

The exact cause of Extrahepatic Biliary Atresia is not known, although some cases may be inherited as an autosomal recessive genetic trait. Infectious agents are also being investigated as a possible cause of this disorder.

In addition to The National Organization for Rare Disorders (NORD) listed in Section III, the following organizations in Section II (Disease Specific) and in Section III (Umbrella) and Section IV (Government Agencies) can provide more information:
American Liver Foundation, *III*
Children's Liver Alliance, *III*
Children's Liver Disease Foundation, *III*
NIH/National Institute of Diabetes, Digestive and Kidney Diseases, *IV*
United Liver Association, *III*

135 BINSWANGER'S DISEASE

Binswanger's Disease is a progressive neurological disorder characterized by degeneration of the white matter of the brain. Affected individuals usually experience a gradual loss of motor, cognitive, and behavioral abilities during a ten year period. In some cases, symptoms and physical findings associated with Binswanger's Disease may stabilize or improve for a brief time; however, in most cases, progression of the disorder usually returns. Affected individuals experience progressive memory loss and deterioration of intellectual abilities (dementia), strokes, paralysis of side of the body (hemiparesis), electrical disturbance in the brain (seizures), and/or an abnormally slow, unsteady walk (abnormal gait). Affected individuals often become depressed, uncaring (apathetic), inactive, unable to make decisions (abulic), hardly speak, and show poor judgment. In addition, affected individuals may exhibit difficulty forming words (dysarthria), swallowing difficulties (dysphagia), and inability to control the release of urine (incontinence). In some cases, affected individuals may demonstrate abnormalities that are similar to those seen in Parkinson Syndrome, such as tremors; short, shuffling steps; loss of trunk mobility; and/or loss of coordination (synergy) between upper limb and trunk movements when walking. Individuals with Binswanger's Disease may be at greater risk to develop narrowing and hardening of blood vessels (arteriosclerosis) and high blood pressure (hypertension) than the general population. The exact cause of Binswanger's Disease is not known.

In addition to The National Organization for Rare Disorders (NORD) listed in Section III, the following organizations in Section II (Disease Specific) and in Section III (Umbrella) and Section IV (Government Agencies) can provide more information:
Alzheimer's Association, *II*
Alzheimer's Disease Education and Referral Center, *II*
NIH/National Institute of Neurological Disorders and Stroke, *IV*
NIH/National Institute on Aging, *IV*
National Association for Continence, *III*

136 BJORNSTAD SYNDROME

Bjornstad Syndrome is an extremely rare inherited disorder characterized by the presence of abnormally flattened, twisted hair shafts (pili torti) and, in most cases, deafness (sensorineural hearing loss). Hearing loss typically affects both ears (bilateral). Individuals with this disorder usually have dry, fragile, lusterless, and/or coarse scalp hair as well as areas of patchy hair loss (alopecia). Bjornstad Syndrome is believed to be inherited as an autosomal dominant genetic trait. However, there may be a form of Bjornstad Syndrome associated with underdevelopment of the ovaries in females and the testes in males (hypogonadism) that is inherited as an autosomal recessive genetic trait.

In addition to The National Organization for Rare Disorders (NORD) listed in Section III, the following organizations in Section II (Disease Specific) and in Section III (Umbrella) and Section IV (Government Agencies) can provide more information:
Alexander Graham Bell Association for the Deaf, Inc., *III*
Better Hearing Institute, *III*
NIH/National Institute of Arthritis and Musculoskeletal and Skin Diseases, *IV*
NIH/National Institute on Deafness and Other Communication Disorders Information Clearinghouse, *IV*
National Information Center on Deafness, *III*

137 BLASTOMYCOSIS

Blastomycosis is a rare infectious multisystem disease that is caused by the fungus Blastomyces dermatitidis. The symptoms vary greatly according the affected organ system. Generalized symptoms may include fever, chills, cough, and/or difficulty breathing (dyspnea). In the chronic phase of the disease, the lungs and skin are most frequently affected. The genitourinary tract and bones may also be involved.

In addition to The National Organization for Rare Disorders (NORD) listed in Section III, the following organizations in Section II (Disease Specific) and in Section III (Umbrella) and Section IV (Government Agencies) can provide more information:
Centers for Disease Control and Prevention, *IV*
NIH/National Institute of Allergy and Infectious Diseases, *IV*
World Health Organization (WHO) Regional Office for the Americas (AMRO), *III*

138 BLEPHAROPHIMOSIS, PTOSIS, EPICANTHUS INVERSUS SYNDROME

Blepharophimosis, Ptosis, Epicanthus Inversus Syndrome (BPES) is a rare disorder that is inherited as an autosomal dominant trait. The main findings of this disorder are eyelids that are abnormally narrow horizontally (blepharophimosis), a vertical fold of skin from the lower eyelid up either side of the nose (epicanthus inversus), and drooping of the upper eyelids (ptosis). There are thought to be two types of the syndrome. Type I BPES, which involves female infertility, is inherited as an autosomal dominant genetic trait and is transmitted by affected males to their offspring. Type II BPES is also transmitted as an autosomal dominant genetic trait. Males and females can transmit the disorder to their offspring, but it is not associated with female infertility.

In addition to The National Organization for Rare Disorders (NORD) listed in Section III, the following organizations in Section II (Disease Specific) and in Section III (Umbrella) and Section IV (Government Agencies) can provide more information:
AboutFace U.S.A., *III*
Blepharophimosis, Ptosis, Epicanthus Inversus Family Network, *II*
Children's Craniofacial Association, *III*
FACES: The National Craniofacial Association, *III*
Forward Face, Inc., *III*
NIH/National Institute of Child Health and Human Development, *IV*

139 BLEPHAROSPASM, BENIGN ESSENTIAL

Benign Essential Blepharospasm is a rare disorder in which the muscles of the eyelids (orbiculares oculi) do not function properly. There are intermittent and involuntary contractions or spasms of the muscles around the eyes. Although the eyes themselves are unaffected, the patient may eventually become functionally blind because of an inability to open the eyelids. Benign Essential Blepharospasm is a form of dystonia, which is a group of neuromuscular disorders characterized by muscle spasms.

In addition to The National Organization for Rare Disorders (NORD) listed in Section III, the following organizations in Section II (Disease Specific) and in Section III (Umbrella) and Section IV (Government Agencies) can provide more information:
Benign Essential Blepharospasm Research Foundation, Inc., *II*
Dystonia Medical Research Foundation, *III*
Dystonia Society, *III*
NIH/National Institute of Neurological Disorders and Stroke, *IV*
WE MOVE, *III*

140 BLOOM SYNDROME

Bloom Syndrome is a rare inherited disorder characterized by short stature, multiple small dilated blood vessels on the face (facial telangiectasia), increased sensitivity to light (photosensitivity), and susceptibility to infections. Later in life, some individuals with Bloom Syndrome may be at an increased risk for certain malignancies. Bloom Syndrome is inherited as an autosomal recessive genetic trait.

In addition to The National Organization for Rare Disorders (NORD) listed in Section III, the following organizations in Section II (Disease Specific) and in Section III (Umbrella) and Section IV (Government Agencies) can provide more information:
Bloom's Syndrome Registry, *II*
Human Growth Foundation, *III*
MAGIC Foundation for Children's Growth, *III*
March of Dimes Birth Defects Foundation, *III*
NIH/National Institute of Child Health and Human Development, *IV*
National Foundation for Jewish Genetic Diseases, *III*

141 BLUE DIAPER SYNDROME

Blue Diaper Syndrome is a rare, inherited metabolic disorder characterized in infants by bluish urine-stained diapers. The incomplete intestinal breakdown of tryptophan, a dietary nutrient, causes this disorder. Symptoms typically include digestive disturbances, fever, and visual difficulties. Some children with Blue Diaper Syndrome may also develop kidney disease. Blue Diaper Syndrome is inherited as an autosomal recessive genetic trait.

In addition to The National Organization for Rare Disorders (NORD) listed in Section III, the following organizations in Section II (Disease Specific) and in Section III (Umbrella) and Section IV (Government Agencies) can provide more information:
Alliance of Genetic Support Groups, *III*
American Kidney Fund, Inc., *III*
March of Dimes Birth Defects Foundation, *III*
Metabolic Information Network, *III*
NIH/National Digestive Diseases Information Clearinghouse, *IV*
National Kidney Foundation, *III*
Research Trust for Metabolic Diseases in Children, *III*

142 BLUE RUBBER BLEB NEVUS

Blue Rubber Bleb Nevus is a very rare congenital blood vessel (vascular) disorder affecting the skin surface as well as the internal organs of the body. Multiple distinctive nodules composed of many blood vessels (hemangiomas) are the primary feature of this disorder. These rubbery skin hemangiomas are blister-like in appearance and vary in color, size, shape, number and site. They may be sensitive to the touch and are usually noncancerous (benign).

In addition to The National Organization for Rare Disorders (NORD) listed in Section III, the following organizations in Section II (Disease Specific) and in Section III (Umbrella) and Section IV (Government Agencies) can provide more information:
NIH/National Arthritis and Musculoskeletal and Skin Diseases Information Clearinghouse, *IV*
Naevus Support Group, *II*
Nevus Network, *II*
Nevus Outreach, Inc., *II*

143 BORJESON SYNDROME

Borjeson Syndrome is a very rare disorder thought to be inherited as an X-linked dominant or X-linked recessive genetic trait with less severe symptoms in females. Major characteristics of this disorder may include an unusual facial appearance, mental retardation, seizures, short stature, delayed sexual development, muscle weakness and/or obesity.

In addition to The National Organization for Rare Disorders (NORD) listed in Section III, the following organizations in Section II (Disease Specific) and in Section III (Umbrella) and Section IV (Government Agencies) can provide more information:
NIH/National Institute of Child Health and Human Development, *IV*

144 BOTULISM

Botulism is a neuromuscular (paralytic) disease cause by a bacterial toxin acting in the intestine (enterotoxin) and causing neuromuscular poisoning (resulting from clostridium botulinum toxin). There are four different forms of botulism; foodborne, wound, infantile, and an undetermined form. The most common form, foodborne botulism, is caused when C. botulinum toxin, produced in contaminated food is ingested. Wound botulism is caused from C. botulinum toxin produced in wounds that are contaminated with this bacterium. Infant botulism is caused by the ingestion of C. botulinum toxin spores and the production of toxin in the intestine of affected infants. There are some documented cases of botulism in older children and adults that is clinically similiar to infant botulism.

In addition to The National Organization for Rare Disorders (NORD) listed in Section III, the following organizations in Section II (Disease Specific) and in Section III (Umbrella) and Section IV (Government Agencies) can provide more information:
Centers for Disease Control and Prevention, *IV*
Food and Drug Administration (FDA) Office of Inquiry & Consumer Information, *IV*
NIH/National Institute of Allergy and Infectious Diseases, *IV*

145 BOWEN HUTTERITE SYNDROME

Bowen Hutterite Syndrome is a very rare disorder inherited as an autosomal recessive genetic trait. Major symptoms may include low birth weight, a small head (microcephaly), a prominent nose, an underdeveloped jaw (micrognathia), "rocker-bottom feet," and failure to thrive.

In addition to The National Organization for Rare Disorders (NORD) listed in Section III, the following organizations in Section II (Disease Specific) and in Section III (Umbrella) and Section IV (Government Agencies) can provide more information:
NIH/National Institute of Child Health and Human Development, *IV*

146 BOWEN'S DISEASE

Bowen's Disease is characterized by a precancerous, slow growing skin malignancy. The major symptom is a red-brown, scaly or crusted patch on the skin which resembles psoriasis or dermatitis. It may occur on any part of the skin or in the mucous membranes.

In addition to The National Organization for Rare Disorders (NORD) listed in Section III, the following organizations in Section II (Disease Specific) and in Section III (Umbrella) and Section IV (Government Agencies) can provide more information:
American Cancer Society, Inc., *III*
NIH/National Arthritis and Musculoskeletal and Skin Diseases Information Clearinghouse, *IV*
Skin Cancer Foundation, *III*

147 BOWENOID PAPULOSIS

Bowenoid Papulosis is a rare sexually transmitted disorder thought to be caused by human papillomavirus type 16. This disorder is characterized by lesions that are found on the genitals of males and females. The lesions are reddish brown or violet in color, small, solid, raised and sometimes velvety.

In addition to The National Organization for Rare Disorders (NORD) listed in Section III, the following organizations in Section II (Disease Specific) and in Section III (Umbrella) and Section IV (Government Agencies) can provide more information:
Centers for Disease Control and Prevention, *IV*
NIH/National Institute of Allergy and Infectious Diseases, *IV*
Sexuality Information and Education Council of the U.S., *III*

148 BRAIN TUMORS, GENERAL

Brain Tumors are abnormal growths in the brain that can be either cancerous (malignant) of noncancerous (benign). The effects on the brain of malignant and benign brain tumors are very similar and can cause the same types of problems depending upon the type of tumor and where it is located in the brain.

In addition to The National Organization for Rare Disorders (NORD) listed in Section III, the following organizations in Section II (Disease Specific) and in Section III (Umbrella) and Section IV (Government Agencies) can provide more information:
American Brain Tumor Association, *III*
American Cancer Society, Inc., *III*
Brain Tumor Foundation for Children, Inc., *III*
Brain Tumor Foundation of Canada, *III*
Brain Tumor Society, *III*
Brain and Pituitary Foundation of America, *III*
Candlelighters Childhood Cancer Foundation, *III*
Candlelighters Childhood Cancer Foundation Canada, *III*
Children's Brain Tumor Foundation, *III*
NIH/National Cancer Institute, *IV*
NIH/Patient Referral Services Unit, *IV*
National Brain Tumor Foundation, *III*
Pituitary Tumor Network Association, *III*

149 BRANCHIO OCULO FACIAL SYNDROME

Branchio-Oculo-Facial Syndrome is a very rare genetic disorder that is apparent at birth (congenital). The disorder may be characterized by low birth weight; presence of an abnormal pit, opening (cleft), or tumor-like skin abnormality (hemangiomatous or atrophic skin lesion) behind both ears (postauricular area); distinctive malformations of the head and facial (craniofacial) area; abnormalities of the eyes; premature graying of the scalp hair during adolescence; and/or other abnormalities. Some individuals with Branchio-Oculo-Facial Syndrome may exhibit incomplete closure of the roof of the mouth (cleft palate) and/or an abnormal groove in the upper lip (cleft lip), while others may have an unusually wide, prominent ridge of the upper lip (philtrum) that resembles a surgically repaired cleft lip (pseudocleft). Additional craniofacial abnormalities may include a broad, misshapen (dysplastic) nose and malformed ears. In individuals with the disorder, characteristic eye (ocular) abnormalities may include unusually small eyes (microphthalmia); clouding of the lenses of the eyes (cataracts); crossing of the eyes at birth (congenital strabismus); widely spaced eyes (ocular hypertelorism); and/or absence of tissue (coloboma) from the colored portion of the eyes (iris), giving the iris a "keyhole" appearance. Branchio-Oculo-Facial Syndrome is inherited as an autosomal dominant genetic trait.

In addition to The National Organization for Rare Disorders (NORD) listed in Section III, the following organizations in Section II (Disease Specific) and in Section III (Umbrella) and Section IV (Government Agencies) can provide more information:
FACES: The National Craniofacial Association, *III*
Let's Face It, Inc., *III*
National Foundation for Facial Reconstruction, *III*

150 BRANCHIO OTO RENAL SYNDROME

Branchio-Oto-Renal Syndrome is a rare disorder inherited as an autosomal dominant genetic trait. This disorder is characterized by pits or car tags in front of the outer ear, abnormal passages from the throat to the outside surface of the neck (branchial fistulas), branchial cysts, hearing loss and/or abnormal development of the kidneys.

In addition to The National Organization for Rare Disorders (NORD) listed in Section III, the following organizations in Section II (Disease Specific) and in Section III (Umbrella) and Section IV (Government Agencies) can provide more information:
American Kidney Fund, Inc., *III*
American Society for Deaf Children, *III*
NIH/National Institute of Child Health and Human Development, *IV*
NIH/National Institute of Diabetes, Digestive and Kidney Diseases, *IV*
National Kidney Foundation, *III*

151 BROAD BETA DISEASE

Broad Beta Disease, or Hyperlipoproteinemia Type III, is one of a group of inherited disorders of fat metabolism known as Hyperlipoproteinemias. It is characterized by the improper transport and storage of cholesterol (beta lipoprotein) in the body. Symptoms include multiple yellowish fatty deposits (xanthomas) under the skin, coronary artery disease, and/or obesity. Other symptoms may include the buildup of fatty substances on the inner walls of large and medium-sized blood vessels (atherosclerosis) and the obstruction of blood vessels by fatty deposits.

In addition to The National Organization for Rare Disorders (NORD) listed in Section III, the following organizations in Section II (Disease Specific) and in Section III (Umbrella) and Section IV (Government Agencies) can provide more information:
American Heart Association, *III*
March of Dimes Birth Defects Foundation, *III*
NIH/National Heart, Lung and Blood Institute Information Center, *IV*
National Lipid Diseases Foundation, *III*

152 BRONCHOPULMONARY DYSPLASIA (BPD)

Bronchopulmonary Dysplasia is a chronic bronchial tube and lung disease that affects infants who have been on a ventilator. The disorder usually occurs when an infant is approximately 28 days old, has certain blood-gas and radiographic (x-ray or gamma ray) abnormalities, and has an apparent lung injury causing a respiratory disorder. Pulmonary Distress Syndrome (lung disease in infants causing difficulty in breathing and collapsed lungs) is often also present.

In addition to The National Organization for Rare Disorders (NORD) listed in Section III, the following organizations in Section II (Disease Specific) and in Section III (Umbrella) and Section IV (Government Agencies) can provide more information:
American Lung Association, *III*
NIH/National Heart, Lung and Blood Institute Information Center, *IV*

153 BROWN SEQUARD SYNDROME

Brown-Sequard Syndrome is a rare spinal motor disease that affects one side of the spinal cord. It is usually caused by an injury to the neck or spinal area. In many cases, affected individuals have received some type of puncture wound to the neck or back that has caused symptoms to appear.

In addition to The National Organization for Rare Disorders (NORD) listed in Section III, the following

organizations in Section II (Disease Specific) and in Section III (Umbrella) and Section IV (Government Agencies) can provide more information:
Amyotrophic Lateral Sclerosis Association, *II*
Families of Spinal Muscular Atrophy, *III*
NIH/National Institute of Neurological Disorders and Stroke, *IV*

154 BROWN SYNDROME

Brown Syndrome is a rare eye disorder characterized by defects in eye movements. This disorder may be present at birth (congenital) or may occur as the result of another underlying disorder (acquired). Muscles control the movements of the eyes. Some of these muscles turn the eyeball up and down, move the eyeball from side to side, or enable the eyeball to rotate slightly in its socket. The superior oblique tendon sheath of the superior oblique muscle surrounds the eyeball. The symptoms of Brown Syndrome are caused by abnormalities of this tendon sheath including shortening, thickening, or inflammation. This results in the inability to move the affected eye upward.

In addition to The National Organization for Rare Disorders (NORD) listed in Section III, the following organizations in Section II (Disease Specific) and in Section III (Umbrella) and Section IV (Government Agencies) can provide more information:
NIH/National Eye Institute, *IV*

155 BRUCELLOSIS

Brucellosis is a widespread infectious disease that affects livestock and may be transmitted to humans. It is caused by one of four different species of the bacteria that belong to the genus Brucella. Brucellosis is rare in the United States but common elsewhere in the world. Initial infection may cause acute flu-like symptoms including fever, muscle pain, headache, loss of appetite, and profuse sweating during the night. In some people, the symptoms occur suddenly, whereas, in others, symptoms may develop over the course of a few months. If Brucellosis is not treated, the disease may take months to resolve once appropriate therapy is begun. Brucellosis may be confined to a certain area of the body (local) or have serious widespread complications that affect the central nervous system, the spine, and other organs of the body. Brucellosis may be prevented if people drink only pasteurized cow's and goat's milk. Pasteurization kills the bacteria that cause the disease. However, farmers and people exposed to butchered meat may also be affected by Brucellosis.

In addition to The National Organization for Rare Disorders (NORD) listed in Section III, the following organizations in Section II (Disease Specific) and in Section III (Umbrella) and Section IV (Government Agencies) can provide more information:
Centers for Disease Control and Prevention, *IV*
Food and Drug Administration (FDA) Office of Inquiry & Consumer Information, *IV*
World Health Organization (WHO) Regional Office for the Americas (AMRO), *III*

156 BUBONIC PLAGUE

Bubonic Plague is an acute, severe infectious disorder caused by the bacterium (bacillus) Yersinia Pestis. These bacteria can be carried by small wild rodents, other wild animals or even household pets. The disease can be transmitted to humans through the bites of fleas or through direct contact with infected animal tissues. The disorder is most common in Southeast Asia, but it also occurs in some areas of the United States. Major symptoms include an abrupt onset with chills, fever, and enlarged lymph nodes (buboes). Treatment must start immediately to avoid severe complications or death. A milder form of Bubonic Plague, Pestis Minor, usually resolves in approximately a week with appropriate treatment.

In addition to The National Organization for Rare Disorders (NORD) listed in Section III, the following organizations in Section II (Disease Specific) and in Section III (Umbrella) and Section IV (Government Agencies) can provide more information:
Centers for Disease Control and Prevention, *IV*
NIH/National Institute of Allergy and Infectious Diseases, *IV*
World Health Organization (WHO) Regional Office for the Americas (AMRO), *III*

157 BUDD CHIARI SYNDROME

Budd-Chiari Syndrome is a rare disorder characterized by narrowing and obstruction (occlusion) of the veins of the liver (hepatic veins). Symptoms associated with Budd Chiari Syndrome include pain in the upper right part of the abdomen, an abnormally large liver (hepatomegaly), and/or accumulation of fluid in the space (peritoneal cavity) between the two layers of the membrane that lines the stomach (ascites). Other findings that may be associated with the disorder include nausea, vomiting, and/or an abnormally large spleen (splenomegaly). The severity of the disorder varies from case to case, depending upon the site and number of affected veins. In some cases, if the major hepatic veins are involved, high blood pressure in the veins carrying blood from the gastrointestinal (GI) tract back to the heart through the liver (portal hypertension) may be present. In most cases, the exact cause of Budd-Chiari Syndrome is not known.

In addition to The National Organization for Rare Disorders (NORD) listed in Section III, the following organizations in Section II (Disease Specific) and in Section III (Umbrella) and Section IV (Government Agencies) can provide more information:

American Liver Foundation, *III*
NIH/National Digestive Diseases Information Clearinghouse, *IV*
United Liver Association, *III*

158 BUERGER'S DISEASE

Buerger's Disease is a very rare disorder that, in most cases, affects young or middle-aged male cigarette smokers. It is characterized by narrowing or blockage (occlusion) of the veins and arteries of the extremities, resulting in reduced blood flow to these areas (peripheral vascular disease). The legs are more often affected than the arms. In most cases, the first symptom is extreme pain of the lower arms and legs while at rest. Affected individuals may also experience cramping in the legs when they walk that, in rare cases, may cause limping (claudication). In addition, affected individuals may have sores (ulcers) on the extremities, numbness and tingling and a lack of normal blood flow to the fingers and/or toes when exposed to cold temperatures (Raynaud's Phenomenon), and/or inflammation and clotting of certain veins (thrombophlebitis). In severe cases, individuals with Buerger's Disease may exhibit tissue death (gangrene) of affected limbs. The exact cause of Buerger's Disease is not known; however, most affected individuals are smokers.

In addition to The National Organization for Rare Disorders (NORD) listed in Section III, the following organizations in Section II (Disease Specific) and in Section III (Umbrella) and Section IV (Government Agencies) can provide more information:

NIH/National Heart, Lung and Blood Institute Information Center, *IV*

159 BULIMIA

Bulimia is a psychiatric disorder consisting of binge eating, often followed by self-induced vomiting or purges by the use of laxatives and diuretics. The majority of patients are female.

In addition to The National Organization for Rare Disorders (NORD) listed in Section III, the following organizations in Section II (Disease Specific) and in Section III (Umbrella) and Section IV (Government Agencies) can provide more information:

American Anorexia and Bulimia Association, Inc., *III*
Anorexia Nervosa & Related Eating Disorders, Inc., *III*
Eating Disorders Awareness and Prevention, Inc., *III*
NIH/National Institute of Mental Health, *IV*
National Alliance for the Mentally Ill, *III*
National Association of Anorexia Nervosa and Associated Disorders, Inc., *III*
National Eating Disorders Organization, *III*
National Mental Health Association, *III*
National Mental Health Consumer Self-Help Clearinghouse, *III*

160 BULLOUS PEMPHIGOID

Bullous Pemphigoid is a rare, chronic skin disorder characterized by blistering. This disorder occurs most frequently in elderly people. Generalized blistering occurs in and under the upper layers of the skin and usually subsides spontaneously within several months or years. However, symptoms may recur. In some rare cases of Bullous Pemphigoid, complications such as pneumonia may develop.

In addition to The National Organization for Rare Disorders (NORD) listed in Section III, the following organizations in Section II (Disease Specific) and in Section III (Umbrella) and Section IV (Government Agencies) can provide more information:

American Autoimmune Related Diseases Association, Inc., *III*
NIH/National Arthritis and Musculoskeletal and Skin Diseases Information Clearinghouse, *IV*
NIH/National Cancer Institute, *IV*
Skin Disease Research Core Centers of the National Institute of Arthritis, *IV*

161 BURNING MOUTH SYNDROME

Burning Mouth Syndrome is characterized by a burning sensation in the mouth and/or tongue. In some cases, this condition may be associated with vitamin B12 deficiency, oral yeast infection (candida albicans), or irritation from dental prosthetics (dentures). The burning sensation may be aggravated by hot spicy foods.

In addition to The National Organization for Rare Disorders (NORD) listed in Section III, the following organizations in Section II (Disease Specific) and in Section III (Umbrella) and Section IV (Government Agencies) can provide more information:

NIH/National Institute of Diabetes, Digestive and Kidney Diseases, *IV*
NIH/National Oral Health Information Clearinghouse, *IV*

162 **C SYNDROME**

C Syndrome is a rare disorder thought to be inherited as an autosomal recessive trait. Patients with this disorder are born with a malformation in which the head is a triangular shape due to premature union of the skull bones (trigonocephaly), a narrow pointed forehead, a flat broad nasal bridge with a short nose, vertical folds over the inner corners of the eyes, an abnormal palate that is deeply furrowed, abnormalities of the ear, crossed eyes (strabismus), joints that are bent or in a fixed position, and loose skin. All recorded patients except one have had mental retardation.

In addition to The National Organization for Rare Disorders (NORD) listed in Section III, the following organizations in Section II (Disease Specific) and in Section III (Umbrella) and Section IV (Government Agencies) can provide more information:

FACES: The National Craniofacial Association, *III*
NIH/National Institute of Child Health and Human Development, *IV*

163 **CHARGE SYNDROME**

CHARGE Syndrome is a rare disorder that results from several defects during early fetal development and affects several organ systems of the body. CHARGE is an acronym that stands for (C)oloboma of the eye, (H)eart defects, (A)tresia of the Choanae, (R)etardation of growth and development, (G)enital and Urinary anomalies, and (E)ar anomalies. Four of these characteristic findings must be present to confirm the diagnosis of CHARGE Syndrome. In addition to these classic findings associated with CHARGE Syndrome, some affected infants may also have other abnormalities including characteristic facial features, paralysis of certain facial nerves (facial palsy), incomplete closure of the roof of the mouth (cleft palate), a vertical groove in the upper lip (cleft lip), an abnormal connection between the windpipe and the tube that carries food from the mouth to the stomach (tracheoesophageal fistula), and/or kidney (renal) malformations. The physical findings and symptoms of individuals with CHARGE Syndrome may vary greatly from case to case. The exact cause of CHARGE Syndrome is not known; most cases are thought to occur randomly, for no apparent reason (sporadic).

In addition to The National Organization for Rare Disorders (NORD) listed in Section III, the following organizations in Section II (Disease Specific) and in Section III (Umbrella) and Section IV (Government Agencies) can provide more information:

American Foundation for the Blind, *III*
CHARGE Syndrome Foundation, Inc., *II*
Congenital Heart Anomalies, Support, Education, & Resources, *III*
NIH/National Institute of Child Health and Human Development, *IV*
National Association for Parents of the Visually Impaired, *III*
The Arc (a national organization on mental retardation), *III*

164 **CAMPTOMELIC SYNDROME**

Camptomelic Syndrome is a rare congenital skeletal disorder that is inherited as an autosomal recessive genetic trait. It is characterized by short stature with bowing and an angular shape of the long bones of the legs. The bones of the shoulder and pelvic area are often abnormal. Eleven pairs of ribs instead of the usual twelve may be present. There are two forms of this disorder the long-limbed form and the short-limbed form. Other abnormalities are associated with both forms of the disorder.

In addition to The National Organization for Rare Disorders (NORD) listed in Section III, the following organizations in Section II (Disease Specific) and in Section III (Umbrella) and Section IV (Government Agencies) can provide more information:

Human Growth Foundation, *III*
Little People of America, *III*
NIH/National Arthritis and Musculoskeletal and Skin Diseases Information Clearinghouse, *IV*
NIH/National Institute of Child Health and Human Development, *IV*
Short Stature Foundation, *III*

165 **CANCER, BREAST**

Breast Cancer is one of approximately 200 different types of cancer. Cancer is a disease in which abnormal cell development occurs, causing destruction of healthy cells. Breast Cancer is one of the most common forms of cancer. Generally, breast cancer is discovered by the patient or physician as a hard, irregularly-shaped mass within the breast. It can also be detected by mammogram (breast x-ray). When detected early, breast cancer is treatable. People who have first degree relatives with breast cancer are at increased risk and should enter a breast cancer screening program on a continuous basis.

In addition to The National Organization for Rare Disorders (NORD) listed in Section III, the following organizations in Section II (Disease Specific) and in Section III (Umbrella) and Section IV (Government Agencies) can provide more information:

American Cancer Society, Inc., *III*
CancerOnline, *III*
NIH/National Cancer Institute, *IV*
NIH/Office of Research on Women's Health, *IV*
National Breast Cancer Coalition, *II*
OncoLink: The University of Pennsylvania Cancer Center Resource, *III*
Sisters Network, Inc., *II*
Y-Me National Breast Cancer Organization, *II*

166 CANCER, COLON

Colon cancer is one of the most common cancers found in the United States. The cause is unknown. It may be related to a high-fat low-fiber diet. In some people, the tendency to develop colon cancer may be inherited. Cancer is a disease in which abnormal cell development occurs, causing destruction of healthy cells. Symptoms of colon cancer may include changes in the shape or color of stools, blood in the stools, constipation and/or diarrhea, abdominal discomfort and sometimes nausea. Surgery is generally performed to correct this type of cancer, usually along with radiation and/or chemotherapy.

In addition to The National Organization for Rare Disorders (NORD) listed in Section III, the following organizations in Section II (Disease Specific) and in Section III (Umbrella) and Section IV (Government Agencies) can provide more information:
American Cancer Society, Inc., *III*
CancerOnline, *III*
Johns Hopkins Hereditary Colorectal Cancer Registry, *III*
OncoLink: The University of Pennsylvania Cancer Center Resource, *III*

167 CANCER, LUNG

Lung Cancer is the most common form of cancer among both men and women in the United States. Those most at risk are smokers, especially heavy smokers. Cancer is a disease in which malignant cell development occurs, causing destruction of healthy cells. Major symptoms of lung cancer may include persistent coughing, chest pain, shortness of breath, coughing up blood from the lungs (hemoptysis), or weight loss. Ninety-five percent of lung cancers are caused by four main types: squamous cell, adenocarcinoma, small (or oat) cell, and large cell lung cancer.

In addition to The National Organization for Rare Disorders (NORD) listed in Section III, the following organizations in Section II (Disease Specific) and in Section III (Umbrella) and Section IV (Government Agencies) can provide more information:
American Cancer Society, Inc., *III*
CancerOnline, *III*
OncoLink: The University of Pennsylvania Cancer Center Resource, *III*

168 CANCER, PROSTATE

Prostate cancer is a prevalent form of cancer affecting only males. Cancer is a disease in which malignant cell development occurs, causing destruction of healthy tissue. The prostate gland, responsible for sperm vitality, is about the size of a walnut and surrounds the part of the male urethra beneath the bladder. Cancer of the prostate gland commonly occurs in older men. Average age of onset is 73 years.

In addition to The National Organization for Rare Disorders (NORD) listed in Section III, the following organizations in Section II (Disease Specific) and in Section III (Umbrella) and Section IV (Government Agencies) can provide more information:
American Cancer Society, Inc., *III*
CancerOnline, *III*
Mathews Foundation for Prostate Cancer Research, *II*
NIH/National Cancer Institute, *IV*
OncoLink: The University of Pennsylvania Cancer Center Resource, *III*
US TOO International, Inc., Prostate Cancer Survivor Support Groups, *II*

169 CANCERS, SKIN, GENERAL

There are many different types of Skin Cancer. Combined together all types of Skin Cancer represent the most prevalent type of cancer. Most skin cancers are characterized by changes in the color or texture of the skin, but some types begin under the skin where they can spread to other parts of the body. Malignant melanoma is the most dangerous of this type of skin cancer.

In addition to The National Organization for Rare Disorders (NORD) listed in Section III, the following organizations in Section II (Disease Specific) and in Section III (Umbrella) and Section IV (Government Agencies) can provide more information:
American Cancer Society, Inc., *III*
CancerOnline, *III*
Candlelighters Childhood Cancer Foundation, *III*
NIH/National Cancer Institute, *IV*
OncoLink: The University of Pennsylvania Cancer Center Resource, *III*
Skin Cancer Foundation, *III*

170 CANDIDIASIS

Candida Albicans is a normally harmless yeast infection found in the mouth, intestinal tract, and vagina. Candidiasis is an infection caused by a fungus called Candida; most commonly the Candida albicans variety. The Candida infection (also known as a yeast infection) usually affects the skin and/or the mucous membranes of the mouth, intestines, or the vagina. Candida infections are rarely serious in otherwise healthy people. In rare cases, it may spread through other parts of the body if the patient's immune system is not functioning properly. In the most severe cases it can affect the blood, the membrane lining the heart muscle (endocardium), or membranes around the brain (meninges).

In addition to The National Organization for Rare Disorders (NORD) listed in Section III, the following organizations in Section II (Disease Specific) and in Section III (Umbrella) and Section IV (Government Agencies) can provide more information:

Centers for Disease Control and Prevention, *IV*
NIH/National Cancer Institute, *IV*
NIH/National Institute of Allergy and Infectious Diseases, *IV*
World Health Organization (WHO) Regional Office for the Americas (AMRO), *III*

171 CARBAMYL PHOSPHATE SYNTHETASE DEFICIENCY

Carbamyl Phosphate Synthetase (CPS) Deficiency is one of several hereditary urea cycle disorders. These disorders are caused by a deficiency of one of the enzymes needed for the synthesis of ammonia into urea, which is normally excreted in the urine. The deficiencies cause an excess of ammonia in the blood and body tissues.

In Carbamyl Phosphate Synthetase Deficiency, the deficient enzyme is carbamyl phosphate synthetase. If left untreated, CPS deficiency manifests itself by an elevated level of toxic ammonia in the blood (hyperammonemia). Untreated, these imbalances may lead to brain damage, coma, and life-threatening complications. Carbamyl Phosphate Synthetase Deficiency is inherited as an autosomal recessive genetic disorder.

In addition to The National Organization for Rare Disorders (NORD) listed in Section III, the following organizations in Section II (Disease Specific) and in Section III (Umbrella) and Section IV (Government Agencies) can provide more information:

American Kidney Fund, Inc., *III*
Metabolic Information Network, *III*
NIH/National Digestive Diseases Information Clearinghouse, *IV*
National Kidney Foundation, *III*
National Urea Cycle Disorders Foundation, *III*
Research Trust for Metabolic Diseases in Children, *III*

172 CARBOHYDRATE DEFICIENT GLYCOPROTEIN SYNDROME TYPE I

Carbohydrate-deficient Glycoprotein Syndrome Type I (CDG1) is an extremely rare inherited metabolic disorder belonging to a group of diseases known as Carbohydrate-deficient Glycoprotein Syndromes (CDGS). These disorders are characterized by the presence of abnormal oligosaccharides, or "sugar chains," on many glycoproteins (e.g., transferrin). Glycoproteins are compounds in which oligosaccharides are "attached" to certain proteins. Oligosaccharides are sugars that are linked together in a very specific manner and may help to define the function of the glycoprotein in the body.

Glycoproteins have several important functions in the body. They play a role in the complex chemical processes that enable the body to function normally. Examples include signalling how cells in the body interact with one another, participating in the transfer of nutrients from one part of the body to another (transport), playing a role in the proper coagulation of blood, functioning as hormones that regulate certain organs or activities in the body (i.e., endocrine activities that help to regulate the rate of growth, sexual development, and/or metabolism), etc.

Carbohydrate-deficient Glycoprotein Syndrome Type I is the most common form of CDGS and affects most systems of the body, particularly the function of the central nervous system (i.e., the brain and spinal cord), the peripheral nervous system (i.e., motor and sensory nerves outside the central nervous system), and the liver, which makes many of the glycoproteins in the blood. Although the severity and range of symptoms may vary from case to case, most affected individuals exhibit severe delays in the acquisition of skills that require the coordination of mental and muscular activity (psychomotor retardation); moderate to severe mental retardation; impaired coordination and balance (cerebellar ataxia) due to underdevelopment (hypoplasia) of certain portions of the brain (cerebellum); impaired nerve transmission to the legs, resulting in progressive, severe muscle thinning and weakness (peripheral neuropathy); skeletal malformations; and/or visual and/or hearing impairment. CDGS Type I is thought to be inherited as an autosomal recessive genetic trait.

In addition to The National Organization for Rare Disorders (NORD) listed in Section III, the following organizations in Section II (Disease Specific) and in Section III (Umbrella) and Section IV (Government Agencies) can provide more information:
Association for Neuro-Metabolic Disorders, *III*
CDG Society (Sweden), *II*
CDGS Family Network, *II*
NIH/National Arthritis and Musculoskeletal and Skin Diseases Information Clearinghouse, *IV*
NIH/National Institute of Child Health and Human Development, *IV*
NIH/National Institute of Neurological Disorders and Stroke, *IV*
National Association for Parents of the Visually Impaired, *III*
National Association for Visually Handicapped, *III*
National Information Center on Deafness, *III*
Research Trust for Metabolic Diseases in Children, *III*
United Leukodystrophy Foundation, *III*
Vaincre Les Maladies Lysosomales, *III*

173 CARBOXYLASE DEFICIENCY, MULTIPLE

Multiple Carboxylase Deficiency is a genetic metabolic disorder that leads to impaired activity of three enzymes that are dependent on the vitamin biotin: propionyl CoA carboxylase, beta-methylcrotonyl CoA carboxylase, and pyruvate carboxylase. This condition results from a defect in cellular biotin transport or metabolism. Symptoms of the disorder include acidity of the blood and body tissues (acidosis), a widespread red skin rash, baldness, and slowed physical development. The disorder occurs in both a neonatal and a late-onset form and is treatable.

In addition to The National Organization for Rare Disorders (NORD) listed in Section III, the following organizations in Section II (Disease Specific) and in Section III (Umbrella) and Section IV (Government Agencies) can provide more information:
Association for Neuro-Metabolic Disorders, *III*
Metabolic Information Network, *III*
NIH/National Digestive Diseases Information Clearinghouse, *IV*
Research Trust for Metabolic Diseases in Children, *III*

174 CARCINOID SYNDROME

Carcinoid Syndrome is a rare, malignant disease affecting the small bowel, stomach and/or pancreas. Slow growing tumors can spread (metastasize) to the liver, lungs and ovaries. Major symptoms include flushing, diarrhea and wheezing. The exact cause of Carcinoid Syndrome is not known.

In addition to The National Organization for Rare Disorders (NORD) listed in Section III, the following organizations in Section II (Disease Specific) and in Section III (Umbrella) and Section IV (Government Agencies) can provide more information:
American Cancer Society, Inc., *III*
National Carcinoid Support Group, Inc., *II*

175 CARCINOMA, RENAL CELL

Renal Cell Carcinoma is a rare malignant kidney disorder. Major symptoms may include loss of kidney function, fever, weight loss, blood problems, high levels of calcium in the system, high blood pressure, blood clots and congestive heart failure. However, the most common feature of the syndrome is the passing of blood in the urine (hematuria).

In addition to The National Organization for Rare Disorders (NORD) listed in Section III, the following organizations in Section II (Disease Specific) and in Section III (Umbrella) and Section IV (Government Agencies) can provide more information:
American Cancer Society, Inc., *III*
American Foundation for Urologic Disease, *III*
CancerOnline, *III*
NIH/National Kidney and Urologic Diseases Information Clearinghouse, *IV*
NIH/Patient Referral Services Unit, *IV*
National Kidney Cancer Association, *II*
National Kidney Foundation, *III*
OncoLink: The University of Pennsylvania Cancer Center Resource, *III*

176 CARCINOMA, SQUAMOUS CELL

Squamous Cell Carcinoma is among the most common types of skin cancer. It usually develops on the tissue of the skin and mucous lining of the body cavities (epithelium) but may occur anywhere on the body. With appropriate treatment, it is usually curable. Squamous Cell Carcinoma most commonly affects individuals who are exposed to large amounts of sunlight. Susceptibility is related to the amount of melanin pigment in the skin, and light-skinned persons are most vulnerable.

In addition to The National Organization for Rare Disorders (NORD) listed in Section III, the following organizations in Section II (Disease Specific) and in Section III (Umbrella) and Section IV (Government Agencies) can provide more information:
American Cancer Society, Inc., *III*
CancerOnline, *III*
OncoLink: The University of Pennsylvania Cancer Center Resource, *III*
Skin Cancer Foundation, *III*

177 CARDIO AUDITORY SYNDROME

Cardio-auditory syndrome is a rare disorder characterized by deafness at birth, fainting spells and prolonged intervals of electrical activity in the ventricles of the heart (prolonged QT) causing seizures and a fast, uneven heartbeat (ventricular fibrillation). Physical activity, excitement or stress may trigger the onset of these symptoms. Cardio-auditory Syndrome is usually detected during early childhood and is inherited as an autosomal recessive trait.

In addition to The National Organization for Rare Disorders (NORD) listed in Section III, the following organizations in Section II (Disease Specific) and in Section III (Umbrella) and Section IV (Government Agencies) can provide more information:

American Heart Association, *III*
Deafness Research Foundation, *III*
EAR (Education and Auditory Research) Foundation, *III*
International Long QT Syndrome Registry, *II*
Long QT Syndrome European Information Center, *II*
NIH/National Heart, Lung and Blood Institute Information Center, *IV*

178 CARDIO FACIO CUTANEOUS SYNDROME

Cardio-Facio-Cutaneous Syndrome is a rare disorder characterized by multiple physical abnormalities and mental retardation. The major symptoms and physical findings associated with the disorder include skin abnormalities; an unusual facial appearance; sparse, curly hair; heart defects; and mental retardation.

In addition to The National Organization for Rare Disorders (NORD) listed in Section III, the following organizations in Section II (Disease Specific) and in Section III (Umbrella) and Section IV (Government Agencies) can provide more information:

American Heart Association, *III*
Cardio-Facial-Cutaneous Syndrome Support Network, *II*
Forward Face, Inc., *III*
Foundation for Ichthyosis & Related Skin Types, *III*
Human Growth Foundation, *III*
MAGIC Foundation for Children's Growth, *III*
NIH/National Institute of Child Health and Human Development, *IV*
National Registry for Ichthyosis and Related Disorders, *III*
THRESHOLD (for uncontrolled seizure disorders), *III*

179 CARNITINE DEFICIENCY SYNDROMES

Carnitine deficiency syndrome is a rare metabolic disorder that may be inherited in some cases, or occur as a result of other metabolic disorders. Carnitine functions in the body as a carrier of fatty acids to the energy centers in muscles (mitochondria). A deficiency of carnitine, normally produced by the liver and kidneys, can result in extreme muscle weakness and other related symptoms.

In addition to The National Organization for Rare Disorders (NORD) listed in Section III, the following organizations in Section II (Disease Specific) and in Section III (Umbrella) and Section IV (Government Agencies) can provide more information:

Alliance of Genetic Support Groups, *III*
Association for Neuro-Metabolic Disorders, *III*
FOD (Fatty Oxidation Disorder) Family Support Group, *III*
March of Dimes Birth Defects Foundation, *III*
Metabolic Information Network, *III*
Muscular Dystrophy Association, *III*
NIH/National Institute of Diabetes, Digestive and Kidney Diseases, *IV*
Organic Acidemia Association, *III*
Research Trust for Metabolic Diseases in Children, *III*
United Mitochondrial Disease Foundation, *III*

180 CARNITINE PALMITOYLTRANSFERASE DEFICIENCY

Carnitine Palmitoyltransferase (CPT) Deficiency is a very rare metabolic disorder that affects the skeletal muscles and their ability to function properly. CPT Deficiency belongs to a group of diseases that involve the defective breakdown (metabolism) of muscle fats (lipids). Prolonged periods of strenuous exercise can trigger an episode of symptoms. These may include muscle aches, stiffness, and weakness. Muscle tissue may break down (rhabdomylosis) and abnormal levels of myoglobulin may be present in the urine (myoglobinuria). The urine may appear dark reddish-brown after prolonged periods of exercise.

Carnitine Palmitoyltransferase (CPT) Deficiency Type 1 typically affects adults and adolescents. Carnitine Palmitoyltransferase (CPT) Deficiency Type 2 may also affect adults; however, a serious form of this type of the disease affects infants.

In addition to The National Organization for Rare Disorders (NORD) listed in Section III, the following organizations in Section II (Disease Specific) and in Section III (Umbrella) and Section IV (Government Agencies) can provide more information:

Association for Neuro-Metabolic Disorders, *III*
FOD (Fatty Oxidation Disorder) Family Support Group, *III*
Muscular Dystrophy Association, *III*
NIH/National Institute of Child Health & Human Development (Preg & Perinat), *IV*

NIH/National Institute of Diabetes, Digestive & Kidney Diseases, *IV*
Research Trust for Metabolic Diseases in Children, *III*

181 CARNOSINEMIA

Carnosinemia is a very rare inherited metabolic disorder characterized by impaired neurological function and developmental delays. Symptoms that begin during infancy may include drowsiness, seizures that may be accompanied by involuntary jerking muscle movements of the arms, legs, or head (myoclonic seizures), and mental retardation.

In addition to The National Organization for Rare Disorders (NORD) listed in Section III, the following organizations in Section II (Disease Specific) and in Section III (Umbrella) and Section IV (Government Agencies) can provide more information:

Association for Neuro-Metabolic Disorders, *III*
March of Dimes Birth Defects Foundation, *III*
Metabolic Information Network, *III*
NIH/National Institute of Child Health and Human Development, *IV*
Research Trust for Metabolic Diseases in Children, *III*
The Arc (a national organization on mental retardation), *III*

182 CAROLI DISEASE

Caroli Disease is a rare inherited disorder characterized by abnormal widening (dilatation) of the ducts that carry bile from the liver (intrahepatic bile ducts). According to the medical literature, there are two forms of Caroli Disease. In most cases, the isolated or simple form Caroli Disease, affected individuals experience recurrent episodes of inflammation of the bile ducts (cholangitis) and unusual accumulation of pus (abscesses) on the liver. A second form of Caroli Disease is associated with abnormal formation bands of fibrous tissue in the portal area of the liver (congenital hepatic fibrosis). The portal area of the liver is a groove (fissure) where the portal vein and the hepatic artery enter the liver. The portal vein is the blood vessel that carries blood from the stomach, intestine, and spleen to the liver and the hepatic artery is the blood vessel that carries blood away from the liver. This form of Caroli Disease is also often associated with high blood pressure of the portal vein (portal hypertension), polycystic kidney disease, and, in severe cases, liver failure. Caroli Disease is thought to be inherited as either an autosomal dominant or recessive genetic trait.

In addition to The National Organization for Rare Disorders (NORD) listed in Section III, the following organizations in Section II (Disease Specific) and in Section III (Umbrella) and Section IV (Government Agencies) can provide more information:

American Liver Foundation, *III*
NIH/National Digestive Diseases Information Clearinghouse, *IV*
United Liver Association, *III*

183 CARPAL TUNNEL SYNDROME

Carpal Tunnel Syndrome (CTS) is a condition caused by compression of peripheral nerves affecting one or both hands. It is characterized by a sensation of numbness, tingling, burning and/or pain in the hand and wrist. Persons affected by this disorder may be awakened at night with the feeling that the hand has "gone to sleep." Strain or injury involving the hand and wrist or various other disorders may cause CTS. The disorder may appear as a symptom of various other diseases or may occur as a single primary condition.

In addition to The National Organization for Rare Disorders (NORD) listed in Section III, the following organizations in Section II (Disease Specific) and in Section III (Umbrella) and Section IV (Government Agencies) can provide more information:

NIH/National Institute of Neurological Disorders and Stroke, *IV*

184 CARPENTER SYNDROME

Carpenter Syndrome is an extremely rare inherited disorder characterized by malformations of the fingers and toes, abnormalities of the head and face (craniofacial) area, short stature, obesity, and, in some cases, mental retardation. In approximately, 50 percent of cases, affected individuals may have congenital heart defects. Malformations of the fingers and toes may include abnormally short fingers (brachydactyly); fifth fingers may be permanently fixed in a bent position (clinodactyly); webbing (syndactyly) of the toes; and/or extra digits on the "big toe" sides of the feet (preaxial polydactyly). Abnormalities of the craniofacial area may include premature closure of the fibrous joints between certain bones in the skull (craniosynostosis), underdevelopment (hypoplasia) of the jaw bones (maxilla and mandible), a highly-arched roof of the mouth (palate), widely spaced eyes (hypertelorism), and/or low-set malformed ears. Carpenter Syndrome is inherited as an autosomal recessive genetic trait.

In addition to The National Organization for Rare Disorders (NORD) listed in Section III, the following organizations in Section II (Disease Specific) and in Section III (Umbrella) and Section IV (Government Agencies) can provide more information:
AboutFace U.S.A., *III*
FACES: The National Craniofacial Association, *III*
Forward Face, Inc., *III*
Let's Face It, Inc., *III*
NIH/National Institute of Child Health and Human Development, *IV*

185 CASTLEMAN'S DISEASE

Castleman's Disease is a rare disorder characterized by non-cancerous (benign) growths (tumors) that may develop in the lymph node tissue throughout the body (i.e., systemic disease [plasma cell type]). Most often, they occur in the chest, stomach, and/or neck (i.e., localized disease [hyaline-vascular type]). Less common sites include the armpit (axilla), pelvis, and pancreas. Usually the growths represent abnormal enlargement of the lymph nodes normally found in these areas (lymphoid hamartoma). There are two main types of Castleman's Disease: hyaline-vascular type and plasma cell type. The hyaline vascular type accounts for approximately 90 percent of the cases. Most individuals exhibit no symptoms of this form of the disorder (asymptomatic) or they may develop non-cancerous growths in the lymph nodes. The plasma cell type of Castleman's Disease may be associated with fever, weight loss, skin rash, early destruction of red blood cells, leading to unusually low levels of circulating red blood cells (hemolytic anemia), and/or abnormally increased amounts of certain immune factors in the blood (hypergammaglobulinemia).

A third type of Castleman's Disease has been reported in the medical literature. This type may affect more than one area of the body (multicentric or generalized Castleman's Disease). Many individuals with Multicentric Castleman's Disease may exhibit an abnormally large liver and spleen (hepatosplenomegaly). Researchers' opinions in the medical literature differ as to whether Multicentric Castleman's Disease is a distinct entity or a multicentric form of the plasma cell type of Castleman's Disease.

In addition to The National Organization for Rare Disorders (NORD) listed in Section III, the following organizations in Section II (Disease Specific) and in Section III (Umbrella) and Section IV (Government Agencies) can provide more information:
American Autoimmune Related Diseases Association, Inc., *III*
American Cancer Society, Inc., *III*
NIH/National Heart, Lung and Blood Institute Information Center, *IV*

186 CAT EYE SYNDROME

Cat Eye Syndrome is an extremely rare chromosomal disorder in which the short arm (p) and a small portion of the long arm (q) of chromosome 22 (22pter-22q11) are present three (trisomy) or four times (tetrasomy) rather than twice in cells of the body. Individuals with a normal chromosomal make-up have two 22nd chromosomes, both of which have a short arm (22p) and a long arm (22q). However, in individuals with Cat Eye Syndrome, a portion of chromosome 22 (i.e., 22pter-22q11) is present in cells of the body three (trisomic) or four times (tetrasomic) rather than the normal two.

Although the symptoms and physical characteristics associated with Cat Eye Syndrome may vary greatly in range and severity from case to case (depending on the mechanism and extent of the duplicated material), abnormalities tend to involve the eyes, ears, the gastrointestinal and/or genital and urinary (genitourinary) tracts, the heart, the kidneys, and/or the skeletal system.

Characteristic features often associated with the disorder may include absence of tissue from the colored portion of one or both eyes (unilateral or bilateral iris coloboma), giving the iris an unusual "keyhole" appearance; downwardly slanted openings between the upper and lower eyelids (palpebral fissures); abnormal outgrowths of skin and small depressions in front of the outer ears (preauricular tags and pits); abnormal obstruction (atresia) of the anus; and/or the presence of abnormal passages (fistulae) from the end portion of the large intestine (rectum) into other surrounding organs. Additional characteristic abnormalities often include congenital cardiac defects; underdevelopment (hypoplasia) and/or absence (agenesis) of one or both kidneys and/or additional renal abnormalities; short stature, abnormal sideways curvature of the spine (scoliosis), and/or other skeletal malformations; and/or mild to moderate mental retardation. Cat Eye Syndrome is usually the result of a spontaneous (de novo) genetic change (mutation) that occurs for unknown reasons (sporadic).

In addition to The National Organization for Rare Disorders (NORD) listed in Section III, the following organizations in Section II (Disease Specific) and in Section III (Umbrella) and Section IV (Government Agencies) can provide more information:

American Heart Association, *III*
American Liver Foundation, *III*
American Pseudo-obstruction & Hirschsprung's Disease Society, Inc., *III*
Big Hearts for Little Hearts, *III*
Children's Liver Alliance, *III*
Children's Liver Disease Foundation, *III*
Congenital Heart Anomalies, Support, Education, & Resources, *III*
Council of Families with Visual Impairment, *III*
Inverted Duplication Exchange, Advocacy and Support, *III*
MAGIC Foundation for Children's Growth, *III*
NIH/National Digestive Diseases Information Clearinghouse, *IV*
NIH/National Heart, Lung and Blood Institute Information Center, *IV*
NIH/National Institute of Child Health and Human Development, *IV*
National Association for Parents of the Visually Impaired, *III*
National Center of Chromosome Inversions, *III*

187 CAT SCRATCH DISEASE

Cat-Scratch Disease (also commonly known as Cat-Scratch Fever) is a self- limiting infectious disease characterized by swelling and pain in the lymph nodes (regional lymphadenitis). Symptoms can vary from mild to severe, and may include achiness and discomfort (malaise), and/or loss of appetite (anorexia). In most cases a scratch, bite, or lick of a cat is considered to be the source of the infection. Symptoms do not appear for several days after exposure and may last for several weeks. Although Cat-Scratch Disease usually subsides without treatment, antibiotic and/or antimicrobial therapy may speed recovery. Approximately 22,000 cases are reported in the United States each year, although more mild cases may go unnoticed and resolve without treatment.

In addition to The National Organization for Rare Disorders (NORD) listed in Section III, the following organizations in Section II (Disease Specific) and in Section III (Umbrella) and Section IV (Government Agencies) can provide more information:

Centers for Disease Control and Prevention, *IV*
NIH/National Institute of Allergy and Infectious Diseases, *IV*

188 CATARACT DENTAL SYNDROME

Cataract-Dental Syndrome is an extremely rare inherited disorder that is apparent at birth (congenital). It is characterized by abnormalities of the teeth; ears that are flared forward (anteverted) and unusually prominent; and/or clouding of the lens of the eyes (congenital cataracts), resulting in poor vision. In addition, the front (anterior), clear portion of the eye through which light passes (cornea) may be unusually small (microcornea), and/or affected individuals may exhibit involuntary, rapid eye movements (nystagmus). In some cases, additional physical abnormalities and/or mental retardation may also be present. The range and severity of symptoms may vary from case to case.

Cataract-Dental Syndrome, which is inherited as an X-linked recessive genetic trait, is fully expressed in males only. However, females who carry a single copy of the disease gene (heterozygotes) may exhibit some of the symptoms associated with the disorder. These may include abnormally small corneas (microcornea) and/or clouding of the lens of the eyes (posterior sutural cataracts). Symptoms are typically less severe than those of affected males, causing only slightly decreased clearness or clarity of vision (visual acuity). In some cases, abnormalities of the teeth may also be present.

In addition to The National Organization for Rare Disorders (NORD) listed in Section III, the following organizations in Section II (Disease Specific) and in Section III (Umbrella) and Section IV (Government Agencies) can provide more information:

Council of Families with Visual Impairment, *III*
Institute for Families of Blind Children, *III*
NIH/National Eye Institute, *IV*
NIH/National Institute of Dental Research, *IV*
National Association for Parents of the Visually Impaired, *III*
National Association for Visually Handicapped, *III*
National Federation of the Blind, *III*
Vision World Wide, Inc., *III*

189 CATARACTS

Cataracts are abnormalities in the lens of the eye that cause a loss of transparency (opacity). They can occur either in one or in both eyes, and are quite common in the elderly. Congenital cataracts affect infants or young children and are considered to be a rare birth defect. Cataracts tend to cause cloudy vision, and, in many cases, may result in blindness when left untreated.

In addition to The National Organization for Rare Disorders (NORD) listed in Section III, the following organizations in Section II (Disease Specific) and in Section III (Umbrella) and Section IV (Government Agencies) can provide more information:

Blind Children's Fund, *III*
NIH/National Eye Institute, *IV*
National Association for Parents of the Visually Impaired, *III*
National Association for Visually Handicapped, *III*
Vision Foundation, Inc., *III*

190 CATEL MANZKE SYNDROME

Catel-Manzke Syndrome is an extremely rare genetic disorder characterized by abnormalities of the fingers and the classic physical characteristics associated with Pierre Robin Syndrome (i.e., an abnormally small jaw [micrognathia], incomplete closure of the roof of the mouth [cleft palate], and displacement of the tongue farther back in the mouth than usual [glossoptosis]). In all reported cases, affected infants have had an extra (supernumerary), irregularly-shaped bone located where the first bones of the index and middle fingers (proximal phalanges) connect with the corresponding bones of the palms (metacarpals). As a result, the index fingers may be fixed in an abnormally bent position (clinodactyly). In some cases, there may be additional abnormalities of the hand. For example, the fifth fingers may also be fixed in a bent position (clinodactyly) and affected individuals may also have an abnormally divided (bifurcated) bone of the lower palm (metacarpal), and/or a single, deep crease across the palms of the hands (simian crease). Due to the presence of cleft palate, glossoptosis, and micrognathia, affected infants may also experience breathing (respiratory) difficulties; episodes characterized by difficulties with spontaneous breathing (asphyxiation); middle ear infections (otitis media); and/or feeding difficulties. In some cases, affected infants may fail to gain the expected amount of weight or may lose weight (failure to thrive) due to such feeding difficulties. In addition, some affected infants may also have abnormalities of the heart that are present at birth (congenital heart defects). The range and severity of symptoms may vary from case to case. Most cases of Catel-Manzke Syndrome appear to occur randomly, for no apparent reason (sporadic).

In addition to The National Organization for Rare Disorders (NORD) listed in Section III, the following organizations in Section II (Disease Specific) and in Section III (Umbrella) and Section IV (Government Agencies) can provide more information:

Cleft Palate Foundation, *III*
Congenital Heart Anomalies, Support, Education, & Resources, *III*
NIH/National Heart, Lung and Blood Institute Information Center, *IV*
NIH/National Institute of Child Health and Human Development, *IV*
Prescription Parents (for parents of children with cleft lip and palate), *III*
Wide Smiles, *III*

191 CAUDAL REGRESSION SYNDROME

Caudal Regression Syndrome is a rare disorder characterized by abnormal development of the lower spine end of the developing fetus. A wide range of abnormalities may occur including partial absence of the tailbone end of the spine causing no apparent symptoms, to extensive abnormalities of the lower vertebrae, pelvis, and spine. Neurological impairment as well as inability to control urination and bowel movements (incontinence) may occur in severe cases.

In addition to The National Organization for Rare Disorders (NORD) listed in Section III, the following organizations in Section II (Disease Specific) and in Section III (Umbrella) and Section IV (Government Agencies) can provide more information:

March of Dimes Birth Defects Foundation, *III*
NIH/National Institute of Arthritis and Musculoskeletal and Skin Diseases, *IV*
NIH/National Institute of Child Health and Human Development, *IV*

192 CAVERNOUS HEMANGIOMA

Cavernous Hemangioma is a rare, often congenital disorder of the venous (veins and arteries) system. The hemangioma is a mass resembling a tumor, consisting of large blood-filled spaces which and can occur at any site in the body.

In addition to The National Organization for Rare Disorders (NORD) listed in Section III, the following organizations in Section II (Disease Specific) and in Section III (Umbrella) and Section IV (Government Agencies) can provide more information:

Hemangioma Support System, *II*
NIH/National Heart, Lung and Blood Institute Information Center, *IV*
National Vascular Malformations Foundation, Inc., *III*
Sturge-Weber Foundation, *II*

193 CAYLER SYNDROME

Cayler Syndrome, also known as "Asymmetric Crying Facies with Cardiac Defects," is an extremely rare disorder characterized by congenital heart defects and the underdevelopment or absence of one of the muscles that control the movements of the lower lip. The disorder is present at birth (congenital) and is usually first noticed when the infant cries or smiles. Half of the lower lip cannot be drawn down and outward because of the incomplete development (hypoplasia) or absence (agenesis) of the depressor anguli oris muscle.

Congenital heart defects associated with Cayler Syndrome may include ventricular septal defects, atrial septal defects, and/or Tetralogy of Fallot. In some rare cases, individuals may have an abnormally small head (microcephaly), unusually small jaw bones (micrognathia), small eyes (microphthalmos), and/or mental retardation. Most cases of Cayler Syndrome are thought to be inherited as an autosomal dominant genetic trait.

In addition to The National Organization for Rare Disorders (NORD) listed in Section III, the following organizations in Section II (Disease Specific) and in Section III (Umbrella) and Section IV (Government Agencies) can provide more information:
American Heart Association, *III*
Congenital Heart Anomalies, Support, Education, & Resources, *III*
NIH/National Institute of Child Health and Human Development, *IV*

194 CELIAC SPRUE

Celiac Sprue is a chronic, hereditary, intestinal malabsorption disorder caused by intolerance to gluten. The illness is characterized by a flat jejunal (part of the intestine) mucosa. Clinical and/or histologic improvement of symptoms follow withdrawal of dietary gluten.

In addition to The National Organization for Rare Disorders (NORD) listed in Section III, the following organizations in Section II (Disease Specific) and in Section III (Umbrella) and Section IV (Government Agencies) can provide more information:
Alliance of Genetic Support Groups, *III*
American Celiac Society-Dietary Support Coalition, *II*
Celiac Sprue Association/USA, Inc., *II*
Gluten Intolerance Group of North America, *II*
NIH/National Digestive Diseases Information Clearinghouse, *IV*

195 CENTRAL CORE DISEASE

Central Core Disease is a rare inherited neuromuscular disorder characterized by muscle weakness (hypotonia), especially of the legs. The symptoms usually begin during the first year of life. Central Core Disease derives its name from characteristic abnormal cores in muscle cells, which are obvious under a microscope.

In addition to The National Organization for Rare Disorders (NORD) listed in Section III, the following organizations in Section II (Disease Specific) and in Section III (Umbrella) and Section IV (Government Agencies) can provide more information:
Malignant Hyperthermia Association of the United States, *II*
March of Dimes Birth Defects Foundation, *III*
Muscular Dystrophy Association, *III*
NIH/National Institute of Neurological Disorders and Stroke, *IV*
North American Malignant Hyperthermia Registry, *II*

196 CENTRAL HYPOVENTILATION SYNDROME, CONGENITAL

Congenital Central Hypoventilation Syndrome is a rare neurological disorder of infancy and childhood characterized by malfunction of the central regulation of breathing during sleep, resulting in a generalized decrease in respiratory function. Many tissues of the body are deprived of oxygen because the lungs do not receive sufficient quantities of air. If left untreated, abnormally shallow breathing and deficient aeration may cause brain damage and/or life-threatening complications. The disorder can improve with age, so early identification and assistive breathing devices during sleep are important to avoid serious long-term effects.

In addition to The National Organization for Rare Disorders (NORD) listed in Section III, the following organizations in Section II (Disease Specific) and in Section III (Umbrella) and Section IV (Government Agencies) can provide more information:
Center for Research in Sleep Disorders, *III*
Congenital Central Hypoventilation Syndrome (CCHS) Family Support Network, *II*
NIH/National Institute of Neurological Disorders and Stroke, *IV*

197 CEREBELLAR AGENESIS

Cerebellar agenesis is a rare disorder thought to be inherited as an autosomal recessive trait. Infants with this disorder are born with partial formation or total absence of the portion of the brain that is located at the base of the skull known as the cerebellum. Infants with partial formation of the cerebellum may have few or no symptoms of the disorder. When total absence of the cerebellum is present, an affected infant may experience low muscle tone, uncontrollable quivering or movements, involuntary movement of the eyes, and/or an inability to coordinate muscle movements.

In addition to The National Organization for Rare Disorders (NORD) listed in Section III, the following organizations in Section II (Disease Specific) and in Section III (Umbrella) and Section IV (Government Agencies) can provide more information:
NIH/National Institute of Neurological Disorders and Stroke, *IV*

198 CEREBELLAR DEGENERATION, SUBACUTE

Subacute cerebellar degeneration is characterized by deterioration of the cerebellum (an area of the brain concerned with muscle coordination and balance). It may also involve the area connecting the spinal cord to the brain such as the medulla oblongata, the cerebral cortex, and possibly the brain stem. There are two subtypes of this disorder. The first is paraneoplastic cerebellar degeneration, which sometimes precedes the diagnosis of cancer. The second is alcoholic or nutritional cerebellar degeneration, caused by a lack of the vitamin B-1 (thiamine) and is not related to cancer.

In addition to The National Organization for Rare Disorders (NORD) listed in Section III, the following organizations in Section II (Disease Specific) and in Section III (Umbrella) and Section IV (Government Agencies) can provide more information:
American Autoimmune Related Diseases Association, Inc., *III*
American Cancer Society, Inc., *III*
NIH/National Institute on Aging, *IV*

199 CEREBRAL PALSY

Cerebral Palsy is a neurological movement disorder characterized by the lack of muscle control and impairment in the coordination of movements. This disorder is usually a result of injury to the brain during early development in the uterus or at birth. Cerebral Palsy is not progressive.

In addition to The National Organization for Rare Disorders (NORD) listed in Section III, the following organizations in Section II (Disease Specific) and in Section III (Umbrella) and Section IV (Government Agencies) can provide more information:
March of Dimes Birth Defects Foundation, *III*
NIH/National Institute of Child Health and Human Development, *IV*
NIH/National Institute of Neurological Disorders and Stroke, *IV*
National Easter Seal Society, Inc., *III*
United Cerebral Palsy Association, *II*
WE MOVE, *III*

200 CEREBRO OCULO FACIO SKELETAL SYNDROME

Cerebro-Oculo-Facio-Skeletal Syndrome is a genetic degenerative disorder of the brain and spinal cord that begins before birth. The disorder is characterized by reduced amounts of white brain matter with gray mottling, lowered muscle tone and diminished or absent reflexes. Abnormalities of the skull, face, eyes, limbs and other parts of the body also occur.

In addition to The National Organization for Rare Disorders (NORD) listed in Section III, the following organizations in Section II (Disease Specific) and in Section III (Umbrella) and Section IV (Government Agencies) can provide more information:
AboutFace U.S.A., *III*
Children's Craniofacial Association, *III*
FACES: The National Craniofacial Association, *III*
Forward Face, Inc., *III*
NIH/National Institute of Neurological Disorders and Stroke, *IV*

201 CEREBROCOSTOMANDIBULAR SYNDROME

Cerebrocostomandibular Syndrome is an extremely rare inherited disorder characterized by an abnormally small jaw (micrognathia), malformations of the roof of the mouth (palate), improper positioning of the tongue (glossoptosis), and abnormal development of the ribs (rib dysplasia). In most cases, such abnormalities contribute to respiratory problems (insufficiency) during early infancy. Although some affected individuals have normal intelligence, others exhibit moderate to severe mental retardation. It is thought that mental retardation may occur as a result of abnormally low levels of circulating oxygen (neonatal hypoxia) due to respiratory difficulties. Although research suggests that Cerebrocostomandibular Syndrome is usually inherited as an autosomal recessive genetic trait, some cases have also been documented in the medical literature that suggest autosomal dominant inheritance.

In addition to The National Organization for Rare Disorders (NORD) listed in Section III, the following organizations in Section II (Disease Specific) and in Section III (Umbrella) and Section IV (Government Agencies) can provide more information:

Cleft Palate Foundation, *III*
NIH/National Heart, Lung and Blood Institute Information Center, *IV*
NIH/National Institute of Child Health and Human Development, *IV*
NIH/National Institute on Deafness and Other Communication Disorders Information Clearinghouse, *IV*
Prescription Parents (for parents of children with cleft lip and palate), *III*
The Arc (a national organization on mental retardation), *III*
Wide Smiles, *III*

202 CHAGAS DISEASE

Chagas Disease is a tropical infectious disease caused by the parasite Trypanosoma cruzi. It is transmitted by the bite of an insect (reduviid bug) or by blood transfusion. Acute Chagas Disease usually affects children and is typically a mild phase of the disease. However, this is generally followed by a low level of parasitic infection (parasitemia). Many years later, about 10 to 30 percent of people with Chagas Disease develop more severe symptoms associated with "chronic" Chagas Disease. The heart and digestive systems are most frequently involved in this phase of the disease. The most common features of late chronic Chagas Disease include abnormal enlargement of the esophagus (megaesophagus) and colon (megacolon), and congestive heart failure. Chagas Disease occurs primarily in Central and South America.

In addition to The National Organization for Rare Disorders (NORD) listed in Section III, the following organizations in Section II (Disease Specific) and in Section III (Umbrella) and Section IV (Government Agencies) can provide more information:
Centers for Disease Control and Prevention, *IV*
NIH/National Institute of Allergy and Infectious Diseases, *IV*
National Dysautonomia Research Foundation, *III*
World Health Organization (WHO) Regional Office for the Americas (AMRO), *III*

203 CHALAZION

Chalazion, also known as meibomian or tarsal cyst, is a round, slowly emerging, localized swelling of the lower or upper eyelid. The usually painless, tumor-like (granulomatous) mass is due to inflammation, obstruction, and retained secretions of one of the glands (meibomian gland) that lubricates the edge of the eyelids. (The meibomian glands of the eyelids secrete sebum, an oily, protective fluid.) In rare cases, if the mass is large, blurred vision may result due to pressure on the cornea, the front, clear portion of the eye through which light passes. In some affected individuals, chalazions may disappear on their own (spontaneously). However, in other cases, treatment may be required. Individuals with chronic inflammation of the eyelids (blepharitis) may be prone to recurrences.

In addition to The National Organization for Rare Disorders (NORD) listed in Section III, the following organizations in Section II (Disease Specific) and in Section III (Umbrella) and Section IV (Government Agencies) can provide more information:
NIH/National Eye Institute, *IV*
Schepens Eye Research Institute, *III*

204 CHANDLER'S SYNDROME

Chandler's Syndrome is a very rare eye disorder that affects females more often that males. It usually becomes apparent during middle age and can cause increased development in the cells lining the cornea, drying up of the iris, corneal swelling, and unusually high pressure in the eye (glaucoma). The disorder may result in vision loss.

In addition to The National Organization for Rare Disorders (NORD) listed in Section III, the following organizations in Section II (Disease Specific) and in Section III (Umbrella) and Section IV (Government Agencies) can provide more information:
NIH/National Eye Institute, *IV*
National Association for Parents of the Visually Impaired, *III*
National Association for Visually Handicapped, *III*
Prevent Blindness America, *III*
Schepens Eye Research Institute, *III*

205 CHARCOT MARIE TOOTH DISEASE

Charcot-Marie-Tooth disease is a hereditary neurological disorder characterized by muscle weakness and atrophy, primarily in the legs. Disappearance of the protective fatty layers surrounding the nerves (segmental demyelination) of peripheral nervous system and associated degeneration of part of the nerve cells (axons) characterize this disorder.

In addition to The National Organization for Rare Disorders (NORD) listed in Section III, the following organizations in Section II (Disease Specific) and in Section III (Umbrella) and Section IV (Government Agencies) can provide more information:
Charcot-Marie-Tooth Association, *II*
Charcot-Marie-Tooth International, *II*
Muscular Dystrophy Association, *III*
NIH/National Institute of Neurological Disorders and Stroke, *IV*

206 CHEDIAK HIGASHI SYNDROME

Chediak-Higashi Syndrome is a rare inherited form of albinism characterized by a decrease in the amount of skin coloration (decreased pigmentation) and visual difficulties. Albinism is a group of rare inherited disorders associated with the absence at birth of color in the skin, hair, and/or eyes. White blood cell (leukocyte) abnormalities associated with Chediak-Higashi Syndrome result in immune deficiencies. Affected individuals may have an increased susceptibility to infections and certain cancers.

In addition to The National Organization for Rare Disorders (NORD) listed in Section III, the following organizations in Section II (Disease Specific) and in Section III (Umbrella) and Section IV (Government Agencies) can provide more information:

International Patient Organization for Primary Immunodeficiencies, *III*
Jeffrey Modell Foundation, *III*
March of Dimes Birth Defects Foundation, *III*
NIH/National Institute of Allergy and Infectious Diseases, *IV*
National Organization for Albinism and Hypopigmentation, *III*

207 CHIARI FROMMEL SYNDROME

Chiari-Frommel Syndrome is a rare endocrine disorder that affects females who have recently given birth (postpartum) and is characterized by the production of breast milk (lactation), lack of ovulation (anovulation), and the absence of regular menstrual periods (amenorrhea). In Chiari-Frommel Syndrome, these symptoms persist long after childbirth. The absence of normal hormonal cycles may result in reduced size of the uterus (atrophy). Some cases of Chiari-Frommel Syndrome resolve completely without treatment (spontaneously); hormone levels and reproductive function return to normal.

In addition to The National Organization for Rare Disorders (NORD) listed in Section III, the following organizations in Section II (Disease Specific) and in Section III (Umbrella) and Section IV (Government Agencies) can provide more information:

NIH/National Institute of Child Health and Human Development, *IV*
Recovery, Inc., *III*

208 CHIKUNGUNYA

Chikungunya is a rare viral infection transmitted by the bite of an infected mosquito. It is characterized by a rash, fever, and severe joint pain (arthralgias). Chikungunya primarily occurs in tropical areas of the world.

In addition to The National Organization for Rare Disorders (NORD) listed in Section III, the following organizations in Section II (Disease Specific) and in Section III (Umbrella) and Section IV (Government Agencies) can provide more information:

Centers for Disease Control and Prevention, *IV*
NIH/National Institute of Allergy and Infectious Diseases, *IV*
World Health Organization (WHO) Regional Office for the Americas (AMRO), *III*

209 CHLAMYDIA

Chlamydia is a sexually-transmitted bacterial infection with symptoms similar to those of gonorrhea. Until recently, it was identified primarily when trachoma (an eye infection) appeared as a symptom. Initially, the symptoms of Chlamydia are usually mild and may not be recognized. Although rarely fatal, Chlamydia may have serious consequences if left untreated. Sexually active people with multiple sex partners are especially at risk. Since many people with Chlamydia do not realize that they have the infection, they may not seek treatment until serious complications occur. Meanwhile, they may have unknowingly spread the disease to others through sexual activity. Treatment with antibiotics is generally successful, but prevention should be the primary course of action.

In addition to The National Organization for Rare Disorders (NORD) listed in Section III, the following organizations in Section II (Disease Specific) and in Section III (Umbrella) and Section IV (Government Agencies) can provide more information:

American Social Health Association, *III*
Centers for Disease Control and Prevention, *IV*

210 CHOLANGITIS, PRIMARY SCLEROSING

Primary sclerosing cholangitis is a rare progressive disorder characterized by inflammation, thickening, and abnormal formation of fibrous tissue (fibrosis) within the passages that carry bile from the liver (bile ducts). This often results in the obstruction or interruption of bile flow from the liver (cholestasis). Symptoms associated with primary sclerosing cholangitis include fatigue and itching (pruritis), followed by yellowing of the skin, mucous membranes, and whites of the eyes (jaundice). In addition, affected individuals may have dark urine, light-colored stools, abdominal pain, and/or nausea. In some cases, an abnormally enlarged liver (hepatomegaly) may also be present. According to the medical literature, approximately 50 to 75 percent of individuals with primary sclerosing cholangitis may also have ulcerative colitis. The exact cause of primary sclerosing cholangitis is not known.

In addition to The National Organization for Rare Disorders (NORD) listed in Section III, the following organizations in Section II (Disease Specific) and in Section III (Umbrella) and Section IV (Government Agencies) can provide more information:
American Liver Foundation, *III*
NIH/National Digestive Diseases Information Clearinghouse, *IV*
United Liver Association, *III*

211 CHOLECYSTITIS

Cholecystitis is inflammation of the gallbladder, the pear-shaped muscular sac that lies below the liver. The gallbladders main function is to store and concentrate bile and to expel the bile through the bile duct during the digestion of fats. (Bile is a greenish-brown liquid produced by the liver that breaks down fats present in the small intestine during digestion.) Cholecystitis may come on suddenly (acute) or may persist over a period of time (chronic). Acute cholecystitis is usually caused by obstruction of the outlet of the gallbladder, which is often due to the development of a stone formed in the biliary tract (gallstone or biliary calculus). Repeated mild episodes of acute cholecystitis may result in chronic cholecystitis, which may be characterized by thickening and shrinking of the gallbladder walls and a resulting inability to store bile. Cholecystitis may cause a variety of symptoms including severe pain in the right side of the abdomen (right upper quadrant) and/or back, nausea, vomiting, indigestion, fever, and persistent yellowing of the skin, mucous membranes, and whites of the eyes (jaundice). In some cases, there may be additional symptoms.

In addition to The National Organization for Rare Disorders (NORD) listed in Section III, the following organizations in Section II (Disease Specific) and in Section III (Umbrella) and Section IV (Government Agencies) can provide more information:
Digestive Disease National Coalition, *III*
NIH/National Digestive Diseases Information Clearinghouse, *IV*

212 CHOLERA

Cholera is an acute infectious disease caused by the bacterium Vibrio cholerae, which lives and multiples (colonizes) in the small intestine but does not destroy or invade the intestinal tissue (noninvasive). The major symptom of cholera is massive watery diarrhea that occurs because of a toxin secreted by the bacteria that stimulates the cells of the small intestine to secrete fluid. There are several strains of V. cholerae and the severity of the disease is based on the particular infectious strain.

Cholera is not a difficult disease to treat and most people recover well with appropriate oral fluid replacement (hydration). However, if the disease goes untreated, it can rapidly lead to shock and life-threatening complications.

In addition to The National Organization for Rare Disorders (NORD) listed in Section III, the following organizations in Section II (Disease Specific) and in Section III (Umbrella) and Section IV (Government Agencies) can provide more information:
Centers for Disease Control and Prevention, *IV*
NIH/National Institute of Allergy and Infectious Diseases, *IV*
World Health Organization (WHO) Regional Office for the Americas (AMRO), *III*

213 CHOLESTASIS

Cholestasis is a relatively rare syndrome that results when the flow of bile from the liver is impaired. Bile is a fluid secreted by the liver into the intestine that helps in the digestion of fats. The many causes of cholestasis produce different symptoms. Common symptoms are dark urine, pale stools, and itchy (pruritus) and yellowed (jaundice) skin.

In addition to The National Organization for Rare Disorders (NORD) listed in Section III, the following organizations in Section II (Disease Specific) and in Section III (Umbrella) and Section IV (Government Agencies) can provide more information:
American Liver Foundation, *III*
Children's Liver Association for Support Services, *III*
NIH/National Institute of Diabetes, Digestive and Kidney Diseases, *IV*
United Liver Association, *III*

214 CHONDROCALCINOSIS, FAMILIAL ARTICULAR

Familial articular chondrocalcinosis is a rare inherited metabolic disorder characterized by deposits of calcium pyrophosphate dihydrate crystals (CPPD) in one or more joints of the body. Symptoms may develop due to decreased activity of the enzyme pyrophosphohydrolase. The symptoms of familial articular chondrocalcinosis mimic those of classical gout and may include swelling, stiffness, and pain, usually in one joint. The knee is most commonly affected. Most cases of familial articular chondrocalcinosis are inherited as an autosomal dominant genetic trait.

In addition to The National Organization for Rare Disorders (NORD) listed in Section III, the following organizations in Section II (Disease Specific) and in Section III (Umbrella) and Section IV (Government Agencies) can provide more information:
Alliance of Genetic Support Groups, *III*
Arthritis Foundation, *III*
Metabolic Information Network, *III*
NIH/National Institute of Arthritis and Musculoskeletal and Skin Diseases, *IV*

215 CHOREA, SYDENHAM'S

Sydenham's Chorea is a non-progressive neurological movement disorder characterized by spontaneous movements, lck of coordination of voluntary movements, and muscular weakness. This disorder may occur following a streptococcal infection such as Rheumatic Fever, Meningitis or Scarlet Fever.

In addition to The National Organization for Rare Disorders (NORD) listed in Section III, the following organizations in Section II (Disease Specific) and in Section III (Umbrella) and Section IV (Government Agencies) can provide more information:
Centers for Disease Control and Prevention, *IV*
NIH/National Institute of Neurological Disorders and Stroke, *IV*
WE MOVE, *III*

216 CHOROIDEREMIA

Choroideremia is a genetic vision disorder that usually affects males. Female carriers may have mild symptoms without loss of vision. Major symptoms include a progressive loss of the central field of vision and night blindness during childhood.

In addition to The National Organization for Rare Disorders (NORD) listed in Section III, the following organizations in Section II (Disease Specific) and in Section III (Umbrella) and Section IV (Government Agencies) can provide more information:
American Council of the Blind, Inc., *III*
American Foundation for the Blind, *III*
Blind Children's Fund, *III*
Council of Families with Visual Impairment, *III*
NIH/National Eye Institute, *IV*
National Association for Parents of the Visually Impaired, *III*
National Association for Visually Handicapped, *III*
National Federation of the Blind, *III*
Vision Foundation, Inc., *III*

217 CHOROIDITIS, SERPIGINOUS

Serpiginous Choroiditis is a rare recurrent eye disorder characterized by irregularly-shaped (serpiginous) lesions involving two layers of the eye surface (the retinal pigment epithelium and the choriocapillaris). No symptoms are apparent unless a specific area of the retina (macula) is damaged. A sudden, painless decrease in vision in one eye may be the first sign of Serpiginous Choroiditis. Both eyes are commonly affected, although the second eye may not develop lesions for weeks to years after the first eye. The exact cause of Serpiginous Choroiditis is not known.

In addition to The National Organization for Rare Disorders (NORD) listed in Section III, the following organizations in Section II (Disease Specific) and in Section III (Umbrella) and Section IV (Government Agencies) can provide more information:
Association for Macular Diseases, Inc., *III*
NIH/National Eye Institute, *IV*
National Association for Visually Handicapped, *III*
Vision Foundation, Inc., *III*

218 CHROMOSOME 10, DISTAL TRISOMY 10Q

Chromosome 10, Distal Trisomy 10q is an extremely rare chromosomal disorder in which the end (distal) portion of the long arm (q) of one chromosome 10 (10q) appears three times (trisomy) rather than twice in cells of the body. The disorder is characterized by unusually slow growth before and after birth (prenatal and postnatal growth retardation); abnormally diminished muscle tone (hypotonia); severe mental retardation; and severe delays in the acquisition of skills requiring coordination of mental and muscular activities (psychomotor retardation). Affected infants and children may also have distinctive malformations of the head and facial (craniofacial) area; defects of the hands and/or feet; and/or skeletal, heart (cardiac), kidney (renal), and/or respiratory (pulmonary) abnormalities. The range and severity of symptoms and physical findings may vary from case to case, depending upon the exact length and location of the duplicated portion of chromosome 10q. In most cases, Chromosome 10, Distal Trisomy 10q is due to a chromosomal balanced translocation in one of the parents.

In addition to The National Organization for Rare Disorders (NORD) listed in Section III, the following organizations in Section II (Disease Specific) and in Section III (Umbrella) and Section IV (Government Agencies) can provide more information:
Children's Craniofacial Association, *III*
Congenital Heart Anomalies, Support, Education, & Resources, *III*

Craniofacial Foundation of America, *III*
FACES: The National Craniofacial Association, *III*
Forward Face, Inc., *III*
NIH/National Heart, Lung and Blood Institute Information Center, *IV*
NIH/National Institute of Child Health and Human Development, *IV*
NIH/National Kidney and Urologic Diseases Information Clearinghouse, *IV*
Support Organization for Trisomy 18, 13, and Related Disorders, *III*
UNIQUE - Rare Chromosome Disorder Support Group, *III*

219 CHROMOSOME 10, MONOSOMY 10P

Chromosome 10, Monosomy 10p is a very rare chromosomal disorder in which the end (distal) portion of the short arm (p) of chromosome 10 is missing. Major physical symptoms may include a small underdeveloped jaw (micrognathia), bulging of bone on the front of the head (frontal bossing), drooping eyes, small ears, an unusually small head (microcephaly), and/or other unusual head and facial features. Delayed development, heart defects, abnormalities of the reproductive organs, and/or urinary tract defects may also be present in infants with this disorder. Mental retardation often occurs. Many reported cases of this disorder occur for no apparent reason (de novo). Genetic testing is standard for the diagnosis of chromosomal disorders such as Chromosome 10, Monosomy 10p.

In addition to The National Organization for Rare Disorders (NORD) listed in Section III, the following organizations in Section II (Disease Specific) and in Section III (Umbrella) and Section IV (Government Agencies) can provide more information:
Chromosome Deletion Outreach, *III*
NIH/National Institute of Child Health and Human Development, *IV*
UNIQUE - Rare Chromosome Disorder Support Group, *III*

220 CHROMOSOME 11, PARTIAL MONOSOMY 11Q

Chromosome 11, Partial Monosomy 11q is a rare chromosomal disorder in which a portion of the long arm (q) of chromosome 11 is missing (deleted or monosomic). The range and severity of symptoms may vary, depending upon the exact size and location of the deletion on 11q. Chromosome 11, Partial Monosomy 11q may be characterized by abnormally slow growth before and after birth (prenatal and postnatal growth retardation), mental retardation, and/or moderate to severe delays in the acquisition of skills requiring the coordination of mental and muscular activity (psychomotor retardation). Characteristic physical abnormalities may include malformations of the head and facial (craniofacial) area, abnormalities of the eyes, malformations of the hands and/or feet, and/or defects of the heart. The exact cause of Chromosome 11, Partial Monosomy 11q is not fully understood.

In addition to The National Organization for Rare Disorders (NORD) listed in Section III, the following organizations in Section II (Disease Specific) and in Section III (Umbrella) and Section IV (Government Agencies) can provide more information:
11Q Research and Resource Group, *II*
Children's Craniofacial Association, *III*
Chromosome Deletion Outreach, *III*
Congenital Heart Anomalies, Support, Education, & Resources, *III*
Craniofacial Foundation of America, *III*
European Chromosome 11q Network, *II*
FACES: The National Craniofacial Association, *III*
NIH/National Heart, Lung and Blood Institute Information Center, *IV*
NIH/National Institute of Child Health and Human Development, *IV*
NIH/National Institute on Deafness and Other Communication Disorders Information Clearinghouse, *IV*
UNIQUE - Rare Chromosome Disorder Support Group, *III*

221 CHROMOSOME 11, PARTIAL TRISOMY 11Q

Chromosome 11, Partial Trisomy 11q is a very rare chromosomal disorder caused by a duplication (trisomy) of the end (distal) portion of the long arm of chromosome 11. This disorder is usually apparent at birth and is characterized by delayed mental and physical development, retarded growth of the fetus during pregnancy and of the child after birth, an unusually small brain (microencephaly), and/or distinctive facial features. Chromosomal analysis is necessary for a definite diagnosis.

In addition to The National Organization for Rare Disorders (NORD) listed in Section III, the following organizations in Section II (Disease Specific) and in Section III (Umbrella) and Section IV (Government Agencies) can provide more information:
European Chromosome 11q Network, *II*
NIH/National Institute of Child Health and Human Development, *IV*
Support Organization for Trisomy 18, 13, and Related Disorders, *III*

UNIQUE - Rare Chromosome Disorder Support Group, *III*

222 CHROMOSOME 13, PARTIAL MONOSOMY 13Q

Chromosome 13, Partial Monosomy 13q is a rare chromosomal disorder in which a portion of the long arm (q) of chromosome 13 is missing (deleted or monosomic). The range and severity of symptoms may vary greatly, depending upon the exact size and location of the deletion on 13q. Chromosome 13, Partial Monosomy 13q is usually apparent at birth and may be characterized by low birth weight, malformations of the head and facial (craniofacial) area, abnormalities of the eyes, defects of the hands and/or feet, genital malformations in affected males, and/or additional physical abnormalities. Affected infants and children may also exhibit delays in the acquisition of skills requiring the coordination of mental and muscular activity (psychomotor retardation) as well as varying degrees of mental retardation. In the majority of cases, Chromosome 13, Partial Monosomy 13q appears to occur randomly, for no apparent reason (sporadic).

In addition to The National Organization for Rare Disorders (NORD) listed in Section III, the following organizations in Section II (Disease Specific) and in Section III (Umbrella) and Section IV (Government Agencies) can provide more information:

Children's Craniofacial Association, *III*
Chromosome Deletion Outreach, *III*
Congenital Heart Anomalies, Support, Education, & Resources, *III*
Craniofacial Foundation of America, *III*
FACES: The National Craniofacial Association, *III*
Institute for Families of Blind Children, *III*
NIH/National Cancer Institute, *IV*
NIH/National Eye Institute, *IV*
NIH/National Institute of Child Health and Human Development, *IV*
National Retinoblastoma Parent Group, *II*
UNIQUE - Rare Chromosome Disorder Support Group, *III*

223 CHROMOSOME 14 RING

Chromosome 14 Ring is a rare chromosomal disorder that is diagnosed through analysis of the chromosomes (cytogenetic studies). Major features of this disorder include growth retardation, mental retardation, seizures, and an unusually small head (microcephaly). Distinct facial features in individuals with Chromosome 14 Ring include a long face, narrow-shaped eyes, and a broad nasal bridge.

In addition to The National Organization for Rare Disorders (NORD) listed in Section III, the following organizations in Section II (Disease Specific) and in Section III (Umbrella) and Section IV (Government Agencies) can provide more information:

Chromosome Deletion Outreach, *III*
Epilepsy Foundation of America, *III*
NIH/National Institute of Child Health and Human Development, *IV*
UNIQUE - Rare Chromosome Disorder Support Group, *III*

224 CHROMOSOME 14, TRISOMY MOSAIC

Chromosome 14, Trisomy Mosaic is a very rare chromosomal disorder in which an extra chromosome 14 is present in some of the cells of the affected individual's body. Characteristic features include delayed growth of the fetus during pregnancy and/or of the child after birth, a wide nasal bridge, unusually small jaws (micrognathia), developmental delays, and mental retardation. Heart disease is present at birth (congenital) in most cases. This disorder is usually apparent at birth and may be diagnosed during pregnancy or after birth (prenatally or postnatally) by chromosomal analysis.

In addition to The National Organization for Rare Disorders (NORD) listed in Section III, the following organizations in Section II (Disease Specific) and in Section III (Umbrella) and Section IV (Government Agencies) can provide more information:

NIH/National Institute of Child Health and Human Development, *IV*
Support Organization for Trisomy 18, 13, and Related Disorders, *III*
UNIQUE - Rare Chromosome Disorder Support Group, *III*

225 CHROMOSOME 15 RING

Chromosome 15 Ring is a rare chromosomal disorder in which the affected infant has a ring formation of chromosome 15 caused by the breakage of the chromosome at both ends and joining of the ends to form a ring. The amount of genetic material lost at the two ends of the chromosome may vary. As a result, an infant with very little absent genetic material may have no apparent symptoms while an infant with a significant part of the chromosomal ends missing may have many symptoms. The most apparent features of this disorder are delayed growth, a small head circumference, triangular shaped face, poor muscle tone, and mental retardation.

In addition to The National Organization for Rare Disorders (NORD) listed in Section III, the following organizations in Section II (Disease Specific) and in Section III (Umbrella) and Section IV (Government Agencies) can provide more information:
Chromosome Deletion Outreach, *III*
NIH/National Institute of Child Health and Human Development, *IV*
UNIQUE - Rare Chromosome Disorder Support Group, *III*

226 **CHROMOSOME 15, DISTAL TRISOMY 15Q**

Chromosome 15, Distal Trisomy 15q is an extremely rare chromosomal disorder in which the end (distal) portion of the long arm (q) of the 15th chromosome (15q) appears three times (trisomy) rather than twice in cells of the body. The disorder is characterized by growth delays before and/or after birth (prenatal and/or postnatal growth retardation); mental retardation; and/or distinctive malformations of the head and facial (craniofacial) area. Additional abnormalities typically include an unusually short neck; malformations of the fingers and/or toes; abnormal sideways curvature of the spine (scoliosis) and/or other skeletal malformations; genital abnormalities, particularly in affected males; and/or, in some cases, heart (cardiac) defects. The range and severity of symptoms and physical findings may vary from case to case, depending upon the length and location of the duplicated portion of chromosome 15q. In most cases, Chromosome 15, Distal Trisomy 15q is due to a chromosomal balanced translocation in one of the parents.

In addition to The National Organization for Rare Disorders (NORD) listed in Section III, the following organizations in Section II (Disease Specific) and in Section III (Umbrella) and Section IV (Government Agencies) can provide more information:
Children's Craniofacial Association, *III*
Congenital Heart Anomalies, Support, Education, & Resources, *III*
NIH/National Institute of Child Health and Human Development, *IV*
NIH/National Institute of Neurological Disorders and Stroke, *IV*
Support Organization for Trisomy 18, 13, and Related Disorders, *III*
UNIQUE - Rare Chromosome Disorder Support Group, *III*

227 **CHROMOSOME 18, MONOSOMY 18P**

Chromosome 18, Monosomy 18p (deletion of the a portion of the short arm of the chromosome 18) is characterized by unusual facial characteristics and mild to severe mental retardation. The affected individual often has an I.Q. averaging between 45 to 50. In some individuals, however, there has been no mental deficiency at all. Language is often affected, and many people with Chromosome 18, Monosomy 18p may not speak simple sentences until seven to nine years of age. Restlessness, emotional "ups and downs," a fear of strangers, and lack of concentration are frequent behavioral characteristics.

In addition to The National Organization for Rare Disorders (NORD) listed in Section III, the following organizations in Section II (Disease Specific) and in Section III (Umbrella) and Section IV (Government Agencies) can provide more information:
Chromosome 18 Registry and Research Society, *III*
Chromosome Deletion Outreach, *III*
NIH/National Institute of Child Health and Human Development, *IV*
Support Organization for Trisomy 18, 13, and Related Disorders, *III*

228 **CHROMOSOME 18, RING**

Chromosome 18, Ring is a rare chromosomal disorder in which an affected infant has a ring formation of chromosome 18 caused by the breakage of the chromosome at both ends and joining of the ends to form a ring. The amount of material lost at the two ends of the chromosome may vary. As a result, an infant with very little absent genetic material may have no apparent symptoms, while an infant with a significant part of the chromosomal ends lost, may have many symptoms. The most apparent features of this disorder are mental retardation, unusual facial features, a small head and poor muscle tone. The diagnosis of Chromosome 18, Ring can only be made through chromosomal analysis (cytogenetic analysis).

In addition to The National Organization for Rare Disorders (NORD) listed in Section III, the following organizations in Section II (Disease Specific) and in Section III (Umbrella) and Section IV (Government Agencies) can provide more information:
Chromosome 18 Registry and Research Society, *III*
Chromosome Deletion Outreach, *III*
NIH/National Institute of Child Health and Human Development, *IV*
UNIQUE - Rare Chromosome Disorder Support Group, *III*

229 **CHROMOSOME 18, TETRASOMY 18P**

Chromosome 18, Tetrasomy 18p is a very rare chromosomal disorder in which the short arm of the 18th chromosome (18p) appears four times (tetrasomy) rather than twice in cells of the body. Individuals with a normal chromosomal make-up (karyotype) have two 18th chromosomes, both of which have a short arm ("18p") and a long arm ("18q"). However, in individuals with Chromosome 18, Tetrasomy 18p, four short arms (18ps) are present in cells of the body rather than the normal two.

The symptoms of Chromosome 18, Tetrasomy 18p may vary from case to case. Many affected individuals may have abnormalities of the head and facial (craniofacial) area; malformations of the spine, hands, and/or feet; neuromuscular abnormalities, such as increased muscle tone (hypertonia), increased reflex reactions (hyperreflexia), and difficulty coordinating movement; kidney (renal) malformations; and/or additional physical abnormalities. In addition, children and adults with Chromosome 18, Tetrasomy 18p often exhibit moderate to severe mental retardation, limitations in speech, and/or behavioral abnormalities. In most cases, Chromosome 18, Tetrasomy 18p is the result of a spontaneous (de novo) genetic change (mutation) early in embryonic development that occurs for unknown reasons (sporadic).

In addition to The National Organization for Rare Disorders (NORD) listed in Section III, the following organizations in Section II (Disease Specific) and in Section III (Umbrella) and Section IV (Government Agencies) can provide more information:
Chromosome 18 Registry and Research Society, *III*
NIH/National Institute of Child Health and Human Development, *IV*
Support Organization for Trisomy 18, 13, and Related Disorders, *III*
UNIQUE - Rare Chromosome Disorder Support Group, *III*

230 CHROMOSOME 18Q- SYNDROME

Chromosome 18q- Syndrome is a rare congenital chromosomal disorder caused by a deletion of a piece of the long arm (q) of chromosome 18. The amount of genetic material that is missing may vary. As a result, affected infant with very little absent genetic material may have no apparent symptoms, while a infant with a significant part of the long arm of chromosome 18 missing may have many symptoms. The most apparent and common symptoms of this disorder are mental retardation, short stature, a flat midface, poor muscle tone, a small head and unusual facial features.

In addition to The National Organization for Rare Disorders (NORD) listed in Section III, the following organizations in Section II (Disease Specific) and in Section III (Umbrella) and Section IV (Government Agencies) can provide more information:
Chromosome 18 Registry and Research Society, *III*
Chromosome Deletion Outreach, *III*
NIH/National Institute of Child Health and Human Development, *IV*
UNIQUE - Rare Chromosome Disorder Support Group, *III*

231 CHROMOSOME 21 RING

Chromosome 21 Ring is a rare chromosomal disorder in which the affected infant has a breakage of chromosome 21 at both ends, and the ends of the chromosome join together to form a ring. The amount of genetic material lost at the two ends of the chromosome may vary. As a result, an infant with very little absent genetic material may have no apparent symptoms while an infant with a significant part of the chromosomal ends missing may have many symptoms. When symptoms of the disorder are present, the affected infant may have mental retardation as well as abnormalities of the face, eyes, skeleton, and/or internal organs.

In addition to The National Organization for Rare Disorders (NORD) listed in Section III, the following organizations in Section II (Disease Specific) and in Section III (Umbrella) and Section IV (Government Agencies) can provide more information:
Chromosome Deletion Outreach, *III*
NIH/National Institute of Child Health and Human Development, *IV*
Scleroderma Info Exchange, Inc., *II*
UNIQUE - Rare Chromosome Disorder Support Group, *III*

232 CHROMOSOME 22 RING

Chromosome 22 Ring is a rare chromosomal disorder in which the affected infant has a breakage of chromosome 22 at both ends, and the ends of the chromosome join together to form a ring. The amount of genetic material lost at the two ends of the chromosome may vary. As a result, an infant with very little absent genetic material may have no apparent symptoms while an infant with a significant part of the chromosomal ends missing may have many symptoms. The most apparent features of this disorder are mental retardation, lack of coordination of voluntary movements, and muscle weakness.

In addition to The National Organization for Rare Disorders (NORD) listed in Section III, the following

organizations in Section II (Disease Specific) and in Section III (Umbrella) and Section IV (Government Agencies) can provide more information:
Chromosome Deletion Outreach, *III*
NIH/National Institute of Child Health and Human Development, *IV*
UNIQUE - Rare Chromosome Disorder Support Group, *III*

233 CHROMOSOME 22, TRISOMY MOSAIC

Chromosome 22, Trisomy Mosaic is a rare chromosomal disorder in which an extra chromosome 22 is present in some of the cells of the affected individual's body. The severity of symptoms may depend on the percentage of cells with the extra chromosome (trisomy). Characteristic features include unequal development of the two sides of the body (hemidystrophy), a shortened limb, and a webbed neck. This disorder is usually apparent at birth, and may be diagnosed during pregnancy or after birth (prenatally or postnatally) through specialized testing. Chromosomal testing is necessary for a definite diagnosis.

In addition to The National Organization for Rare Disorders (NORD) listed in Section III, the following organizations in Section II (Disease Specific) and in Section III (Umbrella) and Section IV (Government Agencies) can provide more information:
NIH/National Institute of Child Health and Human Development, *IV*
Support Organization for Trisomy 18, 13, and Related Disorders, *III*
UNIQUE - Rare Chromosome Disorder Support Group, *III*

234 CHROMOSOME 3, MONOSOMY 3P2

Chromosome 3, Monosomy 3p2 is a very rare chromosomal disorder in which the end of the short arm of chromosome 3 (distal portion) is missing. Major symptoms may include failure of the fetus to grow during pregnancy and/or severely delayed growth of the child after birth. Mental retardation and/or severe to profound delays in development may also occur. Characteristic abnormalities include an unusually small head (microcephaly), eyebrows that grow together (synophrys), and/or excessive growth of the hair (hypertrichosis). Developmental delays and unusual facial characteristics usually make this disorder apparent in the first years of life.

In addition to The National Organization for Rare Disorders (NORD) listed in Section III, the following organizations in Section II (Disease Specific) and in Section III (Umbrella) and Section IV (Government Agencies) can provide more information:
Chromosome Deletion Outreach, *III*
NIH/National Institute of Child Health and Human Development, *IV*
UNIQUE - Rare Chromosome Disorder Support Group, *III*

235 CHROMOSOME 3, TRISOMY 3Q2

Chromosome 3, Trisomy 3q2 is a very rare chromosomal disorder caused by a duplication of a portion of the long arm (q) of chromosome 3. The disorder, usually evident at birth (congenital), may be characterized by mental retardation, developmental delays, and/or multiple craniofacial abnormalities. These may include a low hairline, widely-spaced eyes, connected bushy eyebrows, and/or an elongated or widened head. Malformations of the heart, the kidneys, and/or other internal organs, and/or abnormalities of the limbs, particularly the hands and toes, may also occur. Genetic analysis and chromosomal testing are necessary for a definite diagnosis.

In addition to The National Organization for Rare Disorders (NORD) listed in Section III, the following organizations in Section II (Disease Specific) and in Section III (Umbrella) and Section IV (Government Agencies) can provide more information:
NIH/National Institute of Child Health and Human Development, *IV*
Support Organization for Trisomy 18, 13, and Related Disorders, *III*
UNIQUE - Rare Chromosome Disorder Support Group, *III*

236 CHROMOSOME 4 RING

Chromosome 4 Ring is a rare chromosomal disorder in which the affected infant has a breakage of chromosome 4 at both ends, and the ends of the chromosome join together to form a ring. The amount of genetic material lost at the two ends of the chromosome may vary. As a result, an infant with very little absent genetic material may have fewer symptoms than an infant with a significant part of the chromosomal ends missing. The most consistent features of this disorder are slowed growth and development, an abnormally small head (microcephaly), beaked nose, unusually small jaw bones (micrognathia), and/or incomplete closure of the roof of the mouth (cleft palate).

In addition to The National Organization for Rare Disorders (NORD) listed in Section III, the following organizations in Section II (Disease Specific) and in

Section III (Umbrella) and Section IV (Government Agencies) can provide more information:
Chromosome Deletion Outreach, *III*
NIH/National Institute of Child Health and Human Development, *IV*
UNIQUE - Rare Chromosome Disorder Support Group, *III*

237 CHROMOSOME 4, MONOSOMY 4Q

Chromosome 4, Monosomy 4q is a chromosomal disorder caused by a partial deletion of the long arm of chromosome 4. The patient may have an extremely prominent forehead (frontal bossing), enlargement of the back part of the head, low placement of ears, short broad hands and feet, unusually small size associated with slow or delayed growth, congenital heart defects, and possible mental retardation.

In addition to The National Organization for Rare Disorders (NORD) listed in Section III, the following organizations in Section II (Disease Specific) and in Section III (Umbrella) and Section IV (Government Agencies) can provide more information:
Chromosome Deletion Outreach, *III*
NIH/National Institute of Child Health and Human Development, *IV*
UNIQUE - Rare Chromosome Disorder Support Group, *III*

238 CHROMOSOME 4, MONOSOMY DISTAL 4Q

Chromosome 4, Monosomy Distal 4q is a rare disorder in which there is a deletion of an end piece of the long arm (q) of chromosome 4. The majority of cases of this disorder occur during embryonic development for no apparent reason (de novo). The major symptoms of Chromosome 4, Monosomy Distal 4q are mental retardation and unusual facial features. Heart defects as well as limb deformities may also be present.

In addition to The National Organization for Rare Disorders (NORD) listed in Section III, the following organizations in Section II (Disease Specific) and in Section III (Umbrella) and Section IV (Government Agencies) can provide more information:
Chromosome Deletion Outreach, *III*
Cleft Palate Foundation, *III*
FACES: The National Craniofacial Association, *III*
NIH/National Institute of Child Health and Human Development, *IV*
Wide Smiles, *III*

239 CHROMOSOME 4, PARTIAL TRISOMY DISTAL 4Q

Chromosome 4, Partial Trisomy Distal 4Q is an extremely rare chromosomal disorder caused by a duplication of the end (distal) portion of the long arm (q) of the fourth chromosome. The symptoms of this disorder vary from case to case and may include an abnormally small head (microcephaly); malformations of the arms, legs, and head and facial (craniofacial) area; and/or mental retardation. Chromosome 4, Partial Trisomy Distal 4Q usually occurs because of a balanced translocation between two chromosomes of one of the parents. Some cases have occurred for no apparent reason (de novo) and are not inherited. Chromosomal analysis is necessary for a definite diagnosis.

In addition to The National Organization for Rare Disorders (NORD) listed in Section III, the following organizations in Section II (Disease Specific) and in Section III (Umbrella) and Section IV (Government Agencies) can provide more information:
Children's Craniofacial Association, *III*
Congenital Heart Anomalies, Support, Education, & Resources, *III*
FACES: The National Craniofacial Association, *III*
Forward Face, Inc., *III*
NIH/National Institute of Child Health and Human Development, *IV*
Support Organization for Trisomy 18, 13, and Related Disorders, *III*
UNIQUE - Rare Chromosome Disorder Support Group, *III*

240 CHROMOSOME 4, TRISOMY 4P

Trisomies are rare chromosomal abnormalities. Chromosomes are found in the nucleus of all body cells. They carry the genetic characteristics of each individual. Pairs of human chromosomes are numbered from 1 through 22, with an unequal 23rd pair of X and Y chromosomes for males, and two X chromosomes for females. People with a trisomy have an extra chromosome added to one of the normal pairs. Each chromosome has a short arm designated as "p," and a long arm designated "q." Trisomy 4p is a chromosomal disorder in which there is an additional piece added to the short arm of chromosome 4. Although the symptoms vary depending on the amount of duplication of the short arm "p" of chromosome 4, the most frequent features of this disorder are characteristic facial features, slowed growth after birth, abnormally slow mental and muscular movement (psychomotor retardation), and various other major and minor abnormalities. Trisomy 4p is diagnosed through chromosomal testing.

In addition to The National Organization for Rare Disorders (NORD) listed in Section III, the following

organizations in Section II (Disease Specific) and in Section III (Umbrella) and Section IV (Government Agencies) can provide more information:
NIH/National Institute of Child Health and Human Development, *IV*
Support Organization for Trisomy 18, 13, and Related Disorders, *III*
UNIQUE - Rare Chromosome Disorder Support Group, *III*

241 CHROMOSOME 5, TRISOMY 5P

Chromosome 5, Trisomy 5p is a very rare chromosomal disorder caused by a duplication of all or part of the short arm of chromosome 5. Chromosome 5, Trisomy 5p is characterized by normal birth weight, an abnormally small head (microcephaly), malformations of the face (facial dysmorphism), lack of muscle tone (hypotonia), mental retardation, and/or delayed motor development (psychomotor retardation).

In addition to The National Organization for Rare Disorders (NORD) listed in Section III, the following organizations in Section II (Disease Specific) and in Section III (Umbrella) and Section IV (Government Agencies) can provide more information:
NIH/National Institute of Child Health and Human Development, *IV*
Support Organization for Trisomy 18, 13, and Related Disorders, *III*

242 CHROMOSOME 6 RING

Chromosome 6 Ring is a rare chromosomal disorder in which the affected infant has a breakage of chromosome 6 at both ends, and the ends of the chromosome join together to form a ring. The amount of genetic material lost at the two ends of the chromosome can vary. As a result, an infant with very little absent genetic material may have no apparent symptoms while an infant with a significant part of the chromosomal ends missing may have many symptoms. The most apparent features of this disorder are mild to severe mental retardation, delays in growth and self-controlled muscle movement (psychomotor retardation), a small head circumference and jaw, low-set ears, a flat nasal bridge, and/or abnormalities of the eyes.

In addition to The National Organization for Rare Disorders (NORD) listed in Section III, the following organizations in Section II (Disease Specific) and in Section III (Umbrella) and Section IV (Government Agencies) can provide more information:
Chromosome Deletion Outreach, *III*
NIH/National Institute of Child Health and Human Development, *IV*
Spotlight 6, *III*
UNIQUE - Rare Chromosome Disorder Support Group, *III*

243 CHROMOSOME 6, PARTIAL TRISOMY 6Q

Chromosome 6, Partial Trisomy 6q is an extremely rare chromosomal disorder in which the end (distal) portion of the long arm (q) of the 6th chromosome (6q) appears three times (trisomy) rather than twice in cells of the body. This disorder is characterized by abnormalities of the head and facial (craniofacial) area; an unusually short, webbed neck; and/or joints that are fixed in a bent position (flexion contractures) in the hands, feet, and/or other areas of the body. Many affected individuals also exhibit unusually slow physical development (growth retardation), a delay in the acquisition of skills requiring coordination of muscular and mental activity (psychomotor retardation), and/or mental retardation. The range and severity of symptoms may vary from case to case, depending upon the length and location of the duplicated portion of chromosome 6q. In most cases, Chromosome 6, Partial Trisomy 6q may be the result of an error during very early development of the embryo if one of the parents has a balanced chromosomal rearrangement.

In addition to The National Organization for Rare Disorders (NORD) listed in Section III, the following organizations in Section II (Disease Specific) and in Section III (Umbrella) and Section IV (Government Agencies) can provide more information:
NIH/National Institute of Child Health and Human Development, *IV*
Spotlight 6, *III*
Support Organization for Trisomy 18, 13, and Related Disorders, *III*
UNIQUE - Rare Chromosome Disorder Support Group, *III*

244 CHROMOSOME 7, MONOSOMY 7P2

Chromosome 7, Monosomy 7p2 is an extremely rare chromosomal disorder in which the end portion of the short arm (p) of chromosome 7 is missing. Major symptoms may involve characteristic abnormalities of the head and face (craniofacial area) such as the premature closure of the joints (sutures) that unite the larger craniofacial bones (craniosynostosis). Premature closure of the sutures on the sides of the head (scaphocephaly) may cause the head to appear abnormally long and narrow. In addition, the forehead may have an abnormally triangular-shaped appearance (trigonocephaly). Other abnormalities may include skeletal malformations of the fingers and feet; underdevelopment of the heart, kidneys, and colon; and/or abnormal reproductive organs in both genders. Affected individuals may also exhibit growth delays, developmental delays, and mental retardation. The degree of these abnormalities may vary from moderate to severe. The majority of the documented cases of Chromosome 7, Monosomy 7p2 occur for no apparent reason (de novo). Chromosomal testing and genetic analysis are necessary for a definite diagnosis.

In addition to The National Organization for Rare Disorders (NORD) listed in Section III, the following organizations in Section II (Disease Specific) and in Section III (Umbrella) and Section IV (Government Agencies) can provide more information:
AboutFace U.S.A., *III*
Children's Craniofacial Association, *III*
Chromosome Deletion Outreach, *III*
Congenital Heart Anomalies, Support, Education, & Resources, *III*
FACES: The National Craniofacial Association, *III*
NIH/National Institute of Child Health and Human Development, *IV*
Support Organization for Trisomy 18, 13, and Related Disorders, *III*
UNIQUE - Rare Chromosome Disorder Support Group, *III*

245 CHROMOSOME 8, MONOSOMY 8P2

Chromosome 8, Monosomy 8p2 is a very rare chromosomal disorder in which a portion of the short arm (p) of chromosome 8 is missing. Major physical symptoms and characteristics may include an abnormally small head (microcephaly); extra folds of skin at the inner corners of the eyes (epicanthal folds); a short, nubbed nose; and/or a broad chest with widely- spaced, underdeveloped nipples. Prenatal or postnatal growth delays, congenital heart defects, and/or genital abnormalities particularly in males may also exist. Mental retardation may vary from mild to severe. This disorder may be due to a chromosomal abnormality in one parent (balanced translocation) or occur for no apparent reason (de novo). Genetic analysis and chromosomal testing are necessary for a definite diagnosis.

In addition to The National Organization for Rare Disorders (NORD) listed in Section III, the following organizations in Section II (Disease Specific) and in Section III (Umbrella) and Section IV (Government Agencies) can provide more information:
American Heart Association, *III*
Chromosome Deletion Outreach, *III*
Congenital Heart Anomalies, Support, Education, & Resources, *III*
NIH/National Institute of Child Health and Human Development, *IV*
UNIQUE - Rare Chromosome Disorder Support Group, *III*

246 CHROMOSOME 9 RING

Chromosome 9 Ring is a rare chromosomal disorder in which the affected infant has a breakage of chromosome 9 at both ends, and the ends of the chromosome join together to form a ring. The amount of genetic material lost at the two ends of the chromosome may vary. As a result, an infant with very little absent genetic material may have no apparent symptoms, while an infant with a significant part of the chromosomal ends missing may have more severe symptoms. Symptoms of this disorder may include unusual facial features, heart defects, moderate to severe mental retardation, and skeletal abnormalities.

In addition to The National Organization for Rare Disorders (NORD) listed in Section III, the following organizations in Section II (Disease Specific) and in Section III (Umbrella) and Section IV (Government Agencies) can provide more information:
Chromosome Deletion Outreach, *III*
NIH/National Institute of Child Health and Human Development, *IV*
UNIQUE - Rare Chromosome Disorder Support Group, *III*

247 CHROMOSOME 9, PARTIAL MONOSOMY 9P

Chromosome 9, Partial Monosomy 9p is a rare chromosomal disorder in which the end (distal) portion of the short arm (p) of chromosome 9 is missing (deleted). This disorder is usually apparent at birth and is characterized by distinctive facial features, abnormalities of the hands and feet, genital malformations in affected males and females, additional physical abnormalities, and varying degrees of mental retardation. In the majority of cases, Chromosome 9, Partial Monosomy 9p is the result of a spontaneous (de novo) genetic change very early in embryonic development that occurs for unknown reasons (sporadic).

In addition to The National Organization for Rare Disorders (NORD) listed in Section III, the following organizations in Section II (Disease Specific) and in Section III (Umbrella) and Section IV (Government Agencies) can provide more information:
Children's Craniofacial Association, *III*
Chromosome Deletion Outreach, *III*

NIH/National Institute of Child Health and Human Development, *IV*
Support Group for 9p-, *II*
Support Group for Monosomy 9P, *II*
UNIQUE - Rare Chromosome Disorder Support Group, *III*

248 CHROMOSOME 9, TETRASOMY 9P

Chromosome 9, Tetrasomy 9p is a very rare chromosomal disorder in which the short arm of the ninth chromosome (9p) appears four times (tetrasomy) rather than twice in cells of the body. Individuals with a normal chromosomal make-up (karyotype) have two 9th chromosomes, both of which have a short arm ("9p") and a long arm ("9q"). However, in individuals with Chromosome 9, Tetrasomy 9p, four short arms (9ps) are present in cells of the body rather than the normal two.

The symptoms of Chromosome 9, Tetrasomy 9p can vary from case to case. Affected individuals may exhibit developmental abnormalities, such as mild growth retardation and/or a moderate to severe delay in the attainment of skills requiring the coordination of muscular and mental activity (psychomotor retardation). Moderate to severe mental retardation may also be present. In addition, people with the disorder may display a variety of physical abnormalities, such as malformations of the head and facial (craniofacial) area, abnormalities of the hands and fingers, skeletal malformations, and heart (cardiac) defects. Chromosome 9, Tetrasomy 9p is the result of a spontaneous (de novo) genetic change (mutation) early in embryonic development that occurs for unknown reasons (sporadic).

In addition to The National Organization for Rare Disorders (NORD) listed in Section III, the following organizations in Section II (Disease Specific) and in Section III (Umbrella) and Section IV (Government Agencies) can provide more information:
American Heart Association, *III*
Support Organization for Trisomy 18, 13, and Related Disorders, *III*
Trisomy 9 International Parent Support, *II*
UNIQUE - Rare Chromosome Disorder Support Group, *III*

249 CHROMOSOME 9, TRISOMY 9P (MULTIPLE VARIANTS)

Chromosome 9, Trisomy 9p is a rare chromosomal disorder in which part or all of the short arm (p) of chromosome 9 is present three times (trisomy) rather than twice in the cells of the body. In some cases, an extra (trisomic) segment of the long arm (q) of chromosome 9 may also be present. The symptoms of this disorder are unusually similar among affected infants despite differing lengths of the duplicated segment and are thought to relate to extra chromosomal material on the end (distal) portion of the short arm (9p). Chromosome 9, Trisomy 9p is characterized by mental retardation, characteristic physical abnormalities of the head and facial (craniofacial) area, and/or skeletal malformations. In about 25 percent of infants with this disorder, heart defects are present at birth (congenital). Affected infants may also experience growth retardation and a significant delay in the acquisition of language and communication skills. In some cases of Chromosome 9, Trisomy 9p occurs because of a balanced chromosomal rearrangement between two chromosomes of one of the parents; other cases are the result of a spontaneous (de novo) genetic change early in embryonic development that occurs for unknown reasons. Chromosomal analysis is necessary for definite diagnosis.

In addition to The National Organization for Rare Disorders (NORD) listed in Section III, the following organizations in Section II (Disease Specific) and in Section III (Umbrella) and Section IV (Government Agencies) can provide more information:
NIH/National Institute of Child Health and Human Development, *IV*
Support Organization for Trisomy 13/18 and Related Disorders, UK, *II*
Support Organization for Trisomy 18, 13, and Related Disorders, *III*
Trisomy 9 International Parent Support, *II*
UNIQUE - Rare Chromosome Disorder Support Group, *III*

250 CHROMOSOME 9, TRISOMY MOSAIC

Chromosome 9 Trisomy Mosaic is a rare chromosomal disorder in which an extra chromosome 9 is present in some of the cells of the affected individual's body. The severity of symptoms may depend on the percentage of cells with the extra chromosome (trisomy). Characteristic features include delayed growth of the fetus, heart defects present at birth, facial abnormalities (e.g., low-set and/or malformed ears), an abnormally small head, kidney and/or genital abnormalities, skeletal abnormalities (e.g., fixed and/or dislocated joints), and/or malformations of the brain.

In addition to The National Organization for Rare Disorders (NORD) listed in Section III, the following organizations in Section II (Disease Specific) and in Section III (Umbrella) and Section IV (Government Agencies) can provide more information:
NIH/National Institute of Child Health and Human Development, *IV*
Support Organization for Trisomy 18, 13, and Related Disorders, *III*
Trisomy 9 International Parent Support, *II*
UNIQUE - Rare Chromosome Disorder Support Group, *III*

251 CHRONIC FATIGUE SYNDROME

Chronic Fatigue Syndrome (CFS) is a disorder characterized by profound fatigue and other related symptoms. Standards for the diagnosis of CFS have been defined by researchers and the Centers for Disease Control (CDC). These include excessive fatigue or easy fatigability that does not respond to bed rest. The fatigue is severe enough to reduce the average daily activities of the affected individual by at least 50 percent. The onset of these symptoms is usually sudden, sometimes following a flu-like illness. According to the CDC, the profound fatigue must last for at least six months in order for the diagnosis to be confirmed. The syndrome may persist for months or years, and disappear without treatment.

The many symptoms of Chronic Fatigue Syndrome do not always occur with the same degree of severity or at the same time. There are usually instances when symptoms may disappear for periods of time. Scientists believe Chronic Fatigue Syndrome is not contagious and laboratory tests (blood, urine, etc.) are of little value in diagnosing the syndrome.

In addition to The National Organization for Rare Disorders (NORD) listed in Section III, the following organizations in Section II (Disease Specific) and in Section III (Umbrella) and Section IV (Government Agencies) can provide more information:
Centers for Disease Control and Prevention, *IV*
NIH/National Institute of Allergy and Infectious Diseases, *IV*
National Chronic Fatigue Syndrome & Fibromyalgia Association, *II*

252 CHRONIC INFLAMMATORY DEMYELINATING POLYNEUROPATHY

Chronic inflammatory demyelinating polyneuropathy (CIDP) is a rare disorder in which there is swelling of nerve roots and destruction of the fatty protective covering (myelin sheath) over the nerves. This disorder causes weakness, paralysis and/or impairment in motor function, especially of the limbs. Sensory loss may also be present causing numbness, tingling, or prickling sensations. The motor and sensory impairments are usually symmetrical (on both sides of the body), and the degree of severity may vary. The course of CIDP may also vary. Some affected individuals may follow a slow steady pattern of symptoms while others may have symptoms that wax and wane, with the most severe symptoms occuring after many months or a year or more. One feature that distinguishes this disorder from other similar disorders is that there is typically no preceding viral infection at least three months prior to the appearance of the disorder, and no family history of other similar disorders or polyneuropathy.

In addition to The National Organization for Rare Disorders (NORD) listed in Section III, the following organizations in Section II (Disease Specific) and in Section III (Umbrella) and Section IV (Government Agencies) can provide more information:
American Autoimmune Related Diseases Association, Inc., *III*
NIH/National Institute of Neurological Disorders and Stroke, *IV*

253 CHURG STRAUSS SYNDROME

Churg-Strauss Syndrome is a rare disorder that affects multiple organ systems and is characterized by the formation and accumulation of an abnormally large number of certain white blood cells (eosinophils), inflammation of blood vessels (angiitis or vasculitis), and inflammatory nodular lesions (granulomatosis). Other symptoms of Churg-Strauss Syndrome include fever, a general feeling of weakness and fatigue (malaise), loss of appetite (anorexia) and weight loss. It is often preceded by asthma or allergies. The exact causes of Churg-Strauss Syndrome is not known.

In addition to The National Organization for Rare Disorders (NORD) listed in Section III, the following organizations in Section II (Disease Specific) and in Section III (Umbrella) and Section IV (Government Agencies) can provide more information:
American Lung Association, *III*
Churg-Strauss Syndrome International Support Group, *II*
NIH/National Heart, Lung and Blood Institute Information Center, *IV*
NIH/National Institute of Allergy and Infectious Diseases, *IV*

254 **CIGUATERA FISH POISONING**

Ciguatera fish poisoning is a rare disorder that occurs because of the ingestion of certain contaminated tropical and subtropical fish. When ingested, the toxin (ciguatoxin), which is present at high levels in these contaminated fish, may affect the digestive, muscular, and/or neurological systems. More than 400 different species of fish have been implicated as a cause of ciguatera fish poisoning, including many that are otherwise considered edible (i.e., sea bass, snapper, and perch). These fish typically inhabit low-lying shore areas or coral reefs in tropical or subtropical areas. In the United States, ciguatera fish poisoning has occurred more frequently in the last decade perhaps as a result of a general increase in fish consumption.

In addition to The National Organization for Rare Disorders (NORD) listed in Section III, the following organizations in Section II (Disease Specific) and in Section III (Umbrella) and Section IV (Government Agencies) can provide more information:

Centers for Disease Control and Prevention, *IV*

255 **CIRRHOSIS, PRIMARY BILIARY**

Primary biliary cirrhosis is a chronic progressive liver disorder thought to be related to abnormalities in the immune system. Obstruction of the small bile ducts is accompanied by yellow discoloration of the skin (jaundice). Excessive amounts of copper accumulate in the liver, and fibrous or granular hardening (induration) of the soft liver tissue develops. This disorder occurs mainly in females during the fourth to the seventh decade of life, and is marked by four progressive stages.

In addition to The National Organization for Rare Disorders (NORD) listed in Section III, the following organizations in Section II (Disease Specific) and in Section III (Umbrella) and Section IV (Government Agencies) can provide more information:

American Liver Foundation, *III*
NIH/National Digestive Diseases Information Clearinghouse, *IV*
Primary Biliary Cirrhosis Patient Support Network, *II*
United Liver Association, *III*

256 **CITRULLINEMIA**

Citrullinemia is one of several hereditary urea cycle disorders. These disorders are caused by a deficiency of one of the enzymes needed for the incorporation of ammonia into urea, which is normally excreted in the urine. The deficiencies cause an excess of ammonia in the blood and body tissues.

In citrullinemia the deficient enzyme is argininosuccinic acid synthetase. If left untreated, the disorder manifests itself by an elevated level of toxic ammonia in the blood (hyperammonemia). This imbalance may lead to brain damage and eventually to coma.

In addition to The National Organization for Rare Disorders (NORD) listed in Section III, the following organizations in Section II (Disease Specific) and in Section III (Umbrella) and Section IV (Government Agencies) can provide more information:

American Kidney Fund, Inc., *III*
Metabolic Information Network, *III*
NIH/National Digestive Diseases Information Clearinghouse, *IV*
National Kidney Foundation, *III*
National Urea Cycle Disorders Foundation, *III*
Research Trust for Metabolic Diseases in Children, *III*

257 **CLEFT PALATE AND CLEFT LIP**

Cleft cip and palate are common malformations that are noticeable at birth (congenital). A cleft is an incomplete closure of the palate or lip, or both. This defect is caused when the pair of long bones that form the upper jaw (maxillae) do not fuse properly during the early development of the embryo. The cleft may be barely noticeable or result in severe deformities requiring surgical correction.

In addition to The National Organization for Rare Disorders (NORD) listed in Section III, the following organizations in Section II (Disease Specific) and in Section III (Umbrella) and Section IV (Government Agencies) can provide more information:

AboutFace U.S.A., *III*
Alliance of Genetic Support Groups, *III*
Children's Craniofacial Association, *III*
Cleft Palate Foundation, *III*
Forward Face, Inc., *III*
Let's Face It, Inc., *III*
March of Dimes Birth Defects Foundation, *III*
NIH/National Oral Health Information Clearinghouse, *IV*
Wide Smiles, *III*

258 **CLEIDOCRANIAL DYSPLASIA**

Cleidocranial Dysplasia is a rare craniofacial disorder inherited as an autosomal dominant trait. Major symptoms may include premature closing of the soft spot on the head (coronal), delayed closure of the space between the bones of the skull (fontanels) and complete or partial absence of the collarbones (clavicles). Delayed eruption of teeth, moderately short stature, a high arched palate, a wide pelvic joint, failure of the lower jaw joints to unite, and fingers that are irregular in length may also be present.

In addition to The National Organization for Rare Disorders (NORD) listed in Section III, the following organizations in Section II (Disease Specific) and in Section III (Umbrella) and Section IV (Government Agencies) can provide more information:
Children's Craniofacial Association, *III*
FACES: The National Craniofacial Association, *III*
NIH/National Arthritis and Musculoskeletal and Skin Diseases Information Clearinghouse, *IV*

259 CLUBFOOT

Clubfoot is a general term used to describe a group of deformities of the ankles and/or feet that are usually present at birth. The defect may be mild or severe and may affect one or both of the ankles and/or feet. Different forms of clubfoot may include talipes equinovarus in which the foot is turned inward and downward; calcaneal valgus in which the foot is angled at the heel with the toes pointing upward and outward; and metatarsus varus in which the front of the foot is turned inward. If not corrected, affected individuals may develop an unusual manner of walking (gait). Clubfoot may be caused by a combination of hereditary and other factors (e.g., environment) and may occur as an isolated condition or due to a number of different underlying disorders.

In addition to The National Organization for Rare Disorders (NORD) listed in Section III, the following organizations in Section II (Disease Specific) and in Section III (Umbrella) and Section IV (Government Agencies) can provide more information:
Alliance of Genetic Support Groups, *III*
CHERUB—Association of Families and Friends of Children with Limb Disorders, *III*
NIH/National Institute of Child Health and Human Development, *IV*
Superkids, Inc. (newsletter for families and friends of children with limb differences), *III*

260 COATS' DISEASE

Coats' Disease is a rare eye disorder that usually presents itself during the first ten years of a child's life. This disorder is characterized by a white or yellowish area encompassing the small blind spot on the surface of the retina (optic disk). Inflammation may result from an excess of fluid beneath the retina. Loss of vision and retinal detachment may also occur. Coats' Disease is usually found in one eye only and normally progresses slowly. Hyperlipemic retinitis is the adult form of Coats' Disease.

In addition to The National Organization for Rare Disorders (NORD) listed in Section III, the following organizations in Section II (Disease Specific) and in Section III (Umbrella) and Section IV (Government Agencies) can provide more information:
American Council of the Blind, Inc., *III*
American Foundation for the Blind, *III*
Blind Children's Fund, *III*
Council of Families with Visual Impairment, *III*
Foundation Fighting Blindness, *III*
NIH/National Eye Institute, *IV*
National Association for Parents of the Visually Impaired, *III*
National Association for Visually Handicapped, *III*
National Federation of the Blind, *III*
Retinitis Pigmentosa International, *II*

261 COCHIN JEWISH DISORDER

Cochin Jewish Disorder is a rare inherited disorder characterized by the development of red, scaly thickened patches of skin on the palms of the hands and soles of the feet (palmoplantar hyperkeratosis), frequent pus-producing (pyogenic) skin infections, overgrowth (hypertrophy) of the fingernails and toenails (onychogryphosis), and degeneration of the structures that surround and support the teeth (periodontosis). Periodontosis usually results in the premature loss of teeth. Affected individuals may also have flat feet (pes planus) and abnormally long, slender fingers and toes (arachnodactyly). Most individuals with this disorder experience numbness and tingling and lack normal blood flow to the fingers and/or toes (when exposed to cold temperatures) as well as loss of bone tissue at the ends of the fingers and/or toes (acroosteolysis). Cochin Jewish Disorder is thought to be inherited as an autosomal recessive genetic trait. Some researchers believe that it may be a variant of Papillon-Lefevre Syndrome.

In addition to The National Organization for Rare Disorders (NORD) listed in Section III, the following organizations in Section II (Disease Specific) and in Section III (Umbrella) and Section IV (Government Agencies) can provide more information:
NIH/National Institute of Arthritis and Musculoskeletal and Skin Diseases, *IV*
NIH/National Institute of Dental Research, *IV*

262 COCKAYNE SYNDROME

Cockayne Syndrome is a rare inherited disorder characterized by growth retardation, abnormal sensitivity to light (photosensitivity), and a prematurely aged appearance. In the classical form of Cockayne Syndrome (Type I) the symptoms are progressive and typically become apparent after the age of one year. An early onset or congenital form of Cockayne Syndrome (Type II) is apparent at birth (congenital). There may also be a third form, known as Cockayne Syndrome Type III, which may be a late onset form of the disease.

In addition to The National Organization for Rare Disorders (NORD) listed in Section III, the following organizations in Section II (Disease Specific) and in Section III (Umbrella) and Section IV (Government Agencies) can provide more information:

Human Growth Foundation, *III*
International Progeria Registry, *III*
MAGIC Foundation for Children's Growth, *III*
Metabolic Information Network, *III*
NIH/National Institute of Child Health and Human Development, *IV*
Research Trust for Metabolic Diseases in Children, *III*
Share and Care Cockayne Syndrome Network, *II*

263 COFFIN LOWRY SYNDROME

Coffin-Lowry Syndrome is a rare genetic disorder characterized by mental retardation; abnormalities of the head and facial (craniofacial) area; large, soft hands with short, thin (tapered) fingers; short stature; and/or various skeletal abnormalities. Characteristic facial features may include an underdeveloped upper jaw bone (maxillary hypoplasia), an abnormally prominent brow, downslanting eyelid folds (palpebral fissures), widely spaced eyes (hypertelorism), large ears, and/or unusually thick eyebrows. Skeletal abnormalities may include abnormal front-to-back and side-to-side curvature of the spine (kyphoscoliosis) and unusual prominence of the breastbone (sternum) (pectus carinatum). In most cases, additional abnormalities may be present. Coffin-Lowry Syndrome is thought to be inherited as an X-linked dominant genetic trait; in most cases, certain females (heterozygotes) with Coffin-Lowry Syndrome may exhibit a less severe form of the disorder.

In addition to The National Organization for Rare Disorders (NORD) listed in Section III, the following organizations in Section II (Disease Specific) and in Section III (Umbrella) and Section IV (Government Agencies) can provide more information:

Coffin-Lowry Syndrome Foundation, *II*
NIH/National Arthritis and Musculoskeletal and Skin Diseases Information Clearinghouse, *IV*
NIH/National Institute of Neurological Disorders and Stroke, *IV*
The Arc (a national organization on mental retardation), *III*

264 COFFIN SIRIS SYNDROME

Coffin-Siris Syndrome is an extremely rare genetic disorder that is present at birth and is characterized by mental retardation, short stature, and malformations of the 5th finger. Infants with Coffin-Siris Syndrome have characteristic facial features, feeding problems, muscle weakness, and frequent respiratory infections.

In addition to The National Organization for Rare Disorders (NORD) listed in Section III, the following organizations in Section II (Disease Specific) and in Section III (Umbrella) and Section IV (Government Agencies) can provide more information:

NIH/National Institute of Child Health and Human Development, *IV*
The Arc (a national organization on mental retardation), *III*

265 COGAN REESE SYNDROME

Cogan-Reese Syndrome is an extremely rare eye disorder characterized by a matted or smudged appearance to the surface of the iris; the development of small colored lumps on the iris (nodular iris nevi); the attachment of portions of the iris to the cornea (peripheral anterior synechiae); and/or increased pressure in the eye (glaucoma). Secondary glaucoma may lead to vision loss. This disorder most frequently appears in young and middle-aged females, usually affecting only one eye (unilateral) and developing slowly over time.

In addition to The National Organization for Rare Disorders (NORD) listed in Section III, the following organizations in Section II (Disease Specific) and in Section III (Umbrella) and Section IV (Government Agencies) can provide more information:

Glaucoma Research Foundation, *II*
NIH/National Eye Institute, *IV*
National Association for Visually Handicapped, *III*
Prevent Blindness America, *III*

266 COHEN SYNDROME

Cohen Syndrome is an extremely rare genetic disorder characterized by malformations of the head and facial (craniofacial) area, eye (ocular) abnormalities, diminished muscle tone (hypotonia), obesity, abnormally narrow hands and feet with long fingers and toes, and/or mental retardation. In infants and children with the disorder, characteristic craniofacial malformations may include an unusually small head (microcephaly); abnormal shortness of the groove in the middle of the upper lip (philtrum); a small jaw (micrognathia); an unusually narrow, highly-arched roof of the mouth (palate); prominent front teeth (incisors); a high nasal bridge; down-slanting eyelid folds (palpebral fissures); and/or malformed, protruding ears. Ocular abnormalities often associated with Cohen Syndrome may include diminished vision in bright light (hemeralopia), decreased clarity of vision, narrowed visual fields, degeneration of the nerve-rich membrane lining the eyes (retinitis pigmentosa), and/or gradual deterioration of the nerves of the eyes (optic atrophy). The degree of visual impairment depends upon the severity and/or combination of eye abnormalities present. In infants and children with the disorder, many additional physical abnormalities may also be present. The range and severity of symptoms may vary from case to case. In most cases, Cohen Syndrome is thought to be inherited as an autosomal recessive genetic trait.

In addition to The National Organization for Rare Disorders (NORD) listed in Section III, the following organizations in Section II (Disease Specific) and in Section III (Umbrella) and Section IV (Government Agencies) can provide more information:
Cohen Syndrome Support Group, *II*
NIH/National Institute of Child Health and Human Development, *IV*

267 COLITIS, COLLAGENOUS

Collagenous Colitis is a chronic digestive disease characterized by changes in the lining of the large intestine (colon). The colon is inflamed and contains a thickened layer of the protein collagen in its walls. Chronic diarrhea and weight loss also occur.

In addition to The National Organization for Rare Disorders (NORD) listed in Section III, the following organizations in Section II (Disease Specific) and in Section III (Umbrella) and Section IV (Government Agencies) can provide more information:
Crohn's and Colitis Foundation of America, *III*
Digestive Disease National Coalition, *III*
Gastro-Intestinal Research Foundation, *III*
International Foundation for Functional Gastrointestinal Disorders, *III*
Intestinal Disease Foundation, *III*
NIH/National Digestive Diseases Information Clearinghouse, *IV*
Pediatric Crohn's & Colitis Association, Inc., *III*
Reach Out for Youth with Ileitis and Colitis, Inc., *II*

268 COLITIS, ULCERATIVE

Ulcerative Colitis is an inflammatory bowel disease of unknown cause characterized by diarrhea and bleeding from the rectum. Inflammation typically occurs in the left colon and the membranes that line the rectum. Inflammatory changes in the colon result in scar tissue, abnormal thickening of the walls of the bowel, and/or polyp-like growths in the colon. Ulcerative Colitis is usually a chronic disease with repeated episodes of symptoms and remission (relapsing-remitting). However, some individuals have a chronic, continuous form of Ulcerative Colitis.

In addition to The National Organization for Rare Disorders (NORD) listed in Section III, the following organizations in Section II (Disease Specific) and in Section III (Umbrella) and Section IV (Government Agencies) can provide more information:
Crohn's and Colitis Foundation of America, *III*
Gastro-Intestinal Research Foundation, *III*
International Foundation for Functional Gastrointestinal Disorders, *III*
Intestinal Disease Foundation, *III*
NIH/National Digestive Diseases Information Clearinghouse, *IV*
Pediatric Crohn's & Colitis Association, Inc., *III*
Reach Out for Youth with Ileitis and Colitis, Inc., *II*
United Ostomy Association, Inc., *III*

269 COLORADO TICK FEVER

Colorado Tick Fever is a rare viral disease transmitted by ticks that commonly inhabit the western United States. Major symptoms may include fever, headaches, muscle aches, and/or generalized discomfort (myalgia). The symptoms usually last for about a week and resolve on their own.

In addition to The National Organization for Rare Disorders (NORD) listed in Section III, the following organizations in Section II (Disease Specific) and in Section III (Umbrella) and Section IV (Government Agencies) can provide more information:
Centers for Disease Control and Prevention, *IV*
NIH/National Institute of Allergy and Infectious Diseases, *IV*
World Health Organization (WHO) Regional Office for the Americas (AMRO), *III*

270 CONDYLOMA

Condyloma is a wart caused by the human papilloma virus (HPV) and is usually transmitted by direct sexual contact. These warts can be found on the genitals, mucous membranes of the mouth, near the anus, or in the rectum.

In addition to The National Organization for Rare Disorders (NORD) listed in Section III, the following organizations in Section II (Disease Specific) and in Section III (Umbrella) and Section IV (Government Agencies) can provide more information:

American Social Health Association, *III*
Centers for Disease Control and Prevention, *IV*
NIH/National Institute of Allergy and Infectious Diseases, *IV*
Sexuality Information and Education Council of the U.S., *III*

271 CONE DYSTROPHY

Cone Dystrophy is a rare disorder of the eye that is usually inherited. However, there have been numerous reports of cases appearing for no apparent reason. The cells that receive light stimuli (cone cells and rod cells) in the retina of the eye deteriorate causing impaired vision. This disorder normally occurs during the first to third decades of life.

In addition to The National Organization for Rare Disorders (NORD) listed in Section III, the following organizations in Section II (Disease Specific) and in Section III (Umbrella) and Section IV (Government Agencies) can provide more information:
Association for Macular Diseases, Inc., *III*
Foundation Fighting Blindness, *III*
NIH/National Eye Institute, *IV*
Retinitis Pigmentosa International, *II*

272 CONGENITAL VARICELLA SYNDROME

Congenital Varicella Syndrome is an extremely rare disorder in which affected infants have distinctive abnormalities at birth (congenital) due to the mother's infection with chickenpox (maternal varicella zoster) early during pregnancy (i.e., up to 20 weeks gestation). Affected newborns may have a low birth weight and characteristic abnormalities of the skin; the arms, legs, hands, and/or feet (extremities); the brain; the eyes; and/or, in rare cases, other areas of the body. The range and severity of associated symptoms and physical findings may vary greatly from case to case depending upon when maternal varicella zoster infection occurred during fetal development.

In many cases, newborns with Congenital Varicella Syndrome may be abnormally small and have a low birth weight due to abnormal growth delays during fetal development (intrauterine growth retardation). In addition, distinctive skin abnormalities are often present. Certain areas of the skin may consist of thickened, overgrown (hypertrophic) scar tissue (cicatrix), and surrounding skin may appear abnormally hardened (indurate), red, and inflamed (erythema). Such cicatrix scarring typically occurs on one or more of the arms and/or legs, which may also be malformed, underdeveloped (hypoplastic), and abnormally shortened (reduction deformities). Affected infants may also exhibit incomplete development (hypoplasia) of certain fingers and/or toes (rudimentary digits).

In some cases, newborns with Congenital Varicella Syndrome may have abnormalities of the brain such as degeneration of the outer portion of the brain (cortical atrophy) and/or abnormal enlargement of cavities of the brain (dilated ventricles [ventriculomegaly]). There may also be abnormalities of the part of the nervous system that controls involuntary functions (autonomic nervous system) such as damage to or abnormalities of certain nerve fibers (sympathetic nerve fibers) that pass from the spinal cord to the neck and/or pelvic area. Some affected infants and children may also exhibit abnormal smallness of the head (microcephaly), delays in the acquisition of skills requiring the coordination of mental and physical activities (psychomotor retardation), varying degrees of mental retardation, and/or learning disabilities. In some cases, characteristic eye (ocular) abnormalities may also be present including loss of transparency of the lenses of the eyes (cataracts); abnormal smallness of one or both eyes (unilateral or bilateral microphthalmia); involuntary, rapid, side-to-side movements of the eyes (pendular nystagmus); and/or inflammation and scarring of certain membranes of the eyes (chorioretinitis and chorioretinal scarring). Such ocular abnormalities may result in varying degrees of visual impairment. In rare cases, newborns with Congenital Varicella Syndrome may have additional abnormalities associated with the disorder.

In addition to The National Organization for Rare Disorders (NORD) listed in Section III, the following organizations in Section II (Disease Specific) and in Section III (Umbrella) and Section IV (Government Agencies) can provide more information:
Association of Birth Defect Children, Inc., *III*
CHERUB—Association of Families and Friends of Children with Limb Disorders, *III*
Centers for Disease Control and Prevention, *IV*
NIH/National Eye Institute, *IV*
NIH/National Institute of Allergy and Infectious Diseases, *IV*
NIH/National Institute of Child Health and Human Development, *IV*
NIH/National Institute of Neurological Disorders and

Stroke, *IV*
National Maternal and Child Health Clearinghouse, *IV*
World Health Organization (WHO) Regional Office for the Americas (AMRO), *III*

273 CONJUNCTIVITIS, LIGNEOUS

Ligneous Conjunctivitis is a rare disorder that is characterized by recurrent lesions of the mucous membranes, especially in the eye. This disorder usually presents itself during childhood and may also be found in the mucous membranes of the larynx, vocal chords, nose, trachea, bronchi, vagina, cervix, and gingiva. The lesions in the mucous membranes have a wood-like (ligneous) consistency to them and are thick, firm, knotty and tough. The cause of this disorder is not known although there have been multiple cases of siblings with this condition suggesting an autosomal recessive inheritance.

In addition to The National Organization for Rare Disorders (NORD) listed in Section III, the following organizations in Section II (Disease Specific) and in Section III (Umbrella) and Section IV (Government Agencies) can provide more information:
American Autoimmune Related Diseases Association, Inc., *III*
NIH/National Eye Institute, *IV*

274 CONN SYNDROME

Conn Syndrome is characterized by an increased level of the hormone aldosterone in the blood causing increased sodium levels in the blood. An increase in blood volume (hypervolemia), and a low potassium level (hypokalemic alkalosis) also occur. This disorder is characterized by periods of weakness, unusual sensations such as tingling and warmness, a transient paralysis, and muscle cramps. An increase in blood pressure (hypertension), excessive urination (polyuria), and excessive thirst (polydipsia) can also occur.

In addition to The National Organization for Rare Disorders (NORD) listed in Section III, the following organizations in Section II (Disease Specific) and in Section III (Umbrella) and Section IV (Government Agencies) can provide more information:
NIH/National Heart, Lung and Blood Institute Information Center, *IV*
NIH/National Institute of Diabetes, Digestive and Kidney Diseases, *IV*
National Adrenal Diseases Foundation, *III*
National Hypertension Association, Inc., *II*

275 CONRADI HUNERMANN SYNDROME

Conradi-Hunermann Syndrome is a form of Chondrodysplasia Punctata. It is a rare inherited disease affecting infants and young children. This disorder is marked by mild to moderate growth deficiencies and unusual facial characteristics. Large skin pores and sparse hair that tends to be coarse may also be symptomatic of this condition.

Conradi-Hunermann Syndrome is usually inherited as an autosomal recessive genetic trait. However, X-linked dominant and X-linked recessive forms of the disease have been identified.

In addition to The National Organization for Rare Disorders (NORD) listed in Section III, the following organizations in Section II (Disease Specific) and in Section III (Umbrella) and Section IV (Government Agencies) can provide more information:
Human Growth Foundation, *III*
Little People of America, *III*
Little People's Research Fund, Inc., *III*
MAGIC Foundation for Children's Growth, *III*
NIH/National Arthritis and Musculoskeletal and Skin Diseases Information Clearinghouse, *IV*
NIH/National Eye Institute, *IV*
Short Stature Foundation, *III*
The Arc (a national organization on mental retardation), *III*

276 CONVERSION DISORDER

Conversion disorder is a mental illness characterized by the loss or alteration of physical functioning without any physiological reason. These physical symptoms are the result of emotional conflicts or needs. The symptoms usually appear suddenly and at times of extreme psychological stress. A lack of concern over the debilitating symptoms (la belle indifference) distinguishes this mental illness from other physiological disorders.

In addition to The National Organization for Rare Disorders (NORD) listed in Section III, the following organizations in Section II (Disease Specific) and in Section III (Umbrella) and Section IV (Government Agencies) can provide more information:
NIH/National Institute of Mental Health, *IV*
National Alliance for the Mentally Ill, *III*
National Mental Health Association, *III*
National Mental Health Consumer Self-Help Clearinghouse, *III*

277 COR TRIATRIATUM

Cor triatriatum is an extremely rare heart defect that is present at birth (congenital). The normal human heart has four chambers. Two chambers are called atria, which are separated from each other by a partition called the atrial septum. The other two chambers, known as ventricles, are also separated by a septum. In cor triatriatum there is a small extra chamber above the left atrium of the heart. The pulmonary veins, returning blood from the lungs, drain into this extra "third atrium." The passage of blood from the lungs into the heart (left atrium and ventricle) is slowed by this extra chamber. Features of congestive heart failure and obstruction may eventually develop with cor triatriatum.

In addition to The National Organization for Rare Disorders (NORD) listed in Section III, the following organizations in Section II (Disease Specific) and in Section III (Umbrella) and Section IV (Government Agencies) can provide more information:
American Heart Association, *III*
Congenital Heart Anomalies, Support, Education, & Resources, *III*
NIH/National Heart, Lung and Blood Institute, *IV*

278 CORNEAL DYSTROPHY

Corneal Dystrophies are disorders affecting the outer clear layer of the eyeball known as the cornea. They are caused by faulty metabolism in the tissues in and around the eye. Clarity of vision is usually impaired by clouding of the cornea.

In addition to The National Organization for Rare Disorders (NORD) listed in Section III, the following organizations in Section II (Disease Specific) and in Section III (Umbrella) and Section IV (Government Agencies) can provide more information:
Eye Bank Association of America, *III*
NIH/National Eye Institute, *IV*
National Association for Visually Handicapped, *III*

279 CORNELIA DE LANGE SYNDROME

Cornelia de Lange Syndrome (CDLS) is a very rare disorder characterized by delays in physical development before and after birth (prenatal and postnatal growth retardation); distinctive abnormalities of the head and facial (craniofacial) area; malformations of the hands, feet, arms, and/or legs (limbs); and/or other physical malformations. Affected infants and children may also demonstrate delays in the acquisition of skills requiring the coordination of mental and muscular activity (psychomotor retardation) and/or mild to severe mental retardation. The range and severity of symptoms may vary greatly from case to case.

In infants and children with CDLS, distinctive craniofacial abnormalities typically include an abnormally small head (microcephaly) that may also be unusually short and wide (brachycephaly); a small, broad, upturned nose; thick, defined, arched eyebrows that grow together (synophrys); and/or long, curly eyelashes. Other characteristic features may include thin, downturned lips; an abnormally long groove in the center of the upper lip (philtrum); low-set and/or malformed ears; and/or excessive hair growth (hirsutism) on various areas of the body. Affected individuals may also have small hands and feet, webbing of the toes (syndactyly), and/or other abnormalities of the hands, feet, arms, and/or legs (limb anomalies). Many infants and children with Cornelia de Lange Syndrome may also exhibit hearing loss, abnormal speech development, malformations of the gastrointestinal and/or genitourinary systems, heart (cardiac) abnormalities, increased susceptibility to respiratory infections, and/or other physical abnormalities.

Most cases of Cornelia de Lange Syndrome occur randomly, for no apparent reason (sporadic). However, a pattern of autosomal dominant inheritance has been demonstrated in rare cases.

In addition to The National Organization for Rare Disorders (NORD) listed in Section III, the following organizations in Section II (Disease Specific) and in Section III (Umbrella) and Section IV (Government Agencies) can provide more information:
CHERUB—Association of Families and Friends of Children with Limb Disorders, *III*
Children's Craniofacial Association, *III*
Congenital Heart Anomalies, Support, Education, & Resources, *III*
Congenital Heart Disease Resource Page, *III*
Cornelia de Lange Syndrome Foundation, Inc., *II*
FACES: The National Craniofacial Association, *III*
Forward Face, Inc., *III*
March of Dimes Birth Defects Foundation, *III*
NIH/National Institute of Child Health and Human Development, *IV*
NIH/National Institute on Deafness and Other Communication Disorders Information Clearinghouse, *IV*
Superkids, Inc. (newsletter for families and friends of children with limb differences), *III*
The Arc (a national organization on mental retardation), *III*

280 CORTICOBASAL DEGENERATION

Corticobasal Degeneration is a rare progressive neurological disorder characterized by cell loss and shrinkage (atrophy) in certain areas of the brain (cerebral cortex and substantia nigra). Affected individuals may have sufficient muscle power for manual tasks but often have difficulty directing their movements appropriately. Initial symptoms typically appear in people during their sixties, and may include poor coordination, difficulty accomplishing goal-directed tasks (i.e., buttoning a shirt), and/or difficulty pantomiming actions. Symptoms usually begin on one side of the body (unilateral), but both sides may be affected as the disease progresses. Cognitive impairment (i.e., memory loss) and/or visual-spatial impairments may also occur.

In addition to The National Organization for Rare Disorders (NORD) listed in Section III, the following organizations in Section II (Disease Specific) and in Section III (Umbrella) and Section IV (Government Agencies) can provide more information:
NIH/National Institute of Neurological Disorders and Stroke, *IV*
WE MOVE, *III*

281 COSTELLO SYNDROME

Costello Syndrome is an extremely rare disorder characterized by growth delay after birth (postnatal), leading to short stature; excessive, redundant loose skin on the neck, palms of the hands, fingers, and soles of the feet; development of benign (non-cancerous) growths (papillomata) around the mouth (perioral) and nostrils (nares); mental retardation; and/or characteristic facial appearance. Other physical features may include the development of dry hardened skin on the palms of the hands and the soles of the feet (palmoplantar hyperkeratosis), abnormally deep creases on the palms and soles, and/or abnormally flexible joints of the fingers (hyperextensible). There is an increased incidence of congenital abnormalities of the heart and thickening of the heart muscle called a cardiomyopathy. Characteristic craniofacial features may include an abnormally large head (macrocephaly); low-set ears with large, thick lobes; unusually thick lips; and/or abnormally wide nostrils (nares). Most cases of Costello Syndrome are isolated with no other affected family members (sporadic). The exact cause of Costello Syndrome is unknown.

In addition to The National Organization for Rare Disorders (NORD) listed in Section III, the following organizations in Section II (Disease Specific) and in Section III (Umbrella) and Section IV (Government Agencies) can provide more information:
Human Growth Foundation, *III*
Little People of America, *III*
MAGIC Foundation for Children's Growth, *III*
NIH/National Institute of Child Health and Human Development, *IV*
Short Stature Foundation, *III*

282 COWPOX

Cowpox is a viral disease that normally affects the udders and teats of cows. On rare occasions, it may be transmitted to humans and produce a characteristic red skin rash and abnormally enlarged lymph nodes (lymphadenopathy). Cowpox is caused by the vaccinia virus and has been known to cause systemic reactions (generalized vaccinia) in some people who have been recently vaccinated against cowpox.

Cowpox produces an immunity to a more serious infectious disease known as smallpox. In the 19th century, the vaccinia virus was used in vaccination programs against smallpox. Because of the widespread vaccination, smallpox has been wiped out worldwide.

In addition to The National Organization for Rare Disorders (NORD) listed in Section III, the following organizations in Section II (Disease Specific) and in Section III (Umbrella) and Section IV (Government Agencies) can provide more information:
Centers for Disease Control and Prevention, *IV*
NIH/National Institute of Allergy and Infectious Diseases, *IV*
World Health Organization (WHO) Regional Office for the Americas (AMRO), *III*

283 CRANIOFRONTONASAL DYSPLASIA

Craniofrontonasal Dysplasia is a very rare inherited disorder characterized by abnormalities of the head and face (craniofacial area), hands and feet, and certain skeletal bones. Major symptoms of this disorder may include widely spaced eyes (ocular hypertelorism), a groove (cleft) on the tip of the nose, an unusually wide mouth, malformations of the fingers and toes, and/or underdevelopment of portions of the face (midface hypoplasia), such as the forehead, nose, and chin. In addition, the head may appear unusually wide and short (brachycephaly). The exact mode of inheritance of Craniofrontonasal Dysplasia is unknown. Autosomal dominant and X-linked forms of the disorder have been discussed in the medical literature.

In addition to The National Organization for Rare Disorders (NORD) listed in Section III, the following organizations in Section II (Disease Specific) and in Section III (Umbrella) and Section IV (Government Agencies) can provide more information:

AboutFace U.S.A., *III*
Children's Craniofacial Association, *III*
FACES: The National Craniofacial Association, *III*
Forward Face, Inc., *III*
NIH/National Institute of Child Health and Human Development, *IV*

284 CRANIOMETAPHYSEAL DYSPLASIA

Craniometaphyseal Dysplasia is an extremely rare genetic disorder characterized by distinctive abnormalities of the head and facial (craniofacial) area, impairment of certain nerves (cranial nerves) that emerge from the brain, and malformations of the long bones of the arms and legs. In infants and children with Craniometaphyseal Dysplasia, there may be overgrowth and/or abnormal hardening of certain bones of the skull (cranial hyperostosis and/or sclerosis) and overgrowth (hypertrophy) of craniofacial bones, resulting in widely-spaced eyes (ocular hypetelorism), an abnormally wide nasal bridge, an enlarged lower jaw (mandible), and a "leonine" facial appearance (leontiasis ossea). Compression of certain nerves emerging from the brain (cranial nerves) may result in loss of some motor function (paralysis) in the facial area (cranial nerve palsy) and hearing loss (conductive and/or sensorineural hearing impairment). In addition, in individuals with the disorder, the long bones of the arms and legs may develop abnormally, resulting in unusual "club-like" flaring or broadening of the end portions (metaphyses) of the bones (metaphyseal dysplasia). In some cases, Craniometaphyseal Dysplasia may be inherited as an autosomal dominant genetic trait; in other cases, the disorder may have an autosomal recessive mode of inheritance.

In addition to The National Organization for Rare Disorders (NORD) listed in Section III, the following organizations in Section II (Disease Specific) and in Section III (Umbrella) and Section IV (Government Agencies) can provide more information:

AboutFace U.S.A., *III*
Children's Craniofacial Association, *III*
FACES: The National Craniofacial Association, *III*
Forward Face, Inc., *III*
NIH/National Institute of Child Health and Human Development, *IV*
National Foundation for Facial Reconstruction, *III*

285 CRANIOSYNOSTOSIS, PRIMARY

Primary Craniosynostosis is a rare disorder of the skull that may be inherited as an autosomal dominant or autosomal recessive genetic trait. Premature closure of the bones (sutures) in the skull result in an abnormally shaped head. The severity of symptoms and shape of the skull depend on which skull bones are prematurely closed. This disorder is present at birth.

In addition to The National Organization for Rare Disorders (NORD) listed in Section III, the following organizations in Section II (Disease Specific) and in Section III (Umbrella) and Section IV (Government Agencies) can provide more information:

AboutFace U.S.A., *III*
Children's Craniofacial Association, *III*
Craniofacial Support Group, *III*
FACES: The National Craniofacial Association, *III*
Forward Face, Inc., *III*
Guardians of Hydrocephalus Research Foundation, *II*
Hydrocephalus Association, *II*
NIH/National Institute of Child Health and Human Development, *IV*
National Hydrocephalus Foundation, *II*

286 CREUTZFELDT JAKOB DISEASE

Creutzfeldt-Jakob Disease (CJD) is an extremely rare degenerative brain disorder (i.e., spongiform encephalopathy) characterized by the sudden onset of rapidly progressive neurological and neuromuscular symptoms. Initially, such symptoms may include confusion, depression, behavioral changes, impaired vision, and/or lack of coordination. As the disorder advances, affected individuals experience rapidly progressive loss of intellectual abilities (dementia) in association with neuromuscular problems such as muscle weakness and loss of muscle mass (wasting); repeated, involuntary, shock-like muscle spasms (myoclonus); and/or continual, involuntary writhing movements, particularly of the arms and legs (athetosis). Later stages of the disease may include further loss of physical and intellectual functions, coma, and increased susceptibility to repeated infections of the respiratory tract (e.g., pneumonia). In many cases, life-threatening complications may develop less than a year after the disorder becomes apparent.

In approximately 90 percent of cases, CJD appears to occur randomly for no apparent reason (sporadically), while about 10 percent of affected individuals may inherit the disorder as an autosomal dominant genetic trait. In some extremely rare cases, CJD may take an infectious form. The disorder is thought to result from abnormal changes (mutations) in the gene that regulates (encodes for) the production of the human prion protein or direct contamination (transmission) with abnormal prion protein in infected brain tissue.

In addition to The National Organization for Rare Disorders (NORD) listed in Section III, the following organizations in Section II (Disease Specific) and in Section III (Umbrella) and Section IV (Government Agencies) can provide more information:

Alzheimer's Association, *II*
Alzheimer's Disease Education and Referral Center, *II*
Centers for Disease Control and Prevention, *IV*
Creutzfeldt-Jakob Disease Foundation, Inc., *II*
NIH/National Institute of Allergy and Infectious Diseases, *IV*
NIH/National Institute of Neurological Disorders and Stroke, *IV*
National Hospice Organization, *III*
World Health Organization (WHO) Regional Office for the Americas (AMRO), *III*

287 CRI DU CHAT SYNDROME

Cri du Chat Syndrome, a rare chromosomal disorder that is apparent at birth, is characterized by a distinctive high, shrill, mewing, "kitten-like" cry during infancy. This distinctive cry becomes less pronounced during late infancy. Other findings and symptoms may include low birth weight and failure to grow at the expected rate (failure to thrive); distinctive abnormalities of the head and face (craniofacial area) including an unusually small head (microcephaly), widely spaced eyes (ocular hypertelorism), and an unusually small jaw (micrognathia); and mental retardation. Cri du Chat Syndrome is caused by the absence of genetic material (deletion) on the short arm (p) of chromosome 5.

In addition to The National Organization for Rare Disorders (NORD) listed in Section III, the following organizations in Section II (Disease Specific) and in Section III (Umbrella) and Section IV (Government Agencies) can provide more information:

5p- Society, *II*
Chromosome Deletion Outreach, *III*
Cri Du Chat Syndrome Support Group, *II*
March of Dimes Birth Defects Foundation, *III*
NIH/National Institute of Child Health and Human Development, *IV*
The Arc (a national organization on mental retardation), *III*

288 CRIGLER NAJJAR SYNDROME TYPE I

Crigler-Najjar Syndrome Type I is a very rare inherited metabolic disorder characterized by the complete absence of the enzyme uridine diphosphate glucuronosyltransferase (UDPGT), which is normally found in the liver. This enzyme is required for the conversion (conjugation) and subsequent excretion of bilirubin from the body. When UDP-glucuronosyltransferase activity is absent, these metabolic processes are hampered and abnormally high levels of bilirubin accumulate in the blood (hyperbilirubinemia).

Within the first few days of life, most infants with Crigler-Najjar Syndrome Type I develop persistent yellowing of the skin, mucous membranes, and whites of the eyes (jaundice). In addition, many affected individuals eventually develop kernicterus, a potentially life-threatening neurological condition in which toxic levels of bilirubin accumulate in the brain, causing damage to the central nervous system. Early signs of kernicterus may include lack of energy (lethargy), vomiting, fever, and/or unsatisfactory feedings. More serious signs of kernicterus may develop including abnormal muscle rigidity, resulting in muscle spasms (dystonia) and involuntary movements of the limbs and/or entire body (athetosis). Crigler-Najjar Syndrome Type I is inherited as an autosomal recessive genetic trait.

In addition to The National Organization for Rare Disorders (NORD) listed in Section III, the following organizations in Section II (Disease Specific) and in Section III (Umbrella) and Section IV (Government Agencies) can provide more information:

American Liver Foundation, *III*
NIH/National Digestive Diseases Information Clearinghouse, *IV*
NIH/National Institute of Child Health and Human Development, *IV*
Research Trust for Metabolic Diseases in Children, *III*
United Liver Association, *III*

289 CROHN'S DISEASE

Crohn's Disease is an inflammatory bowel disease characterized by severe, chronic inflammation of the intestinal wall or any portion of the gastrointestinal tract. The lower portion of the small intestine (ileum) and the rectum are most commonly affected by this disorder. Symptoms may include watery diarrhea and abdominal pain. The symptoms of

Crohn's Disease can be difficult to manage and diagnosis is often delayed.

In addition to The National Organization for Rare Disorders (NORD) listed in Section III, the following organizations in Section II (Disease Specific) and in Section III (Umbrella) and Section IV (Government Agencies) can provide more information:

Alliance of Genetic Support Groups, *III*
Crohn's and Colitis Foundation of America, *III*
Gastro-Intestinal Research Foundation, *III*
International Foundation for Functional Gastrointestinal Disorders, *III*
Intestinal Disease Foundation, *III*
March of Dimes Birth Defects Foundation, *III*
NIH/National Digestive Diseases Information Clearinghouse, *IV*
NIH/National Institute of Allergy and Infectious Diseases, *IV*
Pediatric Crohn's & Colitis Association, Inc., *III*
United Ostomy Association, Inc., *III*

290 CRONKHITE CANADA DISEASE

Cronkhite-Canada Disease (Allergic Granulomatous Angiitis) is an extremely rare disorder characterized by multiple benign growths in the mucous lining of the intestines and stomach (generalized polyposis), loss of scalp hair (alopecia), widespread areas of dark spots on the skin (hyperpigmentation), and the loss of fingernails (onycholytic dystrophy).

In addition to The National Organization for Rare Disorders (NORD) listed in Section III, the following organizations in Section II (Disease Specific) and in Section III (Umbrella) and Section IV (Government Agencies) can provide more information:

Intestinal Multiple Polyposis and Colorectal Cancer Registry, *III*
NIH/National Digestive Diseases Information Clearinghouse, *IV*

291 CROUZON DISEASE

Crouzon Disease is a genetic disorder characterized by abnormalities in the skull, face, and brain caused by premature hardening of the skull. The skull is made up of several bony plates initially joined by fibrous connective tissue, which normally fuse together and harden over a period of several years after growth of the brain. Facial deformities are often present at birth and may progress with time. Vision disturbances and deafness can develop in some cases. With treatment, pressure inside the skull may be relieved and major symptoms may improve.

In addition to The National Organization for Rare Disorders (NORD) listed in Section III, the following organizations in Section II (Disease Specific) and in Section III (Umbrella) and Section IV (Government Agencies) can provide more information:

AboutFace U.S.A., *III*
Alliance of Genetic Support Groups, *III*
Children's Craniofacial Association, *III*
Craniofacial Support Group, *III*
Crouzon's/Meniere's Support Network, *III*
FACES: The National Craniofacial Association, *III*
Forward Face, Inc., *III*
Let's Face It, Inc., *III*
NIH/National Institute of Child Health and Human Development, *IV*
The Arc (a national organization on mental retardation), *III*

292 CRYOGLOBULINEMIA, ESSENTIAL MIXED

Essential Mixed Cryoglobulinemia is a rare autoimmune disorder that affects the blood and various other body systems. Major symptoms may include unusual response to cold, skin abnormalities, weakness and blood problems. There may also be joint pain, inflamed blood vessels and kidney problems.

In addition to The National Organization for Rare Disorders (NORD) listed in Section III, the following organizations in Section II (Disease Specific) and in Section III (Umbrella) and Section IV (Government Agencies) can provide more information:

American Autoimmune Related Diseases Association, Inc., *III*
NIH/National Heart, Lung and Blood Institute Information Center, *IV*

293 CRYPTOCOCCOSIS

Cryptococcosis is caused by a fungus known as Filobasidiella Neoformans or Cryptococcosis Neoformans. The infection may be spread to humans through contact with pigeon droppings or unwashed raw fruit. Contact with an infected individual may also spread the infection. Individuals with disorders characterized by lowered immunity are at high risk for contracting these infections.

Cryptococcosis may appear in various forms depending on how the infection is acquired. In most cases, the infection begins in the lungs and may then spread to the brain, urinary tract, skin, and/or bones. In some forms of Cryptococcosis, symptoms may be limited to the lungs. Respiratory symptoms may include coughing and chest pain. In some affected individuals, inflammation of the membranes surrounding the brain and spinal cord (meningitis) may occur as a serious complication. Symptoms associated with meningitis may include dizziness, blurred vision, severe headache, and/or stiffness of the neck. In such cases, immediate treatment is essential to help prevent potentially life-threatening complications.

In addition to The National Organization for Rare Disorders (NORD) listed in Section III, the following organizations in Section II (Disease Specific) and in Section III (Umbrella) and Section IV (Government Agencies) can provide more information:

Centers for Disease Control and Prevention, *IV*
NIH/National Institute of Allergy and Infectious Diseases, *IV*
NIH/National Institute of Neurological Disorders and Stroke, *IV*
World Health Organization (WHO) Regional Office for the Americas (AMRO), *III*

294 CUSHING SYNDROME

Cushing Syndrome is a rare endocrine disorder characterized by a variety of symptoms and physical abnormalities that occur due to excessive amounts of certain hormones (corticosteroids) produced by the adrenal glands.

In addition to The National Organization for Rare Disorders (NORD) listed in Section III, the following organizations in Section II (Disease Specific) and in Section III (Umbrella) and Section IV (Government Agencies) can provide more information:

Brain and Pituitary Foundation of America, *III*
Cushing Support and Research Foundation, Inc., *II*
NIH/National Digestive Diseases Information Clearinghouse, *IV*
National Adrenal Diseases Foundation, *III*

295 CUTIS LAXA

Cutis Laxa is a rare congenital or acquired connective tissue disorder characterized by skin that is loose (lax), hanging, wrinkled, and lacking in elasticity. The affected areas of skin may be thickened and dark. Most cases of Cutis Laxa are inherited as an autosomal recessive genetic trait. Cutis Laxa may be present at birth (congenital) or may be acquired.

In addition to The National Organization for Rare Disorders (NORD) listed in Section III, the following organizations in Section II (Disease Specific) and in Section III (Umbrella) and Section IV (Government Agencies) can provide more information:

American Autoimmune Related Diseases Association, Inc., *III*
British Coalition of Heritable Disorders of Connective Tissue, *III*
NIH/National Arthritis and Musculoskeletal and Skin Diseases Information Clearinghouse, *IV*

296 CUTIS MARMORATA TELANGIECTATICA CONGENITA

Cutis Marmorata Telangiectatica Congenita (CMTC) is a rare congenital skin disorder characterized by discolored patches of skin (livedo reticularis) caused by dilated surface blood vessels (telangiectases) that give the skin a blue or purple marbling or "fishnet" appearance. This condition is often associated with crater-like lesions (ulcers) of the skin. Other congenital abnormalities are found in at least 50 percent of affected individuals.

In addition to The National Organization for Rare Disorders (NORD) listed in Section III, the following organizations in Section II (Disease Specific) and in Section III (Umbrella) and Section IV (Government Agencies) can provide more information:

NIH/National Arthritis and Musculoskeletal and Skin Diseases Information Clearinghouse, *IV*
Nevus Network, *II*

297 CYCLIC VOMITING SYNDROME

Scientists think that Cyclic Vomiting Syndrome is a rare form of "abdominal migraine" disorder in children. Major symptoms may include chronic nausea, vomiting, motion-sickness, abdominal pain and, in some cases, dizziness (vertigo) that may last hours to days. The attacks seem to be similar in onset and duration for each child. All of these symptoms tend to begin in early childhood around the age of three years, but may begin later.

In addition to The National Organization for Rare Disorders (NORD) listed in Section III, the following organizations in Section II (Disease Specific) and in Section III (Umbrella) and Section IV (Government Agencies) can provide more information:

Cyclic Vomiting Syndrome Association, *II*
NIH/National Digestive Diseases Information Clearinghouse, *IV*
National Headache Foundation, *III*

298 CYSTIC FIBROSIS

Cystic Fibrosis is an inherited disorder that affects the exocrine, or outward-secreting, glands of the body. It affects children and young adults. The main consequences are related to the mucus producing glands. The secreted mucus is thick and sticky, clogging and obstructing air passages in the lungs and pancreatic bile ducts. Cystic Fibrosis also causes dysfunction of salivary and sweat glands. There is presently no cure for CF, but with proper treatment, those affected can lead active lives.

In addition to The National Organization for Rare Disorders (NORD) listed in Section III, the following organizations in Section II (Disease Specific) and in Section III (Umbrella) and Section IV (Government Agencies) can provide more information:
Alliance of Genetic Support Groups, *III*
American Lung Association, *III*
Canadian Cystic Fibrosis Foundation, *II*
Cystic Fibrosis Foundation, *II*
Cystic Fibrosis Trust, *II*
March of Dimes Birth Defects Foundation, *III*
NIH/National Digestive Diseases Information Clearinghouse, *IV*

299 CYSTIC HYGROMA

Cystic hygroma is an inborn tumor of the lymphatic system that, in some rare cases, may be inherited as an autosomal recessive genetic trait. This progressive disorder is characterized by a large sac filled with lymph fluid protruding from the skull at the nape of the neck. The hygroma is thought to be caused by a failure of the lymph system to properly connect with the blood vessels in the neck and thus with the appropriate blood circulation system.

In addition to The National Organization for Rare Disorders (NORD) listed in Section III, the following organizations in Section II (Disease Specific) and in Section III (Umbrella) and Section IV (Government Agencies) can provide more information:
American Cancer Society, Inc., *III*
Children Anguished with Lymphatic Malformations, *III*
National Lymphatic and Venous Diseases Foundation, Inc., *III*

300 CYSTICERCOSIS

Cysticercosis is a complication of severe tapeworm infection acquired by eating uncooked pork. The disorder is caused by larval pork tapeworms. The scientific name for this parasite is Taenia solium. Cysticerci are immature tapeworms that normally live in the muscle (meat) of swine. When they develop instead in human muscle and die, they can cause severe inflammatory reactions. Cysticercosis is a rare disorder in the United States, Western Europe, Japan and in non-pork eating cultures.

In addition to The National Organization for Rare Disorders (NORD) listed in Section III, the following organizations in Section II (Disease Specific) and in Section III (Umbrella) and Section IV (Government Agencies) can provide more information:
Centers for Disease Control and Prevention, *IV*
NIH/National Institute of Allergy and Infectious Diseases, *IV*
World Health Organization (WHO) Regional Office for the Americas (AMRO), *III*

301 CYSTINOSIS

Cystinosis is a rare inherited disorder characterized by the impaired transport of cystine out of parts of cells called lysosomes. Cystine is an amino acid found in many different proteins in the body. Lysosomes, which are membrane bound particles within cells, aid in intracellular digestive function. Cystinosis is characterized by the accumulation of cystine in tissues throughout the body, which can cause certain organs to malfunction.

Three distinct forms of Cystinosis are recognized. Infantile Nephropathic Cystinosis is the most severe form of the disease. Symptoms, including abnormal sensitivity to light and loss of color in the retina of the eyes, can appear as early as 6 to 12 months of age. If left untreated, this form of the disease may lead to kidney failure by 10 years of age. In people with Intermediate Cystinosis or Juvenile (Adolescent) Cystinosis, kidney and eye symptoms typically become apparent during the teenage years or early adulthood. In Benign or Adult Cystinosis, crystalline cystine accumulates primarily in the cornea of the eyes.

One of the major complications of Cystinosis is Renal Fanconi Syndrome which is characterized by impaired kidney function including excessive urination (polyuria), excessive thirst (polydipsia), and abnormally low levels of potassium in the blood (hypokalemia).

In addition to The National Organization for Rare Disorders (NORD) listed in Section III, the following organizations in Section II (Disease Specific) and in Section III (Umbrella) and Section IV (Government Agencies) can provide more information:
Alliance of Genetic Support Groups, *III*
American Foundation for Urologic Disease, *III*
Cystinosis Foundation, Inc., *II*
March of Dimes Birth Defects Foundation, *III*
Metabolic Information Network, *III*
NIH/National Kidney and Urologic Diseases Information Clearinghouse, *IV*
Research Trust for Metabolic Diseases in Children, *III*
Vaincre Les Maladies Lysosomales, *III*

302 CYSTINURIA

Cystinuria is an inherited metabolic disorder characterized by the abnormal movement (transport) in the intestines and kidneys, of certain organic chemical compounds (amino acids). These include cystine, lysine, arginine, and ornithine. Excessive amounts of undissolved cystine in the urine (cystinuria) cause the formation of stones (calculi) in the kidney, bladder, and/or ureter.

Four subtypes of Cystinuria are recognized. In Type I Cystinuria, there is a defect in the active transport of cystine and the amino acids (dibasic) lysine, arginine, and ornithine in the kidneys and small intestine. People who are carriers of the gene for this type of the disorder generally have no symptoms. In Type II Cystinuria, cystine and lysine transport is severely impaired in the kidneys and only somewhat impaired in the intestines. In Type III Cystinuria, kidney transport of cystine and lysine is defective; intestinal transport is normal. People who are carriers of the gene for this variety of the disease typically have slightly elevated levels of cystine and lysine in the urine. In Hypercystinuria, there is generally a moderate elevation of cystine in the urine; intestinal absorption of cystine and the dibasic amino acids is normal.

In addition to The National Organization for Rare Disorders (NORD) listed in Section III, the following organizations in Section II (Disease Specific) and in Section III (Umbrella) and Section IV (Government Agencies) can provide more information:
Alliance of Genetic Support Groups, *III*
American Kidney Fund, Inc., *III*
Cystinuria Support Network, *II*
March of Dimes Birth Defects Foundation, *III*
Metabolic Information Network, *III*
National Kidney Foundation, *III*

303 CYTOCHROME C OXIDASE DEFICIENCY

Cytochrome C Oxidase Deficiency is a very rare inherited metabolic disorder characterized by deficiency of the enzyme cytochrome C oxidase (COX), or Complex IV, an essential enzyme that is active in the subcellular structures that help to regulate energy production (mitochondria). Deficiency of COX may be limited (localized) to the tissues of the skeletal muscles or may affect several tissues, such as the heart, kidney, liver, brain, and/or connective tissue (fibroblasts); in other cases, the COX deficiency may be generalized (systemic).

Four distinct forms of Cytochrome C Oxidase Deficiency have been identifed. The first form of this disorder is known as COX Deficiency Type Benign Infantile Mitochondrial Myopathy. Affected infants exhibit many of the same symptoms as those with the more severe infantile form of the disease; however, because the COX deficiency is limited (localized) to tissues of the skeletal muscles, they typically do not have heart or kidney dysfunction.

In the second type of the disease, known as COX Deficiency Type Infantile Mitochondrial Myopathy, because the COX deficiency affects tissues of the skeletal muscles as well as several other tissues, the disorder may be characterized by a generalized weakness of skeletal muscles (myotonia), abnormalities of the heart and kidneys, and/or abnormally high levels of lactic acid in the blood (lactic acidosis).

The third form of COX Deficiency, known as Leigh's Disease (Subacute Necrotizing Encephalomyelopathy), is thought to be a generalized (systemic) form of COX Deficiency. Leigh's Disease is characterized by progressive degeneration of the brain and dysfunction of other organs of the body including the heart, kidneys, muscles, and liver. Symptoms may include loss of previously acquired motor skills, loss of appetite, vomiting, irritability, and/or seizure activity. As Leigh's Disease progresses, symptoms may also include generalized weakness; loss of muscle tone (hypotonia); and/or episodes of lactic acidosis.

In the fourth form of COX Deficiency, known as COX Deficiency French-Canadian Type, the COX deficiency affects tissues of the skeletal muscles, connective tissue, and, in particular, the brain (Leigh's Disease) and the liver. Affected infants and children may demonstrate developmental delays, diminished muscle tone (hypotonia), crossing of the eyes (strabismus), Leigh's Disease, and/or episodes of lactic acidosis.

Many cases of COX Deficiency are inherited as an autosomal recessive genetic trait. However, it is possible that other cases may be inherited due to abnormal changes in genetic material (mutation) found within mitochondria (mtDNA).

In addition to The National Organization for Rare Disorders (NORD) listed in Section III, the following organizations in Section II (Disease Specific) and in Section III (Umbrella) and Section IV (Government Agencies) can provide more information:
Association for Neuro-Metabolic Disorders, *III*
Lactic Acidosis Support Trust, *III*
NIH/National Institute of Child Health and Human Development, *IV*
NIH/National Institute of Diabetes, Digestive & Kidney Diseases, *IV*
Research Trust for Metabolic Diseases in Children, *III*
United Mitochondrial Disease Foundation, *III*

304 CYTOMEGALOVIRUS INFECTION

Cytomegalovirus Infection (CMV) is a viral infection occuring at birth (congenitally), after birth (postnatally), or at any age. CMV ranges in severity from a silent infection without consequences, to a disease manifested by fever, hepatitis, and (in newborns) severe brain damage, and possible life-threatening complications.

In addition to The National Organization for Rare Disorders (NORD) listed in Section III, the following organizations in Section II (Disease Specific) and in Section III (Umbrella) and Section IV (Government Agencies) can provide more information:
Centers for Disease Control and Prevention, *IV*
NIH/National Eye Institute, *IV*
NIH/National Institute of Allergy and Infectious Diseases, *IV*
National Congenital CMV Disease Registry, *II*

305 DOOR SYNDROME

DOOR Syndrome is an extremely rare inherited disorder characterized by hearing impairment, malformations of the nails and certain bones, mental retardation, other abnormalities. "DOOR," an acronym for the characteristic abnormalities associated with the disorder, stands for (D)eafness due to malformation of the inner ears (sensorineural hearing loss); (O)nychodystrophy, malformation of the nails; (O)steodystrophy, malformation of certain bones; and mild to severe mental (R)etardation. In some cases, affected infants may also experience episodes of electrical disturbances in the brain (grand mal seizures [epilepsy]). Distinctive nail abnormalities associated with the disorder may include underdeveloped, misshapen, or absent fingernails and/or toenails, while characteristic bone malformations may consist of an extra small bone in the thumbs and/or great toes (triphalangy) and/or underdevelopment (hypoplasia) of bones in other fingers and/or toes. DOOR Syndrome is inherited as an autosomal recessive genetic trait.

In addition to The National Organization for Rare Disorders (NORD) listed in Section III, the following organizations in Section II (Disease Specific) and in Section III (Umbrella) and Section IV (Government Agencies) can provide more information:
American Society for Deaf Children, *III*
Better Hearing Institute, *III*
Epilepsy Foundation of America, *III*
NIH/National Institute of Arthritis and Musculoskeletal and Skin Diseases, *IV*
NIH/National Institute of Child Health and Human Development, *IV*
NIH/National Institute of Neurological Disorders and Stroke, *IV*

306 DANDY WALKER MALFORMATION

Dandy-Walker Malformation is a rare malformation of the brain that is present at birth (congenital). It is characterized by an abnormally enlarged space at the back of the brain (cystic 4th ventricle) that interferes with the normal flow of cerebrospinal fluid through the openings between the ventricle and other parts of the brain (foramina of Magendia and Luschka). Excessive amounts of fluid accumulate around the brain and cause abnormally high pressure within the skull, swelling of the head (congenital hydrocephalus), and neurological impairment. Motor delays and learning problems may also occur. Dandy-Walker Malformation is a form of "Obstructive" or "Internal Noncommunicating Hydrocephalus," meaning that the normal flow of cerebrospinal fluid is blocked resulting in the widening of the ventricles.

In addition to The National Organization for Rare Disorders (NORD) listed in Section III, the following organizations in Section II (Disease Specific) and in Section III (Umbrella) and Section IV (Government Agencies) can provide more information:
Alliance of Genetic Support Groups, *III*
Dandy-Walker Syndrome Network, *II*
Guardians of Hydrocephalus Research Foundation, *II*
Hydrocephalus Association, *II*
Hydrocephalus Support Group, Inc., *II*
NIH/National Institute of Neurological Disorders and Stroke, *IV*
National Association for Visually Handicapped, *III*
National Hydrocephalus Foundation, *II*

307 DARIER DISEASE

Darier Disease is a rare gradually progressive, hereditary skin disorder. It is characterized by elevated spots (papules) on the scalp, forehead, face, neck, area behind the ears, and middle of the back. Darier Disease is inherited as an autosomal dominant genetic trait.

In addition to The National Organization for Rare Disorders (NORD) listed in Section III, the following organizations in Section II (Disease Specific) and in Section III (Umbrella) and Section IV (Government Agencies) can provide more information:
Foundation for Ichthyosis & Related Skin Types, *III*
NIH/National Arthritis and Musculoskeletal and Skin Diseases Information Clearinghouse, *IV*

308 DE BARSY SYNDROME

De Barsy Syndrome is a rare disorder that is inherited as an autosomal recessive genetic trait. The main characteristics associated with this disorder are degeneration of the elastic tissue in the skin (cutis laxa), involuntary movements of the arms and legs (athetosis), a cloudy cornea of the eye, large prominent ears, loss of muscle tone, unusual flexibility of the small joints, a forehead that protrudes outward (frontal bossing) and/or short stature.

In addition to The National Organization for Rare Disorders (NORD) listed in Section III, the following organizations in Section II (Disease Specific) and in Section III (Umbrella) and Section IV (Government Agencies) can provide more information:
NIH/National Arthritis and Musculoskeletal and Skin Diseases Information Clearinghouse, *IV*

309 DE SANTIS CACCHIONE SYNDROME

De Sanctis-Cacchione Syndrome is an extremely rare disorder characterized by the skin and eye symptoms of Xeroderma Pigmentosum (XP) occurring in association with neurological abnormalities, mental retardation, unusually short stature (dwarfism), and underdevelopment of the testes or ovaries (hypogonadism). Xeroderma Pigmentosum is a group of rare inherited skin disorders characterized by a heightened reaction to ultraviolet light (photosensitivity), skin discolorations, and the possible development of several types of eye disorders and skin cancers. The most common neurological abnormalities associated with De Sanctis- Cacchione Syndrome are low intelligence, an abnormally small head (microcephaly), the loss of ability to coordinate voluntary movement (ataxia), and/or absent (areflexia) or weakened (hyporeflexia) reflexes. De Sanctis-Cacchione Syndrome is inherited as an autosomal recessive genetic trait.

In addition to The National Organization for Rare Disorders (NORD) listed in Section III, the following organizations in Section II (Disease Specific) and in Section III (Umbrella) and Section IV (Government Agencies) can provide more information:
NIH/National Arthritis and Musculoskeletal and Skin Diseases Information Clearinghouse, *IV*
Skin Cancer Foundation, *III*
Skin Disease Research Core Centers of the National Institute of Arthritis, *IV*

310 DEGOS DISEASE

Degos Disease is a rare systemic disorder that affects small and medium sized arteries, causing them to become blocked (occlusive arteriopathy). Degos Disease usually progresses through two stages. During the first stage, characteristic skin lesions appear that may last for a period of time ranging from weeks to years. The second stage of Degos Disease is most frequently characterized by lesions in the small intestine, but other organs may also be affected. Major symptoms may include abdominal pain, diarrhea, and/or weight loss. Intestinal lesions may break through the wall of the bowel (perforation), a potentially life-threatening complication.

In addition to The National Organization for Rare Disorders (NORD) listed in Section III, the following organizations in Section II (Disease Specific) and in Section III (Umbrella) and Section IV (Government Agencies) can provide more information:
Digestive Disease National Coalition, *III*
NIH/National Digestive Diseases Information Clearinghouse, *IV*

311 DEJERINE SOTTAS DISEASE

Dejerine-Sottas Disease is an inherited neurological disorder that progressively affects mobility. Peripheral nerves become enlarged or thickened causing an irregular progression of muscle weakness. Pain, weakness, numbness, and a tingling, prickling or burning sensation can occur in the legs of individuals with this disorder. Many people with Dejerine-Sottas Disease can remain active and usually have a normal life span.

In addition to The National Organization for Rare Disorders (NORD) listed in Section III, the following organizations in Section II (Disease Specific) and in Section III (Umbrella) and Section IV (Government Agencies) can provide more information:
Muscular Dystrophy Association, *III*
NIH/National Institute of Neurological Disorders and Stroke, *IV*

312 DENGUE FEVER

Dengue Fever is an acute viral infection characterized by fever. It is caused by a bite from mosquitoes carrying dengue virus. The primary form of Dengue Fever is characterized by a skin rash and a high fever with severe pain in the head and muscles. Other symptoms may include shaking chills, diarrhea, and vomiting. Bouts of extreme exhaustion may last for months after the initial symptoms.

The secondary forms of this disorder are called Dengue Hemorrhagic Fever and Dengue Shock Syndrome. These usually are caused by a secondary infection with a different type of Dengue virus (Type 2), but may also be caused by the same virus that causes Dengue Fever. Several days after onset other symptoms may include fever, bleeding under the skin, red spots on the legs, and bleeding into the intestines. A marked fall in blood pressure (shock) occurs in very severe cases.

In addition to The National Organization for Rare Disorders (NORD) listed in Section III, the following organizations in Section II (Disease Specific) and in Section III (Umbrella) and Section IV (Government Agencies) can provide more information:

Centers for Disease Control and Prevention, *IV*
NIH/National Institute of Allergy and Infectious Diseases, *IV*
World Health Organization (WHO) Regional Office for the Americas (AMRO), *III*

313 DENTIN DYSPLASIA, CORONAL

Coronal Dentin Dysplasia is a genetic disorder characterized by brownish-blue opalescent baby teeth and permanent teeth that appear normal. The hard calcified tissue beneath the enamel (dentin) is the main substance of the teeth. The baby teeth in children affected by this disorder contain obliterated pulp chambers and reduced root canals. Permanent teeth also have abnormalities.

In addition to The National Organization for Rare Disorders (NORD) listed in Section III, the following organizations in Section II (Disease Specific) and in Section III (Umbrella) and Section IV (Government Agencies) can provide more information:

NIH/National Oral Health Information Clearinghouse, *IV*
National Foundation for Ectodermal Dysplasias, *II*

314 DENTIN DYSPLASIA, RADICULAR

Radicular Dentin Dysplasia is a genetic disorder characterized by atypical formation of the calcified tissue between the enamel pulp of the teeth (dentin). The teeth lack pulp chambers or have half-moon shaped pulp chambers in short or abnormal shaped roots. The color of the teeth is usually normal.

In addition to The National Organization for Rare Disorders (NORD) listed in Section III, the following organizations in Section II (Disease Specific) and in Section III (Umbrella) and Section IV (Government Agencies) can provide more information:

NIH/National Oral Health Information Clearinghouse, *IV*
National Foundation for Ectodermal Dysplasias, *II*

315 DENTINOGENESIS IMPERFECTA TYPE III

Dentinogenesis Imperfecta, Type III is a genetic dental disorder characterized by rapid erosion of crowns of the baby and permanent teeth soon after they erupt. The inside of the teeth (dental pulp), which is filled with blood vessels and nerve endings, is usually exposed. Other genetic traits may accompany these tooth abnormalities.

In addition to The National Organization for Rare Disorders (NORD) listed in Section III, the following organizations in Section II (Disease Specific) and in Section III (Umbrella) and Section IV (Government Agencies) can provide more information:

NIH/National Oral Health Information Clearinghouse, *IV*
National Foundation for Ectodermal Dysplasias, *II*

316 DEPERSONALIZATION DISORDER

Depersonalization Disorder is a psychiatric disorder affecting emotions and behavior. It is characterized by an alteration in how an affected individual perceives or experiences his or her unique sense of self. The usual sense of one's own reality is temporarily lost or changed. A feeling of detachment from, or being an outside observer of one's mental processes, or body occurs such as the sensation of being in a dream.

In addition to The National Organization for Rare Disorders (NORD) listed in Section III, the following organizations in Section II (Disease Specific) and in Section III (Umbrella) and Section IV (Government Agencies) can provide more information:

NIH/National Institute of Mental Health, *IV*
National Alliance for the Mentally Ill, *III*
National Mental Health Association, *III*
National Mental Health Consumer Self-Help Clearinghouse, *III*

317 DERCUM DISEASE

Dercum Disease is a rare disorder characterized by pressure of fatty deposits on nerves, resulting in weakness and pain. This disorder usually occurs in obese females between the ages of 45 and 60 years. Various areas of the body may swell for no apparent reason. The swelling may disappear without treatment, leaving hardened tissue or pendulous skin folds. In some cases, affected individuals may also experience depression, lethargy, and/or confusion. Dercum Disease is thought to be inherited as an autosomal dominant genetic trait.

In addition to The National Organization for Rare Disorders (NORD) listed in Section III, the following organizations in Section II (Disease Specific) and in Section III (Umbrella) and Section IV (Government Agencies) can provide more information:
American Chronic Pain Association, *III*
Dercum's Connection, *II*
NIH/National Institute of Diabetes, Digestive and Kidney Diseases, *IV*

318 DERMATITIS, ATOPIC

Atopic dermatitis is a common chronic inherited form of eczema. Eczema is a skin condition characterized by redness, swelling (edema), oozing, crusting, scaling, burning pain, and itching (pruritus). Scratching or rubbing eczema may lead to thickening and marking of the skin (lichenification). The causes of eczema fall into two classifications: constitutional eczema (atopic dermatitis), and external eczema which is caused by allergies, irritations, or chemical reactions such as in contact dermatitis.

In addition to The National Organization for Rare Disorders (NORD) listed in Section III, the following organizations in Section II (Disease Specific) and in Section III (Umbrella) and Section IV (Government Agencies) can provide more information:
NIH/National Institute of Arthritis and Musculoskeletal and Skin Diseases, *IV*

319 DERMATITIS, CONTACT

Contact dermatitis is an acute or chronic skin inflammation triggered by substances that come in contact with the skin. Affected individuals may have abnormal redness of the skin (erythema) and/or itching (pruritis). Symptoms and physical findings associated with contact dermatitis vary greatly depending upon the cause of the disorder. Causes of contact dermatitis include an allergic reaction or response to a substance or a direct toxic effect of a substance (e.g., chemical irritants, medications, certain plants).

In addition to The National Organization for Rare Disorders (NORD) listed in Section III, the following organizations in Section II (Disease Specific) and in Section III (Umbrella) and Section IV (Government Agencies) can provide more information:
NIH/National Arthritis and Musculoskeletal and Skin Diseases Information Clearinghouse, *IV*
National Eczema Association for Science and Education, *II*

320 DERMATOMYOSITIS

Dermatomyositis is a progressive connective tissue disorder characterized by inflammatory and degenerative changes of the muscles and of the skin. In many cases, a skin rash may precede the development of muscle abnormalities by more than one year. In some cases, the severity of muscle and skin abnormalities may coincide; in other cases, they have no relationship.

The symptoms and physical findings of Dermatomyositis vary widely from case to case. Muscle abnormalities may begin with aches and weakness of the muscles of the upper arms and legs (proximal muscles). Muscles may be stiff, sore, and tender and, eventually, show signs of degeneration (atrophy). Affected individuals may experience difficulty in performing certain functions such as raising their arms and/or climbing stairs. In addition, affected individuals may experience speech and swallowing difficulties.

Skin abnormalities associated with Dermatomyositis typically include a reddish-purple rash on the upper eyelids (Heliotrope rash); reddish-purple, horn-like growths on the surface of the knuckles, elbows, and/or knees (Gottron's sign); and/or a red rash (erythema) affecting the skin of the face, neck, and/or upper torso.

The symptoms of Childhood Dermatomyositis are similar to those associated with the adult form of the disorder. However, onset is usually more sudden. In addition, abnormal accumulations of calcium deposits (calcifications) in muscle and skin tissues, as well as involvement of the digestive (gastrointestinal) tract are more common in the childhood form of Dermatomyositis.

Although the exact cause of Dermatomyositis is not known, it is thought to be an autoimmune disorder.

In addition to The National Organization for Rare Disorders (NORD) listed in Section III, the following

organizations in Section II (Disease Specific) and in Section III (Umbrella) and Section IV (Government Agencies) can provide more information:
American Autoimmune Related Diseases Association, Inc., *III*
Arthritis Foundation, *III*
British Coalition of Heritable Disorders of Connective Tissue, *III*
Muscular Dystrophy Association, *III*
Myositis Association of America, Inc., *III*
NIH/National Institute of Arthritis and Musculoskeletal and Skin Diseases, *IV*
New Onset Juvenile Dermatomyositis (JDMS) Registry, *II*

321 DEVIC DISEASE

Devic Disease is a rare nerve disorder characterized by loss (demyelination) of the fatty sheath surrounding the optic nerve and nerves in the spinal cord. This disorder can begin at any age after puberty. An initial phase consisting of a slight fever, sore throat and/or head cold often occurs. Loss of clear vision is accompanied by mild paralysis (usually of the lower limbs) and loss of bladder and bowel control. Devic Disease can occur spontaneously, or in conjunction with Multiple Sclerosis or Systemic Lupus Erythematosus.

In addition to The National Organization for Rare Disorders (NORD) listed in Section III, the following organizations in Section II (Disease Specific) and in Section III (Umbrella) and Section IV (Government Agencies) can provide more information:
American Autoimmune Related Diseases Association, Inc., *III*
NIH/National Eye Institute, *IV*
NIH/National Institute of Neurological Disorders and Stroke, *IV*

322 DEXTROCARDIA WITH SITUS INVERSUS

Dextrocardia with Situs Inversus is a rare heart condition characterized by abnormal positioning of the heart. In this condition, the tip of the heart (apex) is positioned on the right side of the chest. Additionally, the position of the heart chambers as well as the visceral organs such as the liver and spleen is reversed (situs inversus). However, most affected individuals can live a normal life without associated symptoms or disability.

In addition to The National Organization for Rare Disorders (NORD) listed in Section III, the following organizations in Section II (Disease Specific) and in Section III (Umbrella) and Section IV (Government Agencies) can provide more information:
American Heart Association, *III*
American Lung Association, *III*
Congenital Heart Anomalies, Support, Education, & Resources, *III*
NIH/National Heart, Lung and Blood Institute Information Center, *IV*
NIH/National Institute of Child Health and Human Development, *IV*

323 DIGEORGE SYNDROME

DiGeorge Syndrome is a very rare group of congenital abnormalities that are the result of defects during early fetal developmental. These defects occur in areas known as the 3rd and 4th pharyngeal pouches which later develop into the thymus and parathyroid glands. Developmental abnormalities may also occur in the 4th branchial arch.

Normally the thymus gland is located below the thyroid gland in the neck and front of the chest and is the primary gland of the lymphatic system which is necessary for the normal functioning of the immune system. The parathyroid glands, located on the sides of the thyroid gland, are responsible for the maintenance of normal levels of calcium in the blood. The thymus and parathyroid glands are missing or underdeveloped in children with DiGeorge Syndrome. The symptoms of this disorder vary greatly depending on the extent of the missing thymus and parathyroid tissue. The primary problem caused by DiGeorge Syndrome is repeated infections due to a diminished immune system.

In addition to The National Organization for Rare Disorders (NORD) listed in Section III, the following organizations in Section II (Disease Specific) and in Section III (Umbrella) and Section IV (Government Agencies) can provide more information:
22q and You, *II*
Alliance of Genetic Support Groups, *III*
Immune Deficiency Foundation, *III*
International Patient Organization for Primary Immunodeficiencies, *III*
March of Dimes Birth Defects Foundation, *III*
NIH/National Institute of Child Health and Human Development, *IV*
The Arc (a national organization on mental retardation), *III*

324 DIABETES INSIPIDUS

Diabetes Insipidus is a rare metabolic disease that is not related to diabetes mellitus. It is characterized by a deficiency of the hormone vasopressin (anti-diuretic hormone [ADH]), which is produced in the posterior lobe of the pituitary gland. The lack of effect of this hormone on the kidney causes excretion of excessive quantities of very dilute (but otherwise normal) urine. Excessive thirst and urination are the major symptoms of this disorder.

In addition to The National Organization for Rare Disorders (NORD) listed in Section III, the following organizations in Section II (Disease Specific) and in Section III (Umbrella) and Section IV (Government Agencies) can provide more information:
Alliance of Genetic Support Groups, *III*
Diabetes Insipidus And Related Disorders, *III*
Diabetes Insipidus Foundation, Inc., *III*
Metabolic Information Network, *III*
NIH/National Diabetes Information Clearinghouse, *IV*
Nephrogenic Diabetes Insipidus Parent Support Group of CHOP, *II*
Pituitary Tumor Network Association, *III*

325 DIABETES, INSULIN DEPENDENT

Insulin-dependent diabetes is a disorder in which the body does not produce enough insulin and is, therefore, unable to convert nutrients into the energy necessary for daily activity. The disorder affects females and males in equal numbers. Although the exact causes of Insulin-Dependent Diabetes are not known, genetic and environmental (i.e., viral) factors seem to play a role.

In addition to The National Organization for Rare Disorders (NORD) listed in Section III, the following organizations in Section II (Disease Specific) and in Section III (Umbrella) and Section IV (Government Agencies) can provide more information:
JDF The Diabetes Research Foundation, *II*
Juvenile Diabetes Foundation International, *II*
NIH/National Diabetes Information Clearinghouse, *IV*

326 DIASTROPHIC DYSPLASIA

Diastrophic Dysplasia is a rare inherited disorder characterized by abnormalities of the hands and feet, characteristic facial features, skeletal malformations, and growth retardation before birth (prenatally). In most cases, as affected individuals age, they may exhibit short stature with abnormally short arms and legs (short-limbed dwarfism). Abnormalities of the hands and feet may include abnormally short fingers (brachydactyly), thumbs that are bent toward the body (hitchhikers thumb), and/or the heel of the foot being turned inward toward body while the rest of the foot is bent downward and inward (clubfoot or talipes equinovarus). Facial features may include a narrow bridge of the nose, flared nostrils, and/or abnormally swelling of the outer portions of the ears (pinnae). Skeletal malformations may include abnormal side-to-side curvature of the spine (scoliosis), abnormal front-to-back curvature of the spine (kyphosis), and/or incomplete closure of bones in the spinal column surrounding the spinal cord (spina bifida occulta), leaving a portion of the spinal cord exposed.

In addition to The National Organization for Rare Disorders (NORD) listed in Section III, the following organizations in Section II (Disease Specific) and in Section III (Umbrella) and Section IV (Government Agencies) can provide more information:
Human Growth Foundation, *III*
Little People of America, *III*
Little People's Research Fund, Inc., *III*
MAGIC Foundation for Children's Growth, *III*
NIH/National Institute of Arthritis and Musculoskeletal and Skin Diseases, *IV*
Short Stature Foundation, *III*

327 DIENCEPHALIC SYNDROME

The Diencephalic Syndrome is a very rare neurological disorder. It is normally seen in infancy or early childhood. However, some cases have been reported in older children and even adults. Diencephalic Syndrome is characterized by failure to thrive, abnormal thinness (emaciation), amnesia, intense sleepiness, unusual eye position, and sometimes blindness. The disorder does not affect the linear growth of the child. However, growth hormone levels are usually elevated.

In addition to The National Organization for Rare Disorders (NORD) listed in Section III, the following organizations in Section II (Disease Specific) and in Section III (Umbrella) and Section IV (Government Agencies) can provide more information:
American Cancer Society, Inc., *III*
Guardians of Hydrocephalus Research Foundation, *II*
Hydrocephalus Association, *II*
National Hydrocephalus Foundation, *II*

328 DILATATION OF THE PULMONARY ARTERY, IDIOPATHIC

Idiopathic Dilatation of the Pulmonary Artery (IDPA) is a rare congenital defect characterized by a wider than normal main pulmonary artery in the absence of any apparent anatomical or physiological cause.

In addition to The National Organization for Rare Disorders (NORD) listed in Section III, the following organizations in Section II (Disease Specific) and in Section III (Umbrella) and Section IV (Government Agencies) can provide more information:
American Lung Association, *III*
NIH/National Heart, Lung and Blood Institute, *IV*

329 **DIVERTICULITIS**

Diverticulitis is a common digestive disorder and a frequent complication of diverticulosis. Diverticulosis is characterized by small sac-like protrusions (hernias) of mucous tissue through the wall of the large intestine (colon). These protrusions are known as diverticula and may occur in any part of the colon, but most often in the lowest part (sigmoid). Diverticulitis is characterized by inflammation of one or more of these sacs (diverticula). Symptoms may include abdominal pain, fever, digestive problems, and/or bleeding from part of the large intestine (rectum).

In addition to The National Organization for Rare Disorders (NORD) listed in Section III, the following organizations in Section II (Disease Specific) and in Section III (Umbrella) and Section IV (Government Agencies) can provide more information:

Digestive Disease National Coalition, *III*
Intestinal Disease Foundation, *III*
NIH/National Digestive Diseases Information Clearinghouse, *IV*

330 **DIVERTICULOSIS**

Diverticulosis is characterized by small sac-like protrusions (hernias) of inner intestinal tissue through the muscular wall of the large intestine (colon). These protrusions are called diverticula and may occur in any part of the colon, but most frequently are found in the lowest part (sigmoid).

In addition to The National Organization for Rare Disorders (NORD) listed in Section III, the following organizations in Section II (Disease Specific) and in Section III (Umbrella) and Section IV (Government Agencies) can provide more information:

Digestive Disease National Coalition, *III*
Intestinal Disease Foundation, *III*
NIH/National Digestive Diseases Information Clearinghouse, *IV*

331 **DOWN SYNDROME**

Down Syndrome is the most common and readily identifiable genetic condition associated with mental retardation. Facial, skeletal, and frequently cardiac abnormalities are among the more the 50 features seen in this syndrome. It is rare to find all symptoms or even most of them in one person with Down Syndrome.

In addition to The National Organization for Rare Disorders (NORD) listed in Section III, the following organizations in Section II (Disease Specific) and in Section III (Umbrella) and Section IV (Government Agencies) can provide more information:

Association for Children with Down Syndrome, Inc., *II*
March of Dimes Birth Defects Foundation, *III*
NIH/National Institute of Child Health and Human Development, *IV*
National Down Syndrome Congress, *II*
National Down Syndrome Society, *II*
The Arc (a national organization on mental retardation), *III*

332 **DRACUNCULOSIS**

Dracunculosis is an infection caused by a parasitic worm known as Dracunculus medinensis, the guinea worm. Infected water fleas release the larvae of the worm into drinking water. Ingestion of contaminated water causes the larvae to migrate from the intestines via the abdominal cavity to the tissue under the skin. The larvae mature and release a toxic substance that makes the overlying skin ulcerate. After treatment, symptoms disappear and the worms can be safely removed from the skin.

In addition to The National Organization for Rare Disorders (NORD) listed in Section III, the following organizations in Section II (Disease Specific) and in Section III (Umbrella) and Section IV (Government Agencies) can provide more information:

Centers for Disease Control and Prevention, *IV*
NIH/National Institute of Allergy and Infectious Diseases, *IV*
World Health Organization (WHO) Regional Office for the Americas (AMRO), *III*

333 **DRASH SYNDROME**

Drash Syndrome is a very rare disorder that typically appears for no apparent reason (sporadically). In rare cases, it may be inherited as an autosomal dominant genetic trait. This disorder usually appears early in life. In its complete form, it is characterized by the combination of abnormal kidney function, genital abnormalities (pseudohermaphroditism), and a cancerous tumor of the kidney called a Wilms' tumor. Some affected individuals may have the incomplete form of Drash Syndrome, which consists of abnormal kidney function with either genital abnormalities (pseudohermaphroditism) or Wilms' tumor. This disorder predominantly affects males but a few female cases have been reported.

In addition to The National Organization for Rare Disorders (NORD) listed in Section III, the following organizations in Section II (Disease Specific) and in Section III (Umbrella) and Section IV (Government Agencies) can provide more information:

American Cancer Society, Inc., *III*
American Kidney Fund, Inc., *III*
Candlelighters Childhood Cancer Foundation, *III*

NIH/National Institute of Child Health and Human Development, *IV*
National Kidney Foundation, *III*

334 DUANE SYNDROME

Duane Syndrome is a rare inherited disorder of eye movement characterized by limited motion of the eye from side to side (horizontal motility). This disorder belongs to a group of eye disorders associated with ocular abnormalities that result in a cross-eyed appearance (strabismus). The symptoms of Duane Syndrome, which are present at birth (congenital), may include retraction of the eyeball, impaired ability to move the eye, and compensating face-turning. The exact cause of Duane Syndrome is not known. However, it may occur in association with a variety of other disorders. Three types of Duane Syndrome are recognized, based on the specific form of eye impairment.

In addition to The National Organization for Rare Disorders (NORD) listed in Section III, the following organizations in Section II (Disease Specific) and in Section III (Umbrella) and Section IV (Government Agencies) can provide more information:
NIH/National Eye Institute, *IV*
Schepens Eye Research Institute, *III*

335 DUBIN JOHNSON SYNDROME

Dubin Johnson Syndrome is a rare genetic liver disorder that tends to affect people of Middle Eastern Jewish heritage disproportionately to other groups. It appears to be associated with clotting factor VII in this population. Symptoms may include a yellowish color to the skin (jaundice), and a liver that is sometimes enlarged and tender.

In addition to The National Organization for Rare Disorders (NORD) listed in Section III, the following organizations in Section II (Disease Specific) and in Section III (Umbrella) and Section IV (Government Agencies) can provide more information:
American Liver Foundation, *III*
NIH/National Digestive Diseases Information Clearinghouse, *IV*
National Foundation for Jewish Genetic Diseases, *III*
United Liver Association, *III*

336 DUBOWITZ SYNDROME

Dubowitz Syndrome is a very rare developmental disorder characterized by growth retardation, short stature, and unusual facial and physical characteristics. Symptoms may develop while the fetus is still in the uterus (intrauterine) or immediately after birth (neonatal). Physical characteristics associated with Dubowitz Syndrome include a high nasal bridge, underdevelopment of the bony ridges above the eyes (supraorbital ridges), widely spaced eyes (ocular hypertelorism), and/or droopy eyelids (ptosis). Affected children typically have patchy areas of itchy red skin (eczema) on their face, knees, and elbows. Dubowitz Syndrome is inherited as an autosomal recessive genetic trait.

In addition to The National Organization for Rare Disorders (NORD) listed in Section III, the following organizations in Section II (Disease Specific) and in Section III (Umbrella) and Section IV (Government Agencies) can provide more information:
Learning Disabilities Association of America, *III*
NIH/National Institute of Child Health and Human Development, *IV*
The Arc (a national organization on mental retardation), *III*

337 DUHRING DISEASE

Duhring Disease, also known as Dermatitis Herpetiformis, is a rare chronic skin disorder characterized by the presence of groups of severely itchy (pruritic) blisters and raised skin lesions (papules). The exact cause of this disease is not known although it is frequently associated with the inability to digest gluten (gluten-sensitive enteropathy).

In addition to The National Organization for Rare Disorders (NORD) listed in Section III, the following organizations in Section II (Disease Specific) and in Section III (Umbrella) and Section IV (Government Agencies) can provide more information:
Gluten Intolerance Group of North America, *II*
NIH/National Arthritis and Musculoskeletal and Skin Diseases Information Clearinghouse, *IV*

338 DUODENAL ATRESIA OR STENOSIS

Duodenal Atresia and Duodenal Stenosis are rare congenital digestive disorders that usually occur for no apparent reason (sporadically). However, a few cases of Duodenal Atresia have been inherited as an autosomal recessive genetic trait. Absence or complete closure (atresia) of a portion of the channel (lumen) within the first part of the small intestine (duodenum), or partial obstruction due to narrowing (stenosis) of the duodenum is present. Other associated abnormalities may be found in over half of those affected with Duodenal Atresia or Duodenal Stenosis.

In addition to The National Organization for Rare Disorders (NORD) listed in Section III, the following organizations in Section II (Disease Specific) and in Section III (Umbrella) and Section IV (Government Agencies) can provide more information:

Digestive Disease National Coalition, *III*
NIH/National Digestive Diseases Information Clearinghouse, *IV*

339 DUPUYTREN'S CONTRACTURE

Dupuytren's Contracture is a rare connective tissue disorder characterized by fixation of the joints (e.g., proximal interphalangeal joints and metacarpophalangeal joints) of certain fingers in a permanently flexed position (joint contractures). Due to abnormal thickening and shortening of the bands of fibrous tissue beneath the skin of the palm (palmar fascia), a hardened nodule may develop, eventually forming an abnormal band of hardened (fibrotic) tissue. As a result, the fingers of the affected area begin to be "drawn in" toward the palm over several months or years and cannot be pulled back (contracture). In addition, the skin of the affected area may "pucker." In most cases, the ring and pinky (fourth and fifth) fingers are most affected. In addition, the disorder usually affects both hands (bilateral). Although the exact cause of Dupuytren's Contracture is unknown, the disorder is thought to be inherited as an autosomal dominant genetic trait in some cases. In addition, there appears to be an increased incidence of the disease in individuals with alcoholic liver disease (cirrhosis).

In addition to The National Organization for Rare Disorders (NORD) listed in Section III, the following organizations in Section II (Disease Specific) and in Section III (Umbrella) and Section IV (Government Agencies) can provide more information:
NIH/National Arthritis and Musculoskeletal and Skin Diseases Information Clearinghouse, *IV*

340 DYGGVE MELCHIOR CLAUSEN SYNDROME

Dyggve-Melchior-Clausen Syndrome is a rare disorder inherited through an autosomal recessive trait. Major symptoms may include short stature, mental retardation, bulging of the chest sternum, flattening of the vertebrae and upper border of the pelvis (iliac crest), shortening of the bones in the middle portion of the hand (metacarpals) and changes in the long bones. Patients with the Smith-McCort Dwarfism form of this disorder do not have mental retardation.

In addition to The National Organization for Rare Disorders (NORD) listed in Section III, the following organizations in Section II (Disease Specific) and in Section III (Umbrella) and Section IV (Government Agencies) can provide more information:
Human Growth Foundation, *III*
MAGIC Foundation for Children's Growth, *III*
NIH/National Institute of Child Health and Human Development, *IV*

341 DYSAUTONOMIA, FAMILIAL

Familial Dysautonomia is a rare genetic disorder of the autonomic nervous system (ANS) characterized by diminished sensitivity to pain, lack of overflow tearing in the eyes, a decrease in the number of knob-like projections that cover the tongue (fungiform papillae), unusual fluctuations of body temperature, and unstable blood pressure. Symptoms of this disorder are apparent at birth. The autonomic nervous system controls vital involuntary body functions.

In addition to The National Organization for Rare Disorders (NORD) listed in Section III, the following organizations in Section II (Disease Specific) and in Section III (Umbrella) and Section IV (Government Agencies) can provide more information:
Alliance of Genetic Support Groups, *III*
Dysautonomia Foundation, Inc., *II*
NIH/National Institute of Neurological Disorders and Stroke, *IV*

342 DYSCHONDROSTEOSIS

Dyschondrosteosis is a rare disorder that is inherited through an autosomal dominant trait. Male-to-male transmission has been observed in multiple cases. The major features of this disorder are a deformity of the wrist called Madelung Deformity and abnormally short forearms and lower legs (mesomelic short stature).

In addition to The National Organization for Rare Disorders (NORD) listed in Section III, the following organizations in Section II (Disease Specific) and in Section III (Umbrella) and Section IV (Government Agencies) can provide more information:
Human Growth Foundation, *III*
Little People of America, *III*
Little People's Research Fund, Inc., *III*
MAGIC Foundation for Children's Growth, *III*
NIH/National Institute of Child Health and Human Development, *IV*
Short Stature Foundation, *III*

343 DYSKERATOSIS CONGENITA

Dyskeratosis Congenita is a rare disorder in which three groups of symptoms occur: darkening and/or unusual absence of skin color (hyper/hypopigmentation); progressive nail dystrophy; and slowly changing characteristics of mucous membranes (leukoplakia) in the anus, urethra, lips, mouth and/or eye.

Other symptoms found in some patients with this syndrome may be reduction in red and white blood cells and platelets (pancytopenia), overgrowth of skin on the palms of the hands and soles of the feet, excessive sweating of the palms and soles, sparse or absent hair, fragile bones, underdeveloped testes, and dental abnormalities. Dyskeratosis Congenita is more prevalent among males then females and an X-linked recessive inheritance is the most common form although cases of autosomal recessive and autosomal dominant inheritance have been recorded. This disorder has also occurred sporadically (no known cause) in a significant number of cases.

In addition to The National Organization for Rare Disorders (NORD) listed in Section III, the following organizations in Section II (Disease Specific) and in Section III (Umbrella) and Section IV (Government Agencies) can provide more information:
NIH/National Heart, Lung and Blood Institute Information Center, *IV*
NIH/National Institute of Child Health and Human Development, *IV*
National Foundation for Ectodermal Dysplasias, *II*

344 DYSLEXIA

Dyslexia is a condition in which an individual with normal vision is unable to interpret written language, and therefore is unable to read or may read slowly with great difficulty. Onset is during childhood and males are affected most often.

In addition to The National Organization for Rare Disorders (NORD) listed in Section III, the following organizations in Section II (Disease Specific) and in Section III (Umbrella) and Section IV (Government Agencies) can provide more information:
HEATH Resource Center, *III*
International Dyslexia Association, *II*
Learning Disabilities Association of America, *III*
NIH/National Institute of Neurological Disorders and Stroke, *IV*
National Center for Learning Disabilities, *III*

345 DYSPHONIA, CHRONIC SPASMODIC

Chronic spasmodic dysphonia is a rare voice disorder characterized by stuttering, momentary periods of uncontrolled vocal spasms, tightness in the throat, and/or recurrent hoarseness. At certain times, affected individuals must make a conscious effort to speak. The most frequent sign of this disorder is a sudden, momentary lapse or interruption of the voice. Chronic spasmodic dysphonia is a form of dystonia, a group of neuromuscular disorders characterized by involuntary muscle spasms.

There are two types of Chronic spasmodic dysphonia: Abductor spasmodic dysphonia and the more common adductor spasmodic dysphonia. In the abductor type, the vocal cords draw apart (abduction); in the adductor type, the vocal cords draw together (adduction) and may become locked. The exact cause of chronic spasmodic dysphonia is not known.

In addition to The National Organization for Rare Disorders (NORD) listed in Section III, the following organizations in Section II (Disease Specific) and in Section III (Umbrella) and Section IV (Government Agencies) can provide more information:
Dystonia Medical Research Foundation, *III*
Dystonia Society, *III*
NIH/National Institute on Deafness and Other Communication Disorders (Balance), *IV*
National Spasmodic Dysphonia Association, *II*
WE MOVE, *III*

346 DYSPLASIA, EPIPHYSEALIS HEMIMELICA

Epiphysealis Hemimelica Dysplasia is a disorder that affects bone joints. It is characterized by overgrowth of the cartilage on the end (epiphysis) of one or more of the long bones (carpal or tarsal bones) in the hand or foot. Less often, the cartilage on other bones such as those in the ankle, knee or hip joint can be affected. Usually only one limb is involved. The limbs may be unequal in length.

In addition to The National Organization for Rare Disorders (NORD) listed in Section III, the following organizations in Section II (Disease Specific) and in Section III (Umbrella) and Section IV (Government Agencies) can provide more information:
CHERUB—Association of Families and Friends of Children with Limb Disorders, *III*
NIH/National Arthritis and Musculoskeletal and Skin Diseases Information Clearinghouse, *IV*
NIH/National Institute of Child Health and Human Development, *IV*
Superkids, Inc. (newsletter for families and friends of children with limb differences), *III*

347 DYSPLASIA, FIBROUS

Fibrous Dysplasia is a disease of the medullary bone in which benign cysts occur as a result of irregular bone development. This disorder may involve a single bone (Monostotic

Fibrous dysplasia or Jaffe-Lichtenstein disease) or affect multiple bones (Polyostotic Fibrous dysplasia or McCune Albright syndrome).

Fibrous Dysplasia first appears during childhood and the bone lesions usually stop developing at puberty. These lesions may be painful, deforming and widespread. The bones most often affected are the ribs, skull, facial bones, femur and tibia of the leg.

In addition to The National Organization for Rare Disorders (NORD) listed in Section III, the following organizations in Section II (Disease Specific) and in Section III (Umbrella) and Section IV (Government Agencies) can provide more information:

NIH/National Institute of Arthritis and Musculoskeletal and Skin Diseases, *IV*
Paget Foundation for Paget's Disease of Bone and Related Disorders, *III*

348 DYSPLASTIC NEVUS SYNDROME

Dysplastic Nevus Syndrome is a malignant genetic skin disorder characterized by mole-like tumors. These tumors may appear in different sizes, shapes, and shades of color (usually reddish-brown to pink). The tumors have a variable ability for spreading to adjacent parts of the skin, or through the blood and lymph circulation to other organs. Dysplastic Nevus Syndrome may later evolve into Malignant Melanoma, a common form of skin cancer.

In addition to The National Organization for Rare Disorders (NORD) listed in Section III, the following organizations in Section II (Disease Specific) and in Section III (Umbrella) and Section IV (Government Agencies) can provide more information:

American Cancer Society, Inc., *III*
Naevus Support Group, *II*
Nevus Network, *II*
Nevus Outreach, Inc., *II*
Skin Cancer Foundation, *III*

349 DYSTHYMIA

Dysthymia is a common psychological disorder characterized by a chronic but mild depressive state that has been present in an individual for more than two years. When the depressive state has lasted for several years, it may be difficult to distinguish between a person's usual functioning and the mood disturbance. Dysthymia is a chronic mood disturbance that is classified as a form of neurosis. It must be distinguished from major depression disorders.

In addition to The National Organization for Rare Disorders (NORD) listed in Section III, the following organizations in Section II (Disease Specific) and in Section III (Umbrella) and Section IV (Government Agencies) can provide more information:

NIH/National Institute of Mental Health, *IV*
NIH/National Institute of Mental Health (Depression Hotline), *IV*
National Alliance for the Mentally Ill, *III*
National Foundation for Depressive Illness, Inc., *III*
National Mental Health Association, *III*
National Mental Health Consumer Self-Help Clearinghouse, *III*

350 DYSTONIA, TORSION

Torsion dystonia is a neurological movement disorder characterized by involuntary contortions of muscles in the neck, torso and extremities. Occasionally only one or a few muscles are involved. The disorder is most noticeable when walking. The involvement of several muscle groups may produce a sideways gait and the body may twist as if writhing or distorted. There are several types of dystonias that are characterized by involuntary muscle spasms.

In addition to The National Organization for Rare Disorders (NORD) listed in Section III, the following organizations in Section II (Disease Specific) and in Section III (Umbrella) and Section IV (Government Agencies) can provide more information:

Alliance of Genetic Support Groups, *III*
Dystonia Medical Research Foundation, *III*
Dystonia Society, *III*
March of Dimes Birth Defects Foundation, *III*
NIH/National Institute of Neurological Disorders and Stroke, *IV*
National Foundation for Jewish Genetic Diseases, *III*
WE MOVE, *III*

351 DYSTROPHY, ASPHYXIATING THORACIC

Asphyxiating Thoracic Dystrophy is a very rare genetic disorder affecting the development of the bone structure of the chest area. Major findings include failure of the rib cage to develop correctly, kidney problems, and shortened bones of the arms and legs.

In addition to The National Organization for Rare Disorders (NORD) listed in Section III, the following organizations in Section II (Disease Specific) and in Section III (Umbrella) and Section IV (Government Agencies) can provide more information:

Human Growth Foundation, *III*
MAGIC Foundation for Children's Growth, *III*
NIH/National Arthritis and Musculoskeletal and Skin Diseases Information Clearinghouse, *IV*
NIH/National Institute of Child Health and Human Development, *IV*

352 DYSTROPHY, MYOTONIC

Myotonic Dystrophy is an inherited disorder involving the muscles, vision, and endocrine glands. It can cause mental deficiency and loss of hair. Onset of this rare disorder commonly occurs during young adulthood. However, it can occur at any age and is extremely variable in degree of severity.

In addition to The National Organization for Rare Disorders (NORD) listed in Section III, the following organizations in Section II (Disease Specific) and in Section III (Umbrella) and Section IV (Government Agencies) can provide more information:

Muscular Dystrophy Association, *III*
NIH/National Institute of Arthritis and Musculoskeletal and Skin Diseases, *IV*
NIH/National Institute of Neurological Disorders and Stroke, *IV*

353 EALES DISEASE

Eales Disease is a rare vision disorder that appears to an examining physician as an inflammation and white haze around the outercoat of the veins in the retina. The disorder is most prevalent among young males and normally affects both eyes. There is usually a sudden blurring of vision due to oozing of the clear jelly that fills the eyeball behind the lens of the eye (vitreous hemorrhaging).

In addition to The National Organization for Rare Disorders (NORD) listed in Section III, the following organizations in Section II (Disease Specific) and in Section III (Umbrella) and Section IV (Government Agencies) can provide more information:

NIH/National Eye Institute, *IV*
Schepens Eye Research Institute, *III*
Vision Foundation, Inc., *III*

354 EAR, PATELLA, SHORT STATURE SYNDROME

Ear, Patella, Short Stature Syndrome is an extremely rare inherited disorder characterized by underdevelopment or absence of the outer structures of both ears (pinna) including the external ear canal (microtia), absence of the knee caps (patellae), and/or short stature. Other findings may include various skeletal abnormalities, early feeding difficulties, and/or poor weight gain. In addition, characteristic craniofacial features may be present including a small mouth (microstomia) with full lips, an abnormally small head (microcephaly), and/or underdevelopment (hypoplasia) of the upper (maxillary) and/or lower (mandibular) jaw bones. Ear, Patella, Short Stature Syndrome is thought to be inherited as an autosomal recessive genetic trait.

In addition to The National Organization for Rare Disorders (NORD) listed in Section III, the following organizations in Section II (Disease Specific) and in Section III (Umbrella) and Section IV (Government Agencies) can provide more information:

Better Hearing Institute, *III*
Ear Anomalies Reconstructed: Atresia/Microtia Support Group, *III*
Human Growth Foundation, *III*
Little People of America, *III*
NIH/National Institute of Arthritis and Musculoskeletal and Skin Diseases, *IV*
NIH/National Institute of Child Health and Human Development, *IV*
NIH/National Institute on Deafness and Other Communication Disorders Information Clearinghouse, *IV*
Short Stature Foundation, *III*

355 EATON LAMBERT SYNDROME

Eaton-Lambert Syndrome is a neuromuscular disorder that may be an autoimmune disease. Major symptoms include muscle weakness and fatigue especially of the pelvic and thigh muscles. Other symptoms may include dryness of the mouth, impotence, pain in the thighs, and a pricking, tingling or creeping sensation on the skin (paresthesias) around the affected areas.

In addition to The National Organization for Rare Disorders (NORD) listed in Section III, the following organizations in Section II (Disease Specific) and in Section III (Umbrella) and Section IV (Government Agencies) can provide more information:

American Autoimmune Related Diseases Association, Inc., *III*
Muscular Dystrophy Association, *III*
Myasthenia Gravis Foundation of America, *II*
NIH/National Institute of Neurological Disorders and Stroke, *IV*

356 ECTODERMAL DYSPLASIAS

The Ectodermal Dysplasias are a group of hereditary, non-progressive syndromes in which the affected tissue derives primarily from the ectodermal germ layer. The skin, its derivatives, and some other organs are involved. A predisposition to respiratory infections, due to a somewhat depressed immune system and to defective mucous glands in parts of the respiratory tract, is the most life threatening characteristic of this group of disorders.

In addition to The National Organization for Rare Disorders (NORD) listed in Section III, the following organizations in Section II (Disease Specific) and in

Section III (Umbrella) and Section IV (Government Agencies) can provide more information:
Alliance of Genetic Support Groups, *III*
March of Dimes Birth Defects Foundation, *III*
NIH/National Oral Health Information Clearinghouse, *IV*
National Foundation for Ectodermal Dysplasias, *II*
The Arc (a national organization on mental retardation), *III*

357 ECTRODACTYLY ECTODERMAL DYSPLASIA CLEFT LIP/PALATE

Ectrodactyly-Ectodermal Dysplasia-Cleft Lip/Palate (EEC Syndrome) is a rare form of ectodermal dysplasia inherited as an autosomal dominant genetic trait. It can vary from mild symptoms to severe. The most common symptoms found in patients with EEC Syndrome are: missing or irregular fingers and/or toes (ectrodactyly), abnormalities of the hair and glands, cleft lip and/or palate, or unusual facial features, as well as abnormalities of the eyes and urinary tract.

In addition to The National Organization for Rare Disorders (NORD) listed in Section III, the following organizations in Section II (Disease Specific) and in Section III (Umbrella) and Section IV (Government Agencies) can provide more information:
NIH/National Arthritis and Musculoskeletal and Skin Diseases Information Clearinghouse, *IV*
National Foundation for Ectodermal Dysplasias, *II*

358 EDEMA, IDIOPATHIC

Idiopathic Edema is a common disorder that occurs almost exclusively in women. It is characterized by salt retention in the absence of heart, kidney, or liver disease. The swelling (edema) may be episodic or persistent. Swelling of the face, hands, and feet develops rapidly, frequently accompanied by headache, irritability, and depression. Weight gain also occurs.

In addition to The National Organization for Rare Disorders (NORD) listed in Section III, the following organizations in Section II (Disease Specific) and in Section III (Umbrella) and Section IV (Government Agencies) can provide more information:
NIH/National Digestive Diseases Information Clearinghouse, *IV*

359 EHLERS DANLOS SYNDROME

Ehlers-Danlos Syndrome is a rare inherited connective tissue disorder. It is characterized by the ability of affected individuals to flex their bodies beyond the normal range (articular hypermobility), to abnormally stretch their skin (hyperelasticity of the skin), and widespread tissue fragility (i.e., skin, blood vessels, and other tissues can rupture from even minor trauma). Many forms of Ehlers-Danlos Syndrome are inherited as an autosomal dominant genetic trait, but some forms of the disorder are inherited as either an autosomal recessive or a x-linked recessive genetic trait.

In addition to The National Organization for Rare Disorders (NORD) listed in Section III, the following organizations in Section II (Disease Specific) and in Section III (Umbrella) and Section IV (Government Agencies) can provide more information:
British Coalition of Heritable Disorders of Connective Tissue, *III*
Ehlers-Danlos National Foundation, *III*
Ehlers-Danlos Syndrome Support Group UK, *II*
NIH/National Institute of Arthritis and Musculoskeletal and Skin Diseases, *IV*

360 EISENMENGER SYNDROME

Eisenmenger Syndrome is characterized by a large opening in the wall of the heart which separates the heart chambers (ventricular septal defect). The flow of blood between the heart and lungs meets with resistance (pulmonary vascular resistance, PVR). This resistance increases as the child matures, resulting in high lung (pulmonary) artery pressure. Blood that has lost its oxygen during circulation through the body needs to pass through the lungs to take up oxygen again. The high pulmonary artery pressure in patients with Eisenmenger Syndrome causes increasing difficulty breathing (dyspnea), insufficient levels of oxygen in the blood, and swelling (edema) of lung tissue. Some patients can do well until age 40 or 50 years when their condition may begin to deteriorate.

In addition to The National Organization for Rare Disorders (NORD) listed in Section III, the following organizations in Section II (Disease Specific) and in Section III (Umbrella) and Section IV (Government Agencies) can provide more information:
Congenital Heart Anomalies, Support, Education, & Resources, *III*
NIH/National Heart, Lung and Blood Institute Information Center, *IV*

361 ELEPHANTIASIS

Elephantiasis is a rare disorder of the lymphatic system. Inflammation of the lymphatic vessels causes extreme enlargement of the affected area, most commonly a limb or parts of the head and torso. It occurs most commonly in tropical regions and particularly in parts of Africa.

In addition to The National Organization for Rare Disorders (NORD) listed in Section III, the following organizations in Section II (Disease Specific) and in Section III (Umbrella) and Section IV (Government Agencies) can provide more information:
Centers for Disease Control and Prevention, *IV*
NIH/National Institute of Allergy and Infectious Diseases, *IV*

362 ELLIS VAN CREVELD SYNDROME

Ellis-Van Creveld Syndrome is a rare genetic disorder characterized by short limb dwarfism, additional fingers and/or toes (polydactyly), abnormal development of fingernails and, in over half of the cases, congenital heart defects. This disorder is inherited through an autosomal recessive trait.

In addition to The National Organization for Rare Disorders (NORD) listed in Section III, the following organizations in Section II (Disease Specific) and in Section III (Umbrella) and Section IV (Government Agencies) can provide more information:
Human Growth Foundation, *III*
MAGIC Foundation for Children's Growth, *III*
NIH/National Institute of Child Health and Human Development, *IV*

363 EMPHYSEMA, CONGENITAL LOBAR

Congenital Lobar Emphysema is a respiratory disorder of varying degrees of severity which allows air to enter the lungs but not to escape. It is sometimes apparent at birth or shortly after birth. In others it doesn't become apparent until adulthood or may not cause any breathing difficulties at all. It may be so severe as to cause associated heart problems or be so mild as to never become apparent. Congenital Lobar Emphysema may be caused by hereditary transmission or occur for no apparent reason.

In addition to The National Organization for Rare Disorders (NORD) listed in Section III, the following organizations in Section II (Disease Specific) and in Section III (Umbrella) and Section IV (Government Agencies) can provide more information:
American Lung Association, *III*
NIH/National Heart, Lung and Blood Institute Information Center, *IV*

364 EMPTY SELLA SYNDROME

Empty Sella Syndrome is a genetic brain disorder transmitted through autosomal dominant genes. The disorder is characterized by an empty space filled with cerebrospinal fluid in the "sella turcica" area of the brain. The area fills with fluid as a result of a defect in the sella diaphragm. This disorder affects mostly obese, middle-aged women. Primary and secondary types of the disorder are distinguished by the exact cause.

In addition to The National Organization for Rare Disorders (NORD) listed in Section III, the following organizations in Section II (Disease Specific) and in Section III (Umbrella) and Section IV (Government Agencies) can provide more information:
NIH/National Institute of Neurological Disorders and Stroke, *IV*

365 ENCEPHALITIS, HERPETIC

Encephalitis is a central nervous system infection. Herpetic Encephalitis is caused by a virus known as Herpes Simplex Virus. Primary symptoms include headache, drowsiness, hyperactivity and/or general weakness. This disorder may have some similar symptoms to Meningitis such as a stiff neck, altered reflexes, confusion, possible paralysis and/or speech disorders. Skin lesions usually are not found.

In addition to The National Organization for Rare Disorders (NORD) listed in Section III, the following organizations in Section II (Disease Specific) and in Section III (Umbrella) and Section IV (Government Agencies) can provide more information:
Centers for Disease Control and Prevention, *IV*
NIH/National Institute of Allergy and Infectious Diseases, *IV*
NIH/National Institute of Neurological Disorders and Stroke, *IV*

366 ENCEPHALITIS, JAPANESE

Japanese Encephalitis is a severe viral infection which causes inflammation of the brain. The Japanese B Encephalitis Virus is transmitted by the bite of infected mosquitoes in certain areas of the world, particularly Asia. This disorder most commonly affects children and tends to be more actively spread during the summer. Symptoms include high fever, headaches, weakness, nausea, vomiting, paralysis, personality changes, and coma, possibly leading to neurological damage or death.

In addition to The National Organization for Rare Disorders (NORD) listed in Section III, the following organizations in Section II (Disease Specific) and in Section III (Umbrella) and Section IV (Government Agencies) can provide more information:
Centers for Disease Control and Prevention, *IV*
NIH/National Institute of Allergy and Infectious Diseases, *IV*
World Health Organization (WHO) Regional Office for the Americas (AMRO), *III*

367 ENCEPHALITIS, RASMUSSEN'S

Rasmussen's Encephalitis is a rare central nervous system disorder characterized by chronic inflammation of the brain (encephalitis) and episodes of uncontrolled electrical disturbances in the brain that cause convulsive seizures (epilepsy). Progressive symptoms including paralysis of one side of the body (hemiparesis) and mental retardation may also occur. Although the exact cause of this disorder is not known, it is thought to result from an unidentified viral infection.

In addition to The National Organization for Rare Disorders (NORD) listed in Section III, the following organizations in Section II (Disease Specific) and in Section III (Umbrella) and Section IV (Government Agencies) can provide more information:

Centers for Disease Control and Prevention, *IV*
NIH/National Institute of Neurological Disorders and Stroke, *IV*
Rasmussen's Syndrome and Hemispherectomy Support Network, *II*
The Arc (a national organization on mental retardation), *III*

368 ENCEPHALOCELE

Encephalocele is a rare disorder in which an infant is born with a gap in the skull. The membranes that cover the brain (meninges), and brain tissue, protrude through this gap. This disorder is probably caused by failure of the neural tube to close during development of a fetus.

In addition to The National Organization for Rare Disorders (NORD) listed in Section III, the following organizations in Section II (Disease Specific) and in Section III (Umbrella) and Section IV (Government Agencies) can provide more information:

AboutFace U.S.A., *III*
Children's Craniofacial Association, *III*
FACES: The National Craniofacial Association, *III*
Fighters for Encephaly Support Group, *III*
Forward Face, Inc., *III*
Guardians of Hydrocephalus Research Foundation, *II*
Hydrocephalus Association, *II*
NIH/National Institute of Child Health and Human Development, *IV*
NIH/National Institute of Neurological Disorders and Stroke, *IV*
National Hydrocephalus Foundation, *II*

369 ENCEPHALOMYELITIS, MYALGIC

Myalgic Encephalomyelitis is thought to be an infectious disorder affecting the central, peripheral and autonomic nervous systems and the muscles. Major symptoms may include general exhaustion, headache, muscle pain, weakness, and possible mental changes. The exact cause of this disorder is not known, but researchers believe a virus associated with an immune system abnormality may be responsible. Adults are most commonly affected, with more cases seen in females than in males. Epidemics of Myalgic Encephalomyelitis have occurred worldwide, but cases tend to appear sporadically. Symptoms can resolve in a few weeks but may recur at any time. Other cases may persist for many years.

In addition to The National Organization for Rare Disorders (NORD) listed in Section III, the following organizations in Section II (Disease Specific) and in Section III (Umbrella) and Section IV (Government Agencies) can provide more information:

Centers for Disease Control and Prevention, *IV*
NIH/National Institute of Allergy and Infectious Diseases, *IV*

370 ENDOCARDIAL FIBROELASTOSIS (EFE)

Endocardial Fibroelastosis (EFE) is a rare heart disorder that affects infants and children. It is characterized by a thickening within the muscular lining of the heart chambers due to an increase in the amount of supporting connective tissue (inelastic collagen) and elastic fibers. The normal heart has four chambers. Two chambers, known as atria, are separated from each other by a partition called the atrial septum. The other two chambers, known as ventricles, are also separated by a septum. Valves connect the atria (left and right) to their respective ventricles.

The symptoms of Endocardial Fibroelastosis are related to the overgrowth of fibrous tissues causing abnormal enlargement of the heart (cardiac hypertrophy), especially the left ventricle. Impaired heart and lung function eventually lead to congestive heart failure. Endocardial Fibroelastosis may occur for no apparent reason (sporadic) or may be inherited as an X-linked (EFE2) or autosomal recessive (EFE1) genetic trait.

In addition to The National Organization for Rare Disorders (NORD) listed in Section III, the following organizations in Section II (Disease Specific) and in Section III (Umbrella) and Section IV (Government Agencies) can provide more information:

Alliance of Genetic Support Groups, *III*
American Heart Association, *III*
Big Hearts for Little Hearts, *III*
Congenital Heart Anomalies, Support, Education, & Resources, *III*
NIH/National Heart, Lung and Blood Institute, *IV*

371 ENDOCARDITIS, INFECTIVE

Infective endocarditis is a bacterial infection of the inner lining of the heart muscle (endocardium). This inner lining also covers the heart valves, and it is these valves which are primarily affected by infective endocarditis. If the infection remains untreated, multiplying bacteria may eventually destroy the valves and result in heart failure. Bacteria may also form small clots (emboli) which move through the blood and block small arteries. These clots may lodge in various parts of the body including the brain and cause serious damage.

There are several forms of infective endocarditis. Two types that have similar symptoms but are caused by different bacteria are acute bacterial endocarditis and subacute bacterial endocarditis. Acute bacterial endocarditis may affect normal heart valves, while subacute bacterial endocarditis more commonly affects heart valves which have been previously damaged by disease. A third type of infective endocarditis, prosthetic valvular endocarditis (PVE), may develop in patients who have previously had artificial (prosthetic) valve replacement or tissue valve replacement.

In addition to The National Organization for Rare Disorders (NORD) listed in Section III, the following organizations in Section II (Disease Specific) and in Section III (Umbrella) and Section IV (Government Agencies) can provide more information:

American Heart Association, *III*
Centers for Disease Control and Prevention, *IV*
NIH/National Heart, Lung and Blood Institute Information Center, *IV*

372 ENDOMETRIOSIS

Endometriosis is a prevalent gynecological condition that affects women. It is characterized by an inability to shed the build-up of tissue that normally forms in the uterus (endometrium) before menstruation. As a result the built-up tissue escapes from the uterus and spreads to other parts of the pelvic area, sometimes spreading as far as the lungs. Major symptoms may include lower back pain, pain in the thighs or excessive pain during the menstrual cycle, repeated miscarriages, and infertility. Bleeding from the rectum or bladder may also occur.

In addition to The National Organization for Rare Disorders (NORD) listed in Section III, the following organizations in Section II (Disease Specific) and in Section III (Umbrella) and Section IV (Government Agencies) can provide more information:

Endometriosis Association, *II*
NIH/National Institute of Child Health and Human Development, *IV*
National Women's Health Network, *III*

373 ENDOMYOCARDIAL FIBROSIS

Endomyocardial Fibrosis is a heart disease of unknown origin in which the most characteristic feature is a gross fibrosis of the lining of the heart cavities (the endocardium) of one or both ventricles. Fibrosis progresses towards constriction of the ventricular cavities and involvement of the chordae tendinae and atrioventricular valves. Loeffler's disease is a disease of the heart and small arteries, of unknown origin, characterized by eosinophilia, gross fibrosis of the endocardium, small vessel arteritis and infiltration of other organs. Endomyocardial Fibrosis is thought to be a late stage of Loeffler's disease by some authorities.

In addition to The National Organization for Rare Disorders (NORD) listed in Section III, the following organizations in Section II (Disease Specific) and in Section III (Umbrella) and Section IV (Government Agencies) can provide more information:

American Heart Association, *III*
Centers for Disease Control and Prevention, *IV*
Congenital Heart Anomalies, Support, Education, & Resources, *III*
NIH/Developmental Endocrinology Branch, *IV*
NIH/National Institute of Child Health and Human Development, *IV*

374 ENGELMANN DISEASE

Engelmann Disease is a rare genetic disorder characterized by progressive widening and malformation of the shafts of the long bones (diaphyseal dysplasia). Major symptoms may include bone pain, particularly in the legs; skeletal abnormalities; and/or weakness and underdevelopment (hypoplasia) of various muscles. Pain and weakness of the leg muscles may result in an unusual "waddling" walk (gait). Skeletal malformations may include abnormal side-to-side or inward curvature of the spine (scoliosis or lumbar lordosis) and/or hardening (sclerosis) of the bones near the base of the skull and, in rare cases, the jaw. Engelmann Disease is inherited as an autosomal dominant genetic trait.

In addition to The National Organization for Rare Disorders (NORD) listed in Section III, the following organizations in Section II (Disease Specific) and in Section III (Umbrella) and Section IV (Government

Agencies) can provide more information:
NIH/National Arthritis and Musculoskeletal and Skin Diseases Information Clearinghouse, *IV*

375 ENTEROBIASIS

Enterobiasis or pinworm infection is the most common type of parasitic infection found in children. The infection is contracted by swallowing or inhaling the tiny eggs of the pinworm. Enterobiasis rarely causes any physical problems, except for the main symptom, severe rectal itching.

In addition to The National Organization for Rare Disorders (NORD) listed in Section III, the following organizations in Section II (Disease Specific) and in Section III (Umbrella) and Section IV (Government Agencies) can provide more information:
Centers for Disease Control and Prevention, *IV*
NIH/National Institute of Allergy and Infectious Diseases, *IV*

376 EOSINOPHILIA MYALGIA

Eosinophilia Myalgia Syndrome is a disorder associated with the oral use of large doses of tryptophan (also known as L-Tryptophan), a dietary supplement often sold in health food stores. It is a disease of abrupt onset causing severe, disabling, chronic muscle pain, skin symptoms and other neurotoxic reactions . It can be diagnosed by finding unusually high levels of eosinophils in the blood (white cells).

In addition to The National Organization for Rare Disorders (NORD) listed in Section III, the following organizations in Section II (Disease Specific) and in Section III (Umbrella) and Section IV (Government Agencies) can provide more information:
Centers for Disease Control and Prevention, *IV*
NIH/National Institute of Arthritis and Musculoskeletal and Skin Diseases, *IV*
Scleroderma Federation, Inc., *II*

377 EOSINOPHILIC FASCIITIS

Eosinophilic Fasciitis is a disorder of unknown cause characterized by symmetric and painful inflammation and loss of elasticity in the tissues of the hands, arms, legs and feet. The disorder has been recently recognized as a variant of Scleroderma, a disease in which connective tissue in the body shrinks and hardens. Eosinophilic Fasciitis most commonly affects middle- aged men. It has also been related to ingestion of L-Tryptophan, a food supplement sold in health food stores as a sleeping aid.

In addition to The National Organization for Rare Disorders (NORD) listed in Section III, the following organizations in Section II (Disease Specific) and in Section III (Umbrella) and Section IV (Government Agencies) can provide more information:
American Autoimmune Related Diseases Association, Inc., *III*
Centers for Disease Control and Prevention, *IV*
Eosinophilic Fasciitis (Shulman's Syndrome) Home Page, *II*
NIH/National Institute of Allergy and Infectious Diseases, *IV*
Scleroderma Federation, Inc., *II*

378 EPIDERMAL NEVUS SYNDROME

Epidermal Nevus Syndrome is a rare disorder characterized by distinctive birth marks (nevus) on the skin. Neurological and skeletal abnormalities may also occur. This disorder is usually apparent at birth (due to the skin lesions which are most often seen in the mid-face from the forehead down into the nasal area) and is often associated with seizures, mental deficiency, eye problems, bone malformations and atrophy of the brain. The exact cause of Epidermal Nevus Syndrome is not known although an autosomal dominant trait of inheritance seems to occur in approximately two thirds of the cases.

In addition to The National Organization for Rare Disorders (NORD) listed in Section III, the following organizations in Section II (Disease Specific) and in Section III (Umbrella) and Section IV (Government Agencies) can provide more information:
Foundation for Ichthyosis & Related Skin Types, *III*
HME Contact Group, *II*
NIH/National Arthritis and Musculoskeletal and Skin Diseases Information Clearinghouse, *IV*
Naevus Support Group, *II*
Nevus Network, *II*
Nevus Outreach, Inc., *II*

379 EPIDERMOLYSIS BULLOSA

Epidermolysis Bullosa (EB) refers to a group of rare, hereditary skin diseases. It is characterized by fragile skin in which blisters and raised areas, that usually contain fluid (vesicles), develop following minor trauma. In some forms of EB the mucous membranes are involved. Healing is impaired in some forms, causing multiple scars or damage to underlying muscle tissue (contractures).

In addition to The National Organization for Rare Disorders (NORD) listed in Section III, the following organizations in Section II (Disease Specific) and in Section III (Umbrella) and Section IV (Government Agencies) can provide more information:
Alliance of Genetic Support Groups, *III*
Dystrophic Epidermolysis Bullosa Research Association of America, Inc., *III*

Dystrophic Epidermolysis Bullosa Research Association-United Kingdom, *II*
March of Dimes Birth Defects Foundation, *III*
NIH/National Arthritis and Musculoskeletal and Skin Diseases Information Clearinghouse, *IV*
NIH/National Cancer Institute, *IV*

380 EPIDERMOLYTIC HYPERKERATOSIS

Epidermolytic Hyperkeratosis is a hereditary skin disorder that is characterized by thick, blistery, warty hardening of the skin over most of the body. This disorder is a form of Ichthyosis which is a group of rare skin diseases.

In addition to The National Organization for Rare Disorders (NORD) listed in Section III, the following organizations in Section II (Disease Specific) and in Section III (Umbrella) and Section IV (Government Agencies) can provide more information:
Foundation for Ichthyosis & Related Skin Types, *III*
NIH/National Arthritis and Musculoskeletal and Skin Diseases Information Clearinghouse, *IV*

381 EPIDIDYMITIS

Epididymitis is inflammation of the long, tightly coiled tube behind each testicle (epididymis) that carries sperm from the testicle to the spermatic duct. Affected individuals usually have painful swelling of the one epididymitis and the associated testicle. In some cases, the second testicle may also be tender. In addition, affected individuals have fever, painful swelling and redness (erythema) of the scrotum, and/or inflammation of the tube from which urine is carried from the bladder (urethritis). The two main forms of epididymitis are the sexally-transmitted form and the nonspecific bacterial form.

In addition to The National Organization for Rare Disorders (NORD) listed in Section III, the following organizations in Section II (Disease Specific) and in Section III (Umbrella) and Section IV (Government Agencies) can provide more information:
American Social Health Association, *III*
Centers for Disease Control and Prevention, *IV*
NIH/National Institute of Child Health and Human Development, *IV*

382 EPILEPSY

Epilepsy is a group of disorders of the central nervous system characterized by repeated convulsive (paroxysomal) electrical disturbances in the brain. The major symptoms may include loss of consciousness, convulsions, spasms, sensory confusion and disturbances in the nerves that control involuntary body functions (autonomic nervous system). Episodes of these symptoms are frequently preceded by an "aura." An aura is described as a feeling of uneasiness or sensory discomfort that precedes the onset of a seizure.

Epilepsy may take several different forms including: Grand Mal Epilepsy (Major Epilepsy, Status Epilepticus); Jacksonian Epilepsy (Focal Epilepsy); Myoclonic Progressive Familial Epilepsy (Unverricht Syndrome, Lundborg- Unverricht Disease, Unverricht-Lundborg-Laf Disease); Petit Mal Epilepsy (Minor Epilepsy, Pyknoepilepsy, Akinetic Seizure, Myoclonic seizure); Myoclonic Astatic Petit Mal Epilepsy (Lennox-Gastaut Syndrome, Petit Mal Variant); Febrile Seizures; and Psychomotor Epilepsy (Temporal Lobe Epilepsy, Psychomotor Equivalent, Psychomotor Convulsion with Epilepsia Procursiva, Abdominal Epilepsy).

In addition to The National Organization for Rare Disorders (NORD) listed in Section III, the following organizations in Section II (Disease Specific) and in Section III (Umbrella) and Section IV (Government Agencies) can provide more information:
Alliance of Genetic Support Groups, *III*
Antiepileptic Drug Pregnancy Registry, *II*
Epilepsy Canada, *II*
Epilepsy Foundation of America, *III*
March of Dimes Birth Defects Foundation, *III*
NIH/National Institute of Neurological Disorders and Stroke, *IV*

383 EPILEPSY, MYOCLONIC PROGRESSIVE FAMILIAL

Myoclonic Progressive Familial Epilepsy is a disorder of the central nervous system. It begins in childhood, and is progressive. The main characteristic of this form of myoclonus is jerking involuntary muscle movements may involve muscles in the limbs or the whole body. As the disease progresses, there is impairment of mental capabilities, which may lead to loss of reason (dementia). Myoclonic epilepsy can be a symptom of many central nervous system disorders.

In addition to The National Organization for Rare Disorders (NORD) listed in Section III, the following organizations in Section II (Disease Specific) and in Section III (Umbrella) and Section IV (Government Agencies) can provide more information:
Epilepsy Canada, *II*
Epilepsy Foundation of America, *III*
Myoclonus Research Foundation, *III*
NIH/National Institute of Neurological Disorders and

Stroke, *IV*
National Pediatric Myoclonus Center, *II*
WE MOVE, *III*

384 **EPITHELIOPATHY, ACUTE POSTERIOR MULTIFOCAL PLACOID PIGMENT**

Acute Posterior Multifocal Placoid Pigment Epitheliopathy (APMPPE) is a rare eye disorder of unknown (idiopathic) cause. The disorder is characterized by the impairment of central vision in one eye (unilateral); within a few days, the second eye may also become affected (bilateral). In most cases, the disorder resolves within a few weeks without loss of clearness of vision (acuity). However, in some cases, visual acuity does not improve. In approximately 50 percent of the cases, an influenza-like illness preceded the development of the disorder.

In addition to The National Organization for Rare Disorders (NORD) listed in Section III, the following organizations in Section II (Disease Specific) and in Section III (Umbrella) and Section IV (Government Agencies) can provide more information:
NIH/National Eye Institute, *IV*
National Association for Visually Handicapped, *III*
Vision Foundation, Inc., *III*

385 **ERB'S PALSY**

Erb's Palsy is caused by an injury to one or more nerves that control and supply the muscles of the shoulder and upper extremities (upper brachial plexus). It is usually seen in newborns and occurs as a result of a difficult delivery.

In addition to The National Organization for Rare Disorders (NORD) listed in Section III, the following organizations in Section II (Disease Specific) and in Section III (Umbrella) and Section IV (Government Agencies) can provide more information:
Brachial Plexus Injury (Erb's Palsy Support & Information Network), *II*
Brachial Plexus Palsy Foundation, *II*
Erb's Palsy Group, *II*
NIH/National Institute of Arthritis and Musculoskeletal and Skin Diseases, *IV*
Support Group for Brachial Plexus Injury, *II*

386 **ERDHEIM CHESTER DISEASE**

Erdheim-Chester Disease is an extremely rare lipid storage disorder. It is characterized by hardening of the growth areas of the long bones of the body. Fatty-like (lipid) cell deposits (histiocytes) are found in various vital organs of the body such as: heart, lungs, the lining of the abdominal cavity (peritoneum), the kidneys, and other tissues. Severity of the disease differs with each patient.

In addition to The National Organization for Rare Disorders (NORD) listed in Section III, the following organizations in Section II (Disease Specific) and in Section III (Umbrella) and Section IV (Government Agencies) can provide more information:
NIH/National Arthritis and Musculoskeletal and Skin Diseases Information Clearinghouse, *IV*

387 **ERYSIPELAS**

Erysipelas is a bacterial infection characterized by a spreading inflammation of the skin and its underlying tissue (cellulitis) particularly on the face, arms or legs. It is a type of cellulitis that is due to an acute infection by streptococci or staphylococcus bacteria.

In addition to The National Organization for Rare Disorders (NORD) listed in Section III, the following organizations in Section II (Disease Specific) and in Section III (Umbrella) and Section IV (Government Agencies) can provide more information:
Centers for Disease Control and Prevention, *IV*
NIH/National Institute of Allergy and Infectious Diseases, *IV*

388 **ERYTHEMA MULTIFORME**

Erythema Multiforme is an inflammatory skin disorder characterized by symmetric red and blistery (bullous) lesions of the skin or mucous membranes of the hands, feet and eyelids.

In addition to The National Organization for Rare Disorders (NORD) listed in Section III, the following organizations in Section II (Disease Specific) and in Section III (Umbrella) and Section IV (Government Agencies) can provide more information:
NIH/National Institute of Arthritis and Musculoskeletal and Skin Diseases, *IV*

389 **ERYTHROKERATODERMIA WITH ATAXIA**

Erythrokeratodermia with Ataxia is a hereditary skin disorder characterized by groups of red hardened plaques that develop during infancy and childhood. After these skin lesions heal, a neurological syndrome develops during adulthood. Skin symptoms may improve during the summer months. Erythrokeratodermia with Ataxia is thought to be inherited as an autosomal dominant genetic trait.

In addition to The National Organization for Rare Disorders (NORD) listed in Section III, the following organizations in Section II (Disease Specific) and in Section III (Umbrella) and Section IV (Government Agencies) can provide more information:
Foundation for Ichthyosis & Related Skin Types, *III*

NIH/National Arthritis and Musculoskeletal and Skin Diseases Information Clearinghouse, *IV*
National Registry for Ichthyosis and Related Disorders, *III*

390 ERYTHROMELALGIA

Erythromelalgia is a rare vascular disorder that affects the skin of the feet and/or hands and is characterized by episodes of sudden widening of the blood vessels (paroxysmal vasodilatation) in these areas. Symptoms may include severe burning pain, redness, and/or increased skin temperature.

Primary or Familial Erythromelalgia is an inherited disorder. However, when the disorder occurs as a result of another underlying disease, it is called Secondary Erythromelalgia.

In addition to The National Organization for Rare Disorders (NORD) listed in Section III, the following organizations in Section II (Disease Specific) and in Section III (Umbrella) and Section IV (Government Agencies) can provide more information:
Erythromelalgia and Related Disorders Association of America, *III*
NIH/National Institute of Arthritis and Musculoskeletal and Skin Diseases, *IV*

391 ERYTHROPOIETIC PROTOPORPHYRIA (EPP)

Erythropoietic Protoporphyria (EPP) is a rare inherited metabolic disorder characterized by a deficiency of the enzyme ferrochelatase (FECH). Due to abnormally low levels of this enzyme, excessive amounts of protoporphyrin accumulate in the plasma, red blood cells, and the liver. The major symptom of this disorder is hypersensitivity of the skin to sunlight and some types of artificial light, such as fluorescent lights (photosensitivity). After exposure to light, the skin may become itchy and red. Affected individuals may also experience a burning sensation on their skin. The hands, arms, and face are the most commonly affected areas. Some people with Erythropoietic Protoporphyria may also have complications related to liver and gallbladder function. Erythropoietic Protoporphyria is inherited as an autosomal dominant genetic trait.

Erythropoietic Protoporphyria is one of a group of disorders known as the porphyrias. The porphyrias are all characterized by abnormally high levels of particular chemicals (porphyrins) in the body due to deficiencies of certain enzymes. There are at least seven types of porphyria. The symptoms associated with the various types of porphyria differ, depending upon the specific enzyme that is deficient. It is important to note that people who have one type of porphyria do not develop any of the other types.

In addition to The National Organization for Rare Disorders (NORD) listed in Section III, the following organizations in Section II (Disease Specific) and in Section III (Umbrella) and Section IV (Government Agencies) can provide more information:
American Porphyria Foundation, *III*
Canadian Porphyria Foundation, Inc., *II*
Erythropoietic Protoporphyria Research and Education Fund, *II*
Metabolic Information Network, *III*
NIH/National Digestive Diseases Information Clearinghouse, *IV*
Research Trust for Metabolic Diseases in Children, *III*

392 ESOPHAGEAL ATRESIA AND/OR TRACHEOESOPHAGEAL FISTULA

Esophageal Atresia and Tracheoesophageal Fistula are disorders of the esophagus that may be inherited as an autosomal recessive genetic trait, or may result from developmental problems in a fetus. Esophageal Atresia is a condition in which the patient is born with an abnormality in the part of the digestive tube that runs from below the tongue to the stomach (esophagus). This disorder is commonly associated with Tracheoesophageal Fistula which is an abnormal tubelike passage between the windpipe and esophagus. Symptoms of these disorders may be excessive salivation, choking, the return of swallowed food into the mouth, and/or a swollen abdomen when a Tracheoesophageal Fistula is present.

In addition to The National Organization for Rare Disorders (NORD) listed in Section III, the following organizations in Section II (Disease Specific) and in Section III (Umbrella) and Section IV (Government Agencies) can provide more information:
EA/TEF Child and Family Support Connection, Inc., *III*
NIH/National Digestive Diseases Information Clearinghouse, *IV*
TEF/VATER/VACTRL National Support Network, *II*

393 ESSENTIAL IRIS ATROPHY

Essential Iris Atrophy is a very rare, progressive disorder of the eye characterized by a pupil that is out of place and/or distorted, areas of degeneration on the iris (atrophy), and/or holes in the iris. This disorder most frequently appears in young and middle-aged women, usually affecting only one eye (unilateral) and developing slowly over time. Attachment of portions of the iris to the cornea (peripheral anterior synechiae) and/or abnormalities in the cornea may lead to secondary glaucoma and vision loss.

In addition to The National Organization for Rare Disorders (NORD) listed in Section III, the following organizations in Section II (Disease Specific) and in Section III (Umbrella) and Section IV (Government Agencies) can provide more information:
Glaucoma Research Foundation, *II*
NIH/National Eye Institute, *IV*
National Association for Parents of the Visually Impaired, *III*
National Association for Visually Handicapped, *III*
Prevent Blindness America, *III*

394 EXOSTOSES, MULTIPLE

Multiple Exostoses is a rare disorder that is inherited as an autosomal dominant genetic trait. This disorder is characterized by multiple bony growths or tumors (exostoses) that are covered by cartilage. The bone tumors continue to grow until shortly after puberty and may cause deformities especially of the ankle, knee, and wrist.

In addition to The National Organization for Rare Disorders (NORD) listed in Section III, the following organizations in Section II (Disease Specific) and in Section III (Umbrella) and Section IV (Government Agencies) can provide more information:
MHE (Multiple Hereditary Exostoses) Family Support Group, *II*
NIH/National Arthritis and Musculoskeletal and Skin Diseases Information Clearinghouse, *IV*

395 EXSTROPHY OF THE BLADDER

Exstrophy of the Bladder is a rare developmental abnormality that is present at birth (congenital) and is characterized by the absence of a portion of the lower abdominal wall and the front part of the bladder wall (anterior vesical wall). The rear portion of the bladder wall (posterior vesical wall) turns outward (exstrophy) through the opening in the abdominal wall and urine is excreted through this opening. The exact cause of Exstrophy of the Bladder is not known. The physical characteristics of this disorder are the result of developmental abnormalities during embryonic or fetal growth.

In addition to The National Organization for Rare Disorders (NORD) listed in Section III, the following organizations in Section II (Disease Specific) and in Section III (Umbrella) and Section IV (Government Agencies) can provide more information:
American Foundation for Urologic Disease, *III*
NIH/National Kidney and Urologic Diseases Information Clearinghouse, *IV*
National Association for Continence, *III*

396 FG SYNDROME

FG Syndrome is an uncommon hereditary disorder that affects males. The presence and severity of symptoms vary from patient to patient. Some females may have certain physical characteristics related to FG Syndrome because they are "carriers" of the trait, but they are not affected by the disorder itself.

Males with FG Syndrome may have mental retardation, an absence of an anal opening (imperforate anus) or an abnormally placed anus, constipation, diminished muscle tone (hypotonia), a large head and certain other physical characteristics. Deafness may be present in some patients. Individuals with FG Syndrome seem to have a specific personality type and are often friendly, outgoing, and hyperactive with a short attention span.

In addition to The National Organization for Rare Disorders (NORD) listed in Section III, the following organizations in Section II (Disease Specific) and in Section III (Umbrella) and Section IV (Government Agencies) can provide more information:
NIH/National Institute of Child Health and Human Development, *IV*

397 FABRY DISEASE

Fabry Disease is a rare inherited disorder of lipid metabolism characterized by the abnormal accumulation of certain fatty substances (i.e., glycolipids such as glycosphingolipid) in various organs of the body. Symptoms may include clusters of wart-like discolorations on the skin (angiokeratomas), abdominal pain, and/or visual impairment. Later in the course of the disease, kidney failure, heart problems, and/or neurological symptoms may cause serious complications. Fabry Disease is inherited as an X-linked recessive genetic trait, and affects mostly males. A milder form of the disease has been identified in females.

In addition to The National Organization for Rare Disorders (NORD) listed in Section III, the following organizations in Section II (Disease Specific) and in Section III (Umbrella) and Section IV (Government Agencies) can provide more information:
Association for Neuro-Metabolic Disorders, *III*
Fabry Disease Home Page, *II*
Fabry Support & Information Group, *II*
International Center for Fabry Disease, *II*
Metabolic Information Network, *III*
Morbus Fabry Homepage Germany, *II*
NIH/National Institute of Neurological Disorders and

Stroke, *IV*
National Lipid Diseases Foundation, *III*
National Tay-Sachs and Allied Diseases Association, Inc., *III*
Research Trust for Metabolic Diseases in Children, *III*

398 FACTOR IX DEFICIENCY

Factor IX Deficiency is a severe genetic bleeding disorder that resembles classic Hemophilia A, although it occurs only one-fifth as often as Hemophilia A. Factor IX is a component of the blood clotting substance thromboplastin. It is deficient at birth in patients with this disorder. Factor IX Deficiency varies in severity between families and occurs most often among males. In rare instances, female carriers have been known to exhibit this deficiency in a mild form. Symptoms include prolonged bleeding episodes, and in very severe cases, joint pain and bone deformities.

In addition to The National Organization for Rare Disorders (NORD) listed in Section III, the following organizations in Section II (Disease Specific) and in Section III (Umbrella) and Section IV (Government Agencies) can provide more information:
NIH/National Heart, Lung and Blood Institute Information Center, *IV*
National Hemophilia Foundation, *II*

399 FACTOR XIII DEFICIENCY

Factor XIII Deficiency is an extremely rare inherited blood disorder characterized by abnormal blood clotting that may result in abnormal bleeding. Associated symptoms and findings occur as the result of a deficiency in the blood clotting factor F13A1 (Factor XIII). In affected individuals, the blood fails to clot appropriately, resulting in poor wound healing. Blood may seep into surrounding soft tissues, resulting in local pain and swelling. Internal bleeding may occur; approximately 25 percent of affected individuals experience bleeding in the brain (intracranial hemorrhage). Factor XIII Deficiency may be inherited as an autosomal dominant genetic trait. The disease may also be acquired in association with other disorders such as Sickle Cell Disease or Henoch-Schonlein Purpura.

In addition to The National Organization for Rare Disorders (NORD) listed in Section III, the following organizations in Section II (Disease Specific) and in Section III (Umbrella) and Section IV (Government Agencies) can provide more information:
Alliance of Genetic Support Groups, *III*
March of Dimes Birth Defects Foundation, *III*
NIH/National Heart, Lung and Blood Institute, *IV*
National Hemophilia Foundation, *II*

400 FAHR'S DISEASE

Fahr's Disease is a rare neurological disorder characterized by abnormal calcium deposits in certain areas of the brain. Major symptoms develop when these deposits accumulate including progressive deterioration of mental functioning, loss of previous motor development, spastic paralysis and twisting movements of the hands and feet (athetosis). Mental retardation and optic atrophy can also occur. In many cases, this disorder is inherited, although some cases may appear with no apparent genetic cause.

In addition to The National Organization for Rare Disorders (NORD) listed in Section III, the following organizations in Section II (Disease Specific) and in Section III (Umbrella) and Section IV (Government Agencies) can provide more information:
Association of Birth Defect Children, Inc., *III*
NIH/National Institute of Neurological Disorders and Stroke, *IV*

401 FAIRBANK DISEASE

Fairbank Disease is a mild form of dwarfism inherited as a dominant trait. Symptoms may not be apparent during early childhood, but pain may later occur in hips, knees or ankles due to developmental abnormalities of bones in the hips. Stature may be only slightly shortened while arms, legs, fingers or toes may be unusually short. In some cases, movement may be somewhat restricted.

In addition to The National Organization for Rare Disorders (NORD) listed in Section III, the following organizations in Section II (Disease Specific) and in Section III (Umbrella) and Section IV (Government Agencies) can provide more information:
Human Growth Foundation, *III*
MAGIC Foundation for Children's Growth, *III*
NIH/National Institute of Child Health and Human Development, *IV*
Short Stature Foundation, *III*

402 FARBER'S DISEASE

Farber's Disease is a rare inherited metabolic disorder. Major symptoms may include hoarseness, painful and swollen joints, nodules under the skin, and growths in the lungs and other parts of the body. The heart and lymph nodes may also be involved. Difficulty in breathing may necessitate the implantation of a breathing tube (tracheostomy) in the throat. Farber's Disease is inherited as an autosomal recessive genetic trait

In addition to The National Organization for Rare Disorders (NORD) listed in Section III, the following organizations in Section II (Disease Specific) and in Section III (Umbrella) and Section IV (Government Agencies) can provide more information:
Arthritis Foundation, *III*
Association for Neuro-Metabolic Disorders, *III*
Metabolic Information Network, *III*
NIH/National Arthritis and Musculoskeletal and Skin Diseases Information Clearinghouse, *IV*
Research Trust for Metabolic Diseases in Children, *III*
Vaincre Les Maladies Lysosomales, *III*

403 FASCIOLIASIS

Fascioliasis is a rare infectious disorder caused by parasites. These parasites are liver flukes that live in plant-eating animals. Liver flukes can be found on water plants in certain parts of the world. When the parasite invades the liver, bile passages may be blocked. A subdivision of Fascioliasis called Halzoun Syndrome affects the throat (pharynx). This infection can usually be controlled and/or cured with timely treatment.

In addition to The National Organization for Rare Disorders (NORD) listed in Section III, the following organizations in Section II (Disease Specific) and in Section III (Umbrella) and Section IV (Government Agencies) can provide more information:
American Liver Foundation, *III*
Centers for Disease Control and Prevention, *IV*
NIH/National Institute of Allergy and Infectious Diseases, *IV*
United Liver Association, *III*

404 FELTY SYNDROME

Felty Syndrome is a rare form of Rheumatoid Arthritis, a disorder characterized by painful, stiff, and swollen joints. Major symptoms and physical findings of Felty Syndrome include an unusually large spleen (splenomegaly) and abnormally low levels of certain white blood cells (neutophils [neutropenia]). As a result of neutropenia, affected individuals may have an increased susceptibility to certain infections. Other symptoms associated with Felty Syndrome may include fatigue, fever, weight loss, and/or discoloration of patches of skin (brown pigmentation). The exact cause of Felty Syndrome is unknown. It is believed to be an autoimmune disorder.

In addition to The National Organization for Rare Disorders (NORD) listed in Section III, the following organizations in Section II (Disease Specific) and in Section III (Umbrella) and Section IV (Government Agencies) can provide more information:
Arthritis Foundation, *III*
NIH/National Arthritis and Musculoskeletal and Skin Diseases Information Clearinghouse, *IV*

405 FEMORAL-FACIAL SYNDROME

Femoral-Facial Syndrome is a rare disorder that occurs for no apparent reason (sporadically). However, there have been two reported cases in which the disorder was believed to be inherited as an autosomal dominant genetic trait. The major symptoms of this disorder are underdeveloped thigh bones and unusual facial features.

In addition to The National Organization for Rare Disorders (NORD) listed in Section III, the following organizations in Section II (Disease Specific) and in Section III (Umbrella) and Section IV (Government Agencies) can provide more information:
NIH/National Arthritis and Musculoskeletal and Skin Diseases Information Clearinghouse, *IV*

406 FETAL ALCOHOL SYNDROME

Fetal Alcohol Syndrome (FAS) is a combination of various birth defects involving both physical and mental impairments. Extensive scientific research into the effects of alcohol on a developing fetus has established that use of alcohol during pregnancy poses a serious threat to the health of the unborn child. FAS is characterized by a combination of the following: prenatal or postnatal growth retardation; central nervous system (brain and spinal cord) dysfunction; an unusually small head (microcephaly); abnormal smallness of the eyes (microphthalmia); narrowing of the eyelid folds (palpebral fissures); and an unusually short vertical groove in the thin upper lip (hypoplastic philtrum) and flattening of the maxillary area.

In addition to The National Organization for Rare Disorders (NORD) listed in Section III, the following organizations in Section II (Disease Specific) and in Section III (Umbrella) and Section IV (Government Agencies) can provide more information:
Family Empowerment Network: Supporting Families Affected by FAS/FAE, *II*
Fetal Alcohol Education Program, *II*
NIH/Institute on Alcohol Abuse and Alcoholism, *IV*
NIH/National Institute of Mental Health, *IV*
National Alliance for the Mentally Ill, *III*
National Mental Health Association, *III*
National Mental Health Consumer Self-Help Clearinghouse, *III*
National Organization on Fetal Alcohol Syndrome, *II*
The Arc (a national organization on mental retardation), *III*

407 FETAL HYDANTOIN SYNDROME

Fetal Hydantoin Syndrome is a rare disorder that is caused by exposure of a fetus to phenytoin (Dilantin) which is an anticonvulsant drug prescribed for epilepsy. Major symptoms of this disorder may include abnormalities of the skull and facial features, growth deficiencies, underdeveloped nails of the fingers and toes, and/or developmental delays.

In addition to The National Organization for Rare Disorders (NORD) listed in Section III, the following organizations in Section II (Disease Specific) and in Section III (Umbrella) and Section IV (Government Agencies) can provide more information:

Cleft Palate Foundation, *III*

NIH/National Institute of Child Health and Human Development, *IV*

408 FETAL VALPROATE SYNDROME

Fetal Valproate Syndrome is a rare congenital disorder caused by exposure of the fetus to valproic acid (dalpro, depakene, depakote, depakote sprinkle, divalproex, epival, myproic acid) during the first three months of pregnancy. Valproic acid is an anticonvulsant drug used to control certain types of seizures in the treatment of epilepsy. A small percentage of pregnant women who take this medication can have a child with Fetal Valproate Syndrome. The exact prevalence of this condition remains to be established. Symptoms of this disorder may include spina bifida, distinctive facial features, and other musculoskeletal abnormalities.

In addition to The National Organization for Rare Disorders (NORD) listed in Section III, the following organizations in Section II (Disease Specific) and in Section III (Umbrella) and Section IV (Government Agencies) can provide more information:

NIH/National Institute of Child Health and Human Development, *IV*

Spina Bifida Association of America, *II*

Spina Bifida and Hydrocephalus Association of Canada, *III*

409 FIBER TYPE DISPROPORTION, CONGENITAL

Congenital Fiber Type Disproportion (CFTD) is a rare genetic muscle disease that is apparent at birth. Major symptoms may include loss of muscle tone (hypotonia) and weakness, scoliosis, a drawing up of the muscles, high arched palate, dislocated hips, short stature, and deformities of the feet.

In addition to The National Organization for Rare Disorders (NORD) listed in Section III, the following organizations in Section II (Disease Specific) and in Section III (Umbrella) and Section IV (Government Agencies) can provide more information:

Muscular Dystrophy Association, *III*

NIH/National Institute of Neurological Disorders and Stroke, *IV*

410 FIBRODYSPLASIA OSSIFICANS PROGRESSIVA (FOP)

Fibrodysplasia Ossificans Progressiva (FOP) is a very rare inherited connective tissue disorder characterized by the abnormal development of bone in areas of the body where bone is not normally present (heterotopic ossification), such as the ligaments, tendons, and muscles. Major symptoms may include skeletal malformations and/or abnormally short and malformed toes and fingers. The abnormal development of bone may lead to stiffness in affected areas and may also limit movement in affected joints (e.g., knees, wrists, shoulders, spine, and/or neck). Fibrodysplasia Ossificans Progressiva usually begins during early childhood and progresses throughout life. Most cases of FOP occur randomly (sporadic). However, researchers believe that the defective gene(s) responsible for this disorder may be inherited as an autosomal dominant genetic trait.

In addition to The National Organization for Rare Disorders (NORD) listed in Section III, the following organizations in Section II (Disease Specific) and in Section III (Umbrella) and Section IV (Government Agencies) can provide more information:

British Coalition of Heritable Disorders of Connective Tissue, *III*

International Fibrodysplasia Ossificans Progressiva Association, *II*

NIH/National Arthritis and Musculoskeletal and Skin Diseases Information Clearinghouse, *IV*

411 FIBROMATOSIS, CONGENITAL GENERALIZED

Congenital Generalized Fibromatosis is a rare disorder characterized by multiple noncancerous tumors. It is an invasive and recurring disorder that can involve the bones, internal organs, skin and muscles. These tumors are usually present at, or may occur within a few months of birth.

In addition to The National Organization for Rare Disorders (NORD) listed in Section III, the following organizations in Section II (Disease Specific) and in Section III (Umbrella) and Section IV (Government Agencies) can provide more information:

American Cancer Society, Inc., *III*

NIH/Patient Referral Services Unit, *IV*

412 FIBROMYALGIA

Fibromyalgia is a chronic disorder characterized by pain throughout much of the body. The pain may begin gradually or have a sudden onset. Other symptoms are muscle spasms, fatigue, muscle tissue stiffness and non- restorative (unrefreshing) sleep. The exact cause of this disorder is unknown.

The terms Fibrositis, Fibromyositis, Periarticular Fibrositis and Rheumatoid Myositis are still being used by many to describe this condition. The ending of "itis" on each of these terms is actually incorrect. "Itis" means inflammation, and there is no inflammation in Fibromyalgia. The term Fibromyalgia has now become the accepted term, but many people continue to be diagnosed with the other synonyms. Tension Myalgia is another synonym that is currently being used.

In addition to The National Organization for Rare Disorders (NORD) listed in Section III, the following organizations in Section II (Disease Specific) and in Section III (Umbrella) and Section IV (Government Agencies) can provide more information:

American Chronic Pain Association, *III*
Arthritis Foundation, *III*
Fibromyalgia Alliance of America, Inc., *II*
Myositis Association of America, Inc., *III*
NIH/National Institute of Arthritis and Musculoskeletal and Skin Diseases, *IV*
National Chronic Fatigue Syndrome & Fibromyalgia Association, *II*
Ontario Fibromyalgia Association, *II*

413 FILARIASIS

Filariasis is an infectious tropical disease caused by the round worm parasites Wuchereria bancrofti or Brugia malayi. It is characterized by swollen lymph nodes (lymphadenopathy) and chronic lymphatic obstruction. Over extended periods of time obstruction of the flow of body fluid may cause profoundly swollen areas of the body (elephantiasis), especially the legs and external genitals. The larval form of the parasite is transmitted to humans by the bite of a mosquito. These invade the lymphatic system where they mature and reproduce. Symptoms are primarily a response to adult worms which cause inflammation. Chronic inflammation may progress to hardening of the lymphatic vessels (fibrosis) and obstruction of the lymph flow.

In addition to The National Organization for Rare Disorders (NORD) listed in Section III, the following organizations in Section II (Disease Specific) and in Section III (Umbrella) and Section IV (Government Agencies) can provide more information:

Centers for Disease Control and Prevention, *IV*
NIH/National Institute of Allergy and Infectious Diseases, *IV*
World Health Organization (WHO) Regional Office for the Americas (AMRO), *III*

414 FILIPPI SYNDROME

Filippi Syndrome is a very rare disorder characterized by webbing of the fingers and toes (syndactyly), permanently bent fingers (clinodactyly), an abnormally small head (microcephaly), severe to mild mental and physical retardation, and an unusual facial appearance. This disorder is thought to be inherited as an autosomal recessive genetic trait.

In addition to The National Organization for Rare Disorders (NORD) listed in Section III, the following organizations in Section II (Disease Specific) and in Section III (Umbrella) and Section IV (Government Agencies) can provide more information:

NIH/National Institute of Child Health and Human Development, *IV*

415 FITZ HUGH CURTIS SYNDROME

Fitz-Hugh-Curtis Syndrome is a rare disorder that develops in females as a result of complications of pelvic inflammatory disease. The disorder is characterized by string-like scar tissue (adhesions) that attaches between the liver and other sites in the abdominal lining (peritoneum). Symptoms can mimic those of hepatitis. Severe pain in the upper right area of the abdomen is usually present. Infection occurs, caused by the Chlamydia trachomatis bacteria.

In addition to The National Organization for Rare Disorders (NORD) listed in Section III, the following organizations in Section II (Disease Specific) and in Section III (Umbrella) and Section IV (Government Agencies) can provide more information:

Centers for Disease Control and Prevention, *IV*
NIH/National Institute of Allergy and Infectious Diseases, *IV*
Sexuality Information and Education Council of the U.S., *III*

416 FLOATING-HARBOR SYNDROME

Floating-Harbor Syndrome is a very rare disorder characterized by short stature, delayed language skills, and a triangular shaped face. A broad nose, deep-set eyes and a wide mouth with thin lips give the affected patient a distinct appearance. FHS was named for the first two patients who were seen at Boston Floating Hospital and Harbor General Hospital in California. The cause of this disorder is not known.

In addition to The National Organization for Rare Disorders (NORD) listed in Section III, the following organizations in Section II (Disease Specific) and in Section III (Umbrella) and Section IV (Government Agencies) can provide more information:
Human Growth Foundation, *III*
NIH/National Arthritis and Musculoskeletal and Skin Diseases Information Clearinghouse, *IV*
Short Stature Foundation, *III*

417 FOCAL DERMAL HYPOPLASIA

Focal Dermal Hypoplasia is a rare form of ectodermal dysplasia that is thought to be inherited as an X-linked dominant genetic trait with lethality in males. It is found primarily in females. This disorder is characterized by skin abnormalities in which there are underdeveloped areas of skin that form streaks or lines and tumor-like herniations of fat on the skin. Skeletal, facial, dental, ocular and soft tissue defects are also present.

In addition to The National Organization for Rare Disorders (NORD) listed in Section III, the following organizations in Section II (Disease Specific) and in Section III (Umbrella) and Section IV (Government Agencies) can provide more information:
NIH/National Arthritis and Musculoskeletal and Skin Diseases Information Clearinghouse, *IV*
NIH/National Oral Health Information Clearinghouse, *IV*
National Foundation for Ectodermal Dysplasias, *II*

418 FORBES ALBRIGHT SYNDROME

Forbes-Albright Syndrome is a rare endocrine disorder characterized by the abnormal production of breast milk (lactation), lack of ovulation (anovulation), and the absence of regular menstrual periods (amenorrhea). This disorder is usually caused by a hormone secreting tumor of the pituitary or hypothalamus gland (adenoma) which produces excessive amounts of prolactin.

In addition to The National Organization for Rare Disorders (NORD) listed in Section III, the following organizations in Section II (Disease Specific) and in Section III (Umbrella) and Section IV (Government Agencies) can provide more information:
NIH/National Institute of Child Health and Human Development, *IV*
National Women's Health Network, *III*
National Women's Health Resource Center, *III*

419 FORBES DISEASE

Forbes Disease is a glycogen storage disorder inherited through autosomal recessive genes. Symptoms are caused by a lack of the enzyme amylo-1,6 glucosidase (debrancher enzyme). This enzyme deficiency causes excess amounts of glycogen (the stored form of energy that comes from carbohydrates) to be deposited in the liver, muscles and heart. The heart may be involved in some cases.

In addition to The National Organization for Rare Disorders (NORD) listed in Section III, the following organizations in Section II (Disease Specific) and in Section III (Umbrella) and Section IV (Government Agencies) can provide more information:
Association for Neuro-Metabolic Disorders, *III*
Metabolic Information Network, *III*
Muscular Dystrophy Association, *III*
NIH/National Digestive Diseases Information Clearinghouse, *IV*
Research Trust for Metabolic Diseases in Children, *III*

420 FORESTIER'S DISEASE

Forestier's Disease, also known as diffuse idiopathic skeletal hyperostosis (DISH), is a musculoskeletal disorder that generally affects males and females over the age of 50 years. The disorder is characterized by bony overgrowth (hyperostosis) of the forward, side (anterolateral) portions of bones of the spinal column (vertebrae) and/or sites where tendons join bones (tendon osseous junctions), such as the elbow, knee (patella), and/or heel of the foot. Such overgrowth most often affects vertebrae from below the neck to the middle of the back (thoracic vertebrae). However, in some cases, bony outgrowths (osteophyte formation) may affect the vertebrae of the neck (cervical vertebrae). Individuals with the disorder may experience inflammation, pain, stiffness, and restricted movements of the affected areas. In addition, individuals with neck involvement may have difficulties swallowing (dysphagia). The exact cause of Forestiers Disease is not known.

In addition to The National Organization for Rare Disorders (NORD) listed in Section III, the following organizations in Section II (Disease Specific) and in Section III (Umbrella) and Section IV (Government Agencies) can provide more information:
Arthritis Foundation, *III*
NIH/National Arthritis and Musculoskeletal and Skin Diseases Information Clearinghouse, *IV*

421 FORMALDEHYDE POISONING

Formaldehyde Poisoning is a disorder brought about by breathing the fumes of formaldehyde. This can occur while working directly with formaldehyde, or using equipment cleaned with formaldehyde. Major symptoms may include eye, nose, and throat irritation; headaches; and/or skin rashes.

In addition to The National Organization for Rare Disorders (NORD) listed in Section III, the following organizations in Section II (Disease Specific) and in Section III (Umbrella) and Section IV (Government Agencies) can provide more information:
NIH/National Institute of Environmental Health Sciences Clearinghouse, *IV*

422 FOUNTAIN SYNDROME

Fountain Syndrome is an extremely rare inherited disorder that is characterized by mental retardation; abnormal swelling of the cheeks and lips due to the excessive accumulation of body fluids under the skin (subcutaneous) of the face (edema); skeletal abnormalities; and/or deafness due to malformation of a structure (cochlea) within the inner ear. Fountain Syndrome is thought to be inherited as an autosomal recessive genetic trait.

In addition to The National Organization for Rare Disorders (NORD) listed in Section III, the following organizations in Section II (Disease Specific) and in Section III (Umbrella) and Section IV (Government Agencies) can provide more information:
Epilepsy Foundation of America, *III*
NIH/National Arthritis and Musculoskeletal and Skin Diseases Information Clearinghouse, *IV*
NIH/National Institute of Child Health and Human Development, *IV*
NIH/National Institute on Deafness and Other Communication Disorders Information Clearinghouse, *IV*

423 FOX FORDYCE DISEASE

Fox-Fordyce Disease is a rare disorder that occurs almost solely in women. It is characterized by the development of intense itching usually in the underarm area, the pubic area, and around the nipple of the breast. Perspiration becomes trapped in the sweat gland and in the surrounding area causing intense itching, inflammation, and enlargement of the glands. Skin in the area may become darkened and dry; raised patches develop. Hair follicles in the area dry out resulting in loss or breakage of hair.

In addition to The National Organization for Rare Disorders (NORD) listed in Section III, the following organizations in Section II (Disease Specific) and in Section III (Umbrella) and Section IV (Government Agencies) can provide more information:
NIH/National Arthritis and Musculoskeletal and Skin Diseases Information Clearinghouse, *IV*

424 FRAGILE X SYNDROME

Fragile X Syndrome is a defect of the X chromosome which causes mild mental retardation. The disorder occurs more frequently and severely among males than females. This condition is the leading known familial cause of mental retardation in the United States. Language delays, behavioral problems, autism or autistic-like behavior (including poor eye contact and hand-flapping), enlarged external genitalia (macroorchidism), large or prominent ears, hyperactivity, delayed motor development and/or poor sensory skills are among the wide range of symptoms associated with this disorder.

In addition to The National Organization for Rare Disorders (NORD) listed in Section III, the following organizations in Section II (Disease Specific) and in Section III (Umbrella) and Section IV (Government Agencies) can provide more information:
FRAXA Research Foundation, Inc., *II*
NIH/National Institute on Aging, *IV*
National Fragile X Foundation, *II*
The Arc (a national organization on mental retardation), *III*

425 FRASER SYNDROME

Fraser Syndrome is a rare genetic disorder characterized by partial webbing of the fingers and/or toes (partial syndactyly), kidney (renal) abnormalities, genital malformations, and/or, in some cases, complete fusion of the eyelids (cryptophthalmos) that may be associated with malformation of the eyes, causing blindness. In infants with Fraser Syndrome, renal malformations may include improper development (dysplasia), underdevelopment (hypoplasia), or absence of one or both kidneys (unilateral or bilateral renal agenesis). In affected males, one or both testes may fail to descend into the scrotum (cryptorchidism), the urinary opening (meatus) may be abnormally placed on the underside of the penis (hypospadias), and/or the penis may be abnormally small (micropenis). Affected females may have malformed fallopian tubes, an abnormally enlarged clitoris (clitoromegaly), and/or an abnormally shaped uterus (bicornate uterus). In addition, the folds of skin on either side of the vaginal opening (labia) may be abnormally fused. Infants and children with Fraser Syndrome may also have additional abnormalities including malformations of the middle and outer ear that may result in hearing impairment. Fraser Syndrome is inherited as an autosomal recessive genetic trait.

In addition to The National Organization for Rare Disorders (NORD) listed in Section III, the following organizations in Section II (Disease Specific) and in Section III (Umbrella) and Section IV (Government Agencies) can provide more information:
AboutFace U.S.A., *III*
American Kidney Fund, Inc., *III*
Children's Craniofacial Association, *III*
FACES: The National Craniofacial Association, *III*
Forward Face, Inc., *III*
NIH/National Institute of Child Health and Human Development, *IV*
National Foundation for Facial Reconstruction, *III*
National Kidney Foundation, *III*

426 FREEMAN SHELDON SYNDROME

Freeman-Sheldon Syndrome is a very rare genetic disorder characterized by abnormal muscle and skeletal development and is present at birth. The face, eyes, hands, and feet are most commonly affected. Intelligence is often within the normal range although some mental deficiency may occur.

In addition to The National Organization for Rare Disorders (NORD) listed in Section III, the following organizations in Section II (Disease Specific) and in Section III (Umbrella) and Section IV (Government Agencies) can provide more information:
Freeman-Sheldon Parent Support Group, *II*
NIH/National Arthritis and Musculoskeletal and Skin Diseases Information Clearinghouse, *IV*

427 FREY'S SYNDROME

Frey's Syndrome is a rare neurological disorder that results from injury or surgery near the parotid glands (which manufacture saliva), damaging the facial nerve. The parotid glands are the largest salivary glands and are located on the side of the face below and in front of the ear. This syndrome is characterized by flushing or sweating on one side of the face when certain foods are consumed. The symptoms usually are mild and well tolerated by most individuals. Relief from symptoms may require treatment in some cases.

In addition to The National Organization for Rare Disorders (NORD) listed in Section III, the following organizations in Section II (Disease Specific) and in Section III (Umbrella) and Section IV (Government Agencies) can provide more information:
NIH/National Institute of Neurological Disorders and Stroke, *IV*

428 FROELICH'S SYNDROME

Froelich's Syndrome is a rare endocrine disorder characterized by delayed puberty, small testes, and obesity. This syndrome affects mostly males. In recent years, Froelich's Syndrome has referred only to boys who also have lesions in the hypothalamic gland and exhibit the symptoms. Teen-age boys with this disorder must be distinguished from those who have inherited growth delay disorders or Prader Willi Syndrome.

In addition to The National Organization for Rare Disorders (NORD) listed in Section III, the following organizations in Section II (Disease Specific) and in Section III (Umbrella) and Section IV (Government Agencies) can provide more information:
Human Growth Foundation, *III*
MAGIC Foundation for Children's Growth, *III*
NIH/National Institute of Neurological Disorders and Stroke, *IV*
Short Stature Foundation, *III*
The Arc (a national organization on mental retardation), *III*

429 FRONTOFACIONASAL DYSPLASIA

Frontofacionasal Dysplasia is a very rare disorder in which the patient is born with abnormalities of the skull and face. Cleft lip and palate as well as premature closing of the soft spot (coronal suture) on the top of the head causing excess growth of the head from side to side. A variety of malformations of the eyes, nose and bones of the skull may also be present. Frontofacionasal Dysplasia is inherited as an autosomal recessive genetic trait.

In addition to The National Organization for Rare Disorders (NORD) listed in Section III, the following organizations in Section II (Disease Specific) and in Section III (Umbrella) and Section IV (Government Agencies) can provide more information:
AboutFace U.S.A., *III*
Children's Craniofacial Association, *III*
FACES: The National Craniofacial Association, *III*
Forward Face, Inc., *III*
NIH/National Institute of Child Health and Human Development, *IV*

430 FRONTONASAL DYSPLASIA

Frontonasal Dysplasia, also known as Median Cleft Face Syndrome, is a very rare disorder characterized by abnormalities affecting the head and facial (craniofacial) region. Major physical characteristics may include widely spaced eyes (ocular hypertelorism); a flat broad nose; and/or a vertical groove down the middle of the face. The depth and width of the vertical groove may vary greatly. In some cases, the tip of the nose may be missing; in more severe cases, the nose may separate vertically into two parts. In addition, an abnormal skin-covered gap in the front of the head (anterior cranium occultum) may also be present in some cases. The exact cause of Frontonasal Dysplasia is not known. Most cases occur randomly, for no apparent reason (sporadically). However, some cases are thought to run in families.

In addition to The National Organization for Rare Disorders (NORD) listed in Section III, the following organizations in Section II (Disease Specific) and in Section III (Umbrella) and Section IV (Government Agencies) can provide more information:
AboutFace U.S.A., *III*
Children's Craniofacial Association, *III*
FACES: The National Craniofacial Association, *III*
Forward Face, Inc., *III*

431 FRUCTOSE INTOLERANCE, HEREDITARY

Hereditary Fructose Intolerance is an autosomal recessive genetically caused inability to digest fructose or its precursors sucrose (sugar, sorbitol and brown sugar). This is due to a deficiency of the enzyme 1- phosphofructoaldolase in the liver, kidney cortex and small intestine.

In addition to The National Organization for Rare Disorders (NORD) listed in Section III, the following organizations in Section II (Disease Specific) and in Section III (Umbrella) and Section IV (Government Agencies) can provide more information:
NIH/National Digestive Diseases Information Clearinghouse, *IV*

432 FRUCTOSURIA

Fructosuria is a very rare inherited metabolic disorder. It is characterized by the excretion of fruit sugar (fructose) in the urine. Normally, no fructose is excreted in the urine. This condition is caused by a deficiency of the enzyme fructokinase in the liver. This enzyme is needed for the synthesis of glycogen (the body's form of stored energy) from fructose. The presence of fructose in the blood and urine may lead to an incorrect diagnosis of Diabetes Mellitus.

In addition to The National Organization for Rare Disorders (NORD) listed in Section III, the following organizations in Section II (Disease Specific) and in Section III (Umbrella) and Section IV (Government Agencies) can provide more information:
Metabolic Information Network, *III*
NIH/National Institute of Diabetes, Digestive & Kidney Diseases, *IV*
Research Trust for Metabolic Diseases in Children, *III*

433 FRYNS SYNDROME

Fryns Syndrome is an extremely rare disorder that consists of a group of deformities including unusual facial features, hand and foot abnormalities, poor lung and urogenital development, and, in many cases, diaphragm hernias. There may also be an associated brain cyst known as the Dandy Walker feature.

In addition to The National Organization for Rare Disorders (NORD) listed in Section III, the following organizations in Section II (Disease Specific) and in Section III (Umbrella) and Section IV (Government Agencies) can provide more information:
NIH/National Institute of Child Health and Human Development, *IV*

434 FUCOSIDOSIS

Fucosidosis is an extremely rare inherited lysosomal storage disease characterized by a deficiency of the enzyme alpha-L-fucosidase. This disorder belongs to a group of diseases known as lysosomal storage disorders. Lysosomes are particles bound in membranes within cells that break down certain fats and carbohydrates. Low levels of the alpha-L-fucosidase enzyme lead to the abnormal accumulation of certain fucose-containing complex compounds (i.e., glycosphingolipids, glycolipids, and glycoproteins) in many tissues of the body. Many researchers believe there are two types of Fucosidosis (i.e., Type 1 and Type 2), determined mainly by the severity of the symptoms. Other scientists theorize there are three types, with the age of onset and the disease severity being the determining factors.

The symptoms of Fucosidosis Type 1, the most severe form of the disease, may become apparent as early as six months of age. Symptoms may include progressive deterioration of the brain and spinal cord (central nervous system), mental retardation, loss of previously acquired intellectual skills, and growth retardation leading to short stature. Other physical findings and features become apparent over time including multiple deformities of the bones (dysostosis multiplex), coarse facial features, enlargement of the heart (cardiomegaly), enlargement of the liver and spleen (hepatosplenomegaly), and/or episodes of uncontrolled electrical activity in the brain (seizures). Additional symptoms may include increased or decreased perspiration and/or malfunction of the gallbladder and/or salivary glands.

In Fucosidosis Type 2, deterioration of the

central nervous system becomes apparent in the first few years of life; symptoms progress more slowly than in Type 1. Other symptoms may be similar to but milder than those of Type 1. The most noticeable feature distinguishing Fucosidosis Types 1 from Type 2 is the appearance of horny or warty growths (angiokeratomas) on the skin in those individuals with Type 2. Fucosidosis Types 1 and 2 may be found in the same family.

Many researchers believe that there is no clear distinction between the three proposed types of Fucosidosis and that they actually represent varying clinical expressions of the disorder rather than distinct subtypes. Fucosidosis is inherited as an autosomal recessive genetic trait.

In addition to The National Organization for Rare Disorders (NORD) listed in Section III, the following organizations in Section II (Disease Specific) and in Section III (Umbrella) and Section IV (Government Agencies) can provide more information:
Association for Neuro-Metabolic Disorders, *III*
NIH/National Institute of Child Health and Human Development, *IV*
NIH/National Institute of Neurological Disorders and Stroke, *IV*
National MPS (Mucopolysaccharidoses/Mucolipidoses) Society, Inc., *III*
National Tay-Sachs and Allied Diseases Association, Inc., *III*
Vaincre Les Maladies Lysosomales, *III*

435 GALACTOSEMIA

Galactosemia is an autosomal recessive hereditary disorder of carbohydrate metabolism. It is a rare inability to convert galactose (a sugar contained in milk) to glucose (a different type of sugar). The disorder is caused by a deficiency of the enzyme "galactose-1-phosphate uridyl transferase".

A Duarte and a Negro variant of the Galactosemia gene have been identified. The Duarte variant causes a milder form of the disorder, while the Negro variant causes a more severe form. These variants can be distinguished by differences in galactose metabolism. Since milk is the main staple of an infant's diet, early diagnosis and treatment of this disorder is absolutely essential to avoid serious lifelong disability.

In addition to The National Organization for Rare Disorders (NORD) listed in Section III, the following organizations in Section II (Disease Specific) and in Section III (Umbrella) and Section IV (Government Agencies) can provide more information:
Association for Neuro-Metabolic Disorders, *III*
Children's Liver Alliance, *III*
Galactosaemia Support Group, *II*
Metabolic Information Network, *III*
NIH/National Digestive Diseases Information Clearinghouse, *IV*
Parents of Galactosemic Children, Inc., *II*
Research Trust for Metabolic Diseases in Children, *III*

436 GALLOWAY MOWAT SYNDROME

Galloway-Mowat Syndrome, which is also known as Microcephaly-Hiatal Hernia-Nephrotic Syndrome, is an extremely rare genetic disorder that is characterized by a variety of physical and developmental abnormalities. Physical features may include an unusually small head (microcephaly) and additional abnormalities of the head and facial (craniofacial) area; damage to clusters of capillaries in the kidneys (focal glomerulosclerosis and/or diffuse mesangial sclerosis), resulting in abnormal kidney function (Nephrotic Syndrome); and, in many cases, protrusion of part of the stomach through an abnormal opening (esophageal hiatus) in the diaphragm (hiatal hernia). Additional physical abnormalities are often present. These may include various malformations of the brain, seizures, diminished muscle tone throughout the body (generalized hypotonia), and/or increased reflex reactions (hyperreflexia). Infants and children with Galloway-Mowat Syndrome may also exhibit developmental abnormalities including an inability to perform certain movement (motor) skills normal for their age and a profound delay in the attainment of skills requiring the coordination of muscular and mental activity (psychomotor retardation). Mental retardation may also be present. Galloway-Mowat Syndrome is inherited as an autosomal recessive genetic trait.

In addition to The National Organization for Rare Disorders (NORD) listed in Section III, the following organizations in Section II (Disease Specific) and in Section III (Umbrella) and Section IV (Government Agencies) can provide more information:
Epilepsy Foundation of America, *III*
NIH/National Institute of Child Health & Human Development (Preg & Perinat), *IV*
NIH/National Institute of Neurological Disorders and Stroke, *IV*
NIH/National Kidney and Urologic Diseases Information Clearinghouse, *IV*
National Kidney Foundation, *III*

437 **GARDNER SYNDROME**

Gardner Syndrome is a rare inherited disorder characterized by multiple growths (polyps) in the colon, extra teeth (supernumerary), bony tumors of the skull (osteomas), and fatty cysts (epithelial) and/or fibrous tumors in the skin (fibromas or epithelial cysts). Gardner Syndrome is a variant of Familial Polyposis which is a group of disorders characterized by the growth of multiple polyps in the colon.

In addition to The National Organization for Rare Disorders (NORD) listed in Section III, the following organizations in Section II (Disease Specific) and in Section III (Umbrella) and Section IV (Government Agencies) can provide more information:
American Cancer Society, Inc., *III*
Intestinal Multiple Polyposis and Colorectal Cancer Registry, *III*
March of Dimes Birth Defects Foundation, *III*
NIH/National Institute of Diabetes, Digestive and Kidney Diseases, *IV*
NIH/Patient Referral Services Unit, *IV*
United Ostomy Association, Inc., *III*

438 **GASTRITIS, CHRONIC, EROSIVE**

Chronic, Erosive Gastritis is characterized by many inflamed lesions in the mucous lining of the stomach. It may be a transitory or a chronic condition lasting for years.

In addition to The National Organization for Rare Disorders (NORD) listed in Section III, the following organizations in Section II (Disease Specific) and in Section III (Umbrella) and Section IV (Government Agencies) can provide more information:
Crohn's and Colitis Foundation of America, *III*
Digestive Disease National Coalition, *III*
NIH/National Institute of Diabetes, Digestive and Kidney Diseases, *IV*

439 **GASTRITIS, GIANT HYPERTROPHIC**

Giant Hypertrophic Gastritis is a chronic digestive disorder characterized by large, coiled ridges or folds, in the inner wall of the stomach which resemble polyps. In some cases, inflammation of the stomach may also occur.

In addition to The National Organization for Rare Disorders (NORD) listed in Section III, the following organizations in Section II (Disease Specific) and in Section III (Umbrella) and Section IV (Government Agencies) can provide more information:
NIH/National Digestive Diseases Information Clearinghouse, *IV*

440 **GASTROENTERITIS, EOSINOPHILIC**

Eosinophilic Gastroenteritis is a rare digestive disease characterized by an abnormal infiltration of certain white blood cells (eosinophils) in the lining of the stomach, small intestines and/or large intestine.

In addition to The National Organization for Rare Disorders (NORD) listed in Section III, the following organizations in Section II (Disease Specific) and in Section III (Umbrella) and Section IV (Government Agencies) can provide more information:
Digestive Disease National Coalition, *III*
NIH/National Digestive Diseases Information Clearinghouse, *IV*

441 **GASTROESOPHAGEAL REFLUX**

Gastroesophageal Reflux is characterized by a flowing back (reflux) of stomach or small intestines (duodenum) acids or contents into the mouth, from the tube in the back of the mouth going to the stomach (esophagus) and sometimes the mouth. This condition is a common problem and may be a symptom of other gastrointestinal disorders.

In addition to The National Organization for Rare Disorders (NORD) listed in Section III, the following organizations in Section II (Disease Specific) and in Section III (Umbrella) and Section IV (Government Agencies) can provide more information:
Digestive Disease National Coalition, *III*
NIH/National Digestive Diseases Information Clearinghouse, *IV*
Pediatric/Adolescent Gastroesophageal Reflux Association, Inc., *II*
Tracheo Oesophageal Fistula Support Group, *II*

442 **GASTROSCHISIS**

Gastroschisis is a rare congenital disorder in which the patient is born with a defect in the wall of the abdomen. Typically there is a small abdominal cavity with herniated intestines that usually appear on the right outerside of the abdomen. There is no membranous sac covering the intestines and they may be swollen and look shortened due to exposure to the liquid that surrounds the fetus during pregnancy (amniotic fluid).

In addition to The National Organization for Rare Disorders (NORD) listed in Section III, the following organizations in Section II (Disease Specific) and in Section III (Umbrella) and Section IV (Government Agencies) can provide more information:
Digestive Disease National Coalition, *III*
NIH/National Digestive Diseases Information Clearinghouse, *IV*

443 **GAUCHER DISEASE**

Gaucher disease is the most common of the lipid storage diseases (which include Tay-Sachs, Fabry's, and Neimann-Pick diseases).

Lipids are various fats or fat-like substances in the body. Lipids are stored by the body to be used as energy at a later time. There are three forms of Gaucher disease: Type I (non-neuroleptic); Type II (acute neuroleptic, or infantile cerebral); Type III (subacute neuroleptic). Major symptoms include a swollen abdomen, bone deterioration and acute attacks of bone pain.

In addition to The National Organization for Rare Disorders (NORD) listed in Section III, the following organizations in Section II (Disease Specific) and in Section III (Umbrella) and Section IV (Government Agencies) can provide more information:

Alliance of Genetic Support Groups, *III*
Gauchers Association, *II*
March of Dimes Birth Defects Foundation, *III*
NIH/National Institute of Neurological Disorders and Stroke, *IV*
National Gaucher Foundation, Inc., *II*
The Arc (a national organization on mental retardation), *III*
Vaincre Les Maladies Lysosomales, *III*

444 GERSTMANN SYNDROME

Gerstmann Syndrome is a rare neurological disorder that can occur as the result of a brain injury or as a developmental disorder. The syndrome is characterized by the loss or absence of certain sensory abilities. These include the loss of the ability to express thoughts in writing (agraphia), to perform simple arithmetic problems (acalculia), to recognize or indicate one's own or another's fingers (finger agnosia), and to make a distinction between right and left.

In addition to The National Organization for Rare Disorders (NORD) listed in Section III, the following organizations in Section II (Disease Specific) and in Section III (Umbrella) and Section IV (Government Agencies) can provide more information:

American Brain Tumor Association, *III*
Learning Disabilities Association of America, *III*
NIH/National Institute of Child Health and Human Development, *IV*

445 GIANOTTI CROSTI SYNDROME

Gianotti-Crosti Syndrome is a rare skin disease affecting children between the ages of nine months to nine years. Major symptoms may include blisters on the skin of the legs, buttocks and arms. The disorder is usually preceded by a viral infection.

In addition to The National Organization for Rare Disorders (NORD) listed in Section III, the following organizations in Section II (Disease Specific) and in Section III (Umbrella) and Section IV (Government Agencies) can provide more information:

Centers for Disease Control and Prevention, *IV*
NIH/National Arthritis and Musculoskeletal and Skin Diseases Information Clearinghouse, *IV*
NIH/National Institute of Allergy and Infectious Diseases, *IV*

446 GIARDIASIS

Giardiasis is an infectious disorder of the gastrointestinal tract caused by a genus of protozoan parasite known as Giardia lamblia. This disorder may not cause noticeable symptoms, but when many of these parasites are present, absorption of nutrients is diminished. Additionally, acute gastrointestinal discomfort, chronic or acute diarrhea, and other digestive system abnormalities can occur. This disorder has occurred in epidemics associated with contaminated water in which infected beavers live because parasites in the cyst stage from beavers are infectious to humans. These cysts can survive in cold water for several months.

In addition to The National Organization for Rare Disorders (NORD) listed in Section III, the following organizations in Section II (Disease Specific) and in Section III (Umbrella) and Section IV (Government Agencies) can provide more information:

Centers for Disease Control and Prevention, *IV*
NIH/National Institute of Allergy and Infectious Diseases, *IV*
World Health Organization (WHO) Regional Office for the Americas (AMRO), *III*

447 GILBERT SYNDROME

One of a benign group of metabolic abnormalities, Gilbert Syndrome is a hereditary disorder involving a defect in the clearance of bile pigment (bilirubin) from the liver. This syndrome is common but innocuous and easily controllable. It is marked by a persistent yellow skin coloration (jaundice) which may fluctuate in severity.

In addition to The National Organization for Rare Disorders (NORD) listed in Section III, the following organizations in Section II (Disease Specific) and in Section III (Umbrella) and Section IV (Government Agencies) can provide more information:

Alliance of Genetic Support Groups, *III*
American Liver Foundation, *III*
Children's Liver Disease Foundation, *III*
Metabolic Information Network, *III*
NIH/National Digestive Diseases Information Clearinghouse, *IV*
United Liver Association, *III*

448 GLIOBLASTOMA MULTIFORME

Glioblastoma multiforme is a highly malignant, rapidly infiltrating, primary brain tumor, with tentacles that may invade surrounding tissue. This provides a butterfly-like distribution pattern through the white matter of the cerebral hemispheres. The tumor may invade a membrane covering the brain (the dura), or spread via the spinal fluid through the ventricles of the brain. Spread of the tumor (metastasis) outside the brain and spinal cord is rare.

In addition to The National Organization for Rare Disorders (NORD) listed in Section III, the following organizations in Section II (Disease Specific) and in Section III (Umbrella) and Section IV (Government Agencies) can provide more information:
American Brain Tumor Association, *III*
American Cancer Society, Inc., *III*
Brain Tumor Society, *III*
Candlelighters Childhood Cancer Foundation, *III*
NIH/Patient Referral Services Unit, *IV*
National Brain Tumor Foundation, *III*

449 GLUCOSE GALACTOSE MALABSORPTION

Glucose-Galactose Malabsorption (carbohydrate intolerance) is a genetic disorder characterized by the small intestine's inability to transport and absorb glucose and galactose (sugars which can be broken down no further, or monosaccharides). Glucose and galactose have almost identical chemical structures, and normally the same transport enzyme provides them with entry into specialized cells in the small intestine where they are absorbed and transferred to other cells. At the present time, this transport enzyme has not been identified. However, it is known to be defective in individuals with glucose-galactose malabsorption.

The glucose and galactose which have not been absorbed through the specialized cells of the small intestine are then poorly absorbed much further along in the intestine. This abnormal absorption may interfere with other intestinal absorption processes.

In addition to The National Organization for Rare Disorders (NORD) listed in Section III, the following organizations in Section II (Disease Specific) and in Section III (Umbrella) and Section IV (Government Agencies) can provide more information:
NIH/National Digestive Diseases Information Clearinghouse, *IV*

450 GLUCOSE-6-PHOSPHATE DEHYDROGENASE DEFICIENCY

Glucose-6-Phosphate Dehydrogenase Deficiency is an inherited metabolic disorder characterized by a deficiency of Glucose-6-Phosphate Dehydrogenase, an enzyme that is essential in sugar (glucose) metabolism and provides red blood cells with defense against destruction by certain drugs. A deficiency of this enzyme may result in the premature destruction of red blood cells (hemolytic anemia) when an affected individual is exposed to certain medications or chemicals, experiences certain viral or bacterial infections, and/or inhales the pollen of or consumes fava beans (favism). More than 300 variants of the disorder have been identified, resulting from mutations of the Glucose-6-Phosphate Dehydrogenase gene. The severity of symptoms associated with G6PD Deficiency may vary greatly among affected individuals, depending upon the specific form of the disorder that is present. Glucose- 6-Phosphate Dehydrogenase Deficiency is inherited as an X-linked genetic trait.

In addition to The National Organization for Rare Disorders (NORD) listed in Section III, the following organizations in Section II (Disease Specific) and in Section III (Umbrella) and Section IV (Government Agencies) can provide more information:
Association for Neuro-Metabolic Disorders, *III*
Metabolic Information Network, *III*
NIH/National Institute of Diabetes, Digestive and Kidney Diseases, *IV*
Research Trust for Metabolic Diseases in Children, *III*

451 GLUTARICACIDURIA I

Glutaricaciduria is a rare hereditary metabolic disorder, caused by a deficiency of the enzyme glutaryl-CoA dehydrogenase. One of a group of disorders known as "organic acidemias," it is characterized by decreased muscle tone (hypotonia), vomiting, and excess acid in the blood. Affected individuals may also have involuntary movements of the trunk and limbs (dystonia or athetosis) and mental retardation may also occur.

In addition to The National Organization for Rare Disorders (NORD) listed in Section III, the following organizations in Section II (Disease Specific) and in Section III (Umbrella) and Section IV (Government Agencies) can provide more information:
International Organization of Glutaric Aciduria, *III*
Lactic Acidosis Support Trust, *III*
Metabolic Information Network, *III*
National Urea Cycle Disorders Foundation, *III*
Organic Acidemia Association, *III*
Research Trust for Metabolic Diseases in Children, *III*
The Arc (a national organization on mental retardation), *III*

452 GLUTARICACIDURIA II

There are two forms of Glutaricaciduria II which occur during different stages of life. They are both forms of organic acidemias which are a group of metabolic disorders characterized by excess acid in the blood and urine.

1) Glutaricaciduria IIA (GA IIA), Neonatal Form of Glutaricaciduria II. This neonatal form of Glutaricaciduria II is a very rare, sex-linked hereditary disorder characterized by large amounts of glutaric and other acids in blood and urine. Some researchers believe the disorder is caused by a defect in the breakdown of acyl-CoA compounds.

2) Glutaricaciduria IIB (GA IIB; Ethylmalonic Adipicaciduria), Adult Form of Glutaricaciduria II.

This milder form of the disorder is inherited as an autosomal recessive trait. Acidity of the body tissues (metabolic acidosis), and a low blood sugar level (hypoglycemia) without an elevated level of ketones in body tissues (ketosis), occur during adulthood. Large amounts of glutaric acid in the blood and urine are caused by a deficiency of the enzyme "multiple acyl- CoA dehydrogenase."

In addition to The National Organization for Rare Disorders (NORD) listed in Section III, the following organizations in Section II (Disease Specific) and in Section III (Umbrella) and Section IV (Government Agencies) can provide more information:

FOD (Fatty Oxidation Disorder) Family Support Group, *III*
International Organization of Glutaric Aciduria, *III*
Lactic Acidosis Support Trust, *III*
Metabolic Information Network, *III*
National Urea Cycle Disorders Foundation, *III*
Organic Acidemia Association, *III*
Research Trust for Metabolic Diseases in Children, *III*

453 GLYCOGEN STORAGE DISEASE VIII

Glycogen Storage Disease VIII is an X-linked genetic disorder caused by a deficiency of the enzyme liver phosphorylase kinase. The disorder is characterized by slightly low blood sugar (hypoglycemia). Excess amounts of glycogen (the stored form of energy that comes from carbohydrates) are deposited in the liver, causing enlargement of the liver (hepatomegaly).

In addition to The National Organization for Rare Disorders (NORD) listed in Section III, the following organizations in Section II (Disease Specific) and in Section III (Umbrella) and Section IV (Government Agencies) can provide more information:

Alliance of Genetic Support Groups, *III*
Association for Neuro-Metabolic Disorders, *III*
Children's Liver Alliance, *III*
Metabolic Information Network, *III*
NIH/National Institute of Diabetes, Digestive and Kidney Diseases, *IV*
Research Trust for Metabolic Diseases in Children, *III*

454 GOLDENHAR SYNDROME (OCULO AURICULO VERTEBRAL SPECTRUM)

Goldenhar Syndrome, a term that is often used synonymously with "Oculo-Auriculo-Vertebral (OAV) Spectrum," is a rare disorder that is apparent at birth (congenital). The disorder is characterized by a wide spectrum of symptoms and physical features that may vary greatly in range and severity from case to case. However, such abnormalities tend to involve the cheekbones, jaws, mouth, ears, eyes, and/or bones of the spinal column (vertebrae). In most cases, malformations affect one side of the body. In 10 to 33% of affected individuals malformations occur on both sides of the body with one side more affected than the other (usually the right side).

Due to craniofacial malformations, an affected individual's face may appear smaller on one side than the other (hemifacial microsomia); in addition, if both sides are affected (bilateral), the face may appear dissimilar from one side to the other (facial asymmetry). Craniofacial abnormalities may include underdevelopment of the cheekbones (malar hypoplasia), bones of the upper and lower jaws (maxillary and mandibular hypoplasia), and the bones forming a portion of the lower skull (temporal hypoplasia); incomplete development of certain muscles of the face; an abnormally wide mouth (macrostomia); incomplete closure of the roof of the mouth (cleft palate); an abnormal groove in the upper lip (cleft lip); and/or abnormalities of the tongue and/or teeth. Affected individuals may also exhibit absence and/or malformation of the outer ears; narrow, blind ending, or absent external ear canals; abnormal outgrowths of skin and cartilage on or in front of the ears; and/or abnormalities affecting the middle and/or inner ears, contributing to or resulting in hearing impairment (i.e., conductive and/or sensorineural hearing loss). Eye abnormalities may also be present including the formation of cysts on the eyeballs, partial or total absence of tissue from the upper eyelids, abnormal smallness of the eyes, narrowing of the eyelid folds between the upper and lower eyelids, crossing of the eyes, and/or other eye abnormalities.

Vertebral malformations associated with Goldenhar Syndrome (OAV Spectrum) may include incomplete development (hypoplasia), fusion, and/or absence of certain vertebrae. In addition, many affected individuals may have additional skeletal, neurological, heart (cardiac), lung (pulmonary), kidney (renal), and/or gastrointestinal abnormalities. In approximately five to 15 percent of affected individuals, mild mental retardation may also be present.

In most cases, Goldenhar Syndrome (OAV Spectrum) appears to occur randomly, with no apparent cause (sporadic). However, in some cases, positive family histories have been present that have suggested autosomal dominant or recessive inheritance. In addition, some researchers suggest that the disorder may be caused by the interaction of many genes, possibly in combination with environmental factors (multifactorial inheritance).

In addition to The National Organization for Rare Disorders (NORD) listed in Section III, the following organizations in Section II (Disease Specific) and in Section III (Umbrella) and Section IV (Government Agencies) can provide more information:

Children's Craniofacial Association, *III*
Congenital Heart Anomalies, Support, Education, & Resources, *III*
EA/TEF Child and Family Support Connection, Inc., *III*
Ear Anomalies Reconstructed: Atresia/Microtia Support Group, *III*
International Children's Anophthalmia Network, *III*
NIH/National Eye Institute, *IV*
NIH/National Heart, Lung and Blood Institute Information Center, *IV*
NIH/National Institute of Child Health and Human Development, *IV*
National Association for Parents of the Visually Impaired, *III*
National Kidney Foundation, *III*
The Arc (a national organization on mental retardation), *III*

455 GOODMAN SYNDROME

Goodman Syndrome (Acrocephalopolysyndactyly Type IV) is an extremely rare genetic disorder characterized by marked malformations of the head and face, abnormalities of the hands and feet, and congenital heart disease. The syndrome is inherited as an autosomal recessive trait. Some researchers feel that Goodman Syndrome is a variant of Carpenter Syndrome (Acrocephalopolysyndactyly Type II).

In addition to The National Organization for Rare Disorders (NORD) listed in Section III, the following organizations in Section II (Disease Specific) and in Section III (Umbrella) and Section IV (Government Agencies) can provide more information:

AboutFace U.S.A., *III*
American Heart Association, *III*
Children's Craniofacial Association, *III*
Congenital Heart Anomalies, Support, Education, & Resources, *III*
FACES: The National Craniofacial Association, *III*
Forward Face, Inc., *III*
Let's Face It, Inc., *III*
NIH/National Heart, Lung and Blood Institute Information Center, *IV*
NIH/National Institute of Child Health and Human Development, *IV*
National Foundation for Facial Reconstruction, *III*

456 GOODPASTURE SYNDROME

Goodpasture Syndrome is a rare autoimmune disorder characterized by inflammation of the filtering structures (glomeruli) of the kidneys (glomerulonephritis) and excessive bleeding into the lungs (pulmonary hemorrhaging). Autoimmune syndromes occur when the body's natural defenses (antibodies) against invading or "foreign" organisms begin to attack the body's own tissue, often for unknown reasons. Symptoms of Goodpasture Syndrome include recurrent episodes of coughing up of blood (hemoptysis), difficulty breathing (dyspnea), fatigue, chest pain, and/or abnormally low levels of circulating red blood cells (anemia). In many cases, Goodpasture Syndrome may result in an inability of the kidneys to process waste products from the blood and excrete them in the urine (acute renal failure). In some cases of Goodpasture Syndrome, affected individuals have had an upper respiratory tract infection before the development of the disorder. The exact cause of Goodpasture Syndrome is not known.

In addition to The National Organization for Rare Disorders (NORD) listed in Section III, the following organizations in Section II (Disease Specific) and in

Section III (Umbrella) and Section IV (Government Agencies) can provide more information:
American Autoimmune Related Diseases Association, Inc., *III*
American Lung Association, *III*
Immune Deficiency Foundation, *III*
NIH/National Kidney and Urologic Diseases Information Clearinghouse, *IV*
National Kidney Foundation, *III*

457 GORDON SYNDROME

Gordon Syndrome is an extremely rare disorder that belongs to a group of genetic disorders known as the Distal Arthrogryposes. These disorders typically involve stiffness and impaired mobility of certain joints of the lower arms and legs (distal extremities) including the knees, elbows, wrists, and/or ankles. These joints tend to be permanently fixed in a bent or flexed position (contractures). Gordon Syndrome is characterized by the permanent fixation of several fingers in a flexed position (camptodactyly), abnormal bending inward of the foot (clubfoot or talipes), and, less frequently, incomplete closure of the roof of the mouth (cleft palate). In some cases, additional abnormalities may also be present. The range and severity of symptoms may vary from case to case. Gordon Syndrome is thought to be inherited as an autosomal dominant genetic trait.

In addition to The National Organization for Rare Disorders (NORD) listed in Section III, the following organizations in Section II (Disease Specific) and in Section III (Umbrella) and Section IV (Government Agencies) can provide more information:
AVENUES—A National Support Group for Arthrogryposis Multiplex Congenita, *II*
NIH/National Arthritis and Musculoskeletal and Skin Diseases Information Clearinghouse, *IV*

458 GORHAM'S DISEASE

Gorham's Disease is an extremely rare bone disorder characterized by bone loss often associated with swelling or abnormal blood vessel growth (angiomatous proliferation). Bone loss can occur in just one bone or spread to soft tissue and adjacent bone.

In addition to The National Organization for Rare Disorders (NORD) listed in Section III, the following organizations in Section II (Disease Specific) and in Section III (Umbrella) and Section IV (Government Agencies) can provide more information:
NIH/National Institute of Arthritis and Musculoskeletal and Skin Diseases, *IV*

459 GORLIN CHAUDHRY MOSS SYNDROME

Gorlin-Chaudhry-Moss Syndrome is an extremely rare inherited disorder characterized by premature closure of the fibrous joints (sutures) between certain bones in the skull (craniosynostosis), unusually small eyes (microphthalmia), absence of some teeth (hypodontia), and/or excessive amounts of hair (hypertrichosis) on most areas of the body. Affected individuals may also exhibit a mild delay in physical development (growth retardation); short fingers and/or toes; and/or underdevelopment (hypoplasia) of the two long folds of skin on either side of the vaginal opening (labia majora) in females. In addition, there may be an abnormal opening between the two large blood vessels that carry blood away from the heart (pulmonary artery and aorta), causing inappropriate recirculation of some blood through the lungs, rather than throughout the rest of the body (patent ductus arteriosus). In some cases, mild mental retardation may also be present. It is believed that Gorlin-Chaudhry-Moss Syndrome may be inherited as an autosomal recessive genetic trait.

In addition to The National Organization for Rare Disorders (NORD) listed in Section III, the following organizations in Section II (Disease Specific) and in Section III (Umbrella) and Section IV (Government Agencies) can provide more information:
American Heart Association, *III*
Children's Craniofacial Association, *III*
FACES: The National Craniofacial Association, *III*
Forward Face, Inc., *III*
NIH/National Institute of Child Health and Human Development, *IV*
NIH/National Institute of Dental Research, *IV*

460 GOTTRON'S SYNDROME

Gottron's Syndrome is an extremely rare inherited disorder characterized by premature aging (progeria) and unusually fragile, thin skin due to the absence of fatty tissue directly under the skin (subcutaneous atrophy). Other findings may include abnormally small hands and feet with thin, delicate, and fragile skin and unusually prominent veins on the chest; small stature; and/or abnormally small jaw (micrognathia). Gottrons Syndrome is inherited as an autosomal recessive genetic trait. Approximately 40 cases have been reported in the medical literature.

In addition to The National Organization for Rare Disorders (NORD) listed in Section III, the following organizations in Section II (Disease Specific) and in

Section III (Umbrella) and Section IV (Government Agencies) can provide more information:
Alliance of Genetic Support Groups, *III*
International Progeria Registry, *III*
March of Dimes Birth Defects Foundation, *III*
NIH/National Institute of Child Health and Human Development, *IV*

461 GRAFT VERSUS HOST DISEASE

Graft versus Host Disease (GVHD) is a rare disorder that can strike persons whose immune system is suppressed and have either received a blood transfusion or a bone marrow transplant. Symptoms may include skin rash, intestinal problems similar to colitis, and liver dysfunction.

In addition to The National Organization for Rare Disorders (NORD) listed in Section III, the following organizations in Section II (Disease Specific) and in Section III (Umbrella) and Section IV (Government Agencies) can provide more information:
Caitlin Raymond International Registry of Bone Marrow Donor Banks, *III*
NIH/National Heart, Lung and Blood Institute Information Center, *IV*

462 GRANULOMA ANNULARE

Granuloma annulare is a rare, degenerative skin disorder. The most common form is localized granuloma annulare, which is characterized by the presence of small, firm red or yellow colored bumps (nodules or papules) that appear arranged in a ring on the skin. In most cases, the sizes of the lesions range from one to five centimeters. The most commonly affected sites include the feet, hands, and fingers. In addition to the localized form, there are four less common forms: generalized or disseminated, linear, perforating, and subcutaneous. The lesions associated with granuloma annulare usually disappear without treatment (spontaneous remission). However, the lesions often reappear. The exact cause of granuloma annulare is unknown.

In addition to The National Organization for Rare Disorders (NORD) listed in Section III, the following organizations in Section II (Disease Specific) and in Section III (Umbrella) and Section IV (Government Agencies) can provide more information:
NIH/National Arthritis and Musculoskeletal and Skin Diseases Information Clearinghouse, *IV*

463 GRANULOMATOSIS, LYMPHOMATOID

Lymphomatoid Granulomatosis is a rare, progressive, vascular disease characterized by infiltration and destruction of the veins and arteries by lesions. These lesions can affect various parts of the body, especially the lungs. It can be a benign or malignant condition.

In addition to The National Organization for Rare Disorders (NORD) listed in Section III, the following organizations in Section II (Disease Specific) and in Section III (Umbrella) and Section IV (Government Agencies) can provide more information:
American Autoimmune Related Diseases Association, Inc., *III*
American Cancer Society, Inc., *III*
American Lung Association, *III*

464 GRANULOMATOUS DISEASE, CHRONIC

Chronic Granulomatous Disease is a very rare inherited primary immune deficiency disorder that affects certain white blood corpuscles (lymphocytes). It is characterized by widespread granulomatous tunor-like lesions, and an inability to resist repeated infectious diseases. Life-threatening infections of the skin, lungs, and bones may occur along with swollen areas of inflamed tissues known as granulomas.

In addition to The National Organization for Rare Disorders (NORD) listed in Section III, the following organizations in Section II (Disease Specific) and in Section III (Umbrella) and Section IV (Government Agencies) can provide more information:
Chronic Granulomatous Disease Association, Inc., *II*
Immune Deficiency Foundation, *III*
International Patient Organization for Primary Immunodeficiencies, *III*
Jeffrey Modell Foundation, *III*
NIH/National Institute of Allergy and Infectious Diseases, *IV*

465 GRAVES' DISEASE

Graves' Disease is a disease affecting the thyroid gland. It is thought to occur as a result of an imbalance in the immune system. This disorder causes increased thyroid secretion (hyperthyroidism), enlargement of the thyroid gland (goiter) and protrusion of the eyeballs.

In addition to The National Organization for Rare Disorders (NORD) listed in Section III, the following organizations in Section II (Disease Specific) and in Section III (Umbrella) and Section IV (Government Agencies) can provide more information:
NIH/National Digestive Diseases Information Clearinghouse, *IV*
National Graves' Disease Foundation, *II*
Thyroid Foundation of America, Inc., *III*
Thyroid Foundation of Canada, *III*

466 GREIG CEPHALOPOLYSYNDACTYLY SYNDROME

Greig Cephalopolysyndactyly Syndrome (GCPS) is a very rare inherited disorder characterized by physical abnormalities affecting the fingers and toes (digits) and the head and facial (craniofacial) area. Characteristic digital features may include extra (supernumerary) fingers and/or toes (polydactyly), webbing and/or fusion of the fingers and/or toes (syndactyly), and/or additional abnormalities. Craniofacial malformations associated with this disorder may include a large and/or unusually shaped skull; a high, prominent forehead (frontal bossing); an abnormally broad nasal bridge; widely spaced eyes (ocular hypertelorism); and/or other physical abnormalities. The range and severity of symptoms may vary greatly from case to case. In most cases, GCPS is thought to be inherited as an autosomal dominant genetic trait.

In addition to The National Organization for Rare Disorders (NORD) listed in Section III, the following organizations in Section II (Disease Specific) and in Section III (Umbrella) and Section IV (Government Agencies) can provide more information:

AboutFace U.S.A., *III*
Children's Craniofacial Association, *III*
FACES: The National Craniofacial Association, *III*
Forward Face, Inc., *III*
NIH/National Institute of Child Health and Human Development, *IV*

467 GROVER'S DISEASE

Grover's Disease is a rare temporary skin disorder that consists of small, firm, raised red lesions on the skin. Under a microscope one finds separation of closely connected cells in the skin's outer layers (acantholysis) that can be identified by a dermatologist. Small blisters containing a watery liquid are present. These blisters tend to group and have a swollen red border around them. Grover's Disease is mainly seen in males over the age of forty. Its cause is unknown but it is thought to be related to trauma to sun damaged skin.

In addition to The National Organization for Rare Disorders (NORD) listed in Section III, the following organizations in Section II (Disease Specific) and in Section III (Umbrella) and Section IV (Government Agencies) can provide more information:

NIH/National Arthritis and Musculoskeletal and Skin Diseases Information Clearinghouse, *IV*

468 GROWTH DELAY, CONSTITUTIONAL

Constitutional Growth Delay is a term describing a temporary delay in the skeletal growth and height of a child with no other physical abnormalities causing the delay. Short stature may be the result of a growth pattern inherited from a parent (familial) or occur for no apparent reason (sporadic). Typically there is a period during childhood in which growth slows down, eventually resuming at a normal rate.

In addition to The National Organization for Rare Disorders (NORD) listed in Section III, the following organizations in Section II (Disease Specific) and in Section III (Umbrella) and Section IV (Government Agencies) can provide more information:

Human Growth Foundation, *III*
Little People of America, *III*
Little People's Research Fund, Inc., *III*
MAGIC Foundation for Children's Growth, *III*
NIH/National Institute of Child Health and Human Development, *IV*
Short Stature Foundation, *III*

469 GROWTH HORMONE DEFICIENCY

Growth Hormone is manufactured in the pituitary gland. If it is missing or reduced in quantity during infancy or childhood, it results in growth retardation, short stature and other maturation delays.

Growth Hormone Deficiency (GHD) causes an absence or delay of lengthening and widening of the skeletal bones inappropriate to the chronological age of the child. A sufficient quantity of growth hormone is required during childhood to maintain growth and normalize sexual maturity. In some cases the onset of the disorder occurs prenatally (before birth), and in others the condition occurs months or years later. Laboratory testing is necessary before a diagnosis of Growth Hormone Deficiency is made because growth and maturity delays can be caused by a wide variety of other factors, including normal genetic influences.

In addition to The National Organization for Rare Disorders (NORD) listed in Section III, the following organizations in Section II (Disease Specific) and in Section III (Umbrella) and Section IV (Government Agencies) can provide more information:

Human Growth Foundation, *III*
Little People of America, *III*
Little People's Research Fund, Inc., *III*
MAGIC Foundation for Children's Growth, *III*
NIH/National Institute of Child Health and Human

Development, *IV*
Short Stature Foundation, *III*

470 GUILLAIN BARRE SYNDROME

Guillain-Barre Syndrome (acute idiopathic polyneuritis) is a very rare, rapidly progressive disorder causing inflammation of the nerves (polyneuritis) and paralysis. Although the precise cause of Guillain-Barre Syndrome is unknown, a viral or respiratory infection precedes the onset of the syndrome in about half of the cases. This has led to the theory that Guillain-Barre Syndrome may be an autoimmune disease (caused by the body's own immune system). Damage to the covering of nerve cells (myelin) and nerve axons (the extension of the nerve cell that conducts impulses away from the nerve cell body) results in delayed nerve signal transmission. There is a corresponding weakness in the muscles that are supplied with nerve impulses (innervated) by the affected nerves.

The following subdivisions are recognized: Miller-Fischer syndrome (Fischer syndrome, acute disseminated encephalomyeloradiculopathy); chronic Guillain-Barre Syndrome (chronic idiopathic polyneuritis); relapsing Guillain-Barre Syndrome; chronic inflammatory demyelinating polyradiculoneuropathy; chronic relapsing polyneuropathy; polyneuropathy; and polyradiculoneuropathy.

In addition to The National Organization for Rare Disorders (NORD) listed in Section III, the following organizations in Section II (Disease Specific) and in Section III (Umbrella) and Section IV (Government Agencies) can provide more information:
American Autoimmune Related Diseases Association, Inc., *III*
Guillain-Barre Syndrome Foundation International, *II*
NIH/National Institute of Neurological Disorders and Stroke, *IV*

471 HAGEMAN FACTOR DEFICIENCY

Hageman Factor Deficiency is a genetic blood disorder. It is caused by a lack in activity of the Hageman factor in blood plasma, a single-chain glycoprotein which is also called Factor XII. This factor is needed for blood clotting. However, when it is deficient, other blood clotting factors tend to compensate for Factor XII. This disorder usually presents no symptoms and is only accidentally discovered through pre-operative blood tests that are required by hospitals.

In addition to The National Organization for Rare Disorders (NORD) listed in Section III, the following organizations in Section II (Disease Specific) and in Section III (Umbrella) and Section IV (Government Agencies) can provide more information:
NIH/National Heart, Lung and Blood Institute Information Center, *IV*
National Hemophilia Foundation, *II*

472 HAJDU CHENEY SYNDROME

Hajdu-Cheney Syndrome is a rare connective tissue disorder. Connective tissue is strong fibrous tissue that supports and joins other body tissues and parts. The most distinctive feature of individuals with this disorder is the appearance of ulcerating lesions on the palms of the hands and soles of the feet; this is accompanied by softening and destruction of bones (acroosteolysis). Abnormal development of bones, joints, and teeth also occurs. A decrease in bone mass and changes in the skull and jawbone are also features of this syndrome. The majority of cases are of unknown cause but multiple cases have been reported in families, suggesting autosomal dominant genetic transmission.

In addition to The National Organization for Rare Disorders (NORD) listed in Section III, the following organizations in Section II (Disease Specific) and in Section III (Umbrella) and Section IV (Government Agencies) can provide more information:
NIH/National Institute of Arthritis and Musculoskeletal and Skin Diseases, *IV*

473 HALLERMANN STREIFF SYNDROME

Hallermann-Streiff syndrome, also known as oculomandibulodyscephaly, is a syndrome of bony abnormalities of the roof of the skull (calvaria), face and jaw. Affected persons have a bird-like face with a narrow curved nose, and multiple eye defects including cataracts. Also, the corneas of the eyes and the eyeballs themselves are smaller than normal. Hair can be thinned or absent overlying the lines where the plates of the skull meet, and eyebrows may be absent or underdeveloped. Premature aging (progeria) and atrophy of the elastic tissue of the skin may also occur.

In addition to The National Organization for Rare Disorders (NORD) listed in Section III, the following organizations in Section II (Disease Specific) and in Section III (Umbrella) and Section IV (Government Agencies) can provide more information:
AboutFace U.S.A., *III*
Children's Craniofacial Association, *III*
FACES: The National Craniofacial Association, *III*

Forward Face, Inc., *III*
NIH/National Institute of Child Health and Human Development, *IV*
The Arc (a national organization on mental retardation), *III*

474 HALLERVORDEN SPATZ DISEASE

Hallervorden-Spatz Disease is a rare neurological movement disorder characterized by the progressive degeneration of the nervous system. Symptoms may vary greatly and include slow writhing and distorting muscle contractions (dystonia), muscular rigidity, sudden involuntary muscle spasms (spasticity), progressive confusion, disorientation, and/or deterioration of intellectual abilities (dementia). Hallervorden-Spatz Disease typically develops during childhood, although occasionally the disease may begin during adulthood.

In addition to The National Organization for Rare Disorders (NORD) listed in Section III, the following organizations in Section II (Disease Specific) and in Section III (Umbrella) and Section IV (Government Agencies) can provide more information:
Dystonia Medical Research Foundation, *III*
Metabolic Information Network, *III*
NIH/National Heart, Lung and Blood Institute Information Center, *IV*
Research Trust for Metabolic Diseases in Children, *III*
The Arc (a national organization on mental retardation), *III*

475 HAND FOOT MOUTH SYNDROME

Hand-Foot-Mouth Syndrome is an infectious disease primarily caused by the coxsackie virus A16. The disease most often occurs in young children. It is characterized by a rash of small blister-like sores (lesions). The rash usually occurs on the palms of the hands, soles of the feet, and in the mouth.

In addition to The National Organization for Rare Disorders (NORD) listed in Section III, the following organizations in Section II (Disease Specific) and in Section III (Umbrella) and Section IV (Government Agencies) can provide more information:
Centers for Disease Control and Prevention, *IV*
NIH/National Institute of Allergy and Infectious Diseases, *IV*

476 HANHART SYNDROME

Hanhart Syndromc is a rare birth defect that is characterized by a short, incompletely developed tongue (hypoglossia); absent or partially missing fingers and/or toes (ectrodactylia); malformed arms and/or legs (peromelia); and an extremely small jaw (micrognathia). The severity of these physical abnormalities varies greatly from case to case. Children with this disorder often have some, but not all, of the symptoms. The cause of Hanhart Syndrome is not fully understood.

In addition to The National Organization for Rare Disorders (NORD) listed in Section III, the following organizations in Section II (Disease Specific) and in Section III (Umbrella) and Section IV (Government Agencies) can provide more information:
Association of Children's Prosthetic/Orthotic Clinics, *III*
FACES: The National Craniofacial Association, *III*
Forward Face, Inc., *III*
NIH/National Institute of Child Health and Human Development, *IV*

477 HANTAVIRUS PULMONARY SYNDROME

Hantavirus Pulmonary Syndrome is an infectious disease caused by the Muerto Canyon hantavirus. Transmission occurs when direct or indirect (airborne) contact is made with the saliva or waste products of rodents that carry the virus, most commonly the deer mouse (Peromyscus maniculatus). Initial symptoms may include fever, muscle aches (myalgias), headache, cough, and/or difficulty breathing. Symptoms progress rapidly, and abnormally low blood pressure (hypotension), shock, and/or respiratory failure may occur.

In addition to The National Organization for Rare Disorders (NORD) listed in Section III, the following organizations in Section II (Disease Specific) and in Section III (Umbrella) and Section IV (Government Agencies) can provide more information:
Centers for Disease Control and Prevention, *IV*
NIH/National Institute of Allergy and Infectious Diseases, *IV*
World Health Organization (WHO) Regional Office for the Americas (AMRO), *III*

478 HARTNUP DISEASE

Hartnup Disease is a rare metabolic disorder inherited as a recessive trait. It involves an inborn error of amino acid metabolism as well as niacin deficiency. Factors which precipitate attacks of this disorder may include poor nutrition, exposure to sunlight, sulfonamide medications and/or psychological stress. Hartnup Disease may be marked by skin problems, coordination impairment, vision problems, mild mental retardation, and central nervous system abnormalities. Frequency of attacks usually diminish with age.

In addition to The National Organization for Rare Disorders (NORD) listed in Section III, the following organizations in Section II (Disease Specific) and in

Section III (Umbrella) and Section IV (Government Agencies) can provide more information:
Metabolic Information Network, *III*
NIH/National Institute of Diabetes, Digestive and Kidney Diseases, *IV*
Research Trust for Metabolic Diseases in Children, *III*
The Arc (a national organization on mental retardation), *III*

479 HASHIMOTO'S SYNDROME

Hashimoto's Syndrome is a form of chronic autoimmune thyroiditis. It is a progressive disease of the thyroid that will eventually destroy the thyroid gland and cause a lack of thyroid hormone (hypothyroidism).

In addition to The National Organization for Rare Disorders (NORD) listed in Section III, the following organizations in Section II (Disease Specific) and in Section III (Umbrella) and Section IV (Government Agencies) can provide more information:
NIH/National Digestive Diseases Information Clearinghouse, *IV*
Thyroid Foundation of America, Inc., *III*
Thyroid Foundation of Canada, *III*

480 HAY WELL'S SYNDROME

Hay-Well's Syndrome is one of a group of rare genetic skin disorders known as the Ectodermal Dysplasias. Major characteristics of this disorder include cleft lip and/or palate, fusion of one or both eyelids together, absent or defective nails, coarse, sparse or wiry hair, diminished ability to sweat, and missing, widely spaced, or cone-shaped teeth. Hay-Well's Syndrome is inherited as a autosomal dominant trait.

In addition to The National Organization for Rare Disorders (NORD) listed in Section III, the following organizations in Section II (Disease Specific) and in Section III (Umbrella) and Section IV (Government Agencies) can provide more information:
NIH/National Institute of Arthritis and Musculoskeletal and Skin Diseases, *IV*
National Foundation for Ectodermal Dysplasias, *II*

481 HEADACHE, CLUSTER

Cluster Headaches are a rare form of severe disabling headache. The headaches are deep, non-throbbing, extremely painful ones that tend to recur in the same area of the head or face with each occurrence. They usually come on during sleep and awaken the patient. They are typically associated with watering of the eyes and nose.

In addition to The National Organization for Rare Disorders (NORD) listed in Section III, the following organizations in Section II (Disease Specific) and in Section III (Umbrella) and Section IV (Government Agencies) can provide more information:
American Council for Headache Education, *II*
JAMA Migraine Information Center, *II*
NIH/National Institute of Neurological Disorders and Stroke, *IV*
National Headache Foundation, *III*

482 HEART BLOCK, CONGENITAL

Congenital Heart Block is characterized by interference with the transfer of electrical nerve impulses (conduction) that regulate the normal rhythmic pumping activity of the heart muscle (heart block). The severity of such conduction abnormalities may vary among affected individuals.

The normal heart has four chambers. The two upper chambers are known as the atria and the two lower chambers are known as the ventricles. In the mild form of heart block (First Degree), the two upper chambers of the heart (atria) beat normally, but the contractions of the two lower chambers (ventricles) slightly lag behind. In the more severe forms (Second Degree), only a half to a quarter of the atrial beats are conducted to the ventricles. In complete heart block (Third Degree), the atria and ventricles beat independently. In most cases, infants with First or Second Degree experience no symptoms (asymptomatic). However, infants with complete heart block may experience episodes of unconsciousness (syncope), breathlessness, and/or fatigue.

In addition to The National Organization for Rare Disorders (NORD) listed in Section III, the following organizations in Section II (Disease Specific) and in Section III (Umbrella) and Section IV (Government Agencies) can provide more information:
American Heart Association, *III*
Congenital Heart Anomalies, Support, Education, & Resources, *III*
Congenital Heart Disease Resource Page, *III*
NIH/National Heart, Lung and Blood Institute, *IV*

483 HEAVY METAL POISONING

Heavy Metal Poisoning results from an overexposure to some types of metal. This may occur from industrial exposure, from air or water pollution, or from foods, medicines or improperly coated food containers. Occasionally hemodialysis (filtering of the blood mechanically to treat severe kidney failure) may be a cause.

In addition to The National Organization for Rare Disorders (NORD) listed in Section III, the following organizations in Section II (Disease Specific) and in Section III (Umbrella) and Section IV (Government

Agencies) can provide more information:
Food and Drug Administration (FDA) Office of Inquiry & Consumer Information, *IV*
NIH/National Institute of Environmental Health Sciences Clearinghouse, *IV*
National Lead Information Center, *III*

484 HEMANGIOMA THROMBOCYTOPENIA SYNDROME

Hemangioma-Thrombocytopenia Syndrome (also known as Kasabach-Merritt Syndrome) is a rare disorder characterized by an abnormal blood condition in which the low number of blood platelets causes bleeding (thrombocytopenia). The thrombocytopenia is found in association with a benign tumor consisting of large, blood-filled spaces (cavernous hemangioma). The exact cause of this disorder is not known.

In addition to The National Organization for Rare Disorders (NORD) listed in Section III, the following organizations in Section II (Disease Specific) and in Section III (Umbrella) and Section IV (Government Agencies) can provide more information:
Hemangioma Support System, *II*
NIH/National Heart, Lung and Blood Institute, *IV*

485 HEMATURIA, BENIGN, FAMILIAL

Benign Familial Hematuria, also known as Thin-Basement-Membrane Nephropathy, is a nonprogressive genetic kidney disease that usually begins during childhood. The disorder is characterized by the presence of red blood cells in the urine (hematuria). The blood in the urine may be present in microscopic amounts (microscopic hematuria) and not visible to the eye, present in small amounts that give the urine a "cloudy" or "smoky" appearance, or easily visible. Many individuals with the disorder have abnormalities of the kidneys glomeruli, the clusters of small blood vessels (capillaries) that normally filter the blood passing through the kidneys (glomeruli filtration). In such cases, the membrane (basement membrane) supporting the loops of capillaries that make up the renal glomeruli may be abnormally thin. Benign Familial Hematuria may be inherited as an autosomal dominant genetic trait.

In addition to The National Organization for Rare Disorders (NORD) listed in Section III, the following organizations in Section II (Disease Specific) and in Section III (Umbrella) and Section IV (Government Agencies) can provide more information:
American Foundation for Urologic Disease, *III*
American Kidney Fund, Inc., *III*
NIH/National Kidney and Urologic Diseases Information Clearinghouse, *IV*
National Kidney Foundation, *III*

486 HEMOCHROMATOSIS, HEREDITARY

Hereditary Hemochromatosis is a metabolic disorder characterized by excessive absorption of iron. The high accumulation of iron eventually damages numerous organs. Involvement of the liver, pancreas or heart may lead to serious complications, particularly in older patients. Joints and skin may also become diseased.

In addition to The National Organization for Rare Disorders (NORD) listed in Section III, the following organizations in Section II (Disease Specific) and in Section III (Umbrella) and Section IV (Government Agencies) can provide more information:
Alliance of Genetic Support Groups, *III*
Iron Overload Diseases Association, Inc., *III*
March of Dimes Birth Defects Foundation, *III*
Metabolic Information Network, *III*
NIH/National Institute of Diabetes, Digestive and Kidney Diseases, *IV*

487 HEMOGLOBINURIA, PAROXYSMAL COLD

Paroxysmal Cold Hemoglobinuria is a very rare autoimmune hemolytic disorder characterized by the premature destruction of healthy red blood cells minutes to hours after exposure to cold. Autoimmune diseases occur when the body's natural defenses against invading organisms (e.g., lymphocytes, antibodies) destroy healthy tissue for unknown reasons. Normally, red blood cells have a life span of approximately 120 days before they are removed by the spleen. In an individual affected with Paroxysmal Cold Hemoglobinuria, the red blood cells are destroyed prematurely and suddenly (paroxysmally) upon exposure to temperatures of 10 to 15 degrees Centigrade and below.

In addition to The National Organization for Rare Disorders (NORD) listed in Section III, the following organizations in Section II (Disease Specific) and in Section III (Umbrella) and Section IV (Government Agencies) can provide more information:
American Autoimmune Related Diseases Association, Inc., *III*
NIH/National Institute of Allergy and Infectious Diseases, *IV*

488 HEMOGLOBINURIA, PAROXYSMAL NOCTURNAL

Paroxysmal Nocturnal Hemoglobinuria is a decrease of red blood cells (anemia) caused by a defect in the membrane of the red blood cells. It is characterized by the presence of blood (hemoglobin) in the urine (hemoglobinuria) and plasma (hemoglobinemia) which occurs chiefly at night due to breakdown of red blood cells.

In addition to The National Organization for Rare Disorders (NORD) listed in Section III, the following organizations in Section II (Disease Specific) and in Section III (Umbrella) and Section IV (Government Agencies) can provide more information:
NIH/Hematology Branch, National Heart, Lung and Blood Institute (NHLBI), *IV*
NIH/National Institute of Allergy and Infectious Diseases, *IV*

489 HEMOLYTIC UREMIC SYNDROME

Hemolytic-Uremic Syndrome (HUS) is a very rare disorder that primarily affects young children between the ages of one to 10 years, particularly those under the age of four years. In many cases, the onset of HUS is preceded by a flu-like illness (gastroenteritis) characterized by vomiting, abdominal pain, fever, and diarrhea, which, in some cases, may be bloody. Symptoms of Hemolytic-Uremic Syndrome usually become apparent three to 10 days after the development of gastroenteritis and may include sudden paleness (pallor), irritability, weakness, lack of energy (lethargy), and/or excretion of abnormally diminished amounts of urine (oliguria). The disease typically progresses to include inability of the kidneys to process waste products from the blood and excrete them into the urine (acute renal failure); a decrease in circulating red blood cells (microangiopathic hemolytic anemia); a decrease in circulating blood platelets, which assist in blood clotting functions (thrombocytopenia); and the abnormal accumulation of platelets within certain blood vessels (microthrombi), reducing the blood flow to several organs (e.g., kidneys, pancreas, brain) potentially leading to multiple organ dysfunction or failure. In some cases, neurological problems may be present at the onset of Hemolytic-Uremic Syndrome or may occur at any time during the disorder's progression. Neurological symptoms may include dizziness, seizures (partial or generalized), disorientation or confusion, and/or loss of consciousness (coma). The onset of Hemolytic-Uremic Syndrome is most frequently associated with infection by a particular strain (O157:H7) of Escherichia coli (E. coli) bacterium. Occasionally, adults may be affected by Hemolytic-Uremic Syndrome.

In addition to The National Organization for Rare Disorders (NORD) listed in Section III, the following organizations in Section II (Disease Specific) and in Section III (Umbrella) and Section IV (Government Agencies) can provide more information:
American Kidney Fund, Inc., *III*
Lois Joy Galler Foundation for Hemolytic Uremic Syndrome, Inc., *II*
NIH/National Institute of Allergy and Infectious Diseases, *IV*
NIH/National Institute of Diabetes, Digestive and Kidney Diseases, *IV*
NIH/National Institute of Neurological Disorders and Stroke, *IV*
National Kidney Foundation, *III*
World Health Organization (WHO) Regional Office for the Americas (AMRO), *III*

490 HEMOPHILIA

Hemophilia is a rare inherited blood clotting (coagulation) disorder caused by inactive or deficient blood proteins (usually factor VIII). Factor VIII is one of several proteins that enable the blood to clot. Hemophilia may be classified as mild, moderate, or severe. The level of severity is determined by the percentage of active clotting factor in the blood (normal percentage ranges from 50 to 150 percent). People who have severe hemophilia have less than one percent of active clotting factor in their blood.

There are three major types of Hemophilia: Hemophilia A (also known as classical hemophilia, Factor VIII deficiency or antihemophilic globulin [AHG] deficiency); Hemophilia B (Christmas disease or factor IX deficiency); and Hemophilia C (factor XI deficiency). Hemophilia A and B are inherited as X-linked recessive genetic traits, while Hemophilia C is inherited as an autosomal recessive genetic trait. Therefore, while Hemophilia A and B are fully expressed in males only, Hemophilia C affects males and females in equal numbers.

In addition to The National Organization for Rare Disorders (NORD) listed in Section III, the following organizations in Section II (Disease Specific) and in Section III (Umbrella) and Section IV (Government Agencies) can provide more information:
Alliance of Genetic Support Groups, *III*
March of Dimes Birth Defects Foundation, *III*

NIH/National Heart, Lung and Blood Institute Information Center, *IV*
National Hemophilia Foundation, *II*

491 **HEMORRHAGIC TELANGIECTASIA, HEREDITARY**

Hereditary Hemorrhagic Telangiectasia (HHT or Osler-Weber-Rendu Syndrome) is a hereditary disorder characterized by blood vessel lesions (telangiectases) on the skin, mucous membranes and in many internal organs. Often, patients exhibit signs of anemia caused by bleeding of the telangiectases.

In addition to The National Organization for Rare Disorders (NORD) listed in Section III, the following organizations in Section II (Disease Specific) and in Section III (Umbrella) and Section IV (Government Agencies) can provide more information:
Alliance of Genetic Support Groups, *III*
Hereditary Hemorrhagic Telangiectasia (HHT) Foundation International, Inc., *II*
NIH/National Heart, Lung and Blood Institute, *IV*

492 **HEPATIC FIBROSIS, CONGENITAL**

Congenital Hepatic Fibrosis is a rare disease that affects both the liver and kidneys. The patient is born with this disorder (congenital) and it is thought to be inherited as an autosomal recessive trait. The typical liver abnormalities are an enlarged liver (hepatomegaly), increased pressure in the venous system that carries blood from different organs to the liver (portal hypertension), and fiberlike connective tissue that spreads over the liver (hepatic fibrosis). Many patients with Congenital Hepatic Fibrosis also have polycystic kidney disease, which is characterized by cysts in the kidneys. Bleeding from the gastrointestinal area (stomach and intestines) is the main clinical problem in patients with Congenital Hepatic Fibrosis.

In addition to The National Organization for Rare Disorders (NORD) listed in Section III, the following organizations in Section II (Disease Specific) and in Section III (Umbrella) and Section IV (Government Agencies) can provide more information:
American Kidney Fund, Inc., *III*
American Liver Foundation, *III*
International Patient Advocacy Association, *III*
NIH/National Kidney and Urologic Diseases Information Clearinghouse, *IV*
National Kidney Foundation, *III*

493 **HEPATITIS B**

Hepatitis B Virus (HBV) is one of three viral agents which cause inflammation of the liver known as "hepatitis" or "diffuse hepatocellular inflammatory disease." Hepatitis B is characterized by fever, nausea, vomiting and yellow discoloration of the skin (jaundice). In its most serious form Hepatitis B can become a chronic infection, or may cause liver cancer if left untreated. The hepatitis B virus can be passed from mother to unborn child, and is highly contagious through bodily fluids such as blood, semen and possibly saliva. It is often spread from person to person through intravenous drug use.

In addition to The National Organization for Rare Disorders (NORD) listed in Section III, the following organizations in Section II (Disease Specific) and in Section III (Umbrella) and Section IV (Government Agencies) can provide more information:
American Liver Foundation, *III*
American Social Health Association, *III*
Centers for Disease Control and Prevention, *IV*
Immunization Action Coalition/Hepatitis B Coalition, *III*
NIH/National Institute of Allergy and Infectious Diseases, *IV*
United Liver Association, *III*

494 **HEPATITIS, NEONATAL**

Neonatal Hepatitis, also known as Giant Cell Hepatitis, is a liver disease of infancy. It is the most common cause of interrupted bile flow from the liver (cholestasis) in newborns.

Bile is secreted by the liver and flows through the bile ducts into the small intestine. Bile aids in the digestion of fats. The symptoms of Neonatal Hepatitis may include an abnormal yellow discoloration of the skin (jaundice), pale stools, and/or dark urine. The exact cause of Neonatal Hepatitis is not fully understood. Most cases occur for no apparent reason (sporadic). However, some cases of Neonatal Hepatitis may be inherited as an autosomal recessive genetic trait.

In addition to The National Organization for Rare Disorders (NORD) listed in Section III, the following organizations in Section II (Disease Specific) and in Section III (Umbrella) and Section IV (Government Agencies) can provide more information:
American Liver Foundation, *III*
Children's Liver Alliance, *III*
NIH/National Digestive Diseases Information Clearinghouse, *IV*
United Liver Association, *III*

495 **HEPATITIS, NON-A, NON-B (HEPATITIS C)**

Non-A, Non-B (NANB) Hepatitis (Hepatitis C) is a contagious liver disease that appears to be caused by at least two different viruses.

Diagnosis is usually established by excluding Hepatitis A, Hepatitis B or a variety of other similar liver diseases. The main sources of Non-A, Non-B Hepatitis infection include blood transfusions, intravenous drug use, or rarely personal contact with infected people. This disorder causes symptoms that appear similar to Hepatitis A or Hepatitis B and, in some cases, may cause chronic liver disease such as cirrhosis or hepatocellular carcinoma. The symptoms of NANB Hepatitis may linger on for quite a long time, but they tend to regress in most cases.

In addition to The National Organization for Rare Disorders (NORD) listed in Section III, the following organizations in Section II (Disease Specific) and in Section III (Umbrella) and Section IV (Government Agencies) can provide more information:
American Liver Foundation, *III*
Centers for Disease Control and Prevention, *IV*
NIH/National Institute of Allergy and Infectious Diseases, *IV*
United Liver Association, *III*

496 HEPATORENAL SYNDROME

Hepatorenal Syndrome is a progressive type of kidney (renal) failure that occurs as a result of severe LIVER disease. It is characterized by acute kidney (renal) failure that is NOT caused by primary KIDNEY dysfunction. Symptoms such as yellowing of the skin (jaundice) and urination problems occur in the two types of this liver disease.

In addition to The National Organization for Rare Disorders (NORD) listed in Section III, the following organizations in Section II (Disease Specific) and in Section III (Umbrella) and Section IV (Government Agencies) can provide more information:
American Association of Kidney Patients, *III*
American Foundation for Urologic Disease, *III*
American Kidney Fund, Inc., *III*
American Liver Foundation, *III*
NIH/National Kidney and Urologic Diseases Information Clearinghouse, *IV*

497 HERMANSKY PUDLAK SYNDROME

Hermansky-Pudlak Syndrome is a rare, hereditary disorder that consists of four characteristics: lack of skin pigmentation (albinism), blood platelet dysfunction with prolonged bleeding, visual impairment, and abnormal storage of a fatty-like substance (ceroid) in various tissues of the body.

In addition to The National Organization for Rare Disorders (NORD) listed in Section III, the following organizations in Section II (Disease Specific) and in Section III (Umbrella) and Section IV (Government Agencies) can provide more information:
Blind Children's Fund, *III*
Hermansky-Pudlak Syndrome Network, Inc., *II*
NIH/National Institute of Arthritis and Musculoskeletal and Skin Diseases, *IV*
National Association for Parents of the Visually Impaired, *III*
National Association for Visually Handicapped, *III*

498 HERMAPHRODITISM, TRUE

True Hermaphroditism is a very rare genetic disorder in which an infant is born with the internal reproductive organs (gonads) of both sexes (i.e., female ovaries and male testes). The external sex organs of an affected individual are usually a combination of male and female.

In addition to The National Organization for Rare Disorders (NORD) listed in Section III, the following organizations in Section II (Disease Specific) and in Section III (Umbrella) and Section IV (Government Agencies) can provide more information:
NIH/National Institute of Child Health and Human Development, *IV*

499 HERPES, NEONATAL

Neonatal Herpes is a very rare disorder affecting newborn infants infected with the Herpes simplex virus (HSV), also called Herpesvirus hominis. This disorder can vary from mild to severe. In most cases the disorder is transferred by a parent with oral or genital herpes to an offspring before, during, or shortly after birth.

In the mild form, Neonatal Herpes is caused by type 2 virus. The skin, eyes, and mouth may become infected, and symptoms may recur for some time.

In its severe form, which is caused by type 1 virus, Neonatal Herpes is a serious disease characterized by blistery (vesicular) red lesions of the skin and mucous membranes. Liver, spleen, lungs, brain, kidneys, and adrenal glands may also become infected.

In addition to The National Organization for Rare Disorders (NORD) listed in Section III, the following organizations in Section II (Disease Specific) and in Section III (Umbrella) and Section IV (Government Agencies) can provide more information:
Centers for Disease Control and Prevention, *IV*
NIH/National Institute of Allergy and Infectious Diseases, *IV*

500 HERS DISEASE

Hers Disease is a hereditary glycogen storage disease which usually has milder symptoms than most other types of glycogen storage disorders. It is caused by a deficiency of the enzyme known as liver phosphorylase. Hers Disease is characterized by enlargement of the liver (hepatomegaly), moderately low blood sugar (hypoglycemia), elevated levels of acetone and other ketone bodies in the blood (ketosis), and moderate growth retardation. Symptoms are not always evident during childhood. Children are usually able to lead normal lives. In some cases symptoms may be severe.

In addition to The National Organization for Rare Disorders (NORD) listed in Section III, the following organizations in Section II (Disease Specific) and in Section III (Umbrella) and Section IV (Government Agencies) can provide more information:

Association for Neuro-Metabolic Disorders, *III*
Metabolic Information Network, *III*
NIH/National Institute of Diabetes, Digestive & Kidney Diseases, *IV*
Research Trust for Metabolic Diseases in Children, *III*

501 HICCUPS, CHRONIC

Hiccups are sudden, involuntary, repeated spasms of the diaphragm, followed by an intake of air into the larynx which causes the characteristic "hic" sound. They may occur a few times within a minute or several times a second. Normally, hiccups last for only a few minutes. However, when they persist for days or weeks they can be very serious.

In addition to The National Organization for Rare Disorders (NORD) listed in Section III, the following organizations in Section II (Disease Specific) and in Section III (Umbrella) and Section IV (Government Agencies) can provide more information:

NIH/National Heart, Lung and Blood Institute Information Center, *IV*

502 HIDRADENITIS SUPPURATIVA

Hidradenitis Suppurativa is a bacterial infection that occurs in certain areas of the body producing obstruction and rupture of the apocrine glands (similar to sweat glands). These locally infected areas, seen as swellings or nodules just under the skin, can cause deep painful inflammations that resemble boils.

In addition to The National Organization for Rare Disorders (NORD) listed in Section III, the following organizations in Section II (Disease Specific) and in Section III (Umbrella) and Section IV (Government Agencies) can provide more information:

Hidradenitis Support Group, *II*
NIH/National Institute of Allergy and Infectious Diseases, *IV*
NIH/National Institute of Arthritis and Musculoskeletal and Skin Diseases, *IV*

503 HIRSCHSPRUNG'S DISEASE

Hirschsprung's Disease is a rare disorder of the colon. A person may be born with it (congenital) or it may be acquired later in life.

In congenital Hirschsprung's Disease major symptoms may include constipation, distention of the bowel and vomiting. The disease may be apparent at birth, may not be diagnosed until later in infancy, or may not become apparent until later in childhood.

Acquired Hirschsprung's Disease develops later in life when the entire rectum and colon appear unusually wide (dilated). In this form of the disorder it is usually associated with diseases such as Parkinson's disease, scleroderma, intestinal pseudo-obstruction, Chagas' disease, amyloidosis, and drug-induced or idiopathic (cause unknown) constipation.

In addition to The National Organization for Rare Disorders (NORD) listed in Section III, the following organizations in Section II (Disease Specific) and in Section III (Umbrella) and Section IV (Government Agencies) can provide more information:

American Pseudo-obstruction & Hirschsprung's Disease Society, Inc., *III*
NIH/National Digestive Diseases Information Clearinghouse, *IV*
Pull-thru Network, *III*
United Ostomy Association, Inc., *III*

504 HISTIDINEMIA

Histidinemia is a rare hereditary metabolic disorder characterized by a deficiency of the enzyme histidase, which is necessary for the metabolism of the amino acid histidine. The concentration of histidine is elevated in the blood. Excessive amounts of histidine, imidazole pyruvic acid, and other imidazole metabolism products are excreted in the urine. Mental retardation and a speech defect have been found in some cases of Histidinemia, while in other cases, no obvious symptoms appear to indicate that a person may have this disorder (asymptomatic).

In addition to The National Organization for Rare Disorders (NORD) listed in Section III, the following organizations in Section II (Disease Specific) and in Section III (Umbrella) and Section IV (Government Agencies) can provide more information:

Association for Neuro-Metabolic Disorders, *III*
Metabolic Information Network, *III*
NIH/National Institute of Diabetes, Digestive & Kidney Diseases, *IV*
Research Trust for Metabolic Diseases in Children, *III*

505 HISTIOCYTOSIS X

Histiocytosis-X is a term formerly given to three blood disorders that share basic characteristics and a common origin. As a result of better understanding of this childhood illness, the term Langerhans Cell Histiocytosis (LCH) is now often applied. This group of disorders develop similarly although symptoms vary widely between cases. The most common feature is the abnormal accumulation of a specific type of tissue cell (histiocytes) in various organs. The type of damage caused by accumulations depends on the size and location of the "growth." Bones, skin, the liver, spleen, lungs and brain are most commonly affected. The growths are not cancerous despite the aggressive clinical course and therapies resembling those used for cancer patients. Most cases are sporadic (non-familial). Although more than one case has appeared in the same family, no clear inheritance pattern has been identified.

In addition to The National Organization for Rare Disorders (NORD) listed in Section III, the following organizations in Section II (Disease Specific) and in Section III (Umbrella) and Section IV (Government Agencies) can provide more information:
American Lung Association, *III*
Histiocytosis Association of America, *III*
NIH/National Heart, Lung and Blood Institute Information Center, *IV*

506 HODGKIN'S DISEASE

Hodgkin's Disease is a form of cancer of the lymphatic system, especially the lymph nodes. Tumors occur in the lymph nodes (places where lymphatic vessels unite) and/or the area around the nodes. Fever, night sweats, and weight loss may occur along with swollen lymph nodes.

In addition to The National Organization for Rare Disorders (NORD) listed in Section III, the following organizations in Section II (Disease Specific) and in Section III (Umbrella) and Section IV (Government Agencies) can provide more information:
American Cancer Society, Inc., *III*
NIH/National Cancer Institute, *IV*

507 HOLOPROSENCEPHALY

Holoprosencephaly is the failure of the prosenceplon section of the forebrain (the part of the brain in the fetus that evolves into parts of the adult brain) to develop. This causes defects in the development of the middle of the face and in brain structure and function. Closely set eyes (hypotelorism), missing front teeth (incisors), and an abnormally small head (microcephaly) may occur. Rarely, severely affected infants are born with cyclopia (the eyes fused into one) and a deformed or absent nose.

In addition to The National Organization for Rare Disorders (NORD) listed in Section III, the following organizations in Section II (Disease Specific) and in Section III (Umbrella) and Section IV (Government Agencies) can provide more information:
Fighters for Encephaly Support Group, *III*
Independent Holoprosencephaly Support Site, *II*
NIH/National Institute of Child Health and Human Development, *IV*

508 HOLT ORAM SYNDROME

Holt-Oram Syndrome (HOS) is an extremely rare genetic disorder characterized by distinctive malformations of the bones of the thumbs and forearms (upper limbs) and/or abnormalities of the heart. The symptoms and physical findings associated with Holt-Oram Syndrome vary greatly from case to case. In many infants with the disorder, the thumbs may be absent or underdeveloped (hypoplastic) or have an extra bone (triphalangy). Affected infants may also have additional upper limb malformations such as underdevelopment (hypoplasia) of or extra bones in the wrists (e.g., scaphoid bone); malformations of certain bones of the hands (metacarpals); and/or underdevelopment of the bones of the forearms (radius and ulna) and/or the bones of the upper arms (humerus). The shoulder blades (scapulae), the collarbones (clavicles), and/or other bones may also be malformed.

In most cases, infants with Holt-Oram Syndrome have heart (cardiac) abnormalities that may include structural (anatomical) malformations of the heart and/or abnormal transmission of electrical impulses (signals) that coordinate the heart's muscular contractions (electrocardiographic conduction defects). In individuals with the disorder, atrial and/or ventricular septal defects (ASDs and/or VSDs) are the most common structural heart defects. ASDs are characterized by an abnormal opening in the fibrous partition (septum) that separates the two upper chambers (atria) of the heart. VSDs are characterized by an abnormal opening in the septum that divides the heart's two lower chambers (ventricles). Individuals with Holt-Oram Syndrome may have electrocardiographic conduction defects as a separate finding or in association with structural abnormalities of the heart (e.g., ASDs and/or VSDs). In many affected individuals with conduction defects, there may be an interruption of the normal flow of electrical impulses (heart block) through the heart. Depending upon the nature and combination of structural heart defects and/or conduction abnormalities, the effects of such defects are highly variable, ranging from no apparent symptoms (asymptomatic) in some affected individuals to serious, potentially life-threatening complications in others.

In approximately 60 percent of cases, Holt-Oram Syndrome is inherited as an autosomal dominant genetic trait. In about 40 percent of cases, the disorder appears to occur randomly, for unknown reasons (sporadically).

In addition to The National Organization for Rare Disorders (NORD) listed in Section III, the following organizations in Section II (Disease Specific) and in Section III (Umbrella) and Section IV (Government Agencies) can provide more information:
American Heart Association, *III*
Association of Children's Prosthetic/Orthotic Clinics, *III*
Big Hearts for Little Hearts, *III*
CHERUB—Association of Families and Friends of Children with Limb Disorders, *III*
Congenital Heart Anomalies, Support, Education, & Resources, *III*
Congenital Heart Disease Resource Page, *III*
Holt-Oram Syndrome Support Group, *II*
NIH/National Arthritis and Musculoskeletal and Skin Diseases Information Clearinghouse, *IV*
NIH/National Heart, Lung and Blood Institute Information Center, *IV*
NIH/National Institute of Child Health and Human Development, *IV*
Superkids, Inc. (newsletter for families and friends of children with limb differences), *III*

509 HOMOCYSTINURIA

Homocystinuria is a rare hereditary error of metabolism. The amino acid methionine is not properly metabolized due to a defect in the enzyme cystathionine synthetase. Symptoms associated with Homocystinuria include mental retardation; delays in reaching developmental milestones (e.g., crawling, walking, sitting); displacement of the lens of the eye (ectopia lentis); abnormal thinning and weakness of the bones (osteoporosis); and/or the formation of blood clots (thrombi) in various veins and arteries that may lead to life-threatening complications. Homocystinuria is thought to be inherited as an autosomal recessive genetic trait.

In addition to The National Organization for Rare Disorders (NORD) listed in Section III, the following organizations in Section II (Disease Specific) and in Section III (Umbrella) and Section IV (Government Agencies) can provide more information:
Alliance of Genetic Support Groups, *III*
Association for Neuro-Metabolic Disorders, *III*
March of Dimes Birth Defects Foundation, *III*
Metabolic Information Network, *III*
NIH/National Digestive Diseases Information Clearinghouse, *IV*
Research Trust for Metabolic Diseases in Children, *III*
The Arc (a national organization on mental retardation), *III*

510 HORNER'S SYNDROME

Horner's Syndrome is a disorder that consists of extreme contraction of the pupil of the eye (miosis), drooping of the upper eyelid (ptosis), absence of sweating of the face (anidrosis), and sinking of the eyeball into the bony cavity that protects the eye (enophthalmos). The disorder is caused by a buildup of tissue (lesion or growth) or injury somewhere along the cervical sympathetic chain. The cervical sympathetic chain is a grouping of nerves that involuntarily stimulate the muscles, the heart, and the sweat glands. This chain governs the uncontrolled reflexes our body performs such as contraction of the eye.

In addition to The National Organization for Rare Disorders (NORD) listed in Section III, the following organizations in Section II (Disease Specific) and in Section III (Umbrella) and Section IV (Government Agencies) can provide more information:
NIH/National Eye Institute, *IV*

511 HUMAN GRANULOCYTIC EHRLICHIOSIS (HGE)

Human Granulocytic Ehrlichiosis (HGE) is a rare infectious disease belonging to a group of diseases known as the Human Ehrlichioses. The Ehrlichioses are a group of infectious diseases caused by bacteria belonging to the "Ehrlichia" family. Three forms of Human Ehrlichial infection have been identified including Human Granulocytic Ehrlichiosis (HGE), Sennetsu Fever, and Human Monocytic Ehrlichiosis (HME). Though caused by different strains of Ehrlichia bacteria, the three disorders are all characterized by similar symptoms.

The symptoms of Human Granulocytic Ehrlichiosis (HGE) may include a sudden high fever, headache, muscle aches (myalgia), chills, and a general feeling of weakness and fatigue (malaise) within a week or so after initial infection. In most cases, abnormal laboratory findings may occur including an abnormally low number of circulating blood platelets (thrombocytopenia), a decrease in white blood cells (leukopenia), and an abnormal increase in the level of certain liver enzymes (hepatic transaminases). In some cases, symptoms may progress to include nausea, vomiting, cough, diarrhea, loss of appetite (anorexia), and/or confusion. If Human Granulocytic Ehrlichiosis is left untreated, life-threatening symptoms, such as kidney failure and/or respiratory problems, may develop in some cases. Human Granulocytic Ehrlichiosis is caused by a bacterium of the Ehrlichiosis family that has not yet been named. The Ehrlichial bacterium is carried and transmitted by certain ticks (vectors), such as the deer tick (Ixodes dammini) and the American dog tick (Dermacentor variabilis).

In addition to The National Organization for Rare Disorders (NORD) listed in Section III, the following organizations in Section II (Disease Specific) and in Section III (Umbrella) and Section IV (Government Agencies) can provide more information:

American Lyme Disease Foundation, Inc., *II*
Centers for Disease Control and Prevention, *IV*
NIH/National Institute of Allergy and Infectious Diseases, *IV*
World Health Organization (WHO) Regional Office for the Americas (AMRO), *III*

512 HUMAN MONOCYTIC EHRLICHIOSIS (HME)

Human Monocytic Ehrlichiosis (HME) is a rare infectious disease belonging to a group of diseases known as the Human Ehrlichioses. These diseases are caused by bacteria belonging to the "Ehrlichia" family. Three forms of Human Ehrlichioses have been identified, including Human Monocytic Ehrlichiosis, Sennetsu Fever, and Human Granulocytic Ehrlichiosis. Though caused by different strains of Ehrlichia bacteria, the three disorders are characterized by similar symptoms.

The symptoms of Human Monocytic Ehrlichiosis may include a sudden high fever, headache, muscle aches (myalgia), chills, and a general feeling of weakness and fatigue (malaise) within a few weeks after initial infection. In addition, in many cases, laboratory findings may indicate an abnormally low number of circulating blood platelets (thrombocytopenia), a decrease in white blood cells (leukopenia), and an abnormal increase in the level of certain liver enzymes (hepatic transaminases). In some individuals, symptoms may progress to include nausea, vomiting, diarrhea, weight loss, and/or confusion. If HME is left untreated, life-threatening symptoms, such as kidney failure and respiratory problems, may develop in some cases. Human Monocytic Ehrlichiosis is caused by the bacteria Ehrlichia chaffeensis (or E. chaffeensis). E. chaffeensis is carried and transmitted by certain ticks (vectors), such as the Lone Star tick (Amblyomma americanum) and the American dog tick (Dermacentor variabilis).

In addition to The National Organization for Rare Disorders (NORD) listed in Section III, the following organizations in Section II (Disease Specific) and in Section III (Umbrella) and Section IV (Government Agencies) can provide more information:

Centers for Disease Control and Prevention, *IV*
NIH/National Institute of Allergy and Infectious Diseases, *IV*
World Health Organization (WHO) Regional Office for the Americas (AMRO), *III*

513 HUNTER SYNDROME

Mucopolysaccharidoses (MPS Disorders) are a group of rare genetic disorders caused by the deficiency of one of ten specific lysosomal enzymes resulting in an inability to metabolize complex carbohydrates (mucopolysaccharides) into simpler molecules. The accumulation of these large, undegraded mucopolysaccharides in the cells of the body causes a number of physical symptoms and abnormalities.

The most prevalent form of MPS Type II is called Hunter Syndrome. The disorder can be manifested in a mild or a severe form.

In addition to The National Organization for Rare Disorders (NORD) listed in Section III, the following organizations in Section II (Disease Specific) and in Section III (Umbrella) and Section IV (Government Agencies) can provide more information:

Alliance of Genetic Support Groups, *III*
Canadian Society for Mucopolysaccharide and Related Diseases, Inc., *III*
Metabolic Information Network, *III*
NIH/National Institute of Diabetes, Digestive and Kidney Diseases, *IV*

National MPS (Mucopolysaccharidoses/Mucolipidoses) Society, Inc., *III*
Research Trust for Metabolic Diseases in Children, *III*
The Arc (a national organization on mental retardation), *III*
Vaincre Les Maladies Lysosomales, *III*

514 HUNTINGTON'S DISEASE

Huntington's Disease is an inherited progressively degenerative disorder of the nervous system. This disorder is characterized by involuntary muscle movements (chorea) and the loss of cognitive abilities (dementia).

In addition to The National Organization for Rare Disorders (NORD) listed in Section III, the following organizations in Section II (Disease Specific) and in Section III (Umbrella) and Section IV (Government Agencies) can provide more information:
Alliance of Genetic Support Groups, *III*
Hereditary Disease Foundation, Inc., *III*
Huntington Society of Canada, *II*
Huntington's Disease Society of America, *II*
March of Dimes Birth Defects Foundation, *III*
NIH/National Institute of Neurological Disorders and Stroke, *IV*
WE MOVE, *III*

515 HURLER SYNDROME

Mucopolysaccharidoses (MPS Disorders), are a group of rare genetic disorders caused by the deficiency of one of ten specific lysosomal enzymes, resulting in an inability to metabolize complex carbohydrates (mucopolysaccharides) into simpler molecules. The accumulation of these large, undegraded mucopolysaccharides in the cells of the body causes a number of physical symptoms and abnormalities. Hurler Syndrome is a form of MPS.

In addition to The National Organization for Rare Disorders (NORD) listed in Section III, the following organizations in Section II (Disease Specific) and in Section III (Umbrella) and Section IV (Government Agencies) can provide more information:
Canadian Society for Mucopolysaccharide and Related Diseases, Inc., *III*
Metabolic Information Network, *III*
NIH/National Digestive Diseases Information Clearinghouse, *IV*
National MPS (Mucopolysaccharidoses/Mucolipidoses) Society, Inc., *III*
Research Trust for Metabolic Diseases in Children, *III*
The Arc (a national organization on mental retardation), *III*
Vaincre Les Maladies Lysosomales, *III*

516 HUTCHINSON GILFORD PROGERIA SYNDROME

Hutchinson-Gilford Progeria Syndrome is a very rare progressive disorder of childhood characterized by premature aging (progeria), growth delays occurring in the first year of life resulting in short stature and low weight, deterioration of the layer of fat beneath the skin (subcutaneous adipose tissue), and characteristic craniofacial abnormalities including an abnormally small face, underdeveloped jaw (micrognathia), unusually prominent eyes, and/or a small, "beak-like" nose. In addition, during the first year or two of life, scalp hair, eyebrows, and eyelashes may become sparse, and veins of the scalp may become unusually prominent. Additional symptoms and physical findings may include joint stiffness, repeated nonhealing fractures, a progressive aged appearance of the skin, delays in tooth eruption (dentition), and/or malformation and crowding of the teeth. Individuals with the disorder typically have normal intelligence. In most cases, affected individuals experience premature, widespread thickening and loss of elasticity of artery walls (arteriosclerosis), potentially resulting in life-threatening complications. Hutchinson-Gilford Progeria Syndrome is thought to be due to an autosomal dominant genetic change (mutation) that occurs for unknown reasons (sporadic).

In addition to The National Organization for Rare Disorders (NORD) listed in Section III, the following organizations in Section II (Disease Specific) and in Section III (Umbrella) and Section IV (Government Agencies) can provide more information:
International Progeria Registry, *III*
Metabolic Information Network, *III*
NIH/National Institute of Child Health and Human Development, *IV*
Research Trust for Metabolic Diseases in Children, *III*

517 HYDRANENCEPHALY

Hydranencephaly is a central nervous system disorder inherited through an unknown mode of transmission. This extremely rare form of Porencephaly involves almost total absence of portions of the brain. Results of neurologic examination in newborns may be normal or abnormal. The head can appear enlarged at birth in some children. Vision impairment, lack of growth and intellectual deficits are symptomatic of this disorder.

In addition to The National Organization for Rare Disorders (NORD) listed in Section III, the following

organizations in Section II (Disease Specific) and in Section III (Umbrella) and Section IV (Government Agencies) can provide more information:
Children's Brain Diseases Foundation, *II*
Guardians of Hydrocephalus Research Foundation, *II*
Hydrocephalus Association, *II*
NIH/National Institute of Neurological Disorders and Stroke, *IV*
National Hydrocephalus Foundation, *II*
The Arc (a national organization on mental retardation), *III*

518 HYDROCEPHALUS

Hydrocephalus is a condition in which abnormally widened (dilated) cerebral spaces in the brain (ventricles) inhibit the normal flow of cerebrospinal fluid (CSF). The cerebrospinal fluid accumulates in the skull and puts pressure on the brain tissue. An enlarged head in infants and increased cerebrospinal fluid pressure are frequent findings but are not necessary for the diagnosis of Hydrocephalus. There are several different forms of Hydrocephalus: communicating hydrocephalus, non-communicating hydrocephalus or obstructive hydrocephalus, internal hydrocephalus, normal pressure hydrocephalus, and benign hydrocephalus.

In addition to The National Organization for Rare Disorders (NORD) listed in Section III, the following organizations in Section II (Disease Specific) and in Section III (Umbrella) and Section IV (Government Agencies) can provide more information:
Alliance of Genetic Support Groups, *III*
Association for Spina Bifida and Hydrocephalus, *III*
Guardians of Hydrocephalus Research Foundation, *II*
Hydrocephalus Association, *II*
Hydrocephalus Research Foundation, Inc., *II*
Hydrocephalus Support Group, Inc., *II*
March of Dimes Birth Defects Foundation, *III*
NIH/National Institute of Neurological Disorders and Stroke, *IV*
National Hydrocephalus Foundation, *II*
The Arc (a national organization on mental retardation), *III*

519 HYPER IGM SYNDROME

Hyper-IgM Syndrome (HIGM1) is a rare inherited (primary) immunodeficiency disorder that is typically inherited as an X-linked recessive genetic trait. Symptoms and physical findings associated with the disorder usually become apparent in the first or second year of life. Hyper-IgM Syndrome may be characterized by recurrent pus-producing (pyogenic) bacterial infections of the middle ear (otitis media); the membrane that lines the eyelids and the white portions (sclera) of the eyes (conjunctivitis); the sinuses (sinusitis); the lungs (pneumonitis or pneumonia); the upper respiratory tract; the skin (pyoderma); and/or other areas. Individuals with this disorder are also susceptible to "opportunistic" infections, which are infections caused by microorganisms that usually do not cause disease in non-immunodeficient individuals or widespread (systemic) overwhelming disease by microorganisms that typically cause only localized, mild infection. In individuals with Hyper-IgM Syndrome, such opportunistic infections may include those caused by Pneumocystic carinii, a microorganism that causes a form of pneumonia. In addition, affected individuals are prone to certain autoimmune disorders affecting particular elements of the blood, such as neutropenia, a condition in which there is an abnormal decrease of certain white blood cells (neutrophils).

Additional physical findings often associated with the disorder may include enlargement (hypertrophy) of the tonsils, enlargement of the liver and spleen (hepatosplenomegaly), impaired absorption of nutrients by the intestinal tract (malabsorption) with resulting diarrhea, and/or other symptoms. Individuals with this disorder may also develop disorders of the lymphoid tissues, often with involvement of the gastrointestinal tract.

The range and severity of symptoms and physical features associated with this disorder may vary from case to case. Because approximately 70 percent of reported cases of Hyper-IgM Syndrome are inherited as an X-linked recessive genetic trait, the vast majority of affected individuals are male. However, some cases of autosomal recessive and autosomal dominant genetic inheritance have been reported. In addition, an acquired form of this disorder has been described in the medical literature.

In addition to The National Organization for Rare Disorders (NORD) listed in Section III, the following organizations in Section II (Disease Specific) and in Section III (Umbrella) and Section IV (Government Agencies) can provide more information:
American Autoimmune Related Diseases Association, Inc., *III*
Immune Deficiency Foundation, *III*
International Bone Marrow Transplant Registry, *III*
International Patient Organization for Primary Immunodeficiencies, *III*
Jeffrey Modell Foundation, *III*

NIH/National Arthritis and Musculoskeletal and Skin Diseases Information Clearinghouse, *IV*
NIH/National Heart, Lung and Blood Institute Information Center, *IV*
National Bone Marrow Transplant Link, *III*
National Neutropenia Network, *II*
Neutropenia Support Association, Inc., *II*

520 HYPERCHOLESTEROLEMIA

Hypercholesterolemia means unusually high cholesterol. It is a common disorder characterized by a high accumulation of fats in the blood. It is one of the leading causes of atherosclerosis (fatty obstruction of the blood vessels), heart attack and stroke. High cholesterol is the leading health problem in the United States and other Western countries accounting for 50 percent of all deaths. This disorder appears to get worse with advancing age, although in rare cases children can also be affected.

In addition to The National Organization for Rare Disorders (NORD) listed in Section III, the following organizations in Section II (Disease Specific) and in Section III (Umbrella) and Section IV (Government Agencies) can provide more information:
American Heart Association, *III*
NIH/National Heart, Lung and Blood Institute Information Center, *IV*

521 HYPERCHYLOMICRONEMIA

Hyperchylomicronemia is a rare hereditary inborn error of metabolism characterized by a massive accumulation of fatty droplets (chylomicrons) in blood plasma, and a corresponding increase of the blood plasma concentration of fatty substances called triglycerides. The concentration of another fatty substance called "very low density lipoprotein" (VLDL) is usually normal. The disorder is caused by the absence of the enzyme lipoprotein lipase.

In addition to The National Organization for Rare Disorders (NORD) listed in Section III, the following organizations in Section II (Disease Specific) and in Section III (Umbrella) and Section IV (Government Agencies) can provide more information:
Metabolic Information Network, *III*
NIH/National Digestive Diseases Information Clearinghouse, *IV*
Research Trust for Metabolic Diseases in Children, *III*

522 HYPEREXPLEXIA

Hyperexplexia is a rare hereditary neurological disorder. Individuals with this disorder have an excessive startle reaction to sudden unexpected noise, movement, or touch. Symptoms include extreme muscle tension sometimes causing stiffness (hypertonia), and falling stiffly (like a log) to the ground without loss of consciousness. Exaggeration of reflexes (hyperreflexia), and an unstable gait may also occur.

In addition to The National Organization for Rare Disorders (NORD) listed in Section III, the following organizations in Section II (Disease Specific) and in Section III (Umbrella) and Section IV (Government Agencies) can provide more information:
NIH/National Institute of Neurological Disorders and Stroke, *IV*

523 HYPERHIDROSIS, PRIMARY

Primary Hyperhidrosis is a rare disorder characterized by excessive activity (hyperactivity) of the sweat glands (eccrine) in various parts of the body. Symptoms may include generalized or localized profuse sweating. Sweating may occur on the palms of the hands, on the soles of the feet, in the underarm area (axillary), in the groin area, and/or under the breasts. The exact cause of Primary Hyperhidrosis is not known. When excessive sweating occurs because of an underlying disorder, it is said to be Secondary Hyperhidrosis, which is a more common condition than Primary Hyperhidrosis.

In addition to The National Organization for Rare Disorders (NORD) listed in Section III, the following organizations in Section II (Disease Specific) and in Section III (Umbrella) and Section IV (Government Agencies) can provide more information:
NIH/National Institute of Arthritis and Musculoskeletal and Skin Diseases, *IV*
Skin Disease Research Core Centers of the National Institute of Arthritis, *IV*

524 HYPERKALEMIA

Hyperkalemia is an abnormally high concentration of potassium in the blood. It usually occurs due to another underlying medical condition. The body uses potassium for the contraction of muscles (including the heart) and for the functioning of many complicated proteins (enzymes). Potassium is found primarily in the skeletal muscle and bone, and participates with sodium to contribute to the normal flow between the body fluids and the cells of the body. The concentration of potassium in the body is regulated by the kidneys through excretion in urine. When the kidneys are functioning normally, the amount of potassium eaten in the diet is usually sufficient for use by the body and the excess is excreted. Chemical and hormonal influences also regulate the internal potassium balance. Secretion of the hormone insulin, which is normally stimulated by food, prevents a temporary diet-induced high level of potassium (hyperkalemia) by increasing cell absorption of potassium. The hormone aldosterone also aids in regulating the internal balance of potassium. When hyperkalemia occurs, there is an imbalance resulting from a dysfunction of these normal processes.

In addition to The National Organization for Rare Disorders (NORD) listed in Section III, the following organizations in Section II (Disease Specific) and in Section III (Umbrella) and Section IV (Government Agencies) can provide more information:
Digestive Disease National Coalition, *III*
NIH/National Digestive Diseases Information Clearinghouse, *IV*

525 HYPERLIPOPROTEINEMIA TYPE IV

Hyperlipoproteinemia Type IV is an inherited metabolic disorder. It is characterized by an increased blood level of the fats called triglycerides which are contained in very low-density lipids (VLDL). An abnormally high level of triglycerides or cholesterol can result from diet, from genetic causes, or it may occur secondary to other metabolic disorders or as a side effect of certain drugs.

In addition to The National Organization for Rare Disorders (NORD) listed in Section III, the following organizations in Section II (Disease Specific) and in Section III (Umbrella) and Section IV (Government Agencies) can provide more information:
American Heart Association, *III*
Metabolic Information Network, *III*
NIH/National Heart, Lung and Blood Institute Information Center, *IV*

526 HYPEROSTOSIS FRONTALIS INTERNA

Hyperostosis Frontalis Interna is a disorder in which there is excessive growth or thickening of the frontal bone of the skull. It is not known whether this disorder is actually rare. Some scientists feel that this may be a common abnormality found in as many as 12 percent of the female population. This disorder has been found in association with a variety of conditions such as seizures, headaches, obesity, diabetes insipidus, excessive hair growth and sex gland disturbances. Increased serum alkaline phosphatase and elevated serum calcium may occur.

In addition to The National Organization for Rare Disorders (NORD) listed in Section III, the following organizations in Section II (Disease Specific) and in Section III (Umbrella) and Section IV (Government Agencies) can provide more information:
Children's Craniofacial Association, *III*
FACES: The National Craniofacial Association, *III*
NIH/National Arthritis and Musculoskeletal and Skin Diseases Information Clearinghouse, *IV*

527 HYPEROXALURIA, PRIMARY (TYPE I)

Primary Hyperoxaluria (Type I) is a hereditary disorder characterized by an inborn error of glyoxylic acid metabolism. Excessive formation of oxalic acid occurs in the liver, spleen, and kidneys, resulting in excessive levels of the acid in the urine. Calcium oxalate does not dissolve and consequently "stones" are formed in the urinary tract.

In addition to The National Organization for Rare Disorders (NORD) listed in Section III, the following organizations in Section II (Disease Specific) and in Section III (Umbrella) and Section IV (Government Agencies) can provide more information:
Children's Liver Alliance, *III*
Metabolic Information Network, *III*
NIH/National Digestive Diseases Information Clearinghouse, *IV*
Oxalosis and Hyperoxaluria Foundation, *III*
Research Trust for Metabolic Diseases in Children, *III*

528 HYPERPROLINEMIA TYPE I

Hyperprolinemia Type I is a very rare hereditary disorder characterized by an abnormally high level of the amino acid proline in the blood and urine. The high level of this substance is caused by a deficiency of the enzyme proline oxidase, which normally breaks down proline.

In addition to The National Organization for Rare Disorders (NORD) listed in Section III, the following organizations in Section II (Disease Specific) and in Section III (Umbrella) and Section IV (Government Agencies) can provide more information:
Metabolic Information Network, *III*
NIH/National Institute of Diabetes, Digestive & Kidney Diseases, *IV*
Research Trust for Metabolic Diseases in Children, *III*

529 HYPERPROLINEMIA TYPE II

Hyperprolinemia Type II is a very rare hereditary disorder characterized by an abnormally high level of the amino acid proline in the urine. The high level of this substance is caused by a deficiency of the enzyme delta-1-pyrroline-5- carboxylic acid dehydrogenase.

Mild mental retardation and seizures may occur in some cases.

In addition to The National Organization for Rare Disorders (NORD) listed in Section III, the following organizations in Section II (Disease Specific) and in Section III (Umbrella) and Section IV (Government Agencies) can provide more information:
Metabolic Information Network, *III*
NIH/National Institute of Diabetes, Digestive & Kidney Diseases, *IV*
Research Trust for Metabolic Diseases in Children, *III*
The Arc (a national organization on mental retardation), *III*

530 HYPERTHERMIA

Hyperthermia occurs when the body temperature of an individual increases and the body is not able to reduce its temperature to a normal 98.6 degrees. Most frequently, this occurs during the heat of summer. However, it may also be triggered by other medical conditions or certain medications. The symptoms of hyperthermia may include headache, nausea, fatigue, muscle cramps, thirst and/or profuse sweating. The skin of an affected individual may feel cold and clammy. Without appropriate and prompt treatment to lower body temperature, hyperthermia may lead to serious complications.

In addition to The National Organization for Rare Disorders (NORD) listed in Section III, the following organizations in Section II (Disease Specific) and in Section III (Umbrella) and Section IV (Government Agencies) can provide more information:
NIH/National Institute on Aging, *IV*

531 HYPOCHONDROPLASIA

Hypochrondroplasia is an inherited skeletal disorder. Major symptoms include dwarfism that does not become evident until mid-childhood. The disorder is characterized by a normal sized head and small but normally shaped hands and feet.

In addition to The National Organization for Rare Disorders (NORD) listed in Section III, the following organizations in Section II (Disease Specific) and in Section III (Umbrella) and Section IV (Government Agencies) can provide more information:
Human Growth Foundation, *III*
Little People of America, *III*
Little People's Research Fund, Inc., *III*
MAGIC Foundation for Children's Growth, *III*
NIH/National Institute of Arthritis and Musculoskeletal and Skin Diseases, *IV*
Short Stature Foundation, *III*

532 HYPOGLYCEMIA

Hypoglycemia is a common condition characterized by an abnormally low blood sugar (glucose) level. Glucose is essential for the functioning of many organs and systems in the body, especially the central nervous system.

In addition to The National Organization for Rare Disorders (NORD) listed in Section III, the following organizations in Section II (Disease Specific) and in Section III (Umbrella) and Section IV (Government Agencies) can provide more information:
Hypoglycemia Association, Inc., *II*
NIH/National Digestive Diseases Information Clearinghouse, *IV*
NIH/National Institute of Diabetes, Digestive & Kidney Diseases, *IV*
National Hypoglycemia Association, *II*

533 HYPOKALEMIA

Hypokalemia is a metabolic imbalance characterized by extremely low potassium levels in the blood. It is a symptom of another disease or condition, or a side effect of diuretic drugs. The body needs potassium for the contraction of muscles (including the heart), and for the functioning of many complicated proteins (enzymes). Potassium is found primarily in the skeletal muscle and bone, and participates with sodium to contribute to the normal flow of body fluids between the cells in the body. The normal concentration of potassium in the body is regulated by the kidneys through the excretion of urine. When the kidneys are functioning normally, the amount of potassium in the diet is sufficient for use by the body and the excess is usually excreted through urine and sweat. Body chemicals and hormones such as aldosterone also regulate potassium balance. Secretion of the hormone insulin, which is normally stimulated by food, prevents a temporary diet-induced Hypokalemia by increasing cell absorption of potassium. When Hypokalemia occurs, there is an imbalance resulting from a dysfunction in this normal process, or the rapid loss of urine or sweat without replacement of sufficient potassium.

In addition to The National Organization for Rare Disorders (NORD) listed in Section III, the following organizations in Section II (Disease Specific) and in Section III (Umbrella) and Section IV (Government Agencies) can provide more information:
Digestive Disease National Coalition, *III*
Metabolic Information Network, *III*
NIH/National Institute of Diabetes, Digestive and Kidney Diseases, *IV*
Research Trust for Metabolic Diseases in Children, *III*

534 **HYPOMELANOSIS OF ITO**

Hypomelanosis of Ito is a rare disorder that is characterized by an unusual lack of skin color (hypopigmentation) affecting many areas of the body. It may be associated with other symptoms such as mental retardation, seizures, a lack of sweating on the areas of hypopigmentation, crossed eyes (strabismus), nearsightedness, a cleft along the edge of the eyeball (coloboma), overgrowth of brain tissue, and/or a small head. Hypomelanosis of Ito may occur sporadically or it be inherited as an autosomal dominant trait.

In addition to The National Organization for Rare Disorders (NORD) listed in Section III, the following organizations in Section II (Disease Specific) and in Section III (Umbrella) and Section IV (Government Agencies) can provide more information:

Epilepsy Foundation of America, *III*
NIH/National Institute of Arthritis and Musculoskeletal and Skin Diseases, *IV*

535 **HYPOPARATHYROIDISM**

Hypoparathyroidism is a condition characterized by insufficient production of parathyroid hormones by the parathyroid glands, the small, oval glands located near the thyroid gland in the neck. Parathyroid hormones (along with vitamin D and the hormone calcitonin, which is produced by the thyroid gland) play a role in regulating levels of calcium in the blood. Due to deficiency of parathyroid hormones, affected individuals exhibit abnormally low levels of calcium in the blood (hypocalcemia). Symptoms and findings associated with Hypoparathyroidism may include weakness, muscle cramps, excessive nervousness, headaches, and/or increased excitability (hyperexcitability) of nerves resulting in uncontrollable twitching and cramping spasms of certain muscles such as those of the hands, feet, arms, and/or face (tetany). Hypoparathyroidism may result from absence of the parathyroid glands at birth, occur due to or in association with a number of different underlying disorders, or result from removal of or damage to the parathyroid glands. In rare cases, Hypoparathyroidism may be inherited as an autosomal recessive genetic trait.

In addition to The National Organization for Rare Disorders (NORD) listed in Section III, the following organizations in Section II (Disease Specific) and in Section III (Umbrella) and Section IV (Government Agencies) can provide more information:

Hypoparathyroidism Newsletter, *II*
NIH/National Digestive Diseases Information Clearinghouse, *IV*
Thyroid Foundation of America, Inc., *III*
Thyroid Foundation of Canada, *III*

536 **HYPOPHOSPHATASIA**

Hypophosphatasia is a inborn metabolic disorder of the bones characterized by skeletal defects resembling those of rickets. The symptoms result from a failure of bone mineral to be deposited in young, uncalcified bone (osteoid), and in the cartilage at the end of the long bones (epiphyses) during early years. The activity of the enzyme alkaline phosphatase in blood serum and bone cells is lower than normal. Urinary excretion and blood plasma concentrations of phosphoethanolamine and inorganic pyrophosphate are abnormally high. Unlike other forms of rickets, Hypophosphatasia does not respond to treatment with vitamin D.

In addition to The National Organization for Rare Disorders (NORD) listed in Section III, the following organizations in Section II (Disease Specific) and in Section III (Umbrella) and Section IV (Government Agencies) can provide more information:

MAGIC Foundation for Children's Growth, *III*
Metabolic Information Network, *III*
NIH/National Arthritis and Musculoskeletal and Skin Diseases Information Clearinghouse, *IV*
Research Trust for Metabolic Diseases in Children, *III*

537 **HYPOPLASTIC LEFT HEART SYNDROME**

Hypoplastic Left Heart Syndrome is a term used to describe a group of closely related rare heart defects which are present at birth (congenital). The normal heart has four chambers. Two chambers are called atria which are separated from each other by a partition called the atrial septum. The other two chambers, known as ventricles, are also separated by a septum. Valves connect the atria (left and right) to their respective ventricles. Hypoplastic Left Heart Syndrome is characterized by the underdevelopment (hypoplasia) of the chambers on the left side of the heart (i.e., left atrium and ventricle). In addition, the mitral valve, which connects these chambers to each other, is usually abnormally narrow (stenosis) or closed (atresia) and the aortic valve, which connects the heart to the major vessels that lead from the lungs (ascending aorta), may also be narrow or closed. Infants with Hypoplastic Left Heart Syndrome also have an abnormally narrow ascending aorta.

In addition to The National Organization for Rare Disorders (NORD) listed in Section III, the following organizations in Section II (Disease Specific) and in Section III (Umbrella) and Section IV (Government Agencies) can provide more information:
American Heart Association, *III*
Congenital Heart Anomalies, Support, Education, & Resources, *III*
NIH/National Heart, Lung and Blood Institute, *IV*

538 HYPOTENSION, ORTHOSTATIC

Orthostatic Hypotension is an extreme drop in blood pressure that occurs when a person stands up suddenly. The blood pools in the blood vessels of the legs. Because of this pooling, there is a temporary decrease in the amount of blood carried back to the heart by the veins. Subsequently, less blood is pumped out from the heart, resulting in a sudden drop in blood pressure. Normally, specialized cells in the body (baroreceptors) quickly respond to changes in blood pressure. These baroreceptors then activate the autonomic nervous system's reflexes to increase levels of catecholamine in the body. Increased catecholamine levels rapidly restore the blood pressure. When there is a defect in this reflex action, heart rate and blood pressure do not rise adequately and Orthostatic Hypotension results.

In addition to The National Organization for Rare Disorders (NORD) listed in Section III, the following organizations in Section II (Disease Specific) and in Section III (Umbrella) and Section IV (Government Agencies) can provide more information:
NIH/National Institute of Neurological Disorders and Stroke, *IV*
National Dysautonomia Research Foundation, *III*

539 HYPOTHYROIDISM

Hypothyroidism may be a genetic or acquired condition that occurs alone or as a symptom of another illness. Major symptoms may include the development of an enlarged thyroid gland (goiter) in the neck. A dull facial expression, puffiness and swelling around the eyes, drooping eyelids and thinning hair, which is coarse and dry, may also occur. Intelligence may or may not be affected.

In addition to The National Organization for Rare Disorders (NORD) listed in Section III, the following organizations in Section II (Disease Specific) and in Section III (Umbrella) and Section IV (Government Agencies) can provide more information:
NIH/National Digestive Diseases Information Clearinghouse, *IV*
Thyroid Foundation of America, Inc., *III*

540 HYPOTONIA, BENIGN CONGENITAL

Benign Congenital Hypotonia is a nonprogressive neuromuscular disorder which occurs at birth. This condition is characterized by decreased muscle tone that is manifested as muscle weakness or "floppiness." The condition can occur as a disorder of unknown cause, or as a symptom of other neuromuscular diseases.

In addition to The National Organization for Rare Disorders (NORD) listed in Section III, the following organizations in Section II (Disease Specific) and in Section III (Umbrella) and Section IV (Government Agencies) can provide more information:
Families of Spinal Muscular Atrophy, *III*
Muscular Dystrophy Association, *III*
NIH/National Institute of Neurological Disorders and Stroke, *IV*

541 I CELL DISEASE

I-Cell Disease (Mucolipidosis II) is a rare inherited metabolic disorder characterized by multiple enzyme deficiencies (i.e., beta-N-acetylhexosaminidase, arylsulfatase A, iduronate sulfatase, and glycosidases). This disorder belongs to a group of diseases known as lysosomal storage disorders. Lysosomes are particles bound in membranes within cells that break down certain fats and carbohydrates. Multiple enzyme deficiencies associated with I-Cell Disease lead to the accumulation of certain fatty substances (mucolipids) and certain complex carbohydrates (mucopolysaccharides) within the cells of many tissues of the body.

The symptoms of I-Cell Disease are similar to but more severe than those of Hurler Syndrome. The symptoms associated with this disorder typically become obvious during infancy and may include multiple abnormalities of the skull and face, growth delays, and/or mental retardation. I-Cell Disease is inherited as an autosomal recessive genetic trait.

In addition to The National Organization for Rare Disorders (NORD) listed in Section III, the following organizations in Section II (Disease Specific) and in Section III (Umbrella) and Section IV (Government Agencies) can provide more information:
Canadian Society for Mucopolysaccharide and Related Diseases, Inc., *III*
Metabolic Information Network, *III*
NIH/National Digestive Diseases Information Clearinghouse, *IV*
National Lipid Diseases Foundation, *III*
National MPS (Mucopolysaccharidoses/Mucolipidoses)

Society, Inc., *III*
Research Trust for Metabolic Diseases in Children, *III*
The Arc (a national organization on mental retardation), *III*
Vaincre Les Maladies Lysosomales, *III*

542 ICHTHYOSIS

Ichthyosis is a general term describing a group of skin disorders that are characterized by an excessive accumulation of large amounts of dead skin cells (squames) in the top layer of the skin. The conversion of an abnormally large number of skin cells into squamous cells is thought to be caused by a defect in the metabolism of skin cells known as "corneocytes," or of the fat-rich matrix around these cells. The cells can be thought of as bricks, while the matrix would be the mortar holding these cells together. In general, all forms of Ichthyosis cause dry scaly skin.

In addition to The National Organization for Rare Disorders (NORD) listed in Section III, the following organizations in Section II (Disease Specific) and in Section III (Umbrella) and Section IV (Government Agencies) can provide more information:
Foundation for Ichthyosis & Related Skin Types, *III*
NIH/National Arthritis and Musculoskeletal and Skin Diseases Information Clearinghouse, *IV*
National Registry for Ichthyosis and Related Disorders, *III*

543 ICHTHYOSIS CONGENITA

Ichthyosis Congenita is an inherited skin disorder. It is characterized by generalized, abnormally red (erythroderma), dry and rough skin.

In addition to The National Organization for Rare Disorders (NORD) listed in Section III, the following organizations in Section II (Disease Specific) and in Section III (Umbrella) and Section IV (Government Agencies) can provide more information:
Foundation for Ichthyosis & Related Skin Types, *III*
NIH/National Institute of Child Health and Human Development, *IV*
National Eczema Association for Science and Education, *II*
National Registry for Ichthyosis and Related Disorders, *III*

544 ICHTHYOSIS HYSTRIX, CURTH MACKLIN TYPE

Ichthyosis Hystrix, Curth-Macklin Type is a rare inherited skin disorder. It is characterized by scaling skin (ichthyosis) ranging from mild to severe. Thick, horny skin (keratoderma) on the palms of the hands and the soles of the feet may occur with no other symptoms, or the whole body surface may be covered with scales.

In addition to The National Organization for Rare Disorders (NORD) listed in Section III, the following organizations in Section II (Disease Specific) and in Section III (Umbrella) and Section IV (Government Agencies) can provide more information:
Foundation for Ichthyosis & Related Skin Types, *III*
NIH/National Institute of Allergy and Infectious Diseases, *IV*
National Registry for Ichthyosis and Related Disorders, *III*

545 ICHTHYOSIS VULGARIS

Ichthyosis Vulgaris is an inherited skin disorder characterized by cornification of the skin. Scaly or platelike (squamous) skin forms instead of the normal smooth top layer of the skin. Fine scales usually develop on the patient's back and over muscles near a joint such as an elbow or a knee (extensor muscles).

In addition to The National Organization for Rare Disorders (NORD) listed in Section III, the following organizations in Section II (Disease Specific) and in Section III (Umbrella) and Section IV (Government Agencies) can provide more information:
Foundation for Ichthyosis & Related Skin Types, *III*
NIH/National Arthritis and Musculoskeletal and Skin Diseases Information Clearinghouse, *IV*
National Registry for Ichthyosis and Related Disorders, *III*

546 ICHTHYOSIS, CHILD SYNDROME

CHILD Syndrome (an acronym for Congenital Hemidysplasia with Ichthyosiform erythroderma and Limb Defects) is an inherited disorder characterized by skin abnormalities and limb defects on one side of the body. Abnormalities of other parts of the body may also be present.

In addition to The National Organization for Rare Disorders (NORD) listed in Section III, the following organizations in Section II (Disease Specific) and in Section III (Umbrella) and Section IV (Government Agencies) can provide more information:
Foundation for Ichthyosis & Related Skin Types, *III*
NIH/National Institute of Allergy and Infectious Diseases, *IV*

547 ICHTHYOSIS, CHANARIN DORFMAN SYNDROME

Chanarin Dorfman Syndrome is a rare hereditary disorder of fat (lipid) metabolism. It is characterized by scaly skin (ichthyosis), degeneration of the muscles (myopathy), and abnormal white blood cells with small spaces (vacuoles) filled with fat (lipids).

In addition to The National Organization for Rare Disorders (NORD) listed in Section III, the following organizations in Section II (Disease Specific) and in Section III (Umbrella) and Section IV (Government Agencies) can provide more information:
Foundation for Ichthyosis & Related Skin Types, *III*
NIH/National Institute of Allergy and Infectious Diseases, *IV*

548 ICHTHYOSIS, ERYTHROKERATODERMIA PROGRESSIVA SYMMETRICA

Erythrokeratodermia Progressiva Symmetrica is a rare hereditary skin disorder characterized by red hardened (keratotic) plaques with clear limits. These plaques are distributed symmetrically on the surface of both sides of the body, as well as on the head, buttocks, and extremities. The lesions first appear during infancy. This disorder is a form of Ichthyosis, a group of rare hereditary disorders characterized by scaly skin.

In addition to The National Organization for Rare Disorders (NORD) listed in Section III, the following organizations in Section II (Disease Specific) and in Section III (Umbrella) and Section IV (Government Agencies) can provide more information:
Foundation for Ichthyosis & Related Skin Types, *III*
NIH/National Arthritis and Musculoskeletal and Skin Diseases Information Clearinghouse, *IV*
National Registry for Ichthyosis and Related Disorders, *III*

549 ICHTHYOSIS, ERYTHROKERATODERMIA VARIABILIS

Erythrokeratodermia Variabilis is a form of Ichthyosis, a group of hereditary skin disorders characterized by scaly patches on the skin. In this type of Ichthyosis, sharply defined red areas (erythemas) resemble a geographic map with a shifting configuration. Fixed hardened (keratotic) skin plaques independent of the red areas usually also develop. Skin lesions are localized in most cases, but may spread over the entire body surface.

In addition to The National Organization for Rare Disorders (NORD) listed in Section III, the following organizations in Section II (Disease Specific) and in Section III (Umbrella) and Section IV (Government Agencies) can provide more information:
Foundation for Ichthyosis & Related Skin Types, *III*
NIH/National Arthritis and Musculoskeletal and Skin Diseases Information Clearinghouse, *IV*

550 ICHTHYOSIS, ERYTHROKERATOLYSIS HIEMALIS

Erythrokeratolysis Hiemalis is a form of Ichthyosis, which is a group of hereditary skin disorders. This condition is characterized by periodic attacks of red (erythematous) plaques that are distributed equally on both sides of the body. A layer of skin can be peeled from these plaques. Symptoms usually improve with age.

In addition to The National Organization for Rare Disorders (NORD) listed in Section III, the following organizations in Section II (Disease Specific) and in Section III (Umbrella) and Section IV (Government Agencies) can provide more information:
Foundation for Ichthyosis & Related Skin Types, *III*
NIH/National Arthritis and Musculoskeletal and Skin Diseases Information Clearinghouse, *IV*

551 ICHTHYOSIS, HARLEQUIN TYPE

Harlequin Type Ichthyosis is a rare genetic skin disorder characterized by massive, thick skin plates that usually produce distorted facial features and often deformities in other parts of the body. At birth the chest and abdomen of patients are usually severely constricted. This makes breathing and eating difficult. The skin symptoms can be somewhat controlled with treatment.

In addition to The National Organization for Rare Disorders (NORD) listed in Section III, the following organizations in Section II (Disease Specific) and in Section III (Umbrella) and Section IV (Government Agencies) can provide more information:
Foundation for Ichthyosis & Related Skin Types, *III*
NIH/National Institute of Allergy and Infectious Diseases, *IV*
National Registry for Ichthyosis and Related Disorders, *III*

552 ICHTHYOSIS, KERATOSIS FOLLICULARIS SPINULOSA DECALVANS

Keratosis Follicularis Spinulosa Decalvans is a rare skin disorder. The disorder is characterized by hardening of the skin (keratosis) around the hair follicles, leading to progressive scarring and baldness (alopecia).

In addition to The National Organization for Rare Disorders (NORD) listed in Section III, the following organizations in Section II (Disease Specific) and in Section III (Umbrella) and Section IV (Government Agencies) can provide more information:
Foundation for Ichthyosis & Related Skin Types, *III*
NIH/National Arthritis and Musculoskeletal and Skin Diseases Information Clearinghouse, *IV*

National Registry for Ichthyosis and Related Disorders, *III*

553 ICHTHYOSIS, LAMELLAR RECESSIVE

Lamellar Recessive Ichthyosis is a serious skin disorder. Cornification, which is the conversion of the upper layer of the skin into scaly or platelike (squamous) type skin, is the major symptom. The entire body surface is involved, with large, dark, platelike scales. In serious cases, the eyelids and the lips may turn outward (ectropion).

In addition to The National Organization for Rare Disorders (NORD) listed in Section III, the following organizations in Section II (Disease Specific) and in Section III (Umbrella) and Section IV (Government Agencies) can provide more information:
Foundation for Ichthyosis & Related Skin Types, *III*
NIH/National Arthritis and Musculoskeletal and Skin Diseases Information Clearinghouse, *IV*
National Registry for Ichthyosis and Related Disorders, *III*

554 ICHTHYOSIS, NETHERTON SYNDROME

Netherton Syndrome is a rare hereditary skin disorder occurring almost exclusively in females. This disorder is characterized by scaling of the skin in a distinctive circular pattern (ichthyosis linearis circumflexa). Symptoms affecting the hair include hair shafts held back in the hair root (trichorrhexis invaginata) or a fragile hair condition, called "bamboo hair". Both skin and hair abnormalities are caused by conversion of an abnormally large amount of epidermal skin cells into dead cells (cornification). Another characteristic of Netherton Syndrome is a predisposition to allergies such as asthma, or food allergies which cause skin eruptions.

In addition to The National Organization for Rare Disorders (NORD) listed in Section III, the following organizations in Section II (Disease Specific) and in Section III (Umbrella) and Section IV (Government Agencies) can provide more information:
Foundation for Ichthyosis & Related Skin Types, *III*
NIH/National Arthritis and Musculoskeletal and Skin Diseases Information Clearinghouse, *IV*
National Registry for Ichthyosis and Related Disorders, *III*

555 ICHTHYOSIS, SJOGREN LARSSON SYNDROME

Sjogren Larsson Syndrome is an inherited disorder characterized by scaling skin (ichthyosis), mental retardation, speech abnormalities, and spasticity. Affected infants develop various degrees of reddened skin, and fine scaling skin. Additionally, larger platelike thick scales (hyperkeratosis) usually develop in the outer skin layer (hyperkeratosis). After infancy, skin on the arms, legs and the abdomen often displays dark scales and absence of redness. Speech abnormalities and seizures may accompany skin symptoms. Approximately half of the children affected with this disorder will have degeneration of the pigment in the retina of the eyes.

In addition to The National Organization for Rare Disorders (NORD) listed in Section III, the following organizations in Section II (Disease Specific) and in Section III (Umbrella) and Section IV (Government Agencies) can provide more information:
Foundation for Ichthyosis & Related Skin Types, *III*
NIH/National Arthritis and Musculoskeletal and Skin Diseases Information Clearinghouse, *IV*
The Arc (a national organization on mental retardation), *III*

556 ICHTHYOSIS, TAY SYNDROME

Tay Syndrome is a hereditary disorder characterized by brittle, twisted hair, scaly dry skin (ichthyosis), and abnormal finger and toe nails. Loss of subcutaneous fat results in a prematurely aged-looking face. Physical development is usually slowed and mental retardation may also be present. A wide variety of central nervous system abnormalities may include seizures, tremors, lack of muscle coordination (ataxia), and neurosensory deafness. The reproductive organs are usually underdeveloped. Very small cataracts often develop in the eyes. Abnormalities of the bones and teeth may also occur, as well as an increased susceptibility to infection.

In addition to The National Organization for Rare Disorders (NORD) listed in Section III, the following organizations in Section II (Disease Specific) and in Section III (Umbrella) and Section IV (Government Agencies) can provide more information:
Foundation for Ichthyosis & Related Skin Types, *III*
NIH/National Arthritis and Musculoskeletal and Skin Diseases Information Clearinghouse, *IV*
National Registry for Ichthyosis and Related Disorders, *III*

557 ICHTHYOSIS, X-LINKED

X-Linked Ichthyosis is a genetic skin disorder that affects males. It is an inborn error of metabolism characterized by a deficiency of the enzyme steroid sulfatase. This enzyme defect leads to several biochemical alterations in the steroid sex hormone metabolism, including diminished maternal estrogen production in late pregnancy. Cholesterol sulfate may accumulate in the blood and skin. Normal functioning of sex hormones does not appear to be affected. Corneal opacities may be present, but do not interfere with vision.

In addition to The National Organization for Rare Disorders (NORD) listed in Section III, the following organizations in Section II (Disease Specific) and in Section III (Umbrella) and Section IV (Government Agencies) can provide more information:

Foundation for Ichthyosis & Related Skin Types, *III*
NIH/National Institute of Arthritis and Musculoskeletal and Skin Diseases, *IV*
National Registry for Ichthyosis and Related Disorders, *III*

558 IGA NEPHROPATHY

IgA Nephropathy is a kidney disorder occuring during childhood and young adulthood. It usually follows a viral infection of the upper respiratory or gastrointestinal tracts. The major symptom is the passing of blood in the urine (hematuria). There may be associated pain in the loin area.

In addition to The National Organization for Rare Disorders (NORD) listed in Section III, the following organizations in Section II (Disease Specific) and in Section III (Umbrella) and Section IV (Government Agencies) can provide more information:

American Foundation for Urologic Disease, *III*
American Kidney Fund, Inc., *III*
IgA Nephropathy Support Network, *II*
NIH/National Kidney and Urologic Diseases Information Clearinghouse, *IV*
National Kidney Foundation, *III*

559 IMPERFORATE ANUS

Imperforate anus is a rare inborn abnormality characterized by the absence or abnormal localization of the anus. The rectum or the colon may be connected to the vagina or the bladder by a tunnel (fistula). With surgical correction, normal elimination can become possible.

In addition to The National Organization for Rare Disorders (NORD) listed in Section III, the following organizations in Section II (Disease Specific) and in Section III (Umbrella) and Section IV (Government Agencies) can provide more information:

NIH/National Digestive Diseases Information Clearinghouse, *IV*
Pull-thru Network, *III*
United Ostomy Association, Inc., *III*

560 INCONTINENTIA PIGMENTI

Incontinentia Pigmenti is a genetic dermatological disorder characterized by unusual patterns of discolored skin. These discolorations tend to improve with age. Abnormal deposits of normal skin pigment (melanin) cause these discolorations. Three stages of progression may overlap or even occur simultaneously in some cases. Other oral, visual and/or neurological symptoms may also occur.

In addition to The National Organization for Rare Disorders (NORD) listed in Section III, the following organizations in Section II (Disease Specific) and in Section III (Umbrella) and Section IV (Government Agencies) can provide more information:

Alliance of Genetic Support Groups, *III*
IP Support Network, *II*
NIH/National Institute of Arthritis and Musculoskeletal and Skin Diseases, *IV*
National Incontinentia Pigmenti Foundation, *II*

561 INTERSTITIAL CYSTITIS

Interstitial Cystitis is a slowly progressive inflammatory disease of the bladder characterized by pressure and pain above the pubic area along with frequency and urgency of urination. This occurs because of chronic inflammation of the lining of the bladder and swelling of the interior walls of the bladder. Affected individuals urinate frequently because of a smaller than normal bladder capacity. In a small percentage of cases, people with Interstitial Cystitis also have scarring and ulcerations on the membranes that line the bladder. Interstitial Cystitis typically affects young and middle-aged women.

In addition to The National Organization for Rare Disorders (NORD) listed in Section III, the following organizations in Section II (Disease Specific) and in Section III (Umbrella) and Section IV (Government Agencies) can provide more information:

American Foundation for Urologic Disease, *III*
Interstitial Cystitis Association of America, Inc., *II*
Interstitial Cystitis Information Center, *II*
NIH/National Kidney and Urologic Diseases Information Clearinghouse, *IV*

562 INTESTINAL PSEUDOOBSTRUCTION

Intestinal Pseudoobstruction is a digestive disorder that may be present at birth. The intestinal walls are unable to contract normally in wave-like (peristaltic) motions (hypomotility). This condition resembles a true obstruction, but no such blockage exists. Abdominal pain, vomiting, diarrhea, constipation, malabsorption of nutrients leading to weight loss and/or failure to thrive, enlargement of various parts of the small intestine or bowel also occur.

In addition to The National Organization for Rare Disorders (NORD) listed in Section III, the following organizations in Section II (Disease Specific) and in Section III (Umbrella) and Section IV (Government Agencies) can provide more information:
American Pseudo-obstruction & Hirschsprung's Disease Society, Inc., *III*
NIH/National Institute of Diabetes, Digestive and Kidney Diseases, *IV*
United Ostomy Association, Inc., *III*

563 IRRITABLE BOWEL SYNDROME

Irritable Bowel Syndrome, also known as Spastic Colon or Mucous Colitis, is a digestive disorder characterized by an abnormal increase in the mobility of the intestines (small and large). Symptoms may include abdominal pain, constipation, and diarrhea. This disorder is common; about 50 percent of all gastrointestinal problems are associated with Irritable Bowel Syndrome. There is no organic disease present, only the function of the intestines is affected. However, based on the symptoms, this disease can be confused with other organic bowel diseases.

In addition to The National Organization for Rare Disorders (NORD) listed in Section III, the following organizations in Section II (Disease Specific) and in Section III (Umbrella) and Section IV (Government Agencies) can provide more information:
Crohn's and Colitis Foundation of America, *III*
Digestive Disease National Coalition, *III*
International Foundation for Functional Gastrointestinal Disorders, *III*
Intestinal Disease Foundation, *III*
NIH/National Digestive Diseases Information Clearinghouse, *IV*

564 ISAACS' SYNDROME

Isaacs' Syndrome is a peripheral motor neuron disorder characterized by muscular stiffness and cramping, particularly in the limbs. Continuous fine vibrating muscle movements (myokymia) can be seen. Muscle relaxation may be difficult especially after physical activity involving the particular muscle(s). These symptoms persist even during sleep.

In addition to The National Organization for Rare Disorders (NORD) listed in Section III, the following organizations in Section II (Disease Specific) and in Section III (Umbrella) and Section IV (Government Agencies) can provide more information:
NIH/National Arthritis and Musculoskeletal and Skin Diseases Information Clearinghouse, *IV*

565 IVEMARK SYNDROME

Ivemark Syndrome is a rare progressive disorder usually evident at birth. It is characterized by the absence of a spleen, malformations of the cardiovascular system and abnormal displacement of the abdomen and intestines.

In addition to The National Organization for Rare Disorders (NORD) listed in Section III, the following organizations in Section II (Disease Specific) and in Section III (Umbrella) and Section IV (Government Agencies) can provide more information:
Ivemark Syndrome Association, *II*
NIH/National Institute of Child Health and Human Development, *IV*

566 JACKSON-WEISS SYNDROME

Jackson-Weiss Syndrome is a rare disorder inherited as an autosomal dominant genetic trait. This disorder is characterized by permanent premature closure of the bones of the skull (craniosynostosis) along with abnormalities of bones in the face and feet. Typically the deformities of the feet include fusion of the bones of the upper foot along with malformed great toes. Symptoms of this disorder can vary within a family from mild to severe.

In addition to The National Organization for Rare Disorders (NORD) listed in Section III, the following organizations in Section II (Disease Specific) and in Section III (Umbrella) and Section IV (Government Agencies) can provide more information:
AboutFace U.S.A., *III*
Children's Craniofacial Association, *III*
FACES: The National Craniofacial Association, *III*
Forward Face, Inc., *III*
NIH/National Institute of Child Health and Human Development, *IV*

567 JANSEN TYPE METAPHYSEAL CHONDRODYSPLASIA

Jansen Type Metaphyseal Chondrodysplasia is an extremely rare progressive disorder in which portions of the bones of the arms and legs develop abnormally with unusual cartilage formations and subsequent abnormal bone formation at the large (bulbous) end portions (metaphyses) of these long bones (metaphyseal chondrodysplasia). As a result, affected individuals exhibit unusually short arms and legs and short stature (short-limbed dwarfism), findings that typically become apparent during childhood. Abnormal cartilage and bone development may also affect other bones of the body, particularly those of the hands and feet (i.e., metacarpals and metatarsals). Infants with Jansen Type Metaphyseal

Chondrodysplasia may also have characteristic facial abnormalities and additional skeletal malformations. During childhood, affected individuals may begin to exhibit progressive stiffening and swelling of many joints and/or an unusual "waddling gait" and squatting stance. In addition, affected adults may eventually develop abnormally hardened (sclerotic) bones especially in the back of the head (cranial bones), which, in some cases, may lead to deafness. The range and severity of symptoms may vary from case to case. Jansen Type Metaphyseal Chondrodysplasia is thought to be inherited as an autosomal dominant genetic trait.

In addition to The National Organization for Rare Disorders (NORD) listed in Section III, the following organizations in Section II (Disease Specific) and in Section III (Umbrella) and Section IV (Government Agencies) can provide more information:
Craniofacial Foundation of America, *III*
Human Growth Foundation, *III*
Little People of America, *III*
MAGIC Foundation for Children's Growth, *III*
NIH/National Arthritis and Musculoskeletal and Skin Diseases Information Clearinghouse, *IV*
NIH/National Institute of Child Health and Human Development, *IV*
NIH/National Institute on Deafness and Other Communication Disorders Information Clearinghouse, *IV*
National Information Center on Deafness, *III*
Short Stature Foundation, *III*

568 JARCHO LEVIN SYNDROME

Jarcho-Levin Syndrome is a rare genetic disorder characterized by distinctive malformations of bones of the spinal column (vertebrae) and the ribs, respiratory insufficiency, and/or other abnormalities. In infants with Jarcho-Levin Syndrome, the trunk may appear abnormally short due to fusion of many vertebrae, incomplete development (dysplasia) of one side of certain vertebrae (hemivertebrae), fusion of certain ribs, and/or other rib malformations. In addition, abnormalities of vertebrae within the neck area (cervical vertebrae) may cause shortness of the neck, limited neck motion, and an abnormally low hairline. In many infants with the disorder, the abdomen may be abnormally prominent and the arms and legs may appear unusually long, although they may actually be of normal length. In addition, in most cases, infants with Jarcho-Levin Syndrome experience respiratory insufficiency and are prone to repeated respiratory infections (pneumonia) that may result in life-threatening complications. Jarcho-Levin Syndrome is thought to be inherited as an autosomal recessive genetic trait.

In addition to The National Organization for Rare Disorders (NORD) listed in Section III, the following organizations in Section II (Disease Specific) and in Section III (Umbrella) and Section IV (Government Agencies) can provide more information:
NIH/National Institute of Child Health and Human Development, *IV*

569 JEJUNAL ATRESIA

Jejunal Atresia is a rare genetic disorder. Patients with this disorder are born with a partial absence of the fold of the stomach membrane that connects the small intestine to the back wall of the abdomen. As a result, one of the three portions of the small intestine (the jejunal) twists around one of the arteries of the colon called the marginal artery and causes a blockage (atresia). Symptoms in individuals with this disorder include vomiting, a swollen abdomen, and constipation.

In addition to The National Organization for Rare Disorders (NORD) listed in Section III, the following organizations in Section II (Disease Specific) and in Section III (Umbrella) and Section IV (Government Agencies) can provide more information:
NIH/National Digestive Diseases Information Clearinghouse, *IV*

570 JOB SYNDROME

Job Syndrome is a rare disorder present at birth (congenital) in which there are large bacterial infections, particularly of the skin, with some swelling and redness (cold staphylococcal abscesses); a defect in the attraction of white blood cells (leukocytes) that destroy bacteria, fungi, and viruses to chemical stimuli (granulocyte chemotactic defect); an abundance of one of the antibodies that are concentrated in the lungs, skin and cells of mucous membranes (immunoglobulinemia E); inflammation, redness, pain or itching of the skin (chronic-eczematoid dermatitis); and a mild increase in the number of leukocyte white blood cells (mild eosinophilia). Job Syndrome is often inherited as an autosomal recessive trait.

In addition to The National Organization for Rare Disorders (NORD) listed in Section III, the following organizations in Section II (Disease Specific) and in Section III (Umbrella) and Section IV (Government Agencies) can provide more information:
Immune Deficiency Foundation, *III*
International Patient Organization for Primary Immunodeficiencies, *III*

NIH/National Institute of Allergy and Infectious Diseases, *IV*

571 JOHANSON BLIZZARD SYNDROME

Johanson-Blizzard Syndrome (JBS) is an extremely rare inherited disorder characterized by an unusually small nose that appears "beak shaped" due to absence (aplasia) or underdevelopment (hypoplasia) of the nostrils (nasal alae); abnormally small, malformed primary (deciduous) teeth and misshapen or absent secondary (permanent) teeth; and/or unusually sparse, dry, coarse scalp hair that tends to have a distinctive "upsweep" in the forehead area. In addition, affected infants may have a low birth weight, demonstrate signs of insufficient intestinal absorption (malabsorption) of fats and other nutrients due to abnormal development of the pancreas (exocrine pancreatic insufficiency), and fail to grow and gain weight at the expected rate (failure to thrive) during the first years of life, contributing to short stature.

Approximately one third of infants with Johanson-Blizzard Syndrome also demonstrate abnormally decreased activity of the thyroid gland and underproduction of thyroid hormones (hypothyroidism), causing generalized weakness and contributing to growth retardation as well as abnormal delays in the acquisition of skills requiring the coordination of mental and physicial activity (psychomotor retardation). In many cases, affected infants may also exhibit hearing impairment of both ears at birth due to abnormalities of the inner ear (congenital bilateral sensorineural hearing loss) and may experience associated, severe speech impairment. In addition, approximately 60 percent of affected children have moderate mental retardation; however, others may have normal intelligence or mild retardation. In many cases, additional abnormalities may also be present. The range and severity of symptoms may vary greatly from case to case. Johanson-Blizzard Syndrome is thought to be inherited as an autosomal recessive genetic trait.

In addition to The National Organization for Rare Disorders (NORD) listed in Section III, the following organizations in Section II (Disease Specific) and in Section III (Umbrella) and Section IV (Government Agencies) can provide more information:

Congenital Heart Anomalies, Support, Education, & Resources, *III*
FACES: The National Craniofacial Association, *III*
MAGIC Foundation for Children's Growth, *III*
NIH/National Digestive Diseases Information Clearinghouse, *IV*
NIH/National Institute of Child Health and Human Development, *IV*
NIH/National Institute of Dental Research, *IV*
Pull-thru Network, *III*
Short Stature Foundation, *III*

572 JOSEPH'S DISEASE

Joseph's Disease is a rare inherited neurological disorder of the central nervous system characterized by the slow degeneration of certain areas of the brain. Symptoms begin during adulthood. Neurological impairment and loss of feeling in the arms and legs (peripheral sensory loss) typically occur. There are three forms of Joseph's Disease: Types I, II, III. This disorder mainly affects people of Portuguese ancestry.

In addition to The National Organization for Rare Disorders (NORD) listed in Section III, the following organizations in Section II (Disease Specific) and in Section III (Umbrella) and Section IV (Government Agencies) can provide more information:

International Joseph Diseases Foundation, Inc., *II*
March of Dimes Birth Defects Foundation, *III*
NIH/National Institute of Neurological Disorders and Stroke, *IV*

573 JOUBERT SYNDROME

Joubert Syndrome is a very rare neurological disorder involving a malformation of the area of the brain that controls balance and coordination. Generally motor activity is slowed (psychomotor retardation) and there are abnormal eye movements. Respiratory irregularities, including rapid panting, may occur during infancy.

In addition to The National Organization for Rare Disorders (NORD) listed in Section III, the following organizations in Section II (Disease Specific) and in Section III (Umbrella) and Section IV (Government Agencies) can provide more information:

Alliance of Genetic Support Groups, *III*
Children's Brain Diseases Foundation, *II*
Joubert Syndrome Parents-In-Touch Network, *II*
March of Dimes Birth Defects Foundation, *III*
NIH/National Institute of Neurological Disorders and Stroke, *IV*
The Arc (a national organization on mental retardation), *III*

574 JUBERG MARSIDI SYNDROME

Juberg-Marsidi Syndrome is an extremely rare X-linked inherited disorder that affects males only and is apparent at birth (congenital) or during the first few weeks of life (neonatal period). Affected children exhibit severe mental retardation; delays in reaching developmental milestones (e.g., crawling, walking, etc.); muscle weakness; diminished muscle tone (hypotonia); and/or delayed bone growth as well as growth retardation, resulting in short stature. Affected infants also exhibit hearing loss; underdevelopment of the genitals (microgenitalism); and/or abnormalities of the head and facial (craniofacial) area such as an abnormally small head (microcephaly), a flat (depressed) nasal bridge, eye (ocular) abnormalities, and/or, in some cases, additional physical abnormalities. The range and severity of symptoms may vary from case to case. Juberg-Marsidi Syndrome is inherited as an X-linked recessive genetic trait.

In addition to The National Organization for Rare Disorders (NORD) listed in Section III, the following organizations in Section II (Disease Specific) and in Section III (Umbrella) and Section IV (Government Agencies) can provide more information:
NIH/National Eye Institute, *IV*
NIH/National Institute of Child Health and Human Development, *IV*
NIH/National Institute on Deafness and Other Communication Disorders Information Clearinghouse, *IV*
Short Stature Foundation, *III*

575 JUMPING FRENCHMEN OF MAINE

"Jumping Frenchmen" is a disorder characterized by an unusually extreme startle reaction. The startle reaction is a natural response to an unexpected noise or sight. This disorder was first identified during the late nineteenth century in Maine and the Canadian province of Quebec. Lumberjacks of French Canadian descent were originally associated with this phenomenon but it has since been observed in other societies in many parts of the world as well. "Jumping Frenchmen" is suspected to be a genetic disorder and/or an extreme conditioned response to a particular situation possibly influenced by cultural factors. Symptoms tend to improve with age.

In addition to The National Organization for Rare Disorders (NORD) listed in Section III, the following organizations in Section II (Disease Specific) and in Section III (Umbrella) and Section IV (Government Agencies) can provide more information:
NIH/National Institute of Neurological Disorders and Stroke, *IV*

576 KBG SYNDROME

KBG Syndrome is a very rare genetic disorder characterized by short stature, moderate to severe degrees of mental retardation, developmental abnormalities of the limbs, vertebrae, extremities, and/or underdevelopment of the bones of the skeleton. Abnormalities of the head and face (craniofacial dysmorphism) and malformations of the teeth and jaws (dentoskeletal dysplasia) may also be present. KBG Syndrome is thought to be inherited as an autosomal dominant genetic trait with variable degree of penetrance.

In addition to The National Organization for Rare Disorders (NORD) listed in Section III, the following organizations in Section II (Disease Specific) and in Section III (Umbrella) and Section IV (Government Agencies) can provide more information:
NIH/National Institute of Child Health and Human Development, *IV*

577 KABUKI MAKE-UP SYNDROME

Kabuki Make-Up Syndrome is a rare disorder characterized by mental retardation, short stature, unusual facial features, abnormalities of the skeleton and unusual skin ridge patterns on the fingers, toes, palms of the hands and soles of the feet. The majority of the reported cases of this disorder have occurred for no apparent reason (sporadic). However several cases have been cases have been reported to be inherited as an autosomal dominant trait.

In addition to The National Organization for Rare Disorders (NORD) listed in Section III, the following organizations in Section II (Disease Specific) and in Section III (Umbrella) and Section IV (Government Agencies) can provide more information:
NIH/National Institute of Neurological Disorders and Stroke, *IV*

578 KALLMANN SYNDROME

Kallmann Syndrome is a rare inherited disorder in which the organ that produces sex cells does not function properly (hypogonadism) and there is a loss of the sense of smell (anosmia). The impaired production of hormones as well as sperm and egg cells often causes delayed puberty, growth and infertility. This disorder affects both males and females, although it is more common in males.

In addition to The National Organization for Rare Disorders (NORD) listed in Section III, the following organizations in Section II (Disease Specific) and in Section III (Umbrella) and Section IV (Government Agencies) can provide more information:
NIH/National Institute of Child Health and Human Development, *IV*

579 KARTAGENER SYNDROME

Kartagener Syndrome is a genetic disorder combining three major symptoms. These include chronic enlargement of the bronchial tubes (bronchiectasis), chronic inflammation of the lining of the sinuses (sinusitis), and abnormal cross-positioning of body organs during prenatal development (situs inversus).

In addition to The National Organization for Rare Disorders (NORD) listed in Section III, the following organizations in Section II (Disease Specific) and in Section III (Umbrella) and Section IV (Government Agencies) can provide more information:

American Lung Association, *III*

580 KAWASAKI SYNDROME

Kawasaki Syndrome is an inflammatory disease of childhood characterized by fever, skin rash, swollen lymph nodes (lymphadenopathy), inflammation of arteries (polyarteritis), and inflammation of the blood vessels (vasculitis). Inflammatory changes cause destructive lesions in blood vessels and may lead to complications involving the liver, gall bladder, and especially the heart. Kawasaki Syndrome is the main cause of acquired heart disease in children. The exact cause of Kawasaki Syndrome is unclear although it may be related to two previously unknown strains of staphylococcus and streptococcus bacteria.

In addition to The National Organization for Rare Disorders (NORD) listed in Section III, the following organizations in Section II (Disease Specific) and in Section III (Umbrella) and Section IV (Government Agencies) can provide more information:

Centers for Disease Control and Prevention, *IV*
Kawasaki Families' Network, *II*
NIH/National Institute of Allergy and Infectious Diseases, *IV*

581 KEARNS SAYRE SYNDROME (KSS)

Kearns-Sayre Syndrome is a rare neuromuscular disorder characterized by three primary findings: progressive paralysis of certain eye muscles (chronic progressive external ophthalmoplegia [CPEO]); abnormal accumulation of colored (pigmented) material on the nerve-rich membrane lining the eyes (atypical retinitis pigmentosa), leading to chronic inflammation, progressive degeneration, and wearing away of certain eye structures (pigmentary degeneration of the retina); and heart disease (cardiomyopathy) such as heart block. Other findings may include muscle weakness, short stature, hearing loss, and/or the loss of ability to coordinate voluntary movements (ataxia) due to problems affecting part of the brain (cerebellum). In some cases, Kearns-Sayre Syndrome may be associated with other disorders and/or conditions.

Kearns-Sayre Syndrome belongs (in part) to a group of rare neuromuscular disorders known as mitochondrial encephalomyopathies. Mitochondrial encephalomyopathies are disorders in which a defect in genetic material arises from a part of the cell structure that releases energy (mitochondria), causing the brain and muscles to function improperly (encephalomyopathies). In these disorders, abnormally high numbers of defective mitochondria are present. In approximately 80 percent of cases of Kearns-Sayre Syndrome, tests will reveal missing genetic material (deletion) involving the unique DNA in mitochondria (mtDNA).

In addition to The National Organization for Rare Disorders (NORD) listed in Section III, the following organizations in Section II (Disease Specific) and in Section III (Umbrella) and Section IV (Government Agencies) can provide more information:

Alliance of Genetic Support Groups, *III*
American Heart Association, *III*
Foundation Fighting Blindness, *III*
NIH/National Arthritis and Musculoskeletal and Skin Diseases Information Clearinghouse, *IV*
NIH/National Eye Institute, *IV*
NIH/National Institute of Child Health and Human Development, *IV*
NIH/National Institute of Neurological Disorders and Stroke, *IV*
National Association for Visually Handicapped, *III*
United Mitochondrial Disease Foundation, *III*

582 KENNEDY DISEASE

Kennedy Disease is a rare, slowly progressive muscular disorder that affects males only and is inherited as an X-linked genetic trait. Uncontrollable twitching (fasciculations) followed by weakness and wasting of the muscles becomes apparent some time after the age of fifteen. The muscles of the face, lips, tongue, mouth, throat, vocal chords, trunk and limbs may be affected. Swelling of the breasts, difficulty swallowing, and very large calves may also be found in some patients with this disorder.

In addition to The National Organization for Rare Disorders (NORD) listed in Section III, the following organizations in Section II (Disease Specific) and in Section III (Umbrella) and Section IV (Government Agencies) can provide more information:

Families of Spinal Muscular Atrophy, *III*
NIH/National Institute of Neurological Disorders and Stroke, *IV*
National Ataxia Foundation, *III*

583 **KENNY CAFFE SYNDROME**

Kenny-Caffe Syndrome is an extremely rare hereditary skeletal disorder characterized by thickening of the long bones, thin marrow cavities in the bones (medullary stenosis), and abnormalities affecting the head and eyes. Most cases are obvious at birth (congenital). The primary outcome of Kenny-Caffe Syndrome is short stature. Mental abilities are rarely affected. Individuals with Kenny-Caffe Syndrome may also have recurrent episodes of low levels of calcium in the blood stream (hypocalcemia) that is caused by insufficient production of parathyroid hormones (Hypoparathyroidism). Most cases of Kenny-Caffe Syndrome are thought to be inherited as autosomal dominant genetic traits. Some cases may be autosomal recessive; X-linked autosomal recessive genetic inheritance has not been ruled out.

In addition to The National Organization for Rare Disorders (NORD) listed in Section III, the following organizations in Section II (Disease Specific) and in Section III (Umbrella) and Section IV (Government Agencies) can provide more information:
Human Growth Foundation, *III*
Hypoparathyroidism Newsletter, *II*
Little People of America, *III*
Little People's Research Fund, Inc., *III*
NIH/National Institute of Child Health and Human Development, *IV*
Short Stature Foundation, *III*

584 **KERATITIS ICHTHYOSIS DEAFNESS SYNDROME**

Keratitis Ichthyosis Deafness (KID) Syndrome is a very rare disorder that occurs most often for no apparent reason but has also been linked to an autosomal recessive trait. It is characterized by inflammation of the eyes corneas (keratitis), fixed hardened skin scales (plaques) on the extremities and face, thick hardened skin on the palms of the hands and the soles of the feet, and deafness.

In addition to The National Organization for Rare Disorders (NORD) listed in Section III, the following organizations in Section II (Disease Specific) and in Section III (Umbrella) and Section IV (Government Agencies) can provide more information:
Foundation for Ichthyosis & Related Skin Types, *III*
NIH/National Arthritis and Musculoskeletal and Skin Diseases Information Clearinghouse, *IV*
NIH/National Eye Institute, *IV*

585 **KERATOCONJUNCTIVITIS, VERNAL**

Vernal Keratoconjunctivitis is a non-contagious, seasonal allergic disorder usually occuring during the spring or warm weather. Major symptoms include inflammation of the conjunctiva of the eyes, sensitivity to light and intense itching.

In addition to The National Organization for Rare Disorders (NORD) listed in Section III, the following organizations in Section II (Disease Specific) and in Section III (Umbrella) and Section IV (Government Agencies) can provide more information:
NIH/National Eye Institute, *IV*
NIH/National Institute of Allergy and Infectious Diseases, *IV*

586 **KERATOCONUS**

Keratoconus is a slowly progressive enlargement of the curved transparent outer layer of fibrous tissue covering the eyeball (cornea). The resulting conical shape of the cornea causes blurred vision and other vision problems. Inherited forms of this disorder usually begin after puberty. Keratoconus can also occur in conjunction with a variety of other disorders.

In addition to The National Organization for Rare Disorders (NORD) listed in Section III, the following organizations in Section II (Disease Specific) and in Section III (Umbrella) and Section IV (Government Agencies) can provide more information:
Eye Bank Association of America, *III*
NIH/National Eye Institute, *IV*
National Association for Visually Handicapped, *III*
National Keratoconus Foundation, *II*
The Arc (a national organization on mental retardation), *III*
Vision Foundation, Inc., *III*

587 **KERATOMALACIA**

Keratomalacia is an eye disease caused by a deficiency of vitamin A. Vitamin A (retinol) is found mainly in fish liver oils, liver, egg yolk, cream and butter. The human body stores vitamin A mainly in the liver. Once it is released by the liver, vitamin A is converted to light sensitive pigments in the retina that are involved in night, day and color vision. Vitamin A also helps maintain healthy body tissue.

Keratomalacia is very rare in North America and Western Europe, but is a leading cause of blindness in Southeast Asia, parts of Africa and Central and South America. In these areas vitamin A deficiency is usually caused by general malnutrition in infants and young children.

In addition to The National Organization for Rare Disorders (NORD) listed in Section III, the following organizations in Section II (Disease Specific) and in Section III (Umbrella) and Section IV (Government Agencies) can provide more information:
Blind Children's Center, *III*
NIH/National Eye Institute, *IV*
National Association for Visually Handicapped, *III*
National Eye Research Foundation, *III*
Prevent Blindness America, *III*
Vision Foundation, Inc., *III*

588 KERATOSIS, SEBORRHEIC

Seborrheic Keratosis is a skin disorder usually characterized by discolored lesions that appear to be "stuck on" the skin surface. Warts may appear and skin is often oily or greasy. These skin lesions are sometimes mistaken for cancerous growths and tend to appear predominately during middle age. Itching, irritation, inflammations or unsightliness of lesions may require surgical removal of affected skin areas.

In addition to The National Organization for Rare Disorders (NORD) listed in Section III, the following organizations in Section II (Disease Specific) and in Section III (Umbrella) and Section IV (Government Agencies) can provide more information:
NIH/National Arthritis and Musculoskeletal and Skin Diseases Information Clearinghouse, *IV*

589 KERNICTERUS

Kernicterus is a rare neurological disorder characterized by excessive levels of bilirubin in the blood (hyperbilirubinemia) during infancy. Bilirubin is an orange-yellow bile pigment that is a byproduct of the natural breakdown of hemoglobin in red blood cells (hemolysis). Toxic levels of bilirubin may accumulate in the brain, potentially resulting in a variety of symptoms and physical findings. These symptoms may include lack of energy (lethargy), poor feeding habits, fever, and vomiting. Affected infants may also experience the absence of certain reflexes (e.g., Moro reflex, etc.); mild to severe muscle spasms including those in which the head and heels are bent backward and the body bows forward (opisthotonus); and/or uncontrolled involuntary muscle movements (spasticity). In some cases, infants with kernicterus may develop life-threatening complications.

In addition to The National Organization for Rare Disorders (NORD) listed in Section III, the following organizations in Section II (Disease Specific) and in Section III (Umbrella) and Section IV (Government Agencies) can provide more information:
Alliance of Genetic Support Groups, *III*
American Liver Foundation, *III*
NIH/National Institute of Child Health and Human Development, *IV*
NIH/National Institute of Diabetes, Digestive and Kidney Diseases, *IV*
United Liver Association, *III*

590 KIENBOCK DISEASE

Kienbock Disease is an acquired bone disorder. Abnormalities of the lunate bone in the wrist develops following an injury or inflammation. Recurrent pain and stiffness occur in conjunction with thickening, swelling and tenderness in soft tissue overlying the lunate bone. The range of motion in the wrist may become limited.

In addition to The National Organization for Rare Disorders (NORD) listed in Section III, the following organizations in Section II (Disease Specific) and in Section III (Umbrella) and Section IV (Government Agencies) can provide more information:
NIH/National Arthritis and Musculoskeletal and Skin Diseases Information Clearinghouse, *IV*

591 KIKUCHI'S DISEASE

Kikuchi's Disease is a rare noncancerous disorder in which there are lesions that typically affect the lymph nodes in the neck of young adults. This disorder is often mistaken for malignant Lymphoma because the symptoms are very similar. The lesions, or tissue abnormalities in this disorder cause the lymph nodes to become enlarged, inflamed and painful. The exact cause of Kikuchi's Disease is not known.

In addition to The National Organization for Rare Disorders (NORD) listed in Section III, the following organizations in Section II (Disease Specific) and in Section III (Umbrella) and Section IV (Government Agencies) can provide more information:
NIH/National Institute of Allergy and Infectious Diseases, *IV*

592 KINSBOURNE SYNDROME

Kinsbourne Syndrome is a rare neurological disorder that usually affects infants and young children. The disorder is characterized by the sudden onset of brief, repeated, shock-like spasms of several muscles within the arms, legs, or entire body (polymyoclonus), an impaired ability to control voluntary movements (ataxia), and continual, involuntary, rapid eye movements in both horizontal and vertical directions (opsoclonus).

In approximately 50 percent of affected individuals, a malignant tumor, usually a tumor of embryonic nerve cells (neuroblastoma), is responsible for the symptoms associated with Kinsbourne Syndrome. In most other cases, Kinsbourne Syndrome may be due to a viral infection such as Coxsackievirus B3, poliovirus, or St. Louis encephalitis virus. Rarely, the disorder may result due to other underlying causes such as a tumor within the skull (intracranial tumors) or hydrocephalus, a condition in which inhibition of the normal flow of cerebrospinal fluid (CSF) and abnormal widening (dilatation) of the cerebral spaces of the brain (ventricles) causes accumulation of CSF in the skull and potentially increased pressure on brain tissue.

In addition to The National Organization for Rare Disorders (NORD) listed in Section III, the following organizations in Section II (Disease Specific) and in Section III (Umbrella) and Section IV (Government Agencies) can provide more information:
Dancing Eye Syndrome Support Trust, *II*
Myoclonus Research Foundation, *III*
NIH/National Institute of Neurological Disorders and Stroke, *IV*
National Pediatric Myoclonus Center, *II*
Opsoclonus-Myoclonus Support Network, Inc., *II*

593 KLEINE LEVIN SYNDROME

Kleine-Levin Syndrome is a rare disorder characterized by the need for excessive amounts of sleep (hypersomnolence), (i.e., up to 20 hours a day); excessive food intake (compulsive hyperphagia); and an abnormally uninhibited sexual drive. The disorder primarily affects adolescent males. When awake, affected individuals may exhibit irritability, lack of energy (lethargy), and/or lack of emotions (apathy). They may also appear confused (disoriented) and experience hallucinations. Symptoms of Kleine-Levin Syndrome are cyclical. An affected individual may go for weeks or months without experiencing symptoms. When present, symptoms may persist for days to weeks. In most cases, the symptoms associated with Kleine-Levin Syndrome eventually disappear with advancing age. The exact cause of Kleine-Levin Syndrome is not known. However, researchers believe that in some cases, the disorder may be inherited as an autosomal dominant genetic trait. It is thought that symptoms of Kleine-Levin Syndrome may be related to malfunction of the portion of the brain that helps to regulate functions such as sleep, appetite, and body temperature (hypothalamus).

In addition to The National Organization for Rare Disorders (NORD) listed in Section III, the following organizations in Section II (Disease Specific) and in Section III (Umbrella) and Section IV (Government Agencies) can provide more information:
NIH/National Institute of Mental Health, *IV*
NIH/National Institute of Neurological Disorders and Stroke, *IV*
National Mental Health Association, *III*
National Mental Health Consumer Self-Help Clearinghouse, *III*
National Sleep Foundation, *III*

594 KLINEFELTER SYNDROME

The classic form of Klinefelter Syndrome causes impaired function of the testes (primary hypogonadism) in males. This rare disorder is characterized by the presence of an extra X chromosome. Klinefelter Syndrome may not be diagnosed until puberty because the symptoms may be very subtle until that age and secondary sex characteristics are not apparent before puberty.

In addition to The National Organization for Rare Disorders (NORD) listed in Section III, the following organizations in Section II (Disease Specific) and in Section III (Umbrella) and Section IV (Government Agencies) can provide more information:
49XXXXY, *II*
Klinefelter Syndrome and Associates, *II*
March of Dimes Birth Defects Foundation, *III*
NIH/National Institute of Child Health and Human Development, *IV*

595 KLIPPEL FEIL SYNDROME

Klippel-Feil Syndrome is a rare, congenital disorder of the spine. Major symptoms may include a short neck, low hairline at the back of the head and restricted mobility of the upper spine. There may also be associated hearing loss, neurologic, heart, kidney and breathing problems.

In addition to The National Organization for Rare Disorders (NORD) listed in Section III, the following organizations in Section II (Disease Specific) and in Section III (Umbrella) and Section IV (Government Agencies) can provide more information:
KFS (Klippel-Feil Syndrome) Network Online, *II*
NIH/National Arthritis and Musculoskeletal and Skin Diseases Information Clearinghouse, *IV*

NIH/National Institute of Child Health and Human Development, *IV*

596 KLIPPEL TRENAUNAY SYNDROME

Klippel-Trenaunay Syndrome, a rare disorder that is present at birth (congenital), is characterized by abnormal benign growths on the skin (cutaneous) consisting of masses of blood vessels (hemangiomas), excessive growth (hypertrophy) of the soft tissue and bone of a leg and/or arm (limb), and varicose veins. (In individuals with the disorder, such hypertrophy typically affects one side of the body [hemihypertrophy].) In many cases, hemangiomas may consist of distinctive purplish-reddish birthmarks ("port wine stain" or nevus flammeus) on certain areas of the skin. The symptoms and findings associated with the disorder may vary in range and severity from case to case.

In addition to The National Organization for Rare Disorders (NORD) listed in Section III, the following organizations in Section II (Disease Specific) and in Section III (Umbrella) and Section IV (Government Agencies) can provide more information:

Alliance of Genetic Support Groups, *III*
Klippel-Trenaunay Support Group, *II*
March of Dimes Birth Defects Foundation, *III*
NIH/National Institute of Neurological Disorders and Stroke, *IV*
National Vascular Malformations Foundation, Inc., *III*
Nevus Network, *II*
Sturge-Weber Foundation, *II*

597 KLUVER BUCY SYNDROME

Kluver-Bucy Syndrome is a very rare cerebral neurological disorder. Major symptoms may include an urge to put all kinds of objects into the mouth, memory loss, extreme sexual behavior, placidity, and visual distractibility.

In addition to The National Organization for Rare Disorders (NORD) listed in Section III, the following organizations in Section II (Disease Specific) and in Section III (Umbrella) and Section IV (Government Agencies) can provide more information:

Alzheimer's Association, *II*
Alzheimer's Disease Education and Referral Center, *II*
NIH/National Institute of Neurological Disorders and Stroke, *IV*
NIH/National Institute on Deafness and Other Communication Disorders (Balance), *IV*

598 KNIEST SYNDROME

Kniest Syndrome is a type of dwarfism that is characterized by unusually short arms and legs, a round face with hollow or depressed areas, swelling and stiffness of the joints, and a stiff drawing up (contractures) of the fingers. Cleft palate, abnormal curvature of the spine (scoliosis), and vision and/or hearing problems may also occur. Intellect is usually normal in people with this syndrome.

In addition to The National Organization for Rare Disorders (NORD) listed in Section III, the following organizations in Section II (Disease Specific) and in Section III (Umbrella) and Section IV (Government Agencies) can provide more information:

Human Growth Foundation, *III*
Kniest Syndrome Group, *II*
Little People of America, *III*
Little People's Research Fund, Inc., *III*
MAGIC Foundation for Children's Growth, *III*
NIH/National Institute of Child Health and Human Development, *IV*
Short Stature Foundation, *III*

599 KOHLER DISEASE

Kohler Disease is a rare bone disorder of the foot characterized by a painful, swollen foot, eventually causing the individual to limp. It generally occurs in children between the ages of three and five and affects males more often than females. Recovery usually occurs in less than a year.

In addition to The National Organization for Rare Disorders (NORD) listed in Section III, the following organizations in Section II (Disease Specific) and in Section III (Umbrella) and Section IV (Government Agencies) can provide more information:

NIH/National Institute of Arthritis and Musculoskeletal and Skin Diseases, *IV*
NIH/National Institute of Child Health and Human Development, *IV*

600 KORSAKOFF'S SYNDROME

Korsakoff's Syndrome is a deficiency of vitamin B-1 (or thiamine) which causes cardiovascular, central and peripheral nervous system disturbances. The disease results from either inadequate dietary intake or from impaired absorption or utilization of vitamin B-1. It is common in the Orient where excessive milling of rice reduces its thiamine content.

In addition to The National Organization for Rare Disorders (NORD) listed in Section III, the following organizations in Section II (Disease Specific) and in Section III (Umbrella) and Section IV (Government Agencies) can provide more information:

NIH/National Digestive Diseases Information Clearinghouse, *IV*

601 KUFS DISEASE

The chief characteristics of Kufs Disease are neurologic symptoms that may mimic mental illness, and dermatologic abnormalities resembling ichthyosis. Symptoms of Kufs Disease may be linked to excess accumulations of pigments (lipofuscins) dissolved in fat tissues that are found throughout the central nervous system. Kufs Disease, Batten Disease and Bielchowsky Disease are different forms of the same disorder and are differentiated by the age of onset (see the Related Disorders section of this report). Both major forms of this disorder may be extremely difficult to differentiate from other progressive degenerative diseases of the central nervous system.

In addition to The National Organization for Rare Disorders (NORD) listed in Section III, the following organizations in Section II (Disease Specific) and in Section III (Umbrella) and Section IV (Government Agencies) can provide more information:

Children's Brain Diseases Foundation, *II*
NIH/National Institute of Neurological Disorders and Stroke, *IV*
National Tay-Sachs and Allied Diseases Association, Inc., *III*
The Arc (a national organization on mental retardation), *III*

602 KUGELBERG WELANDER SYNDROME

Kugelberg-Welander Syndrome is a rare inherited disorder. Major symptoms may include wasting and weakness in the muscles of the arms and legs, twitching, clumsiness in walking, and eventual loss of reflexes. Kugelberg- Welander Syndrome is not apparent at birth, it usually appears during the first 10 to 20 years of life.

In addition to The National Organization for Rare Disorders (NORD) listed in Section III, the following organizations in Section II (Disease Specific) and in Section III (Umbrella) and Section IV (Government Agencies) can provide more information:

Families of Spinal Muscular Atrophy, *III*
Jennifer Trust for Spinal Muscular Atrophy, *II*
Muscular Dystrophy Association, *III*
NIH/National Institute of Neurological Disorders and Stroke, *IV*

603 LADD SYNDROME

LADD Syndrome is a rare genetic disorder inherited through an autosomal dominant trait. The major feature of this syndrome is malformations of the upper limbs. Other symptoms of the disorder may include: malformations in the network of structures of the eye that secretes tears and drains them from the surface of the eyeball (lacrimal malformations); abnormalities of the teeth; small cupped ears; absent or underdeveloped salivary glands; hearing loss; abnormalities of the sexual and urinary system of the body (genitourinary) and/or unusual skin ridge patterns.

In addition to The National Organization for Rare Disorders (NORD) listed in Section III, the following organizations in Section II (Disease Specific) and in Section III (Umbrella) and Section IV (Government Agencies) can provide more information:

NIH/National Arthritis and Musculoskeletal and Skin Diseases Information Clearinghouse, *IV*

604 LEOPARD SYNDROME

LEOPARD Syndrome is an extremely rare inherited disorder characterized by abnormalities of the skin, the structure and function of the heart, the inner ear, the head and facial (craniofacial) area, and/or the genitals. In individuals with the disorder, the range and severity of symptoms and physical characteristics may vary from case to case. "LEOPARD," an acronym for the characteristic abnormalities associated with the disorder, stands for (L)entigines, multiple black or dark brown "freckle-like" spots on the skin; (E)lectrocardiographic conduction defects, abnormalities of the electrical activity—and the coordination of proper contractions—of the heart; (0)cular hypertelorism, widely-spaced eyes; (P)ulmonary stenosis, obstruction of the normal outflow of blood from the lower right chamber (ventricle) of the heart; (A)bnormalities of the genitals; (R)etarded growth resulting in short stature; and (D)eafness or hearing loss due to malfunction of the inner ear (sensorineural deafness). Some individuals with LEOPARD Syndrome may also exhibit mild mental retardation, speech difficulties, and/or, in some cases, additional physical abnormalities. In most cases, LEOPARD Syndrome appears to occur randomly for unknown reasons (sporadically). However, in other cases, the disorder is thought to be inherited as an autosomal dominant genetic trait.

In addition to The National Organization for Rare Disorders (NORD) listed in Section III, the following organizations in Section II (Disease Specific) and in Section III (Umbrella) and Section IV (Government Agencies) can provide more information:

American Heart Association, *III*
Big Hearts for Little Hearts, *III*
Congenital Heart Anomalies, Support, Education, & Resources, *III*
Human Growth Foundation, *III*
MAGIC Foundation for Children's Growth, *III*
NIH/National Heart, Lung and Blood Institute

Information Center, *IV*
NIH/National Institute of Child Health and Human Development, *IV*
Short Stature Foundation, *III*

605 **LABAND SYNDROME**

Laband Syndrome is an extremely rare inherited disorder characterized by abnormalities of the head and facial (craniofacial) area and the hands and feet. Most children with this disorder have abnormally large gums (gingival fibromatosis). Overgrown gums may affect the ability to chew, swallow, and/or speak. In addition, affected infants may exhibit abnormally long, thin fingers and toes and/or deformed (dysplastic) or absent nails at birth. In some cases, mental retardation may also be present. Laband Syndrome is believed to be inherited as an autosomal dominant genetic trait.

In addition to The National Organization for Rare Disorders (NORD) listed in Section III, the following organizations in Section II (Disease Specific) and in Section III (Umbrella) and Section IV (Government Agencies) can provide more information:
NIH/National Institute of Arthritis and Musculoskeletal and Skin Diseases, *IV*
NIH/National Institute of Child Health and Human Development, *IV*
NIH/National Institute of Dental Research, *IV*

606 **LACTOSE INTOLERANCE**

Lactose is a sugar found in milk and milk products. People with lactose intolerance cannot properly digest lactose. This disorder is an inborn error of carbohydrate metabolism characterized by the impaired ability to absorb nutrients from the small intestine (malabsorption syndrome).

In addition to The National Organization for Rare Disorders (NORD) listed in Section III, the following organizations in Section II (Disease Specific) and in Section III (Umbrella) and Section IV (Government Agencies) can provide more information:
March of Dimes Birth Defects Foundation, *III*
NIH/National Institute of Diabetes, Digestive and Kidney Diseases, *IV*

607 **LANDAU KLEFFNER SYNDROME**

Landau-Kleffner Syndrome is a rare neurological disorder of childhood and is characterized by aphasia or loss of the ability to understand speech and deterioration of previously acquired speech skills. Most children with Landau-Kleffner Syndrome experience convulsive epileptic seizures. Some affected children also lose the ability to identify environmental sounds and show a general lack of attention to sounds (auditory agnosia). The exact cause of this disorder is not known. Symptoms, which develop due to brain dysfunction, vary greatly among affected individuals.

In addition to The National Organization for Rare Disorders (NORD) listed in Section III, the following organizations in Section II (Disease Specific) and in Section III (Umbrella) and Section IV (Government Agencies) can provide more information:
American Autoimmune Related Diseases Association, Inc., *III*
C.A.N.D.L.E., *III*
NIH/National Institute of Neurological Disorders and Stroke, *IV*
NIH/National Institute on Deafness and Other Communication Disorders (Balance), *IV*
National Aphasia Association, *II*

608 **LARON DWARFISM**

Laron Dwarfism is a rare genetic disorder that results from the body's inability to use the growth hormone that it produces. People with this disorder produce normal levels of growth hormone but the levels in their plasma may be high because the body does not use the hormone properly. The Laron form of dwarfism is characterized by very small stature, peculiar facial features, and high levels of growth hormone in plasma.

In addition to The National Organization for Rare Disorders (NORD) listed in Section III, the following organizations in Section II (Disease Specific) and in Section III (Umbrella) and Section IV (Government Agencies) can provide more information:
Human Growth Foundation, *III*
Little People of America, *III*
Little People's Research Fund, Inc., *III*
MAGIC Foundation for Children's Growth, *III*
NIH/National Institute of Child Health and Human Development, *IV*
Short Stature Foundation, *III*

609 **LARSEN SYNDROME**

Larsen Syndrome is a multi-system genetic disorder that is present at birth. It is characterized by multiple bone dislocations and abnormalities, an extremely high arch of the foot, non-tapering cylindrically shaped fingers, and an unusual facial appearance. In some cases, short stature, heart problems, cleft palate or lips, deafness, or mental retardation may also occur.

In addition to The National Organization for Rare Disorders (NORD) listed in Section III, the following organizations in Section II (Disease Specific) and in

Section III (Umbrella) and Section IV (Government Agencies) can provide more information:
NIH/National Arthritis and Musculoskeletal and Skin Diseases Information Clearinghouse, *IV*
NIH/National Institute of Child Health and Human Development, *IV*
The Arc (a national organization on mental retardation), *III*

610 LAURENCE MOON SYNDROME

Laurence-Moon Syndrome is a rare inherited disorder characterized by diminished hormone production by the testes or ovaries (hypogonadism), progressive loss of vision (retinitis pigmentosa), mental retardation, and paralysis of the legs and lower part of the body accompanied by involuntary muscle contractions (spastic paraplegia). Confusion exists in the medical literature regarding the difference between Laurence-Moon Syndrome and Bardet-Biedl Syndrome. Some researchers believe that Bardet-Biedl Syndrome is a subdivision of Laurence-Moon Syndrome which they term "Laurence-Moon-Biedl Syndrome."

In addition to The National Organization for Rare Disorders (NORD) listed in Section III, the following organizations in Section II (Disease Specific) and in Section III (Umbrella) and Section IV (Government Agencies) can provide more information:
Alliance of Genetic Support Groups, *III*
American Council of the Blind, Inc., *III*
American Foundation for the Blind, *III*
Blind Children's Fund, *III*
Council of Families with Visual Impairment, *III*
Laurence Moon Bardet Biedl Syndrome, *II*
March of Dimes Birth Defects Foundation, *III*
NIH/National Institute of Child Health and Human Development, *IV*
NIH/National Institute of Neurological Disorders and Stroke, *IV*
National Association for Parents of the Visually Impaired, *III*
National Association for Visually Handicapped, *III*
Prevent Blindness America, *III*
The Arc (a national organization on mental retardation), *III*
Vision Foundation, Inc., *III*

611 LEBER'S CONGENITAL AMAUROSIS

Leber's Congenital Amaurosis (LCA) is a rare genetic eye disorder. Affected infants are often blind at birth or loss their sight within the first few of years of life. Other symptoms may include crossed eyes (strabismus); rapid, involuntary eye movements (nystagmus); unusual sensitivity to light (photophobia); clouding of the lenses of the eyes (cataracts); and/or abnormal protrusion of the front (anterior), clear portion of the eye through which light passes (cornea) (keratoconus). In addition, some infants may exhibit hearing loss, mental retardation, and/or a delay in the acquisition of skills that require the coordination of mental and muscular activity (psychomotor retardation). Lebers Congenital Amaurosis is inherited as an autosomal recessive genetic trait.

In addition to The National Organization for Rare Disorders (NORD) listed in Section III, the following organizations in Section II (Disease Specific) and in Section III (Umbrella) and Section IV (Government Agencies) can provide more information:
American Council of the Blind, Inc., *III*
American Foundation for the Blind, *III*
Blind Children's Fund, *III*
Foundation Fighting Blindness, *III*
NIH/National Eye Institute, *IV*
National Association for Parents of the Visually Impaired, *III*
National Association for Visually Handicapped, *III*
Retinitis Pigmentosa International, *II*

612 LEBER'S OPTIC ATROPHY

Lebers Optic Atrophy is a rare inherited disorder of the eye that is characterized by the slow, painless, progressive loss of vision in one eye. Within a few weeks or months, the other eye often becomes involved. In most cases, visual loss is permanent. In some cases, affected individuals may experience recurrent headaches and gradual deterioration of the nerves of the eye (optic atrophy). Lebers Optic Atrophy is inherited due to abnormal changes in genetic material (mutation[s]) found within the unique DNA of mitochondria (mtDNA). Mitochondria, which are found by the hundreds in the cells of the body, particularly in muscle and nerve tissue, carry the blueprints for regulating energy production.

In addition to The National Organization for Rare Disorders (NORD) listed in Section III, the following organizations in Section II (Disease Specific) and in Section III (Umbrella) and Section IV (Government Agencies) can provide more information:
American Council of the Blind, Inc., *III*
American Foundation for the Blind, *III*
Blind Children's Center, *III*
Council of Families with Visual Impairment, *III*
Guiding Eyes for the Blind, Inc., *III*
NIH/National Eye Institute, *IV*
National Association for Parents of the Visually Impaired, *III*
National Association for Visually Handicapped, *III*
National Federation of the Blind, *III*

United Mitochondrial Disease Foundation, *III*
Vision Foundation, Inc., *III*

613 LEGG CALVE PERTHES DISEASE

Legg-Calve-Perthes Disease (LCPD) is one of a group of disorders known as the Osteochondroses. The Osteochondroses typically are characterized by degeneration (avascular necrosis) and subsequent regeneration of the growing end of a bone (epiphyses). In Legg-Calve-Perthes Disease, the growing end (epiphysis) of the upper portion (capital) of the thigh bone (femur) is affected. Researchers believe that an unexplained interruption of the blood supply (ischemia) to the capital femoral epiphysis results in degeneration (avascular necrosis) and deformity of the thigh bone in this area. Symptoms may include a limp with or without pain in the hip, knee, thigh, and/or groin; muscle spasms; delayed maturation of the femur (delayed bone age); mild short stature; and/or limited movements of the affected hip. The disease process seems to be self-limiting as new blood supplies are established (revascularization) and new healthy bone forms (reossifies) in the affected area. Most cases of Legg-Calve-Perthes Disease occur randomly for no apparent reason (sporadically). Other cases are thought to be inherited as an autosomal dominant genetic trait.

In addition to The National Organization for Rare Disorders (NORD) listed in Section III, the following organizations in Section II (Disease Specific) and in Section III (Umbrella) and Section IV (Government Agencies) can provide more information:
NIH/National Institute of Arthritis and Musculoskeletal and Skin Diseases, *IV*
NIH/National Institute of Child Health and Human Development, *IV*

614 LEGIONNAIRE'S DISEASE

Legionnaire's Disease is recognized as an acute respiratory pneumonia caused by the aerobic gram-negative microorganism, Legionella pneumophila, and other species. This microorganism may also affect other body systems. Afflicted patients may have pulmonary (lung and bronchi), gastrointestinal tract, and central nervous system complications. Renal insufficiency may occur occasionally and can be severe enough to require dialysis.

In addition to The National Organization for Rare Disorders (NORD) listed in Section III, the following organizations in Section II (Disease Specific) and in Section III (Umbrella) and Section IV (Government Agencies) can provide more information:
Centers for Disease Control and Prevention, *IV*
NIH/National Institute of Allergy and Infectious Diseases, *IV*
World Health Organization (WHO) Regional Office for the Americas (AMRO), *III*

615 LEIGH'S DISEASE

Leigh's Disease is a rare inherited neurometabolic disorder. It is characterized by the degeneration of the central nervous system (i.e., brain, spinal cord, and optic nerve). The symptoms of Leigh's Disease usually begin between the ages of three months and two years. Symptoms are associated with progressive neurological deterioration and may include loss of previously acquired motor skills, loss of appetite, vomiting, irritability, and/or seizure activity. As Leigh's Disease progresses, symptoms may also include generalized weakness, lack of muscle tone, and episodes of lactic acidosis, which may lead to impairment of respiratory and kidney function. In most cases, Leigh's Disease is inherited as an autosomal recessive genetic trait. However, autosomal dominant, X-linked recessive, and mitochondrial inheritance have also been noted. There appear to be several different types of genetically determined enzyme defects that can cause Leigh's Disease.

In addition to The National Organization for Rare Disorders (NORD) listed in Section III, the following organizations in Section II (Disease Specific) and in Section III (Umbrella) and Section IV (Government Agencies) can provide more information:
Alliance of Genetic Support Groups, *III*
Association for Neuro-Metabolic Disorders, *III*
Children's Brain Diseases Foundation, *II*
Lactic Acidosis Support Trust, *III*
Metabolic Information Network, *III*
NIH/National Institute of Neurological Disorders and Stroke, *IV*
Research Trust for Metabolic Diseases in Children, *III*
The Arc (a national organization on mental retardation), *III*
United Mitochondrial Disease Foundation, *III*

616 LEINER DISEASE

Leiner Disease is a skin disorder that usually first appears during the first two months of life. A reddish skin patch of thickened skin appears first on the buttocks and spreads to other parts of the infant's body. Scaling and peeling may occur with anemia, itching and diarrhea. The redness and scaliness usually decrease after a few weeks with treatment.

In addition to The National Organization for Rare Disorders (NORD) listed in Section III, the following organizations in Section II (Disease Specific) and in Section III (Umbrella) and Section IV (Government Agencies) can provide more information:
NIH/National Arthritis and Musculoskeletal and Skin Diseases Information Clearinghouse, *IV*

617 LENNOX GASTAUT SYNDROME

Lennox-Gastaut Syndrome is a very rare childhood seizure disorder. It is usually apparent in infancy or early childhood. It is characterized by drop attacks (from simple dropping of the head to collapse of the entire body) and other seizures that occur many times a day.

In addition to The National Organization for Rare Disorders (NORD) listed in Section III, the following organizations in Section II (Disease Specific) and in Section III (Umbrella) and Section IV (Government Agencies) can provide more information:
Epilepsy Foundation of America, *III*
NIH/National Institute of Neurological Disorders and Stroke, *IV*
THRESHOLD (for uncontrolled seizure disorders), *III*

618 LENZ MICROPHTHALMIA SYNDROME

Lenz Microphthalmia Syndrome is an extremely rare inherited disorder characterized by abnormal smallness of one or both eyes (unilateral or bilateral microphthalmos) and/or droopy eyelids (blepharoptosis), resulting in visual impairment. In rare cases, affected infants may exhibit complete absence of the eyes (anophthalmia). Most affected infants also exhibit developmental delay and mental retardation, ranging from mild to severe. Additional physical abnormalities are often associated with this disorder such as an unusually small head (microcephaly) and/or malformations of the teeth, ears, and/or fingers and/or toes (digits). The range and severity of findings may vary from case to case.

Lenz Microphthalmia Syndrome, which is inherited as an X-linked recessive genetic trait, is fully expressed in males only. However, females who carry one copy of the disease gene (heterozygotes) may exhibit some of the symptoms associated with the disorder, such as an abnormally small head (microcephaly), short stature, and/or malformations of the fingers and/or toes.

In addition to The National Organization for Rare Disorders (NORD) listed in Section III, the following organizations in Section II (Disease Specific) and in Section III (Umbrella) and Section IV (Government Agencies) can provide more information:
Council of Families with Visual Impairment, *III*
International Children's Anophthalmia Network, *III*
NIH/National Eye Institute, *IV*
NIH/National Institute of Child Health and Human Development, *IV*
National Association for Parents of the Visually Impaired, *III*
National Association for Visually Handicapped, *III*
National Federation of the Blind, *III*
Vision Foundation, Inc., *III*

619 LEPRECHAUNISM

Leprechaunism is a progressive hereditary endocrine disorder characterized by overdevelopment (hyperplasia) of the pancreas, insulin resistance, and excessive amounts of estrogens. It may be associated with abnormal carbohydrate metabolism, and a large quantity of iron in the liver (hepatic siderosis). Physical and sometimes mental retardation occurs with facial abnormalities and abnormal external genitalia.

In addition to The National Organization for Rare Disorders (NORD) listed in Section III, the following organizations in Section II (Disease Specific) and in Section III (Umbrella) and Section IV (Government Agencies) can provide more information:
Alliance of Genetic Support Groups, *III*
Metabolic Information Network, *III*
NIH/National Institute of Diabetes, Digestive and Kidney Diseases, *IV*
Research Trust for Metabolic Diseases in Children, *III*
The Arc (a national organization on mental retardation), *III*

620 LEPROSY

Leprosy is a progressive, chronic infectious disease caused by the bacteria, Mycobacterium leprae. This disease affects the nerves that are located outside the central nervous system (peripheral nerves), and the skin, mucous membranes, and eyes. In severe cases of Leprosy, loss of sensation, disfigurement, and/or blindness may occur.

There are several forms of Leprosy: Tuberculoid (Minor and Major, and Benign Hansen's Disease), Lepromatous (Malignant Hansen's Disease), Dimorphous (Borderline Leprosy), and Indeterminate Leprosy. This disease is rare in the United States but prevalent in third world countries.

In addition to The National Organization for Rare Disorders (NORD) listed in Section III, the following organizations in Section II (Disease Specific) and in Section III (Umbrella) and Section IV (Government Agencies) can provide more information:
American Leprosy Missions, *II*
Centers for Disease Control and Prevention, *IV*
NIH/National Institute of Allergy and Infectious Diseases, *IV*

621 LEPTOSPIROSIS

Leptospirosis is an inclusive term for all bacterial infections caused by any Leptospira bacteria, regardless of the type. A single type of bacteria may cause various clinical symptoms, or a single syndrome such as aseptic meningitis may be caused by many types of this bacteria.

In addition to The National Organization for Rare Disorders (NORD) listed in Section III, the following organizations in Section II (Disease Specific) and in Section III (Umbrella) and Section IV (Government Agencies) can provide more information:
Centers for Disease Control and Prevention, *IV*
NIH/National Institute of Allergy and Infectious Diseases, *IV*
World Health Organization (WHO) Regional Office for the Americas (AMRO), *III*

622 LERI PLEONOSTEOSIS

Leri Pleonosteosis is an extremely rare inherited disorder characterized by unusual, flattened facial features, abnormalities of the hands and feet, skeletal malformations, short stature, and/or limitation of joint movements. Characteristic abnormalities of the hands and feet may include unusually broad and/or short thumbs and great toes (brachydactyly) that may be bent outward from the body (valgus position); as a result, the hands may have a "spade-shaped" appearance. Skeletal malformations may include knees that are bent backward (genu recurvitum) and abnormal enlargement of the cartilaginous structures that surround the upper portion of the spinal cord (posterior neural arches of the cervical vertebrae). In addition, affected individuals may develop thickened tissue on the palms (palmar) and forearms. Symptoms may vary from case to case. Leri Pleonosteosis is inherited as an autosomal dominant genetic trait.

In addition to The National Organization for Rare Disorders (NORD) listed in Section III, the following organizations in Section II (Disease Specific) and in Section III (Umbrella) and Section IV (Government Agencies) can provide more information:
Human Growth Foundation, *III*
Little People of America, *III*
Little People's Research Fund, Inc., *III*
NIH/National Institute of Arthritis and Musculoskeletal and Skin Diseases, *IV*
NIH/National Institute of Child Health and Human Development, *IV*
Short Stature Foundation, *III*

623 LESCH NYHAN SYNDROME

Lesch-Nyhan Syndrome is a rare inborn error of purine metabolism characterized by the absence of the enzyme hypoxanthine-guanine phosphoribosyltransferase (HPRT). Purine, a nitrogen-containing compound found in many foods (e.g., organ meats, poultry, and legumes), is not broken down properly, due to the absence of HPRT. Uric acid levels are abnormally high in people with Lesch-Nyhan Syndrome, and they form sodium urate crystals that are deposited in the joints, kidneys, central nervous system, and other tissues of the body. Lesch-Nyhan Syndrome is inherited as an X-linked recessive genetic disorder that effects only males.

The symptoms of Lesch-Nyhan Syndrome include impaired kidney function, joint pain, and self-mutilating behaviors such as lip and finger biting and/or head banging. Other symptoms may include muscle weakness (hypotonia), uncontrolled spastic muscle movements, and neurological impairment.

In addition to The National Organization for Rare Disorders (NORD) listed in Section III, the following organizations in Section II (Disease Specific) and in Section III (Umbrella) and Section IV (Government Agencies) can provide more information:
Association for Neuro-Metabolic Disorders, *III*
International Lesch-Nyhan Disease Association, *II*
Metabolic Information Network, *III*
Purine Research Society, *III*
Research Trust for Metabolic Diseases in Children, *III*
The Arc (a national organization on mental retardation), *III*

624 LEUKEMIA, CHRONIC LYMPHOCYTIC

Chronic Lymphocytic Leukemia is a malignant blood disorder in which there is an increased number of white blood cells formed in the lymphoid tissue. This uncontrolled buildup and enlargement of lymphoid tissue can occur in various sites of the body such as the lymph nodes, spleen, bone marrow, and lungs. There are many different forms of Leukemia which are all characterized by an overabundance of white blood cells. In Chronic

Lymphocytic Leukemia the disease occurs in the lymphoid tissue.

The lymph vessels, which return fluids to the circulatory system, and the lymph nodes, which are a mass of tissue separated into compartments by connective tissue, make up the immune system. The lymph nodes serve as filters, removing foreign particles, tissue debris, and bacterial cells from the circulation. When this system is not working properly, the body's defenses cannot fight off foreign particles.

In the majority of cases, Chronic Lymphocytic Leukemia is the result of a rapid production of B lymphocyte cells (a short-lived type of white blood cell that is responsible for the production of vertebrate serum proteins that include antibodies). A small percentage of Chronic Lymphocytic Leukemia cases stem from the overproduction of T lymphocyte cells (a type of white blood cell that have a long life and are important in the resistance of disease).

In addition to The National Organization for Rare Disorders (NORD) listed in Section III, the following organizations in Section II (Disease Specific) and in Section III (Umbrella) and Section IV (Government Agencies) can provide more information:
American Cancer Society, Inc., *III*
Leukemia Society of America, Inc., *II*
NIH/Patient Referral Services Unit, *IV*
National Leukemia Research Association, Inc., *II*

625 LEUKEMIA, CHRONIC MYELOGENOUS

Chronic myelogenous leukemia is characterized by an excessive amount of white blood cells in the bone marrow, spleen, liver and blood. As the disease progresses, the leukemic cells invade other areas of the body including the intestinal tract, kidneys, lungs, gonads and lymph nodes.

There are two phases to chronic myelogenous leukemia. The first phase, or chronic phase, is characterized by an overproduction of white blood cells. An advanced phase is called the acute phase or blast crisis. At this point, over 50 percent of the cells in the bone marrow are immature malignant cells (blast cells or promelocytes). In the acute phase, the leukemia is very aggressive and does not respond well to therapy. Approximately 85 percent of all individuals with chronic myelogenous leukemia enter the acute phase.

In addition to The National Organization for Rare Disorders (NORD) listed in Section III, the following organizations in Section II (Disease Specific) and in Section III (Umbrella) and Section IV (Government Agencies) can provide more information:
American Cancer Society, Inc., *III*
Leukemia Society of America, Inc., *II*
MPD (Myeloproliferative Disease) Research Center, Inc., *III*
National Leukemia Research Association, Inc., *II*

626 LEUKEMIA, HAIRY CELL

Hairy cell leukemia is a rare type of blood cancer characterized by the presence of abnormal mononuclear blood cells called "hairy cells," and by a deficiency of other blood cell elements (pancytopenia), including an abnormal decrease of certain white blood cells (neutrophils [neutropenia]) and certain red blood cells (platelets [thrombocytopenia]). Affected individuals usually exhibit fatigue, weakness, fever, weight loss, and/or abdominal discomfort due to an abnormally enlarged spleen (splenomegaly). In addition, affected individuals may have a slightly enlarged liver (hepatomegaly) and may be unusually susceptible to bruising and/or severe infection. The exact cause of hairy cell leukemia is not known.

In addition to The National Organization for Rare Disorders (NORD) listed in Section III, the following organizations in Section II (Disease Specific) and in Section III (Umbrella) and Section IV (Government Agencies) can provide more information:
American Cancer Society, Inc., *III*
Leukemia Society of America, Inc., *II*
NIH/National Cancer Institute, *IV*
NIH/Patient Referral Services Unit, *IV*
National Leukemia Research Association, Inc., *II*

627 LEUKODYSTROPHY

Leukodystrophy is the name given to a group of very rare, progressive, metabolic, genetic diseases that affect the brain, spinal cord and often the peripheral nerves. Each of the leukodystrophies will affect one of the chemicals that make up the myelin sheath or white matter of the brain, causing the various types of leukodystrophy. The myelin sheath, which acts as insulation of the nervous system, is composed of different lipids (fatty substances). Thus defects in production and degradation of these lipids can lead to the many ways in which these diseases can manifest themselves.

In addition to The National Organization for Rare Disorders (NORD) listed in Section III, the following organizations in Section II (Disease Specific) and in Section III (Umbrella) and Section IV (Government Agencies) can provide more information:
Association for Neuro-Metabolic Disorders, *III*
Metabolic Information Network, *III*
NIH/National Institute of Neurological Disorders and Stroke, *IV*
National Tay-Sachs and Allied Diseases Association, Inc., *III*
United Leukodystrophy Foundation, *III*

628 LEUKODYSTROPHY, CANAVAN'S

Canavan's Leukodystrophy is a rare inherited neurological disorder characterized by spongy degeneration of the brain and spinal cord (central nervous system). Symptoms may include progressive mental decline accompanied by the loss of muscle tone, poor head control, an abnormally enlarged head (megalocephaly), and/or blindness. Canavan's Leukodystrophy is caused by a deficiency of the enzyme aspartoacylase. Symptoms appear in early infancy and usually progress rapidly.

In addition to The National Organization for Rare Disorders (NORD) listed in Section III, the following organizations in Section II (Disease Specific) and in Section III (Umbrella) and Section IV (Government Agencies) can provide more information:
Association for Neuro-Metabolic Disorders, *III*
March of Dimes Birth Defects Foundation, *III*
NIH/National Institute of Neurological Disorders and Stroke, *IV*
NIH/Patient Referral Services Unit, *IV*
National Foundation for Jewish Genetic Diseases, *III*
National Tay-Sachs and Allied Diseases Association, Inc., *III*
United Leukodystrophy Foundation, *III*

629 LEUKODYSTROPHY, KRABBE'S

Krabbe's Leukodystrophy is a very rare hereditary lipid storage disorder caused by a deficiency of the enzyme galactoside beta-galactosidase (galactosyl-ceramidase). This causes the myelin sheath surrounding nerves in the brain to degenerate (demyelination). Characteristic globoid cells appear in affected areas of the brain. This metabolic disorder is characterized by progressive neurological dysfunction such as mental retardation, paralysis, blindness, deafness and pseudobulbar palsy.

In addition to The National Organization for Rare Disorders (NORD) listed in Section III, the following organizations in Section II (Disease Specific) and in Section III (Umbrella) and Section IV (Government Agencies) can provide more information:
Association for Neuro-Metabolic Disorders, *III*
Metabolic Information Network, *III*
NIH/National Institute of Neurological Disorders and Stroke, *IV*
NIH/Patient Referral Services Unit, *IV*
Research Trust for Metabolic Diseases in Children, *III*
The Arc (a national organization on mental retardation), *III*
United Leukodystrophy Foundation, *III*

630 LEUKODYSTROPHY, METACHROMATIC

Metachromatic Leukodystrophy (MLD), the most common form of leukodystrophy, is a rare inherited neurometabolic disorder affecting the white matter of the brain (leukoencephalopathy). It is characterized by the accumulation of a fatty substance known as sulfatide (a sphingolipid) in the brain and other areas of the body (i.e., liver, gall bladder, kidneys, and/or spleen). The fatty protective covering on the nerve fibers (myelin) is lost from areas of the central nervous system (CNS) due to the buildup of sulfatide. Symptoms of Metachromatic Leukodystrophy may include convulsions, seizures, personality changes, spasticity, progressive dementia, motor disturbances progressing to paralysis, and/or visual impairment leading to blindness.

Metachromatic Leukodystrophy is inherited as an autosomal recessive trait. There are three forms of the disease that have similar symptoms. However, they are distinguished by the age of onset: infantile, juvenile, and adult forms of Metachromatic Leukodystrophy.

In addition to The National Organization for Rare Disorders (NORD) listed in Section III, the following organizations in Section II (Disease Specific) and in Section III (Umbrella) and Section IV (Government Agencies) can provide more information:
Association for Neuro-Metabolic Disorders, *III*
Metabolic Information Network, *III*
NIH/National Institute of Neurological Disorders and Stroke, *IV*
National Lipid Diseases Foundation, *III*
National Tay-Sachs and Allied Diseases Association, Inc., *III*
United Leukodystrophy Foundation, *III*

631 LICHEN PLANUS

Lichen Planus is a rare skin disorder characterized by recurrent, itchy, inflammatory eruptions (lesions) of the skin. These euptions may appear as small separate, angular spots; eventually they may coalesce into rough scaly patches. This disorder is frequently accompanied by oral lesions of the mucous membranes that line the mouth. Females are most commonly affected by the disorder. The exact cause of Lichen Planus is not known.

In addition to The National Organization for Rare Disorders (NORD) listed in Section III, the following organizations in Section II (Disease Specific) and in Section III (Umbrella) and Section IV (Government Agencies) can provide more information:
NIH/National Institute of Arthritis and Musculoskeletal and Skin Diseases, *IV*
Skin Disease Research Core Centers of the National Institute of Arthritis, *IV*

632 LICHEN SCLEROSUS

Lichen Sclerosus is a chronic skin disorder that most commonly affects females after menopause; however, cases have been identified among younger females (pre-menopausal). This disorder is characterized by skin changes of the external genitalia (i.e., vulva), although other parts of the body may also be affected. In some very rare cases, males have also been affected (known as Balanitis Xerotica Obliteran). Lichen Sclerosus can develop concurrently with other skin abnormalities.

In addition to The National Organization for Rare Disorders (NORD) listed in Section III, the following organizations in Section II (Disease Specific) and in Section III (Umbrella) and Section IV (Government Agencies) can provide more information:
American Autoimmune Related Diseases Association, Inc., *III*
NIH/National Institute of Arthritis and Musculoskeletal and Skin Diseases, *IV*
National Vulvodynia Association, *III*
National Women's Health Network, *III*
National Women's Health Resource Center, *III*

633 LIPODYSTROPHY

Lipodystrophies are a group of rare metabolic disorders which can be either inherited or acquired. They are characterized by abnormalities in fatty (adipose) tissue associated with total or partial loss of body fat, abnormalities of carbohydrate and lipid metabolism, severe resistance to naturally occurring and synthetic insulin, and immune system dysfunction. These disorders are differentiated by degrees of severity, and by areas or systems of the body affected. Lipodystrophies can also be associated with other disorders and various developmental abnormalities.

In addition to The National Organization for Rare Disorders (NORD) listed in Section III, the following organizations in Section II (Disease Specific) and in Section III (Umbrella) and Section IV (Government Agencies) can provide more information:
Metabolic Information Network, *III*
NIH/National Digestive Diseases Information Clearinghouse, *IV*
Research Trust for Metabolic Diseases in Children, *III*
The Arc (a national organization on mental retardation), *III*

634 LISSENCEPHALY

Lissencephaly is a brain formation disorder characterized by the lack of normal convolutions or folds in the brain. It is thought to be inherited. Two major subdivisions including Miller-Dieker Syndrome and Norman-Roberts Syndrome have been identified, although as many as eight variants of Lissencephaly may exist. An abnormally small head and an unusual facial appearance, as well as abnormalities of the brain, kidney, heart and gastrointestinal tract may occur. This disorder may occur alone or as a symptom of other medical conditions.

In addition to The National Organization for Rare Disorders (NORD) listed in Section III, the following organizations in Section II (Disease Specific) and in Section III (Umbrella) and Section IV (Government Agencies) can provide more information:
Lissencephaly Contact Grmup, *II*
Lissencephaly Network, Inc., *II*
NIH/National Institute of Neurological Disorders and Stroke, *IV*

635 LISTERIOSIS

Listeriosis is a disorder caused by a bacterial infection (Listeria monocytogenes) transmitted to humans through contaminated food products, usually improperly pasteurized milk or cheese. Some cases have been transmitted through contact with other infected persons or animals. Cases range in severity from a transient carrier state with no apparent symptoms, to acute suddenly occurring (fulminant) spread of bacteria throughout the blood stream (septicemia). Many factors may contribute to development of symptoms which are not well understood. However, prompt recognition and treatment of the disease is necessary to avoid complications.

In addition to The National Organization for Rare Disorders (NORD) listed in Section III, the following organizations in Section II (Disease Specific) and in

Section III (Umbrella) and Section IV (Government Agencies) can provide more information:
Centers for Disease Control and Prevention, *IV*
Food and Drug Administration (FDA) Office of Inquiry & Consumer Information, *IV*
NIH/National Institute of Allergy and Infectious Diseases, *IV*

636 LOCKED IN SYNDROME

Locked-In Syndrome is characterized by complete paralysis except for voluntary eye movements. It is usually caused by lesions in the nerve centers that control muscle contractions, or a blood clot that blocks circulation of oxygen to the brain stem.

In addition to The National Organization for Rare Disorders (NORD) listed in Section III, the following organizations in Section II (Disease Specific) and in Section III (Umbrella) and Section IV (Government Agencies) can provide more information:
Brain and Pituitary Foundation of America, *III*
NIH/National Institute of Neurological Disorders and Stroke, *IV*
WE MOVE, *III*

637 LOKEN SENIOR SYNDROME

Loken-Senior Syndrome is a rare disorder inherited as an autosomal recessive genetic trait. This disorder is characterized by progressive wasting of the filtering unit of the kidney (nephronophthisis), with or without medullary Cystic Disease, and progressive eye disease. Typically this disorder becomes apparent during the first year of life.

In addition to The National Organization for Rare Disorders (NORD) listed in Section III, the following organizations in Section II (Disease Specific) and in Section III (Umbrella) and Section IV (Government Agencies) can provide more information:
American Foundation for Urologic Disease, *III*
American Kidney Fund, Inc., *III*
Blind Children's Center, *III*
Blind Children's Fund, *III*
Foundation Fighting Blindness, *III*
NIH/National Eye Institute, *IV*
NIH/National Kidney and Urologic Diseases Information Clearinghouse, *IV*
National Association for Parents of the Visually Impaired, *III*
National Association for Visually Handicapped, *III*
National Kidney Foundation, *III*
Retinitis Pigmentosa International, *II*

638 LONG CHAIN ACYL COA DEHYDROGENASE DEFICIENCY (LCAD)

Long-Chain Acyl-CoA Dehydrogenase Deficiency is a very rare inherited metabolic disorder characterized by a deficiency of the enzyme long-chain acyl-CoA dehydrogenase, which is needed to break down fatty acids. Symptoms develop due to the inherited enzyme deficiency. Characteristic features usually begin during infancy or early childhood and may continue to affect the individual into adulthood. Major symptoms may include recurrent episodes of abnormally low blood glucose after fasting, without accumulation of ketone bodies in blood and body tissues (nonketotic hypoglycemia). Coma may also occur after fasting. In the first few weeks of life infants with this disorder may feed poorly, vomit frequently, and not gain weight appropriately. Other symptoms during acute episodes may include muscle weakness (hypotonia) and/or heart problems due to enlargement of the muscles of the heart (hypertrophic cardiomyopathy).

In addition to The National Organization for Rare Disorders (NORD) listed in Section III, the following organizations in Section II (Disease Specific) and in Section III (Umbrella) and Section IV (Government Agencies) can provide more information:
Association for Neuro-Metabolic Disorders, *III*
FOD (Fatty Oxidation Disorder) Family Support Group, *III*
NIH/National Digestive Diseases Information Clearinghouse, *IV*
Organic Acidemia Association, *III*
Research Trust for Metabolic Diseases in Children, *III*
United Mitochondrial Disease Foundation, *III*

639 LOWE'S SYNDROME

Lowe's Syndrome, also known as oculo-cerebro-renal syndrome, is a rare inherited metabolic disease that affects males. This disorder is characterized by lack of muscle tone (hypotonia), multiple abnormalities of the eyes and bones, the presence at birth of clouding of the lenses of the eyes (cataracts), mental retardation, and kidney problems. Other findings may include protrusion of the eyeball from the eye socket (enophthalmos); failure to gain weight and grow at the expected rate; weak or absent deep tendon reflexes; and multiple kidney problems (e.g., renal tubular dysfunction, renal hyperaminoaciduria, etc.). Lowe's Syndrome is inherited as an X-linked genetic trait and symptoms may develop due to lack of the enzyme inositol-polyphosphate-5-phosphatase.

In addition to The National Organization for Rare Disorders (NORD) listed in Section III, the following organizations in Section II (Disease Specific) and in Section III (Umbrella) and Section IV (Government

Agencies) can provide more information:
Blind Children's Fund, *III*
Lowe Syndrome Association, *II*
March of Dimes Birth Defects Foundation, *III*
Metabolic Information Network, *III*
NIH/National Institute of Child Health and Human Development, *IV*
National Association for Visually Handicapped, *III*
The Arc (a national organization on mental retardation), *III*

640 LUPUS

Lupus (Systemic Lupus Erythematosus) is an inflammatory disease of the connective tissue. Tissue damage occurs when the body's own immune system attacks healthy tissue causing inflammation and malfunction of various organ systems. Many different symptoms are associated with Lupus, and most patients do not get all of the symptoms.

In addition to The National Organization for Rare Disorders (NORD) listed in Section III, the following organizations in Section II (Disease Specific) and in Section III (Umbrella) and Section IV (Government Agencies) can provide more information:
American Juvenile Arthritis Organization, *II*
Lupus Canada, *II*
Lupus Foundation of America, Inc., *II*
NIH/National Arthritis and Musculoskeletal and Skin Diseases Information Clearinghouse, *IV*

641 LYELLES SYNDROME

Lyelles Syndrome is a serious skin disorder characterized by severe redness, blisters and peeling. Onset can begin during any stage of life. The infantile form may follow an infection. In adults the disorder is often caused by a drug reaction. Treatment of cases caused by infection may differ from those caused by drug reactions.

In addition to The National Organization for Rare Disorders (NORD) listed in Section III, the following organizations in Section II (Disease Specific) and in Section III (Umbrella) and Section IV (Government Agencies) can provide more information:
Dystrophic Epidermolysis Bullosa Research Association of America, Inc., *III*
NIH/National Arthritis and Musculoskeletal and Skin Diseases Information Clearinghouse, *IV*

642 LYME DISEASE

Lyme Disease is an infectious tick-transmitted inflammatory disorder characterized by an early focal skin lesion, and subsequently a growing red area on the skin (erythema migrans or EM). The disorder may be followed weeks later by neurological, heart, or joint abnormalities.

In addition to The National Organization for Rare Disorders (NORD) listed in Section III, the following organizations in Section II (Disease Specific) and in Section III (Umbrella) and Section IV (Government Agencies) can provide more information:
American Lyme Disease Foundation, Inc., *II*
Centers for Disease Control and Prevention, *IV*
Lyme Disease Resource Center, *II*
NIH/National Arthritis and Musculoskeletal and Skin Diseases Information Clearinghouse, *IV*

643 LYMPHADENOPATHY, ANGIOIMMUNOBLASTIC WITH DYSPROTEINEMIA

Angioimmunoblastic Lymphadenopathy with Dysproteinemia (AILD) is a progressive immune system disorder possibly caused by viral infections, chronic stimulation of immune responses or drug treatments prescribed for other conditions. This disorder occurs mostly among persons over 50 years of age. Fever, chills, sweating, a general feeling of discomfort, weight loss, and/or skin rashes are the major symptoms. In some cases, AILD may evolve into a severe form of lymphoma (a type of cancer).

In addition to The National Organization for Rare Disorders (NORD) listed in Section III, the following organizations in Section II (Disease Specific) and in Section III (Umbrella) and Section IV (Government Agencies) can provide more information:
Immune Deficiency Foundation, *III*
International Patient Organization for Primary Immunodeficiencies, *III*
NIH/National Institute of Allergy and Infectious Diseases, *IV*

644 LYMPHANGIOLEIOMYOMATOSIS

Lymphangioleiomyomatosis (LAM) is a very rare progressive lung disease (airway and interstitial) that affects females of childbearing age. The disease is characterized by the abnormal growth of smooth muscle, leading to airway obstruction and cystic lesions (blebs) in the lungs. The symptoms of Lymphangioleiomyomatosis may include shortness of breath, coughing, and/or difficulty breathing (dyspnea), especially following periods of exercise or exertion. Affected individuals may experience repeated episodes of chest pain due to fluid accumulation around the lungs (pleural effusion). Collapse of a lung (pneumothorax) is also common in females with this disorder. The exact cause of Lymphangioleiomyomatosis is not known.

In addition to The National Organization for Rare Disorders (NORD) listed in Section III, the following

organizations in Section II (Disease Specific) and in Section III (Umbrella) and Section IV (Government Agencies) can provide more information:
American Lung Association, *III*
LAM Foundation, *II*
NIH/National Heart, Lung and Blood Institute Information Center, *IV*
Second Wind Lung Transplant Association, Inc., *III*

645 LYMPHANGIOMA, CAVERNOUS

Cavernous Lymphangioma is a congenital disorder of the lymph vessels. It is characterized by a mass of lymphoid tissue under the skin. Lymphangioma is usually present at birth but may develop later in life as well.

In addition to The National Organization for Rare Disorders (NORD) listed in Section III, the following organizations in Section II (Disease Specific) and in Section III (Umbrella) and Section IV (Government Agencies) can provide more information:
American Cancer Society, Inc., *III*
National Lymphatic and Venous Diseases Foundation, Inc., *III*

646 LYMPHEDEMA, HEREDITARY

Hereditary Lymphedema is a rare inherited disorder of the lymphatic system that is characterized by abnormal swelling of certain parts of the body. The lymphatic system is a network of vessels, ducts, and nodes that filter and distribute certain fluid (lymph) and blood cells throughout the body. Lymphatic fluid collects in the soft tissues under the skin (subcutaneous) due to the obstruction, malformation, or underdevelopment (hypoplasia) of various lymphatic vessels.

There are three forms of Hereditary Lymphedema: Congenital Hereditary Lymphedema or Milroy Disease, Lymphedema Praecox or Meige Disease, and Lymphedema Tarda. In most cases, Hereditary Lymphedema is inherited as an autosomal dominant genetic trait.

In addition to The National Organization for Rare Disorders (NORD) listed in Section III, the following organizations in Section II (Disease Specific) and in Section III (Umbrella) and Section IV (Government Agencies) can provide more information:
NIH/National Heart, Lung and Blood Institute, *IV*
National Lymphatic and Venous Diseases Foundation, Inc., *III*
National Lymphedema Network, *III*

647 LYMPHOCYTIC INFILTRATE OF JESSNER

Lymphocytic Infiltrate of Jessner is a skin disorder characterized by benign accumulations of lymph cells in the skin. These small lesions are solid, pink or red in color, and appear on the face, neck, and/or back. Skin surrounding these lesions is itchy and reddened. The lesions may remain unchanged for several years and then spontaneously disappear leaving no scars.

In addition to The National Organization for Rare Disorders (NORD) listed in Section III, the following organizations in Section II (Disease Specific) and in Section III (Umbrella) and Section IV (Government Agencies) can provide more information:
NIH/National Institute of Arthritis and Musculoskeletal and Skin Diseases, *IV*

648 LYMPHOMA, GASTRIC, NON-HODGKINS TYPE

Non-Hodgkins Type Gastric Lymphoma is a rare form of stomach cancer characterized by unrestrained growth of certain lymphoid cells of the stomach. This form of cancer is thought to arise from certain white blood cells (lymphocytes) within lymphoid tissue of the stomachs mucous membrane (mucosa). Non-Hodgkins Type Gastric Lymphoma may be a primary disease process (primary lymphoma) or may develop due to another underlying lymphoma. Symptoms and findings associated with Non-Hodgkins Type Gastric Lymphoma may include pain, bleeding, obstruction of, and/or the development of a hole in the wall of the stomach (perforation). In many affected individuals, an abnormal mass may be felt (palpable) in the upper middle (epigastric) region of the abdomen. Non-Hodgkins Type Gastric Lymphoma affects males more often than females and usually appears to occur during middle age. According to the medical literature, Non-Hodgkins Type Gastric Lymphoma tends to occur an average of approximately 10 years earlier than gastric adenocarcinoma, a more common form of stomach cancer.

In addition to The National Organization for Rare Disorders (NORD) listed in Section III, the following organizations in Section II (Disease Specific) and in Section III (Umbrella) and Section IV (Government Agencies) can provide more information:
American Cancer Society, Inc., *III*
Leukemia Society of America, Inc., *II*

649 LYNCH SYNDROMES

The Lynch Syndromes are rare hereditary disorders that usually cause cancer to develop either in the colorectal area or in other sites. Primary cancers may develop in the female genital tract, stomach, brain, breasts, or urological system. The cancers of the colorectal area associated with the Lynch Syndromes usually develop at a younger age than is normally found in other persons with colorectal cancer.

In addition to The National Organization for Rare Disorders (NORD) listed in Section III, the following organizations in Section II (Disease Specific) and in Section III (Umbrella) and Section IV (Government Agencies) can provide more information:

American Cancer Society, Inc., *III*
NIH/Patient Referral Services Unit, *IV*

650 MASA SYNDROME

MASA Syndrome is an extremely rare inherited disorder that is one of several disorders known as X-linked Mental Retardation (XLMR) syndromes. The acronym MASA stands for (M)ental retardation, (A)phasia, a diminished ability to communicate by speech, writing, and/or signs, (S)huffling manner of walking (gait), and (A)dducted thumbs, thumbs that are flexed inward toward the palm. Shuffling gait may be due to impaired control of voluntary movements and progressive rigidity of muscles in the legs (spastic paraplegia). Adduction of the thumbs may be due to absence or underdevelopment (hypoplasia) of certain muscles (extensor pollicis longus and/or brevis muscles) of the hand near the thumb.

The symptoms and physical findings associated with MASA Syndrome vary greatly from case to case. Affected individuals may not experience all of the main characteristics described above and may exhibit various other symptoms and physical findings such as abnormal widening (dilatation) of cavities (ventricles) within the brain and accumulation of excessive cerebrospinal fluid in the skull (hydrocephalus), mild short stature, abnormally increased inward curvature of the lower spine (exaggerated lumbar lordosis), and/or other skeletal abnormalities. According to the medical literature, mental retardation is the only feature that has been present in all documented cases of the disorder.

MASA Syndrome is thought to be inherited as an X-linked recessive genetic trait. Therefore, the disorder is usually fully expressed in males only. However, some females who carry one copy of the gene (heterozygotes) do appear to fully express the disease, while others may exhibit only some milder symptoms associated with the disorder such as dull intelligence and/or adducted thumbs.

In addition to The National Organization for Rare Disorders (NORD) listed in Section III, the following organizations in Section II (Disease Specific) and in Section III (Umbrella) and Section IV (Government Agencies) can provide more information:

C.A.N.D.L.E., *III*
Guardians of Hydrocephalus Research Foundation, *II*
Hydrocephalus Association, *II*
NIH/National Institute of Child Health and Human Development, *IV*
NIH/National Institute of Neurological Disorders and Stroke, *IV*
NIH/National Institute on Deafness and Other Communication Disorders Information Clearinghouse, *IV*
National Aphasia Association, *II*
National Hydrocephalus Foundation, *II*
WE MOVE, *III*

651 MELAS SYNDROME

MELAS Syndrome is one of a group of rare muscular disorders that are called mitochondrial encephalomyopathies. Mitochondrial encephalomyopathies are disorders in which a defect in genetic material arises from a part of the cell structure that releases energy (mitochondria) resulting in disease of the brain and muscles (encephalomyopathies). This mitochondrial defect as well as "ragged red fibers" (an abnormality of muscle tissue when viewed under a microscope) are typically present. The most characteristic symptom of MELAS Syndrome is recurring, stroke-like episodes in which there are sudden headaches followed by vomiting and seizures. Short stature, an accumulation of lactic acid in the blood (lactic acidosis), and muscular weakness on one side of the body (hemiparesis) are typically present. Visual symptoms may include: impaired vision or blindness in one half of the visual field (hemianopsia), and/or blindness due to lesions in the area of the brain concerned with vision (cortical blindness). Although the exact cause of MELAS Syndrome is not fully understood, it has been found to run in families (familial).

In addition to The National Organization for Rare Disorders (NORD) listed in Section III, the following organizations in Section II (Disease Specific) and in Section III (Umbrella) and Section IV (Government Agencies) can provide more information:
Epilepsy Foundation of America, *III*
Lactic Acidosis Support Trust, *III*
NIH/National Institute of Neurological Disorders and Stroke, *IV*
Research Trust for Metabolic Diseases in Children, *III*
United Mitochondrial Disease Foundation, *III*

652 MERRF SYNDROME

MERRF Syndrome (Myoclonus Epilepsy Associated with Ragged-Red Fibers) is one of a group of rare muscular disorders that are called mitochondrial encephalomyopathies. Mitochondrial encephalomyopathies are disorders in which a defect in the genetic material arises from a part of the cell structure that releases energy (mitochondria). This can cause a dysfunction of the brain and muscles (encephalomyopathies). The mitochondrial defect as well as "ragged-red fibers" (an abnormality of tissue when viewed under a microscope) are always present. The most characteristic symptom of MERRF Syndrome is myoclonic seizures which are usually sudden, brief, jerking, spasms that can affect the limbs or the entire body. An impairment in the ability to coordinate movements (ataxia), as well as an accumulation of lactic acid in the blood (lactic acidosis) are also be present in affected individuals. Difficulty speaking (dysarthria), optic atrophy, short stature, hearing loss, dementia, and involuntary jerking of the eyes (nystagmus) may also occur.

In addition to The National Organization for Rare Disorders (NORD) listed in Section III, the following organizations in Section II (Disease Specific) and in Section III (Umbrella) and Section IV (Government Agencies) can provide more information:
Epilepsy Foundation of America, *III*
Lactic Acidosis Support Trust, *III*
NIH/National Institute of Neurological Disorders and Stroke, *IV*
Research Trust for Metabolic Diseases in Children, *III*
United Mitochondrial Disease Foundation, *III*

653 MURCS ASSOCIATION

MURCS Association is a very rare developmental disorder that affects only females. The acronym MURCS stands for (MU)llerian, (R)enal, (C)ervicothoracic (S)omite abnormalities. This rare disorder is characterized by the absence of the uterus, cervix, and upper part of the vagina (Mullerian Aplasia); kidney (renal) abnormalities, including absent (agenic) and/or improperly positioned (ectopic) kidneys; and/or malformations of the spinal column, ribs, and/or arms. Some affected females may exhibit additional physical abnormalities, such as malformations of the head and facial (craniofacial) area. In individuals with MURCS Association, symptoms vary from case to case.

MURCS Association appears to occur randomly, with no apparent cause (sporadic). Some researchers suggest that the malformations associated with this disorder may result from abnormal changes in cellular material (blastema) in portions of the embryo that later develop into the arms, certain bones (vertebrae) in the spinal column, the kidneys, and adjacent structures (e.g., fallopian tubes).

In addition to The National Organization for Rare Disorders (NORD) listed in Section III, the following organizations in Section II (Disease Specific) and in Section III (Umbrella) and Section IV (Government Agencies) can provide more information:
NIH/National Institute of Child Health and Human Development, *IV*
NIH/National Kidney and Urologic Diseases Information Clearinghouse, *IV*
National Kidney Foundation, *III*

654 MACROGLOSSIA

Macroglossia is the abnormal enlargement of the tongue. In rare cases, macroglossia occurs as an isolated finding that is present at birth (congenital). In many cases, macroglossia may occur secondary to a primary disorder or a tumor of the tongue. Symptoms and physical findings associated with macroglossia may include noisy, high-pitched breathing (stridor), snoring, and/or feeding difficulties. In some cases, the tongue may protrude from the mouth. Macroglossia is thought to be inherited as an autosomal dominant genetic trait.

In addition to The National Organization for Rare Disorders (NORD) listed in Section III, the following organizations in Section II (Disease Specific) and in Section III (Umbrella) and Section IV (Government Agencies) can provide more information:
Association for Neuro-Metabolic Disorders, *III*
NIH/National Oral Health Information Clearinghouse, *IV*
Smell and Taste Center, *III*

655 MACULAR DEGENERATION

Macular degeneration is a common hereditary eye (retinal) disorder with several subdivisions:

Behr 1 (infantile optic atrophyataxia) Behr 2 (adult or presenile macula lutea retinae degeneration) Stargardt's disease (juvenile macular degeneration) Macular Degeneration, senile Macular Degeneration, disciform

This disorder is characterized by a gradual bilateral decrease of vision. Although usually inherited as a dominant trait, a recessive type (Stargardt's disease) is a possible form of central Retinitis Pigmentosa with macular degeneration. Ordinary RP does not affect the macula. X-linked hereditary macular dystrophy can be observed in males with color blindness.

Macular degeneration can be a static condition for many years but then becomes slowly progressive. Senile macular degeneration patients may be mislabeled as colorblind. This form of the disease could also be associated with neurological dysfunction.

In addition to The National Organization for Rare Disorders (NORD) listed in Section III, the following organizations in Section II (Disease Specific) and in Section III (Umbrella) and Section IV (Government Agencies) can provide more information:

American Council of the Blind, Inc., *III*
American Foundation for the Blind, *III*
Association for Macular Diseases, Inc., *III*
Council of Families with Visual Impairment, *III*
Macular Degeneration Foundation, Inc., *III*
Macular Degeneration International, *III*
NIH/National Eye Institute, *IV*
National Association for Visually Handicapped, *III*
Vision Foundation, Inc., *III*
Vision World Wide, Inc., *III*

656 MACULAR DEGENERATION, POLYMORPHIC

Polymorphic Macular degeneration is a dominant hereditary vision disorder that includes Best Disease and Sorsby Disease. Best disease is also called vitelline macular dystrophy. The disorder affects both eyes and is usually diagnosed between five and fifteen years of age. Sorsby disease is also called macular cyst, or cystoid macular degeneration. Symptoms usually begin between 20 and 40 years of age. This form of the disorder is marked by impairment of vision, possible color vision abnormality, and can be progressive in nature.

In addition to The National Organization for Rare Disorders (NORD) listed in Section III, the following organizations in Section II (Disease Specific) and in Section III (Umbrella) and Section IV (Government Agencies) can provide more information:

American Council of the Blind, Inc., *III*
American Foundation for the Blind, *III*
Association for Macular Diseases, Inc., *III*
Council of Families with Visual Impairment, *III*
Macular Degeneration International, *III*
NIH/National Eye Institute, *IV*
National Association for Parents of the Visually Impaired, *III*
National Association for Visually Handicapped, *III*
Vision Foundation, Inc., *III*

657 MADELUNG'S DISEASE

Madelung's Disease is a disorder of fat metabolism (lipid storage) that results in an unusual accumulation of fat deposits around the neck and shoulder areas. Adult alcoholic males are most often affected, although women and those who do not drink alcohol can also get Madelung's Disease.

In addition to The National Organization for Rare Disorders (NORD) listed in Section III, the following organizations in Section II (Disease Specific) and in Section III (Umbrella) and Section IV (Government Agencies) can provide more information:

NIH/National Institute of Diabetes, Digestive and Kidney Diseases, *IV*

658 MAFFUCCI SYNDROME

Maffucci Syndrome is a rare genetic disorder characterized by benign overgrowths of cartilage (enchondromas), skeletal deformities, and dark red irregularly shaped patches of skin (hemangiomas). Enchondromas are most often found in certain bones (phalanges) of the hands and feet. Skeletal malformations may include legs that are disproportionate in length and/or abnormal side-to-side curvature of the spine (scoliosis). In many cases, bones may tend to fracture easily. In most cases, hemangiomas appear at birth or during early childhood and may be progressive. Maffucci Syndrome is inherited as an autosomal dominant genetic trait.

In addition to The National Organization for Rare Disorders (NORD) listed in Section III, the following organizations in Section II (Disease Specific) and in Section III (Umbrella) and Section IV (Government Agencies) can provide more information:

American Cancer Society, Inc., *III*
NIH/National Arthritis and Musculoskeletal and Skin Diseases Information Clearinghouse, *IV*
NIH/National Heart, Lung and Blood Institute, *IV*

NIH/Patient Referral Services Unit, *IV*
Ollier/Maffucci Self-Help Group, *II*

659 MAL DE MELEDA

Mal de Meleda is an extremely rare inherited skin disorder characterized by the slowly progressive development of dry, thick patches of skin on the palms of the hands and soles of the feet (palmoplantar hyperkeratosis). Affected skin may be unusually red (erythema) and become abnormally thick and scaly (symmetrical cornification). Affected children may also exhibit various abnormalities of the nails; excessive sweating (hyperhidrosis) associated with an unpleasant odor; and/or, in some cases, development of small, firm raised lesions (lichenoid plaques). The range and severity of symptoms may vary from case to case. Mal de Meleda is thought to be inherited as an autosomal recessive genetic trait.

In addition to The National Organization for Rare Disorders (NORD) listed in Section III, the following organizations in Section II (Disease Specific) and in Section III (Umbrella) and Section IV (Government Agencies) can provide more information:
NIH/National Arthritis and Musculoskeletal and Skin Diseases Information Clearinghouse, *IV*

660 MALARIA

Malaria is a communicable parasitic disorder spread through the bite of the Anopheles mosquito. Major symptoms may vary depending on which species of parasite causes the infection and the stage of development of the parasite. Chills and fever commonly occur, although not every case follows the same pattern. Each recurrence becomes milder. Although the disorder was once thought to be under control throughout the world, Malaria is a wide spread infection especially in the tropics where certain types of mosquitos are becoming resistant to pesticides. The annual number of cases reported in the United States has increased in recent years.

In addition to The National Organization for Rare Disorders (NORD) listed in Section III, the following organizations in Section II (Disease Specific) and in Section III (Umbrella) and Section IV (Government Agencies) can provide more information:
Centers for Disease Control and Prevention, *IV*
NIH/National Institute of Allergy and Infectious Diseases, *IV*
World Health Organization (WHO) Regional Office for the Americas (AMRO), *III*

661 MALIGNANT HYPERTHERMIA

Malignant Hyperthermia is hereditary disorder in which a person does not react appropriately to certain drugs due to a genetic abnormality. The patient develops a rapid, high fever after the administration of general anesthesia or certain muscle relaxants. Drugs that could cause this response include halothane, cyclopropane, or succinylcholine.

In addition to The National Organization for Rare Disorders (NORD) listed in Section III, the following organizations in Section II (Disease Specific) and in Section III (Umbrella) and Section IV (Government Agencies) can provide more information:
Alliance of Genetic Support Groups, *III*
Malignant Hyperthermia Association, *II*
Malignant Hyperthermia Association of the United States, *II*
March of Dimes Birth Defects Foundation, *III*
NIH/National Institute of General Medical Sciences, *IV*
North American Malignant Hyperthermia Registry, *II*

662 MALLORY WEISS SYNDROME

Mallory-Weiss Syndrome is characterized by a laceration of the mucous membrane in the junction between the esophagus and the stomach (gastroesophageal). It is usually caused by severe vomiting and can lead to rupturing and loss of blood (hemorrhaging) from certain blood vessels of the gastrointestinal tract.

In addition to The National Organization for Rare Disorders (NORD) listed in Section III, the following organizations in Section II (Disease Specific) and in Section III (Umbrella) and Section IV (Government Agencies) can provide more information:
Digestive Disease National Coalition, *III*
NIH/National Digestive Diseases Information Clearinghouse, *IV*

663 MANIC DEPRESSION, BIPOLAR

Bipolar Manic Depression is a mental illness in which intense mood swings occur, usually with remissions and recurrences. Depressive symptoms may be most common and can last at least a full day and perhaps several weeks or longer. Manic symptoms may involve hyperactivity and feelings of invincibility, happiness and restlessness.

In addition to The National Organization for Rare Disorders (NORD) listed in Section III, the following organizations in Section II (Disease Specific) and in Section III (Umbrella) and Section IV (Government Agencies) can provide more information:
Alliance of Genetic Support Groups, *III*
Depression and Related Affective Disorders Association, *III*
NIH/National Institute of Mental Health, *IV*
NIH/National Institute of Mental Health (Depression

Hotline), *IV*
National Alliance for the Mentally Ill, *III*
National Depressive and Manic-Depressive Association, *II*
National Foundation for Depressive Illness, Inc., *III*
National Mental Health Association, *III*
National Mental Health Consumer Self-Help Clearinghouse, *III*

664 MANNOSIDOSIS

Mannosidosis is a genetic disorder characterized by a lysosomal enzyme deficiency resulting in progressive mental and physical deterioration. A deficiency of the enzyme alpha-D-mannosidase causes the symptoms of this disorder which can vary in severity. Symptoms of the most severe form may begin within the first year of life while a milder form may begin during juvenile or adult years.

In addition to The National Organization for Rare Disorders (NORD) listed in Section III, the following organizations in Section II (Disease Specific) and in Section III (Umbrella) and Section IV (Government Agencies) can provide more information:
Metabolic Information Network, *III*
NIH/National Digestive Diseases Information Clearinghouse, *IV*
National MPS (Mucopolysaccharidoses/Mucolipidoses) Society, Inc., *III*
Research Trust for Metabolic Diseases in Children, *III*
The Arc (a national organization on mental retardation), *III*
Vaincre Les Maladies Lysosomales, *III*

665 MAPLE SYRUP URINE DISEASE

Maple Syrup Urine Disease is an extremely rare inherited metabolic disorder characterized by a distinctive sweet odor of the urine and sweat. Symptoms develop because of the body's inability to properly break down (metabolize) leucine, isoleucine, and valine. These are organic substances found in proteins (branched chain amino acids). Life-threatening complications that may occur in a newborn include the abnormal accumulation of acid in the blood and other tissues of the body (metabolic acidosis) and seizures. If left untreated, Maple Syrup Urine Disease may progress to coma.

In addition to The National Organization for Rare Disorders (NORD) listed in Section III, the following organizations in Section II (Disease Specific) and in Section III (Umbrella) and Section IV (Government Agencies) can provide more information:
Alliance of Genetic Support Groups, *III*
Association for Neuro-Metabolic Disorders, *III*
Maple Syrup Urine Disease Family Support Group, *II*
March of Dimes Birth Defects Foundation, *III*
Metabolic Information Network, *III*
NIH/National Digestive Diseases Information Clearinghouse, *IV*
Research Trust for Metabolic Diseases in Children, *III*
The Arc (a national organization on mental retardation), *III*

666 MARCUS GUNN PHENOMENON

Marcus Gunn Phenomenon is a rare genetic disorder that is usually present at birth. It is characterized by the rapid rising motion of the upper eyelid of one eye upon movement of the jaw. Other eye abnormalities and vision difficulties may also occur. The exact cause of this phenomenon is not known.

In addition to The National Organization for Rare Disorders (NORD) listed in Section III, the following organizations in Section II (Disease Specific) and in Section III (Umbrella) and Section IV (Government Agencies) can provide more information:
NIH/National Eye Institute, *IV*

667 MARDEN WALKER SYNDROME

Marden-Walker Syndrome is a rare connective tissue disorder that is inherited as an autosomal recessive trait. Patients with this disorder typically have a distinct face, a cleft or high-arched palate, bone joints in a fixed position, growth delay and limited control of muscle movement. Marden-Walker Syndrome affects males more often than females.

In addition to The National Organization for Rare Disorders (NORD) listed in Section III, the following organizations in Section II (Disease Specific) and in Section III (Umbrella) and Section IV (Government Agencies) can provide more information:
British Coalition of Heritable Disorders of Connective Tissue, *III*

668 MARFAN SYNDROME

Marfan Syndrome is an inherited disorder that affects the connective tissues of the heart and blood vessels (cardiovascular system). The musculoskeletal system (ligaments and muscles) is also affected. Major symptoms also include unusual height, large hands and feet, and involvement of the lungs and the eyes.

In addition to The National Organization for Rare Disorders (NORD) listed in Section III, the following organizations in Section II (Disease Specific) and in Section III (Umbrella) and Section IV (Government Agencies) can provide more information:
Alliance of Genetic Support Groups, *III*
British Coalition of Heritable Disorders of Connective Tissue, *III*
Canadian Marfan Association, *II*
European Marfan Support Network, *II*
March of Dimes Birth Defects Foundation, *III*

Marfan Association UK, *II*
NIH/National Arthritis and Musculoskeletal and Skin Diseases Information Clearinghouse, *IV*
National Marfan Foundation, *II*

669 MARINESCO SJOGREN SYNDROME

Marinesco-Sjogren Syndrome is a rare disorder that is inherited through autosomal recessive genes. The major features of this disorder are a loss of muscle coordination as a result of disease in the cerebellum (cerebellar ataxia), loss of clearness in the eyes' lenses (cataract), increased muscle tension (spasticity), progressive muscle weakness, and mental deficiency.

In addition to The National Organization for Rare Disorders (NORD) listed in Section III, the following organizations in Section II (Disease Specific) and in Section III (Umbrella) and Section IV (Government Agencies) can provide more information:
NIH/National Arthritis and Musculoskeletal and Skin Diseases Information Clearinghouse, *IV*
NIH/National Institute of Neurological Disorders and Stroke, *IV*
National Ataxia Foundation, *III*
National Scoliosis Foundation, *II*

670 MAROTEAUX LAMY SYNDROME

Mucopolysaccharidoses are a group of rare genetic disorders caused by the deficiency of one of ten specific lysosomal enzymes, resulting in an inability to metabolize complex carbohydrates (mucopolysaccharides) into simpler molecules. The accumulation of these large, undegraded mucopolysaccharides in the cells of the body causes a number of physical symptoms and abnormalities.

Maroteaux-Lamy Syndrome (MPS Type VI) occurs in three types: a classic severe type, an intermediate type, and a mild type. The syndrome is characterized by a deficiency in the enzyme arylsulfatase B (also called N-acetylgalactosamine-4-sulfatase), which leads to an excess of dermatan sulfate in the urine.

In general, growth retardation occurs from two to three years of age, with coarsening of facial features and abnormalities in the bones of hands and spine. Joint stiffness also occurs. The intellect is usually normal.

In addition to The National Organization for Rare Disorders (NORD) listed in Section III, the following organizations in Section II (Disease Specific) and in Section III (Umbrella) and Section IV (Government Agencies) can provide more information:
Blind Children's Fund, *III*
Canadian Society for Mucopolysaccharide and Related Diseases, Inc., *III*
Metabolic Information Network, *III*
NIH/National Digestive Diseases Information Clearinghouse, *IV*
National Association for Visually Handicapped, *III*
National MPS (Mucopolysaccharidoses/Mucolipidoses) Society, Inc., *III*
Research Trust for Metabolic Diseases in Children, *III*
Vaincre Les Maladies Lysosomales, *III*

671 MARSHALL SMITH SYNDROME

Marshall-Smith Syndrome is characterized by unusually quick physical growth and bone development (maturation), usually starting before birth. Other symptoms can include respiratory difficulties, mental retardation, and certain physical characteristics. (Note: Marshall-Smith Syndrome is not to be confused with "Marshall" Syndrome, which is very different from "Marshall-Smith" Syndrome.)

In addition to The National Organization for Rare Disorders (NORD) listed in Section III, the following organizations in Section II (Disease Specific) and in Section III (Umbrella) and Section IV (Government Agencies) can provide more information:
Human Growth Foundation, *III*
Little People of America, *III*
Little People's Research Fund, Inc., *III*
MAGIC Foundation for Children's Growth, *III*
NIH/National Institute of Child Health and Human Development, *IV*

672 MARSHALL SYNDROME

Marshall Syndrome is a rare genetic disorder. Major symptoms may include a distinct face with a flattened nasal bridge and nostrils that are tilted upward, widely spaced eyes, nearsightedness, cataracts and hearing loss. Marshall Syndrome is inherited as an autosomal dominant trait.

In addition to The National Organization for Rare Disorders (NORD) listed in Section III, the following organizations in Section II (Disease Specific) and in Section III (Umbrella) and Section IV (Government Agencies) can provide more information:
American Society for Deaf Children, *III*
Children's Craniofacial Association, *III*
Let's Face It, Inc., *III*
NIH/National Eye Institute, *IV*
NIH/National Institute of Child Health and Human Development, *IV*
National Foundation for Facial Reconstruction, *III*

673 MASTOCYTOSIS

Mastocytosis is a rare disorder characterized by abnormal accumulations of specific cells (mast cells) normally found in connective tissue. The liver, spleen, lungs, bone, skin, and sometimes the membrane surrounding the brain and spine (meninges) may be affected. Cases beginning during adulthood tend to involve the inner organs more than the skin, whereas during childhood, the condition is often marked by skin manifestations with minimal organ involvement.

In addition to The National Organization for Rare Disorders (NORD) listed in Section III, the following organizations in Section II (Disease Specific) and in Section III (Umbrella) and Section IV (Government Agencies) can provide more information:
Mastocytosis Society, Inc., *II*
NIH/National Arthritis and Musculoskeletal and Skin Diseases Information Clearinghouse, *IV*

674 MAXILLOFACIAL DYSOSTOSIS

Maxillofacial Dysostosis is a rare disorder inherited as an autosomal dominant trait. Major characteristics include an underdeveloped upper jaw, delayed speech as well as poor articulation, down-slanting of the eyelids, and malformations of the external ear.

In addition to The National Organization for Rare Disorders (NORD) listed in Section III, the following organizations in Section II (Disease Specific) and in Section III (Umbrella) and Section IV (Government Agencies) can provide more information:
AboutFace U.S.A., *III*
Children's Craniofacial Association, *III*
FACES: The National Craniofacial Association, *III*
Forward Face, Inc., *III*
Let's Face It, Inc., *III*
NIH/National Institute of Child Health and Human Development, *IV*

675 MAXILLONASAL DYSPLASIA, BINDER TYPE

Binder Type Maxillonasal Dysplasia is a rare disorder that may occur for no apparent reason (sporadically) or may be inherited as an autosomal dominant or autosomal recessive genetic trait. Individuals affected with this disorder have distinct facial features that typically include a small, flat, low-set nose and a protruding chin. Crossed eyes, cleft lip and palate, as well as abnormalities of the cervical spine have also been found in some affected affected individuals.

In addition to The National Organization for Rare Disorders (NORD) listed in Section III, the following organizations in Section II (Disease Specific) and in Section III (Umbrella) and Section IV (Government Agencies) can provide more information:
AboutFace U.S.A., *III*
Children's Craniofacial Association, *III*
FACES: The National Craniofacial Association, *III*
NIH/National Institute of Arthritis and Musculoskeletal and Skin Diseases, *IV*
National Foundation for Facial Reconstruction, *III*

676 MAY HEGGLIN ANOMALY

May-Hegglin Anomaly is a rare inherited blood platelet disorder characterized by abnormally large and misshapen platelets and defects of specialized white blood cells known as leukocytes. Some people with this disorder may have no symptoms while others may have various bleeding abnormalities. In mild cases treatment for May-Hegglin Anomaly is not usually necessary. In more severe cases transfusions of blood platelets may be necessary.

In addition to The National Organization for Rare Disorders (NORD) listed in Section III, the following organizations in Section II (Disease Specific) and in Section III (Umbrella) and Section IV (Government Agencies) can provide more information:
March of Dimes Birth Defects Foundation, *III*
NIH/National Heart, Lung and Blood Institute Information Center, *IV*

677 MCARDLE DISEASE

McArdle Disease is a glycogen storage disease. Symptoms of this hereditary metabolic disorder are caused by an inborn lack of the enzyme myophosphorylase. This enzyme is needed for the breakdown of glycogen (the body's form of stored energy) into sugar (glucose) in muscle tissues. In McArdle Disease the breakdown of glucose cannot take place. Severe muscle cramps occur as a result of heavy exercise.

In addition to The National Organization for Rare Disorders (NORD) listed in Section III, the following organizations in Section II (Disease Specific) and in Section III (Umbrella) and Section IV (Government Agencies) can provide more information:
Association for Glycogen Storage Disease, *III*
Metabolic Information Network, *III*
Muscular Dystrophy Association, *III*
NIH/National Digestive Diseases Information Clearinghouse, *IV*
Research Trust for Metabolic Diseases in Children, *III*
Vaincre Les Maladies Lysosomales, *III*

678 MCCUNE ALBRIGHT SYNDROME

McCune-Albright Syndrome (MAS) is a rare multisystem disorder characterized by the displacement of normal bone tissue with areas of abnormal fibrous growth (polyostotic fibrous dysplasia). Such fibrous bony areas (lesions) may develop in many bones of the body, causing impaired mobility, pain, and/or, in some cases, hearing and/or visual impairment. MAS is also characterized by patches of abnormal skin pigmentation (i.e., large, light brown discolorations on the skin [cafe-au-lait spots] with jagged borders) and/or abnormalities of certain hormone-producing glands that help to regulate the rate of growth, sexual development, and certain metabolic functions (multiple endocrine dysfunction). For example, in many affected individuals, endocrine dysfunction may result in premature development of secondary sexual characteristics (precocious puberty). McCune-Albright Syndrome is due to a genetic change (mutation) that occurs randomly, for no apparent reason (sporadic). In individuals with the disorder, this sporadic genetic mutation is present in only some of the body's cells (mosaic pattern). The symptoms and physical characteristics associated with the disorder may vary greatly from case to case, depending upon the specific body cells and tissues that are affected by the genetic mutation. Because this mutation occurs after fertilization (postzygotic somatic mutation), it is not inherited from the parents.

In addition to The National Organization for Rare Disorders (NORD) listed in Section III, the following organizations in Section II (Disease Specific) and in Section III (Umbrella) and Section IV (Government Agencies) can provide more information:

MAGIC Foundation for Children's Growth, *III*
NIH/National Arthritis and Musculoskeletal and Skin Diseases Information Clearinghouse, *IV*
Paget Foundation for Paget's Disease of Bone and Related Disorders, *III*

679 MCKUSICK TYPE METAPHYSEAL CHONDRODYSPLASIA

McKusick Type Metaphyseal Chondrodysplasia is a rare progressive inherited disorder characterized by unusually fine, sparse hair and short stature with abnormally short arms and legs (short-limbed dwarfism). Portions of the long bones of the arms and legs develop abnormally with unusual cartilage formations and subsequent abnormal bone formation at the large (bulbous) end portions (metaphyses) of these long bones (metaphyseal chondrodysplasia). In addition, most individuals with McKusick Type Metaphyseal Chondrodysplasia may exhibit impairment of specialized cells (T-cells) that play an important role in helping the body's immune system to fight infection (cellular immunodeficiency). Affected individuals may also have abnormally low levels of certain white blood cells (neutropenia and lymphopenia); low levels of circulating red blood cells (anemia); and/or increased susceptibility to certain infections, such as chickenpox. In some cases, affected infants may also exhibit improper intestinal absorption of certain necessary nutrients (malabsorption) and/or dental abnormalities such as unusually small teeth (microdontia). Some individuals with the disorder may also have additional physical abnormalities. The range and severity of symptoms vary widely from case to case. McKusick Type Metaphyseal Chondrodysplasia is inherited as an autosomal recessive genetic trait.

In addition to The National Organization for Rare Disorders (NORD) listed in Section III, the following organizations in Section II (Disease Specific) and in Section III (Umbrella) and Section IV (Government Agencies) can provide more information:

Human Growth Foundation, *III*
Immune Deficiency Foundation, *III*
Little People of America, *III*
MAGIC Foundation for Children's Growth, *III*
NIH/National Heart, Lung and Blood Institute Information Center, *IV*
NIH/National Institute of Child Health & Human Development (Preg & Perinat), *IV*
Short Stature Foundation, *III*

680 MEASLES

Measles is a highly contagious disease occurring primarily in children. This disease is characterized by fever, cough, acute nasal mucous membrane discharge (coryza), inflammation of the lining of the eyelids (conjunctivitis), a spreading rash, and eruption of small, irregular, bright red spots (Koplik's spots) on the inner cheeks in the mouth with a minute bluish or white speck in the center of each.

Because measles can be contracted from someone whose symptoms have not yet appeared, it is often difficult to avoid exposure. Measles ceases to be contagious four days after appearance of the rash.

Although concerted efforts have been made to eliminate measles in the United States, increasing numbers of cases have been reported recently in some areas. This may be due in part to a drastic rise in the cost of vaccine, shortage of supplies due to liability insurance problems, or fear by the public of possible side effects of vaccines. This is in spite of strict observance of immunization/attendance requirements by school officials. However, parents may underestimate the need for this immunization. Usually measles and the danger of its complications can be avoided by timely immunization.

In addition to The National Organization for Rare Disorders (NORD) listed in Section III, the following organizations in Section II (Disease Specific) and in Section III (Umbrella) and Section IV (Government Agencies) can provide more information:
Centers for Disease Control and Prevention, *IV*
NIH/National Institute of Allergy and Infectious Diseases, *IV*

681 MECKEL SYNDROME

Meckel Syndrome is a rare inherited disorder. Major symptoms may include, congenital deformities of the brain resulting in mental retardation. Malformations of the hands and feet, and bone deformities of the arms and legs may also occur. In males genitals may fail to develop properly. Kidney, pancreas and liver may also be abnormal.

In addition to The National Organization for Rare Disorders (NORD) listed in Section III, the following organizations in Section II (Disease Specific) and in Section III (Umbrella) and Section IV (Government Agencies) can provide more information:
NIH/National Institute of Child Health and Human Development, *IV*

682 MEDITERRANEAN FEVER, FAMILIAL

Familial Mediterranean Fever is a rare inflammatory disease characterized by recurrent attacks of fever accompanied by acute inflammation of the membranes that line the abdominal cavity (peritonitis) and/or the lungs (pleuritis). Sometimes individuals with Mediterranean Fever also have swollen and painful joints (arthritis). These recurring episodes of inflammation usually resolve within a few days (self-limiting).

In addition to The National Organization for Rare Disorders (NORD) listed in Section III, the following organizations in Section II (Disease Specific) and in Section III (Umbrella) and Section IV (Government Agencies) can provide more information:
Alliance of Genetic Support Groups, *III*
March of Dimes Birth Defects Foundation, *III*
NIH/National Digestive Diseases Information Clearinghouse, *IV*
NIH/National Institute of Arthritis and Musculoskeletal and Skin Diseases, *IV*

683 MEDIUM CHAIN ACYL COA DEHYDROGENASE DEFICIENCY

Medium Chain Acyl-CoA Dehydrogenase (MCAD) Deficiency is a very rare inherited metabolic disorder characterized by a deficiency of the enzyme medium chain acyl-CoA dehydrogenase. This enzyme is found to be most active in the liver, certain white blood cells (leukocytes), and certain connective tissue cells (fibroblasts) and is necessary for the breakdown (oxidation) of certain fats (medium chain fatty acids). Failure to break down these fats can lead to the abnormal accumulation of fatty acids in the liver and the brain. Abnormally low levels of the MCAD enzyme may also hamper or interrupt other processes associated with the metabolism of fatty acids.

In infants with MCAD Deficiency, symptoms may include recurrent episodes of unusually low levels of a certain sugar (glucose) in the blood (hypoglycemia), lack of energy (lethargy), vomiting, and/or liver malfunction. These symptoms are most frequently triggered when an affected infant does not eat for an extended period of time (fasting). In some cases, a viral illness (e.g., upper respiratory infection) that limits food intake may cause the symptoms to occur. MCAD Deficiency is the most common disease in a group of disorders that involve abnormalities of fatty acid metabolism. Medium Chain Acyl-CoA Dehydrogenase Deficiency is inherited as an autosomal recessive genetic trait.

In addition to The National Organization for Rare Disorders (NORD) listed in Section III, the following organizations in Section II (Disease Specific) and in Section III (Umbrella) and Section IV (Government Agencies) can provide more information:
Association for Neuro-Metabolic Disorders, *III*
FOD (Fatty Oxidation Disorder) Family Support Group, *III*
Lactic Acidosis Support Trust, *III*
MCAD (Medium Chain Acyl-CoA Dehydrogenase Deficiency) Family Support Group, *II*
Metabolic Information Network, *III*
NIH/National Institute of Diabetes, Digestive & Kidney Diseases, *IV*
Organic Acidemia Association, *III*
Research Trust for Metabolic Diseases in Children, *III*
United Mitochondrial Disease Foundation, *III*

684 MEDULLARY CYSTIC DISEASE

Medullary Cystic Disease is a rare inherited kidney disease (nephropathy) characterized by excessive amounts of urea and other waste products in the urine (uremia). Impairment of kidney function occurs due to the development of numerous cysts deep within the kidneys (medulla). In most cases, the first symptoms of this disorder appear during childhood or adolescence (Familial Juvenile Nephronophthisis). This form of the disease is inherited as an autosomal recessive genetic trait. Other affected individuals may not experience any symptoms or onset of symptoms may occur later in adulthood. This type of the disease is inherited as an autosomal dominant genetic trait.

People with Medullary Cystic Disease typically pass large volumes of urine (polyuria) that contain abnormally high levels of salt (sodium-wasting). Medullary Cystic Disease is the second most common cause of chronic kidney failure during childhood.

Approximately 15 percent of people with Medullary Cystic Disease also experience visual impairment caused by degeneration of the retina of the eyes (Renal-Retinal Dysplasia).

In addition to The National Organization for Rare Disorders (NORD) listed in Section III, the following organizations in Section II (Disease Specific) and in Section III (Umbrella) and Section IV (Government Agencies) can provide more information:

American Foundation for Urologic Disease, *III*
American Kidney Fund, Inc., *III*
NIH/National Kidney and Urologic Diseases Information Clearinghouse, *IV*
National Kidney Foundation, *III*

685 MEDULLARY SPONGE KIDNEY

Medullary Sponge Kidney is a rare inherited disorder characterized by the abnormal widening (dilatation) of the tubular structures within the kidneys (tubules) that collect urine. The initial symptoms of this disorder may include excessive urination (polyuria) and/or burning and pain while urinating. Calcium stones may form within the kidneys (nephrolithiasis) and blood may be present in the urine (hematuria). The exact cause of Medullary Sponge Kidney is not known.

In addition to The National Organization for Rare Disorders (NORD) listed in Section III, the following organizations in Section II (Disease Specific) and in Section III (Umbrella) and Section IV (Government Agencies) can provide more information:

American Foundation for Urologic Disease, *III*
American Kidney Fund, Inc., *III*
NIH/National Kidney and Urologic Diseases Information Clearinghouse, *IV*
National Kidney Foundation, *III*

686 MEDULLOBLASTOMA

A Medulloblastoma is a tumor in the cerebellum (a part of the brain), located in the lower rear portion of the skull (posterior fossa). About half of medulloblastomas are confined to the connecting bridge between the two halves of the cerebellum (vermis), and the other half actually invade the cerebellum or the brainstem (pons and medulla).

In addition to The National Organization for Rare Disorders (NORD) listed in Section III, the following organizations in Section II (Disease Specific) and in Section III (Umbrella) and Section IV (Government Agencies) can provide more information:

American Brain Tumor Association, *III*
American Cancer Society, Inc., *III*
Brain Tumor Society, *III*
Candlelighters Childhood Cancer Foundation, *III*
NIH/Patient Referral Services Unit, *IV*
National Brain Tumor Foundation, *III*

687 MEGALOCORNEA MENTAL RETARDATION SYNDROME

Megalocornea-Mental Retardation Syndrome is an extremely rare genetic disorder characterized by distinctive abnormalities of the eyes, diminished muscle tone that is apparent at birth (congenital hypotonia), and varying degrees of mental retardation. In some cases, additional abnormalities may also be present. The range and severity of symptoms and physical findings may vary from case to case.

In most infants with Megalocornea-Mental Retardation Syndrome, the front, clear portion of the eyes through which light passes may be abnormally large (megalocornea). Both eyes are usually affected (bilateral involvement). Many affected infants also have additional eye (ocular) abnormalities including underdevelopment of the colored portion of the eyes (iris hypoplasia), abnormal "unsteadiness" of the irises during eye movements (iridodonesis), and/or other ocular abnormalities, potentially leading to varying degrees of visual impairment. In addition to abnormally diminished muscle tone (hypotonia), most affected infants also have additional neuromuscular abnormalities including abnormal delays in the acquisition of skills requiring the coordination of mental and muscular activities (psychomotor retardation) and/oran impaired ability to coordinate voluntary movements (ataxia). In most cases, affected infants and children also have moderate to severe mental retardation.

In some cases, infants and children with Megalocornea-Mental Retardation Syndrome may have additional abnormalities including short stature; episodes of uncontrolled electrical disturbances in the brain (seizures); and/or certain distinctive abnormalities of the head and facial (craniofacial) area. Such craniofacial malformations may include an unusually prominent forehead (frontal bossing), widely spaced eyes (ocular hypertelorism), a long upper lip, an abnormally small lower jaw (hypoplastic mandible), and/or unusually large and/or "cup-shaped" ears. In most cases, Megalocornea-Mental Retardation Syndrome appears to occur randomly for unknown reasons (sporadically). In other cases, the disorder is thought to be inherited as an autosomal recessive genetic trait.

In addition to The National Organization for Rare Disorders (NORD) listed in Section III, the following organizations in Section II (Disease Specific) and in Section III (Umbrella) and Section IV (Government Agencies) can provide more information:
Children's Craniofacial Association, *III*
Council of Families with Visual Impairment, *III*
Craniofacial Foundation of America, *III*
Glaucoma Research Foundation, *II*
Human Growth Foundation, *III*
NIH/National Eye Institute, *IV*
NIH/National Institute of Child Health and Human Development, *IV*
NIH/National Institute of Neurological Disorders and Stroke, *IV*
National Association for Parents of the Visually Impaired, *III*
National Association for Visually Handicapped, *III*
Short Stature Foundation, *III*
Vision Foundation, Inc., *III*

688 MEIGE SYNDROME

Meige Syndrome is a rare neurological movement disorder (dyskinesia) characterized by spasms of the muscles of the eyelids and associated loss of tone in these eyelid muscles. Symptoms may include excessive blinking (blepharospasm) or involuntary eyelid closure. On occasion, the muscles of the face may also be involved. The exact cause of Meige Syndrome is not known. This disorder generally affects people during late middle age.

In addition to The National Organization for Rare Disorders (NORD) listed in Section III, the following organizations in Section II (Disease Specific) and in Section III (Umbrella) and Section IV (Government Agencies) can provide more information:
Benign Essential Blepharospasm Research Foundation, Inc., *II*
Dystonia Medical Research Foundation, *III*
NIH/National Institute of Neurological Disorders and Stroke, *IV*
WE MOVE, *III*

689 MELANOMA, MALIGNANT

Malignant Melanoma is a common skin cancer that arises from the melanin cells of the upper layer of the skin (epidermis) or from similar cells that can be found in moles (nevi). This type of skin cancer may send down roots into deeper layers of the skin. Some of these microscopic roots can spread (metastasize) causing new tumor growths in vital organs of the body.

In addition to The National Organization for Rare Disorders (NORD) listed in Section III, the following organizations in Section II (Disease Specific) and in Section III (Umbrella) and Section IV (Government Agencies) can provide more information:
American Cancer Society, Inc., *III*
Skin Cancer Foundation, *III*

690 MELKERSSON ROSENTHAL SYNDROME

Melkersson-Rosenthal Syndrome is a rare neurological disorder. Recurrent swelling (edema) of the face, especially the lip, is accompanied by intermittent paralysis and a fissured tongue (lingua plicata). This disorder usually begins during childhood.

In addition to The National Organization for Rare Disorders (NORD) listed in Section III, the following organizations in Section II (Disease Specific) and in Section III (Umbrella) and Section IV (Government Agencies) can provide more information:
American Autoimmune Related Diseases Association, Inc., *III*
NIH/National Institute of Neurological Disorders and Stroke, *IV*

691 MELNICK NEEDLES SYNDROME

Melnick-Needles Syndrome is a genetic disorder characterized by abnormal bone development. Prominent eyes, an extremely small lower jaw, bowing of the bones in the arms and legs, and other bone abnormalities may occur.

In addition to The National Organization for Rare Disorders (NORD) listed in Section III, the following organizations in Section II (Disease Specific) and in

Section III (Umbrella) and Section IV (Government Agencies) can provide more information:
Melnick-Needles Syndrome Support Group, *II*
NIH/National Institute of Child Health and Human Development, *IV*

692 MENIERE DISEASE

Meniere's Disease is a disorder characterized by recurrent prostrating dizziness (vertigo), possible hearing loss and ringing sounds (tinnitus). It is associated with dilation of the membranous labyrinth (endolymphatic hydrops) in the ear.

In addition to The National Organization for Rare Disorders (NORD) listed in Section III, the following organizations in Section II (Disease Specific) and in Section III (Umbrella) and Section IV (Government Agencies) can provide more information:
American Tinnitus Association, *II*
Better Hearing Institute, *III*
Crouzon's/Meniere's Support Network, *III*
EAR (Education and Auditory Research) Foundation, *III*
Meniere's Australia, Inc., *II*
Meniere's Disease and Dizziness Support Group, *II*
Meniere's Network, *II*
NIH/National Institute on Deafness and Other Communication Disorders (Balance), *IV*
Vestibular Disorders Association, *III*

693 MENINGIOMA

Meningiomas are benign, slow-growing tumors, classified as brain tumors, but actually growing in the three protective membranes that surround the brain (meninges). Sometimes they cause thickening or thinning of adjoining skull bones. Meningiomas do not spread to other areas of the body.

In addition to The National Organization for Rare Disorders (NORD) listed in Section III, the following organizations in Section II (Disease Specific) and in Section III (Umbrella) and Section IV (Government Agencies) can provide more information:
American Brain Tumor Association, *III*
American Cancer Society, Inc., *III*
Brain Tumor Society, *III*
NIH/Patient Referral Services Unit, *IV*
National Brain Tumor Foundation, *III*

694 MENINGITIS

Meningitis is characterized by inflammation of the membranes (meninges) around the brain or spinal cord. The disorder can occur in three different forms: adult, infantile, and neonatal. This inflammation may be caused by different types of bacteria, viruses, fungi, or malignant tumors. Chemical reactions to certain injections into the spinal canal can also cause Meningitis. This inflammation can begin suddenly (acute) or develop gradually (subacute). Adult forms of Meningitis are characterized by fever, headache, and a stiff neck, sometimes with aching muscles. Nausea, vomiting and other symptoms may occur. Treatment with antibiotics is usually effective against the infection.

In addition to The National Organization for Rare Disorders (NORD) listed in Section III, the following organizations in Section II (Disease Specific) and in Section III (Umbrella) and Section IV (Government Agencies) can provide more information:
Centers for Disease Control and Prevention, *IV*
NIH/National Institute of Allergy and Infectious Diseases, *IV*
The Arc (a national organization on mental retardation), *III*
World Health Organization (WHO) Regional Office for the Americas (AMRO), *III*

695 MENINGITIS, BACTERIAL

Bacterial Meningitis is a central nervous system disease caused by certain types of bacteria. Meningitis is characterized by inflammation of the membranes (meninges) around the brain or spinal cord. Inflammation can begin suddenly (acute) or develop gradually (subacute). Major symptoms may include fever, headache, and a stiff neck, sometimes with aching muscles. Nausea, vomiting and other symptoms may occur.

In addition to The National Organization for Rare Disorders (NORD) listed in Section III, the following organizations in Section II (Disease Specific) and in Section III (Umbrella) and Section IV (Government Agencies) can provide more information:
Centers for Disease Control and Prevention, *IV*
NIH/National Institute of Allergy and Infectious Diseases, *IV*
World Health Organization (WHO) Regional Office for the Americas (AMRO), *III*

696 MENINGITIS, MENINGOCOCCAL

Meningococcal Meningitis is a form of meningitis caused by a specific bacteria known as Neisseria meningitidis. Meningitis is characterized by inflammation of the membranes (meninges) around the brain or spinal cord. This inflammation can begin suddenly (acute) or develop gradually (subacute). Symptoms may include fever, headache, and a stiff neck, sometimes with aching muscles. Nausea, vomiting and other symptoms may occur. Skin rashes occur in about half of all patients with Meningococcal Meningitis. Treatment with antibiotics and other drugs is usually effective against this infection.

In addition to The National Organization for Rare Disorders (NORD) listed in Section III, the following organizations in Section II (Disease Specific) and in Section III (Umbrella) and Section IV (Government Agencies) can provide more information:
Centers for Disease Control and Prevention, *IV*
NIH/National Institute of Allergy and Infectious Diseases, *IV*
World Health Organization (WHO) Regional Office for the Americas (AMRO), *III*

697 MENINGITIS, TUBERCULOUS

Tuberculous Meningitis (TBM) is a form of meningitis caused by a specific bacteria known as Mycobacterium Tuberculosis. Meningitis is characterized by inflammation of the membranes (meninges) around the brain or spinal cord. This inflammation can begin suddenly (acute) or develop gradually (subacute). In Tuberculous Meningitis, the disorder develops gradually. Symptoms may include fever, headache, and a stiff neck, sometimes with aching muscles. Nausea, vomiting and other symptoms may occur. Treatment with antibiotics and other drugs is usually effective against the infection.

In addition to The National Organization for Rare Disorders (NORD) listed in Section III, the following organizations in Section II (Disease Specific) and in Section III (Umbrella) and Section IV (Government Agencies) can provide more information:
Centers for Disease Control and Prevention, *IV*
NIH/National Institute of Allergy and Infectious Diseases, *IV*

698 MENINGOCOCCEMIA

Meningococcemia is an infectious disease that occurs rarely. However, there are years when epidemics of the illness occur. Major symptoms may include upper respiratory tract infection, fever, skin rash and lesions, eye and ear problems and possibly shock (a sudden state of extreme physical depression which could cause a life-threatening situation).

In addition to The National Organization for Rare Disorders (NORD) listed in Section III, the following organizations in Section II (Disease Specific) and in Section III (Umbrella) and Section IV (Government Agencies) can provide more information:
Centers for Disease Control and Prevention, *IV*
NIH/National Institute of Allergy and Infectious Diseases, *IV*

699 MENKES DISEASE

Menkes Disease is a genetic disorder of copper metabolism beginning before birth. Copper accumulates in excessive amounts in the liver, and is deficient in most other tissues of the body. Structural changes occur in the hair, brain, bones, liver and arteries.

In addition to The National Organization for Rare Disorders (NORD) listed in Section III, the following organizations in Section II (Disease Specific) and in Section III (Umbrella) and Section IV (Government Agencies) can provide more information:
NIH/National Institute of Neurological Disorders and Stroke, *IV*

700 MESENTERITIS, RETRACTILE

Retractile Mesenteritis, also known as Mesenteric Panniculitis, is a disorder that affects the digestive tract membranes. It is characterized by infection, inflammation and intestinal obstructions. Major symptoms include abdominal pain, nausea, vomiting, weight loss, and fever.

In addition to The National Organization for Rare Disorders (NORD) listed in Section III, the following organizations in Section II (Disease Specific) and in Section III (Umbrella) and Section IV (Government Agencies) can provide more information:
Digestive Disease National Coalition, *III*
NIH/National Digestive Diseases Information Clearinghouse, *IV*

701 METATROPIC DYSPLASIA I

Metatropic Dysplasia I is a rare genetic disorder characterized by extremely small stature, with short arms and legs. Other characteristics of this disorder are a narrow thorax, short ribs, and kyphoscoliosis which develops into short trunk dwarfism.

In addition to The National Organization for Rare Disorders (NORD) listed in Section III, the following organizations in Section II (Disease Specific) and in Section III (Umbrella) and Section IV (Government Agencies) can provide more information:
Human Growth Foundation, *III*
Little People of America, *III*
Little People's Research Fund, Inc., *III*
MAGIC Foundation for Children's Growth, *III*
Metatropic Dysplasia Dwarf Registry, *II*
NIH/National Institute of Child Health and Human Development, *IV*

702 MICROVILLUS INCLUSION DISEASE

Microvillus Inclusion Disease is an extremely rare inherited intestinal disorder (enteropathy) that is typically apparent within hours or days after birth. The disorder is characterized by chronic, severe, watery diarrhea and insufficient absorption (malabsorption) of necessary nutrients due to incomplete development (hypoplasia) and/or degeneration (atrophy) of certain cells of the wall of the small intestine (e.g., hypoplastic villus atrophy, defective brush-border assembly and differentiation). In infants with Microvillus Inclusion Disease, chronic diarrhea and malabsorption may result in severe dehydration, deficiency of necessary nutrients (malnutrition), a failure to grow and gain weight at the expected rate (failure to thrive), and/or disturbance of the bodys balance of acids and bases, which is essential in regulating the bodys composition of bodily fluids (acidosis). Microvillus Inclusion Disease is inherited as an autosomal recessive genetic trait.

In addition to The National Organization for Rare Disorders (NORD) listed in Section III, the following organizations in Section II (Disease Specific) and in Section III (Umbrella) and Section IV (Government Agencies) can provide more information:
NIH/National Institute of Diabetes, Digestive and Kidney Diseases, *IV*

703 MIKULICZ SYNDROME

Mikulicz Syndrome is a chronic benign condition characterized by the abnormal enlargement of glands in the head and neck, including those in front of the ears (parotids) and those around the eyes (lacrimal) and mouth (salivary). The tonsils and other glands in the soft tissue of the face and neck may also be involved. Some people with Mikulicz Syndrome may experience recurring fevers. These may be accompanied by swollen eyes (lacrimal adenitis), diminished tear production (lacrimation), and inflammation of various parts of the eyes (uveitis).

The exact cause of Mikulicz Syndrome is not known. This disease always occurs in association with another underlying disorder such as Tuberculosis, Leukemia, Syphilis, Hodgkin's Disease, Lymphosarcoma, Sjogren's Syndrome, or Lupus (SLE).

In addition to The National Organization for Rare Disorders (NORD) listed in Section III, the following organizations in Section II (Disease Specific) and in Section III (Umbrella) and Section IV (Government Agencies) can provide more information:
American Autoimmune Related Diseases Association, Inc., *III*
NIH/National Oral Health Information Clearinghouse, *IV*
National Sjogren's Syndrome Association, *II*
Sjogren's Syndrome Foundation, Inc., *II*

704 MILLER SYNDROME

Miller Syndrome, also known as postaxial acrofacial dysostosis, is an extremely rare genetic disorder that is apparent at birth (congenital). The disorder is characterized by distinctive craniofacial malformations occurring in association with abnormalities of the outer aspects of the forearms and lower legs (postaxial limb deficiency). Craniofacial malformations may include underdevelopment of the cheekbones (malar hypoplasia); an abnormally small jaw (micrognathia); incomplete closure of the roof of the mouth (cleft palate); small, protruding, "cup-shaped" ears; and/or absence of tissue from (colobomas) and/or drooping of the lower eyelids, exposing the conjunctivae, the thin, delicate mucous membranes that line the eyelids as well as a portion of the eyeballs (ectropion). In infants and children with Miller Syndrome, limb abnormalities may include incomplete development (hypoplasia), webbing (syndactyly), and/or absence of certain fingers and/or toes (e.g., the fifth digits and, in some cases, the fourth and third digits) and/or underdevelopment (hypoplasia) of the bones on the "pinky" side (ulna) and, in some cases, the thumb side of the forearms (radius), causing the forearms to appear unusually short. Additional physical abnormalities may be present in some cases. Miller Syndrome is thought to be inherited as an autosomal recessive genetic trait.

In addition to The National Organization for Rare Disorders (NORD) listed in Section III, the following organizations in Section II (Disease Specific) and in Section III (Umbrella) and Section IV (Government Agencies) can provide more information:
American Society for Deaf Children, *III*
Children's Craniofacial Association, *III*
FACES: The National Craniofacial Association, *III*
Foundation for Nager and Miller Syndromes, *III*
NIH/National Institute of Child Health and Human Development, *IV*

705 MITRAL VALVE PROLAPSE SYNDROME

Mitral Valve Prolapse Syndrome is a heart disorder. The exact cause is unknown. It can be a symptom of other disorders such as connective tissue diseases or muscular dystrophy, or it may occur by itself. Major symptoms include chest pain and/or palpitations, accompanied by a heart murmur. Shortness of breath, fatigue, light-headedness and dizzy spells may, in some cases, progress to an inability to breathe except when sitting in an upright position. There is a characteristic click heard through a stethoscope upon physical examination. Blood may flow back through the heart valve (mitral regurgitation) causing other complications.

In addition to The National Organization for Rare Disorders (NORD) listed in Section III, the following organizations in Section II (Disease Specific) and in Section III (Umbrella) and Section IV (Government Agencies) can provide more information:

American Heart Association, *III*
NIH/National Heart, Lung and Blood Institute Information Center, *IV*
National Dysautonomia Research Foundation, *III*

706 MIXED CONNECTIVE TISSUE DISEASE (MCTD)

Mixed Connective Tissue Disease is a collagen disorder. MCTD is often used to describe what may be an overlapping group of connective tissue disorders that cannot be diagnosed in more specific terms. The syndrome is characterized by arthritic, cardiac, pulmonary and skin manifestations, kidney disease, muscle weakness, and dysfunction of the esophagus.

In addition to The National Organization for Rare Disorders (NORD) listed in Section III, the following organizations in Section II (Disease Specific) and in Section III (Umbrella) and Section IV (Government Agencies) can provide more information:

American Autoimmune Related Diseases Association, Inc., *III*
Arthritis Foundation, *III*
British Coalition of Heritable Disorders of Connective Tissue, *III*
Lupus Foundation of America, Inc., *II*
NIH/National Institute of Arthritis and Musculoskeletal and Skin Diseases, *IV*
National Marfan Foundation, *II*
Scleroderma Info Exchange, Inc., *II*
Scleroderma Research Foundation, *II*
Sjogren's Syndrome Foundation, Inc., *II*
United Scleroderma Foundation, Inc., *II*

707 MOEBIUS SYNDROME

Moebius Syndrome is a rare developmental disorder that may have a number of different causes and is characterized by facial paralysis at birth. Facial nerve development is absent or diminished causing abnormalities of the facial muscles and jaw. Other central nervous system dysfunctions may cause abnormalities in the hands, hips, and feet. This disorder is thought to be genetic and is present at birth. Mental retardation occurs in approximately ten percent of cases.

In addition to The National Organization for Rare Disorders (NORD) listed in Section III, the following organizations in Section II (Disease Specific) and in Section III (Umbrella) and Section IV (Government Agencies) can provide more information:

AboutFace U.S.A., *III*
Alliance of Genetic Support Groups, *III*
Children's Craniofacial Association, *III*
FACES: The National Craniofacial Association, *III*
Forward Face, Inc., *III*
Moebius Syndrome Foundation, *II*
Moebius Syndrome Support Group, *II*
NIH/National Institute of Neurological Disorders and Stroke, *IV*
The Arc (a national organization on mental retardation), *III*

708 MONILETHRIX

Monilethrix is a rare inherited disorder characterized by sparse, dry, and/or brittle hair that often breaks before reaching more than a few inches in length. The hair may lack luster, and there may be patchy areas of hair loss (alopecia). Another common symptom may be the appearance of elevated spots (papules) surrounding the hair follicles that may be covered with gray or brown crusts or scales (perifollicular hyperkeratosis). When viewed under a microscope, the hair shaft resembles a string of evenly-spaced beads. In most cases, Monilethrix is believed to be inherited as an autosomal dominant genetic trait.

709 MORQUIO SYNDROME

Mucopolysaccharidoses (MPS Disorders) are a group of rare genetic disorders caused by the deficiency of one of ten specific lysosomal enzymes, resulting in an inability to metabolize complex carbohydrates (mucopolysaccharides) into simpler molecules. The accumulation of these large, undegraded mucopolysaccharides in the cells of the body causes a number of physical symptoms and abnormalities.

Morquio Syndrome (MPS IV) exists in two forms: Morquio Syndromes A and B are due to a deficiency in the enzyme N-acetyl- galactosamine-6-sulfatase and beta-galactosidase, respectively. Deficiency of either enzyme leads to an accumulation of keratan sulfate and bony abnormalities of the head, chest, hands, knees and spine may occur as a result of this metabolic defect, with preservation of intellect. The skeletal abnormalities in MPS IV-B are usually milder that in MPS IV-A.

In addition to The National Organization for Rare Disorders (NORD) listed in Section III, the following organizations in Section II (Disease Specific) and in Section III (Umbrella) and Section IV (Government Agencies) can provide more information:
Canadian Society for Mucopolysaccharide and Related Diseases, Inc., *III*
Metabolic Information Network, *III*
NIH/National Digestive Diseases Information Clearinghouse, *IV*
National MPS (Mucopolysaccharidoses/Mucolipidoses) Society, Inc., *III*
Research Trust for Metabolic Diseases in Children, *III*
Vaincre Les Maladies Lysosomales, *III*

710 MOTOR NEURON DISEASE

Motor Neuron Disease is a group of serious disorders characterized by progressive degeneration of motor neurons (neurons combine to form nerves). Motor neurons control the behavior of muscles. Motor Neuron Diseases may affect the upper motor neurons, nerves that lead from the brain to the medulla (a part of the brain stem) or to the spinal cord, or the lower motor neurons, nerves that lead from the spinal cord to the muscles of the body, or both. Spasms and exaggerated reflexes indicate damage to the upper motor neurons. A progressive wasting (atrophy) and weakness of muscles which have lost their nerve supply indicate damage to the lower motor neurons.

In addition to The National Organization for Rare Disorders (NORD) listed in Section III, the following organizations in Section II (Disease Specific) and in Section III (Umbrella) and Section IV (Government Agencies) can provide more information:
Amyotrophic Lateral Sclerosis Association, *II*
Families of Spinal Muscular Atrophy, *III*
International Alliance of ALS/MND Associations, *III*
Motor Neurone Disease Association, *III*
Muscular Dystrophy Association, *III*
NIH/National Institute of Neurological Disorders and Stroke, *IV*

711 MOUNTAIN SICKNESS, ACUTE

Acute Mountain Sickness is a group of symptoms that may occur in some people who ascend rapidly to altitudes higher than 8200 ft. (2500 m). Major symptoms may include headaches, nausea, vomiting, and insomnia.

In addition to The National Organization for Rare Disorders (NORD) listed in Section III, the following organizations in Section II (Disease Specific) and in Section III (Umbrella) and Section IV (Government Agencies) can provide more information:
NIH/National Institute of Environmental Health Sciences Clearinghouse, *IV*

712 MOYAMOYA DISEASE

Moyamoya Disease is a progressive disease that affects the blood vessels in the brain (cerebrovascular). It is characterized by narrowing and/or closing of the main artery to the brain (carotid). This lack of blood may cause paralysis of the feet, legs or the upper extremities. Headaches, various vision problems, mental retardation, and psychiatric problems may also occur.

In addition to The National Organization for Rare Disorders (NORD) listed in Section III, the following organizations in Section II (Disease Specific) and in Section III (Umbrella) and Section IV (Government Agencies) can provide more information:
Families with Moyamoya Support Network, *II*
NIH/National Institute of Neurological Disorders and Stroke, *IV*

713 MUCHA HABERMANN DISEASE

Mucha-Habermann Disease is an uncommon skin disorder characterized by recurrent red, round and elevated lesions (papules), hemorrhages under the skin (purpura), and blister-like lesions (vesicles). It occurs most often in young adults and children.

In addition to The National Organization for Rare Disorders (NORD) listed in Section III, the following organizations in Section II (Disease Specific) and in Section III (Umbrella) and Section IV (Government Agencies) can provide more information:
American Autoimmune Related Diseases Association, Inc., *III*
NIH/National Arthritis and Musculoskeletal and Skin Diseases Information Clearinghouse, *IV*
Skin Disease Research Core Centers of the National Institute of Arthritis, *IV*

714 MUCOLIPIDOSIS IV

Mucolipidosis IV is a rare inherited metabolic disorder believed to be characterized by a deficiency of the enzyme ganglioside sialidase (neuraminidase). However, it has not been confirmed that this is the primary enzyme defect associated with this disorder. Mucolipidosis IV belongs to a group of diseases known as lysosomal storage disorders. Lysosomes are particles bound in membranes within cells that break down certain fats and carbohydrates. A deficiency of ganglioside sialidase may lead to the accumulation of certain fatty substances (mucolipids) and certain complex carbohydrates (mucopolysaccharides) within the cells of many tissues of the body.

Mucolipidosis IV is characterized by mental retardation; severe impairment in the acquisition of skills requiring the coordination of muscular and mental activities (psychomotor retardation); diminished muscle tone (hypotonia); clouding (opacity) of the clear portion of the eyes through which light passes (cornea); and/or degeneration of the nerve-rich membrane lining the eyes (retinal degeneration). Mucolipidosis IV is thought to be inherited as an autosomal recessive genetic trait.

In addition to The National Organization for Rare Disorders (NORD) listed in Section III, the following organizations in Section II (Disease Specific) and in Section III (Umbrella) and Section IV (Government Agencies) can provide more information:

Alliance of Genetic Support Groups, *III*
Association for Neuro-Metabolic Disorders, *III*
Canadian Society for Mucopolysaccharide and Related Diseases, Inc., *III*
ML 4 (Mucolipidosis Type IV Foundation), *II*
March of Dimes Birth Defects Foundation, *III*
Metabolic Information Network, *III*
NIH/National Digestive Diseases Information Clearinghouse, *IV*
National Lipid Diseases Foundation, *III*
National MPS (Mucopolysaccharidoses/Mucolipidoses) Society, Inc., *III*
Research Trust for Metabolic Diseases in Children, *III*
The Arc (a national organization on mental retardation), *III*

715 MUCOPOLYSACCHARIDOSIS

The Mucopolysaccharidoses are a group of hereditary diseases of lysosomal storage. They are characterized by deposits of mucopolysaccharides in the arteries, skeleton, eyes, joints, ears, skin and teeth. These deposits may also be found in the respiratory system, liver, spleen, central nervous system, blood cells and bone marrow.

In addition to The National Organization for Rare Disorders (NORD) listed in Section III, the following organizations in Section II (Disease Specific) and in Section III (Umbrella) and Section IV (Government Agencies) can provide more information:

Canadian Society for Mucopolysaccharide and Related Diseases, Inc., *III*
NIH/National Institute of Diabetes, Digestive and Kidney Diseases, *IV*
National MPS (Mucopolysaccharidoses/Mucolipidoses) Society, Inc., *III*
Vaincre Les Maladies Lysosomales, *III*

716 MULIBREY NANISM SYNDROME (PERHEENTUPA SYNDROME)

Mulibrey Nanism Syndrome (Perheentupa Syndrome) is an extremely rare inherited disorder characterized by profound growth delays (dwarfism) and distinctive abnormalities of the muscles, liver, brain, and eyes. The acronym MULIBREY stands for (MU)scle, (LI)ver, (BR)ain, and (EY)e. "Nanism" is another word for "dwarfism." Characteristic symptoms may include low birth weight, short stature, and severe progressive growth delays. Muscles are usually underdeveloped and lack normal tone (hypotonia). Some infants with this disorder may have an abnormally large liver (hepatomegaly). Other findings may include abnormal widening (dilation) of the spaces surrounding the brain (cerebral ventricles) and the excessive accumulation of fluid (cerebrospinal) around the brain (hydrocephalus). Infants with Mulibrey Nanism typically have yellow discolorations in their eyes. In addition, a portion of the inner layer of the eyes may be underdeveloped (choriocapillaris hypoplasia). Vision may also be impaired (amblyopia).

Infants with Mulibrey Nanism Syndrome may also experience symptoms related to overgrowth of the fibrous sac that surrounds the heart (constrictive pericarditis). Symptoms may include excessive fluid in the lungs (pulmonary effusion) and abnormal fluid accumulation in the abdomen (ascites). Other related symptoms may include unusual swelling of the arms and/or legs (peripheral edema) and/or enlargement of the heart. Mulibrey Nanism Syndrome is inherited as an autosomal recessive genetic trait.

In addition to The National Organization for Rare Disorders (NORD) listed in Section III, the following organizations in Section II (Disease Specific) and in Section III (Umbrella) and Section IV (Government Agencies) can provide more information:

American Heart Association, *III*
Human Growth Foundation, *III*
Hydrocephalus Association, *II*
Hydrocephalus Research Foundation, Inc., *II*
Hydrocephalus Support Group, Inc., *II*
Little People of America, *III*
Little People's Research Fund, Inc., *III*
NIH/National Eye Institute, *IV*
NIH/National Institute of Child Health and Human Development, *IV*
Short Stature Foundation, *III*

717 MULLERIAN APLASIA

Mullerian Aplasia is a rare disorder that affects only females. It is characterized by the absence of the uterus, the cervix, and the upper part of the vagina in a female who has normal ovarian function and normal external genitalia. Although females with this disorder develop normal secondary sexual characteristics during puberty (e.g., breast development and pubic hair), the failure of menstrual cycles to begin (primary amenorrhea) is usually the initial symptom. The exact cause of Mullerian Aplasia is not known. The unusual physical characteristics associated with this disorder seem to result from developmental abnormalities during embryonic or fetal growth.

In addition to The National Organization for Rare Disorders (NORD) listed in Section III, the following organizations in Section II (Disease Specific) and in Section III (Umbrella) and Section IV (Government Agencies) can provide more information:
American Kidney Fund, Inc., *III*
NIH/National Institute of Child Health and Human Development, *IV*
NIH/National Kidney and Urologic Diseases Information Clearinghouse, *IV*
National Kidney Foundation, *III*

718 MULTIPLE SCLEROSIS

Multiple Sclerosis is a chronic disorder of the central nervous system (CNS) that causes the destruction of the covering (myelin sheath) over the nerves. The course of this disease is variable; it may advance, relapse, remit, or stabilize. The demyelinating plaques or patches scattered throughout the central nervous system interfere with the ability of the nerves to communicate (neurotransmission) and can cause a wide range of neurological symptoms.

In addition to The National Organization for Rare Disorders (NORD) listed in Section III, the following organizations in Section II (Disease Specific) and in Section III (Umbrella) and Section IV (Government Agencies) can provide more information:
NIH/National Institute of Neurological Disorders and Stroke, *IV*
National Multiple Sclerosis Society, *II*

719 MULTIPLE SULFATASE DEFICIENCY

Multiple Sulfatase Deficiency is a very rare hereditary metabolic disorder characterized by impairment of all known sulfatase enzymes. Major symptoms include coarse facial features, deafness, and an enlarged liver and spleen (hepatosplenomegaly). Abnormalities of the skeleton may occur such as curvature of the spine (lumbar kyphosis) and in the breast bone. The skin is usually dry and scaly (ichthyosis). Before symptoms are noticeable, children with this disorder usually develop more slowly than normal. They may not learn to walk or speak as quickly as other children.

In addition to The National Organization for Rare Disorders (NORD) listed in Section III, the following organizations in Section II (Disease Specific) and in Section III (Umbrella) and Section IV (Government Agencies) can provide more information:
Metabolic Information Network, *III*
NIH/National Institute of Neurological Disorders and Stroke, *IV*
National Tay-Sachs and Allied Diseases Association, Inc., *III*
Research Trust for Metabolic Diseases in Children, *III*
Vaincre Les Maladies Lysosomales, *III*

720 MULVIHILL SMITH SYNDROME

Mulvihill-Smith Syndrome is an extremely rare inherited disorder characterized by low birth weight; growth delays, leading to short stature (dwarfism); and/or a prematurely aged facial appearance. Other findings may include additional abnormalities of the head and facial (craniofacial) area, multiple deeply-colored skin lesions (pigmented nevi), hearing impairment, and/or mental retardation. Eventually, some affected individuals may develop diminished capabilities to resist and fight off repeated infections (primary immunodeficiency). The range and severity of symptoms varies from case to case. Mulvihill-Smith Syndrome is thought to occur randomly, for no apparent reason (sporadically).

In addition to The National Organization for Rare Disorders (NORD) listed in Section III, the following organizations in Section II (Disease Specific) and in Section III (Umbrella) and Section IV (Government Agencies) can provide more information:
NIH/National Arthritis and Musculoskeletal and Skin Diseases Information Clearinghouse, *IV*
NIH/National Eye Institute, *IV*
NIH/National Institute of Child Health and Human Development, *IV*

721 MUMPS

Mumps is an acute viral illness that causes a painful inflammation and swelling of the saliva glands. These glands include the parotid, submaxillary, sublingual and buccal salivary glands. Mumps used to be a common infectious disease of childhood until a vaccine was developed in 1967 to immunize children against the virus that causes the disorder. However, recent outbreaks of mumps among adolescents and young adults have raised questions about lifetime immunity from the vaccine.

In addition to The National Organization for Rare Disorders (NORD) listed in Section III, the following organizations in Section II (Disease Specific) and in Section III (Umbrella) and Section IV (Government Agencies) can provide more information:
Centers for Disease Control and Prevention, *IV*
NIH/National Institute of Allergy and Infectious Diseases, *IV*

722 MUSCULAR DYSTROPHY, BECKER

Becker Muscular Dystrophy is a rare inherited muscle wasting disease usually beginning during the second or third decade of life. This slowly progressive disorder affects males almost exclusively. Muscles of the hips and shoulders are weakened, walking abnormalities develop, and mild mental retardation may be present. Eventually, other more severe symptoms may involve the heart and lungs.

In addition to The National Organization for Rare Disorders (NORD) listed in Section III, the following organizations in Section II (Disease Specific) and in Section III (Umbrella) and Section IV (Government Agencies) can provide more information:
Muscular Dystrophy Association, *III*
Muscular Dystrophy Group of Great Britain and Northern Ireland, *III*
NIH/National Institute of Neurological Disorders and Stroke, *IV*
Society for Muscular Dystrophy Information International, *III*

723 MUSCULAR DYSTROPHY, DUCHENNE

Duchenne Muscular Dystrophy is a rare inherited neuromuscular disorder and one of the most prevalent types of muscular dystrophy. This disorder is characterized by rapid progression of muscle degeneration which occurs early in life. Almost all affected children are male.

In addition to The National Organization for Rare Disorders (NORD) listed in Section III, the following organizations in Section II (Disease Specific) and in Section III (Umbrella) and Section IV (Government Agencies) can provide more information:
Alliance of Genetic Support Groups, *III*
March of Dimes Birth Defects Foundation, *III*
Muscular Dystrophy Association, *III*
Muscular Dystrophy Association of Canada, *III*
Muscular Dystrophy Group of Great Britain and Northern Ireland, *III*
NIH/National Institute of Neurological Disorders and Stroke, *IV*
Society for Muscular Dystrophy Information International, *III*

724 MUSCULAR DYSTROPHY, EMERY DREIFUSS

Emery-Dreifuss Muscular Dystrophy is a rare, often slowly progressive form of muscular dystrophy affecting the muscles of the arms, legs, face, neck, spine and heart. Major symptoms may include muscle wasting and weakness particularly in the elbows, Achilles tendons, and upper back muscles as well as the heart.

In addition to The National Organization for Rare Disorders (NORD) listed in Section III, the following organizations in Section II (Disease Specific) and in Section III (Umbrella) and Section IV (Government Agencies) can provide more information:
Muscular Dystrophy Association, *III*
Muscular Dystrophy Group of Great Britain and Northern Ireland, *III*
NIH/National Institute of Neurological Disorders and Stroke, *IV*
Society for Muscular Dystrophy Information International, *III*

725 MUSCULAR DYSTROPHY, FUKUYAMA TYPE

Fukuyama Type Muscular Dystrophy is a rare form of Muscular Dystrophy that is inherited as an autosomal recessive trait. Symptoms of this disorder begin before the age of nine months and include mental retardation, loss of muscle tone or tension and weakness of the muscles. This disorder is predominantly found in Japan.

In addition to The National Organization for Rare Disorders (NORD) listed in Section III, the following organizations in Section II (Disease Specific) and in Section III (Umbrella) and Section IV (Government Agencies) can provide more information:
Muscular Dystrophy Association, *III*
Muscular Dystrophy Group of Great Britain and Northern Ireland, *III*
NIH/National Institute of Neurological Disorders and Stroke, *IV*
Society for Muscular Dystrophy Information International, *III*

726 MUSCULAR DYSTROPHY, LANDOUZY DEJERINE

Landouzy-Dejerine Muscular Dystrophy is a neuromuscular disorder inherited as an autosomal dominant trait. Weakness of the facial muscles giving a mask-like appearance as well as weakness of the shoulder girdle typically appear anytime during the first two decades of life. The amount of muscle weakness can vary from slight to severe. A more severe form of Landouzy-Dejerine Muscular

Dystrophy is apparent during infancy and has a rapid progression.

In addition to The National Organization for Rare Disorders (NORD) listed in Section III, the following organizations in Section II (Disease Specific) and in Section III (Umbrella) and Section IV (Government Agencies) can provide more information:
Facio-Scapulo-Humeral Society, Inc., *II*
Muscular Dystrophy Association, *III*
Muscular Dystrophy Group of Great Britain and Northern Ireland, *III*
NIH/National Institute of Neurological Disorders and Stroke, *IV*
Organic Acidemia Association, *III*
Society for Muscular Dystrophy Information International, *III*

727 MUSCULAR DYSTROPHY, LIMB GIRDLE

Limb-Girdle Muscular Dystrophy is a rare disorder that may be inherited as an autosomal recessive or, in rare cases, an autosomal dominant trait. This disorder is characterized by weakness and wasting of the muscles of the hip and shoulders. The symptoms of Limb-Girdle Muscular Dystrophy may first occur during childhood, the second decade of life or during middle age. The muscle weakness may spread from the upper limbs to the lower limbs or vice versa, and it typically progresses slowly although some patients experience a rapid progression of the disorder.

In addition to The National Organization for Rare Disorders (NORD) listed in Section III, the following organizations in Section II (Disease Specific) and in Section III (Umbrella) and Section IV (Government Agencies) can provide more information:
Muscular Dystrophy Association, *III*
Muscular Dystrophy Group of Great Britain and Northern Ireland, *III*
NIH/National Institute of Neurological Disorders and Stroke, *IV*
Society for Muscular Dystrophy Information International, *III*

728 MUSCULAR DYSTROPHY, OCULO-GASTROINTESTINAL

Oculo-Gastrointestinal Muscular Dystrophy is a very rare form of muscular dystrophy that affects females more often than males. It is inherited as an autosomal recessive trait. The major characteristics of this disorder are droopy eyelids (ptosis), loss of movement of the external muscles of the eye (external ophthalmoplegia), and a progressive condition in which the intestinal walls are unable to contract normally causing abdominal pain, diarrhea, constipation, and malabsorption of nutrients (progressive intestinal pseudo-obstruction).

In addition to The National Organization for Rare Disorders (NORD) listed in Section III, the following organizations in Section II (Disease Specific) and in Section III (Umbrella) and Section IV (Government Agencies) can provide more information:
American Pseudo-obstruction & Hirschsprung's Disease Society, Inc., *III*
American Society of Adults with Pseudo-obstruction, Inc., *II*
Muscular Dystrophy Association, *III*
Muscular Dystrophy Group of Great Britain and Northern Ireland, *III*
NIH/National Institute of Neurological Disorders and Stroke, *IV*
Society for Muscular Dystrophy Information International, *III*
United Ostomy Association, Inc., *III*

729 MUTISM, SELECTIVE

Selective Mutism is a rare psychiatric condition primarily occuring during childhood. It is characterized by the refusal to speak in social situations. Ability to understand spoken language and to speak is usually not impaired. Symptoms include excessive shyness, anxiety, depression, and controlling manipulative behavior.

In addition to The National Organization for Rare Disorders (NORD) listed in Section III, the following organizations in Section II (Disease Specific) and in Section III (Umbrella) and Section IV (Government Agencies) can provide more information:
NIH/National Institute of Mental Health, *IV*
National Alliance for the Mentally Ill, *III*
National Mental Health Association, *III*
National Mental Health Consumer Self-Help Clearinghouse, *III*
Selective Mutism Foundation, Inc., *II*
Selective Mutism Group Web Site, *II*

730 MYASTHENIA GRAVIS

Myasthenia Gravis is a chronic neuromuscular disease characterized by weakness and abnormally rapid fatigue of muscles, particularly those that are controlled by the brain stem (bulbar-innervated). The symptoms of Myasthenia Gravis typically improve following a period of rest. Any muscle may be affected by this disorder. However, the muscles around the eyes (extraocular) and those used in swallowing are most frequently affected by Myasthenia Gravis.

In addition to The National Organization for Rare Disorders (NORD) listed in Section III, the following organizations in Section II (Disease Specific) and in Section III (Umbrella) and Section IV (Government

Agencies) can provide more information:
Muscular Dystrophy Association, *III*
Myasthenia Gravis Foundation of America, *II*
Myasthenia Gravis Links, *II*
NIH/National Institute of Neurological Disorders and Stroke, *IV*

731 MYCOSIS FUNGOIDES

Mycosis Fungoides is a rare form of T-cell lymphoma of the skin (cutaneous); the disease is typically slowly progressive and chronic. In individuals with Mycosis Fungoides, the skin becomes infiltrated with plaques and nodules that are composed of lymphocytes. In advanced cases, ulcerated tumors and infiltration of lymph nodes by diseased cells may occur. The disorder may spread to other parts of the body including the gastrointestinal system, liver, spleen, or brain.

In addition to The National Organization for Rare Disorders (NORD) listed in Section III, the following organizations in Section II (Disease Specific) and in Section III (Umbrella) and Section IV (Government Agencies) can provide more information:
American Cancer Society, Inc., *III*
Cutaneous Lymphoma Network, *II*
Skin Cancer Foundation, *III*

732 MYELITIS

Myelitis is a disorder of the spine marked by inflammation of the spinal cord. When inflammation is very limited, the condition may be called a "myelopathy." Injury to the spine, benign tissue growths, or blood vessel abnormalities may also cause this disorder. Major symptoms may initially include pain, followed by gradual paralysis and/or other central nervous system disturbances.

In addition to The National Organization for Rare Disorders (NORD) listed in Section III, the following organizations in Section II (Disease Specific) and in Section III (Umbrella) and Section IV (Government Agencies) can provide more information:
NIH/National Institute of Allergy and Infectious Diseases, *IV*
NIH/National Institute of Neurological Disorders and Stroke, *IV*
Spinal Cord Society, *III*
Transverse Myelitis Association, *II*
WE MOVE, *III*

733 MYELOFIBROSIS, IDIOPATHIC

Myelofibrosis is a condition characterized by formation of fibrous tissue (fibrosis) within the bone marrow. Myelofibrosis may occur as a secondary characteristic to other disorders such as polycythemia vera, certain metabolic disorders, and/or chronic myeloid leukemia. In many cases, the cause of Myelofibrosis may be unknown (idiopathic).

In Idiopathic Myelofibrosis the ability of the bone marrow to produce red blood cells may be impaired. Symptoms of Idiopathic Myelofibrosis may include abnormally low levels of circulating red blood cells (anemia), an abnormally large spleen (splenomegaly), an abnormally large liver (hepatomegaly), weight loss, weakness and fatigue due to replacement of normal bone marrow cells, and/or episodes of severe pain in the abdomen, bones, and joints. In many cases, Myelofibrosis occurs in association with increased bone density and the formation of small sharp pieces of bone (spicules) within the marrow cavity and increased bone density (osteosclerosis).

In addition to The National Organization for Rare Disorders (NORD) listed in Section III, the following organizations in Section II (Disease Specific) and in Section III (Umbrella) and Section IV (Government Agencies) can provide more information:
American Cancer Society, Inc., *III*
MPD (Myeloproliferative Disease) Research Center, Inc., *III*
NIH/National Heart, Lung and Blood Institute Information Center, *IV*

734 MYELOMA, MULTIPLE

Multiple Myeloma is a rare condition characterized by excessive production (proliferation) and improper function of certain cells (plasma cells) of the bone marrow. Major symptoms may include weakness; fatigue; pain in the back and the ribs, worsened by movement; low levels of circulating red blood cells (anemia); and/or renal failure. In most cases, affected individuals are more susceptible to bacterial infections such as pneumonia. If the bones of the spine are involved, they may collapse, resulting in spinal cord compression. The exact cause of Multiple Myeloma is not known.

In addition to The National Organization for Rare Disorders (NORD) listed in Section III, the following organizations in Section II (Disease Specific) and in Section III (Umbrella) and Section IV (Government Agencies) can provide more information:
American Cancer Society, Inc., *III*
American Kidney Fund, Inc., *III*
International Myeloma Foundation, *II*
Leukemia Society of America, Inc., *II*
NIH/Hematology Branch, National Heart, Lung and Blood Institute (NHLBI), *IV*

NIH/Patient Referral Services Unit, *IV*
National Kidney Foundation, *III*

735 **MYHRE SYNDROME**

Myhre Syndrome is an extremely rare inherited disorder characterized by mental retardation, short stature, unusual facial features, and various bone (skeletal) abnormalities. Characteristic facial features may include abnormally narrow skin folds (palpebral fissures) between the upper and lower eyelids (blepharophimosis), underdevelopment of the upper jaw bone (maxillary hypoplasia), and an unusually prominent jaw (prognathism). Other findings may include hearing impairment, abnormal enlargement of the muscles (muscular hypertrophy), and/or joint stiffness. Myhre Syndrome is thought to be inherited as an autosomal dominant genetic trait.

In addition to The National Organization for Rare Disorders (NORD) listed in Section III, the following organizations in Section II (Disease Specific) and in Section III (Umbrella) and Section IV (Government Agencies) can provide more information:
Human Growth Foundation, *III*
Little People of America, *III*
NIH/National Institute of Child Health & Human Development (Preg & Perinat), *IV*
Short Stature Foundation, *III*

736 **MYOCLONUS, GENERAL**

Myoclonus is a neurological movement disorder characterized by sudden, involuntary contractions of skeletal muscles. Based on the various symptoms, there are three types of Myoclonus: Intention Myoclonus, Rhythmical Myoclonus, and Arrhythmic Myoclonus.

Intention Myoclonus (Action Myoclonus) includes Postanoxic Myoclonus and Postencephalitic Myoclonus.

Arrhythmic Myoclonus (stimulus-sensitive myoclonus) includes: Hereditary Essential Myoclonus (paramyoclonus multiplex), Hyperexplexia (Essential Startle Disease), Opsoclonus (Infantile Myoclonic Encephalopathy, Polymyoclonia Familial Arrhythmic Myoclonus), Progressive Myoclonic Epilepsy, Ramsay Hunt Syndrome (Dyssynergia Cerebellaris Myoclonia).

Rhythmical Myoclonus includes (Segmental Myoclonus), Nocturnal Myoclonus, Palatal Myoclonus, and Respiratory Myoclonus.

In addition to The National Organization for Rare Disorders (NORD) listed in Section III, the following organizations in Section II (Disease Specific) and in Section III (Umbrella) and Section IV (Government Agencies) can provide more information:
Alliance of Genetic Support Groups, *III*
Epilepsy Canada, *II*
Epilepsy Foundation of America, *III*
March of Dimes Birth Defects Foundation, *III*
Moving Forward, *III*
Myoclonus Research Foundation, *III*
NIH/National Institute of Neurological Disorders and Stroke, *IV*
National Pediatric Myoclonus Center, *II*
Opsoclonus-Myoclonus Support Network, Inc., *II*
WE MOVE, *III*

737 **MYOPATHY, CONGENITAL, BATTEN TURNER TYPE**

Batten Turner Type Congenital Myopathy is an extremely rare, inherited muscle disease (myopathy) and is characterized by the lack of muscle tone or floppiness at birth (congenital hypotonia). The symptoms of Batten Turner Type Congenital Myopathy are slowly progressive during infancy and childhood. However, this disorder is not progressive in adulthood.

In addition to The National Organization for Rare Disorders (NORD) listed in Section III, the following organizations in Section II (Disease Specific) and in Section III (Umbrella) and Section IV (Government Agencies) can provide more information:
March of Dimes Birth Defects Foundation, *III*
NIH/National Institute of Neurological Disorders and Stroke, *IV*

738 **MYOPATHY, DESMIN STORAGE**

Desmin Storage Myopathy is a rare inherited muscle disorder which may be apparent at birth or may not appear until as late as age 40. There have been three forms of this disorder described in the medical literature. The symptoms and age of onset depend on which form affects the individual. Symptoms of late onset Desmin Storage Myopathy may include weakness of the muscles at the base of the thumb and/or weakness of the muscles used to flex the hand. Muscle weakness in the face, shoulder, and/or pelvic area, a spine that curves backward and to one side, and/or heart disease may occur in the congenital form of the disorder. The third form of Desmin Storage Myopathy is characterized by heart disease (cardiomyopathy) which has a variable age of onset and may lead to life-threatening complications.

In addition to The National Organization for Rare Disorders (NORD) listed in Section III, the following organizations in Section II (Disease Specific) and in Section III (Umbrella) and Section IV (Government Agencies) can provide more information:
American Heart Association, *III*
NIH/National Heart, Lung and Blood Institute Information Center, *IV*

739 MYOPATHY, MYOTUBULAR

Myotubular Myopathy is a rare muscle wasting disorder that occurs in three forms. The most severe form is present at birth, inherited as an X- Linked genetic trait, and presents itself with severe respiratory muscle weakness. A less severe form of Myotubular Myopathy is present at birth or early childhood, progresses slowly and is inherited as an autosomal recessive genetic trait. The least severe of the three forms of Myotubular Myopathy is inherited as an autosomal dominant genetic trait, presents itself between the first and third decades of life and is slowly progressive.

In addition to The National Organization for Rare Disorders (NORD) listed in Section III, the following organizations in Section II (Disease Specific) and in Section III (Umbrella) and Section IV (Government Agencies) can provide more information:
Muscular Dystrophy Association, *III*
Myotubular Myopathy Resource Group, *II*
NIH/National Institute of Child Health and Human Development, *IV*
NIH/National Institute of Neurological Disorders and Stroke, *IV*

740 MYOPATHY, SCAPULOPERONEAL

Scapuloperoneal Myopathy is a genetic disorder characterized by a weakness and wasting of muscles. Symptoms are usually limited to the shoulder blade area (scapula) and the smaller of the two leg muscle groups below the knee (peroneal). Facial muscles may be affected in a few cases. The leg symptoms often appear before the shoulder muscles become weakened. Progression rates vary between cases. This condition can also occur in combination with several other disorders.

In addition to The National Organization for Rare Disorders (NORD) listed in Section III, the following organizations in Section II (Disease Specific) and in Section III (Umbrella) and Section IV (Government Agencies) can provide more information:
Alliance of Genetic Support Groups, *III*
Muscular Dystrophy Association, *III*
NIH/National Institute of Arthritis and Musculoskeletal and Skin Diseases, *IV*
Scapuloperoneal Disease Association, *II*

741 MYOSITIS, INCLUSION BODY

Inclusion Body Myositis (IBM) is a rare muscular disorder that usually becomes apparent during adulthood. The disorder is characterized by slowly progressive inflammation of the muscles (myositis) of the arms and legs (i.e., those nearest [proximal] to and/or farthest [distal] from the trunk). Muscle tissues of the fingers, wrists, knees, and/or feet are also often affected. Individuals with Inclusion Body Myositis may experience weakness, pain, tenderness, and/or degeneration (atrophy) of affected muscles as well as diminished involuntary muscle contractions (deep tendon reflexes). In addition, in some cases, affected individuals may also have impaired nerve transmission to certain muscles (peripheral neuropathy), contributing to muscle thinning and weakness. In individuals with the disorder, removal (biopsy) and examination of samples of muscle tissue under a microscope may reveal abnormal levels of inflammatory cells as well as abnormal membrane-bound cavities (vacuolated inclusion bodies) within muscle tissue. In many cases, the cause of Inclusion Body Myositis is unknown. However, some familial cases of the disorder have been reported in the medical literature. In such cases, Inclusion Body Myositis appears to be inherited as an autosomal dominant genetic trait.

In addition to The National Organization for Rare Disorders (NORD) listed in Section III, the following organizations in Section II (Disease Specific) and in Section III (Umbrella) and Section IV (Government Agencies) can provide more information:
Muscular Dystrophy Association, *III*
Myositis Association of America, Inc., *III*
NIH/National Arthritis and Musculoskeletal and Skin Diseases Information Clearinghouse, *IV*

742 MYOTONIA CONGENITA

Myotonia Congenita is an extremely rare inherited disorder in which an abnormality of the skeletal muscle membranes causes an unusually exaggerated response to stimulation (hyperexcitability). As a result, affected individuals have difficulty relaxing certain muscles after contracting them (myotonia), and affected muscles may be abnormally stiff and rigid. Such symptoms tend to occur when affected individuals attempt to move certain muscles after rest. In many cases, individuals with Myotonia Congenita also exhibit abnormal enlargement of the muscles (hypertrophy) and unusually distinct muscle definition, resulting in a "herculean" or "body-builder like" appearance.

There are two forms of Myotonia Congenita: Thomsen Type and Becker Type. In individuals with Thomsen Type Myotonia Congenita, symptoms such as myotonia, associated muscle stiffness, and abnormal muscle enlargement may become apparent from infancy to approximately two to three years of life. After onset, symptoms stabilize and do not progress with age. In many cases, muscles of the eyelids, hands, and legs may be most affected. However, other muscle groups may be involved as well. In rare cases, some individuals with this form of Myotonia Congenita may also experience weakness in affected muscles. Thomsen Type Myotonia Congenita is inherited as an autosomal dominant genetic trait.

In individuals with Becker Type Myotonia Congenita, symptoms typically become apparent between the ages of four to 12 years; however, in rare cases, onset may occur as late as approximately 18 years of age. As in Thomsen Type Myotonia Congenita, affected individuals develop myotonia, associated muscle stiffness and rigidity, and abnormal muscle enlargement (hypertrophy). However, such symptoms tend to be more severe, and muscle hypertrophy may be particularly striking. In addition, individuals with Becker Type Myotonia Congenita exhibit weakness of affected muscles and may experience muscle pain. This form of the disease, contrary to Thomsen Type, is a progressive disorder that tends to initially affect muscles in the legs. Within a few years, muscles of the arms are affected, and, eventually, the muscles of the jaw (masticatory) and face become involved. This disorder is inherited as an autosomal recessive genetic trait.

In addition to The National Organization for Rare Disorders (NORD) listed in Section III, the following organizations in Section II (Disease Specific) and in Section III (Umbrella) and Section IV (Government Agencies) can provide more information:

Malignant Hyperthermia Association of the United States, *II*
Muscular Dystrophy Association, *III*
NIH/National Arthritis and Musculoskeletal and Skin Diseases Information Clearinghouse, *IV*
NIH/National Institute of Child Health and Human Development, *IV*
NIH/National Institute of Neurological Disorders and Stroke, *IV*
WE MOVE, *III*

743 N-ACETYL GLUTAMATE SYNTHETASE DEFICIENCY

N-Acetyl Glutamate Synthetase (NAGS) Deficiency is one of several hereditary urea cycle disorders. These disorders are caused by a deficiency of one of the enzymes needed for the breakdown of ammonia into urea, which is normally excreted in the urine. The deficiencies cause an excess of ammonia in the blood (hyperammonemia).

In NAGS Deficiency the deficient enzyme is N-acetyl glutamate synthetase. If left untreated, NAGS deficiency manifests itself by an elevated level of toxic ammonia in the blood (hyperammonemia). Untreated this imbalance may lead to brain damage, coma, and life-threatening complications.

In addition to The National Organization for Rare Disorders (NORD) listed in Section III, the following organizations in Section II (Disease Specific) and in Section III (Umbrella) and Section IV (Government Agencies) can provide more information:

American Kidney Fund, Inc., *III*
Association for Neuro-Metabolic Disorders, *III*
Metabolic Information Network, *III*
NIH/National Digestive Diseases Information Clearinghouse, *IV*
National Kidney Foundation, *III*
National Urea Cycle Disorders Foundation, *III*
Research Trust for Metabolic Diseases in Children, *III*

744 NAGER SYNDROME

Nager Syndrome is a rare disorder that may or may not be genetic. Major symptoms may include underdevelopment of the cheek and jaw area of the face. Down-sloping of the opening of the eyes, a smaller than normal jaw, lack or absence of the lower eyelashes, lack of development of the internal and external ear with related hearing problems and cleft palate may also occur. There may be underdevelopment or absence of the thumb, shortened forearms and poor movement in the elbow. Breathing and feeding problems may be present in infants with this syndrome.

In addition to The National Organization for Rare Disorders (NORD) listed in Section III, the following organizations in Section II (Disease Specific) and in Section III (Umbrella) and Section IV (Government Agencies) can provide more information:

American Society for Deaf Children, *III*
Children's Craniofacial Association, *III*
FACES: The National Craniofacial Association, *III*

Forward Face, Inc., *III*
Foundation for Nager and Miller Syndromes, *III*
Let's Face It, Inc., *III*
NIH/National Institute of Child Health and Human Development, *IV*

745 NAIL PATELLA SYNDROME

Nail-Patella Syndrome is an extremely rare inherited disorder that is usually apparent at birth or during early childhood. Although the symptoms and physical characteristics associated with Nail-Patella Syndrome may vary, characteristic abnormalities tend to include improper development (dysplasia) of the fingernails and toenails; absence (aplasia) and/or underdevelopment (hypoplasia) of the knee caps (patellae); underdevelopment of certain bones and/or webbing of skin at the bend of the elbow(s); and/or abnormal projections of bone from the upper (superior) portion of both sides of the hipbone (bilateral iliac horns). In addition, in many affected individuals, the inner margin (pupillary margin) of the colored portion of the eye (iris) may appear abnormally dark (hyperpigmentation) and "cloverleaf shaped" (Lester iris). Approximately 30 to 40 percent of individuals with Nail-Patella Syndrome may also experience abnormalities in kidney function (nephropathy) that may be apparent during childhood or later in life. Nail-Patella Syndrome is inherited as an autosomal dominant genetic trait.

In addition to The National Organization for Rare Disorders (NORD) listed in Section III, the following organizations in Section II (Disease Specific) and in Section III (Umbrella) and Section IV (Government Agencies) can provide more information:
American Association of Kidney Patients, *III*
American Foundation for Urologic Disease, *III*
American Kidney Fund, Inc., *III*
NIH/National Arthritis and Musculoskeletal and Skin Diseases Information Clearinghouse, *IV*
NIH/National Kidney and Urologic Diseases Information Clearinghouse, *IV*
Nail-Patella Syndrome (NPS) Web Site, *II*
Nail-Patella Syndrome (NPS) Web Site (United Kingdom), *II*
Nail-Patella Syndrome Web Site, *II*
National Kidney Foundation, *III*

746 NARCOLEPSY

Narcolepsy is a rare disorder characterized by chronic, excessive drowsiness during the day, sudden extreme muscle weakness (cataplexy), hallucinations, paralysis while sleeping, and disrupted sleep during the night. Although the exact cause of Narcolepsy is not known, many researchers suspect that the disorder is inherited.

In addition to The National Organization for Rare Disorders (NORD) listed in Section III, the following organizations in Section II (Disease Specific) and in Section III (Umbrella) and Section IV (Government Agencies) can provide more information:
Alliance of Genetic Support Groups, *III*
Center for Research in Sleep Disorders, *III*
NIH/National Institute of Neurological Disorders and Stroke, *IV*
Narcolepsy Network, Inc., *II*
Narcolepsy and Cataplexy Foundation of America, *III*
National Narcolepsy Registry, *II*

747 NELSON SYNDROME

Nelson Syndrome is a disorder characterized by abnormal hormone secretion and enlargement of the pituitary gland (hypophysis). It occurs in 5 to 10 percent of affected individuals following surgical removal of the adrenal glands for Cushing Disease. Symptoms associated with Nelson Syndrome include intense skin discoloration (hyperpigmentation), headaches, visual field disturbances, and the cessation of menstrual periods in women.

In addition to The National Organization for Rare Disorders (NORD) listed in Section III, the following organizations in Section II (Disease Specific) and in Section III (Umbrella) and Section IV (Government Agencies) can provide more information:
Brain and Pituitary Foundation of America, *III*
NIH/National Institute of Neurological Disorders and Stroke, *IV*

748 NEMALINE MYOPATHY

Nemaline Myopathy is a rare inherited neuromuscular disease that is usually apparent at birth (congenital) and characterized by extreme muscle weakness (hypotonia). Laboratory examination of muscle tissue samples from people with Nemaline Myopathy reveal the presence of fine fibrous threads known as nemaline rods that interfere with the muscle function.

In addition to The National Organization for Rare Disorders (NORD) listed in Section III, the following organizations in Section II (Disease Specific) and in Section III (Umbrella) and Section IV (Government Agencies) can provide more information:
Alliance of Genetic Support Groups, *III*
March of Dimes Birth Defects Foundation, *III*
Muscular Dystrophy Association, *III*
NIH/National Institute of Neurological Disorders and Stroke, *IV*
Nemaline Myopathy Newsletter, *II*

749 **NEU-LAXOVA SYNDROME**
Neu-Laxova Syndrome is a very rare life-threatening disorder thought to be inherited as an autosomal recessive genetic trait. Major characteristics of this disorder are generalized swelling especially of the scalp, hands, and feet; unusual facial features; a small head; restricted limb movement due to fixed joints; fetal growth retardation; abnormalities of the central nervous system; and abnormal skin changes.

In addition to The National Organization for Rare Disorders (NORD) listed in Section III, the following organizations in Section II (Disease Specific) and in Section III (Umbrella) and Section IV (Government Agencies) can provide more information:
NIH/National Institute of Neurological Disorders and Stroke, *IV*

750 **NEURASTHENIA**
Neurasthenia is a mental disorder triggered by stress or anxiety. Symptoms may include weakness or fatigue, which may be accompanied by chest pain. Additional findings may include rapid intense heartbeat that may be irregular (palpitations, tachycardia); cold, clammy hands and feet; abnormally rapid breathing (hyperventilating); dizziness or faintness; periodic sighing; and/or sweating for no apparent reason.

In addition to The National Organization for Rare Disorders (NORD) listed in Section III, the following organizations in Section II (Disease Specific) and in Section III (Umbrella) and Section IV (Government Agencies) can provide more information:
NIH/National Institute of Mental Health, *IV*
National Alliance for the Mentally Ill, *III*
National Mental Health Association, *III*
National Mental Health Consumer Self-Help Clearinghouse, *III*

751 **NEUROACANTHOCYTOSIS**
Neuroacanthocytosis is a very rare disorder inherited as an autosomal recessive or possibly an autosomal dominant genetic trait. Onset of Neuroacanthocytosis is usually during adolescence or early adult life. Major symptoms of this disorder are wasting of muscles with uncontrolled rapid muscular movements (amyotropic chorea) and abnormal red blood cells (acanthocytosis).

In addition to The National Organization for Rare Disorders (NORD) listed in Section III, the following organizations in Section II (Disease Specific) and in Section III (Umbrella) and Section IV (Government Agencies) can provide more information:
NIH/National Institute of Neurological Disorders and Stroke, *IV*

752 **NEUROFIBROMATOSIS TYPE 1 (NF-1)**
Neurofibromatosis Type 1 (NF-1) is a rare inherited disorder of the nervous system and is characterized by the development of tumors on the covering of nerves. The symptoms of Neurofibromatosis Type 1 include brown spots (cafe-au-lait) and freckles on the skin, as well as multiple benign tumors on the covering of nerves. These tumors can grow on any nerve and may appear at any time, including childhood, adolescence, or adulthood. Neurofibromatosis Type 1 is inherited as an autosomal dominant genetic trait. Approximately 50 percent of individuals with NF-1 do not have a family history of Neurofibromatosis; these cases represent spontaneous genetic changes (mutations).

The term "Neurofibromatosis" is also used in a general way to describe two genetically distinct disorders: Neurofibromatosis Type 1 (NF-1) and Neurofibromatosis Type 2 (NF-2). Neurofibromatosis Type 2 is characterized by benign tumors on both auditory nerves (acoustic neuromas of 8th cranial nerves) and tumors primarily on the central nervous system (brain and spine). Acoustic Neuromas generally cause a loss of hearing.

In addition to The National Organization for Rare Disorders (NORD) listed in Section III, the following organizations in Section II (Disease Specific) and in Section III (Umbrella) and Section IV (Government Agencies) can provide more information:
Alliance of Genetic Support Groups, *III*
March of Dimes Birth Defects Foundation, *III*
NIH/National Institute of Neurological Disorders and Stroke, *IV*
National Neurofibromatosis Foundation, Inc., *II*
Neurofibromatosis, Inc., *II*

753 **NEUROFIBROMATOSIS TYPE 2 (NF-2)**
Neurofibromatosis Type 2 (NF-2) is a rare inherited disorder characterized by the development of benign tumors on both auditory nerves (acoustic neuromas). Other tumors of the central nervous system may also develop (e.g., neurofibromas, meningiomas, gliomas, and/or schwannomas). Symptoms may include balance problems, ringing in the ears (tinnitis), and/or hearing loss. Neurofibromatosis Type 2 is inherited as an autosomal

dominant genetic trait.

The term "Neurofibromatosis" is also used in a general way to describe two genetically distinct disorders: Neurofibromatosis Type 1 (NF-1) and Neurofibromatosis Type 2 (NF-2). Neurofibromatosis Type 1 is characterized by the development of multiple benign tumors on the covering of nerve fibers.

In addition to The National Organization for Rare Disorders (NORD) listed in Section III, the following organizations in Section II (Disease Specific) and in Section III (Umbrella) and Section IV (Government Agencies) can provide more information:
Acoustic Neuroma Association, *II*
Acoustic Neuroma Association of Canada, *II*
Better Hearing Institute, *III*
NIH/National Institute of Neurological Disorders and Stroke, *IV*
NIH/National Institute on Deafness and Other Communication Disorders (Balance), *IV*
National Association of the Deaf, *III*
National Neurofibromatosis Foundation, Inc., *II*
Neurofibromatosis, Inc., *II*

754 NEUROLEPTIC MALIGNANT SYNDROME

Neuroleptic Malignant Syndrome is a potentially fatal reaction to any of a group of antipsychotic drugs or major tranquilizers (neuroleptics). These drugs are commonly prescribed for the treatment of schizophrenia and other neurological, mental, or emotional disorders. Phenothiazines are one type of neuroleptic and may occasionally be prescribed as a treatment for nausea and vomiting. Several of the most commonly prescribed neuroleptics include thioridazine, haloperidol, chlorpromazine, fluphenazine and perphenazine.

Major tranquilizers or neuroleptics have a strong effect on thought disturbances associated with paranoid thinking, delusions, anxiety, and agitation. Neuroleptic Malignant Syndrome occurs when a person taking these drugs reacts with a high fever and other heart, respiratory, and muscle symptoms.

In addition to The National Organization for Rare Disorders (NORD) listed in Section III, the following organizations in Section II (Disease Specific) and in Section III (Umbrella) and Section IV (Government Agencies) can provide more information:
Malignant Hyperthermia Association of the United States, *II*
NIH/National Institute of Mental Health, *IV*
National Alliance for the Mentally Ill, *III*
National Mental Health Association, *III*
National Mental Health Consumer Self-Help Clearinghouse, *III*
North American Malignant Hyperthermia Registry, *II*

755 NEUROPATHY, CONGENITAL HYPOMYELINATION

Congenital Hypomyelination Neuropathy is a neurological disorder present at birth. Major symptoms may include respiratory difficulty, muscle weakness and incoordination, poor muscle tone, absence of reflexes, difficulty in walking, and/or impaired abilities to feel or move part of the body.

In addition to The National Organization for Rare Disorders (NORD) listed in Section III, the following organizations in Section II (Disease Specific) and in Section III (Umbrella) and Section IV (Government Agencies) can provide more information:
American Autoimmune Related Diseases Association, Inc., *III*
NIH/National Institute of Neurological Disorders and Stroke, *IV*

756 NEUROPATHY, GIANT AXONAL

Giant Axonal Neuropathy is a genetic disorder that first appears during infancy. Major symptoms and findings may include kinky hair, unusual leg posture, poor vision, impaired muscle coordination (ataxia) and weakness, and degenerative mental functioning (dementia).

In addition to The National Organization for Rare Disorders (NORD) listed in Section III, the following organizations in Section II (Disease Specific) and in Section III (Umbrella) and Section IV (Government Agencies) can provide more information:
NIH/National Institute of Neurological Disorders and Stroke, *IV*

757 NEUROPATHY, HEREDITARY SENSORY, TYPE I

Hereditary Sensory Neuropathy Type I is a rare genetic disorder. Major symptoms include a loss of sensation usually affecting the feet and legs more severely than the hands and forearms, and perforating ulcers (open sores) on the feet. The loss of sensation is caused by abnormal functioning of the autonomic nervous system, which controls responses to pain and temperature as well as other involuntary or automatic body processes.

In addition to The National Organization for Rare Disorders (NORD) listed in Section III, the following organizations in Section II (Disease Specific) and in Section III (Umbrella) and Section IV (Government Agencies) can provide more information:

NIH/National Institute of Neurological Disorders and Stroke, *IV*

758 NEUROPATHY, HEREDITARY SENSORY, TYPE II

Hereditary Sensory Neuropathy Type II is a rare genetic disorder that usually begins in childhood. Major symptoms include inflammation of the fingers or toes especially around the nails, usually accompanied by pus and infection (paronychia, whitlows), ulcers (open sores) of the fingers and on the soles of the feet, and a loss of sensation noticeable in both arms and legs.

In addition to The National Organization for Rare Disorders (NORD) listed in Section III, the following organizations in Section II (Disease Specific) and in Section III (Umbrella) and Section IV (Government Agencies) can provide more information:
NIH/National Institute of Neurological Disorders and Stroke, *IV*

759 NEUROPATHY, PERIPHERAL

Peripheral Neuropathy is a general term that denotes a disorder of the peripheral nervous system. The peripheral nervous system consists of all the motor and sensory nerves that connect the brain and spinal cord to the rest of the body (i.e., the nerves outside the central nervous system). The symptoms and physical findings associated with peripheral neuropathies may be extremely complex and vary greatly from case to case. Common findings associated with Peripheral Neuropathy may include muscle weakness; pain; numbness; redness; and/or burning or tingling sensations in the affected areas, especially the arms and legs (extremitics). Symptoms and physical findings result from disease of a single nerve (mononeuropathy or mononeuritis), several nerves in asymmetric areas of the body (mononeuritis multiplex), or many nerves simultaneously (polyneuropathy, polyneuritis, or multiple peripheral neuritis). There are many different causes of Peripheral Neuropathy including trauma, fracture, penetrating injuries, and/or an underlying disease process.

In addition to The National Organization for Rare Disorders (NORD) listed in Section III, the following organizations in Section II (Disease Specific) and in Section III (Umbrella) and Section IV (Government Agencies) can provide more information:
NIH/National Institute of Neurological Disorders and Stroke, *IV*
Neuropathy Assocation, *II*

760 NEUTROPENIA, CHRONIC

Chronic Neutropenia is a blood disorder in which the number of certain white blood cells (neutrophils) falls to an abnormally low level. Neutrophils are essential to assist the body in fighting infections. Therefore, with low levels of neutrophils, affected individuals may be more susceptible to recurring infections. Chronic Neutropenia may last for months or years. It can affect both children and adults.

In addition to The National Organization for Rare Disorders (NORD) listed in Section III, the following organizations in Section II (Disease Specific) and in Section III (Umbrella) and Section IV (Government Agencies) can provide more information:
NIH/National Heart, Lung and Blood Institute Information Center, *IV*
National Neutropenia Network, *II*
Neutropenia Support Association, Inc., *II*
Severe Chronic Neutropenia International Registry, *II*
Severe Chronic Neutropenia International Registry Australia, *II*

761 NEUTROPENIA, CYCLIC

Cyclic Neutropenia is a rare blood disorder characterized by regular recurrences of neutropenia, a condition in which there are abnormally low levels of a type of white blood cells called neutrophils. Neutrophils are instrumental in fighting off infection. Therefore, low levels of neutrophils often make individuals more susceptible to recurrent infections.

In addition to The National Organization for Rare Disorders (NORD) listed in Section III, the following organizations in Section II (Disease Specific) and in Section III (Umbrella) and Section IV (Government Agencies) can provide more information:
NIH/National Heart, Lung and Blood Institute Information Center, *IV*
National Neutropenia Network, *II*
Neutropenia Support Association, Inc., *II*
Severe Chronic Neutropenia International Registry, *II*
Severe Chronic Neutropenia International Registry Australia, *II*

762 NEVOID BASAL CELL CARCINOMA SYNDROME

Nevoid Basal Cell Carcinoma Syndrome is a form of cancer characterized by the appearance of lesions and the development of multiple cysts and bony formations of the face and head. The lesions may be found on the first layer of the skin (epidermis) or in the mucous membranes of the mouth. The connective tissues and the nervous and vascular (blood vessel) systems of the body may also be affected. The skin lesions are limited in size, but not in number, and are not usually due to any external causes.

In addition to The National Organization for Rare Disorders (NORD) listed in Section III, the following organizations in Section II (Disease Specific) and in Section III (Umbrella) and Section IV (Government Agencies) can provide more information:

American Cancer Society, Inc., *III*
CancerOnline, *III*
Nevoid Basal Cell Carcinoma Syndrome (NBCCS) Support Network, *II*
OncoLink: The University of Pennsylvania Cancer Center Resource, *III*
Skin Cancer Foundation, *III*

763 NEZELOF'S SYNDROME

Nezelof's Syndrome is an extremely rare immune deficiency disorder characterized by the impairment of cellular immunity against infections, especially by those agents that do not normally cause serious illness (opportunistic infections). In cell-mediated immune responses, specialized white blood cells known as T lymphocytes or "killer cells" help B lymphocytes respond to infectious foreign agents that invade the body. Nezelof's Syndrome may also include some abnormalities in humoral immunity. In this form of immune response, antibodies that are produced by specialized cells (i.e., B lymphocytes) circulate in the lymphatic fluid and blood. Antibodies fight off bacteria, viruses, and other foreign substances that threaten the body. B lymphocytes enable the body to produce and maintain circulating antibodies. In a subgroup of people with Nezelof's Syndrome, immune deficiency may be caused by a lack of the enzyme purine nucleoside phosphorylase (PNP).

In addition to The National Organization for Rare Disorders (NORD) listed in Section III, the following organizations in Section II (Disease Specific) and in Section III (Umbrella) and Section IV (Government Agencies) can provide more information:

Alliance of Genetic Support Groups, *III*
Immune Deficiency Foundation, *III*
International Patient Organization for Primary Immunodeficiencies, *III*
Jeffrey Modell Foundation, *III*
March of Dimes Birth Defects Foundation, *III*
NIH/National Institute of Allergy and Infectious Diseases, *IV*

764 NIEMANN PICK DISEASE

Niemann-Pick Disease is a group of rare inherited disorders of fat metabolism. Excessive amounts of cholesterol and a fatty substance found mostly in the brain and nervous system (sphingomyelin) accumulate in many organs of the body. Symptoms occur as a result of a deficiency of the enzyme sphingomyelinase, which breaks down sphingomyelin.

In addition to The National Organization for Rare Disorders (NORD) listed in Section III, the following organizations in Section II (Disease Specific) and in Section III (Umbrella) and Section IV (Government Agencies) can provide more information:

Alliance of Genetic Support Groups, *III*
Association for Neuro-Metabolic Disorders, *III*
March of Dimes Birth Defects Foundation, *III*
Metabolic Information Network, *III*
NIH/National Institute of Neurological Disorders and Stroke, *IV*
National Lipid Diseases Foundation, *III*
National Niemann-Pick Disease Foundation, Inc., *II*
National Tay-Sachs and Allied Diseases Association, Inc., *III*
Research Trust for Metabolic Diseases in Children, *III*

765 NOCARDIOSIS

Nocardiosis is an infectious pulmonary disease characterized by abscesses in the lungs. These abscesses may extend through the chest wall. The infection is spread through the bloodstream by a microorganism called Nocardia asteroides.

In addition to The National Organization for Rare Disorders (NORD) listed in Section III, the following organizations in Section II (Disease Specific) and in Section III (Umbrella) and Section IV (Government Agencies) can provide more information:

Centers for Disease Control and Prevention, *IV*
NIH/National Institute of Allergy and Infectious Diseases, *IV*

766 NON-KETOTIC HYPERGLYCINEMIA

Non-Ketotic Hyperglycinemia is a genetic disorder characterized by an error of amino acid metabolism. Large amounts of the amino acid glycine tend to accumulate in body fluids particularly in the cerebrospinal fluid. The metabolic block occurs in the conversion of glycine into smaller molecules. Severe illness usually occurs soon after birth and many patients become mentally retarded and/or develop seizure disorders.

In addition to The National Organization for Rare Disorders (NORD) listed in Section III, the following organizations in Section II (Disease Specific) and in Section III (Umbrella) and Section IV (Government Agencies) can provide more information:

Metabolic Information Network, *III*
NIH/National Digestive Diseases Information Clearinghouse, *IV*

Non-Ketotic Hyperglycinemia (NKH) Parent Network, *II*
Organic Acidemia Association, *III*
Research Trust for Metabolic Diseases in Children, *III*
The Arc (a national organization on mental retardation), *III*
Vaincre Les Maladies Lysosomales, *III*

767 NOONAN SYNDROME

Noonan Syndrome is a genetic disorder that can affect both males and females. The condition is characterized by a lack of sexual development, short stature, possible mental retardation, a webbed neck, skeletal and/or heart defects, and various other inborn deformities. Persons with Noonan Syndrome have normal chromosomes (karyotype is normal), while their physical appearance is different from their peers.

In addition to The National Organization for Rare Disorders (NORD) listed in Section III, the following organizations in Section II (Disease Specific) and in Section III (Umbrella) and Section IV (Government Agencies) can provide more information:
Human Growth Foundation, *III*
MAGIC Foundation for Children's Growth, *III*
NIH/National Institute of Child Health and Human Development, *IV*
Noonan Syndrome Support Group, Inc., *II*
The Arc (a national organization on mental retardation), *III*

768 NORRIE SYNDROME

Norrie Syndrome is a rare inherited neurodevelopmental disorder characterized by blindness in both eyes (bilateral) at birth. Some children with this disorder may experience varying degrees of mental retardation. Other symptoms may include mild to profound hearing loss, growth delays, and/or diabetes. The lens of the eyes may become cloudy (cataracts) during early infancy and the eyeball may shrink (phthisis bulbi). The gene responsible for Norrie Syndrome is inherited as an X-linked recessive genetic trait.

In addition to The National Organization for Rare Disorders (NORD) listed in Section III, the following organizations in Section II (Disease Specific) and in Section III (Umbrella) and Section IV (Government Agencies) can provide more information:
American Council of the Blind, Inc., *III*
American Foundation for the Blind, *III*
American Society for Deaf Children, *III*
Blind Children's Center, *III*
Blind Children's Fund, *III*
Council of Families with Visual Impairment, *III*
Deafness Research Foundation, *III*
Foundation Fighting Blindness, *III*
NIH/National Eye Institute, *IV*
National Association for Parents of the Visually Impaired, *III*
National Association for Visually Handicapped, *III*
National Association of the Deaf, *III*
National Federation of the Blind, *III*
National Information Center on Deafness, *III*
Norrie Disease Association, *II*
Retinitis Pigmentosa International, *II*
The Arc (a national organization on mental retardation), *III*
Vision Foundation, Inc., *III*

769 NYSTAGMUS, BENIGN PAROXYSMAL POSITIONAL

Benign Paroxysmal Positional Nystagmus is a disorder of the vestibular system in the middle ear that causes dizziness due to altered function of the semicircular canals, usually the posterior canal. The disorder is paroxysmal because the dizziness takes place without warning; it is positional because the symptoms increase with certain movements of the head or body. Abnormal eye movements or nystagmus accompanies the dizziness.

In addition to The National Organization for Rare Disorders (NORD) listed in Section III, the following organizations in Section II (Disease Specific) and in Section III (Umbrella) and Section IV (Government Agencies) can provide more information:
EAR (Education and Auditory Research) Foundation, *III*
NIH/National Institute of Neurological Disorders and Stroke, *IV*
Vestibular Disorders Association, *III*

770 OBSESSIVE COMPULSIVE DISORDER

Obsessive Compulsive Disorder is characterized by recurrent habitual obsessive or compulsive thoughts or actions. These obsessions and compulsions may become very distressing and time-consuming. In severe cases they can significantly interfere with a person's normal routine, occupational functioning, usual social activities or relationships with others.

In addition to The National Organization for Rare Disorders (NORD) listed in Section III, the following organizations in Section II (Disease Specific) and in Section III (Umbrella) and Section IV (Government Agencies) can provide more information:
NIH/National Institute of Mental Health, *IV*
National Mental Health Association, *III*
Obsessive-Compulsive Foundation, Inc., *II*
Tourette Syndrome Association, Inc., *II*

771 **OCHOA SYNDROME**

Ochoa Syndrome, also known as Hydronephrosis With Peculiar Facial Expression, is an extremely rare inherited disorder that may be apparent at birth (congenital). The first characteristic feature that may be apparent is an unusual "inverted" facial expression (e.g., a peculiar "grimace") that becomes obvious when affected infants laugh or smile.

Ochoa Syndrome is also characterized by abnormalities of certain organs within the urinary tract. Failure of nerve signals between the muscular organ that collects urine (bladder) and the spinal cord results in improper, incomplete emptying of the bladder (mild occult neuropathic bladder). This may, in turn, lead to the backflow (reflux) of urine into the tubes that normally bring urine to the bladder (ureters); abnormal swelling (distention) of and accumulation of urine in the ureters (hydroureter) and the kidneys (hydronephrosis); and/or ureter blockage (obstruction). In some cases, these and additional, associated abnormalities of the urinary tract may result in urinary tract damage and repeated urinary tract infections, potentially leading to chronic kidney (renal) failure. Many affected individuals may also exhibit additional physical abnormalities. In most cases, Ochoa Syndrome is thought to be inherited as an autosomal recessive genetic trait.

In addition to The National Organization for Rare Disorders (NORD) listed in Section III, the following organizations in Section II (Disease Specific) and in Section III (Umbrella) and Section IV (Government Agencies) can provide more information:

American Association of Kidney Patients, *III*
American Kidney Fund, Inc., *III*
NIH/National Kidney and Urologic Diseases Information Clearinghouse, *IV*
National Kidney Foundation, *III*

772 **OCULO DENTO DIGITAL DYSPLASIA**

Oculo-Dento-Digital Dysplasia is a rare disorder that may be inherited as an autosomal dominant trait or be caused by a new change in the genes that occurs for no apparent reason (mutation). Major symptoms of Oculo-Dento-Digital Dysplasia are webbing of the fourth and fifth fingers, an abnormally small transparent part of the eye (microcornea), a slender nose with narrow nostrils, underdevelopment of the outer flaring wall of each nostril (alae), defective enamel and dry hair that grows slowly.

In addition to The National Organization for Rare Disorders (NORD) listed in Section III, the following organizations in Section II (Disease Specific) and in Section III (Umbrella) and Section IV (Government Agencies) can provide more information:

NIH/National Arthritis and Musculoskeletal and Skin Diseases Information Clearinghouse, *IV*
NIH/National Oral Health Information Clearinghouse, *IV*
National Association for Visually Handicapped, *III*
National Foundation for Ectodermal Dysplasias, *II*

773 **OCULOCEREBRAL SYNDROME WITH HYPOPIGMENTATION**

Oculocerebral Syndrome with Hypopigmentation is an extremely rare inherited disorder characterized by the lack of normal color (hypopigmentation) of the skin and hair and abnormalities of the central nervous system that affect the eyes and certain parts of the brain (oculocerebral). Physical findings at birth include unusually light skin color and silvery-gray hair. Abnormal findings associated with the central nervous system may include abnormal smallness of one or both eyes (microphthalmia); clouding (opacities) of the front, clear portion of the eye through which light passes (cornea); and/or rapid, involuntary eye movements (nystagmus). Additional symptoms that may develop during infancy include involuntary muscle contractions, associated loss of muscle function (spastic paraplegia), developmental delays, and/or mental retardation. Oculocerebral Syndrome with Hypopigmentation is believed to be inherited as an autosomal recessive genetic trait.

In addition to The National Organization for Rare Disorders (NORD) listed in Section III, the following organizations in Section II (Disease Specific) and in Section III (Umbrella) and Section IV (Government Agencies) can provide more information:

NIH/National Arthritis and Musculoskeletal and Skin Diseases Information Clearinghouse, *IV*
NIH/National Eye Institute, *IV*
NIH/National Institute of Child Health and Human Development, *IV*
National Association for Parents of the Visually Impaired, *III*
National Association for Visually Handicapped, *III*

774 **OCULOCEREBROCUTANEOUS SYNDROME**

Oculocerebrocutaneous Syndrome is a rare congenital disorder that may occur for no apparent reason (sporadically) or may be inherited as an autosomal dominant trait. Affected individuals may have cysts in the orbit of the eye, malformations of the brain including cysts in the cavities, small brown or flesh colored tags of skin in the orbit of the eyes and front of the ears, skin lesions on the head and trunk, and seizures.

In addition to The National Organization for Rare Disorders (NORD) listed in Section III, the following organizations in Section II (Disease Specific) and in Section III (Umbrella) and Section IV (Government Agencies) can provide more information:
Agenesis of Corpus Callosum (ACC) Network, *II*
Epilepsy Foundation of America, *III*
March of Dimes Birth Defects Foundation, *III*
NIH/National Institute of Neurological Disorders and Stroke, *IV*

775 OLIVOPONTOCEREBELLAR ATROPHY

Olivopontocerebellar Atrophy (OPCA) is a group of inherited forms of Ataxia characterized by progressive neurological degeneration affecting the olivopontocerebellar area of the brain. These inherited forms include Menzel type I, Fickler-Winkler type II, retinal degeneration type III, Schut-Haymaker type IV, and ophthalmoplegia (paralysis of facial and eye muscles) type 5 OPCA. However, cases have occurred that have defied classification in any of these five categories.

In addition to The National Organization for Rare Disorders (NORD) listed in Section III, the following organizations in Section II (Disease Specific) and in Section III (Umbrella) and Section IV (Government Agencies) can provide more information:
NIH/National Institute of Neurological Disorders and Stroke, *IV*
National Ataxia Foundation, *III*
WE MOVE, *III*

776 OLLIER DISEASE

Ollier Disease is a rare skeletal disorder characterized by abnormal bone development (skeletal dysplasia). This disorder is present at birth (congenital); however it may not be apparent until early childhood when certain symptoms, such as deformities or improper limb growth, are observed. Ollier Disease primarily affects the long bones and cartilage in the joints of the arms and legs, specifically the area where the shaft and head of a long bone meet (metaphyses). The pelvis is often involved; in rare cases, the ribs, breast bone (sternum), and/or skull may also be affected. Deformities may also develop in the wrists and ankles.

In Ollier Disease an overgrowth of cartilage in the long bones of the arms and legs results in abnormal bone growth and thinning of the outer layer (cortex) of the bone. These masses of cartilage are benign (non-cancerous) tumors known as enchondromas. The growth of enchondromas can occur anytime. After puberty these growths stabilize as cartilage is replaced by bone. In rare cases, the enchondromas may undergo malignant changes (e.g., chondrosarcomas). The exact cause of Ollier Disease is not known although some cases may be inherited as an autosomal dominant genetic trait.

In addition to The National Organization for Rare Disorders (NORD) listed in Section III, the following organizations in Section II (Disease Specific) and in Section III (Umbrella) and Section IV (Government Agencies) can provide more information:
NIH/National Institute of Arthritis and Musculoskeletal and Skin Diseases, *IV*
Ollier/Maffucci Self-Help Group, *II*

777 OPITZ SYNDROME

Opitz Syndrome is an uncommon hereditary disorder characterized by widely set eyes (hypertelorism), undescended testicles (cryptorchidism) and abnormal placement of the urinary opening (meatus) on the underside of the penis in males (hypospadias), incomplete closure of the roof of the mouth (cleft palate) and/or an abnormal groove in the upper lip (cleft lip), and/or swallowing difficulties (choking, aspiration). In some cases, affected individuals may exhibit absence of the anal opening (imperforate anus), partial or total absence of the thick band of nerve fibers that connects the left and right hemispheres of the brain (hypoplasia or agenesis of the corpus callosum), and/or additional abnormalities.

In addition to The National Organization for Rare Disorders (NORD) listed in Section III, the following organizations in Section II (Disease Specific) and in Section III (Umbrella) and Section IV (Government Agencies) can provide more information:
22q and You, *II*
International Opitz Frias Syndrome Association, *II*
NIH/National Institute of Child Health and Human Development, *IV*
Opitz Family Network, *II*

778 OPPORTUNISTIC INFECTIONS

Opportunistic infections are mild to severe infectious diseases in a compromised host. The infections are caused by microorganisms that normally do not cause serious disease in healthy people. These infections may occur in individuals whose immune system or other physiological defenses are impaired or compromised in some way. The inability to resist such opportunistic infections is usually caused by an underlying disease or trauma, or from procedures and/or drugs that are used to treat another medical condition.

Opportunistic infections may be caused by bacteria, fungi, viruses, or parasites. Symptoms vary according to the microorganism involved and the extent of involvement. Treatment or medical management of opportunistic infections may be difficult because some of these microorganisms may be resistant to standard antibiotic therapy. In some cases an affected individual may have a dysfunctional immune system (compromised) that is not able to fight the infection.

In addition to The National Organization for Rare Disorders (NORD) listed in Section III, the following organizations in Section II (Disease Specific) and in Section III (Umbrella) and Section IV (Government Agencies) can provide more information:

Centers for Disease Control and Prevention, *IV*
NIH/National Institute of Allergy and Infectious Diseases, *IV*

779 ORAL FACIAL DIGITAL SYNDROME

Oral-Facial-Digital Syndrome (OFD) is a genetic disorder. Major symptoms include many episodic neuromuscular disturbances, congenital malformations such as cleft palate, other facial deformities, malformation of the hands and feet, shortened limbs and various degrees of mental retardation.

In addition to The National Organization for Rare Disorders (NORD) listed in Section III, the following organizations in Section II (Disease Specific) and in Section III (Umbrella) and Section IV (Government Agencies) can provide more information:

AboutFace U.S.A., *III*
Children's Craniofacial Association, *III*
FACES: The National Craniofacial Association, *III*
Forward Face, Inc., *III*
Let's Face It, Inc., *III*
NIH/National Oral Health Information Clearinghouse, *IV*
National Foundation for Facial Reconstruction, *III*
Prescription Parents (for parents of children with cleft lip and palate), *III*
The Arc (a national organization on mental retardation), *III*

780 ORGANIC MOOD SYNDROME

Organic Mood Syndrome is a mental disorder due to physical causes. Either "manic" symptoms of unusual euphoria or irritability, or "depressive" symptoms of despondency, fear, anxiety, or suspiciousness may be present. Other symptoms may be present as well.

In addition to The National Organization for Rare Disorders (NORD) listed in Section III, the following organizations in Section II (Disease Specific) and in Section III (Umbrella) and Section IV (Government Agencies) can provide more information:

NIH/National Institute of Mental Health, *IV*
National Alliance for the Mentally Ill, *III*
National Mental Health Association, *III*
National Mental Health Consumer Self-Help Clearinghouse, *III*

781 ORGANIC PERSONALITY SYNDROME

Organic Personality Syndrome is a mental disorder characterized by a persistent personality disturbance due to an organic cause. Significant changes in the personality may endure for a short or long time, depending on the cause. The degree of impairment varies in each case.

In addition to The National Organization for Rare Disorders (NORD) listed in Section III, the following organizations in Section II (Disease Specific) and in Section III (Umbrella) and Section IV (Government Agencies) can provide more information:

NIH/National Institute of Mental Health, *IV*
National Alliance for the Mentally Ill, *III*
National Mental Health Association, *III*
National Mental Health Consumer Self-Help Clearinghouse, *III*

782 ORNITHINE TRANSCARBAMYLASE DEFICIENCY

Ornithine Transcarbamylase Deficiency is a rare inborn error of metabolism and one of six inherited disorders of the urea cycle. The urea cycle is a series of chemical reactions in the liver that break down ammonia into urea. Ammonia is toxic to the body. Urea cycle disorders are caused by deficiencies of certain proteins (enzymes) that act to break down the ammonia into urea that is then eliminated from the body. These enzyme deficiencies cause an abnormal accumulation of ammonia in the blood and body tissues.

In addition to The National Organization for Rare Disorders (NORD) listed in Section III, the following organizations in Section II (Disease Specific) and in Section III (Umbrella) and Section IV (Government Agencies) can provide more information:

Metabolic Information Network, *III*

NIH/National Digestive Diseases Information Clearinghouse, *IV*
National Kidney Foundation, *III*
National Urea Cycle Disorders Foundation, *III*
Research Trust for Metabolic Diseases in Children, *III*

783 OROCRANIODIGITAL SYNDROME

Orocraniodigital Syndrome is an extremely rare inherited disorder characterized by multiple malformations of the head and face (craniofacial area) and the fingers and toes (digits). Major characteristics may include a vertical groove in the upper lip (cleft lip) and/or the inside, upper portion of the mouth (cleft palate), an abnormally small head (microcephaly), widely-spaced eyes (ocular hypertelorism), improper development (hypoplasia) of the thumbs and/or toes, and/or webbing (syndactyly) of the toes. In some cases, malformations of certain skeletal bones may also be present. Mental retardation has occurred in the majority of cases. Orocraniodigital Syndrome may be inherited as an autosomal recessive genetic trait.

In addition to The National Organization for Rare Disorders (NORD) listed in Section III, the following organizations in Section II (Disease Specific) and in Section III (Umbrella) and Section IV (Government Agencies) can provide more information:
AboutFace U.S.A., *III*
Children's Craniofacial Association, *III*
Cleft Palate Foundation, *III*
FACES: The National Craniofacial Association, *III*
Forward Face, Inc., *III*
NIH/National Institute of Child Health and Human Development, *IV*
Wide Smiles, *III*

784 OSGOOD SCHLATTER'S DISEASE

Osgood-Schlatter's Disease is characterized by abnormal bone and cartilage formation in the bone located between the knee and the ankle (tibia). Affected individuals may experience pain, swelling, and tenderness of the knee and ankle.

In addition to The National Organization for Rare Disorders (NORD) listed in Section III, the following organizations in Section II (Disease Specific) and in Section III (Umbrella) and Section IV (Government Agencies) can provide more information:
Arthritis Foundation, *III*
NIH/National Arthritis and Musculoskeletal and Skin Diseases Information Clearinghouse, *IV*

785 OSTEOGENESIS IMPERFECTA

Osteogenesis Imperfecta is characterized by unusually fragile bones that break or fracture easily. There are generally considered to be 4 types of this disorder, some with subtypes. The congenital form, type II, is the most severe; affected infants are either stillborn or die shortly after birth of respiratory insufficiency. Other forms of Osteogenesis Imperfecta range from mild to severe.

In addition to The National Organization for Rare Disorders (NORD) listed in Section III, the following organizations in Section II (Disease Specific) and in Section III (Umbrella) and Section IV (Government Agencies) can provide more information:
Alliance of Genetic Support Groups, *III*
Canadian Osteogenesis Imperfecta Society, *II*
March of Dimes Birth Defects Foundation, *III*
NIH/National Institute of Arthritis and Musculoskeletal and Skin Diseases, *IV*
NIH/National Institute of Child Health and Human Development, *IV*
Osteogenesis Imperfecta Foundation, Inc., *II*

786 OSTEOMYELITIS

Osteomyelitis is a common inflammation of the bone caused by bacteria, frequently Staphylococcus. This disorder is usually due to an infection in another part of the body that is transported through the bloodstream to a bone in a distant location. It can be an acute or chronic condition.

In addition to The National Organization for Rare Disorders (NORD) listed in Section III, the following organizations in Section II (Disease Specific) and in Section III (Umbrella) and Section IV (Government Agencies) can provide more information:
NIH/National Arthritis and Musculoskeletal and Skin Diseases Information Clearinghouse, *IV*

787 OSTEONECROSIS

Osteonecrosis is the destruction of a bone (necrosis) often due to an inadequate supply of blood to a bone. It most commonly affects the joints and bones of the hips, knees and shoulder. It often occurs as a result of bone injuries or in conjunction with other diseases and conditions.

In addition to The National Organization for Rare Disorders (NORD) listed in Section III, the following organizations in Section II (Disease Specific) and in Section III (Umbrella) and Section IV (Government Agencies) can provide more information:
Arthritis Foundation, *III*
NIH/National Arthritis and Musculoskeletal and Skin Diseases Information Clearinghouse, *IV*

788 OSTEOPETROSIS

Osteopetrosis may be inherited as either a dominant or recessive trait and is marked by increased bone density, brittle bones, and in some cases, skeletal abnormalities. Although symptoms may not initially be apparent in people with mild forms of this disorder, trivial injuries may cause bone fractures due to abnormalities of the bone. The dominantly transmitted form is milder than the recessive form of Osteopetrosis, and may not be diagnosed until adolescence or adulthood when symptoms first appear. More serious complications occur in the recessive form that may be diagnosed from examination of skeletal x-rays during infancy or childhood.

In addition to The National Organization for Rare Disorders (NORD) listed in Section III, the following organizations in Section II (Disease Specific) and in Section III (Umbrella) and Section IV (Government Agencies) can provide more information:
FROST: Friends of the Osteopetrosis Support Trust, *II*
Metabolic Information Network, *III*
NIH/National Arthritis and Musculoskeletal and Skin Diseases Information Clearinghouse, *IV*
Osteoporosis and Related Bone Diseases National Resource Center, *III*
Paget Foundation for Paget's Disease of Bone and Related Disorders, *III*
Research Trust for Metabolic Diseases in Children, *III*

789 OTO PALATO DIGITAL SYNDROME TYPE I AND II

Oto-Palato-Digital Syndrome Type I and II are rare genetic disorders in which complete expression of the disease shows up only in males. Females may be mildly affected with some of the symptoms. Type I OPD is inherited through an X-linked recessive trait with variable expression in females while Type II OPD is inherited through an X-linked semi-dominant trait.

OPD Type I is typically a milder disorder with fewer symptoms. Some of the characteristics of both disorders may include cleft palate, a downward slant of the opening between the upper and lower eyelids, hearing loss, and short fingers and toes.

In addition to The National Organization for Rare Disorders (NORD) listed in Section III, the following organizations in Section II (Disease Specific) and in Section III (Umbrella) and Section IV (Government Agencies) can provide more information:
Children's Craniofacial Association, *III*
FACES: The National Craniofacial Association, *III*
Let's Face It, Inc., *III*
NIH/National Institute of Child Health and Human Development, *IV*
National Foundation for Facial Reconstruction, *III*

790 PEPCK DEFICIENCY, MITOCHONDRIAL

Mitochondrial PEPCK Deficiency is an extremely rare disorder of carbohydrate metabolism inherited as an autosomal recessive trait. A deficiency of the enzyme phosphoenolpyruvate carboxykinase, which is a key enzyme in the conversion of proteins and fat to glucose (gluconeogenesis), causes an excess of acid in the circulating blood (acidemia). Characteristics of this disorder are low blood sugar (hypoglycemia), loss of muscle tone, an abnormal enlargement of the liver and failure to gain weight and grow normally.

In addition to The National Organization for Rare Disorders (NORD) listed in Section III, the following organizations in Section II (Disease Specific) and in Section III (Umbrella) and Section IV (Government Agencies) can provide more information:
Lactic Acidosis Support Trust, *III*
NIH/National Digestive Diseases Information Clearinghouse, *IV*
Research Trust for Metabolic Diseases in Children, *III*
United Mitochondrial Disease Foundation, *III*

791 POEMS SYNDROME

POEMS Syndrome is an acronym for Polyneuropathy (a disease of many nerves), Organomegaly (the enlargement of an organ), Endocrinopathy (a functional disorder of an endocrine gland), M protein (monoclonal immunoglobin, a type of antibody), and Skin changes. The exact cause of POEMS Syndrome is not known.

In addition to The National Organization for Rare Disorders (NORD) listed in Section III, the following organizations in Section II (Disease Specific) and in Section III (Umbrella) and Section IV (Government Agencies) can provide more information:
American Autoimmune Related Diseases Association, Inc., *III*
NIH/Developmental Endocrinology Branch, *IV*
NIH/National Arthritis and Musculoskeletal and Skin Diseases Information Clearinghouse, *IV*
NIH/National Institute of Neurological Disorders and Stroke, *IV*

792 PACHYDERMOPERIOSTOSIS

Pachydermoperiostosis is a rare disorder thought to be inherited as an autosomal dominant trait. This disorder typically appears during childhood or adolescence and progresses slowly for about ten years. Symptoms of Pachydermoperiostosis may be enlargement of the fingers and toes (clubbing), a condition in which there is a fibrous covering on the ends of the long bones (periostosis), coarse facial features, increased bulk of the skin on the scalp forming folds, depressions or furrows (cutis verticis gyrata), and/or excessive sweating of the hands and feet.

In addition to The National Organization for Rare Disorders (NORD) listed in Section III, the following organizations in Section II (Disease Specific) and in Section III (Umbrella) and Section IV (Government Agencies) can provide more information:
NIH/National Arthritis and Musculoskeletal and Skin Diseases Information Clearinghouse, *IV*

793 PAGET'S DISEASE

Paget's disease of the bone is a chronic, slowly progressive skeletal condition of abnormally rapid bone destruction (osteolytic) and reformation (osteoblastic). The new bone is structurally abnormal, dense and fragile. The bones most frequently affected are in the spine, skull, pelvis and lower legs.

In addition to The National Organization for Rare Disorders (NORD) listed in Section III, the following organizations in Section II (Disease Specific) and in Section III (Umbrella) and Section IV (Government Agencies) can provide more information:
NIH/National Arthritis and Musculoskeletal and Skin Diseases Information Clearinghouse, *IV*
Osteoporosis and Related Bone Diseases National Resource Center, *III*
Paget Foundation for Paget's Disease of Bone and Related Disorders, *III*

794 PAGET'S DISEASE OF THE BREAST

Paget's Disease of the Breast is a very rare form of cancer. It is characterized by skin changes resembling eczema around the nipple and breast. It may also occur in the skin areas of the genitals and rectum. When it spreads to these areas of the body Paget's Disease of the Breast is called Extramammary Paget's Disease. Paget's Disease of the Breast often signals the existence of other internal cancer. It can occur in men as well as women. Paget's Disease of the Breast is not Paget's Disease of the bones.

In addition to The National Organization for Rare Disorders (NORD) listed in Section III, the following organizations in Section II (Disease Specific) and in Section III (Umbrella) and Section IV (Government Agencies) can provide more information:
American Cancer Society, Inc., *III*
Skin Cancer Foundation, *III*

795 PALLISTER HALL SYNDROME

Pallister-Hall Syndrome is a very rare developmental disorder characterized by a benign (non-cancerous) tumor in a specific area of the brain (hypothalamic hamartomablastoma), extra fingers and/or toes (postaxial polydactyly), an absent or extremely small anal opening (imperforate anus), and decreased pituitary function (hypopituitarism). Unusual facial features, mental retardation, fluid accumulation around the brain (hydrocephalus), and/or increased pressure in the skull (cranial pressure) may also occur. Symptoms are apparent at birth (congenital), and newborns must be monitored closely for signs of hypopituitarism that can lead to life-threatening complications if left untreated.

In addition to The National Organization for Rare Disorders (NORD) listed in Section III, the following organizations in Section II (Disease Specific) and in Section III (Umbrella) and Section IV (Government Agencies) can provide more information:
American Brain Tumor Association, *III*
Hydrocephalus Association, *II*
Hydrocephalus Research Foundation, Inc., *II*
Hydrocephalus Support Group, Inc., *II*
NIH/National Institute of Child Health and Human Development, *IV*
Pallister-Hall Foundation, *II*

796 PALLISTER KILLIAN MOSAIC SYNDROME

Pallister-Killian Mosaic Syndrome is a rare chromosomal disorder that occurs for no apparent reason. Major symptoms may include a coarse face with a high forehead, sparse hair on the scalp, an abnormally wide space between the eyes, a fold of the skin over the inner corner of the eyes, and a broad nasal bridge with a highly arched palate. Mental retardation, loss of muscle tone, and streaks of skin lacking color are often present.

In addition to The National Organization for Rare Disorders (NORD) listed in Section III, the following organizations in Section II (Disease Specific) and in Section III (Umbrella) and Section IV (Government Agencies) can provide more information:
NIH/National Institute of Child Health and Human Development, *IV*
Pallister-Killian Family Support Group, *II*
The Arc (a national organization on mental retardation), *III*

797 PALLISTER W SYNDROME

Pallister-W Syndrome is a rare genetic disorder characterized by unusual facial features such as clefting of the palate and the upper lip, a broad flat nose, widely spaced slanted eyes, and/or downslanting eyelid folds (palpebral fissures). Other symptoms may include mental retardation, speech problems, bone deformities of the arms and legs, and/or seizures. The exact cause of Pallister W Syndrome is not known.

In addition to The National Organization for Rare Disorders (NORD) listed in Section III, the following organizations in Section II (Disease Specific) and in Section III (Umbrella) and Section IV (Government Agencies) can provide more information:

AboutFace U.S.A., *III*
Children's Craniofacial Association, *III*
FACES: The National Craniofacial Association, *III*
Forward Face, Inc., *III*
Let's Face It, Inc., *III*
NIH/National Institute of Child Health and Human Development, *IV*
National Foundation for Facial Reconstruction, *III*

798 PANCREATIC ISLET CELL TUMOR

Pancreatic-islet cell tumors appear in one of two forms. They may be nonfunctioning or functioning tumors. Nonfunctioning tumors may cause obstruction in the shortest part of the small intestine (duodenum) or in the biliary tract, which connects the liver to the duodenum and includes the gall bladder. These nonfunctioning tumors may erode and bleed into the stomach and/or the intestines, or they may cause an abdominal mass.

Functioning tumors secrete excessive amounts of hormones, which may lead to various syndromes including low blood sugar (hypoglycemia), multiple bleeding ulcers (Zollinger-Ellison Syndrome), pancreatic cholera (Verner-Morrison Syndrome), carcinoid syndrome or diabetes.

Islet cells are small, isolated masses of cells that make up the Islet of Langerhans in the pancreas. When functioning normally, they secrete the protein hormones insulin and glucagon. Tumors composed of irregular islet cells may occur alone or in a group of many tumors. Approximately 90% of islet-cell tumors are noncancerous (benign). They usually range in size from 0.5 to 2 cm in diameter.

In addition to The National Organization for Rare Disorders (NORD) listed in Section III, the following organizations in Section II (Disease Specific) and in Section III (Umbrella) and Section IV (Government Agencies) can provide more information:

American Cancer Society, Inc., *III*
International Tremor Foundation, *III*
NIH/National Digestive Diseases Information Clearinghouse, *IV*

799 PANIC ANXIETY SYNDROME

Panic-Anxiety Syndrome is a psychiatric disorder characterized by recurrent and unpredictable anxiety attacks with no apparent cause for the symptoms, such as threat of danger or attack. Panic-Anxiety Syndrome is believed to be caused by biochemical factors, though the specific cause of the disorder is not yet known.

In addition to The National Organization for Rare Disorders (NORD) listed in Section III, the following organizations in Section II (Disease Specific) and in Section III (Umbrella) and Section IV (Government Agencies) can provide more information:

Anxiety Disorders Association of America, *III*
Depression and Related Affective Disorders Association, *III*
NIH/National Institute of Mental Health, *IV*
National Alliance for the Mentally Ill, *III*
National Mental Health Association, *III*
National Mental Health Consumer Self-Help Clearinghouse, *III*

800 PANNICULITIS, IDIOPATHIC NODULAR

Idiopathic nodular panniculitis is a rare spectrum of skin disorders characterized by single or multiple, tender or painful bumps below the surface of the skin (subcutaneous nodules) that usually lead to inflammation of the subcutaneous layer of fat (panniculitis). These nodules tend to be 1-2 centimeters large and most often affect the legs and feet (lower extremities). In most cases, idiopathic nodular panniculitis is associated with fever, a general feeling of ill health (malaise), muscle pain (myalgia), and/or abdominal pain. These symptoms may subside after a few days or weeks and may recur weeks, months, or years later. The exact cause of this disorder is not known (idiopathic).

In addition to The National Organization for Rare Disorders (NORD) listed in Section III, the following organizations in Section II (Disease Specific) and in Section III (Umbrella) and Section IV (Government Agencies) can provide more information:

NIH/National Arthritis and Musculoskeletal and Skin Diseases Information Clearinghouse, *IV*
NIH/National Institute of Allergy and Infectious Diseases, *IV*
NIH/Patient Referral Services Unit, *IV*

801 PAPILLITIS

Papillitis, an eye (ocular) condition, is characterized by progressive inflammation of the optic disk. Also referred to as the "blind spot," the optic disk (optic papilla) is that portion of the optic nerve that enters the eye and joins with the nerve-rich membrane lining the eye (retina). The optic nerves are the pair of nerves (second cranial nerves) that transmit impulses from the retinas to the brain. Individuals with Papillitis experience loss of vision in one eye that may occur within several hours of onset. The severity of visual impairment may vary from case to case, ranging from slight visual deficiency to complete loss of light perception. In addition, affected individuals experience a reduction in color perception. In some cases, spontaneous recovery may occur. However, in other cases, permanent visual impairment may result if the underlying cause is not detected or treated. Papillitis may occur for unknown reasons, after a viral illness, or due to or in association with a number of different underlying disorders or other factors.

In addition to The National Organization for Rare Disorders (NORD) listed in Section III, the following organizations in Section II (Disease Specific) and in Section III (Umbrella) and Section IV (Government Agencies) can provide more information:
NIH/National Eye Institute, *IV*
National Association for Visually Handicapped, *III*
Vision Foundation, Inc., *III*

802 PAPILLON LEFEVRE SYNDROME

Papillon-Lefevre Syndrome is an extremely rare inherited disorder characterized by the development of dry scaly patches of the skin on the palms of the hands and the soles of the feet (palmar-plantar hyperkeratosis) and severe inflammation and degeneration of the structures that surround and support the teeth (periodontium), resulting in premature tooth loss (periodontoclasia). Affected individuals may also have frequent pus producing (pyogenic) skin infections and abnormalities of the nails (nail dystrophy). They may also perspire heavily and frequently (hyperhidrosis). Papillon-Lefevre Syndrome is believed to be inherited as an autosomal recessive genetic trait.

In addition to The National Organization for Rare Disorders (NORD) listed in Section III, the following organizations in Section II (Disease Specific) and in Section III (Umbrella) and Section IV (Government Agencies) can provide more information:
NIH/National Arthritis and Musculoskeletal and Skin Diseases Information Clearinghouse, *IV*
NIH/National Institute of Dental Research, *IV*

803 PARACOCCIDIOIDOMYCOSIS

Paracoccidioidomycosis (PCM) is a chronic infectious tropical disease caused by the fungus Paracoccidioides brasiliensis. The initial infection usually occurs in the lungs, but may also spread to the skin, mucous membranes, and other parts of the body. Specialized cells that line the walls of blood and lymphatic vessels and dispose of cellular waste (reticuloendothelial system) may also be affected by Paracoccidioidomycosis. If left untreated, life-threatening complications can occur. Most cases of this disease occur in South and Central America.

In addition to The National Organization for Rare Disorders (NORD) listed in Section III, the following organizations in Section II (Disease Specific) and in Section III (Umbrella) and Section IV (Government Agencies) can provide more information:
Centers for Disease Control and Prevention, *IV*
NIH/National Institute of Allergy and Infectious Diseases, *IV*
World Health Organization (WHO) Regional Office for the Americas (AMRO), *III*

804 PARAMYOTONIA CONGENITA

Paramyotonia Congenita is a rare muscular disorder inherited as an autosomal dominant trait. This nonprogressive disorder is characterized by a condition in which the muscles do not relax after contracting (myotonia). Symptoms can be triggered by exposure to the cold. There are also intermittent periods of a type of paralysis in which there is no muscle tone (flaccid paresis). This condition does not necessarily coincide with exposure to cold temperatures or myotonia. There is no wasting (atrophy) or increase in bulk (hypertrophy) of muscles with this disorder.

In addition to The National Organization for Rare Disorders (NORD) listed in Section III, the following organizations in Section II (Disease Specific) and in Section III (Umbrella) and Section IV (Government Agencies) can provide more information:
Muscular Dystrophy Association, *III*
NIH/National Arthritis and Musculoskeletal and Skin Diseases Information Clearinghouse, *IV*
WE MOVE, *III*

805 PARAPLEGIA, HEREDITARY SPASTIC

Hereditary Spastic Paraplegia is an inherited neurological disorder characterized by slow progressive degeneration of the corticospinal and other nerve cells in the spinal cord. Abnormal narrowness of the passage inside of the vertebral canal can cause compression of the spinal cord and is one possible cause of this condition. This may cause paralysis. The severity of symptoms depends upon how much the nerves are compressed and damaged. Occasionally associated with other conditions, symptoms are usually first noticed during early childhood although they can begin at any age. Weakness, stiffness and muscle spasms first develop in the legs and may later spread to other parts of the body.

In addition to The National Organization for Rare Disorders (NORD) listed in Section III, the following organizations in Section II (Disease Specific) and in Section III (Umbrella) and Section IV (Government Agencies) can provide more information:
Association Strumpell-Lorrain, *II*
Hereditary Spastic Paraplegia (HSP)/Familial Spastic Paraparesis (FSP) Page, *II*
NIH/National Institute of Neurological Disorders and Stroke, *IV*
The Arc (a national organization on mental retardation), *III*

806 **PARKINSON'S DISEASE**

Parkinson's disease is a slowly progressive neurologic condition characterized by involuntary trembling (tremor), muscular stiffness or inflexibility (rigidity), slowness of movement and difficulty carrying out voluntary movements. Degenerative changes occur in areas deep within the brain (substantia nigra and other pigmented regions of the brain), causing a decrease in dopamine levels in the brain. Dopamine is a neurotransmitter, which is a chemical that sends a signal in the brain. Parkinsonian symptoms can also develop secondary to hydrocephalus (a condition in which the head is enlarged and areas of the brain accumulate excessive fluids, resulting in an increase in pressure on the brain), head trauma, inflammation of the brain (encephalitis), obstructions (infarcts) or tumors deep within the cerebral hemispheres and the upper brain stem (basal ganglia), or exposure to certain drugs and toxins. Parkinson's disease is slowly progressive and may not become incapacitating for many years.

In addition to The National Organization for Rare Disorders (NORD) listed in Section III, the following organizations in Section II (Disease Specific) and in Section III (Umbrella) and Section IV (Government Agencies) can provide more information:
Awakenings (Parkinson's Disease Information and News), *II*
International Tremor Foundation, *III*
NIH/National Institute of Neurological Disorders and Stroke, *IV*
Parkinson's Disease Foundation, Inc., *II*
United Parkinson Foundation, *II*
WE MOVE, *III*

807 **PARRY ROMBERG SYNDROME**

Parry-Romberg Syndrome is a slowly progressive wasting (atrophy) of the soft tissues of the face. The disorder is usually limited to half of the face. Pain may occur in the affected area, and changes of the eyes and facial hair can accompany soft tissue changes. Parry-Romberg Syndrome may also be associated with other disorders. It can begin without warning, usually during the second decade of life. Facial atrophy may cease abruptly or progress slowly and then become stationary.

In addition to The National Organization for Rare Disorders (NORD) listed in Section III, the following organizations in Section II (Disease Specific) and in Section III (Umbrella) and Section IV (Government Agencies) can provide more information:
FACES: The National Craniofacial Association, *III*
NIH/National Institute of Neurological Disorders and Stroke, *IV*
NIH/National Oral Health Information Clearinghouse, *IV*

808 **PARS PLANITIS**

Pars Planitis is a vision disorder characterized by inflammation of the peripheral retina and pars plana (a section of the ciliary body connected to the retina) sections of the eye. Fluid and cells can infiltrate the clear gelatin-like substance (vitreous humor) near the retina and/or pars plana. Swelling inside the eye can also occur. These abnormalities may appear in one or both eyes.

In addition to The National Organization for Rare Disorders (NORD) listed in Section III, the following organizations in Section II (Disease Specific) and in Section III (Umbrella) and Section IV (Government Agencies) can provide more information:
American Autoimmune Related Diseases Association, Inc., *III*
Association for Macular Diseases, Inc., *III*
NIH/National Eye Institute, *IV*

809 **PARSONAGE TURNER SYNDROME**

Parsonage-Turner Syndrome, also known as Brachial Plexus Neuritis or Neuralgic Amyotrophy, is a common condition characterized by inflammation of a network of nerves that control and supply (innervate) the muscles of the chest, shoulders, and arms (brachial plexus). Individuals with the condition first experience a sudden onset of severe pain across the shoulder and upper arm. Within a few hours or days, the muscles of the affected shoulder may be affected by weakness, wasting (atrophy), and paralysis (atrophic paralysis). Although individuals with the condition may experience paralysis of the affected areas for months or, in some cases, years, recovery is usually complete. The exact cause of Parsonage-Turner Syndrome is not known.

In addition to The National Organization for Rare Disorders (NORD) listed in Section III, the following organizations in Section II (Disease Specific) and in Section III (Umbrella) and Section IV (Government Agencies) can provide more information:

American Autoimmune Related Diseases Association, Inc., *III*
NIH/National Arthritis and Musculoskeletal and Skin Diseases Information Clearinghouse, *IV*

810 PATULOUS EUSTACHIAN TUBE

In Patulous Eustachian Tube dysfunction, the eustachian tube abnormally remains open constantly. This results from reduced soft tissue mass around this tube. Symptoms of this disorder occur when the patient's head has been erect for several hours.

In addition to The National Organization for Rare Disorders (NORD) listed in Section III, the following organizations in Section II (Disease Specific) and in Section III (Umbrella) and Section IV (Government Agencies) can provide more information:

Better Hearing Institute, *III*
HEAR Now, *III*
NIH/National Institute on Deafness and Other Communication Disorders (Balance), *IV*

811 PEELING SKIN SYNDROME

Peeling Skin Syndrome is an extremely rare inherited disorder characterized by continual, spontaneous skin peeling (exfoliation). Other findings may include itching (pruritis), short stature, and/or newly formed hairs that can be plucked more easily than normal. In some cases, affected individuals have the ability to manually remove sheets of skin. Peeling Skin Syndrome is thought to be inherited as an autosomal recessive genetic trait.

In addition to The National Organization for Rare Disorders (NORD) listed in Section III, the following organizations in Section II (Disease Specific) and in Section III (Umbrella) and Section IV (Government Agencies) can provide more information:

Foundation for Ichthyosis & Related Skin Types, *III*
NIH/National Arthritis and Musculoskeletal and Skin Diseases Information Clearinghouse, *IV*

812 PELIZAEUS MERZBACHER BRAIN SCLEROSIS

Pelizaeus-Merzbacher Brain Sclerosis is a rare inherited disease of the central nervous system that is associated with the progressive deterioration of the white matter of the brain. Symptoms develop due to the loss of the fatty covering on nerve fibers (myelin sheath) and the accumulation of the breakdown products of myelin. Many areas of the central nervous system may be affected including the deep portions of the cerebrum (subcortical), cerebellum, and/or brain stem. Symptoms may include the impaired ability to coordinate movement (ataxia), loss of motor abilities, and the progressive deterioration of intellectual function. The symptoms of Pelizaeus-Merzbacher Brain Sclerosis are usually slowly progressive.

There are three forms of the disease: Classical X-Linked Pelizaeus- Merzbacher Brain Sclerosis, Acute Infantile Pelizaeus-Merzbacher Brain Sclerosis, and Autosomal Dominant or Late Onset Pelizaeus-Merzbacher Brain Sclerosis. It is not clear if the acute infantile and late onset forms of the disease represent the same genetic defect or if they will come to be recognized as separate distinct disorders.

In addition to The National Organization for Rare Disorders (NORD) listed in Section III, the following organizations in Section II (Disease Specific) and in Section III (Umbrella) and Section IV (Government Agencies) can provide more information:

March of Dimes Birth Defects Foundation, *III*
Metabolic Information Network, *III*
NIH/National Institute of Neurological Disorders and Stroke, *IV*
Research Trust for Metabolic Diseases in Children, *III*
United Leukodystrophy Foundation, *III*

813 PEMPHIGOID, BENIGN MUCOSAL

Benign Mucosal Pemphigoid is a rare skin disease characterized by blisters on the mucous membranes (the thin moist layer lining the body's cavities). Mucous membranes of the mouth and the conjunctiva (the eyelids) are commonly affected areas.

In addition to The National Organization for Rare Disorders (NORD) listed in Section III, the following organizations in Section II (Disease Specific) and in Section III (Umbrella) and Section IV (Government Agencies) can provide more information:

American Autoimmune Related Diseases Association, Inc., *III*

NIH/National Arthritis and Musculoskeletal and Skin Diseases Information Clearinghouse, *IV*

814 PEMPHIGUS

Pemphigus is a group of rare autoimmune skin disorders characterized by the development of blisters in the outer layer of the skin (epidermis) and mucous membranes (thin moist layers that line the body's internal surfaces). The location and type of blisters vary according to the type of Pemphigus. If left untreated Pemphigus can be a serious illness.

In addition to The National Organization for Rare Disorders (NORD) listed in Section III, the following organizations in Section II (Disease Specific) and in Section III (Umbrella) and Section IV (Government Agencies) can provide more information:

American Autoimmune Related Diseases Association, Inc., *III*
March of Dimes Birth Defects Foundation, *III*
NIH/National Arthritis and Musculoskeletal and Skin Diseases Information Clearinghouse, *IV*
NIH/National Cancer Institute, *IV*
National Pemphigus Vulgaris Foundation, *II*

815 PENTA X SYNDROME

Penta X Syndrome is a chromosomal disorder that affects females. It is caused by the presence of extra X chromosomes. Major symptoms may include mental and growth deficiencies, upward slanting eyes with excess skin over the inner corners of the eyes (epicanthal folds), and an unclosed blood vessel that connects the lung's left artery to the heart's main artery (patent ductus arteriosus).

In addition to The National Organization for Rare Disorders (NORD) listed in Section III, the following organizations in Section II (Disease Specific) and in Section III (Umbrella) and Section IV (Government Agencies) can provide more information:

NIH/National Institute of Child Health and Human Development, *IV*
National Information Center For Children and Youth with Disabilities, *III*
Support Organization for Trisomy 18, 13, and Related Disorders, *III*

816 PENTALOGY OF CANTRELL

Pentalogy of Cantrell is a very rare disorder characterized by a combination of severe defects of the middle of the chest, sternum, diaphragm, heart, and abdominal wall. This defect can affect males or females and is apparent at birth or shortly after.

In addition to The National Organization for Rare Disorders (NORD) listed in Section III, the following organizations in Section II (Disease Specific) and in Section III (Umbrella) and Section IV (Government Agencies) can provide more information:

CHERUBS - The Association of Congenital Diaphragmatic Hernia Research, Advocacy and Support, *II*
NIH/National Institute of Child Health and Human Development, *IV*

817 PERNIOSIS

Perniosis is an inflammatory disease of the skin of the arms and legs and is triggered by prolonged exposure to cold temperature. The disorder is characterized by painful, itchy skin lesions on the lower legs, hands, toes, feet, ears and face. The lesions usually last for two to three weeks.

In addition to The National Organization for Rare Disorders (NORD) listed in Section III, the following organizations in Section II (Disease Specific) and in Section III (Umbrella) and Section IV (Government Agencies) can provide more information:

NIH/National Heart, Lung and Blood Institute, *IV*

818 PERTUSSIS

Pertussis is a highly contagious acute respiratory disease caused by the bacteria Bordetella pertussis. This disease has 3 stages: catarrhal, paroxysmal, and convalescent. The symptoms of the catarrhal stage are mild and may go unnoticed. The paroxysmal stage of Pertussis is characterized by episodes of coughing with a distinctive "whooping" sound when breathing in (inspiration). This characteristic cough gives the disease its common name, Whooping Cough. During the convalescent stage, episodes of coughing are less frequent and symptoms improve. The incidence of Pertussis has diminished greatly with widespread use of the DPT vaccine (Diphtheria Pertussis Tetanus), but in certain areas of the United States outbreaks have occurred periodically in recent years.

In addition to The National Organization for Rare Disorders (NORD) listed in Section III, the following organizations in Section II (Disease Specific) and in Section III (Umbrella) and Section IV (Government Agencies) can provide more information:

Centers for Disease Control and Prevention, *IV*
NIH/National Institute of Allergy and Infectious Diseases, *IV*
World Health Organization (WHO) Regional Office for the Americas (AMRO), *III*

819 PEUTZ JEGHERS SYNDROME

Peutz-Jeghers Syndrome is a rare inherited disorder characterized by multiple benign nodular growths (hamartomas) on the mucous lining of the intestinal wall. Affected individuals also have dark skin discolorations, especially around the lips and mucous membranes of the mouth.

In addition to The National Organization for Rare Disorders (NORD) listed in Section III, the following organizations in Section II (Disease Specific) and in Section III (Umbrella) and Section IV (Government Agencies) can provide more information:
Alliance of Genetic Support Groups, *III*
American Cancer Society, Inc., *III*
March of Dimes Birth Defects Foundation, *III*
NIH/National Digestive Diseases Information Clearinghouse, *IV*
NIH/Patient Referral Services Unit, *IV*

820 PEYRONIE DISEASE

Peyronie Disease is a rare connective tissue disorder characterized by the development of fibrous plaques in the soft tissue of the penis of adult males. Affected individuals may experience pain, have cord-like lesions on the penis, and/or exhibit abnormal curvature of the penis when erect. In some cases, these conditions may make it impossible for many affected individuals to have normal sexual intercourse unless treated. Symptoms may be chronic, or may spontaneously resolve in some cases. The exact cause of Peyronie Disease is not known.

In addition to The National Organization for Rare Disorders (NORD) listed in Section III, the following organizations in Section II (Disease Specific) and in Section III (Umbrella) and Section IV (Government Agencies) can provide more information:
American Foundation for Urologic Disease, *III*
NIH/National Kidney and Urologic Diseases Information Clearinghouse, *IV*

821 PFEIFFER SYNDROME

Pfeiffer Syndrome is a very rare genetic disorder primarily affecting the bones. The disorder is characterized by a short, pointed or conical head (acro-brachycephaly) and abnormalities of the face, jaws and teeth. Webbed fingers or toes (syndactyly) and other abnormalities of the thumbs and big toes may also occur. Symptoms may vary, ranging from mild to severe.

In addition to The National Organization for Rare Disorders (NORD) listed in Section III, the following organizations in Section II (Disease Specific) and in Section III (Umbrella) and Section IV (Government Agencies) can provide more information:
AboutFace U.S.A., *III*
Children's Craniofacial Association, *III*
Craniofacial Support Group, *III*
FACES: The National Craniofacial Association, *III*
Forward Face, Inc., *III*
Let's Face It, Inc., *III*
NIH/National Institute of Child Health and Human Development, *IV*

822 PHENYLKETONURIA

Phenylketonuria (PKU) is a rare metabolic disorder of infancy caused by a deficiency of the liver enzyme phenylalanine hydroxylase. Impairment in the metabolism of the amino acid phenylalanine results in excess accumulation of phenylalanine in the fluids of the body. Phenylketonuria is a severe progressive disorder that can produce mental retardation if it is not treated early. With a carefully controlled diet, people with Phenylketonuria can avoid irreversible mental retardation.

In addition to The National Organization for Rare Disorders (NORD) listed in Section III, the following organizations in Section II (Disease Specific) and in Section III (Umbrella) and Section IV (Government Agencies) can provide more information:
Alliance of Genetic Support Groups, *III*
Children's PKU Network, *II*
March of Dimes Birth Defects Foundation, *III*
Metabolic Information Network, *III*
NIH/National Institute of Neurological Disorders and Stroke, *IV*
National PKU Foundation, *II*
National PKU News, *II*
Phenylalanine Hydroxylase Locus Database (PAHdb) Home Page, *II*
The Arc (a national organization on mental retardation), *III*

823 PHEOCHROMOCYTOMA

Pheochromocytoma is a rare type of tumor that arises in certain cells (chromaffin) of the sympathetic nervous system. The sympathetic nervous system controls certain involuntary activities in the body (e.g., regulating the heart beat or breathing rate). Symptoms associated with Pheochromocytomas include high blood pressure (hypertension), headaches, excessive sweating, and/or heart palpitations. In most cases, Pheochromocytomas occur randomly, for unknown reasons (sporadically). In approximately 5 percent of cases, Pheochromocytomas may be inherited as an autosomal dominant genetic trait.

In addition to The National Organization for Rare Disorders (NORD) listed in Section III, the following organizations in Section II (Disease Specific) and in Section III (Umbrella) and Section IV (Government Agencies) can provide more information:
American Cancer Society, Inc., *III*
National Adrenal Diseases Foundation, *III*

824 PHOCOMELIA SYNDROME

Phocomelia Syndrome is a birth defect that may occur sporadically or be genetically transmitted in some cases. In other cases it may be caused by toxins (such as certain drugs) taken by a pregnant woman. Major symptoms may include growth and mental deficiencies, defects in the eyes, ears, and nose, and characteristic deficient limb development affecting the arms and possibly the legs.

In addition to The National Organization for Rare Disorders (NORD) listed in Section III, the following organizations in Section II (Disease Specific) and in Section III (Umbrella) and Section IV (Government Agencies) can provide more information:

Association of Children's Prosthetic/Orthotic Clinics, *III*
CHERUB—Association of Families and Friends of Children with Limb Disorders, *III*
NIH/National Institute of Child Health and Human Development, *IV*
National Rehabilitation Information Center, *III*
Superkids, Inc. (newsletter for families and friends of children with limb differences), *III*

825 PHOSPHOGLYCERATE KINASE DEFICIENCY

Phosphoglycerate Kinase Deficiency is an extremely rare inherited metabolic disorder characterized by deficiency of the enzyme phosphoglycerate kinase. Symptoms and findings associated with the disorder may include low levels of circulating red blood cells (hemolytic anemia); varying degrees of mental retardation; rapidly changing emotions (emotional lability); an impaired ability to communicate through and/or to comprehend speech or writing (aphasia); muscle weakness after exercise; and/or paralysis of one side of the body (hemiplegia). In most cases, Phosphoglycerate Kinase Deficiency is inherited as an X-linked genetic trait. In such cases, the disorder is fully expressed in males only; however, some females who carry one copy of the disease gene (heterozygotes) may have hemolytic anemia.

In addition to The National Organization for Rare Disorders (NORD) listed in Section III, the following organizations in Section II (Disease Specific) and in Section III (Umbrella) and Section IV (Government Agencies) can provide more information:

Association for Neuro-Metabolic Disorders, *III*
Muscular Dystrophy Association, *III*
NIH/National Institute of Child Health and Human Development, *IV*
NIH/National Institute of Diabetes, Digestive & Kidney Diseases, *IV*
Research Trust for Metabolic Diseases in Children, *III*

826 PICA

Pica is an eating disorder that is characterized by the repeated eating of non-nutritive substances over a period of one month or longer. Patients may eat non-edible objects such as paint, plaster, dirt, ice, or laundry starch. Pica generally affects small children, pregnant women, and people whose cultural environment is most compatible with the eating of non-food items.

In addition to The National Organization for Rare Disorders (NORD) listed in Section III, the following organizations in Section II (Disease Specific) and in Section III (Umbrella) and Section IV (Government Agencies) can provide more information:

Centers for Disease Control and Prevention, *IV*
Federation of Families for Children's Mental Health, *III*
NIH/National Institute of Diabetes, Digestive and Kidney Diseases, *IV*
NIH/National Institute of Mental Health, *IV*
National Alliance for the Mentally Ill, *III*
National Mental Health Association, *III*
National Mental Health Consumer Self-Help Clearinghouse, *III*

827 PICK'S DISEASE

Pick's Disease is a very rare progressive disease that affects certain areas of the brain (i.e., temporal and frontal lobes). Symptoms of this disorder may include loss of intellectual abilities and changes in behavior (e.g., lack of inhibition) and personality. Affected individuals may exhibit confusion and a general lack of concern about their surroundings. Other symptoms may include unusual speech patterns and the repetition of another's words (echolalia). In the majority of cases, the exact cause of Pick's Disease is not known; however, about 10 to 20 percent of cases are thought to be inherited as an autosomal dominant genetic trait.

In addition to The National Organization for Rare Disorders (NORD) listed in Section III, the following organizations in Section II (Disease Specific) and in Section III (Umbrella) and Section IV (Government Agencies) can provide more information:

Alzheimer's Association, *II*
Alzheimer's Disease Education and Referral Center, *II*
NIH/National Institute of Neurological Disorders and Stroke, *IV*
NIH/National Institute on Aging, *IV*

828 PIERRE ROBIN SYNDROME

Pierre Robin Syndrome is characterized by a combination of three features, possibly due to the underdevelopment of the lower jaw. The lower jaw is abnormally small (micrognathia), the tongue is displaced downwards (glossoptosis), and there is an abnormal opening in the roof of the mouth (cleft soft palate).

In addition to The National Organization for Rare Disorders (NORD) listed in Section III, the following organizations in Section II (Disease Specific) and in Section III (Umbrella) and Section IV (Government Agencies) can provide more information:
Congenital Heart Anomalies, Support, Education, & Resources, *III*
FACES: The National Craniofacial Association, *III*
NIH/National Institute of Child Health and Human Development, *IV*
Prescription Parents (for parents of children with cleft lip and palate), *III*
Wide Smiles, *III*

829 PINTA

Pinta is an infectious disease characterized by skin rashes and discoloration. It is caused by the spiral-shaped bacterium Treponema carateum, which is transmitted by direct, nonsexual contact. This disease is most common in tropical areas such as the lowlands of South and Central America. Pinta is rare in the United States.

In addition to The National Organization for Rare Disorders (NORD) listed in Section III, the following organizations in Section II (Disease Specific) and in Section III (Umbrella) and Section IV (Government Agencies) can provide more information:
Centers for Disease Control and Prevention, *IV*
NIH/National Institute of Allergy and Infectious Diseases, *IV*
World Health Organization (WHO) Regional Office for the Americas (AMRO), *III*

830 PITYRIASIS RUBRA PILARIS

Pityriasis Rubra Pilaris is a mildly itchy chronic skin disorder that is possibly caused by an inherited metabolic defect. Initially, the disorder is characterized by elevated spots (papules) on the skin. These spots grow and become connected, producing red plaques over large areas.

In addition to The National Organization for Rare Disorders (NORD) listed in Section III, the following organizations in Section II (Disease Specific) and in Section III (Umbrella) and Section IV (Government Agencies) can provide more information:
Foundation for Ichthyosis & Related Skin Types, *III*
NIH/National Institute of Arthritis and Musculoskeletal and Skin Diseases, *IV*

831 PNEUMONIA, EOSINOPHILIC

Eosinophilic pneumonia is a disorder characterized by an inflammation of the lungs and an abnormal increase in the number of certain white blood cells (eosinophils) in the lymph nodes, lungs and blood. This disorder is usually associated with allergic conditions and various parasitic infections.

In addition to The National Organization for Rare Disorders (NORD) listed in Section III, the following organizations in Section II (Disease Specific) and in Section III (Umbrella) and Section IV (Government Agencies) can provide more information:
Centers for Disease Control and Prevention, *IV*
NIH/National Institute of Allergy and Infectious Diseases, *IV*

832 PNEUMONIA, INTERSTITIAL

Interstitial Pneumonia, involving the spaces and tissue (interstices) of the lungs, is a type of primary pneumonia. It involves an abnormal increase in the interstitial tissue and a decrease and hardening (induration) of other lung tissue. Major symptoms may include shortness of breath on exertion, cough (which may or may not be present) and loss of appetite.

In addition to The National Organization for Rare Disorders (NORD) listed in Section III, the following organizations in Section II (Disease Specific) and in Section III (Umbrella) and Section IV (Government Agencies) can provide more information:
American Lung Association, *III*
NIH/National Heart, Lung and Blood Institute Information Center, *IV*

833 POLAND SYNDROME

Poland Syndrome is an extremely rare developmental disorder that is present at birth (congenital). It is characterized by absence (agenesis) or underdevelopment (hypoplasia) of certain muscles of the chest (e.g., pectoralis major, pectoralis minor, and/or other nearby muscles), and abnormally short, webbed fingers (symbrachydactyly). Additional findings may include underdevelopment or absence of one nipple (including the darkened area around the nipple [areola]) and/or patchy hair growth under the arm (axilla). In females, one breast may also be underdeveloped (hypoplastic) or absent (amastia). In some cases, affected individuals may also exhibit underdeveloped upper ribs and/or an abnormally short arm with underdeveloped forearm bones (i.e., ulna and radius) on the affected side (ipsilateral). In most cases, physical abnormalities are confined to one side of the body (unilateral). In approximately 75 percent of the cases, the right side of the body is affected. The range and severity of symptoms may vary from case to case. The exact cause of Poland Syndrome is not known.

In addition to The National Organization for Rare Disorders (NORD) listed in Section III, the following organizations in Section II (Disease Specific) and in Section III (Umbrella) and Section IV (Government Agencies) can provide more information:
CHERUB—Association of Families and Friends of Children with Limb Disorders, *III*
NIH/National Arthritis and Musculoskeletal and Skin Diseases Information Clearinghouse, *IV*
NIH/National Institute of Child Health and Human Development, *IV*

834 POLYARTERITIS NODOSA

Polyarteritis Nodosa, a rare multisystem disorder that usually becomes apparent between the ages of 40 to 50 years, is characterized by widespread inflammation, weakening, and degeneration of small- and medium-sized arteries. Blood vessels in any organ or organ system may be affected including arteries supplying the kidneys, heart, intestine, nervous system, and/or skeletal muscles. Damage to affected arteries may result in abnormally increased blood pressure (hypertension), "ballooning" (aneurysm) of an arterial wall, the formation of blood clots (thrombosis), obstruction of blood supply to certain tissues, and/or tissue damage and loss (necrosis) in certain affected areas. In many cases, affected individuals experience weight loss, fever, a general feeling of ill health (malaise), fatigue, weakness, headache, muscle aches (myalgias), and/or abdominal pain. Other symptoms and findings are often present and depend upon which areas of the body are affected. Although the exact cause of Polyarteritis Nodosa is not known, many researchers suspect that the disorder is due to disturbances of the bodys immune system.

In addition to The National Organization for Rare Disorders (NORD) listed in Section III, the following organizations in Section II (Disease Specific) and in Section III (Umbrella) and Section IV (Government Agencies) can provide more information:
American Autoimmune Related Diseases Association, Inc., *III*
NIH/National Institute of Allergy and Infectious Diseases, *IV*

835 POLYCHONDRITIS

Polychondritis is a rare degenerative disease characterized by recurrent inflammation of the cartilage in the body. Deterioration of the cartilage may affect any site of the body where cartilage is present. Ears, larynx and trachea may become "floppy," and the bridge of the nose can collapse into a "saddlenose" shape. The aortic heart valve may also be affected.

In addition to The National Organization for Rare Disorders (NORD) listed in Section III, the following organizations in Section II (Disease Specific) and in Section III (Umbrella) and Section IV (Government Agencies) can provide more information:
Arthritis Foundation, *III*
NIH/National Arthritis and Musculoskeletal and Skin Diseases Information Clearinghouse, *IV*

836 POLYCYSTIC KIDNEY DISEASES

Polycystic Kidney Diseases are inherited renal disorders characterized by the presence of multiple cysts in both kidneys (bilateral renal cysts). Normal kidney tissue is replaced by fluid-filled sacs or cysts of varying sizes that become larger as the disease progresses. Symptoms of Polycystic Kidney Diseases include abnormally high blood pressure (hypertension) and the progressive loss of kidney function, leading to end-stage renal failure. Other symptoms may include enlarged kidneys, vomiting, and/or failure to thrive. Most infants with Autosomal Recessive Polycystic Kidney Disease also have unusual facial features (Potter's face).

There are two major subdivisions of Polycystic Kidney Diseases. Autosomal Recessive Polycystic Kidney Disease (ARPKD) includes four subdivisions: Perinatal, Neonatal, Infantile, and Juvenile. The different forms of the disease are based on the age at onset, which frequently correlates with the rate of progression and severity of the symptoms.

The second major subdivision is Autosomal Dominant Polycystic Kidney Disease (ADPKD). This form of the disease affects adults, and the symptoms typically progress more slowly than in Autosomal Recessive Polycystic Kidney Disease.

In addition to The National Organization for Rare Disorders (NORD) listed in Section III, the following organizations in Section II (Disease Specific) and in Section III (Umbrella) and Section IV (Government Agencies) can provide more information:
Alliance of Genetic Support Groups, *III*
American Foundation for Urologic Disease, *III*
American Kidney Fund, Inc., *III*
International Patient Advocacy Association, *III*
NIH/National Kidney and Urologic Diseases Information Clearinghouse, *IV*

National Hypertension Association, Inc., *II*
National Kidney Foundation, *III*
PKR (Polycystic Kidney Research) Foundation, *II*

837 POLYCYSTIC LIVER DISEASE

Polycystic Liver Disease (PLD) is an inherited disorder characterized by many cysts in the liver. Abdominal discomfort from swelling of the liver may occur; however, most affected individuals do not have any symptoms. In some cases, Polycystic Liver Disease appears to occur randomly, with no apparent cause (sporadically). Other cases are thought to be inherited as an autosomal dominant genetic trait.

In addition to The National Organization for Rare Disorders (NORD) listed in Section III, the following organizations in Section II (Disease Specific) and in Section III (Umbrella) and Section IV (Government Agencies) can provide more information:
American Liver Foundation, *III*
NIH/National Institute of Diabetes, Digestive and Kidney Diseases, *IV*
United Liver Association, *III*

838 POLYCYTHEMIA VERA

Polycythemia vera is a rare chronic myeloproliferative disorder characterized by overproduction of red blood cells and elements of the bone marrow involved in the formation of red blood cells (hematopoietic elements). In most cases, affected individuals may experience headaches, weakness, dizziness (vertigo), and/or a ringing noise in the ear (tinnitus). In some cases, individuals with polycythemia vera experience itching (pruritis), especially after a hot bath. Affected individuals often have an abnormally enlarged spleen (splenomegaly) and/or liver (hepatomegaly). In some cases, affected individuals may have associated conditions including high blood pressure (hypertension), the formation of blood clots (thrombosis), rupturing of and loss of blood (hemorrhaging) from certain blood vessels, and/or Budd-Chiari Syndrome, a rare disorder characterized by obstruction (occlusion) of veins of the liver (hepatic veins). The exact cause of polycythemia vera is not known.

In addition to The National Organization for Rare Disorders (NORD) listed in Section III, the following organizations in Section II (Disease Specific) and in Section III (Umbrella) and Section IV (Government Agencies) can provide more information:
MPD (Myeloproliferative Disease) Research Center, Inc., *III*
NIH/National Heart, Lung and Blood Institute, *IV*

839 POLYGLUCOSAN BODY DISEASE, ADULT

Adult Polyglucosan Body Disease is a rare progressive neurological disorder characterized by the accumulation of microscopic material (polyglucosan bodies), predominantly in skeletal muscle nerve cells (motor neurons). The disorder typically affects both upper and lower motor neurons, resulting in nerve damage within the brain and/or spinal cord (central nervous system). Symptoms usually begin during middle age or later and may include muscle weakness, loss of sensation, and/or wasting of muscles (atrophy) in the arms and/or legs. Impaired bladder control (neurogenic bladder) and/or mental confusion (dementia) may also occur.

In addition to The National Organization for Rare Disorders (NORD) listed in Section III, the following organizations in Section II (Disease Specific) and in Section III (Umbrella) and Section IV (Government Agencies) can provide more information:
Amyotrophic Lateral Sclerosis Association, *II*
Association for Neuro-Metabolic Disorders, *III*
NIH/National Institute of Neurological Disorders and Stroke, *IV*

840 POLYMYALGIA RHEUMATICA

Polymyalgia Rheumatica is a rare inflammatory disease characterized by muscle pain, stiffness, and other generalized systemic symptoms such as fatigue, low-grade fever, and/or a general feeling of ill health (malaise). Polymyalgia Rheumatica can be a relatively benign condition that is extremely responsive to treatment. In some rare cases, permanent muscle weakness, loss of muscle mass (atrophy), and disability may occur. The exact cause of Polymyalgia Rheumatica is not known, although immunological factors and familial tendencies (genetic predisposition) have been mentioned in the medical literature.

Polymyalgia Rheumatica and Giant Cell Arteritis, a chronic inflammatory disease characterized by progressive inflammation of many arteries of the body, are known to be associated and have been described in the medical literature as possible variants of the same disease process. The exact nature of the association is not fully understood.

In addition to The National Organization for Rare Disorders (NORD) listed in Section III, the following organizations in Section II (Disease Specific) and in Section III (Umbrella) and Section IV (Government Agencies) can provide more information:

Arthritis Foundation, *III*
NIH/National Institute of Arthritis and Musculoskeletal and Skin Diseases, *IV*

841 POLYMYOSITIS

Polymyositis is a systemic connective tissue disorder characterized by inflammatory and degenerative changes in the muscles, leading to symmetric weakness and some degree of muscle atrophy. The areas principally affected are the hip, shoulders, arms, pharynx and neck.

In addition to The National Organization for Rare Disorders (NORD) listed in Section III, the following organizations in Section II (Disease Specific) and in Section III (Umbrella) and Section IV (Government Agencies) can provide more information:
Arthritis Foundation, *III*
British Coalition of Heritable Disorders of Connective Tissue, *III*
Muscular Dystrophy Association, *III*
Myositis Association of America, Inc., *III*
NIH/National Institute of Child Health and Human Development, *IV*

842 POLYPOSIS, FAMILIAL

Familial Polyposis is a group of rare inherited disorders of the gastrointestinal system. Initially the disorder is characterized by benign growths (adenomatous polyps) in the mucous lining of the gastrointestinal tract. If left untreated, affected individuals usually develop cancer of the colon and/or rectum.

In addition to The National Organization for Rare Disorders (NORD) listed in Section III, the following organizations in Section II (Disease Specific) and in Section III (Umbrella) and Section IV (Government Agencies) can provide more information:
Alliance of Genetic Support Groups, *III*
American Cancer Society, Inc., *III*
Intestinal Multiple Polyposis and Colorectal Cancer Registry, *III*
March of Dimes Birth Defects Foundation, *III*
NIH/National Digestive Diseases Information Clearinghouse, *IV*
NIH/Patient Referral Services Unit, *IV*
Roswell Park Family Cancer Registry, *III*
Steve Antanas Stavro Familial Gastrointestinal Cancer Registry, *II*
Strang-Cornell Hereditary Colon Cancer Program, *II*
United Ostomy Association, Inc., *III*

843 POMPE DISEASE

Pompe Disease is a glycogen storage disease. This hereditary metabolic disorder is caused by an inborn lack of the enzyme alpha-1,4 glucosidase (lysosomal glucosidase; acid maltase). This enzyme deficiency causes excess amounts of glycogen to accumulate in the lysosomes of all body tissues, due to an inability to break down the glycogen. The glycogen accumulates in the lysosomes, which swell and cause cell damage.

In addition to The National Organization for Rare Disorders (NORD) listed in Section III, the following organizations in Section II (Disease Specific) and in Section III (Umbrella) and Section IV (Government Agencies) can provide more information:
Acid Maltase Deficiency Association, Inc., *II*
Association for Glycogen Storage Disease, *III*
Association for Neuro-Metabolic Disorders, *III*
Metabolic Information Network, *III*
Muscular Dystrophy Association, *III*
NIH/National Institute of Diabetes, Digestive and Kidney Diseases, *IV*
Research Trust for Metabolic Diseases in Children, *III*
Vaincre Les Maladies Lysosomales, *III*

844 POPLITEAL PTERYGIUM SYNDROME

Popliteal Pterygium Syndrome is an extremely rare inherited disorder that is apparent at birth (congenital). It is characterized by webbed skin (pterygium) on the backs of both legs (popliteal) and between the legs (intercrural), characteristic facial abnormalities, and malformations of the genitalia. Facial abnormalities may include incomplete closure of the roof of mouth (cleft palate), a vertical groove in the upper lip (cleft lip), and/or depressions or "pits" near the center (paramedian) of the lower lip. Other physical findings may include underdevelopment (hypoplasia) of the genitals and/or webbing or fusion of the fingers and/or toes (syndactyly). The range and severity of the symptoms associated with Popliteal Pterygium Syndrome vary greatly from case to case. Popliteal Pterygium Syndrome is believed to be inherited as an autosomal dominant genetic trait.

In addition to The National Organization for Rare Disorders (NORD) listed in Section III, the following organizations in Section II (Disease Specific) and in Section III (Umbrella) and Section IV (Government Agencies) can provide more information:
AboutFace U.S.A., *III*
Children's Craniofacial Association, *III*
Cleft Palate Foundation, *III*
Forward Face, Inc., *III*
NIH/National Arthritis and Musculoskeletal and Skin Diseases Information Clearinghouse, *IV*
NIH/National Institute of Child Health and Human Development, *IV*
Wide Smiles, *III*

845 **PORPHYRIA**

Porphyria is a group of at least seven metabolic disorders characterized by excess accumulation of the natural chemicals "porphyrins" or "porphyrin precursors" in the body. The different types vary in their clinical presentation. Clinical findings associated with the disorders generally include skin (cutaneous) or nervous system manifestations. Sometimes these symptoms are so ill-defined that proper diagnosis is delayed. The urine of some patients is a purple-red color or changes to that color when exposed to light.

In addition to The National Organization for Rare Disorders (NORD) listed in Section III, the following organizations in Section II (Disease Specific) and in Section III (Umbrella) and Section IV (Government Agencies) can provide more information:
American Porphyria Foundation, *III*
Canadian Porphyria Foundation, Inc., *II*
NIH/National Digestive Diseases Information Clearinghouse, *IV*

846 **PORPHYRIA CUTANEA TARDA**

Porphyria Cutanea Tarda (PCT) is the most common of the porphyrias. It results from a deficiency of the enzyme uroporphyrinogen decarboxylase (URO-D). The disorder can be caused by either inherited or acquired factors. PCT is one of the "hepatic" porphyrias, and large amounts of porphyrins can build up in the liver when the disease is active. When inherited, the enzyme deficiency is inherited as an autosomal dominant trait. In most individuals with the inherited enzyme deficiency, the disease remains latent and may never be symptomatic.

The porphyrias are a group of at least seven disorders. The common feature in all porphyrias is the excess accumulation in the body of "porphyrins" or "porphyrin precursors." These are natural chemicals that normally do not accumulate in the body. Precisely which one of these porphyrin chemicals builds up depends upon the type of porphyria that a patient has.

Porphyrias can also be classified into two groups: the "hepatic" and "erythropoietic" types. Porphyrins and related substances originate in excess amounts from the liver in the hepatic types, and mostly from the bone marrow in the erythropoietic types.

The porphyrias with skin manifestations are sometimes called "cutaneous porphyrias." The "acute porphyrias" are characterized by sudden attacks of pain and other neurological manifestations. These "acute" symptoms can be both rapidly appearing and severe. An individual may be considered in a "latent" condition if he or she has the characteristic enzyme deficiency but has never developed symptoms. There can be a wide spectrum of severity between the "latent" and "active" cases of any particular type of porphyria. The symptoms and treatments of the different types of porphyrias are not the same.

In addition to The National Organization for Rare Disorders (NORD) listed in Section III, the following organizations in Section II (Disease Specific) and in Section III (Umbrella) and Section IV (Government Agencies) can provide more information:
American Porphyria Foundation, *III*
Canadian Porphyria Foundation, Inc., *II*
Metabolic Information Network, *III*
NIH/National Digestive Diseases Information Clearinghouse, *IV*
Research Trust for Metabolic Diseases in Children, *III*

847 **PORPHYRIA, ALA-D**

ALA-D porphyria, a recently described form of acute porphyria, is inherited as an autosomal recessive trait and seems to be extremely rare. This form of porphyria is one of the "hepatic" porphyrias.

The Porphyrias are a group of at least seven disorders. The common feature in all porphyrias is the excess accumulation in the body of "porphyrins" or "porphyrin precursors." These are natural chemicals that normally do not accumulate in the body. Precisely which one of these porphyrin chemicals builds up depends upon the type of porphyria that a patient has.

Porphyrias can also be classified into two groups: the "hepatic" and "erythropoietic" types. Porphyrins and related substances originate in excess amounts from the liver in the hepatic types, and mostly from the bone marrow in the erythropoietic types.

The porphyrias with skin manifestations are sometimes called "cutaneous porphyrias." The "acute porphyrias" are characterized by sudden attacks of pain and other neurological manifestations. These acute symptoms can be both rapidly-appearing and severe. An individual may be considered in a "latent" condition if he or she has the characteristic enzyme deficiency, but has never developed symptoms. There can be a wide spectrum of severity between the "latent" and "active" cases of any particular type of this disorder. The symptoms and treatments of the different types of porphyrias are not the same.

In addition to The National Organization for Rare Disorders (NORD) listed in Section III, the following organizations in Section II (Disease Specific) and in Section III (Umbrella) and Section IV (Government Agencies) can provide more information:
American Porphyria Foundation, *III*
Canadian Porphyria Foundation, Inc., *II*
Metabolic Information Network, *III*
NIH/National Digestive Diseases Information Clearinghouse, *IV*
Research Trust for Metabolic Diseases in Children, *III*

848 PORPHYRIA, ACUTE INTERMITTENT

Acute Intermittent Porphyria (AIP) is one of a group of hereditary hepatic Porphyrias. It is inherited as an autosomal dominant trait. The deficient enzyme is porphobilinogen deaminase (PBG-D), also known as uroporphyrinogen I-synthase. This enzyme deficiency by itself is not sufficient to produce symptoms of the disease. Other factors must also be present such as hormones, drugs and dietary changes that trigger the appearance of symptoms.

The Porphyrias are a group of at least seven disorders. The common feature in all porphyrias is the excess accumulation in the body of "porphyrins" or "porphyrin precursors." These are natural chemicals that normally do not accumulate in the body. Precisely which one of these porphyrin chemicals builds up depends upon the type of Porphyria that a patient has.

Porphyrias can also be classified into two groups: the "hepatic" and "erythropoietic" types. In the hepatic types of Porphyria porphyrins and related substances originate in excess amounts from the liver, and mostly from the bone marrow in the erythropoietic types.

The Porphyrias with skin manifestations are sometimes called "cutaneous Porphyrias." The "acute Porphyrias" are characterized by sudden attacks of pain and other neurological symptoms. These "acute" symptoms can be both rapidly-appearing and severe. An individual may be considered in a "latent" condition if he or she has the characteristic enzyme deficiency but has never developed symptoms. There can be a wide spectrum of severity between the "latent" and "active" cases of any particular type of Porphyria. The symptoms and treatments of the different types of Porphyrias are not the same.

In addition to The National Organization for Rare Disorders (NORD) listed in Section III, the following organizations in Section II (Disease Specific) and in Section III (Umbrella) and Section IV (Government Agencies) can provide more information:
Alliance of Genetic Support Groups, *III*
American Porphyria Foundation, *III*
Canadian Porphyria Foundation, Inc., *II*
Metabolic Information Network, *III*
NIH/National Digestive Diseases Information Clearinghouse, *IV*
Research Trust for Metabolic Diseases in Children, *III*

849 PORPHYRIA, CONGENITAL ERYTHROPOIETIC

Congenital Erythropoietic Porphyria (CEP) is extremely rare and is inherited through an autosomal recessive trait. It is also known as Guenther Porphyria. The deficient enzyme is uroporphyrinogen III cosynthase. As is characteristic of the erythropoietic porphyrias, symptoms usually begin during infancy. CEP is manifested by markedly increased levels of porphyrins in bone marrow, red blood cells, plasma, urine and feces. Porphyrins are also deposited in the teeth and bones.

The Porphyrias are a group of at least seven disorders. The common feature in all porphyrias is the excess accumulation in the body of "porphyrins" or "porphyrin precursors." These are natural chemicals that normally do not accumulate in the body. Precisely which one of these porphyrin chemicals builds up depends upon the type of porphyria that a patient has.

Porphyrias can also be classified into two groups: the "hepatic" and "erythropoietic" types. Porphyrins and related substances originate in excess amounts from the liver in the hepatic types, and mostly from the bone marrow in the erythropoietic types.

The porphyrias with skin manifestations are sometimes called "cutaneous porphyrias." The "acute porphyrias" are those characterized by sudden attacks of pain and other neurological manifestations. These acute symptoms can be both rapidly-appearing and severe. An individual may be considered in a "latent" condition if he or she has the characteristic enzyme deficiency, but has never developed symptoms. There can be a wide spectrum of severity between the "latent" and "active" cases of any particular type of this disorder. The symptoms and treatments of the different types of porphyrias are not the same.

In addition to The National Organization for Rare Disorders (NORD) listed in Section III, the following organizations in Section II (Disease Specific) and in Section III (Umbrella) and Section IV (Government Agencies) can provide more information:
American Porphyria Foundation, *III*
Canadian Porphyria Foundation, Inc., *II*
Metabolic Information Network, *III*
NIH/National Digestive Diseases Information Clearinghouse, *IV*
Research Trust for Metabolic Diseases in Children, *III*

850 PORPHYRIA, HEREDITARY COPROPORPHYRIA

Hereditary Coproporphyria is an autosomal dominant form of hepatic porphyria that is very similar to Acute Intermittent Porphyria, although it is usually a less severe disease. It is caused by an enzyme deficiency. Some patients develop skin photosensitivity, and must avoid sunlight. The diagnosis is established by finding excess coproporphyrin in urine and stool (other types of porphyrins show little or no increase). Urinary ALA and PBG are increased during acute attacks, but may become normal on recovery.

The Porphyrias are a group of at least seven disorders. The common feature in all porphyrias is the excess accumulation in the body of "porphyrins" or "porphyrin precursors." These are natural chemicals that normally do not accumulate in the body. Precisely which one of these porphyrin chemicals builds up depends upon the type of porphyria that a patient has.

Porphyrias can also be classified into two groups: the "hepatic" and "erythropoietic" types. Porphyrins and related substances originate in excess amounts from the liver in the hepatic types, and mostly from the bone marrow in the erythropoietic types.

The porphyrias with skin manifestations are sometimes called "cutaneous porphyrias." The "acute porphyrias" are characterized by sudden attacks of pain and other neurological manifestations. These acute symptoms can be both rapidly-appearing and severe. An individual may be considered in a "latent" condition if he or she has the characteristic enzyme deficiency, but has never developed symptoms. There can be a wide spectrum of severity between the "latent" and "active" cases of any particular type of this disorder. The symptoms and treatments of the different types of porphyrias are not the same.

In addition to The National Organization for Rare Disorders (NORD) listed in Section III, the following organizations in Section II (Disease Specific) and in Section III (Umbrella) and Section IV (Government Agencies) can provide more information:
American Porphyria Foundation, *III*
Canadian Porphyria Foundation, Inc., *II*
Metabolic Information Network, *III*
NIH/National Digestive Diseases Information Clearinghouse, *IV*
Research Trust for Metabolic Diseases in Children, *III*

851 PORPHYRIA, VARIEGATE

Variegate Porphyria (VP), a form of hepatic porphyria, is most common in the South African white population and is much less frequent elsewhere. It is an autosomal dominant disorder and may produce acute attacks (as in acute intermittent porphyria) as well as skin photosensitivity. This form of porphyria is also due to an enzyme deficiency.

The diagnosis may be made by finding excess coproporphyrin in urine and both coproporphyrin and protoporphyrin in feces. In patients with photosensitive skin changes alone, it is important to distinguish Varigate Porphyria or hereditary coproporphyria (HCP) from porphyria cutanea tarda (PCT), because treatment by phlebotomy or low-dose chloroquine is not successful in VP and HCP. Acute attacks are managed and may be prevented as in AIP.

The Porphyrias are a group of at least seven disorders. The common feature in all porphyrias is the excess accumulation in the body of "porphyrins" or "porphyrin precursors." These are natural chemicals that normally do not accumulate in the body. Precisely which one of these porphyrin chemicals builds up depends upon the type of porphyria that a patient has.

Porphyrias can also be classified into two groups: the "hepatic" and "erythropoietic" types. Porphyrins and related substances originate in excess amounts from the liver in the hepatic types, and mostly from the bone marrow in the erythropoietic types.

The porphyrias with skin manifestations are sometimes called "cutaneous porphyrias." The "acute porphyrias" are characterized by sudden attacks of pain and other neurological manifestations. These acute symptoms can be both rapidly-appearing and severe. An individual may be considered in a "latent" condition if he or she has the characteristic enzyme deficiency, but has never developed symptoms. There can be a wide spectrum of severity between the "latent" and "active" cases of any particular type of this disorder. The symptoms and treatments of the different types of porphyrias are not the same.

In addition to The National Organization for Rare Disorders (NORD) listed in Section III, the following organizations in Section II (Disease Specific) and in Section III (Umbrella) and Section IV (Government Agencies) can provide more information:

American Porphyria Foundation, *III*
Canadian Porphyria Foundation, Inc., *II*
Metabolic Information Network, *III*
NIH/National Digestive Diseases Information Clearinghouse, *IV*
Research Trust for Metabolic Diseases in Children, *III*

852 POST POLIO SYNDROME

Post-Polio Syndrome is characterized by a history of Poliomyelitis at least ten years previously, and partial recovery of function followed by development of progressive weakness in previously affected muscles for which there is no other definite cause. The exact cause of Post-Polio Syndrome is not fully understood.

In addition to The National Organization for Rare Disorders (NORD) listed in Section III, the following organizations in Section II (Disease Specific) and in Section III (Umbrella) and Section IV (Government Agencies) can provide more information:

Centers for Disease Control and Prevention, *IV*
International Polio Network, *II*
Polio Society, *II*

853 POSTERIOR UVEITIS

Posterior Uveitis is a vision disorder characterized by inflammation of the layer of blood vessels underlying the retina, and usually of the retina as well. Major symptoms include blurred vision, distortion of the size or shape of objects (metamorphopsia), and floating black spots in the visual field. The resulting scars may impair clear vision and cause dimness of vision (amblyopia). In many cases, this disorder occurs as a complication of Toxoplasmosis or other infections. In other cases, the cause cannot be determined.

In addition to The National Organization for Rare Disorders (NORD) listed in Section III, the following organizations in Section II (Disease Specific) and in Section III (Umbrella) and Section IV (Government Agencies) can provide more information:

American Autoimmune Related Diseases Association, Inc., *III*
NIH/National Eye Institute, *IV*
NIH/National Institute of Allergy and Infectious Diseases, *IV*
Vision Foundation, Inc., *III*

854 PRADER WILLI SYNDROME

Prader-Willi syndrome is a complex multisystem disorder that is diagnosed more often in males than females. This disorder is characterized by muscular weakness in the infant (infantile hypotonia), failure to thrive, abnormally decreased function of the testes or ovaries (hypogonadism), short stature and impaired intellectual and behavioral functioning. Hyperphagia (eating excessive amounts of food) leads to severe obesity in early childhood and adolescence.

In addition to The National Organization for Rare Disorders (NORD) listed in Section III, the following organizations in Section II (Disease Specific) and in Section III (Umbrella) and Section IV (Government Agencies) can provide more information:

Alliance of Genetic Support Groups, *III*
March of Dimes Birth Defects Foundation, *III*
NIH/National Institute of Child Health and Human Development, *IV*
Prader-Willi Connection, *II*
Prader-Willi Syndrome Association, *II*
Prader-Willi Syndrome Association, National Headquarters, *II*

855 PRECOCIOUS PUBERTY

Precocious Puberty means an abnormally early onset of puberty. A sequence of events occurs during which a child develops into a young adult beginning at an unexpectedly early age. Glands that secrete growth and sex hormones begin to function abnormally early in life resulting in this condition. The exact cause of Precocious Puberty is not known.

In addition to The National Organization for Rare Disorders (NORD) listed in Section III, the following organizations in Section II (Disease Specific) and in Section III (Umbrella) and Section IV (Government Agencies) can provide more information:
Brain and Pituitary Foundation of America, *III*
NIH/National Institute of Child Health and Human Development, *IV*
National Adrenal Diseases Foundation, *III*

856 PRIMARY LATERAL SCLEROSIS

Primary Lateral Sclerosis is a rare neurological disease affecting the central motor neurons. The disorder causes progressive muscle weakness in the facial area, hands, arms, legs and feet; spasticity; and hyperactive deep-tendon reflexes of the muscles in these areas.

In addition to The National Organization for Rare Disorders (NORD) listed in Section III, the following organizations in Section II (Disease Specific) and in Section III (Umbrella) and Section IV (Government Agencies) can provide more information:
Amyotrophic Lateral Sclerosis Association, *II*
NIH/National Institute of Neurological Disorders and Stroke, *IV*

857 PROCTITIS

Proctitis is a chronic inflammatory disease arising in the rectum and characterized by bloody diarrhea. There are two types of Proctitis, Ulcerative and Gonnoreal, which are differentiated by the means in which they are contracted. Gonnoreal Proctitis is transmitted through sexual contact.

In addition to The National Organization for Rare Disorders (NORD) listed in Section III, the following organizations in Section II (Disease Specific) and in Section III (Umbrella) and Section IV (Government Agencies) can provide more information:
NIH/National Digestive Diseases Information Clearinghouse, *IV*
Sexuality Information and Education Council of the U.S., *III*

858 PROGRESSIVE OSSEOUS HETEROPLASIA (POH)

Progressive Osseous Heteroplasia (POH) is an extremely rare disorder characterized by abnormal development of bone in areas of the body where bone is not normally present (heterotopic ossification). The disorder first appears as areas of patchy bone formation (ossification) on the skin during infancy; heterotopic ossification progresses to involve superficial and deep connective tissues, areas of fat beneath the skin (subcutaneous fat), muscles, tendons, ligaments, and the bands of fibrous tissues that support muscle (fascia). This abnormal formation of bone may restrict the movement of affected joints and/or hinder the growth of affected limbs. The course of the disease is unpredictable; some areas of the body may become severely affected while others may remain unaffected. The exact cause of Progressive Osseous Heteroplasia is not known.

In addition to The National Organization for Rare Disorders (NORD) listed in Section III, the following organizations in Section II (Disease Specific) and in Section III (Umbrella) and Section IV (Government Agencies) can provide more information:
NIH/National Arthritis and Musculoskeletal and Skin Diseases Information Clearinghouse, *IV*
Progressive Osseous Heteroplasia Association, *II*

859 PROGRESSIVE SUPRANUCLEAR PALSY

Progressive Supranuclear Palsy (PSP) is a rare neurologic disorder characterized by spastic weakness of muscles affected by the cranial nerves (i.e., muscles of the face, throat, tongue). Symptoms may include falling, difficulty walking (ataxia), vision disturbances, and difficulty in speech (dysarthia) and swallowing. The exact cause of this disorder is unknown.

In addition to The National Organization for Rare Disorders (NORD) listed in Section III, the following organizations in Section II (Disease Specific) and in Section III (Umbrella) and Section IV (Government Agencies) can provide more information:
NIH/National Institute of Neurological Disorders and Stroke, *IV*
Society for Progressive Supranuclear Palsy, *III*
WE MOVE, *III*

860 PROSTATITIS

Prostatitis is a common infection of the prostate gland, the gland near the penis that is situated at the base of the male urethra. The prostate secretes an alkaline fluid that is the major ingredient of ejaculatory fluid. Prostatitis is classified into four subcategories: acute bacterial, chronic bacterial, nonbacterial and prostatodynia.

In addition to The National Organization for Rare Disorders (NORD) listed in Section III, the following organizations in Section II (Disease Specific) and in Section III (Umbrella) and Section IV (Government Agencies) can provide more information:
American Foundation for Urologic Disease, *III*
NIH/National Kidney and Urologic Diseases Information Clearinghouse, *IV*

861 PROTEUS SYNDROME

Proteus Syndrome is a very rare hereditary disorder characterized by multiple lesions of the lymph vessels (lipolymphohemangiomas), overgrowth of one side of the body (hemihypertrophy), an abnormally large head (macrocephaly), partial gigantism of the feet, and abnormal coffee-colored (cafe-au-lait) spots on the skin.

In addition to The National Organization for Rare Disorders (NORD) listed in Section III, the following organizations in Section II (Disease Specific) and in Section III (Umbrella) and Section IV (Government Agencies) can provide more information:

HME Contact Group, *II*
NIH/National Arthritis and Musculoskeletal and Skin Diseases Information Clearinghouse, *IV*
Proteus Syndrome Foundation, *II*

862 PRUNE BELLY SYNDROME

Prune-Belly Syndrome, also known as Eagle-Barrett Syndrome, is a rare disorder characterized by partial or complete absence of the stomach (abdominal) muscles, failure of both testes to descend into the scrotum (bilateral cryptorchidism), and/or urinary tract malformations, such as abnormal widening (dilation) of the tubes that bring urine to the bladder (ureters), accumulation of urine in the ureters (hydroureter) and the kidneys (hydronephrosis), and/or backflow of urine from the bladder into the ureters (vesicoureteral reflux). Complications associated with Prune-Belly Syndrome may include underdevelopment of the lungs (pulmonary hypoplasia) and/or chronic renal failure. The exact cause of Prune-Belly Syndrome is not known.

In addition to The National Organization for Rare Disorders (NORD) listed in Section III, the following organizations in Section II (Disease Specific) and in Section III (Umbrella) and Section IV (Government Agencies) can provide more information:

Digestive Disease National Coalition, *III*
NIH/National Arthritis and Musculoskeletal and Skin Diseases Information Clearinghouse, *IV*
NIH/National Digestive Diseases Information Clearinghouse, *IV*
National Prune Belly Syndrome Network, *II*

863 PSEUDO HURLER POLYDYSTROPHY

The Mucolipidoses are a family of hereditary disorders in which enzyme deficiencies cause both complex carbohydrates (mucopolysaccharides) and certain fatty substances (mucolipids) to accumulate in body tissues without excess mucopolysaccharides in the urine. Pseudo-Hurler Polydystrophy (Mucolipidosis III) is a rare inherited metabolic disorder characterized by childhood onset, painless joint stiffness, decreased mobility, short stature, some coarseness of the facial features, mild mental retardation, evidence of multiple defective bone formations (dysostosis multiplex), and aortic valve disease. Pseudo-Hurler Polydystrophy is, in general, a milder form of I-cell disease (ML II), a rare inherited metabolic disorder characterized by multiple abnormalities of the skull and face, growth delays, and/or mental retardation.

In addition to The National Organization for Rare Disorders (NORD) listed in Section III, the following organizations in Section II (Disease Specific) and in Section III (Umbrella) and Section IV (Government Agencies) can provide more information:

Canadian Society for Mucopolysaccharide and Related Diseases, Inc., *III*
Metabolic Information Network, *III*
NIH/National Digestive Diseases Information Clearinghouse, *IV*
National MPS (Mucopolysaccharidoses/Mucolipidoses) Society, Inc., *III*
Research Trust for Metabolic Diseases in Children, *III*
The Arc (a national organization on mental retardation), *III*
Vaincre Les Maladies Lysosomales, *III*

864 PSEUDOCHOLINESTERASE DEFICIENCY

Pseudocholinesterase Deficiency is a rare genetic disorder. Individuals with this disorder have a deficiency or absence of the plasma enzyme pseudocholinesterase, which can cause respiratory difficulty during surgery if the muscle-relaxing drug succinylcholine is used.

In addition to The National Organization for Rare Disorders (NORD) listed in Section III, the following organizations in Section II (Disease Specific) and in Section III (Umbrella) and Section IV (Government Agencies) can provide more information:

Malignant Hyperthermia Association of the United States, *II*
NIH/National Institute of General Medical Sciences, *IV*
North American Malignant Hyperthermia Registry, *II*

865 PSEUDOHYPOPARATHYROIDISM

Pseudohypoparathyroidism is a hereditary disorder characterized by an inadequate response to the parathyroid hormone, although the hormone is present in normal amounts. This inadequate response affects bone growth in individuals with Pseudohypoparathyroidism. Affected individuals may also experience headaches, unusual sensations, weakness, easy fatigue, lack of energy, blurred vision, and/or abnormal sensitivity (hypersensitivity) to light. Additional symptoms and findings may include stiffness or cramps in the arms and/or legs, palpitations, and/or abdominal pain. In addition, individuals with Pseudohypoparathyroidism may have an abnormally round face, thick short stature, unusually short fourth fingers, and mental retardation. Hormonal and calcium replacement therapy is often helpful, but the lack of growth may persist.

In addition to The National Organization for Rare Disorders (NORD) listed in Section III, the following organizations in Section II (Disease Specific) and in Section III (Umbrella) and Section IV (Government Agencies) can provide more information:
NIH/National Digestive Diseases Information Clearinghouse, *IV*

866 PSEUDOMYXOMA PERITONEI

Pseudomyxoma Peritonei is a rare malignant growth characterized by the progressive accumulation of mucus-secreting (mucinous) tumor cells within the abdomen and pelvis. The disorder develops after a small growth (polyp) located within the appendix bursts through the wall of the appendix, and spreads mucus-producing tumor cells throughout the surrounding surfaces (e.g., the membrane that lines the abdominal cavity [peritoneum]). As mucinous tumor cells accumulate, the abdominal area becomes swollen and digestive (gastrointestinal) function becomes impaired. Pseudomyxoma Peritonei develops at a variable rate, but may grow at a slower rate (indolent) than other malignancies within the abdomen.

In addition to The National Organization for Rare Disorders (NORD) listed in Section III, the following organizations in Section II (Disease Specific) and in Section III (Umbrella) and Section IV (Government Agencies) can provide more information:
American Cancer Society, Inc., *III*
NIH/National Cancer Institute, *IV*

867 PSEUDOTUMOR CEREBRI

Pseudotumor cerebri is a condition characterized by increased pressure inside the skull (intracranial pressure), headache, nausea, vomiting, and swelling of the optic disk (papilledema), the portion of the optic nerve that enters the eye and joins the nerve-rich membrane lining the eye (retina). (The optic nerves are the pair of nerves [second cranial nerves] that transmit impulses from the retinas to the brain.) In some cases, papilledema may cause progressive visual loss and/or impairment of one of the cranial nerve pairs (sixth cranial nerves [nervus abducens]) arising from the brain (cranial nerve palsy). The sixth cranial nerves control the muscles (lateral rectus muscles) that turn the eyes outward. Although the symptoms and findings associated with Pseudotumor cerebri are similar to those that may occur due to certain brain tumors, no tumor is involved in individuals with Pseudotumor cerebri.

Pseudotumor cerebri most commonly occurs in young, obese females. In most cases, the exact cause of Pseudotumor cerebri is unknown. However, in some cases, the condition appears to occur in association with pregnancy, use of sex hormones, certain parathyroid or adrenal gland disorders, or other underlying disorders, conditions, or other factors.

In addition to The National Organization for Rare Disorders (NORD) listed in Section III, the following organizations in Section II (Disease Specific) and in Section III (Umbrella) and Section IV (Government Agencies) can provide more information:
Brain and Pituitary Foundation of America, *III*
NIH/National Institute of Neurological Disorders and Stroke, *IV*
Pseudotumor Cerebri Society, *II*

868 PSEUDOXANTHOMA ELASTICUM (PXE)

Pseudoxanthoma Elasticum (PXE) is a rare connective tissue disease that is inherited and progressive and affects the elastic tissues of the body. Abnormal accumulations of calcium salts (calcifications) within elastic fibers of the skin, eyes, and cardiovascular system (i.e., heart and blood vessels) result in the physical abnormalities and features associated with Pseudoxanthoma Elasticum. Small, raised yellowish bumps (papules) initially develop on the skin of the sides of the neck and then gradually involve the skin under the arms (axillae), folds of the arms, groin, and behind the knees. After many years, affected skin may become thickened and folded, especially under the arms. Soon after the skin lesions appear, eye abnormalities develop, usually beginning with colored (pigmented) "mottling" (peau d'orange) on the nerve-rich membrane lining the eyes (retina), followed by the development of "vessel-like" angioid streaks. Later in life, the angioid streaks may be the site of retinal hemorrhages (bleeding) that often lead to loss of central vision but never cause total loss of vision. Cardiovascular abnormalities may include calcification of the walls of certain arteries (arteriosclerosis), which leads to narrowing or blockage (occlusion) of affected arteries and prevents proper blood flow to certain areas of the body, most often in the arms and legs. In addition, arteriosclerosis may lead to abnormally high blood pressure (hypertension) and/or rupturing of and loss of blood (hemorrhaging) from certain blood vessels, especially in the stomach. The range and severity of symptoms vary greatly from case to case. The classic form of Pseudoxanthoma Elasticum is inherited as an autosomal recessive genetic trait. There is a less common autosomal dominant form.

In addition to The National Organization for Rare Disorders (NORD) listed in Section III, the following organizations in Section II (Disease Specific) and in Section III (Umbrella) and Section IV (Government Agencies) can provide more information:

Arthritis Foundation, *III*
British Coalition of Heritable Disorders of Connective Tissue, *III*
NIH/National Eye Institute, *IV*
NIH/National Heart, Lung and Blood Institute Information Center, *IV*
NIH/National Institute of Arthritis and Musculoskeletal and Skin Diseases, *IV*
National Association for Pseudoxanthoma Elasticum, *II*
PXE International, Inc., *II*

869 PSITTACOSIS

Psittacosis is a common infectious disorder found in birds that is transmissible to humans. It rarely occurs in humans but when it does it can spread and become epidemic. In humans it can have very serious and complicated effects. The most prominent symptom is usually pneumonia with associated breathing problems. Other major symptoms may include chills, fever, headache, nausea, vomiting, and muscle pain in the neck and back. These symptoms can mimic many other diseases. A definite diagnosis is necessary for appropriate treatment to begin.

In addition to The National Organization for Rare Disorders (NORD) listed in Section III, the following organizations in Section II (Disease Specific) and in Section III (Umbrella) and Section IV (Government Agencies) can provide more information:

Centers for Disease Control and Prevention, *IV*
NIH/National Institute of Allergy and Infectious Diseases, *IV*

870 PSORIASIS

Psoriasis is a common chronic and recurrent skin disorder characterized by dry, well-circumscribed silvery gray scaling spots (papules) or plaques that usually appear on the scalp, elbows, or knees. Although the exact cause of Psoriasis is not known, a family history of the disorder is common. In such cases, it is thought that the disorder is inherited as an autosomal dominant genetic trait.

In addition to The National Organization for Rare Disorders (NORD) listed in Section III, the following organizations in Section II (Disease Specific) and in Section III (Umbrella) and Section IV (Government Agencies) can provide more information:

NIH/National Arthritis and Musculoskeletal and Skin Diseases Information Clearinghouse, *IV*
National Psoriasis Foundation, *II*
Psoriatic Arthropathy Alliance, *II*

871 PTERYGIUM SYNDROME, MULTIPLE

Multiple Pterygium Syndrome is a very rare disorder that may occur for no apparent reason (sporadically) or be inherited as an autosomal recessive or autosomal dominant genetic trait. This disorder is characterized by multiple joints in a fixed position (contractures), permanently bent fingers (camptodactyly), webbing of the skin, short stature, vertebral abnormalities, drooping eyelids, and/or eyes that slant downward. An abnormally long groove in the middle of the upper lip, a small jaw, cleft palate, low-set ears, a downturned mouth and fusion of vertebrae in the neck may also be found in patients with Multiple Pterygium Syndrome.

In addition to The National Organization for Rare Disorders (NORD) listed in Section III, the following organizations in Section II (Disease Specific) and in Section III (Umbrella) and Section IV (Government Agencies) can provide more information:

NIH/National Arthritis and Musculoskeletal and Skin Diseases Information Clearinghouse, *IV*

872 PULMONARY ALVEOLAR PROTEINOSIS

Pulmonary Alveolar Proteinosis is a rare lung disorder characterized by the filling of the air sacs of the lungs (alveoli) with grainy material consisting mostly of protein and fat. Breathing becomes progressively difficult. The disorder occurs in different forms, ranging from mild to severe.

In addition to The National Organization for Rare Disorders (NORD) listed in Section III, the following organizations in Section II (Disease Specific) and in Section III (Umbrella) and Section IV (Government Agencies) can provide more information:
American Lung Association, *III*
NIH/National Heart, Lung and Blood Institute Information Center, *IV*

873 PULMONARY HYPERTENSION, PRIMARY

Primary Pulmonary Hypertension is a very rare and progressive vascular disease. It is characterized by excessively high pulmonary artery pressure, and multiple lesions that affect the small size arteries (arterioles) that lead to the capillaries of the lungs. These lesions are widespread in the lung. Eventually, there is a reduction in the amount of blood able to be forced out by the right ventricle of the heart.

In addition to The National Organization for Rare Disorders (NORD) listed in Section III, the following organizations in Section II (Disease Specific) and in Section III (Umbrella) and Section IV (Government Agencies) can provide more information:
American Heart Association, *III*
American Lung Association, *III*
Foundation for Pulmonary Hypertension, Inc., *II*
NIH/National Heart, Lung and Blood Institute Information Center, *IV*
Pulmonary Hypertension Association, *II*

874 PULMONARY HYPERTENSION, SECONDARY

Secondary Pulmonary Hypertension is a disorder of the blood vessels in the lungs. It usually is the result of other lung diseases or related diseases in other organs. The disorder is characterized by breathing difficulties, especially after exertion.

In addition to The National Organization for Rare Disorders (NORD) listed in Section III, the following organizations in Section II (Disease Specific) and in Section III (Umbrella) and Section IV (Government Agencies) can provide more information:
American Heart Association, *III*
American Lung Association, *III*
Foundation for Pulmonary Hypertension, Inc., *II*
NIH/National Heart, Lung and Blood Institute Information Center, *IV*
Pulmonary Hypertension Association, *II*

875 PURE RED CELL APLASIA, ACQUIRED

Acquired Pure Red Cell Aplasia is a rare blood disorder characterized by the sudden decline of red blood cells (erythrocytes) produced by the bone marrow. Affected individuals may experience fatigue, lethargy, and/or abnormal paleness of the skin (pallor). Acquired Pure Red Cell Aplasia may occur for unknown reasons (idiopathic) or as a primary autoimmune disorder. It is also believed that Acquired Pure Red Cell Aplasia may occur secondary to a tumor of the thymus gland (thyoma), viral infections, or certain drugs.

In addition to The National Organization for Rare Disorders (NORD) listed in Section III, the following organizations in Section II (Disease Specific) and in Section III (Umbrella) and Section IV (Government Agencies) can provide more information:
American Autoimmune Related Diseases Association, Inc., *III*
Aplastic Anemia Foundation of America, Inc., *II*
NIH/National Heart, Lung and Blood Institute, *IV*

876 PURPURA, HENOCH SCHONLEIN

Henoch-Schonlein Purpura is a rare inflammatory disease of the small blood vessels (capillaries) and is usually a self-limited disease. It is the most common form of childhood vascular inflammation (vasculitis) and results in inflammatory changes in small blood vessels. The symptoms of Henoch-Schonlein Purpura usually begin suddenly and may include headache, fever, loss of appetite, cramping abdominal pain, and joint pain. Red or purple spots typically appear on the skin (petechial purpura). Inflammatory changes associated with Henoch-Schonlein Purpura can also develop in the joints, kidneys, digestive system, and, in rare cases, the brain and spinal cord (central nervous system).

In one form of the disorder, termed Schonlein's Purpura, the skin and joints are affected but the gastrointestinal tract is not. In another form, known as Henoch's Purpura, affected individuals have purpura spots on the skin and acute abdominal problems. People with Henoch's Purpura are not affected by joint disease.

The exact cause of Schonlein-Henoch Purpura is not fully understood, although research suggests that it may be an autoimmune disease or, in some rare cases, an extreme allergic reaction to certain offending substances (e.g., foods or drugs).

In addition to The National Organization for Rare Disorders (NORD) listed in Section III, the following organizations in Section II (Disease Specific) and in Section III (Umbrella) and Section IV (Government

Agencies) can provide more information:
American Autoimmune Related Diseases Association, Inc., *III*
American Kidney Fund, Inc., *III*
NIH/National Heart, Lung and Blood Institute Information Center, *IV*
NIH/National Institute of Allergy and Infectious Diseases, *IV*
National Kidney Foundation, *III*

877 PURPURA, IDIOPATHIC THROMBOCYTOPENIC

Idiopathic Thrombocytopenic Purpura (ITP) is characterized by an abnormal decrease of a certain type of blood cell, called platelets (thrombocytopenia) without a readily apparent cause or underlying disease. The disorder is characterized by abnormal bleeding into the skin. Bleeding from mucous membranes also occurs, and may subsequently result in anemia.

In addition to The National Organization for Rare Disorders (NORD) listed in Section III, the following organizations in Section II (Disease Specific) and in Section III (Umbrella) and Section IV (Government Agencies) can provide more information:
ITP Association, *II*
ITP People Place, *II*
ITP Society, *II*
NIH/Hematology Branch, National Heart, Lung and Blood Institute (NHLBI), *IV*
NIH/National Heart, Lung and Blood Institute Information Center, *IV*

878 PURPURA, THROMBOTIC THROMBOCYTOPENIC

Thrombotic Thrombocytopenia Purpura (TTP) is a rare, serious blood disease. Major symptoms may include a severe decrease in the number of blood platelets (thrombocytopenia), abnormal destruction of red blood cells (hemolytic anemia), and disturbances in the nervous system. Kidney dysfunction and fever are also common.

In addition to The National Organization for Rare Disorders (NORD) listed in Section III, the following organizations in Section II (Disease Specific) and in Section III (Umbrella) and Section IV (Government Agencies) can provide more information:
NIH/National Heart, Lung and Blood Institute Information Center, *IV*

879 PYKNODYSOSTOSIS

Pyknodysostosis is a rare disorder that is inherited as an autosomal recessive genetic trait. This disorder is characterized by short stature; a large skull with a protruding forehead and bulge on the back of the skull; unusually broad hands and feet with abnormally short, brittle nails; a bluish discoloration of the whites of the eyes (sclera); an unusually small face; a receding chin; abnormalities of the teeth; and fragile bones that may fracture easily.

In addition to The National Organization for Rare Disorders (NORD) listed in Section III, the following organizations in Section II (Disease Specific) and in Section III (Umbrella) and Section IV (Government Agencies) can provide more information:
AboutFace U.S.A., *III*
Children's Craniofacial Association, *III*
NIH/National Arthritis and Musculoskeletal and Skin Diseases Information Clearinghouse, *IV*

880 PYODERMA GANGRENOSUM

Pyoderma Gangrenosum is a rare skin disorder of unknown origin. Major symptoms include small pustules that develop into large ulcers at various sites on the body. It may or may not be associated with other illnesses.

In addition to The National Organization for Rare Disorders (NORD) listed in Section III, the following organizations in Section II (Disease Specific) and in Section III (Umbrella) and Section IV (Government Agencies) can provide more information:
American Autoimmune Related Diseases Association, Inc., *III*
Crohn's and Colitis Foundation of America, *III*
NIH/National Arthritis and Musculoskeletal and Skin Diseases Information Clearinghouse, *IV*

881 PYRUVATE CARBOXYLASE DEFICIENCY

Pyruvate Carboxylase Deficiency is a rare genetic metabolic disorder that is present at birth. It is classified as a lactic acidemia in which the conversion of pyruvate to oxaloacetate is blocked, impairing gluconeogenesis and resulting in an overabundance of lactic acid in the blood.

Major symptoms may include delayed development, muscle weakness (hypotonia), impaired ability to control voluntary movements (ataxia), seizures, and vomiting.

In addition to The National Organization for Rare Disorders (NORD) listed in Section III, the following organizations in Section II (Disease Specific) and in Section III (Umbrella) and Section IV (Government Agencies) can provide more information:
Association for Neuro-Metabolic Disorders, *III*
Lactic Acidosis Support Trust, *III*
NIH/National Institute of Diabetes, Digestive & Kidney Diseases, *IV*
NIH/National Institute of Neurological Disorders and Stroke, *IV*

Research Trust for Metabolic Diseases in Children, *III*
United Mitochondrial Disease Foundation, *III*

882 PYRUVATE DEHYDROGENASE DEFICIENCY

Pyruvate Dehydrogenase Deficiency is a rare disorder of carbohydrate metabolism inherited as an X-linked recessive genetic trait. Symptoms are caused by a deficiency of the enzyme pyruvate dehydrogenase resulting in persistent or recurrent metabolic acidosis (acidemia). The disorder is manifested by mental retardation and other neurological symptoms.

In addition to The National Organization for Rare Disorders (NORD) listed in Section III, the following organizations in Section II (Disease Specific) and in Section III (Umbrella) and Section IV (Government Agencies) can provide more information:
Association for Neuro-Metabolic Disorders, *III*
Lactic Acidosis Support Trust, *III*
Metabolic Information Network, *III*
NIH/National Institute of Neurological Disorders and Stroke, *IV*
Organic Acidemia Association, *III*
Research Trust for Metabolic Diseases in Children, *III*
The Arc (a national organization on mental retardation), *III*
United Mitochondrial Disease Foundation, *III*

883 PYRUVATE KINASE DEFICIENCY

Pyruvate Kinase Deficiency is a hereditary blood disorder characterized by a deficiency of the enzyme pyruvate kinase. Physical findings associated with the disorder may include reduced levels of oxygen-carrying hemoglobulin in the blood due to premature destruction of red blood cells (hemolytic anemia); abnormally increased levels of bilirubin in the blood (hyperbilirubinemia); abnormal enlargement of the spleen (splenomegaly); and/or other abnormalities. Pyruvate Kinase Deficiency is inherited as an autosomal recessive genetic trait.

In addition to The National Organization for Rare Disorders (NORD) listed in Section III, the following organizations in Section II (Disease Specific) and in Section III (Umbrella) and Section IV (Government Agencies) can provide more information:
Lactic Acidosis Support Trust, *III*
NIH/National Heart, Lung and Blood Institute, *IV*

884 Q FEVER

Q Fever is an infectious disease that is caused by contact with animals that have the parasitic Rickettsia bacteria, Coxiella burnetii. Major symptoms may include headache, fever, chills, muscle aches, and a general feeling of ill health (malaise).

In addition to The National Organization for Rare Disorders (NORD) listed in Section III, the following organizations in Section II (Disease Specific) and in Section III (Umbrella) and Section IV (Government Agencies) can provide more information:
Centers for Disease Control and Prevention, *IV*
NIH/National Institute of Allergy and Infectious Diseases, *IV*
World Health Organization (WHO) Regional Office for the Americas (AMRO), *III*

885 RABIES

Rabies is an infectious disease that can affect all species of warmblooded animals, including man. This disorder is transmitted by the saliva of an infected animal and is caused by a virus (Neurotropic lyssavirus) that affects the salivary glands and the central nervous system. The symptoms may lead to serious complications if the virus is not treated immediately.

In addition to The National Organization for Rare Disorders (NORD) listed in Section III, the following organizations in Section II (Disease Specific) and in Section III (Umbrella) and Section IV (Government Agencies) can provide more information:
Centers for Disease Control and Prevention, *IV*
NIH/National Institute of Allergy and Infectious Diseases, *IV*
World Health Organization (WHO) Regional Office for the Americas (AMRO), *III*

886 RADIATION SYNDROMES

Radiation syndromes describe the harmful effects—acute, delayed, or chronic—produced by exposure to ionizing radiations. Tissues vary in response to immediate radiation injury according to the following descending order of sensitivity: (1) lymph cells (2) reproductive organs (3) proliferating cells of the bone marrow (4) epithelial cells of the bowel (5) top layer (epidermis) of the skin (6) liver cells (7) epithelium of the little lung sacs (alveoli) and bile passages (8) kidney epithelial cells (9) endothelial cells of the membranes around the lungs, lining the chest cavity (pleura) and the abdominal cavity (peritoneum) (10) nerve cells (11) bone cells (12) muscle and connective tissue. Generally, the more rapid the turnover of the cell, the greater the radiation sensitivity.

In addition to The National Organization for Rare Disorders (NORD) listed in Section III, the following organizations in Section II (Disease Specific) and in Section III (Umbrella) and Section IV (Government

Agencies) can provide more information:
American Cancer Society, Inc., *III*
Leukemia Society of America, Inc., *II*
National Council on Radiation Protection and Measurements, *III*

887 **RAPP HODGKINS SYNDROME**

Rapp-Hodgkins Syndrome, an extremely rare inherited multisystem disorder that is apparent at birth (congenital) or during infancy, belongs to a group of diseases known as Ectodermal Dysplasias. Ectodermal Dysplasias typically affect the skin, teeth, hair, and/or nails. Rapp-Hodgkins Syndrome is characterized by an impaired ability to sweat (hypohidrosis or anhidrosis), causing susceptibility to abnormally increased body temperatures (hyperthermia); incomplete closure of the roof of the mouth (cleft palate) and/or an abnormal groove in the upper lip (cleft lip); and/or absence (hypodontia or partial adontia) and/or abnormal smallness (microdontia) of certain primary (deciduous) and secondary (permanent) teeth. Infants and children with the disorder also have abnormally sparse, coarse, wiry scalp hair that is often lost prematurely during adulthood (alopecia); unusually slow-growing, improperly developed nails (dysplastic); and, in some cases, additional physical abnormalities. Rapp-Hodgkins Syndrome is inherited as an autosomal dominant genetic trait.

In addition to The National Organization for Rare Disorders (NORD) listed in Section III, the following organizations in Section II (Disease Specific) and in Section III (Umbrella) and Section IV (Government Agencies) can provide more information:
AboutFace U.S.A., *III*
Children's Craniofacial Association, *III*
Forward Face, Inc., *III*
NIH/National Arthritis and Musculoskeletal and Skin Diseases Information Clearinghouse, *IV*
National Foundation for Ectodermal Dysplasias, *II*

888 **RAYNAUD'S DISEASE AND PHENOMENON**

Raynaud's Disease is a common vascular disorder characterized by episodes of constriction of very small arteries (arteriole vasospasm) in the fingers and skin. Symptoms in the fingers include unusual paleness, absence of color (pallor), and/or a red or bluish color to the skin (cyanosis) usually occurring with exposure to cold temperatures or stress. Occasionally other parts of the body are affected including the nose, ears, and/or tongue. Raynaud's Disease is a common benign condition and does not usually occur in association with any other underlying disorder. A secondary form of the disease, known as Raynaud's Phenomenon, affects a small number of individuals. This form of the disorder is usually found in association with another underlying systemic disorder.

In addition to The National Organization for Rare Disorders (NORD) listed in Section III, the following organizations in Section II (Disease Specific) and in Section III (Umbrella) and Section IV (Government Agencies) can provide more information:
American Heart Association, *III*
NIH/National Heart, Lung and Blood Institute Information Center, *IV*
Scleroderma Info Exchange, Inc., *II*

889 **RECURRENT RESPIRATORY PAPILLOMATOSIS**

Recurrent Respiratory Papillomatosis is a rare viral disease characterized by multiple benign growths (papillomas) in the middle and lower respiratory tract. Symptoms usually begin with hoarseness and/or a change in voice. The growths may be surgically removed, but frequently recur and may require additional surgery. Affected individuals may experience long periods without recurrence (remission), and/or the disease may disappear completely. Children under 5 years of age are most commonly affected, although adults represent about one-third of all documented cases. People with Recurrent Respiratory Papillomatosis may have difficulty breathing (dyspnea) and/or experience other life-threatening complications if the papillomas block the airway.

In addition to The National Organization for Rare Disorders (NORD) listed in Section III, the following organizations in Section II (Disease Specific) and in Section III (Umbrella) and Section IV (Government Agencies) can provide more information:
American Laryngeal Papilloma Foundation, *II*
NIH/National Heart, Lung and Blood Institute Information Center, *IV*
NIH/National Institute of Allergy and Infectious Diseases, *IV*
Recurrent Respiratory Papillomatosis Foundation, *II*

890 **REFLEX SYMPATHETIC DYSTROPHY SYNDROME (RSDS)**

Reflex Sympathetic Dystrophy Syndrome (RSDS) is a rare disorder of the sympathetic nervous system that is characterized by chronic, severe pain. The sympathetic nervous system is that part of the autonomic nervous system that regulates involuntary, bodily functions such as increasing heart rate, constricting blood vessels, and increasing blood pressure. Excessive or abnormal responses of portions of the sympathetic nervous system are thought to be responsible for the pain associated with Reflex Sympathetic Dystrophy Syndrome.

The symptoms of Reflex Sympathetic Dystrophy Syndrome typically begin with burning pain, especially in an arm, finger(s), palm of the hand(s), and/or shoulder(s). In some individuals, RSDS may occur in one or both legs or it may be localized to one knee or hip. Frequently, RSDS may be misdiagnosed as a painful nerve injury. The skin over the affected area(s) may become swollen (edema) and inflamed. Affected skin may be extremely sensitive to touch and to hot or cold temperatures (cutaneous hypersensitivity). The affected limb(s) may perspire excessively and be warm to the touch (vasomotor instability). The exact cause of RSDS is not fully understood, although it may be associated with injury to the nerves, trauma, surgery, atherosclerotic cardiovascular disease, infection, or radiation therapy.

In addition to The National Organization for Rare Disorders (NORD) listed in Section III, the following organizations in Section II (Disease Specific) and in Section III (Umbrella) and Section IV (Government Agencies) can provide more information:

American Chronic Pain Association, *III*
Arthritis Foundation, *III*
NIH/National Arthritis and Musculoskeletal and Skin Diseases Information Clearinghouse, *IV*
RSDHope Group, *II*
Reflex Sympathetic Dystrophy Network, *II*
Reflex Sympathetic Dystrophy Syndrome Association of America, *II*
Worldwide Congress on Pain, *III*

891 REFSUM SYNDROME

Refsum Syndrome is a rare disorder of lipid metabolism inherited as a recessive trait. Symptoms may include a degenerative nerve disease (peripheral neuropathy), failure of muscle coordination (ataxia), retinitis pigmentosa (a progressive vision disorder), and bone and skin changes. This disorder is believed to be due to the absence of phytanic acid hydroxylase in the blood, an enzyme needed for the metabolism of phytanic acid (found in dairy products, beef, lamb and some seafoods). Refsum Syndrome is characterized by a marked accumulation of phytanic acid in the plasma and tissues. Prolonged treatment with a diet deficient in phytanic acid can be beneficial. This slowly progressive disorder is most common in children and young adults of Scandinavian heritage. Phytanic Acid is a derivative of phytol, a component of chlorophyll.

In addition to The National Organization for Rare Disorders (NORD) listed in Section III, the following organizations in Section II (Disease Specific) and in Section III (Umbrella) and Section IV (Government Agencies) can provide more information:

Association for Neuro-Metabolic Disorders, *III*
Blind Children's Fund, *III*
Foundation Fighting Blindness, *III*
Metabolic Information Network, *III*
NIH/National Institute of Neurological Disorders and Stroke, *IV*
National Association for Visually Handicapped, *III*
National Registry for Ichthyosis and Related Disorders, *III*
Research Trust for Metabolic Diseases in Children, *III*
Retinitis Pigmentosa International, *II*
United Leukodystrophy Foundation, *III*

892 REIFENSTEIN SYNDROME

Reifenstein Syndrome (Partial Androgen Insensitivity) is a hereditary form of male pseudohermaphroditism, a condition in which the male has testes but possesses both male and female sexual characteristics. The severity of androgen (male hormone) insensitivity determines how this syndrome will present itself. In mild cases of androgen resistance, infertility may be the only symptom. More severe cases may result in hardening of the tubules in the testes, failure of one or both testes to descend, an abnormal penis in which the urethra opens on the underside, and development of male breasts. The degree of feminization at puberty is not as marked as in other forms of pseudohermaphroditism.

In addition to The National Organization for Rare Disorders (NORD) listed in Section III, the following organizations in Section II (Disease Specific) and in Section III (Umbrella) and Section IV (Government Agencies) can provide more information:

NIH/National Institute of Child Health and Human Development, *IV*

893 REITER'S SYNDROME

Reiter's Syndrome is a rare disorder characterized by arthritis, inflammation of the urinary tract (nongonococcal urethritis), and inflammation of the mucous membranes that line the eyes (conjunctivitis). Painful and swollen joints occur because of an underlying infection (reactive arthritis). Sores (lesions) may also occur on the skin and the mucous membranes of the mouth. In most cases, Reiter's Syndrome is transmitted through sexual contact (venereal). However, occasionally there is an underlying infection of the small bowel (enteric) that may contribute to the onset of Reiter's Syndrome. All the symptoms of the disease may not appear at once, and they may also disappear and then recur.

In addition to The National Organization for Rare Disorders (NORD) listed in Section III, the following organizations in Section II (Disease Specific) and in Section III (Umbrella) and Section IV (Government Agencies) can provide more information:
Centers for Disease Control and Prevention, *IV*
NIH/National Arthritis and Musculoskeletal and Skin Diseases Information Clearinghouse, *IV*
Sexuality Information and Education Council of the U.S., *III*

894 RENAL AGENESIS, BILATERAL

Bilateral Renal Agenesis is the absence of both kidneys at birth. It is a genetic disorder characterized by a failure of the kidneys to develop in a fetus. This absence of kidneys causes a deficiency of amniotic fluid (Oligohydramnios) in a pregnant woman. Normally, the amniotic fluid acts as a cushion for the developing fetus. When there is an insufficient amount of this fluid, compression of the fetus may occur resulting in further malformations of the baby.

This disorder is more common in infants born of a parent who has a kidney malformation, particularly the absence of one kidney (unilateral renal agenesis). Studies have proven that unilateral renal agenesis and bilateral renal agenesis are genetically related.

In addition to The National Organization for Rare Disorders (NORD) listed in Section III, the following organizations in Section II (Disease Specific) and in Section III (Umbrella) and Section IV (Government Agencies) can provide more information:
American Association of Kidney Patients, *III*
American Foundation for Urologic Disease, *III*
American Kidney Fund, Inc., *III*
NIH/National Institute of Diabetes, Digestive and Kidney Diseases, *IV*
National Kidney Foundation, *III*

895 RENAL GLYCOSURIA

Renal Glycosuria is a rare metabolic disorder in which the body excretes abnormal amounts of sugar into the urine. One type of renal glycosuria may be related to defects of the renal (kidney) tubes that cause an excess of amino acids (aminoaciduria) and an accumulation of acids (acidosis). Blood sugar levels are usually low or within normal limits despite high levels of glucose in the urine. In most cases symptoms can be controlled with a proper diet.

In addition to The National Organization for Rare Disorders (NORD) listed in Section III, the following organizations in Section II (Disease Specific) and in Section III (Umbrella) and Section IV (Government Agencies) can provide more information:
American Association of Kidney Patients, *III*
American Foundation for Urologic Disease, *III*
American Kidney Fund, Inc., *III*
Metabolic Information Network, *III*
NIH/National Digestive Diseases Information Clearinghouse, *IV*
National Kidney Foundation, *III*
Research Trust for Metabolic Diseases in Children, *III*

896 RESPIRATORY DISTRESS SYNDROME, ADULT

Adult Respiratory Distress Syndrome is a lung disorder caused by direct injury to the lungs or acute illness. Major symptoms may include breathing difficulties (dyspnea), rapid breathing (tachypnea), excessively deep and rapid breathing (hyperventilation) and insufficient levels of oxygen in the circulating blood (hypoxemia).

In addition to The National Organization for Rare Disorders (NORD) listed in Section III, the following organizations in Section II (Disease Specific) and in Section III (Umbrella) and Section IV (Government Agencies) can provide more information:
American Lung Association, *III*
NIH/National Heart, Lung and Blood Institute Information Center, *IV*

897 RESPIRATORY DISTRESS SYNDROME, INFANT

Infant Respiratory Distress Syndrome is a lung disorder that tends to affect premature infants. Major symptoms include difficulty in breathing and collapsed lungs, potentially requiring mechanical ventilation or positive end-expiratory pressure (PEEP).

In addition to The National Organization for Rare Disorders (NORD) listed in Section III, the following organizations in Section II (Disease Specific) and in Section III (Umbrella) and Section IV (Government Agencies) can provide more information:
American Lung Association, *III*
NIH/National Heart, Lung and Blood Institute Information Center, *IV*

898 **RESTLESS LEGS SYNDROME**

Restless Legs Syndrome is a neurological movement disorder characterized by unusual sensations (e.g., crawling, creeping, burning) in the legs that typically occur during sleep or rest. These feelings cause affected individuals to constantly move their feet and legs to relieve the uncomfortable sensations. Restless Legs Syndrome may be hereditary or may be a complication of alcoholism, iron deficiency anemia, pregnancy, or Diabetes.

In addition to The National Organization for Rare Disorders (NORD) listed in Section III, the following organizations in Section II (Disease Specific) and in Section III (Umbrella) and Section IV (Government Agencies) can provide more information:

Alliance of Genetic Support Groups, *III*
NIH/National Institute of Neurological Disorders and Stroke, *IV*
Restless Legs Syndrome Foundation, Inc., *II*
WE MOVE, *III*

899 **RETINITIS PIGMENTOSA**

Retinitis Pigmentosa (RP) is one of a group of inherited visual disorders that causes the degeneration of the retina of the eyes. Vision gradually decreases and may eventually be lost. Retinitis Pigmentosa can be associated with deafness and other malfunctions, central nervous system and metabolic disorders, and chromosomal abnormalities.

In addition to The National Organization for Rare Disorders (NORD) listed in Section III, the following organizations in Section II (Disease Specific) and in Section III (Umbrella) and Section IV (Government Agencies) can provide more information:

Alliance of Genetic Support Groups, *III*
American Council of the Blind, Inc., *III*
American Foundation for the Blind, *III*
American Printing House for the Blind, *III*
Blind Children's Center, *III*
Council of Families with Visual Impairment, *III*
Foundation Fighting Blindness, *III*
March of Dimes Birth Defects Foundation, *III*
NIH/National Eye Institute, *IV*
National Association for Parents of the Visually Impaired, *III*
National Association for Visually Handicapped, *III*
National Federation of the Blind, *III*
Retinitis Pigmentosa International, *II*
Vision World Wide, Inc., *III*

900 **RETINOBLASTOMA**

Retinoblastoma is an extremely rare malignant tumor that develops in the nerve-rich layers of one eye or both eyes, most commonly in children under the age of three years. The most typical finding associated with retinoblastoma is the appearance of a distinctive white mass in the pupil area behind the lens of the eye or so called "cat's eye reflex" (leukokoria). In addition, the eyes may appear crossed (strabismus). In some affected children, the eye(s) may become red and/or painful. The presence of the tumor may cause a rise in the pressure in the eyeball (glaucoma). In most cases, retinoblastomas occur spontaneously for no apparent reason (sporadic); however, approximately 20 percent of cases are transmitted as an autosomal dominant genetic trait.

In addition to The National Organization for Rare Disorders (NORD) listed in Section III, the following organizations in Section II (Disease Specific) and in Section III (Umbrella) and Section IV (Government Agencies) can provide more information:

Alliance of Genetic Support Groups, *III*
American Cancer Society, Inc., *III*
Candlelighters Childhood Cancer Foundation, *III*
Institute for Families of Blind Children, *III*
NIH/National Eye Institute, *IV*
National Retinoblastoma Parent Group, *II*

901 **RETINOPATHY, ARTERIOSCLEROTIC**

Arteriosclerotic Retinopathy is a series of changes in the retina that are caused by arteriosclerosis. It is characterized by bleeding in the retina, thick fluid oozing from the retina, impaired oxygenation of the retina, an abrupt reduction of blood flow to the heart muscle that may cause dying off of tissue (myocardial infarction), and hardening of the walls of the little arteries (arterioles) in the eye. These degenerative changes can cause vision impairment.

In addition to The National Organization for Rare Disorders (NORD) listed in Section III, the following organizations in Section II (Disease Specific) and in Section III (Umbrella) and Section IV (Government Agencies) can provide more information:

American Council of the Blind, Inc., *III*
American Foundation for the Blind, *III*
American Heart Association, *III*
Council of Families with Visual Impairment, *III*
NIH/National Eye Institute, *IV*
National Association for Visually Handicapped, *III*
National Eye Research Foundation, *III*
Schepens Eye Research Institute, *III*

902 **RETINOPATHY, DIABETIC**

Diabetic Retinopathy is a disorder of the light sensitive tissue of the eye (retina) caused by diabetes. This condition is characterized by pathologic changes in the blood vessels of the retina. Unchecked, it may lead to visual impairment or blindness.

In addition to The National Organization for Rare Disorders (NORD) listed in Section III, the following organizations in Section II (Disease Specific) and in Section III (Umbrella) and Section IV (Government Agencies) can provide more information:
American Foundation for the Blind, *III*
Juvenile Diabetes Foundation International, *II*
NIH/National Eye Institute, *IV*
National Association for Visually Handicapped, *III*
Vision Foundation, Inc., *III*

903 RETINOPATHY, HYPERTENSIVE

Hypertensive Retinopathy is a syndrome of changes in the retina caused by high blood pressure (hypertension). It is characterized by progressive changes in the little arteries (arterioles) of the eye and swelling (edema), resulting in impairment of vision.

In addition to The National Organization for Rare Disorders (NORD) listed in Section III, the following organizations in Section II (Disease Specific) and in Section III (Umbrella) and Section IV (Government Agencies) can provide more information:
American Council of the Blind, Inc., *III*
American Foundation for the Blind, *III*
American Heart Association, *III*
Council of Families with Visual Impairment, *III*
NIH/National Eye Institute, *IV*
National Association for Visually Handicapped, *III*
National Eye Research Foundation, *III*
Schepens Eye Research Institute, *III*

904 RETINOSCHISIS

Retinoschisis means splitting of the eye's retina into two layers. The various forms of this disorder can be inherited or acquired. The disorder is characterized by a slow progressive loss of parts of the field of vision corresponding to the areas of the retina that have become split. Often, Retinoschisis is associated with the development of saclike blisters (cysts) in the retina.

In addition to The National Organization for Rare Disorders (NORD) listed in Section III, the following organizations in Section II (Disease Specific) and in Section III (Umbrella) and Section IV (Government Agencies) can provide more information:
American Council of the Blind, Inc., *III*
American Foundation for the Blind, *III*
Association for Macular Diseases, Inc., *III*
Blind Children's Fund, *III*
Council of Families with Visual Impairment, *III*
Foundation Fighting Blindness, *III*
NIH/National Eye Institute, *IV*
National Association for Parents of the Visually Impaired, *III*
National Association for Visually Handicapped, *III*
Retinitis Pigmentosa International, *II*
Vision Foundation, Inc., *III*

905 RETROLENTAL FIBROPLASIA

Retrolental Fibroplasia is a bilateral eye disorder characterized by abnormality of the retinal vessels. It occurs in premature infants with immature retinas who are exposed to oxygen in an incubator, and possibly to bright lights. The degree of sight impairment appears to be relative to the oxygen levels in incubators. Oxygen levels of 30% or more can cause more severe vision impairment.

In addition to The National Organization for Rare Disorders (NORD) listed in Section III, the following organizations in Section II (Disease Specific) and in Section III (Umbrella) and Section IV (Government Agencies) can provide more information:
NIH/National Eye Institute, *IV*
National Association for Parents of the Visually Impaired, *III*
National Association for Visually Handicapped, *III*
The Arc (a national organization on mental retardation), *III*

906 RETROPERITONEAL FIBROSIS

Retroperitoneal Fibrosis is a rare disorder in which there is a formation of fiber-like tissue behind the membrane that lines the cavity of the abdomen (peritoneum). This abnormal tissue growth usually affects the tubes that carry the urine from the kidney to the bladder (ureters). Often these tubes are blocked by the excess tissue. In most cases the cause of this disorder is unknown.

In addition to The National Organization for Rare Disorders (NORD) listed in Section III, the following organizations in Section II (Disease Specific) and in Section III (Umbrella) and Section IV (Government Agencies) can provide more information:
NIH/National Digestive Diseases Information Clearinghouse, *IV*
National Kidney Foundation, *III*

907 RETT SYNDROME

Rett Syndrome is a rare neurological disorder that begins during early childhood and is characterized by progressive degeneration of the tissue of the brain (encephalopathy). The disorder affects females exclusively. Some symptoms are similar to those of Autism and may include the loss of previously acquired intellectual and motor skills, developmental regression, and other neurological impairment. The classic symptoms of Rett Syndrome include repetitive sighing while breathing and certain repetitive involuntary (stereotypical) hand movements (e.g., rubbing, "handwashing," etc.).

In addition to The National Organization for Rare Disorders (NORD) listed in Section III, the following organizations in Section II (Disease Specific) and in Section III (Umbrella) and Section IV (Government Agencies) can provide more information:

Alliance of Genetic Support Groups, *III*
Canadian Rett Syndrome Association and Resource Centre, *II*
International Rett Syndrome Association, *II*
NIH/National Institute of Neurological Disorders and Stroke, *IV*
Research for Rett Foundation, *II*
The Arc (a national organization on mental retardation), *III*

908 REYE SYNDROME

Reye Syndrome is a rare disease of childhood characterized by liver failure, low levels of glucose in the blood (hypoglycemia), and brain damage (encephalopathy). This syndrome usually follows a viral infection, such as influenza or chickenpox (varicella), and is strongly associated with the use of salicylates (i.e., aspirin). Deficiencies of certain enzymes that eliminate harmful ammonia from the body (urea cycle enzymes) may be involved in the development of Reye Syndrome.

In addition to The National Organization for Rare Disorders (NORD) listed in Section III, the following organizations in Section II (Disease Specific) and in Section III (Umbrella) and Section IV (Government Agencies) can provide more information:

Centers for Disease Control and Prevention, *IV*
NIH/National Institute of Neurological Disorders and Stroke, *IV*
National Reye's Syndrome Foundation, Inc., *II*

909 RH DISEASE

Rh Disease or Rh incompatibility (also known as Erythroblastosis Fetalis) occurs when a woman with Rh-negative blood conceives a child with Rh-positive blood. Red blood cells are destroyed (hemolysis) because of this incompatibility, leading to anemia and other symptoms in the infant. Symptoms vary in severity among affected infants and may include an unusual yellowish coloration of the skin (jaundice); swelling of the chest and abdomen due to the accumulation of fluid (edema); and/or a pale appearance of the skin. In more severe cases, affected infants may have experience life-threatening complications. Rh Disease occurs only when a mother's blood is Rh-negative and her baby's blood is Rh-positive.

In addition to The National Organization for Rare Disorders (NORD) listed in Section III, the following organizations in Section II (Disease Specific) and in Section III (Umbrella) and Section IV (Government Agencies) can provide more information:

NIH/National Heart, Lung and Blood Institute Information Center, *IV*
NIH/National Institute of Child Health and Human Development, *IV*

910 RHEUMATIC FEVER

Rheumatic Fever is an inflammatory syndrome that can occur following streptococcal infections of the throat (strep throat). Patients initially experience moderate fever, a general feeling of ill health (malaise), a sore throat, and fatigue. Major complications can include heart disease, joint pain and arthritis, involuntary abrupt limb movements with characteristic grimaces (chorea), and possible skin symptoms. Treatment should begin as soon as possible and be maintained for months or even years to help control serious complications. Rheumatic fever can be avoided if strep throat is vigorously treated and cured with antibiotics.

In addition to The National Organization for Rare Disorders (NORD) listed in Section III, the following organizations in Section II (Disease Specific) and in Section III (Umbrella) and Section IV (Government Agencies) can provide more information:

Centers for Disease Control and Prevention, *IV*
NIH/National Institute of Allergy and Infectious Diseases, *IV*
World Health Organization (WHO) Regional Office for the Americas (AMRO), *III*

911 RICKETS, HYPOPHOSPHATEMIC

Hypophosphatemic Rickets is a rare genetic form of Rickets characterized by impaired transport of phosphate and diminished Vitamin-D metabolism in the kidneys. Additionally, calcium and phosphate are not absorbed properly in the intestines which can lead to softening of bones. Major symptoms include skeletal changes, weakness and slowed growth. Cases affecting females are usually less severe than those affecting males. One rare acquired form of this disorder may be associated with a benign tumor.

In addition to The National Organization for Rare Disorders (NORD) listed in Section III, the following organizations in Section II (Disease Specific) and in Section III (Umbrella) and Section IV (Government Agencies) can provide more information:

NIH/National Digestive Diseases Information Clearinghouse, *IV*

912 RICKETS, VITAMIN D DEFICIENCY

Vitamin-D Deficiency Rickets, a disorder that becomes apparent during infancy or childhood, is characterized by insufficient amounts of vitamin D in the body. The vitamin deficiency may be caused by poor nutrition, a lack of exposure to the sun, or malabsorption syndromes in which the intestines do not adequately absorb nutrients from foods. Vitamin D is needed for the metabolism of calcium and phosphorus in the body, which, in turn affects how calcium is deposited in the bones. Major symptoms of Vitamin-D Deficiency Rickets include bone disease, restlessness, and slow growth. This disorder is rare in the United States but is not uncommon in certain areas of the world.

In addition to The National Organization for Rare Disorders (NORD) listed in Section III, the following organizations in Section II (Disease Specific) and in Section III (Umbrella) and Section IV (Government Agencies) can provide more information:
NIH/National Digestive Diseases Information Clearinghouse, *IV*

913 RIEGER SYNDROME

Rieger Syndrome is a rare autosomal dominant genetic disorder characterized by absence (hypodontia or partial adontia) and/or malformation of certain teeth; mild craniofacial abnormalities; and various eye abnormalities. The eye abnormalities (referred to as Rieger Eye Malformations) may be present alone or as a part of Rieger Syndrome.

In addition to The National Organization for Rare Disorders (NORD) listed in Section III, the following organizations in Section II (Disease Specific) and in Section III (Umbrella) and Section IV (Government Agencies) can provide more information:
Blind Children's Fund, *III*
NIH/National Eye Institute, *IV*
National Association for Parents of the Visually Impaired, *III*
National Association for Visually Handicapped, *III*
National Foundation for Ectodermal Dysplasias, *II*
Vision Foundation, Inc., *III*

914 ROBERTS SYNDROME

Roberts Syndrome is an extremely rare genetic disorder characterized by growth delays before and after birth (prenatal and postnatal growth retardation); distinctive abnormalities of the head and facial (craniofacial) area, the eyes, and/or the arms and legs (limbs); and/or other symptoms and findings. In many cases, craniofacial abnormalities may include an unusually small, broad head (microbrachycephaly); abnormal grooves on either side of the upper lip and incomplete development of both sides of the roof of the mouth (bilateral cleft lip and palate); thin, small nostrils (hypoplastic nasal alae); low-set and/or malformed (dysplastic) ears; and/or benign tumors consisting of a mass of small blood vessels (capillary hemangiomas) on the forehead, midface, and/or ears. In infants and children with the disorder, characteristic eye (ocular) abnormalities may include the abnormal development of blood vessels within the front, clear portion of the eyes (corneal vascularization) and/or abnormal clouding of the corneas (corneal opacities), potentially causing blindness. In addition, in affected infants and children, all four limbs may be incompletely developed (limb reduction abnormalities), although the arms are usually more severely affected. Such limb reduction abnormalities may include malformation of the hands and absence of certain fingers (oligodactyly); abnormal shortness, underdevelopment (hypoplasia), or absence (aplasia) of the bones on the thumb or pinky side of the forearms (radius or ulna); and/or incomplete development or absence of certain bones (e.g., fibula) of the lower legs. In approximately half of affected individuals, mental retardation may also be present. The range and severity of symptoms vary from case to case. Roberts Syndrome is inherited as an autosomal recessive genetic trait.

In addition to The National Organization for Rare Disorders (NORD) listed in Section III, the following organizations in Section II (Disease Specific) and in Section III (Umbrella) and Section IV (Government Agencies) can provide more information:
AboutFace U.S.A., *III*
Association of Children's Prosthetic/Orthotic Clinics, *III*
Children's Craniofacial Association, *III*
FACES: The National Craniofacial Association, *III*
Forward Face, Inc., *III*
NIH/National Institute of Child Health and Human Development, *IV*

915 ROBINOW SYNDROME

Robinow Syndrome is an extremely rare inherited disorder characterized by mild to moderate short stature (dwarfism) due to growth delays after birth (postnatal growth retardation); distinctive abnormalities of the head and facial (craniofacial) area; additional skeletal malformations; and/or genital abnormalities. The facial features of infants with Robinow Syndrome resemble those of an eight-week-old fetus; within the medical literature, this condition is often referred to as "fetal face." Characteristic craniofacial features may include an abnormally large head (macrocephaly) with a bulging forehead (frontal bossing); widely spaced eyes (ocular hypertelorism) that are abnormally prominent; a small, upturned nose with nostrils that are flared forward (anteverted); and/or a sunken (depressed) nasal bridge. Skeletal malformations may include forearm bones (radius and ulna) that are unusually short (forearm brachymelia), abnormally short fingers and toes, permanent fixation of the fifth fingers in a bent position (clinodactyly), unusually small hands with broad thumbs, malformation of the ribs, abnormal side-to-side curvature of the spine (scoliosis), and/or underdevelopment of one side of the bones in the middle (thoracic) portion of the spinal column (hemivertebrae). Genital abnormalities associated with Robinow Syndrome may include an abnormally small penis (micropenis) and failure of the testes to descend into the scrotum (cryptorchidism) in affected males and underdevelopment (hypoplasia) of the clitoris and the outer, elongated folds of skin on either side of the vaginal opening (labia majora) in affected females. The range and severity of symptoms vary from case to case.

In some cases, Robinow Syndrome may be inherited as an autosomal dominant genetic trait; in other cases, the disorder may have an autosomal recessive mode of inheritance. According to the medical literature, individuals with the recessive form of Robinow Syndrome may have more numerous abnormalities of the ribs and the bones of the spinal column (vertebrae) than in the dominant form of the disorder. In addition, the symptoms and physical findings associated with the recessive form tend to be more severe.

In addition to The National Organization for Rare Disorders (NORD) listed in Section III, the following organizations in Section II (Disease Specific) and in Section III (Umbrella) and Section IV (Government Agencies) can provide more information:
Children's Craniofacial Association, *III*
Congenital Heart Anomalies, Support, Education, & Resources, *III*
Craniofacial Foundation of America, *III*
Human Growth Foundation, *III*
Little People of America, *III*
MAGIC Foundation for Children's Growth, *III*
NIH/National Arthritis and Musculoskeletal and Skin Diseases Information Clearinghouse, *IV*
NIH/National Institute of Child Health and Human Development, *IV*
Robinow Syndrome Foundation, *II*
Short Stature Foundation, *III*

916 ROCKY MOUNTAIN SPOTTED FEVER

Rocky Mountain Spotted Fever is an acute infectious disorder. This disorder is transmitted to humans through the bite of an infected tick, usually in wooded areas of the midwest, eastern and southeastern U.S. The illness can occur in other areas of the world where ticks are infected with the rickettsial parasite. Fever, rash and gastrointestinal problems are among major symptoms. Early diagnosis and treatment are vital in avoiding serious complications of this disease.

In addition to The National Organization for Rare Disorders (NORD) listed in Section III, the following organizations in Section II (Disease Specific) and in Section III (Umbrella) and Section IV (Government Agencies) can provide more information:
Centers for Disease Control and Prevention, *IV*
NIH/National Institute of Allergy and Infectious Diseases, *IV*
World Life Foundation, *III*

917 ROMANO WARD SYNDROME

Romano-Ward Syndrome is a genetic heart disorder. Symptoms usually begin during infancy or early childhood, although onset during adulthood is possible. Recurrent symptoms such as fainting, convulsive seizures and/or heart beat irregularities with chest pain may occur. Physical exertion, excitement or stress may trigger onset of symptoms.

In addition to The National Organization for Rare Disorders (NORD) listed in Section III, the following organizations in Section II (Disease Specific) and in Section III (Umbrella) and Section IV (Government Agencies) can provide more information:
American Heart Association, *III*
International Long QT Syndrome Registry, *II*
Long QT Syndrome European Information Center, *II*
NIH/National Heart, Lung and Blood Institute Information Center, *IV*

918 ROSENBERG CHUTORIAN SYNDROME

Rosenberg-Chutorian Syndrome is a very rare syndrome thought to be inherited as an X-linked semidominant genetic trait. Symptoms of Rosenberg-Chutorian Syndrome become apparent during infancy or puberty. Sensorineural hearing loss, optic atrophy resulting in loss of vision, and noninflammatory degenerative nerve disease (polyneuropathy) of the upper and/or lower limbs are the major characteristics found in affected individuals.

In addition to The National Organization for Rare Disorders (NORD) listed in Section III, the following organizations in Section II (Disease Specific) and in Section III (Umbrella) and Section IV (Government Agencies) can provide more information:
NIH/National Institute of Neurological Disorders and Stroke, *IV*
National Association for Visually Handicapped, *III*

919 ROSEOLA INFANTUM

Roseola Infantum is an acute infectious disorder of infants or very young children. Characterized by high fever and the appearance of a red skin rash, this disorder may resemble Rubella after the fever has disappeared. Seizures may also occur.

In addition to The National Organization for Rare Disorders (NORD) listed in Section III, the following organizations in Section II (Disease Specific) and in Section III (Umbrella) and Section IV (Government Agencies) can provide more information:
Centers for Disease Control and Prevention, *IV*
NIH/National Institute of Allergy and Infectious Diseases, *IV*

920 ROTHMUND THOMSON SYNDROME

Rothmund-Thomson Syndrome is an extremely rare inherited multisystem disorder that is usually apparent during early infancy. The disorder is typically characterized by distinctive abnormalities of the skin, defects of the hair, clouding of the lenses of the eyes (juvenile cataracts), short stature and other skeletal abnormalities, malformations of the head and facial (craniofacial) area, and other physical abnormalities. In rare cases, mental retardation may be present. The range and severity of symptoms may vary from case to case.

During early infancy, individuals with Rothmund-Thomson Syndrome develop abnormally red, inflamed patches (plaques) on the skin (erythema) accompanied by abnormal accumulations of fluid between layers of tissue under the skin (edema). Such plaques typically first appear on the cheeks. In most cases, additional areas of the skin may then become involved to a lesser degree (e.g., the skin of the ears, forehead, chin, hands, forearms, lower legs, etc.). Inflammation eventually tends to recede and the skin of affected areas develops a condition known as poikiloderma, characterized by abnormal widening (dilation) of groups of small blood vessels (telangiectasia); skin tissue degeneration (atrophy); and patchy areas of abnormally decreased and/or unusually increased pigmentation (depigmentation and hyperpigmentation). In many cases, additional skin abnormalities may also occur.

Many infants and children with Rothmund-Thomson Syndrome also have additional physical abnormalities including hair that is gray and abnormally sparse; the development of abnormal clouding of the lenses of the eyes (juvenile cataracts); growth delays leading to mild to severe short stature (dwarfism); and/or additional skeletal abnormalities such as unusually small, short hands and feet, underdeveloped (hypoplastic) or absent thumbs, and/or underdeveloped (hypoplastic) or missing forearm bones (ulna and radii). Affected infants and children may also have characteristic abnormalities of the craniofacial area including a prominent forehead (frontal bossing), a sunken nasal bridge (saddle nose), a protruding lower jaw (prognathism), and/or dental abnormalities. In some cases, affected individuals may have additional physical abnormalities including deficient activity of the ovaries in females or testes in males (hypogonadism), resulting in irregular menstruation in affected females and delayed sexual development in affected males and females. Rothmund-Thomson Syndrome is inherited as an autosomal recessive genetic trait.

In addition to The National Organization for Rare Disorders (NORD) listed in Section III, the following organizations in Section II (Disease Specific) and in Section III (Umbrella) and Section IV (Government Agencies) can provide more information:
Human Growth Foundation, *III*
Little People of America, *III*
MAGIC Foundation for Children's Growth, *III*
NIH/National Arthritis and Musculoskeletal and Skin Diseases Information Clearinghouse, *IV*
NIH/National Eye Institute, *IV*
NIH/National Institute of Child Health and Human Development, *IV*
NIH/National Institute of Dental Research, *IV*
National Association for Parents of the Visually Impaired, *III*
National Association for Visually Handicapped, *III*
Short Stature Foundation, *III*

921 **ROUSSY LEVY SYNDROME**

Roussy-Levy Syndrome, also known as hereditary areflexic dystasia, is a rare genetic neuromuscular disorder that typically becomes apparent during early childhood. The disorder is characterized by incoordination, poor judgment of movements (sensory ataxia), and absence of reflexes (areflexia) of the lower legs and, eventually, the hands; weakness and degeneration (atrophy) of muscles of the lower legs; abnormally high arches of the feet with increased extension of the toes (pes cavus or "clawfoot"); and tremors of the hands. Many affected individuals also have an abnormal front-to-back and sideways curvature of the spine (kyphoscoliosis). In individuals with Roussy-Levy Syndrome, there is a failed communication of certain nerve signals to muscles of the lower legs (denervation). Roussy-Levy Syndrome is inherited as an autosomal dominant genetic trait.

In addition to The National Organization for Rare Disorders (NORD) listed in Section III, the following organizations in Section II (Disease Specific) and in Section III (Umbrella) and Section IV (Government Agencies) can provide more information:
Charcot-Marie-Tooth Association, *II*
NIH/National Institute of Neurological Disorders and Stroke, *IV*

922 **RUBELLA**

Rubella is a contagious viral disease characterized by sore throat, fever, swelling of lymph glands, and a rash. Maternal infection with Rubella during the early months of pregnancy may cause miscarriage or severe congenital defects in a newborn infant.

In addition to The National Organization for Rare Disorders (NORD) listed in Section III, the following organizations in Section II (Disease Specific) and in Section III (Umbrella) and Section IV (Government Agencies) can provide more information:
Centers for Disease Control and Prevention, *IV*
NIH/National Institute of Allergy and Infectious Diseases, *IV*

923 **RUBELLA, CONGENITAL**

Congenital Rubella is a syndrome that occurs when a fetus has been infected with the Rubella virus while in the uterus. It is primarily characterized by abnormalities of the cardiovascular system, the eyes and the ears. Women who contract Rubella during pregnancy have a high risk of having a baby with Congenital Rubella.

In addition to The National Organization for Rare Disorders (NORD) listed in Section III, the following organizations in Section II (Disease Specific) and in Section III (Umbrella) and Section IV (Government Agencies) can provide more information:
NIH/National Institute of Child Health and Human Development, *IV*
The Arc (a national organization on mental retardation), *III*

924 **RUBINSTEIN TAYBI SYNDROME**

Rubinstein-Taybi Syndrome is a rare genetic multi-system disorder that affects many organ systems of the body. The group of findings (constellation) associated with this syndrome include growth retardation and delayed bone age; mental retardation; distinctive abnormalities of the head and face (craniofacial dysmorphism), including widely spaced eyes (hypertelorism), a depressed nasal bridge, and an abnormally large or "beak-shaped" nose; abnormally broad thumbs and great toes (halluces); and/or breathing and swallowing difficulties. In addition, most affected children experience delays in attaining developmental milestones (e.g., sitting, crawling, walking, talking, etc.) and/or delays in the acquisition of skills requiring coordination of muscular and mental activity (psychomotor retardation). Additional craniofacial abnormalities may include an abnormally small head (microcephaly); a highly-arched roof of the mouth (palate); an unusually small (hypoplastic) lower jaw (micrognathia); crossed eyes (strabismus); deep-set eyes; droopy eyelids (ptosis); downwardly slanting eyelid folds (palpebral fissures); and/or an extra fold of skin on either side of the nose that may cover the eyes' inner corners (epicanthal folds). In addition, many individuals with Rubinstein-Taybi Syndrome may have malformations of the heart, kidneys, urogenital system, and/or skeletal system. In most cases, the skin is also affected. The range and severity of symptoms and physical findings may vary widely from case to case. Most cases of Rubinstein-Taybi Syndrome occur randomly, for no apparent reason (sporadic).

In addition to The National Organization for Rare Disorders (NORD) listed in Section III, the following organizations in Section II (Disease Specific) and in Section III (Umbrella) and Section IV (Government Agencies) can provide more information:
Children's Craniofacial Association, *III*
Congenital Heart Anomalies, Support, Education, & Resources, *III*
FACES: The National Craniofacial Association, *III*

NIH/National Institute of Arthritis and Musculoskeletal and Skin Diseases, *IV*
NIH/National Institute of Child Health and Human Development, *IV*
Rubinstein-Taybi Parent Group, *II*
The Arc (a national organization on mental retardation), *III*

925 RUSSELL SILVER SYNDROME (RSS)

Russell-Silver Syndrome is a very rare genetic disorder characterized by growth delays before birth (prenatal or intrauterine growth retardation); overgrowth of one side of the body (hemihypertrophy or asymmetry); unusual characteristic facial features; and other physical abnormalities. Growth delays before birth affect both weight and linear growth. As a result, although carried to full term (normal gestational age), affected infants may be abnormally small and have low birth weight. In addition, growth delays and immature bone development (growth retardation and delayed bone age) continue after birth (postnatally). As a result, affected children may exhibit short stature and may be unusually small and thin for their age. In most cases (65 to 80 percent), asymmetry or overgrowth of one side of the body is obvious at birth. Asymmetry may affect the head, trunk, arms, and/or legs. The extent and severity of asymmetry vary greatly among affected children. Characteristic facial features may include a triangular-shaped face with a small, pointed chin; an abnormally prominent forehead (frontal bossing); bluish discoloration of the tough, outer membranes covering the eyeballs (blue sclera); an unusually small, wide mouth; downturned corners of the mouth; and/or an abnormally small jaw (micrognathia). The range and severity of symptoms associated with Russell-Silver Syndrome vary greatly from case to case.

Other physical findings associated with this disorder may include permanent fixation of the fifth fingers in a bent position (clinodactyly); webbing of the second and third toes (syndactyly); underdevelopment (hypoplasia) of certain bones of the fingers (phalanges); development of smooth, coffee-colored patches on the skin (cafe-au-lait spots); and/or abnormalities of the kidney and urinary tract.

Most cases of Russell-Silver Syndrome are the result of new genetic changes (mutations) that occur randomly for no apparent reason (sporadic). If this mutation were to be inherited, it would do so as an autosomal dominant genetic trait. In rare cases, it is thought that the disorder may be inherited as an autosomal recessive genetic trait. In addition, a rare form of Russell-Silver Syndrome is thought to be inherited as an X-linked dominant genetic trait.

In addition to The National Organization for Rare Disorders (NORD) listed in Section III, the following organizations in Section II (Disease Specific) and in Section III (Umbrella) and Section IV (Government Agencies) can provide more information:
Human Growth Foundation, *III*
Little People of America, *III*
MAGIC Foundation for Children's Growth, *III*
NIH/National Institute of Arthritis and Musculoskeletal and Skin Diseases, *IV*
NIH/National Institute of Child Health and Human Development, *IV*
Short Stature Foundation, *III*
The Arc (a national organization on mental retardation), *III*

926 RUVALCABA SYNDROME

Ruvalcaba Syndrome is a very rare malformation disorder thought to be inherited as an autosomal dominant genetic trait with reduced penetrance. The major characteristics of this disorder are short stature, unusual facial features, skeletal abnormalities and varying degrees of mental retardation in over fifty percent of affected individuals.

In addition to The National Organization for Rare Disorders (NORD) listed in Section III, the following organizations in Section II (Disease Specific) and in Section III (Umbrella) and Section IV (Government Agencies) can provide more information:
Centers for Disease Control and Prevention, *IV*
NIH/National Institute of Child Health and Human Development, *IV*

927 SHORT SYNDROME

SHORT Syndrome is a very rare disorder thought to be inherited as an autosomal recessive trait. Individuals affected with this disorder are usually born with a low birth weight. Short stature, and a congenital condition in which there is a loss of fat under the skin (lipoatrophy) of the arms and face are almost always apparent. Other distinguishing symptoms of SHORT Syndrome are defective development of the anterior chamber of the eye (Rieger Anomaly) and a delay in teething and speech.

In addition to The National Organization for Rare Disorders (NORD) listed in Section III, the following organizations in Section II (Disease Specific) and in Section III (Umbrella) and Section IV (Government Agencies) can provide more information:
Human Growth Foundation, *III*
Little People of America, *III*
Little People's Research Fund, Inc., *III*
MAGIC Foundation for Children's Growth, *III*
NIH/National Arthritis and Musculoskeletal and Skin Diseases Information Clearinghouse, *IV*
NIH/National Eye Institute, *IV*
Short Stature Foundation, *III*

928 SAETHRE CHOTZEN SYNDROME

Saethre-Chotzen Syndrome (Acrocephalosyndactyly Type III) is a rare inherited disorder characterized by various malformations of the head, face, and/or skeletal system. Physical features may include an unusually short and broad head (brachycephaly), an unbalanced appearance to the head (cranial asymmetry), widely spaced eyes, and/or droopy eyelids (ptosis). Abnormalities of the fingers and/or toes such as unusually short fingers (brachydactyly) and mild webbing of some fingers (syndactyly) may also be present. Growth delays may occur, leading to less than average adult height. Intelligence is usually normal, but mild to moderate mental retardation may occur. Saethre-Chotzen Syndrome is believed to be inherited as an autosomal dominant genetic trait.

In addition to The National Organization for Rare Disorders (NORD) listed in Section III, the following organizations in Section II (Disease Specific) and in Section III (Umbrella) and Section IV (Government Agencies) can provide more information:
AboutFace U.S.A., *III*
Alliance of Genetic Support Groups, *III*
Children's Craniofacial Association, *III*
Craniofacial Support Group, *III*
FACES: The National Craniofacial Association, *III*
Forward Face, Inc., *III*
Let's Face It, Inc., *III*
NIH/National Institute of Child Health and Human Development, *IV*
The Arc (a national organization on mental retardation), *III*

929 SAKATI SYNDROME

Sakati Syndrome (Acrocephalopolysyndactyly Type III) is an extremely rare inherited disorder characterized by malformations of the head and face; abnormalities of the hands, feet, and legs; and congenital heart disease. Sakati Syndrome is thought to be caused by a genetic change (mutation) in mature parents that occurs for no apparent reason (sporadic).

In addition to The National Organization for Rare Disorders (NORD) listed in Section III, the following organizations in Section II (Disease Specific) and in Section III (Umbrella) and Section IV (Government Agencies) can provide more information:
AboutFace U.S.A., *III*
American Heart Association, *III*
Children's Craniofacial Association, *III*
Congenital Heart Anomalies, Support, Education, & Resources, *III*
FACES: The National Craniofacial Association, *III*
Forward Face, Inc., *III*
Let's Face It, Inc., *III*
NIH/National Institute of Child Health and Human Development, *IV*
National Foundation for Facial Reconstruction, *III*

930 SANDHOFF DISEASE

Sandhoff Disease is a rare inherited lipid storage disorder resulting in the progressive deterioration of the central nervous system. A deficiency of the enzyme hexosaminidase (beta-subunit) results in the accumulation of certain fats (lipids or fatty acids) in the brain and other organs of the body. Sandhoff Disease is a severe form of Tay-Sachs Disease and is not limited to any particular ethnic group.

In addition to The National Organization for Rare Disorders (NORD) listed in Section III, the following organizations in Section II (Disease Specific) and in Section III (Umbrella) and Section IV (Government Agencies) can provide more information:
Alliance of Genetic Support Groups, *III*
Blind Children's Fund, *III*
March of Dimes Birth Defects Foundation, *III*
NIH/National Institute of Neurological Disorders and Stroke, *IV*
National Association for Visually Handicapped, *III*
National Tay-Sachs and Allied Diseases Association, Inc., *III*

931 SANFILIPPO SYNDROME

Mucopolysaccharidoses (MPS Disorders) are a group of rare genetic disorders caused by the deficiency of one of the lysosomal enzymes, resulting in an inability to metabolize complex carbohydrates (mucopolysaccharides) into simpler molecules. The accumulation of these large, undegraded mucopolysaccharides in the cells of the body causes a number of physical symptoms and abnormalities.

Sanfilippo Syndrome (MPS III), an autosomal recessive hereditary disorder, is characterized by severe mental deterioration, mild physical defects and the excretion of heparan sulfate in the urine. There are four types of Sanfilippo Syndrome; types A and B are the most common forms.

In addition to The National Organization for Rare Disorders (NORD) listed in Section III, the following organizations in Section II (Disease Specific) and in Section III (Umbrella) and Section IV (Government Agencies) can provide more information:
Canadian Society for Mucopolysaccharide and Related Diseases, Inc., *III*
Metabolic Information Network, *III*
NIH/National Digestive Diseases Information Clearinghouse, *IV*
National MPS (Mucopolysaccharidoses/Mucolipidoses) Society, Inc., *III*
Research Trust for Metabolic Diseases in Children, *III*
The Arc (a national organization on mental retardation), *III*
Vaincre Les Maladies Lysosomales, *III*

932 SANTAVUORI DISEASE

Santavuori Disease, an extremely rare inherited disorder, belongs to a group of progressive degenerative neurometabolic diseases known as the neuronal ceroid lipofuscinoses (NCL). These diseases share certain similar symptoms and are distinguished in part by the age at which such symptoms appear. Santavuori Disease is considered the infantile form of the neuronal ceroid lipofuscinoses.

In most cases, infants with Santavuori Disease appear to develop normally until approximately nine to 19 months of age. They may then begin to exhibit a delay in the acquisition of skills that require the coordination of mental and muscular activity (psychomotor retardation). In addition, affected infants begin to lose previously acquired physical and mental abilities (developmental regression). Affected infants may then experience a variety of symptoms including episodes of uncontrolled electrical disturbances in the brain (seizures), impaired ability to coordinate voluntary movements (cerebellar ataxia), abnormally diminished muscle tone (hypotonia), and repeated, brief, shock-like muscle spasms of the arms, legs, or entire body (myoclonic seizures). Affected infants also experience progressive visual impairment due to deterioration of the nerves of the eyes (optic nerves) that transmit impulses from the nerve-rich membranes lining the eyes (retina) to the brain (optic atrophy). Neurological impairment continues to progress and may be characterized by an inability to move voluntarily (immobility); sudden involuntary muscle spasms (spasticity); and lack of response to stimuli in the environment. Life-threatening complications may develop by the end of the first decade. The symptoms and physical characteristics of Santavuori Disease result due to abnormal accumulation of certain fatty, granular substances (i.e., pigmented lipids [lipopigments] ceroid and lipofuscin) within nerve cells (neurons) of the brain as well as other tissues of the body. Santavuori Disease is inherited as an autosomal recessive genetic trait.

In addition to The National Organization for Rare Disorders (NORD) listed in Section III, the following organizations in Section II (Disease Specific) and in Section III (Umbrella) and Section IV (Government Agencies) can provide more information:
Association for Neuro-Metabolic Disorders, *III*
Batten Disease Support and Research Association, *II*
Children's Brain Diseases Foundation, *II*
Epilepsy Foundation of America, *III*
Myoclonus Research Foundation, *III*
NIH/National Eye Institute, *IV*
NIH/National Institute of Neurological Disorders and Stroke, *IV*
National Tay-Sachs and Allied Diseases Association, Inc., *III*
Vaincre Les Maladies Lysosomales, *III*

933 SARCOIDOSIS

Sarcoidosis is a multisystem disorder characterized by the formation of granular, inflammatory nodules or tubercles (granulomas) consisting of cells that ingest microorganisms and other particle fragments (modified macrophages or epithelioid cells). These epithelioid granulomas most commonly affect the lungs, but the upper respiratory system, lymph nodes, skin, and eyes are often involved. In addition, the liver, bone marrow and spleen, musculoskeletal system, heart, salivary glands, nervous system, and/or other organs may sometimes be affected.

The onset of this disorder may appear in an acute form, in which symptoms appear suddenly, sometimes severely, and subside in a relatively short period of time; a subacute form, in which an affected person may exhibit no symptoms (asymptomatic) even though there is organ involvement; or in a chronic form, in which the symptoms may appear slowly and subtly and may persist or recur over a long time span. The range and severity of symptoms associated with this disorder vary greatly and their manifestation is dependent upon the organ(s) involved and the degree of the involvement.

Acute sarcoidosis is often characterized by fatigue, fever, generalized muscle aches, difficulty in breathing (dyspnea), joint pain, swollen glands, skin eruptions, eye irregularities, and/or other symptoms. Initial symptoms of the more chronic form of this disorder may include dyspnea, dry cough, limited airflow, and other respiratory abnormalities. Symptoms associated with other organ involvement may follow.

Sarcoidosis appears to affect slightly more women than men and most often affects individuals between 20 and 40 years of age (although it may appear at any age).

While the exact cause of Sarcoidosis is not known, many researchers believe the symptoms of this disorder result from an overzealous response of the immune system elicited by one or more substances, or antigens. These antigens then react with the specialized white cells and/or antibodies produced by this immune response, thus triggering the process leading to granuloma formation. Paradoxically, while specialized cells of the immune response system are proliferating in the affected organs, the circulation of similar cells is reduced in the blood and other sites.

In addition to The National Organization for Rare Disorders (NORD) listed in Section III, the following organizations in Section II (Disease Specific) and in Section III (Umbrella) and Section IV (Government Agencies) can provide more information:

American Autoimmune Related Diseases Association, Inc., *III*
American Lung Association, *III*
NIH/National Eye Institute, *IV*
NIH/National Heart, Lung and Blood Institute Information Center, *IV*
NIH/National Institute of Allergy and Infectious Diseases, *IV*
NIH/National Institute of Arthritis and Musculoskeletal and Skin Diseases, *IV*
National Sarcoidosis Resource Center, *II*
Sarcoid Networking Association, *II*
Sarcoidosis Network Foundation, Inc., *II*
Sarcoidosis Research Institute, *II*

934 SARCOMA, EWING'S

Ewing's Sarcoma is a malignant tumor of bone (i.e., primitive small round cell tumor) that may invade surrounding soft tissues. In many cases, Ewing's Sarcoma affects the shafts of the long bones (diaphyses) of the legs or arms. Ewing's Sarcoma may also develop in bones of the foot, the hand, the spinal column (vertebrae), the pelvis, the lower jaw (mandible), the skull, and/or other locations. Individuals with Ewing's Sarcoma often experience associated pain and swelling, fever, and abnormally increased levels of circulating white blood cells (leukocytosis). Ewing's Sarcoma affects males more often than females and usually develops between the ages of 10 and 20 years. The exact cause of Ewing's Sarcoma is not known.

In addition to The National Organization for Rare Disorders (NORD) listed in Section III, the following organizations in Section II (Disease Specific) and in Section III (Umbrella) and Section IV (Government Agencies) can provide more information:

American Cancer Society, Inc., *III*

935 SCHINDLER DISEASE

Schindler Disease is an extremely rare inherited metabolic disorder characterized by a deficiency of the lysosomal enzyme alpha-N-acetylgalactosaminidase (alpha-NAGA). This disorder belongs to a group of diseases known as lysosomal storage disorders. Lysosomes are particles bound in membranes within cells that break down certain fats and carbohydrates. Low levels of the alpha-NAGA enzyme lead to the abnormal accumulation of certain complex compounds (glycosphingolipids) consisting of fatty materials and carbohydrates (glycolipids) in many tissues of the body.

There are two forms of Schindler Disease. Schindler Disease, Type I, which is considered the classic form of the disease, has an infantile onset. Affected children develop normally until approximately 1 year of age, when they begin to lose previously acquired physical and mental abilities (developmental regression). Neurological symptoms then begin to appear, which may include muscular weakness, visual impairment, and/or seizures. Neurological impairment continues to progress in affected children and may include sudden involuntary muscle spasms (spasticity), an inability to move voluntarily (immobility), severe mental retardation, and a lack of response to stimuli in the environment. Schindler Disease, Type I is inherited as an autosomal recessive genetic trait.

In the adult-onset form of Schindler Disease (also known as Schindler Disease, Type II or Kanzaki Disease), symptoms may not appear until the second or third decade of life. In this milder form of Schindler Disease, symptoms may include the appearance of clusters of wart-like discolorations on the skin (angiokeratomas), the widening of groups of blood vessels (telangiectasia) in certain areas of the body, slightly coarse facial features, and/or mild intellectual impairment. Progressive neurological degeneration, as seen in Schindler Disease, Type I, has not occurred in this adult-onset form of the disorder. Schindler Disease, Type II is inherited as an autosomal recessive genetic trait.

In addition to The National Organization for Rare Disorders (NORD) listed in Section III, the following organizations in Section II (Disease Specific) and in Section III (Umbrella) and Section IV (Government Agencies) can provide more information:

Association for Neuro-Metabolic Disorders, *III*
NIH/National Institute of Neurological Disorders and Stroke, *IV*
National Lipid Diseases Foundation, *III*
National Tay-Sachs and Allied Diseases Association, Inc., *III*
Research Trust for Metabolic Diseases in Children, *III*
Vaincre Les Maladies Lysosomales, *III*

936 SCHINZEL GIEDION SYNDROME

Schinzel-Giedion Syndrome is a very rare disorder thought to be inherited as an autosomal recessive genetic trait. One of the major symptoms of this disorder is an obstruction of the tube that carries urine from the kidney into the bladder (ureter) causing the pelvis and kidney duct to become swollen with an accumulation of urine (hydronephrosis). Other symptoms characteristic of Schinzel-Giedion Syndrome are excessive growth of hair (hypertrichosis), a flat midface, seizures or abnormal brain activity, apneic spella, abnormalities of the skeleton, mental retardation, and short arms and legs.

In addition to The National Organization for Rare Disorders (NORD) listed in Section III, the following organizations in Section II (Disease Specific) and in Section III (Umbrella) and Section IV (Government Agencies) can provide more information:

NIH/National Institute of Child Health and Human Development, *IV*

937 SCHINZEL SYNDROME

Schinzel Syndrome, also known as Ulnar-Mammary Syndrome (UMS), is an extremely rare inherited disorder characterized by abnormalities affecting the bones of the forearms and hands and/or underdevelopment (hypoplasia) and dysfunction of certain sweat (apocrine) glands and/or the breasts (mammary glands). Abnormalities affecting the hands and/or forearms may range from underdevelopment (hypoplasia) of the bone in the tip of the fifth finger (hypoplastic terminal phalanx) to underdevelopment or complete absence of the bone on the outer aspect of the forearm (ulna) and certain fingers (e.g., third, fourth, fifth). In addition, affected infants may have additional finger (digital) malformations with or without ulnar and/or digital abnormalities on the other side of the body (contralateral limb deficiencies), such as extra fingers on the "pinky" side of the hand (postaxial polydactyly). In addition, certain sweat glands (apocrine glands), such as those located under the arms, may be underdeveloped or absent, resulting in diminished ability or inability to sweat (perspire). In some cases, the breasts (mammary glands) may also be underdeveloped or absent; as a result, affected females exhibit a diminished ability or an inability to produce milk (lactate). Other abnormalities associated with Schinzel Syndrome may include absent or incorrectly positioned (ectopic) teeth, delayed growth, and/or abnormally low levels of testicular function in males (hypogenitalism), resulting in delayed development of secondary sexual characteristics (puberty). The range and severity of physical abnormalities associated with Schinzel Syndrome may vary greatly among affected individuals; some cases may be very mild, while others may be more severe. Schinzel Syndrome is inherited as an autosomal dominant genetic trait.

In addition to The National Organization for Rare Disorders (NORD) listed in Section III, the following organizations in Section II (Disease Specific) and in Section III (Umbrella) and Section IV (Government Agencies) can provide more information:

Association of Children's Prosthetic/Orthotic Clinics, *III*
CHERUB—Association of Families and Friends of Children with Limb Disorders, *III*
NIH/National Institute of Arthritis and Musculoskeletal and Skin Diseases, *IV*
NIH/National Institute of Child Health and Human Development, *IV*

Superkids, Inc. (newsletter for families and friends of children with limb differences), *III*

938 SCHMID TYPE METAPHYSEAL CHONDRODYSPLASIA

Schmid Type Metaphyseal Chondrodysplasia is a very rare inherited disorder characterized by short stature with abnormally short arms and legs (short-limbed dwarfism). Other physical characteristics may include outward "flaring" of the bones of the lower rib cage, bowed legs (genu varum), pain in the legs, and/or hip deformities in which the thigh bone is angled toward the center of the body (coxa vara). Such abnormalities of the legs and hips typically result in an unusual "waddling" walk (gait). Schmid Type Metaphyseal Chondrodysplasia is thought to be inherited as an autosomal dominant genetic trait.

In addition to The National Organization for Rare Disorders (NORD) listed in Section III, the following organizations in Section II (Disease Specific) and in Section III (Umbrella) and Section IV (Government Agencies) can provide more information:

NIH/National Institute of Child Health and Human Development, *IV*

939 SCHMIDT SYNDROME

Schmidt Syndrome is a rare disorder in which there are multiple deficiencies in the glands that secrete hormones. This syndrome is characterized by the presence of Addison's disease and hypothyroidism. Insulin-Dependent Diabetes and failure of additional hormone secreting (endocrine) glands such as the gonads, parathyroids, and pancreas may also occur along with autoimmune type abnormalities. Most cases of this disorder are sporadic although some scientists believe that there could be a familial or hereditary trait associated with Schmidt Syndrome.

In addition to The National Organization for Rare Disorders (NORD) listed in Section III, the following organizations in Section II (Disease Specific) and in Section III (Umbrella) and Section IV (Government Agencies) can provide more information:

American Autoimmune Related Diseases Association, Inc., *III*
Celiac Sprue Association/USA, Inc., *II*
Juvenile Diabetes Foundation International, *II*
Myasthenia Gravis Foundation of America, *II*
NIH/National Digestive Diseases Information Clearinghouse, *IV*
National Adrenal Diseases Foundation, *III*
National Foundation for Vitiligo and Pigment Disorders, *III*
Thyroid Foundation of America, Inc., *III*

940 SCHWARTZ JAMPEL SYNDROME

Schwartz-Jampel Syndrome is an extremely rare inherited disorder characterized by abnormalities of the skeletal muscles, including muscle weakness and stiffness (myotonic myopathy); skeletal malformations, such as a sideways and front-to-back curvature of the spine (kyphoscoliosis), permanently flexed, fixed joints (contractures), and/or improper development of the hip (hip dysplasia); and/or growth delays resulting in abnormally short stature (dwarfism). Affected individuals also have small, fixed facial features and exhibit various abnormalities of the eyes, some of which may cause impaired vision. The range and severity of symptoms may vary from case to case. Schwartz-Jampel Syndrome is believed to be inherited as an autosomal recessive genetic trait.

In addition to The National Organization for Rare Disorders (NORD) listed in Section III, the following organizations in Section II (Disease Specific) and in Section III (Umbrella) and Section IV (Government Agencies) can provide more information:

International Children's Anophthalmia Network, *III*
Malignant Hyperthermia Association of the United States, *II*
NIH/National Arthritis and Musculoskeletal and Skin Diseases Information Clearinghouse, *IV*
NIH/National Eye Institute, *IV*
NIH/National Institute of Child Health and Human Development, *IV*
National Association for Parents of the Visually Impaired, *III*
National Association for Visually Handicapped, *III*

941 SCLERODERMA

Scleroderma is a rare connective tissue disorder characterized by abnormal thickening of the skin. Connective tissue is composed of collagen, which supports and binds other body tissues. There are several types of Scleroderma. Some types affect certain, specific parts of the body, while other types can affect the whole body and internal organs (systemic).

In addition to The National Organization for Rare Disorders (NORD) listed in Section III, the following organizations in Section II (Disease Specific) and in Section III (Umbrella) and Section IV (Government Agencies) can provide more information:

British Coalition of Heritable Disorders of Connective Tissue, *III*
NIH/National Arthritis and Musculoskeletal and Skin Diseases Information Clearinghouse, *IV*

942 SCOTT CRANIODIGITAL SYNDROME WITH MENTAL RETARDATION

Scott Craniodigital Syndrome With Mental Retardation is an extremely rare inherited disorder characterized by mental retardation and various physical abnormalities affecting the head and facial (craniofacial) area and the fingers and/or toes (digits). Characteristic craniofacial features may include a short, wide head (brachycephaly); a small, narrow nose; widely spaced eyes (ocular hypertelorism); and/or an abnormally small lower jaw (mandible). In addition, some children may have a "startled" expression to their faces. Other characteristic features may include webbing of some of the fingers and toes (syndactyly); uncommon skin ridge patterns (dermatoglyphic patterns) on the palms of the hands; and/or abnormal inward turning of the heel of the foot (talipes varus). In addition, individuals with this disorder may have thick scalp hair with an extended hairline; long, dark eyelashes; abnormally thick eyebrows; and/or excessive hair growth on other areas of the body (hirsutism). Scott Craniodigital Syndrome With Mental Retardation is thought to be inherited as an X-linked recessive genetic trait.

In addition to The National Organization for Rare Disorders (NORD) listed in Section III, the following organizations in Section II (Disease Specific) and in Section III (Umbrella) and Section IV (Government Agencies) can provide more information:

Children's Craniofacial Association, *III*
Craniofacial Foundation of America, *III*
FACES: The National Craniofacial Association, *III*
Forward Face, Inc., *III*
NIH/National Institute of Child Health and Human Development, *IV*

943 SECKEL SYNDROME

Seckel Syndrome is an extremely rare inherited disorder characterized by growth delays prior to birth (intrauterine growth retardation) resulting in low birth weight. Growth delays continue after birth (postnatal) resulting in short stature (dwarfism). Other symptoms and physical features associated with Seckel Syndrome include an abnormally small head (microcephaly); varying degrees of mental retardation; and/or unusual characteristic facial features including "beak-like" protrusion of the nose. Other facial features may include abnormally large eyes, a narrow face, malformed ears, and/or an unusually small jaw (micrognathia). In addition, some affected infants may exhibit permanent fixation of the fifth fingers in a bent position (clinodactyly), malformation (dysplasia) of the hips, dislocation of a bone in the forearm (radial dislocation), and/or other physical abnormalities. Seckel Syndrome is thought to be inherited as an autosomal recessive genetic trait.

In addition to The National Organization for Rare Disorders (NORD) listed in Section III, the following organizations in Section II (Disease Specific) and in Section III (Umbrella) and Section IV (Government Agencies) can provide more information:

AboutFace U.S.A., *III*
Children's Craniofacial Association, *III*
Craniofacial Foundation of America, *III*
Forward Face, Inc., *III*
Human Growth Foundation, *III*
Little People of America, *III*
NIH/National Institute of Child Health and Human Development, *IV*
Short Stature Foundation, *III*
The Arc (a national organization on mental retardation), *III*

944 SEITELBERGER DISEASE (INFANTILE NEUROAXONAL DYSTROPHY)

Seitelberger Disease, also known as Infantile Neuroaxonal Dystrophy, is an extremely rare inherited degenerative disorder of the nervous system characterized by abnormalities of nerve endings (axons) within the brain and spinal cord (central nervous system) and outside the central nervous system (peripheral nerves). In most cases, infants and children with Seitelberger Disease appear to develop normally until approximately 14 to 18 months of age, when they may begin to experience progressively increased difficulties in walking. In other cases, symptoms may begin at approximately six to eight months of age, at which time infants may experience delays or an arrest in the acquisition of skills requiring the coordination of mental and physical activities (delayed psychomotor development). Affected infants and children may then begin to lose previously acquired skills (psychomotor regression) including sitting and standing and may demonstrate progressive neuromuscular impairment characterized by generalized muscle weakness, severely diminished muscle tone (hypotonia), abnormally exaggerated reflex responses (hyperreflexia), and/or unusually weak, depressed, or absent reflexes. In some cases, as the disorder progresses, affected children may also experience invluntary movements of the face and hands, sudden invluntary muscle spasms(spasticity) of the lower arms and legs (limbs), and progressive paralysis of the legs and lower part of the body (paraplegia). Progressive mental retardation occurs in association with gradual motor impairment.

Children with Seitelberger Disease also experience progressive neurological impairment including involuntary, rapid, side-to-side movements of the eyes (pendular nystagmus); crossing of the eyes (strabismus); gradual deterioration of the nerves of the eyes (optic atrophy), progressing to blindness; and/or hearing impairment. As neurological impairment progresses, affected children may experience disorientation and loss of intellectual function (dementia); impaired response to touch (tactile stimulation); uncontrolled, rigid extensions and rotations of the arms, legs, fingers, and toes due to progressively degenerative brain abnormalities (decerebrate rigidity); and increased susceptibility to repeated infections of the respiratory tract. Life-threatening complications may develop by the end of the first decade.

The symptoms and physical characteristics associated with Seitelberger Disease occur due to swelling and degeneration of nerve endings (dystrophic axonal swellings or "spheroids") in certain areas of the brain and spinal cord (central nervous system or neuroaxis) and outside the central nervous system (peripheral nerves). In most cases, Seitelberger Disease is inherited as an autosomal recessive genetic trait.

In addition to The National Organization for Rare Disorders (NORD) listed in Section III, the following organizations in Section II (Disease Specific) and in Section III (Umbrella) and Section IV (Government Agencies) can provide more information:

Alliance of Genetic Support Groups, *III*
NIH/National Eye Institute, *IV*
NIH/National Institute of Child Health and Human Development, *IV*
NIH/National Institute of Neurological Disorders and Stroke, *IV*
United Leukodystrophy Foundation, *III*

945 SENNETSU FEVER

Sennetsu Fever is a rare infectious disease belonging to a group of diseases known as the Human Ehrlichioses. These diseases are caused by bacteria belonging to the "Ehrlichia" family. Three forms of Human Ehrlichial infection have been identified including Sennetsu Fever, Human Monocytic Ehrlichiosis (HME), and Human Granulocytic Ehrlichiosis (HGE). Though caused by different strains of Ehrlichia bacteria, the three disorders are all characterized by similar symptoms.

The symptoms of Sennetsu Fever may include a sudden high fever, headache, and muscle aches (myalgia) within a few weeks after initial infection. In some cases, affected individuals may also experience nausea, vomiting, and/or loss of appetite (anorexia). In addition, in many cases, abnormal laboratory findings may include a decrease in white blood cells (leukopenia) and/or an abnormal increase in the level of certain liver enzymes (hepatic transaminases). Sennetsu Fever is caused by the bacterium Ehrlichia sennetsu. The vector (or carrier) for this bacterium has not yet been determined; however, some researchers believe that infection may result from the ingestion of raw fish.

In addition to The National Organization for Rare Disorders (NORD) listed in Section III, the following organizations in Section II (Disease Specific) and in Section III (Umbrella) and Section IV (Government Agencies) can provide more information:

Centers for Disease Control and Prevention, *IV*
NIH/National Institute of Allergy and Infectious Diseases, *IV*
World Health Organization (WHO) Regional Office for the Americas (AMRO), *III*

946 SEPTO OPTIC DYSPLASIA

Septo-Optic Dysplasia (De Morsier Syndrome) is a rare disorder that may be apparent in early infancy, during childhood, or, in some cases, as late as adolescence. The disorder is characterized by abnormal development (dysplasia) of certain structures within the central portion (midline) of the brain, affecting structures of the eyes; the hypothalamus, an area of the brain that plays a role in coordinating hormone function (i.e., endocrine system); and/or other portions of the brain. Resulting characteristic findings may include underdevelopment (hypoplasia) of the optic nerves, the pair of nerves (second cranial nerves) that transmit impulses from the nerve-rich membranes lining the eyes (retina) to the brain; absence (agenesis) of a certain membrane in the brain (septum pellucidum); and diminished activity of the pituitary gland, the hormone-producing gland at the base of the brain, due to improper function of the hypothalamus (hypothalamic hypopituitarism). As a result of such abnormalities, affected individuals may experience partial or complete blindness or mild to severe visual impairment; delays in the acquisition of skills that require the coordination of mental and muscular activity (psychomotor retardation); deficiencies of certain hormones resulting in growth retardation, short stature, and/or other symptoms; and/or, in some cases, additional abnormalities. Although some children with the disorder have normal intelligence, most may exhibit dimished intellectual capabilities ranging from learning disabilities to mental retardation. The cause of Septo-Optic Dysplasia is not fully understood. Most cases are thought to occur randomly for unknown reasons (sporadic).

In addition to The National Organization for Rare Disorders (NORD) listed in Section III, the following organizations in Section II (Disease Specific) and in Section III (Umbrella) and Section IV (Government Agencies) can provide more information:

American Foundation for the Blind, *III*
Blind Children's Center, *III*
Blind Children's Fund, *III*
Brain and Pituitary Foundation of America, *III*
Council of Families with Visual Impairment, *III*
Diabetes Insipidus Foundation, Inc., *III*
Foundation Fighting Blindness, *III*
Human Growth Foundation, *III*
MAGIC Foundation for Children's Growth, *III*
NIH/National Digestive Diseases Information Clearinghouse, *IV*
NIH/National Institute of Child Health and Human Development, *IV*
National Association for Parents of the Visually Impaired, *III*
National Federation of the Blind, *III*
Short Stature Foundation, *III*
The Arc (a national organization on mental retardation), *III*

947 SETLEIS SYNDROME

Setleis Syndrome is an extremely rare inherited disorder that belongs to a group of diseases known as Ectodermal Dysplasias. Ectodermal Dysplasias typically affect the hair, teeth, nails, and/or skin. Setleis Syndrome is characterized by distinctive abnormalities of the facial area that may be apparent at birth (congenital). Most affected infants have multiple, scar-like, circular depressions on both temples (bitemporal). These marks closely resemble those made when forceps are used to assist delivery. In addition, affected infants may have puffy, wrinkled skin around the eyes (periorbital) and/or abnormalities of the eyelashes, eyebrows, and eyelids. Infants with Setleis Syndrome may be missing eyelashes on both the upper and lower lids, or they may have multiple rows of lashes on the upper lids but none on the lower lids. In addition, in some cases, the bridge of the nose may appear flat, while the tip may appear unusually rounded (bulbous). Affected infants often have loose, excessive (redundant) skin, particularly in the area of the nose and the chin. Due to such facial abnormalities, infants with Setleis Syndrome may have an aged and/or "leonine" (lion-like) appearance. The range and severity of symptoms may vary from case to case. Most cases of Setleis Syndrome are thought to be inherited as an autosomal recessive genetic trait.

In addition to The National Organization for Rare Disorders (NORD) listed in Section III, the following organizations in Section II (Disease Specific) and in Section III (Umbrella) and Section IV (Government Agencies) can provide more information:

Children's Craniofacial Association, *III*
Craniofacial Foundation of America, *III*
Forward Face, Inc., *III*
NIH/National Institute of Arthritis and Musculoskeletal and Skin Diseases, *IV*
NIH/National Institute of Child Health and Human Development, *IV*
National Foundation for Ectodermal Dysplasias, *II*

948 SEVERE COMBINED IMMUNODEFICIENCY

Severe Combined Immunodeficiency (SCID) is a group of rare congenital syndromes characterized by little if any immune responses. This results in frequent recurring infections. Cellular immune responses involve specialized white blood cells known as T lymphocytes or "killer cells." These cells assist other white blood cells (B lymphocytes) to respond to infectious, foreign agents that invade the body (i.e., bacteria or viruses). The B lymphocytes maintain immunity by enabling the body to produce and preserve circulating antibodies.

People with Severe Combined Immunodeficiency are unusually susceptible to recurrent infections with bacteria, viruses, fungi, and other infectious agents that can be life-threatening.

There are several types of Severe Combined Immunodeficiencies. These include: Autosomal Recessive Severe Combined Immunodeficiency, X-Linked Recessive Severe Combined Immunodeficiency, Adenosine Deaminase Deficiency (ADA), Bare Lymphocyte Syndrome, Severe Combined Immunodeficiency with Leukopenia (Reticular Dysgenesis), and Swiss-type Agammaglobulinemia. Each type of Severe Combined Immune Deficiency is caused by a different genetic defect, but the primary symptom is reduced or absent immune functions, and all types are hereditary.

In addition to The National Organization for Rare Disorders (NORD) listed in Section III, the following organizations in Section II (Disease Specific) and in Section III (Umbrella) and Section IV (Government Agencies) can provide more information:

Alliance of Genetic Support Groups, *III*
Immune Deficiency Foundation, *III*
International Patient Organization for Primary Immunodeficiencies, *III*
Jeffrey Modell Foundation, *III*
March of Dimes Birth Defects Foundation, *III*
NIH/National Institute of Allergy and Infectious Diseases, *IV*

949 SHEEHAN SYNDROME

Sheehan Syndrome is caused by abnormal diminishment or cessation of pituitary gland functioning (hypopituitarism). The disorder affects females and is caused by necrosis (death of cells) of the anterior pituitary gland secondary to profound blood loss during and after childbirth, with vascular collapse and shock (postpartum collapse).

In addition to The National Organization for Rare Disorders (NORD) listed in Section III, the following organizations in Section II (Disease Specific) and in Section III (Umbrella) and Section IV (Government Agencies) can provide more information:

Brain and Pituitary Foundation of America, *III*
NIH/National Digestive Diseases Information Clearinghouse, *IV*
Thyroid Foundation of America, Inc., *III*

950 SHORT CHAIN ACYL COA DEHYDROGENASE DEFICIENCY (SCAD)

Short-Chain Acyl-CoA Dehydrogenase Deficiency is an extremely rare inherited disorder of fat metabolism belonging to a group of diseases known as organic acidemias. Excessive amounts of acids and ammonia accumulate in the blood and body tissues due to a deficiency of an enzyme known as Short-Chain CoA Dehydrogenase. This enzyme is needed to break down fatty acids in the blood.

There are two distinct types of Short-Chain Acyl-CoA Dehydrogenase Deficiency. The more severe generalized form is present at birth (congenital) and characterized by progressive muscle weakness (hypotonia) and the accumulation of acidic waste product in the blood (organic acidemia). The symptoms in infants associated with organic acidemia may include poor feeding, frequent vomiting, and/or lethargy. Congenital Short-Chain Acyl-CoA Dehydrogenase Deficiency may lead to life-threatening complications. The milder adult onset form of this disorder affects the skeletal muscles and is characterized by muscle weakness.

In addition to The National Organization for Rare Disorders (NORD) listed in Section III, the following organizations in Section II (Disease Specific) and in Section III (Umbrella) and Section IV (Government Agencies) can provide more information:

FOD (Fatty Oxidation Disorder) Family Support Group, *III*
NIH/National Institute of Diabetes, Digestive & Kidney Diseases, *IV*
Organic Acidemia Association, *III*
Research Trust for Metabolic Diseases in Children, *III*
United Mitochondrial Disease Foundation, *III*

951 SHWACHMAN SYNDROME

Shwachman Syndrome is an extremely rare inherited disorder with multiple and varied manifestations. In most cases, the disorder may be characterized by signs of insufficient absorption (malabsorption) of fats and other nutrients due to abnormal development of the pancreas (pancreatic insufficiency); abnormal bone development affecting the rib cage and/or bones in the arms and/or legs (metaphyseal dysostosis); short stature; and/or improper functioning of the bone marrow (bone marrow dysfunction), resulting in low levels of circulating blood cells (hematologic abnormalities).

Due to improper bone changes, individuals with Shwachman Syndrome may exhibit abnormal thickening of the ribs and their supporting connective tissue (costochondral thickening), resulting in abnormally short, flared ribs. In addition, improper bone development (abnormal ossification) within the arms and/or legs (limbs) may cause growth delay in particular bones. Children with Shwachman Syndrome may also be smaller than expected for their ages, with below average height (short stature) and weight. Although malabsorption due to pancreatic insufficiency may itself cause problems with growth and nutrition, short stature appears to be one of the many primary manifestations of Shwachman Syndrome.

In addition, as a result of bone marrow dysfunction, individuals with Shwachman Syndrome may exhibit a decrease in any or all types of blood cells. Therefore, they may have low levels of certain white blood cells (neutropenia), platelets (thrombocytopenia), red blood cells (anemia), and/or all types of blood cells (pancytopenia). Neutropenia is the most common blood abnormality associated with Shwachman Syndrome. Because neutrophils, a type of white blood cell, play an essential role in fighting bacterial infections, many affected individuals are prone to repeated bacterial infections (e.g., recurrent respiratory infections [pneumonia] and infections of the middle ear [otitis media]); in some cases, infections may be severe.

In some cases, affected individuals may also exhibit additional physical and/or developmental abnormalities. Shwachman Syndrome is believed to be inherited as an autosomal recessive genetic trait.

In addition to The National Organization for Rare Disorders (NORD) listed in Section III, the following organizations in Section II (Disease Specific) and in Section III (Umbrella) and Section IV (Government Agencies) can provide more information:

NIH/National Arthritis and Musculoskeletal and Skin Diseases Information Clearinghouse, *IV*
NIH/National Digestive Diseases Information Clearinghouse, *IV*
NIH/National Heart, Lung and Blood Institute Information Center, *IV*
National Neutropenia Network, *II*
Shwachman Syndrome Support International, *II*

952 SHY DRAGER SYNDROME

Shy-Drager Syndrome is a rare neurological disorder characterized by progressive failure of the autonomic nervous system. The autonomic nervous system is the part of the nervous system that controls a variety of vital involuntary body functions. These include regulation of heart rate, blood pressure, sweating, bowel and bladder control, as well as a variety of other bodily functions. Symptoms of Shy-Drager Syndrome include unusually low blood pressure while standing upright (orthostatic hypotension), loss of bladder and bowel control, and/or lack of sweating.

The exact cause of Shy-Drager Syndrome is not known. Symptoms develop due to the degeneration of certain groups of nerve cells in the spinal column. Progressive neurological degeneration may also occur in other areas of the nervous system and can produce other symptoms that are frequently confused with other disorders, especially Parkinson's Disease. The course of Shy-Drager Syndrome is variable, and some people with this disease may have mild symptoms for several years.

In addition to The National Organization for Rare Disorders (NORD) listed in Section III, the following organizations in Section II (Disease Specific) and in Section III (Umbrella) and Section IV (Government Agencies) can provide more information:

Association for Neuro-Metabolic Disorders, *III*
NIH/National Institute of Neurological Disorders and Stroke, *IV*
National Dysautonomia Research Foundation, *III*
Shy Drager Syndrome Support Group, *II*
WE MOVE, *III*

953 SIALADENITIS

Sialadenitis is a condition characterized by inflammation and enlargement of the salivary glands, the three pairs of glands that secrete saliva into the mouth. Sialadenitis is often associated with pain, tenderness, redness, and gradual, localized swelling of the affected area. The exact cause of Sialadenitis is not known.

In addition to The National Organization for Rare Disorders (NORD) listed in Section III, the following organizations in Section II (Disease Specific) and in Section III (Umbrella) and Section IV (Government Agencies) can provide more information:

NIH/National Oral Health Information Clearinghouse, *IV*

954 SIALIDOSIS

Sialidosis is a very rare inherited metabolic disorder characterized by a deficiency of the enzyme alpha-neuraminidase. This disorder belongs to a group of diseases known as lysosomal disorders. Lysosomes are particles bound in membranes within cells that break down certain fats and carbohydrates. The deficiency of alpha-neuraminidase that characterizes Sialidosis leads to the abnormal accumulation of certain complex carbohydrates (mucopolysaccharides) and certain fatty substances (mucolipids) in many tissues of the body. Previously known as Mucolipidosis I, Sialidosis belongs to a subgroup of lysosomal diseases known as Mucolipidoses.

The symptoms of Sialidosis Type I, which typically begin during the 2nd decade of life, may include sudden involuntary muscle contractions (myoclonus), the appearance of red spots (cherry-red macules) in the eyes, and/or other neurological findings. Sialidosis Type II may begin during infancy or later. It is characterized by the same visual characteristics as Sialidosis Type I, as well as other symptoms such as mildly coarse facial features, skeletal malformations, and/or mild mental retardation. Sialidosis is inherited as an autosomal recessive genetic trait.

In addition to The National Organization for Rare Disorders (NORD) listed in Section III, the following organizations in Section II (Disease Specific) and in Section III (Umbrella) and Section IV (Government Agencies) can provide more information:
Canadian Society for Mucopolysaccharide and Related Diseases, Inc., *III*
Metabolic Information Network, *III*
NIH/National Digestive Diseases Information Clearinghouse, *IV*
National MPS (Mucopolysaccharidoses/Mucolipidoses) Society, Inc., *III*
Research Trust for Metabolic Diseases in Children, *III*
The Arc (a national organization on mental retardation), *III*
Vaincre Les Maladies Lysosomales, *III*

955 SICKLE CELL DISEASE

Sickle Cell Disease is a rare inherited blood disorder. It is characterized by the presence of sickle or crescent shaped red blood cells (erythrocytes) in the bloodstream. These abnormally shaped cells become rigid and lodge themselves in the very tiny blood vessels (capillaries) of the peripheral blood system (blood vessels outside of the heart). The capillaries become clogged, preventing the normal flow of oxygen to tissues. Sickle Cell Disease has several recognized forms including Sickle Cell Anemia, Sickle Cell Hemoglobin C Disease and Sickle Cell Thalassemia Disease.

In addition to The National Organization for Rare Disorders (NORD) listed in Section III, the following organizations in Section II (Disease Specific) and in Section III (Umbrella) and Section IV (Government Agencies) can provide more information:
Alliance of Genetic Support Groups, *III*
Canadian Sickle Cell Society, *II*
Cooley's Anemia Foundation, Inc., *II*
March of Dimes Birth Defects Foundation, *III*
NIH/National Heart, Lung and Blood Institute Information Center, *IV*
Sickle Cell Disease Association of America, Inc., *II*
Triad Sickle Cell Anemia Foundation, *II*

956 SIMIAN B VIRUS INFECTION

Simian B Virus Infection is caused by a type of herpesvirus. It is an infectious disorder contracted chiefly by laboratory workers exposed to infected monkeys and/or simian tissue cultures. It is characterized by a viral invasion of the brain (Encephalitis) and the membranes (meninges) surrounding the brain. Occasionally, the infection affects the spinal cord structures as well (Encephalomyelitis). Neurological damage may result from this infection. Without treatment, some cases of Simian B Virus may be life- threatening.

In addition to The National Organization for Rare Disorders (NORD) listed in Section III, the following organizations in Section II (Disease Specific) and in Section III (Umbrella) and Section IV (Government Agencies) can provide more information:
Centers for Disease Control and Prevention, *IV*
NIH/National Institute of Allergy and Infectious Diseases, *IV*
World Health Organization (WHO) Regional Office for the Americas (AMRO), *III*

957 SIMPSON DYSMORPHIA SYNDROME

Simpson Dysmorphia Syndrome is a rare X-linked recessive inherited disorder. Major symptoms and physical findings may include abnormally increased growth before and after birth (prenatally and postnatally); a broad, stocky appearance; a large protruding jaw; a short, broad nose; incomplete closure of the roof of the mouth (cleft palate); and broad, short hands and fingers. Individuals usually reach an above-average height. The general distinguishing features typically become less apparent in adulthood.

In addition to The National Organization for Rare Disorders (NORD) listed in Section III, the following organizations in Section II (Disease Specific) and in Section III (Umbrella) and Section IV (Government Agencies) can provide more information:
Beckwith Wiedemann Support Network, *II*
Children's Craniofacial Association, *III*
FACES: The National Craniofacial Association, *III*
NIH/National Arthritis and Musculoskeletal and Skin Diseases Information Clearinghouse, *IV*

958 SINGLETON MERTEN SYNDROME

Singleton-Merten Syndrome is an extremely rare disorder characterized by abnormalities of the teeth (dental dysplasia), accumulation of calcium deposits (calcifications) in the major artery of the body (aorta) and certain valves of the heart (i.e., aortic and mitral valves), and/or progressive thinning and loss of protein of the bones (osteoporosis). Dental abnormalities may include malformed (dysplastic) teeth and/or premature loss of primary (deciduous) teeth. Abnormal accumulations of calcium deposits in the aorta may lead to narrowing (stenosis) of the aorta, resulting in life-threatening complications (e.g., heart block, heart failure, etc.). Other physical findings associated with Singleton-Merten Syndrome may include generalized muscle weakness; progressive loss or wasting away of muscle tissue (atrophy); growth retardation, possibly resulting in short stature; delays in motor development; a skin condition characterized by thickened patches of red, scaly skin, particularly on the fingers; and/or malformation of the hips and/or feet. Singleton-Merten Syndrome appears to occur randomly for no apparent reason (sporadic).

In addition to The National Organization for Rare Disorders (NORD) listed in Section III, the following organizations in Section II (Disease Specific) and in Section III (Umbrella) and Section IV (Government Agencies) can provide more information:

Congenital Heart Anomalies, Support, Education, & Resources, *III*
Congenital Heart Disease Resource Page, *III*
NIH/National Heart, Lung and Blood Institute Information Center, *IV*
NIH/National Institute of Arthritis and Musculoskeletal and Skin Diseases, *IV*
NIH/National Institute of Child Health and Human Development, *IV*
Osteoporosis and Related Bone Diseases National Resource Center, *III*

959 SIRENOMELIA SEQUENCE

Sirenomelia Sequence is a birth defect in which affected infants are born with a single lower extremity or with two legs that are fused together. Due to the wide range of possible physical deformities that may occur, the symptoms and physical findings associated with Sirenomelia Sequence vary greatly from case to case.

In addition to The National Organization for Rare Disorders (NORD) listed in Section III, the following organizations in Section II (Disease Specific) and in Section III (Umbrella) and Section IV (Government Agencies) can provide more information:

NIH/National Institute of Child Health and Human Development, *IV*

960 SJOGREN SYNDROME

Sjogren Syndrome is an autoimmune disorder characterized by degeneration of the mucus-secreting glands, particularly the tear ducts of the eyes (lacrimal) and saliva glands of the mouth. Autoimmune disorders are caused when the body's natural defenses (antibodies, lymphocytes, etc.) against invading organisms suddenly begin to attack healthy tissue. Sjogren Syndrome is also associated with inflammatory disorders such as arthritis or Lupus.

In addition to The National Organization for Rare Disorders (NORD) listed in Section III, the following organizations in Section II (Disease Specific) and in Section III (Umbrella) and Section IV (Government Agencies) can provide more information:

Arthritis Foundation, *III*
NIH/National Arthritis and Musculoskeletal and Skin Diseases Information Clearinghouse, *IV*
NIH/National Oral Health Information Clearinghouse, *IV*
National Sjogren's Syndrome Association, *II*
Sjogren's Syndrome Foundation, Inc., *II*
Swedish Sjogren's Syndrome Association, *II*

961 SLY SYNDROME

Sly Syndrome (Mucopolysaccharidosis Type VII [MPS VII]) is an extremely rare inherited metabolic disorder characterized by a deficiency of the enzyme beta-glucuronidase, a lysosomal enzyme. Sly Syndrome belongs to a group of disorders known as the Mucopolysaccharidoses, which are lysosomal storage diseases. Lysosomes are particles bound in membranes within cells that break down certain fats and carbohydrates. In Sly Syndrome, the deficiency of beta-glucuronidase leads to the accumulation of certain complex carbohydrates (mucopolysaccharides) in many tissues and organs of the body. Excessive levels of dermatan and keratan sulfate are also present in the urine of people with this disorder.

The symptoms of Sly Syndrome are similar to those of Hurler Syndrome (MPS I) and the other Mucopolysaccharidoses. Symptoms may include mental retardation, short stature with an unusually short trunk, and/or abnormalities of the intestines, corneas of the eyes, and/or the skeletal system. Sly Syndrome is inherited as an autosomal recessive genetic trait.

In addition to The National Organization for Rare Disorders (NORD) listed in Section III, the following organizations in Section II (Disease Specific) and in Section III (Umbrella) and Section IV (Government Agencies) can provide more information:

Canadian Society for Mucopolysaccharide and Related Diseases, Inc., *III*
Metabolic Information Network, *III*
NIH/National Digestive Diseases Information Clearinghouse, *IV*
National MPS (Mucopolysaccharidoses/Mucolipidoses) Society, Inc., *III*
Research Trust for Metabolic Diseases in Children, *III*
The Arc (a national organization on mental retardation), *III*
Vaincre Les Maladies Lysosomales, *III*

962 SMITH LEMLI OPITZ SYNDROME

Smith-Lemli-Opitz syndrome is a hereditary developmental disorder. It is characterized by nostrils that tilt forward (anteverted nares), drooping eyelids, webbing between the second and third toes, male genital abnormalities, mental retardation, and small stature.

In addition to The National Organization for Rare Disorders (NORD) listed in Section III, the following organizations in Section II (Disease Specific) and in Section III (Umbrella) and Section IV (Government Agencies) can provide more information:

NIH/National Institute of Child Health and Human Development, *IV*
Smith Lemli-Opitz/RSH Advocacy and Exchange, *II*
The Arc (a national organization on mental retardation), *III*

963 SMITH MAGENIS SYNDROME

Smith-Magenis Syndrome is a rare chromosomal disorder characterized by abnormalities of the head and facial (craniofacial) area, delays in the acquisition of skills requiring the coordination of mental and muscular activities (psychomotor retardation), mental retardation, speech delays, and/or behavioral abnormalities. Characteristic craniofacial abnormalities may include an abnormally short, broad head (brachycephaly); an abnormally broad, flat midface; a broad nasal bridge; an unusually prominent jaw (prognathism); incomplete closure of the roof of the mouth (cleft palate); and/or malformed, abnormally positioned ears. In addition, most affected individuals experience speech delays that may occur in association with hearing impairment and have an abnormally hoarse, deep voice. Behavioral abnormalities associated with the disorder may include hyperactivity and self-destructive behavior including head-banging, wrist-biting, inserting foreign objects into the nose and ears (polyembolokoilamania), and/or pulling out the fingernails and toenails (onychotillomania). Many individuals with Smith-Magenis Syndrome also experience sleep disturbances including difficulties falling asleep and staying asleep. Smith-Magenis Syndrome occurs due to deletion of a portion of the short arm (p) of chromosome 17 (17p11.2). The chromosomal deletion occurs due to a spontaneous (de novo) genetic change (mutation) that occurs for unknown reasons (sporadic).

In addition to The National Organization for Rare Disorders (NORD) listed in Section III, the following organizations in Section II (Disease Specific) and in Section III (Umbrella) and Section IV (Government Agencies) can provide more information:

American Society for Deaf Children, *III*
Chromosome Deletion Outreach, *III*
NIH/National Institute of Child Health and Human Development, *IV*
PRISMS (Parents & Researchers Interested in Smith-Magenis Syndrome), *II*
Smith-Magenis Syndrome Contact Group, *II*
Vision Foundation, Inc., *III*

964 SNEDDON SYNDROME

Sneddon Syndrome is a rare progressive disorder of the blood vessels that may be inherited as an autosomal dominant trait. Characteristics include multiple episodes of reduced blood flow to the brain (cerebral ischemia) and bluish net-like patterns of discoloration on the skin surrounding normal- appearing skin (livedo reticularis). Major symptoms may include headache, dizziness, abnormally high blood pressure (hypertension), heart disease, mini-strokes, and/or stroke. Lesions (infarcts) may develop within the central nervous system as a result of reduced blood flow to the brain and may cause reduced mental capacity, memory loss, and/or other neurological symptoms.

In addition to The National Organization for Rare Disorders (NORD) listed in Section III, the following organizations in Section II (Disease Specific) and in Section III (Umbrella) and Section IV (Government Agencies) can provide more information:

NIH/National Heart, Lung and Blood Institute Information Center, *IV*
NIH/National Institute of Neurological Disorders and Stroke, *IV*
National Stroke Association, *II*

965 SOTOS SYNDROME

Sotos Syndrome is a rare genetic disorder characterized by excessive growth that occurs prior to and after birth (prenatally and postnatally). At birth, affected infants have unusually increased body length that is abnormal in proportion to weight, which may also be above average; in addition, newborns typically demonstrate advanced bone growth, abnormally large hands and/or feet, and characteristic facial features. Abnormally rapid growth continues after birth until approximately four or five years of age, at which time growth may slow to a normal rate. An affected individual's final height often is within normal range. Affected infants and children may also demonstrate developmental abnormalities including delays in reaching developmental milestones (e.g., sitting, crawling, walking); delays in the acquisition of skills requiring the coordination of muscular and mental activity (psychomotor retardation); delayed language skills; and mild to severe mental retardation. Characteristic facial abnormalities may include an unusually large head (macrocephaly) that may appear elongated (dolichocephalic) with an abnormally prominent forehead (frontal bossing); widely-spaced eyes (ocular hypertelorism); downwardly slanting eyelid folds (palpebral fissures); a highly-arched roof of the mouth (palate); protrusion of the lower jaw (prognathism); and/or a pointed chin. Most cases of Sotos Syndrome occur randomly, for no known reason (sporadically). In rare cases, however, when a positive family history is found, the disorder may be inherited as an autosomal dominant genetic trait.

In addition to The National Organization for Rare Disorders (NORD) listed in Section III, the following organizations in Section II (Disease Specific) and in Section III (Umbrella) and Section IV (Government Agencies) can provide more information:

NIH/National Institute of Child Health and Human Development, *IV*
Sotos Syndrome Support Association, *II*
The Arc (a national organization on mental retardation), *III*

966 SPASMODIC TORTICOLLIS

Spasmodic Torticollis is a tonic or intermittent spasm of the neck muscles resulting in rotation and tilting of the head that is often painful. There are three different varieties of the disorder: Tonic, causing sustained turning of the head to one side, due to increased asymmetric muscle tone in one or more neck muscles; Clonic, causing shaking movements of the head; and Mixed Tonic and Clonic, involving both kinds of movement. The cause of this disorder is usually unknown.

In addition to The National Organization for Rare Disorders (NORD) listed in Section III, the following organizations in Section II (Disease Specific) and in Section III (Umbrella) and Section IV (Government Agencies) can provide more information:

Dystonia Medical Research Foundation, *III*
NIH/National Institute of Neurological Disorders and Stroke, *IV*
National Spasmodic Torticollis Association, *II*
WE MOVE, *III*

967 SPINA BIFIDA

Spina Bifida is characterized by incomplete closure of certain bones of the spinal column (vertebrae), leaving a portion of the spinal cord exposed. Part of the contents of the spinal canal may protrude through this opening. In the most severe form, rachischisis, the opening is extensive. Spina Bifida may cause difficulties with bladder control and walking and/or other abnormalities, depending on the severity of associated symptoms.

In addition to The National Organization for Rare Disorders (NORD) listed in Section III, the following organizations in Section II (Disease Specific) and in Section III (Umbrella) and Section IV (Government Agencies) can provide more information:

Association for Spina Bifida and Hydrocephalus, *III*
March of Dimes Birth Defects Foundation, *III*
NIH/National Institute of Neurological Disorders and Stroke, *IV*
National Easter Seal Society, Inc., *III*
Spina Bifida Association of America, *II*
Spina Bifida and Hydrocephalus Association of Canada, *III*

968 SPLIT HAND DEFORMITY

Split-hand deformity is a genetic disorder characterized by the absence of fingers or parts of fingers, commonly occurring with a cleft of the hand. This combination often gives the hand a clawlike appearance. When a cleft does occur, it usually affects both hands and both feet.

There are many types and combinations of deformities that appear in Split-hand deformity. It is believed that they are all the result of a common genetic defect that ranges widely in severity.

In addition to The National Organization for Rare Disorders (NORD) listed in Section III, the following

organizations in Section II (Disease Specific) and in Section III (Umbrella) and Section IV (Government Agencies) can provide more information:
Association of Children's Prosthetic/Orthotic Clinics, *III*
NIH/National Arthritis and Musculoskeletal and Skin Diseases Information Clearinghouse, *IV*

969 SPONDYLOEPIPHYSEAL DYSPLASIA TARDA

Spondyloepiphyseal Dysplasia Tarda is a rare hereditary disorder and affects males more frequently than females. Physical characteristics may include multiple skeletal abnormalities including dwarfism, spinal deformities, and an unusually short trunk.

In addition to The National Organization for Rare Disorders (NORD) listed in Section III, the following organizations in Section II (Disease Specific) and in Section III (Umbrella) and Section IV (Government Agencies) can provide more information:
Human Growth Foundation, *III*
Little People of America, *III*
Little People's Research Fund, Inc., *III*
MAGIC Foundation for Children's Growth, *III*
NIH/National Institute of Child Health and Human Development, *IV*
Short Stature Foundation, *III*

970 SPONDYLOEPIPHYSEAL DYSPLASIA, CONGENITAL

Congenital Spondyloepiphyseal Dysplasia is a rare inherited disorder characterized by growth deficiency before birth (prenatally), spinal malformations, and/or abnormalities of the eyes. As affected individuals age, growth deficiency eventually results in short stature (dwarfism) due, in part, to a disproportionately short neck and trunk, and a hip deformity in which the thigh bone is angled toward the center of the body (coxa vara). In most cases, affected individuals may have diminished muscle tone (hypotonia), abnormal front-to-back and side-to-side curvature of the spine (kyphoscoliosis), abnormal inward curvature of the spine (lumbar lordosis), and/or unusual protrusion of the breast bone (sternum) (pectus carinatum). Affected individuals also have abnormalities affecting the eyes including nearsightedness (myopia) and, in approximately 50 percent of cases, detachment of the nerve-rich membrane lining the eye (retina). Congenital Spondyloepiphyseal Dysplasia is inherited as an autosomal dominant genetic trait.

In addition to The National Organization for Rare Disorders (NORD) listed in Section III, the following organizations in Section II (Disease Specific) and in Section III (Umbrella) and Section IV (Government Agencies) can provide more information:
Human Growth Foundation, *III*
Little People of America, *III*
Little People's Research Fund, Inc., *III*
MAGIC Foundation for Children's Growth, *III*
NIH/National Institute of Child Health & Human Development (Preg & Perinat), *IV*
Short Stature Foundation, *III*

971 SPRENGEL DEFORMITY

Sprengel Deformity is a rare congenital disorder in which the shoulder blade has an upward displacement. The elevated shoulder blade causes a lump in the back of the base of the neck and may limit movement of the arm on the affected side. This disorder typically appears at birth for no apparent reason although there have been cases in which the disorder was inherited as an autosomal dominant trait. Other skeletal and muscular abnormalities have been found in association with Sprengel Deformity.

In addition to The National Organization for Rare Disorders (NORD) listed in Section III, the following organizations in Section II (Disease Specific) and in Section III (Umbrella) and Section IV (Government Agencies) can provide more information:
NIH/National Arthritis and Musculoskeletal and Skin Diseases Information Clearinghouse, *IV*

972 STEIN LEVANTHAL SYNDROME

Stein-Levanthal Syndrome, a rare disorder that affects females, is characterized by the presence of multiple cysts on the ovaries (polycystic ovaries), the absence of menstruation (amenorrhea) or irregular and abnormal menstruation, excessive amounts of body hair (hirsutism), excessive body weight (obesity), and infertility. In many cases, the disorder may be inherited as a dominant genetic trait.

In addition to The National Organization for Rare Disorders (NORD) listed in Section III, the following organizations in Section II (Disease Specific) and in Section III (Umbrella) and Section IV (Government Agencies) can provide more information:
NIH/National Institute of Child Health and Human Development, *IV*
National Women's Health Network, *III*
Recovery, Inc., *III*

973 STENOSIS, SPINAL

Spinal stenosis is a rare condition characterized by abnormal narrowing (stenosis) of the spaces within the spinal canal, spinal nerve root canals, or the bones of the spinal column (vertebrae). Affected individuals may experience pain in the lower back and/or the legs. In some cases, affected individuals may have difficulty walking. Spinal stenosis may occur as a result of spinal injury, surgery, abnormal bone growth, or deterioration. In some cases, spinal stenosis may be inherited as an autosomal dominant genetic trait.

In addition to The National Organization for Rare Disorders (NORD) listed in Section III, the following organizations in Section II (Disease Specific) and in Section III (Umbrella) and Section IV (Government Agencies) can provide more information:
NIH/National Institute of Arthritis and Musculoskeletal and Skin Diseases, *IV*
National Scoliosis Foundation, *II*
National Spinal Cord Injury Hotline, *III*

974 STEVENS JOHNSON SYNDROME

Stevens-Johnson Syndrome is a rare disorder characterized by inflammation of the mucous membranes of the mouth, throat, anogenital region, intestinal tract and membrane lining the eyelids (conjunctiva). Affected individuals may have abnormalities (lesions) of the skin and mucous membranes that are purplish or red in color. The abnormalities may be flat (macules) or small and raised (papules). In some cases, the lesions may develop raised fluid-filled centers (bullae or blisters). Affected individuals may also have blisters and/or bleeding in the mucous membranes of the lips, eyes, mouth, nasal passage, and genitals. In addition, abnormalities of the eyes may develop as a result of the lesions caused by Stevens-Johnson Syndrome (ocular sequelae). Such abnormalities may include infection of the delicate membrane of the eye and eyelids (conjunctiva) and inflammation associated with an abnormal discharge from the conjunctiva (purulent conjunctivitis).

Some researchers believe that Stevens-Johnson Syndrome is a severe form of Erythema Multiforme, an inflammatory disorder of the skin and mucous membranes (mucocutaneous) that is triggered by an allergic reaction. Other researchers believe that Stevens-Johnson Syndrome is an independent syndrome. It is uncertain exactly what causes the allergic reaction, but researchers think it may be triggered by an allergic reaction to certain drugs such as antibiotics, including sulfonamides, tetracyclines, amoxicillin, and ampicillin. In some cases, nonsteroidal anti-inflammatory medications and anticonvulsants, such as Tegretol and phenobarbitals, have also been implicated. In some cases, it is also possible that the disorder may be triggered by an infection.

In addition to The National Organization for Rare Disorders (NORD) listed in Section III, the following organizations in Section II (Disease Specific) and in Section III (Umbrella) and Section IV (Government Agencies) can provide more information:
NIH/National Eye Institute, *IV*
NIH/National Institute of Allergy and Infectious Diseases, *IV*
NIH/National Institute of Arthritis and Musculoskeletal and Skin Diseases, *IV*

975 STICKLER SYNDROME

Stickler Syndrome is a genetic disorder inherited as a dominant trait. This disorder is characterized by congenital abnormalities of the eye, a small jaw, and a cleft palate. Degenerative changes in some joints with bone abnormalities may occur early in life.

In addition to The National Organization for Rare Disorders (NORD) listed in Section III, the following organizations in Section II (Disease Specific) and in Section III (Umbrella) and Section IV (Government Agencies) can provide more information:
NIH/National Eye Institute, *IV*
Stickler Involved People, *II*
Stickler Syndrome Support Group, *II*

976 STIFF MAN SYNDROME

Stiff-Man Syndrome is an extremely rare progressive neurological disorder characterized by persistent stiffness (rigidity) and spasms of certain voluntary muscles, especially those of the legs and the feet. In some cases, muscles of the neck, trunk, and shoulders may also be involved. Stiff-Man Syndrome may begin as recurring (intermittent) episodes of stiffness and spasms, often precipitated by surprise or minor physical contact. The exact cause of Stiff-Man Syndrome is not known.

In addition to The National Organization for Rare Disorders (NORD) listed in Section III, the following organizations in Section II (Disease Specific) and in Section III (Umbrella) and Section IV (Government Agencies) can provide more information:
American Autoimmune Related Diseases Association, Inc., *III*
NIH/National Institute of Neurological Disorders and Stroke, *IV*

977 STREPTOCOCCUS, GROUP B

Group B Streptococcus is a bacterial infection in which groups of streptococcus bacteria reproduce and multiply (colonize) in the mucous membranes. This bacteria is found most often in the vagina and rectum of females. Group B Streptococci can be transmitted sexually, as well as to a fetus as the infant passes through the birth canal.

The main groups at risk of developing disease from GBS are newborn children of an infected mother, women after childbirth, females after gynecologic surgery and older male and female patients with other serious diseases.

In addition to The National Organization for Rare Disorders (NORD) listed in Section III, the following organizations in Section II (Disease Specific) and in Section III (Umbrella) and Section IV (Government Agencies) can provide more information:
Centers for Disease Control and Prevention, *IV*
Group B Strep Association, *II*
NIH/National Institute of Allergy and Infectious Diseases, *IV*

978 STURGE WEBER SYNDROME

Sturge-Weber Syndrome is composed of three major symptoms. Excessive blood vessel growths (leptomeningeal angiomas) are accompanied by accumulations of calcium inside the brain, and seizures. Facial birth marks (nevus flammeus) appear usually on one side of the face. Angiomas similar to those found in the brain can develop inside the eye, often with secondary glaucoma.

In addition to The National Organization for Rare Disorders (NORD) listed in Section III, the following organizations in Section II (Disease Specific) and in Section III (Umbrella) and Section IV (Government Agencies) can provide more information:
Alliance of Genetic Support Groups, *III*
NIH/National Institute of Neurological Disorders and Stroke, *IV*
Nevus Network, *II*
Nevus Outreach, Inc., *II*
Sturge-Weber Foundation, *II*
The Arc (a national organization on mental retardation), *III*

979 SUBACUTE SCLEROSING PANENCEPHALITIS

Subacute Sclerosing Panencephalitis (SSPE) is a progressive neurological disorder characterized by inflammation of the brain (encephalitis). The disease may develop due to reactivation of the measles virus or an inappropriate immune response to the measles virus. SSPE usually develops 2 to 10 years after the original viral attack. Initial symptoms may include memory loss, irritability, seizures, involuntary muscle movements, and/or behavioral changes, leading to neurological deterioration.

In addition to The National Organization for Rare Disorders (NORD) listed in Section III, the following organizations in Section II (Disease Specific) and in Section III (Umbrella) and Section IV (Government Agencies) can provide more information:
NIH/National Institute of Allergy and Infectious Diseases, *IV*
National Subacute Sclerosing Panencephalitis Registry, *II*
WE MOVE, *III*

980 SUCROSE ISOMALTOSE MALABSORPTION, CONGENITAL

Congenital sucrose-isomaltose malabsorption is a rare inherited metabolic disorder characterized by the deficiency or absence of the enzymes sucrase and isomaltase. This enzyme complex (sucrase-isomaltase) assists in the breakdown of a certain sugar (i.e., sucrose) and certain products of starch digestion (dextrins). The sucrase-isomaltase enzyme complex is normally found within the tiny, finger-like projections or microvilli (brush border) lining the small intestine. When this enzyme complex is deficient, appropriate absorption of the nutrients from ingested sucrose and starch is hampered.

Symptoms of this disorder become evident soon after sucrose or starches are ingested by an affected infant. Breast-fed infants or those on lactose-only formula manifest no symptoms until such time as sucrose (found in fruit juices, solid foods, and/or some medications) is introduced into the diet. Symptoms are variable among affected individuals and may include watery diarrhea, abdominal swelling (distension) and/or discomfort, abnormally low levels of body fluids (dehydration), malnutrition, delay in growth and weight gain (failure to thrive), irritability, colic, abrasion and/or irritation (excoriation) of the skin on the buttocks, and/or vomiting. Intolerance to starch often disappears within the first few years of life and the symptoms of sucrose intolerance usually improve as the affected child ages. Congenital sucrose-isomaltose malabsorption is inherited as an autosomal recessive genetic trait.

In addition to The National Organization for Rare Disorders (NORD) listed in Section III, the following organizations in Section II (Disease Specific) and in Section III (Umbrella) and Section IV (Government Agencies) can provide more information:

Alliance of Genetic Support Groups, *III*
March of Dimes Birth Defects Foundation, *III*
Metabolic Information Network, *III*
NIH/National Digestive Diseases Information Clearinghouse, *IV*
Research Trust for Metabolic Diseases in Children, *III*

981 SUDDEN INFANT DEATH SYNDROME

Sudden Infant Death Syndrome (SIDS) is the sudden death of any infant that is unexpected by history and in which no adequate cause for death can be found. The disorder occurs in infants under the age of one year.

In addition to The National Organization for Rare Disorders (NORD) listed in Section III, the following organizations in Section II (Disease Specific) and in Section III (Umbrella) and Section IV (Government Agencies) can provide more information:
American Sudden Infant Death Syndrome Institute, *II*
NIH/National Institute of Neurological Disorders and Stroke, *IV*
National Sudden Infant Death Syndrome Resource Center, *II*
Sudden Infant Death Syndrome Alliance, Inc., *II*

982 SUMMITT SYNDROME

Summitt Syndrome is an extremely rare genetic disorder characterized by malformations of the head, abnormalities of the hands and/or feet, and obesity. The syndrome is inherited as an autosomal recessive genetic trait. Some researchers believe that Summitt Syndrome may be a variant of Carpenter Syndrome (Acrocephalopolysyndactyly Type II), a rare genetic disorder that is also characterized by malformations of the head, hands, and/or feet.

In addition to The National Organization for Rare Disorders (NORD) listed in Section III, the following organizations in Section II (Disease Specific) and in Section III (Umbrella) and Section IV (Government Agencies) can provide more information:
AboutFace U.S.A., *III*
Children's Craniofacial Association, *III*
FACES: The National Craniofacial Association, *III*
Forward Face, Inc., *III*
Let's Face It, Inc., *III*
NIH/National Institute of Child Health and Human Development, *IV*
National Foundation for Facial Reconstruction, *III*

983 SUTTON'S DISEASE II

Sutton's Disease II is characterized by the recurring eruption of painful inflamed ulcers in the mouth (stomatitis). There may be multiple ulcers of varying sizes. These ulcers in the mouth are commonly called canker sores. Sutton's Disease II is also known as Recurrent Aphthous Stomatitis. The exact cause of this disease is not fully understood, although it may be due to an abnormal immune response to the bacteria that are normally in the mouth.

In addition to The National Organization for Rare Disorders (NORD) listed in Section III, the following organizations in Section II (Disease Specific) and in Section III (Umbrella) and Section IV (Government Agencies) can provide more information:
NIH/National Oral Health Information Clearinghouse, *IV*

984 SWEET SYNDROME

Sweet Syndrome is a rare skin disorder characterized by painful red eruptions usually on the arms, face, neck, and legs. The exact cause of this disorder is not known, although it may be associated with an injury to the skin.

In addition to The National Organization for Rare Disorders (NORD) listed in Section III, the following organizations in Section II (Disease Specific) and in Section III (Umbrella) and Section IV (Government Agencies) can provide more information:
NIH/National Arthritis and Musculoskeletal and Skin Diseases Information Clearinghouse, *IV*
Skin Disease Research Core Centers of the National Institute of Arthritis, *IV*

985 SYPHILIS, ACQUIRED

Syphilis is a chronic infectious disease caused by a microorganism (treponema pallidum). It is transmitted by direct contact with an infected lesion, usually through sexual intercourse. When untreated, Syphilis progresses through primary, secondary and latent stages. Symptoms can remain dormant for years. Eventually any tissue or vascular organ in the body may be affected.

Syphilis may also be acquired by the fetus in the uterus (Congenital Syphilis). Syphilis can be cured with appropriate treatment.

In addition to The National Organization for Rare Disorders (NORD) listed in Section III, the following organizations in Section II (Disease Specific) and in Section III (Umbrella) and Section IV (Government Agencies) can provide more information:
Centers for Disease Control and Prevention, *IV*
NIH/National Institute of Allergy and Infectious Diseases, *IV*
Sexuality Information and Education Council of the U.S., *III*

986 SYPHILIS, CONGENITAL

Congenital Syphilis is a chronic infectious disease caused by a spirochete (treponema pallidum) acquired by the fetus in the uterus before birth. Symptoms of this disease may not become apparent until several weeks or months after birth and in some cases may take years to appear. Congenital Syphilis is passed on to the child from the mother who acquired the disease prior to or during pregnancy. The infant is more likely to have congenital syphilis when the mother has been infected during pregnancy although it is not uncommon for an infant to acquire congenital syphilis from a mother that was infected prior to pregnancy. Symptoms of early Congenital Syphilis include fever, skin problems and low birth weight. In Late Congenital Syphilis the symptoms of the disease do not usually become apparent until two to five years of age. In rare cases the disease may remain latent for years with symptoms not being diagnosed until well into adulthood.

In addition to The National Organization for Rare Disorders (NORD) listed in Section III, the following organizations in Section II (Disease Specific) and in Section III (Umbrella) and Section IV (Government Agencies) can provide more information:

Centers for Disease Control and Prevention, *IV*
NIH/National Institute of Allergy and Infectious Diseases, *IV*

987 SYRINGOBULBIA

Syringobulbia is a neurological disorder characterized by a fluid-filled cavity (syrinx) within the spinal cord that extends to involve the brain stem. The cavity is a congenital lesion, but for unknown reasons it often expands during adolescence or the young adult years. Syringobulbia usually occurs as a slitlike gap within the lower brainstem that may affect the lower cranial nerves including sensory and motor nerve pathways by disruption or compression.

In addition to The National Organization for Rare Disorders (NORD) listed in Section III, the following organizations in Section II (Disease Specific) and in Section III (Umbrella) and Section IV (Government Agencies) can provide more information:

American Syringomyelia Alliance Project, Inc., *II*
NIH/National Institute of Neurological Disorders and Stroke, *IV*
National Spinal Cord Injury Association, *III*
National Spinal Cord Injury Hotline, *III*

988 SYRINGOMYELIA

Syringomyelia is a neurological disorder characterized by a fluid-filled cavity (syrinx) within the spinal cord. The cavity is a congenital lesion, but for unknown reasons it often expands during adolescence or the young adult years. The syrinx is situated near the middle of the spine. It usually begins in the neck (cervical) area, but may extend across the spinal cord or virtually along its whole length.

In addition to The National Organization for Rare Disorders (NORD) listed in Section III, the following organizations in Section II (Disease Specific) and in Section III (Umbrella) and Section IV (Government Agencies) can provide more information:

American Syringomyelia Alliance Project, Inc., *II*
Canadian Syringomyelia Network, *II*
National Spinal Cord Injury Hotline, *III*

989 TORCH SYNDROME

TORCH Syndrome is a combination of 4 infectious diseases. The syndrome can occur in newborn babies, children, or adults with an impaired immune system. The four infections are: (To)xoplasmosis, (R)ubella [German Measles], (C)ytomegalovirus Infection, and Neonatal (H)erpes. The infectious TORCH Syndrome is caused by the Toxoplasmosis parasite and the 3 viruses causing Rubella, Cytomegalovirus infection, and Neonatal Herpes.

In addition to The National Organization for Rare Disorders (NORD) listed in Section III, the following organizations in Section II (Disease Specific) and in Section III (Umbrella) and Section IV (Government Agencies) can provide more information:

Centers for Disease Control and Prevention, *IV*
NIH/National Institute of Allergy and Infectious Diseases, *IV*
NIH/National Institute of Neurological Disorders and Stroke, *IV*

990 TANGIER DISEASE

Tangier Disease is an inherited blood disorder involving decreased concentrations of fat compounds in the blood called high density lipoproteins. Large amounts of these compounds may accumulate in certain organs of the body causing tissue discoloration. In later stages, these accumulations may cause organ enlargement and/or blood circulation problems.

In addition to The National Organization for Rare Disorders (NORD) listed in Section III, the following organizations in Section II (Disease Specific) and in Section III (Umbrella) and Section IV (Government Agencies) can provide more information:

NIH/National Institute of Neurological Disorders and Stroke, *IV*
National Tay-Sachs and Allied Diseases Association, Inc., *III*

991 **TARDIVE DYSKINESIA**

Tardive Dyskinesia (TD) is an involuntary movement disorder resulting from use of neuroleptic drugs that are used to control psychiatric or gastrointestinal problems. Long-term use of these drugs may produce biochemical abnormalities in the area of the brain known as the striatum.

In addition to The National Organization for Rare Disorders (NORD) listed in Section III, the following organizations in Section II (Disease Specific) and in Section III (Umbrella) and Section IV (Government Agencies) can provide more information:

Dystonia Medical Research Foundation, *III*
NIH/National Institute of Mental Health, *IV*
NIH/National Institute of Neurological Disorders and Stroke, *IV*
National Mental Health Association, *III*
Tardive Dyskinesia/Tardive Dystonia National Association, *II*
WE MOVE, *III*

992 **TARSAL TUNNEL SYNDROME**

Tarsal Tunnel Syndrome involves pressure on nerves to the foot causing pain. Persons with this disorder may notice a painful burning or tingling sensation in and around the ankles, sometimes extending to the toes. The disorder usually affects people who stand on their feet for long periods of time.

In addition to The National Organization for Rare Disorders (NORD) listed in Section III, the following organizations in Section II (Disease Specific) and in Section III (Umbrella) and Section IV (Government Agencies) can provide more information:

NIH/National Arthritis and Musculoskeletal and Skin Diseases Information Clearinghouse, *IV*

993 **TARUI DISEASE**

Tarui Disease is a glycogen storage disease. Symptoms of this hereditary metabolic disorder are caused by a lack of the enzyme phosphofructokinase in muscle and a partial deficiency of the enzyme in red blood cells. The enzyme deficiency prevents the breakdown of glucose into energy. Tarui Disease is characterized by pain and cramps in muscles during heavy exercise.

In addition to The National Organization for Rare Disorders (NORD) listed in Section III, the following organizations in Section II (Disease Specific) and in Section III (Umbrella) and Section IV (Government Agencies) can provide more information:

Association for Neuro-Metabolic Disorders, *III*
Metabolic Information Network, *III*
Muscular Dystrophy Association, *III*
NIH/National Digestive Diseases Information Clearinghouse, *IV*
Research Trust for Metabolic Diseases in Children, *III*
Vaincre Les Maladies Lysosomales, *III*

994 **TAY SACHS DISEASE**

Tay-Sachs disease is a rare inherited disorder that results in the progressive destruction of the central nervous system. The body is unable to properly metabolize certain fats (lipids) due to the absence of an enzyme (hexosaminidase A). This results in the accumulation of these fats in the brain (GM2 gangliosidosis). The disease is generally found among children of East European Jewish heritage. Sandhoff disease is another form of Tay-Sachs disease that is not limited to any particular ethnic group.

In addition to The National Organization for Rare Disorders (NORD) listed in Section III, the following organizations in Section II (Disease Specific) and in Section III (Umbrella) and Section IV (Government Agencies) can provide more information:

Alliance of Genetic Support Groups, *III*
Association for Neuro-Metabolic Disorders, *III*
March of Dimes Birth Defects Foundation, *III*
Metabolic Information Network, *III*
NIH/National Institute of Child Health and Human Development, *IV*
NIH/National Institute of Neurological Disorders and Stroke, *IV*
National Foundation for Jewish Genetic Diseases, *III*
National Tay-Sachs and Allied Diseases Association, Inc., *III*
Research Trust for Metabolic Diseases in Children, *III*

995 **TELECANTHUS WITH ASSOCIATED ABNORMALITIES**

Telecanthus With Associated Abnormalities is a very rare genetic disorder affecting the eyes and other parts of the body. Major symptoms include very widely spaced eyes (hypertelorism), urinary tract anomalies, and abnormalities in the development of the mouth and the lips.

In addition to The National Organization for Rare Disorders (NORD) listed in Section III, the following organizations in Section II (Disease Specific) and in Section III (Umbrella) and Section IV (Government Agencies) can provide more information:

AboutFace U.S.A., *III*
Children's Craniofacial Association, *III*
FACES: The National Craniofacial Association, *III*
Forward Face, Inc., *III*
NIH/National Institute of Child Health and Human Development, *IV*
The Arc (a national organization on mental retardation), *III*

996 TEMPOROMANDIBULAR JOINT DYSFUNCTION (TMJ)

Temporomandibular Joint Dysfunction (TMJ) is a painful disorder of the jaw joint that is made worse during or after eating or yawning. It can cause limited jaw movement and clicks and pops during chewing. In severe cases pain can radiate into the neck, shoulders and back.

In addition to The National Organization for Rare Disorders (NORD) listed in Section III, the following organizations in Section II (Disease Specific) and in Section III (Umbrella) and Section IV (Government Agencies) can provide more information:
NIH/National Oral Health Information Clearinghouse, *IV*
TMJ Association, Ltd., *II*

997 TETHERED SPINAL CORD SYNDROME

Tethered Spinal Cord Syndrome is a disorder characterized by progressive neurological deterioration due to unnatural stretching of the spinal cord caused by adhesions on the vertebrae. It most commonly results from defective closure of the neural tube during embryonic development (Spina Bifida).

In addition to The National Organization for Rare Disorders (NORD) listed in Section III, the following organizations in Section II (Disease Specific) and in Section III (Umbrella) and Section IV (Government Agencies) can provide more information:
Association of Birth Defect Children, Inc., *III*
Lipomyelomeningocele Family Support Network, *II*
NIH/National Institute of Child Health and Human Development, *IV*
NIH/National Institute of Neurological Disorders and Stroke, *IV*
Spina Bifida Association of America, *II*
Spina Bifida and Hydrocephalus Association of Canada, *III*

998 TETRAHYDROBIOPTERIN DEFICIENCY

Tetrahydrobiopterin Deficiency is a rare genetic, neurological disorder present at birth. It is caused by an inborn error of metabolism. Tetrahydrobiopterin is a natural substance (coenzyme) that enhances the action of enzymes. When Tetrahydrobiopterin is deficient, an abnormally high blood level of the amino acid phenylalanine occurs and low levels of some neurotransmitters are found. To avoid irreversible neurological damage, diagnosis and treatment of this progressive disorder are essential early in life.

In addition to The National Organization for Rare Disorders (NORD) listed in Section III, the following organizations in Section II (Disease Specific) and in Section III (Umbrella) and Section IV (Government Agencies) can provide more information:
Association for Neuro-Metabolic Disorders, *III*
Metabolic Information Network, *III*
NIH/National Institute of Neurological Disorders and Stroke, *IV*
Research Trust for Metabolic Diseases in Children, *III*
The Arc (a national organization on mental retardation), *III*

999 TETRALOGY OF FALLOT

Tetralogy of Fallot is the most common form of cyanotic congenital heart disease. Cyanosis is the abnormal bluish discoloration of the skin that occurs because of low levels of circulating oxygen in the blood. The normal heart has 4 chambers. The 2 upper chambers, known as atria, are separated from each other by a fibrous partition known as the atrial septum. The two lower chambers are known as ventricles and are separated from each other by the ventricular septum. Valves connect the atria (left and right) to their respective ventricles. The aorta, the main vessel of arterial circulation, carries blood from the left ventricle and away from the heart.

Tetralogy of Fallot consists of a combination of 4 different heart defects: a ventricular septal defect; obstructed outflow of blood from the right ventricle to the lungs (pulmonary stenosis); a displaced aorta, which causes blood to flow into the aorta from both the right and left ventricles (dextroposition or overriding aorta); and abnormal enlargement of the right ventricle (right ventricular hypertrophy). The severity of the symptoms is related to the degree of blood flow obstruction from the right ventricle.

If infants with Tetralogy of Fallot are not treated, the symptoms usually become progressively more severe. Blood flow to the lungs may be further decreased and severe cyanosis may cause life-threatening complications. The exact cause of Tetralogy of Fallot is not known.

In addition to The National Organization for Rare Disorders (NORD) listed in Section III, the following organizations in Section II (Disease Specific) and in Section III (Umbrella) and Section IV (Government Agencies) can provide more information:
American Heart Association, *III*
Congenital Heart Anomalies, Support, Education, &

Resources, *III*
NIH/National Heart, Lung and Blood Institute Information Center, *IV*

1000 THALAMIC SYNDROME (DEJERINE ROUSSY)

Thalamic Syndrome (Dejerine-Roussy) is a rare neurological disorder that occurs as a result of damage to the thalamus, a part of the brain that affects sensation. Primary symptoms are pain and loss of sensation usually in the face, arm, or leg.

In addition to The National Organization for Rare Disorders (NORD) listed in Section III, the following organizations in Section II (Disease Specific) and in Section III (Umbrella) and Section IV (Government Agencies) can provide more information:
NIH/National Institute of Neurological Disorders and Stroke, *IV*

1001 THALASSEMIA MAJOR

Thalassemia Major is a rare blood disorder characterized by a marked increase in F hemoglobin and a decrease in the production of certain oxygen carrying proteins in red blood cells (beta polypeptide chains in the hemoglobin molecule). Thalassemia Major is the most severe form of chronic familial anemias that result from the premature destruction of red blood cells (hemolytic). This disease was originally found in people living near the Mediterranean Sea. People with this disorder also have a reduced number of circulating red blood cells (erythrocytes).

In addition to The National Organization for Rare Disorders (NORD) listed in Section III, the following organizations in Section II (Disease Specific) and in Section III (Umbrella) and Section IV (Government Agencies) can provide more information:
Alliance of Genetic Support Groups, *III*
Children's Blood Foundation, *III*
Cooley's Anemia Foundation, Inc., *II*
March of Dimes Birth Defects Foundation, *III*
NIH/National Heart, Lung and Blood Institute Information Center, *IV*
Sickle Cell Disease Association of America, Inc., *II*

1002 THALASSEMIA MINOR

Thalassemia Minor is a rare blood disorder characterized by a moderately low level of hemoglobin in red blood cells (anemia). This disorder is inherited. People with Thalassemia Minor have one of a pair (heterozygous) of the thalassemia gene. If a person has two copies of the gene, they will have Thalassemia Major, which is a more serious disease.

In addition to The National Organization for Rare Disorders (NORD) listed in Section III, the following organizations in Section II (Disease Specific) and in Section III (Umbrella) and Section IV (Government Agencies) can provide more information:
Alliance of Genetic Support Groups, *III*
Cooley's Anemia Foundation, Inc., *II*
March of Dimes Birth Defects Foundation, *III*
NIH/National Heart, Lung and Blood Institute, *IV*
Sickle Cell Disease Association of America, Inc., *II*

1003 THREE M SYNDROME

Three M Syndrome is an extremely rare inherited disorder characterized by low birth weight, short stature (dwarfism), characteristic abnormalities of the head and facial (craniofacial) area, distinctive skeletal malformations, and/or other physical abnormalities. Characteristic craniofacial malformations typically include a long, narrow head (dolichocephaly), an unusually prominent forehead (frontal bossing), and a triangular-shaped face with a prominent, pointed chin, large ears, and/or abnormally flat cheeks. In addition, in some affected children, the teeth may be abnormally crowded together; as a result, the upper and lower teeth may not meet properly (malocclusion). Skeletal abnormalities associated with the disorder include unusually thin bones, particularly the shafts of the long bones of the arms and legs (diaphyses); abnormally long, thin bones of the spinal column (vertebrae); and/or distinctive malformations of the ribs and shoulder blades (scapulae). Affected individuals may also have additional abnormalities including permanent fixation of certain fingers in a bent position (clinodactyly), unusually short fifth fingers, and/or increased flexibility (hyperextensibility) of the joints. The range and severity of symptoms and physicial features may vary from case to case. Three M Syndrome is thought to be inherited as an autosomal recessive genetic trait.

In addition to The National Organization for Rare Disorders (NORD) listed in Section III, the following organizations in Section II (Disease Specific) and in Section III (Umbrella) and Section IV (Government Agencies) can provide more information:
Alliance of Genetic Support Groups, *III*
Children's Craniofacial Association, *III*
Craniofacial Foundation of America, *III*
Little People of America, *III*
MAGIC Foundation for Children's Growth, *III*
March of Dimes Birth Defects Foundation, *III*
NIH/National Arthritis and Musculoskeletal and Skin Diseases Information Clearinghouse, *IV*

NIH/National Institute of Child Health and Human Development, *IV*
Short Stature Foundation, *III*

1004 THROMBASTHENIA OF GLANZMANN AND NAEGELI

Thrombasthenia of Glanzmann and Naegeli is a rare inherited blood clotting (coagulation) disorder characterized by the impaired function of specialized red blood cells (platelets) that are essential for proper blood clotting. Symptoms of this disorder may include abnormal bleeding and/or hemorrhage. The symptoms are not progressive and may improve with age. However, prolonged untreated or unsuccessfully treated hemorrhaging associated with Thrombasthenia of Glanzmann and Naegeli may be life-threatening.

In addition to The National Organization for Rare Disorders (NORD) listed in Section III, the following organizations in Section II (Disease Specific) and in Section III (Umbrella) and Section IV (Government Agencies) can provide more information:
March of Dimes Birth Defects Foundation, *III*
NIH/National Heart, Lung and Blood Institute Information Center, *IV*

1005 THROMBOCYTHEMIA, ESSENTIAL

Essential Thrombocythemia is a rare disorder of blood platelet production. Major symptoms may include overproduction of platelets in the bone marrow, accompanied by active bleeding or an enlarged spleen (splenomegaly).

In addition to The National Organization for Rare Disorders (NORD) listed in Section III, the following organizations in Section II (Disease Specific) and in Section III (Umbrella) and Section IV (Government Agencies) can provide more information:
MPD (Myeloproliferative Disease) Research Center, Inc., *III*
NIH/National Heart, Lung and Blood Institute Information Center, *IV*

1006 THROMBOCYTOPENIA ABSENT RADIUS SYNDROME

Thrombocytopenia-Absent Radius (TAR) Syndrome is a genetic disorder characterized by a very low level of the number of blood platelets (thrombocytopenia) and the absence or underdevelopment of one of the short bones (radius) in the arm. TAR Syndrome is inherited as an autosomal recessive genetic trait.

In addition to The National Organization for Rare Disorders (NORD) listed in Section III, the following organizations in Section II (Disease Specific) and in Section III (Umbrella) and Section IV (Government Agencies) can provide more information:
NIH/National Heart, Lung and Blood Institute Information Center, *IV*
TAR Syndrome Association, *II*

1007 THROMBOCYTOPENIA, ESSENTIAL

Essential Thrombocytopenia is a rare blood disease affecting the clotting factor (platelets) of the blood. It is characterized by an abnormally low platelet count and a shorter than normal (ten days) platelet survival time. Major symptoms include a tendency to bleed excessively into the skin or mucous membranes, especially during menstruation. There are many different reasons for the development of decreased marrow production or platelet destruction that causes this disorder. These can sometimes be determined by examination of bone marrow. Other forms of Thrombocytopenia may be associated with hereditary factors.

In addition to The National Organization for Rare Disorders (NORD) listed in Section III, the following organizations in Section II (Disease Specific) and in Section III (Umbrella) and Section IV (Government Agencies) can provide more information:
NIH/National Heart, Lung and Blood Institute Information Center, *IV*
TAR Syndrome Association, *II*

1008 TIETZE SYNDROME

Tietze Syndrome is a rare, inflammatory disorder characterized by chest pain and swelling of the cartilage of one or more of the upper ribs (costochondral junction). Onset of pain may be gradual or sudden; pain may spread to affect the arms and/or shoulders. The exact cause of Tietze Syndrome is not known.

In addition to The National Organization for Rare Disorders (NORD) listed in Section III, the following organizations in Section II (Disease Specific) and in Section III (Umbrella) and Section IV (Government Agencies) can provide more information:
NIH/National Arthritis and Musculoskeletal and Skin Diseases Information Clearinghouse, *IV*

1009 TINNITUS

Tinnitus is a common condition characterized by the sensation of sound for which there is no external source outside the individual. In other words, people with Tinnitus perceive sound when no environmental or external sounds are present. These sounds have been described as clicking, buzzing, and/or ringing. Tinnitus commonly occurs as a side effect of certain drugs and because of other underlying disorders (secondary), especially those of the middle and inner ear (i.e., cochlea). In rare cases, no underlying cause can be found and the condition is termed "idiopathic" Tinnitus. Infection, obstruction of blood vessels near the ear, and/or environmental factors have also been implicated as a cause of Tinnitus.

In addition to The National Organization for Rare Disorders (NORD) listed in Section III, the following organizations in Section II (Disease Specific) and in Section III (Umbrella) and Section IV (Government Agencies) can provide more information:

American Hearing Research Foundation, *III*
American Tinnitus Association, *II*
Better Hearing Institute, *III*
Meniere's Network, *II*
NIH/National Institute on Deafness and Other Communication Disorders (Balance), *IV*
Vestibular Disorders Association, *III*

1010 TOLOSA HUNT SYNDROME

Tolosa-Hunt Syndrome is a rare neurological disorder characterized by severe headaches and pain often preceding weakness and painful paralysis (ophthalmoplegia) of certain eye muscles. Symptoms usually affect only one side of the head (unilateral). In most cases, affected individuals experience intense sharp pain and paralysis of muscles around the eye. Symptoms subside without intervention (spontaneous remission) and recur without a distinct pattern (randomly). In addition, affected individuals may exhibit paralysis (palsy) of certain facial nerves and drooping of the upper eyelid (ptosis). Other symptoms may include double vision, fever, chronic fatigue, headaches, a feeling that one's surroundings are spinning (vertigo), pain in the joints (arthralgia), and/or abnormal protrusion of one or both eyeballs (exophthalmos). The exact cause of Tolosa-Hunt Syndrome is not known, but the disorder is thought to be associated with inflammation of the areas behind the eyes (cavernous sinus and superior orbital fissure).

In addition to The National Organization for Rare Disorders (NORD) listed in Section III, the following organizations in Section II (Disease Specific) and in Section III (Umbrella) and Section IV (Government Agencies) can provide more information:

American Autoimmune Related Diseases Association, Inc., *III*
NIH/National Institute of Neurological Disorders and Stroke, *IV*
National Association for Visually Handicapped, *III*
National Headache Foundation, *III*

1011 TONGUE CARCINOMA

Tongue Carcinoma is an oral cancer that is characterized by an ulcerating malignant tumor, usually on the side of the tongue, consisting of scaly (squamous) cells. The tumor may spread to the lymph nodes on the same side of the neck.

In addition to The National Organization for Rare Disorders (NORD) listed in Section III, the following organizations in Section II (Disease Specific) and in Section III (Umbrella) and Section IV (Government Agencies) can provide more information:

American Cancer Society, Inc., *III*
CancerOnline, *III*
OncoLink: The University of Pennsylvania Cancer Center Resource, *III*

1012 TONGUE, FISSURED

Fissured tongue is a rare inherited disorder characterized by grooves or depressions (fissures) on the tongue. Fissures may differ in size and depth. In rare cases, fissured tongue may be associated with incomplete closure of the roof of the mouth (cleft palate). In some cases, fissured tongue is thought to be inherited as an autosomal dominant genetic trait.

In addition to The National Organization for Rare Disorders (NORD) listed in Section III, the following organizations in Section II (Disease Specific) and in Section III (Umbrella) and Section IV (Government Agencies) can provide more information:

NIH/National Oral Health Information Clearinghouse, *IV*
Smell and Taste Center, *III*

1013 TONGUE, GEOGRAPHIC

Geographic Tongue is an inflammation of the tongue (glossitis) that may go into remission and recur. This form of inflammation is characterized by irregular, migrating denuded smooth areas (excoriations) on the tongue that may feel slightly sore and itchy.

In addition to The National Organization for Rare Disorders (NORD) listed in Section III, the following organizations in Section II (Disease Specific) and in Section III (Umbrella) and Section IV (Government Agencies) can provide more information:

NIH/National Oral Health Information Clearinghouse, *IV*
Smell and Taste Center, *III*

1014 TONGUE, HAIRY

Hairy Tongue is a disorder characterized by yellowish, brownish, blackish, or bluish discoloration of the tongue, with excessive growth of the threadlike elevations in front of the taste buds (filiform papillae). These elevations are arranged in a V-form towards the back of the tongue. A bad taste in the mouth usually also occurs.

In addition to The National Organization for Rare Disorders (NORD) listed in Section III, the following organizations in Section II (Disease Specific) and in Section III (Umbrella) and Section IV (Government Agencies) can provide more information:

NIH/National Oral Health Information Clearinghouse, *IV*
Smell and Taste Center, *III*

1015 TOOTH AND NAIL SYNDROME

Tooth and Nail Syndrome is a rare genetic disorder that belongs to a group of diseases known as Ectodermal Dysplasias. Ectodermal Dysplasias typically affect the teeth, nails, hair, and/or skin. Tooth and Nail Syndrome is primarily characterized by absence (hypodontia) and/or malformation of certain primary (deciduous) and secondary (permanent) teeth occurring in association with improper development (dysplasia) of the nails, particularly the toenails.

In individuals with Tooth and Nail Syndrome, certain primary teeth and/or several secondary teeth may either be absent or widely spaced and/or conical in shape (coniform). In addition, in infants with the disorder, certain nails may be absent at birth and may grow extremely slowly, particularly during the first two to three years of life. The nails may be unusually small and underdeveloped (hypoplastic), with distinctive, abnormal hollowing that causes them to appear spoon shaped. The toenails are usually more severely affected than the fingernails. In rare cases, additional symptoms and findings may be present. Tooth and Nail Syndrome is inherited as an autosomal dominant genetic trait.

In addition to The National Organization for Rare Disorders (NORD) listed in Section III, the following organizations in Section II (Disease Specific) and in Section III (Umbrella) and Section IV (Government Agencies) can provide more information:

NIH/National Institute of Child Health and Human Development, *IV*
NIH/National Institute of Dental Research, *IV*
NIH/National Oral Health Information Clearinghouse, *IV*
National Foundation for Ectodermal Dysplasias, *II*

1016 TOURETTE SYNDROME

Tourette Syndrome is a hereditary neurologic movement disorder that is characterized by repetitive motor and vocal tics. Symptoms may include involuntary movements of the extremities, shoulders, and face accompanied by uncontrollable sounds and sometimes inappropriate words. Tourette Syndrome is not a progressive nor degenerative disorder; rather, symptoms tend to be variable and follow a chronic waxing and waning course throughout an otherwise normal life span.

In addition to The National Organization for Rare Disorders (NORD) listed in Section III, the following organizations in Section II (Disease Specific) and in Section III (Umbrella) and Section IV (Government Agencies) can provide more information:

March of Dimes Birth Defects Foundation, *III*
NIH/National Institute of Neurological Disorders and Stroke, *IV*
Tourette Syndrome Association, Inc., *II*
Tourette Syndrome Foundation of Canada, *II*
WE MOVE, *III*

1017 TOWNES BROCKS SYNDROME

Townes-Brocks Syndrome is a rare genetic disorder present at birth. Symptoms of the disorder and the severity of these symptoms vary from person to person. Major characteristics may include an absence of an anal opening in association with hand, foot and ear abnormalities. Hearing loss or deafness due to lesions or dysfunctions of part of the internal ear or its nerve tracts and centers (sensorineural hearing loss or deafness) is present in some patients.

In addition to The National Organization for Rare Disorders (NORD) listed in Section III, the following organizations in Section II (Disease Specific) and in Section III (Umbrella) and Section IV (Government Agencies) can provide more information:

NIH/National Institute of Child Health and Human Development, *IV*

1018 TOXIC SHOCK SYNDROME

Toxic Shock Syndrome is a rare multisystem disease with many widespread symptoms. It is caused by a toxin that is produced and secreted by the bacterium Staphylococcus aureus. The symptoms of Toxic Shock Syndrome may include a sudden high fever, nausea, vomiting, diarrhea, abnormally low blood pressure (hypotension), and a characteristic skin rash that resembles a bad sunburn. Most cases of Toxic Shock Syndrome occur in menstruating females in association with the use of tampons. Other cases may occur in association with minor postoperative wound infections or nasal packing.

In addition to The National Organization for Rare Disorders (NORD) listed in Section III, the following organizations in Section II (Disease Specific) and in Section III (Umbrella) and Section IV (Government Agencies) can provide more information:
Centers for Disease Control and Prevention, *IV*
NIH/National Institute of Allergy and Infectious Diseases, *IV*
World Health Organization (WHO) Regional Office for the Americas (AMRO), *III*

1019 TOXOCARIASIS

Toxocariasis, an infectious parasitic disorder that primarily affects children, is caused by human ingestion of soil contaminated with the eggs of a common roundworm (nematode) excreted by dogs (Toxocara canis) or, less often, cats (Toxocara cati). The eggs hatch inside an affected individual's small intestine and the released larvae spread throughout the body, potentially affecting numerous organs (Visceral Larva Migrans) or solely the eyes (Ocular Larva Migrans). In most cases, affected individuals exhibit few or no symptoms (asymptomatic).

In Visceral Larva Migrans, the liver is most often affected and abnormal enlargement of the liver is common (hepatomegaly). Affected individuals may also experience fever, wheezing, coughing, unusually pale skin (pallor), loss of appetite (anorexia), weight loss, recurrent stomach (abdominal) pain, fatigue, and/or a general feeling of ill health (malaise). In some cases, affected individuals may have serious respiratory complications including recurrent attacks of labored or difficult breathing and wheezing (asthma), inflammation of the lungs (pneumonia), inflammation of the throat (pharyngitis), and, in rare cases, severe respiratory distress. In rare cases, the larvae may spread to the brain, potentially resulting in dizziness, behavior abnormalities, sleep disturbances, and/or periods of uncontrolled electrical disturbances in the brain (seizures). In addition, affected individuals often experience headaches, which may or may not be due to brain involvement. In rare cases, the larvae may spread to the heart. Involvement of the lungs, brain, and/or heart may, in extremely rare cases, result in life-threatening complications without appropriate treatment.

In most individuals with Ocular Larva Migrans, associated symptoms and physical findings are limited to the eye. The presence of larvae in the eye may lead to the formation of an inflammatory mass (e.g., granuloma) consisting of certain granular white blood cells (eosinophils) and/or widespread inflammation of the ocular cavities and surrounding structures (endophthalmitis). The most common symptom associated with Ocular Larva Migrans is severely decreased clearness or clarity of vision (visual acuity). In some cases, if left untreated, Ocular Larva Migrans may progress to cause blindness in the affected eye.

In addition to The National Organization for Rare Disorders (NORD) listed in Section III, the following organizations in Section II (Disease Specific) and in Section III (Umbrella) and Section IV (Government Agencies) can provide more information:
Centers for Disease Control and Prevention, *IV*
NIH/National Eye Institute, *IV*
NIH/National Institute of Allergy and Infectious Diseases, *IV*
World Health Organization (WHO) Regional Office for the Americas (AMRO), *III*

1020 TOXOPLASMOSIS

Toxoplasmosis is an infectious disease that can be caused by contact with a microscopic parasitic organism called Toxoplasma gondii. This parasitic infection, found worldwide, can be either acquired or be present at birth (congenital). The congenital type is a result of a maternal infection during pregnancy that is transmitted to the fetus and involves lesions of the central nervous system. These lesions may lead to blindness, brain defects and more serious conditions. The disorder may be most severe when it is transmitted to the fetus during the second through sixth month of pregnancy. Twenty to 80 percent of those affected will show the presence of toxoplasmosis antibodies when tested.

The acquired form includes these two types of Toxoplasmosis: 1) Lymphadenopathic Toxoplasmosis is a form of the disorder that resembles mononucleosis. 2) Disseminated Toxoplasmosis is a form of the disorder in which lesions involve chiefly the lungs, liver, heart, skin, muscle, brain, and spinal cord membranes. It is characterized by inflammation of the lungs (pneumonitis), hepatitis, inflammation of the muscular walls of the heart (myocarditis), and inflammation of the brain and meninges (meningoencephalitis), all in varying degrees.

In addition to The National Organization for Rare Disorders (NORD) listed in Section III, the following organizations in Section II (Disease Specific) and in Section III (Umbrella) and Section IV (Government Agencies) can provide more information:

Centers for Disease Control and Prevention, *IV*
NIH/National Institute of Allergy and Infectious Diseases, *IV*
The Arc (a national organization on mental retardation), *III*

1021 TREACHER COLLINS SYNDROME

Treacher Collins Syndrome is a rare inherited disorder characterized by distinctive abnormalities of the head and facial (craniofacial) area due to underdevelopment (hypoplasia) of certain portions of the skull (e.g., supraorbital rims and zygomatic arches). Although the symptoms and physical characteristics associated with Treacher Collins Syndrome may vary greatly in severity from case to case, craniofacial abnormalities tend to involve the cheekbones, jaws, mouth, ears, and/or eyes.

Craniofacial malformations associated with Treacher Collins Syndrome may include underdeveloped (hypoplastic) or absent cheek (malar) bones; an incompletely developed, abnormally small lower jaw (mandibular hypoplasia and micrognathia); an unusually large mouth (macrostomia); malformations of the roof of the mouth (palate); and/or dental abnormalities such as misaligned teeth (malocclusion). Affected infants may also have underdeveloped (hypoplastic) and/or malformed (dysplastic) ears (pinnae) with blind ending or absent external ear canals (microtia), resulting in hearing impairment (conductive hearing loss). In addition, infants with Treacher Collins Syndrome may exhibit abnormally downwardly slanted openings between the upper and lower eyelids (palpebral fissures), partial or total absence of tissue (colobomas) from the outer third of the lower eyelids, and/or additional eye (ocular) abnormalities, resulting in varying degrees of visual impairment in some cases. Some individuals with the disorder may have additional physical abnormalities. In approximately 40 percent of cases, Treacher Collins Syndrome is thought to be inherited as an autosomal dominant genetic trait. However, in about 60 percent of cases, a positive family history is not found. Research suggests that such cases represent new genetic changes (mutations) that occur randomly, with no apparent cause (sporadic).

In addition to The National Organization for Rare Disorders (NORD) listed in Section III, the following organizations in Section II (Disease Specific) and in Section III (Umbrella) and Section IV (Government Agencies) can provide more information:

AboutFace U.S.A., *III*
American Society for Deaf Children, *III*
Children's Craniofacial Association, *III*
Council of Families with Visual Impairment, *III*
Craniofacial Foundation of America, *III*
Ear Anomalies Reconstructed: Atresia/Microtia Support Group, *III*
FACES: The National Craniofacial Association, *III*
Forward Face, Inc., *III*
Let's Face It, Inc., *III*
NIH/National Institute of Child Health and Human Development, *IV*
NIH/National Institute on Deafness and Other Communication Disorders Information Clearinghouse, *IV*
Treacher Collins Foundation, *II*
Vision Foundation, Inc., *III*

1022 TRICHO DENTO OSSEOUS SYNDROME

Tricho-Dento-Osseous (TDO) Syndrome is an extremely rare inherited multisystem disorder that belongs to a group of diseases known as Ectodermal Dysplasias. Ectodermal Dysplasias typically affect the hair, teeth, nails, and/or skin. TDO Syndrome is characterized by extremely kinky or curly hair; underdeveloped (hypoplastic) tooth enamel and other dental abnormalities; unusual hardening (sclerosis), thickening, and/or denseness of the top portion of the skull (calvaria) and/or the long bones (i.e., bones in the arms and legs); and/or abnormally thin, brittle nails. In some cases, affected individuals may also exhibit premature closure (fusion) of the fibrous joints between certain bones in the skull (craniosynostosis), causing the head to appear abnormally long and narrow (dolicocephaly).

It is believed that there may be three distinct types of TDO Syndrome. Some researchers suggest that these variants may be differentiated mainly by whether the calvaria and/or long bones exhibit abnormal hardening (sclerosis), thickening, and/or density. Other symptoms may vary among the three disorder types. Tricho-Dento-Osseous Syndrome is inherited as an autosomal dominant genetic trait.

In addition to The National Organization for Rare Disorders (NORD) listed in Section III, the following organizations in Section II (Disease Specific) and in Section III (Umbrella) and Section IV (Government Agencies) can provide more information:
AboutFace U.S.A., *III*
Children's Craniofacial Association, *III*
Craniofacial Foundation of America, *III*
FACES: The National Craniofacial Association, *III*
NIH/National Institute of Arthritis and Musculoskeletal and Skin Diseases, *IV*
NIH/National Oral Health Information Clearinghouse, *IV*
National Foundation for Ectodermal Dysplasias, *II*

1023 TRICHORHINOPHALANGEAL SYNDROME TYPE I

Trichorhinophalangeal Syndrome Type I (TRPS1) is an extremely rare inherited multisystem disorder that belongs to a group of diseases known as Ectodermal Dysplasias. Ectodermal Dysplasias typically affect the hair, teeth, nails, and/or skin. TRPS1 is characterized by thin, sparse scalp hair, unusual facial features, abnormalities of the fingers and/or toes, and multiple abnormalities of the "growing ends" (epiphyses) of the bones (skeletal dysplasia), especially in the hands and feet. Characteristic facial features may include a rounded (bulbous) "pear-shaped" nose, an abnormally small jaw (micrognathia), dental anomalies, and/or unusually large (prominent) ears. In most cases, the fingers and/or toes may be abnormally short (brachydactyly) and curved. In addition, affected individuals may exhibit short stature (dwarfism). The range and severity of symptoms may vary from case to case. In most cases, Trichorhinophalangeal Syndrome Type I is thought to be inherited as an autosomal dominant genetic trait. However, some cases may be inherited as an autosomal recessive genetic trait.

In addition to The National Organization for Rare Disorders (NORD) listed in Section III, the following organizations in Section II (Disease Specific) and in Section III (Umbrella) and Section IV (Government Agencies) can provide more information:
Human Growth Foundation, *III*
Little People of America, *III*
NIH/National Institute of Arthritis and Musculoskeletal and Skin Diseases, *IV*
NIH/National Institute of Child Health and Human Development, *IV*
National Foundation for Ectodermal Dysplasias, *II*

1024 TRICHORHINOPHALANGEAL SYNDROME TYPE II

Trichorhinophalangeal Syndrome Type II (TRPS2), also known as Langer-Giedion Syndrome, is an extremely rare inherited multisystem disorder that belongs to a group of diseases known as Ectodermal Dysplasias. Ectodermal Dysplasias typically affect the hair, teeth, nails, and/or skin. TRPS2 is characterized by fine, thin hair; unusual facial features; progressive growth retardation resulting in short stature (dwarfism); abnormally short fingers and toes (brachydactyly); "cone-shaped" formation of the "growing ends" of certain bones (epiphyseal coning); and/or development of multiple bony growths (exostoses) projecting outward from the surfaces of various bones of the body. In addition, affected individuals may exhibit unusually flexible (hyperextensible) joints, diminished muscle tone (hypotonia), excess folds of skin (redundant skin), and/or discolored elevated spots on the skin (maculopapular nevi). Affected individuals may also exhibit mild to severe mental retardation, hearing loss (sensorineural deafness), and/or delayed speech development. The range and severity of symptoms may vary from case to case. Most cases of Trichorhinophalangeal Syndrome Type II appear to be due to spontaneous genetic change(s) [mutation(s)] that occur for unknown reasons (sporadically).

In addition to The National Organization for Rare Disorders (NORD) listed in Section III, the following organizations in Section II (Disease Specific) and in Section III (Umbrella) and Section IV (Government Agencies) can provide more information:
Langer-Giedion Syndrome Association, *II*
Little People of America, *III*
NIH/National Institute of Arthritis and Musculoskeletal and Skin Diseases, *IV*
NIH/National Institute of Child Health and Human Development, *IV*
NIH/National Institute on Deafness and Other Communication Disorders Information Clearinghouse, *IV*
National Foundation for Ectodermal Dysplasias, *II*

1025 TRICHORHINOPHALANGEAL SYNDROME TYPE III

Trichorhinophalangeal Syndrome Type III (TRPS3) is an extremely rare inherited multisystem disorder that belongs to a group of diseases known as Ectodermal Dysplasias. Ectodermal Dysplasias typically affect the hair, teeth, nails, and/or skin. TRPS3 is characterized by fine, thin light-colored hair; unusual facial features; abnormalities of the fingers and/or toes; and multiple abnormalities of the "growing ends" (epiphyses) of the bones (skeletal dysplasia), especially in the hands and feet. Characteristic facial features may include a pear-shaped or rounded (bulbous) nose; an abnormally long prominent groove (philtrum) in the upper lip; and/or abnormalities such as delayed eruption of teeth. In addition, affected individuals also exhibit severe shortening of the fingers and toes (brachydactyly) due to improper development of bones in the hands and feet (metacarpalphalangeal shortening). Additional features often include short stature (dwarfism) and/or additional skeletal abnormalities. The range and severity of symptoms may vary from case to case. Trichorhinophalangeal Syndrome Type III is thought to be inherited as an autosomal dominant genetic trait.

In addition to The National Organization for Rare Disorders (NORD) listed in Section III, the following organizations in Section II (Disease Specific) and in Section III (Umbrella) and Section IV (Government Agencies) can provide more information:

Human Growth Foundation, *III*
Little People of America, *III*
NIH/National Institute of Arthritis and Musculoskeletal and Skin Diseases, *IV*
NIH/National Institute of Child Health and Human Development, *IV*
National Foundation for Ectodermal Dysplasias, *II*

1026 TRICHOTILLOMANIA

Trichotillomania is a mental illness characterized by an overwhelming urge to pull out one's own hair. This results in patches of baldness; most often, areas on the head and face are involved, such as eyelashes, eyebrows, beard, or scalp area. In some cases, affected individuals ingest the hair they have pulled out (trichophagy).

In addition to The National Organization for Rare Disorders (NORD) listed in Section III, the following organizations in Section II (Disease Specific) and in Section III (Umbrella) and Section IV (Government Agencies) can provide more information:

Federation of Families for Children's Mental Health, *III*
NIH/National Institute of Mental Health, *IV*
National Alliance for the Mentally Ill, *III*
National Mental Health Association, *III*
National Mental Health Consumer Self-Help Clearinghouse, *III*
Obsessive-Compulsive Foundation, Inc., *II*

1027 TRIGEMINAL NEURALGIA (TIC DOULOUREUX)

Trigeminal Neuralgia, also known as Tic Douloureux, is a disorder of the fifth cranial nerve (trigeminal nerve) characterized by attacks of intense, stabbing pain affecting the mouth, cheek, nose, and/or other areas on one side of the face. The exact cause of Trigeminal Neuralgia is not fully understood.

In addition to The National Organization for Rare Disorders (NORD) listed in Section III, the following organizations in Section II (Disease Specific) and in Section III (Umbrella) and Section IV (Government Agencies) can provide more information:

NIH/National Institute of Neurological Disorders and Stroke, *IV*
NIH/National Oral Health Information Clearinghouse, *IV*
Trigeminal Neuralgia Association, *II*

1028 TRIMETHYLAMINURIA

Trimethylaminuria is a very rare metabolic disorder that may be inherited as an autosomal dominant genetic trait. It may also be acquired as a result of treatment with large doses of the amino acid derivative L-carnitine (levocarnitine). This disorder occurs when there is an impairment in the ability of a liver enzyme (trimethylamine-N-oxide synthetase) to break down trimethylamine from choline and trimethylamine-oxide in the diet. When trimethylamine is not properly metabolized it is excreted in the urine, sweat and breath, causing a strong fishy odor.

In addition to The National Organization for Rare Disorders (NORD) listed in Section III, the following organizations in Section II (Disease Specific) and in Section III (Umbrella) and Section IV (Government Agencies) can provide more information:

Association for Neuro-Metabolic Disorders, *III*
NIH/National Institute of Child Health and Human Development, *IV*
Research Trust for Metabolic Diseases in Children, *III*

1029 TRIPLO X SYNDROME

Triplo X Syndrome is a rare chromosomal disorder that affects females. Females normally have two X chromosomes; however, those with Triplo X Syndrome carry three X chromosomes in the cells of their body (somatic). The symptoms of this disorder can vary greatly from case to case. Some affected females exhibit very few symptoms. Others may have a variety of physical deformities, such as eyes that are spaced widely apart (ocular hypertelorism), a head that is abnormally short (brachycephaly) or unusually small (microcephaly), and/or malformations of the reproductive and urinary (genitourinary) tracts. Other symptoms may include moderate to severe mental retardation, delayed speech and motor skills, and/or behavioral abnormalities. The cause of this disorder is not completely understood.

In addition to The National Organization for Rare Disorders (NORD) listed in Section III, the following organizations in Section II (Disease Specific) and in Section III (Umbrella) and Section IV (Government Agencies) can provide more information:
Learning Disabilities Association of America, *III*
NIH/National Institute of Child Health and Human Development, *IV*
National Center for Learning Disabilities, *III*
National Information Center For Children and Youth with Disabilities, *III*
UNIQUE - Rare Chromosome Disorder Support Group, *III*

1030 TRIPLOID SYNDROME

Triploid Syndrome is an extremely rare chromosomal disorder. A complete extra set of chromosomes totaling sixty-nine, rather than the normal forty-six, is found in the infant. Babies with Triploid Syndrome usually are lost through early miscarriage. However, some infants have been born and survived as long as five months. The infant shows severely retarded fetal growth and many other prenatal abnormalities.

In addition to The National Organization for Rare Disorders (NORD) listed in Section III, the following organizations in Section II (Disease Specific) and in Section III (Umbrella) and Section IV (Government Agencies) can provide more information:
NIH/National Institute of Child Health and Human Development, *IV*
National Adrenal Diseases Foundation, *III*
UNIQUE - Rare Chromosome Disorder Support Group, *III*

1031 TRISMUS PSEUDOCAMPTODACTYLY SYNDROME

Trismus-Pseudocamptodactyly Syndrome is a very rare inherited disorder characterized by the inability to completely open the mouth (trismus), causing difficulty with chewing (mastication) and/or the presence of abnormally short muscle-tendon units in the fingers, causing the fingers to curve or bend (camptodactyly) when the hand is bent back at the wrist (dorsiflexion). Because the fingers are not permanently bent or curved, this particular finding is termed "pseudocamptodactyly" (pseudo meaning false). In addition, the muscle-tendon units of the forearms and/or the legs may also be abnormally short, resulting in limited movements and various deformities of the feet. Individuals with this disorder are slightly shorter than would otherwise be expected. The severity of these physical findings varies from individual to individual. Trismus-Pseudocamptodactyly Syndrome is thought to be inherited as an autosomal dominant genetic trait.

In addition to The National Organization for Rare Disorders (NORD) listed in Section III, the following organizations in Section II (Disease Specific) and in Section III (Umbrella) and Section IV (Government Agencies) can provide more information:
NIH/National Arthritis and Musculoskeletal and Skin Diseases Information Clearinghouse, *IV*
NIH/National Institute of Child Health and Human Development, *IV*

1032 TRISOMY

Trisomies are very rare genetic disorders characterized by a chromosome aberration. Chromosomes are found in the nucleus of all body cells. They carry the genetic characteristics of each individual. Pairs of human chromosomes are numbered from 1 through 22, with an unequal 23rd pair of X and Y chromosomes for males, and two X chromosomes for females. People with a Trisomy have an extra chromosome added to one of the normal pairs. Each chromosome has a short arm that is designated "p" and a long arm identified by the letter "q." The triplication of the chromosome may be partial; i.e., with only a portion of the chromosome duplicated. Defects are classified by the name of the abnormal chromosome pair and which portion of the chromosome is affected. For example, 22p+ means that there is an extra short arm added to the 22nd pair of chromosomes. In general, the most common symptom of the trisomies is mental retardation.

In addition to The National Organization for Rare Disorders (NORD) listed in Section III, the following organizations in Section II (Disease Specific) and in Section III (Umbrella) and Section IV (Government Agencies) can provide more information:
National Down Syndrome Congress, *II*
Support Organization for Trisomy 18, 13, and Related Disorders, *III*
The Arc (a national organization on mental retardation), *III*
Trisomy 9 International Parent Support, *II*

1033 TRISOMY 13 SYNDROME

Trisomy 13 Syndrome is a rare chromosomal disorder characterized by the presence of an extra chromosome 13. Characteristic features may include major developmental defects along the center of the brain and face (midline); cleft lip and cleft palate; extra fingers or toes (polydactyly) and other skeletal abnormalities; mental retardation; and/or congenital heart defects. Other symptoms may include deafness, visual impairment, cysts in the kidneys, and/or genital abnormalities. The symptoms and physical characteristics of Trisomy 13 Syndrome develop due to the presence of an additional chromosome 13 (complete trisomy). The exact cause of this disorder is not known.

In addition to The National Organization for Rare Disorders (NORD) listed in Section III, the following organizations in Section II (Disease Specific) and in Section III (Umbrella) and Section IV (Government Agencies) can provide more information:

Alliance of Genetic Support Groups, *III*
NIH/National Institute of Child Health and Human Development, *IV*
Support Organization for Trisomy 13/18 and Related Disorders, UK, *II*
Support Organization for Trisomy 18, 13, and Related Disorders, *III*
The Arc (a national organization on mental retardation), *III*
UNIQUE - Rare Chromosome Disorder Support Group, *III*

1034 TRISOMY 18 SYNDROME

Trisomy 18 Syndrome is a rare chromosomal disorder characterized by the presence of an extra chromosome 18. Normally humans have two of each chromosome, but in this disorder they have 3 of the 18th chromosome. The unusual physical characteristics and other abnormalities associated with this disorder develop during fetal growth in the uterus. Infants with Trisomy 18 Syndrome have multiple birth defects (congenital anomalies). Most affected infants experience failure to thrive and are unusually thin due to poor sucking ability. Infants with Trisomy 18 Syndrome also have generalized muscle rigidity (hypertonicity), especially when bending their arms and legs. Mental retardation is also present. The exact cause of this disorder is not known.

In addition to The National Organization for Rare Disorders (NORD) listed in Section III, the following organizations in Section II (Disease Specific) and in Section III (Umbrella) and Section IV (Government Agencies) can provide more information:

NIH/National Institute of Child Health and Human Development, *IV*
Support Organization for Trisomy 13/18 and Related Disorders, UK, *II*
Support Organization for Trisomy 18, 13, and Related Disorders, *III*
The Arc (a national organization on mental retardation), *III*
UNIQUE - Rare Chromosome Disorder Support Group, *III*

1035 TROPICAL SPRUE

Tropical Sprue is a rare digestive disease characterized by an impairment in the ability to properly absorb nutrients in the small intestine (malabsorption), many nutritional deficiencies, and abnormalities in the mucous lining of the small intestine. The exact cause of this disorder is not known. Tropical Sprue is an acquired disease and may be related to environmental and nutritional conditions. This disease is most common in the islands of the Caribbean, India, southern Africa, and southeast Asia.

In addition to The National Organization for Rare Disorders (NORD) listed in Section III, the following organizations in Section II (Disease Specific) and in Section III (Umbrella) and Section IV (Government Agencies) can provide more information:

Centers for Disease Control and Prevention, *IV*
NIH/National Digestive Diseases Information Clearinghouse, *IV*

1036 TRUNCUS ARTERIOSUS, PERSISTENT

Persistent Truncus Arteriosus is a major heart defect that is present at birth (congenital). The truncus arteriosus is a vascular structure present in the developing fetus that normally divides into the aorta and pulmonary artery. In Persistent Truncus Arteriosus the structure fails to divide properly and is said to "persist." Blood from both ventricles of the heart is mixed and affects blood flow to and from the heart and lungs. The delivery of oxygen to all parts of the body is diminished. Persistent Truncus Arteriosus is usually associated with a ventricular septal defect. The most common life-threatening complication of this disorder in infancy is congestive heart failure and extremely high blood pressure in the lungs (pulmonary hypertension), which may result in severe breathing difficulties (pulmonary vascular obstructive disease).

In addition to The National Organization for Rare Disorders (NORD) listed in Section III, the following

organizations in Section II (Disease Specific) and in Section III (Umbrella) and Section IV (Government Agencies) can provide more information:
American Heart Association, *III*
NIH/National Heart, Lung and Blood Institute Information Center, *IV*

1037 TUBERCULOSIS

Tuberculosis (TB) is an acute or chronic bacterial infection found most commonly in the lungs. The infection is spread like a cold, mainly through airborne droplets breathed into the air by a person infected with TB. The bacteria causes formation of small tissue masses called tubercles. In the lungs these tubercles produce breathing impairment, coughing and release of sputum. TB may recur after long periods of inactivity (latency) if not treated adequately. Many variations of TB exist and are distinguished by the area of the body affected, degree of severity and affected population. This disease today is considered curable and preventable. It is very rare in the United States but is on an upsurge.

In addition to The National Organization for Rare Disorders (NORD) listed in Section III, the following organizations in Section II (Disease Specific) and in Section III (Umbrella) and Section IV (Government Agencies) can provide more information:
American Lung Association, *III*
Centers for Disease Control and Prevention, *IV*
NIH/National Institute of Allergy and Infectious Diseases, *IV*

1038 TUBEROUS SCLEROSIS

Tuberous Sclerosis is a rare genetic multisystem disorder characterized by the appearance of characteristic benign tumors in various areas of the body, seizures, and mental retardation. Other findings and symptoms may include developmental delays; characteristic skin lesions (e.g., adenoma sebaceum); lesions in the eyes (ocular); uncontrollable involuntary muscle spasms (myoclonic jerking); and/or learning disabilities. The range and severity of associated symptoms and findings may vary greatly from case to case. Tuberous Sclerosis is inherited as an autosomal dominant genetic trait. Two genes have been identified that may cause this disorder. One disease gene, the TSC1 gene, is located on the long arm of chromosome 9 (9q34). The other gene, the TSC2 gene, has been located on the short arm of chromosome 16 (16p13.3). Approximately 65 percent of the cases of Tuberous Sclerosis occur as a result of a spontaneous genetic change (new mutation).

In addition to The National Organization for Rare Disorders (NORD) listed in Section III, the following organizations in Section II (Disease Specific) and in Section III (Umbrella) and Section IV (Government Agencies) can provide more information:
Alliance of Genetic Support Groups, *III*
Epilepsy Foundation of America, *III*
March of Dimes Birth Defects Foundation, *III*
NIH/National Institute of Neurological Disorders and Stroke, *IV*
National Tuberous Sclerosis Association, *II*
The Arc (a national organization on mental retardation), *III*
Tuberous Sclerosis Association, *II*
Tuberous Sclerosis Canada, *II*

1039 TURNER SYNDROME

Turner Syndrome is a rare chromosomal disorder of females characterized by short stature and the lack of sexual development at puberty. Other physical features may include a webbed neck, heart defects, kidney abnormalities, and/or various other malformations. Normally, females have two X chromosomes. In some cases of Turner Syndrome, however, one X chromosome is missing from the cells (45,X); research studies suggest that approximately 40 percent of these individuals may have some Y chromosomal material in addition to the one X chromosome. In other affected females, both X chromosomes may be present, but one may have genetic defects. In still other cases, some cells may have the normal pair of X chromosomes while other cells do not (45,X/46,XX mosaicism). Although the exact cause of Turner Syndrome is not known, it is believed that the disorder may result from an error during the division (meiosis) of a parent's sex cells.

In addition to The National Organization for Rare Disorders (NORD) listed in Section III, the following organizations in Section II (Disease Specific) and in Section III (Umbrella) and Section IV (Government Agencies) can provide more information:
Alliance of Genetic Support Groups, *III*
Human Growth Foundation, *III*
March of Dimes Birth Defects Foundation, *III*
NIH/National Institute of Child Health and Human Development, *IV*
Turner's Syndrome Society, *II*
Turner's Syndrome Society of the United States, *II*

1040 TWIN-TWIN TRANSFUSION SYNDROME

Twin-Twin Transfusion Syndrome (TTTS) is a rare disorder that sometimes occurs when women are pregnant with identical (monozygotic) twins. It is a rare disease of the placenta, the organ that joins the mother to her offspring and provides nourishment to the developing fetuses. During the development of identical twins, there are often blood vessels in the fetuses' shared placenta that connect their blood circulations (placental anastomoses). In most cases, the blood flows properly through these vessels. However, in Twin-Twin Transfusion Syndrome, the blood begins to flow unevenly, with one fetal twin receiving too much blood (recipient) and one receiving too little (donor). The recipient twin may experience heart failure due to continual strain on its heart and blood vessels (cardiovascular system). The donor twin, on the other hand, may experience life-threatening anemia due to its inadequate supply of blood. Such an imbalance in blood flow (i.e., twin-twin transfusion) can occur at any time during the pregnancy, including during delivery.

The effects of Twin-Twin Transfusion Syndrome can vary in severity from case to case, depending upon when during pregnancy the syndrome occurs, when it is diagnosed, and any treatment that may be given. The cause of Twin-Twin Transfusion Syndrome is not fully understood, although it is known that placental characteristics play an important role.

In addition to The National Organization for Rare Disorders (NORD) listed in Section III, the following organizations in Section II (Disease Specific) and in Section III (Umbrella) and Section IV (Government Agencies) can provide more information:
NIH/National Institute of Child Health and Human Development, *IV*
Twin Hope (Twin-Twin Transfusion Syndrome), *III*
Twin to Twin Transfusion Syndrome Foundation, *II*

1041 TYPHOID

Typhoid fever is a bacterial infection that is rare in the United States. However, it is not rare in many other countries. Major symptoms may include unusually high fever, headache, loss of appetite, fatigue, abdominal pain and diarrhea.

In addition to The National Organization for Rare Disorders (NORD) listed in Section III, the following organizations in Section II (Disease Specific) and in Section III (Umbrella) and Section IV (Government Agencies) can provide more information:
Centers for Disease Control and Prevention, *IV*
NIH/National Institute of Allergy and Infectious Diseases, *IV*
World Health Organization (WHO) Regional Office for the Americas (AMRO), *III*

1042 TYROSINEMIA, HEREDITARY

Tyrosinemia is a rare inborn error of metabolism involving the amino acid tyrosine associated with a lack of the enzyme fumarylacetoacetase parahydroxyphenylpyruvic acid (p-HPPA) oxidase. The disorder is characterized by elevated levels of tyrosine and its metabolites (including succinylacetone) in the urine. It causes developmental delay and profound liver dysfunction, kidney problems, and liver cell cancer. There are often neurologic problems causing peripheral nerve palsy and paralysis.

In addition to The National Organization for Rare Disorders (NORD) listed in Section III, the following organizations in Section II (Disease Specific) and in Section III (Umbrella) and Section IV (Government Agencies) can provide more information:
Association for Neuro-Metabolic Disorders, *III*
Children's Liver Alliance, *III*
Metabolic Information Network, *III*
NIH/National Institute of Diabetes, Digestive and Kidney Diseases, *IV*
Research Trust for Metabolic Diseases in Children, *III*
The Arc (a national organization on mental retardation), *III*

1043 URTICARIA PIGMENTOSA

Urticaria Pigmentosa is a rare skin disorder that is a localized (cutaneous) form of Mastocytosis. Mast cells are specialized cells of connective tissue that store substances such as histamine and heparin. When mast cells cluster and multiply excessively (proliferate), histamine and heparin are released into the skin (Mastocytosis). The characteristic skin lesions of Urticaria Pigmentosa appear in these areas. Urticaria Pigmentosa is generally benign and is usually self-limited. The exact cause of the disease is not known, although some cases may be inherited.

In addition to The National Organization for Rare Disorders (NORD) listed in Section III, the following organizations in Section II (Disease Specific) and in Section III (Umbrella) and Section IV (Government Agencies) can provide more information:
NIH/National Institute of Allergy and Infectious Diseases, *IV*

1044 URTICARIA, CHOLINERGIC

Cholinergic Urticaria is a disorder of the immune system characterized by an immediate skin reaction (hypersensitivity) to heat, emotional stress, and/or exercise. Symptoms of the disorder include the appearance of distinctive small skin eruptions (hives) with well-defined borders and pale centers, surrounded by patches of red skin (wheal-and-flare reaction). These red areas are typically intensely itchy (pruritus). Occasionally, Cholinergic Urticaria may be associated with systemic symptoms such as fever and/or difficulty breathing.

The symptoms of Cholinergic Urticaria may develop due to the reaction of specific immune system antibodies (IgE) to certain antigens, leading to a hypersensitivity response (Type I) and the wheal-and-flare reaction that is typical of Cholinergic Urticaria.

In addition to The National Organization for Rare Disorders (NORD) listed in Section III, the following organizations in Section II (Disease Specific) and in Section III (Umbrella) and Section IV (Government Agencies) can provide more information:
NIH/National Institute of Allergy and Infectious Diseases, *IV*

1045 URTICARIA, COLD

Cold Urticaria is a chronic, reactive skin disorder. It is probably the most common form of physical urticaria. Major symptoms may include abnormal reddening of the skin (erythema), hives and itching after exposure of the skin to cold temperatures.

In addition to The National Organization for Rare Disorders (NORD) listed in Section III, the following organizations in Section II (Disease Specific) and in Section III (Umbrella) and Section IV (Government Agencies) can provide more information:
American Autoimmune Related Diseases Association, Inc., *III*
Asthma and Allergy Foundation of America, Inc., *III*
NIH/National Institute of Allergy and Infectious Diseases, *IV*

1046 URTICARIA, PAPULAR

Papular Urticaria, more commonly known as "hives," is characterized by local elevated ridges (wheals) and redness (erythema) of the skin. This condition is usually triggered by allergic reactions to insect bites, sensitivity to drugs, or other environmental causes. The first symptom of Papular Urticaria is usually itching (pruritus), followed by the appearance of small or large wheals. In some cases, swelling of the soft tissues of the face, neck, and hands (angioedema) may also occur. Papular Urticaria may be caused by drug allergies, insect stings or bites, desensitization injections (allergy shots), or ingestion of certain foods (particularly eggs, shellfish, nuts, or fruits) by individuals who are allergic to these substances.

In addition to The National Organization for Rare Disorders (NORD) listed in Section III, the following organizations in Section II (Disease Specific) and in Section III (Umbrella) and Section IV (Government Agencies) can provide more information:
NIH/National Institute of Allergy and Infectious Diseases, *IV*

1047 URTICARIA, PHYSICAL

Physical Urticaria is a condition in which red (erythematous) allergic skin lesions and itching (pruritus) are produced by exposure to cold temperatures, water, or mild trauma. The disorder occurs most commonly in infants.

In addition to The National Organization for Rare Disorders (NORD) listed in Section III, the following organizations in Section II (Disease Specific) and in Section III (Umbrella) and Section IV (Government Agencies) can provide more information:
NIH/National Institute of Allergy and Infectious Diseases, *IV*

1048 USHER'S SYNDROME

Usher's Syndrome is a genetic disorder primarily characterized by deafness accompanied by Retinitis Pigmentosa, a disorder that causes progressive loss of vision. The age at which the disorder appears as well as severity of symptoms distinguishes the four types of Usher's Syndrome.

In addition to The National Organization for Rare Disorders (NORD) listed in Section III, the following organizations in Section II (Disease Specific) and in Section III (Umbrella) and Section IV (Government Agencies) can provide more information:
Alexander Graham Bell Association for the Deaf, Inc., *III*
American Council of the Blind, Inc., *III*
American Foundation for the Blind, *III*
American Society for Deaf Children, *III*
Blind Children's Center, *III*
Blind Children's Fund, *III*
Council of Families with Visual Impairment, *III*
Deafness Research Foundation, *III*
Foundation Fighting Blindness, *III*
NIH/National Eye Institute, *IV*
NIH/National Institute on Deafness and Other Communication Disorders (Balance), *IV*
National Association for Parents of the Visually Impaired, *III*
National Association for Visually Handicapped, *III*
National Federation of the Blind, *III*
National Information Center on Deafness, *III*
Retinitis Pigmentosa International, *II*
Usher Family Support, *II*

1049 VACTERL ASSOCIATION

VACTERL Association is an acronym for (V)ertebral anomalies, (A)nal atresia, congenital (C)ardiac disease, (T)racheo(E)sophageal fistula, (R)enal anomalies, radial dysplasia, and other (L)imb defects. Abnormalities are present at birth. Symptoms occur in various combinations and can be manifestations of several recognized disorders. Related disorders such as the VATER Association and the REAR Syndrome, which are composed of some of the same symptoms, have been expanded into the VACTERL Association. Nearly all cases have occurred sporadically, although some familial cases have been identified. Occasionally, other abnormalities may accompany this association of symptoms.

In addition to The National Organization for Rare Disorders (NORD) listed in Section III, the following organizations in Section II (Disease Specific) and in Section III (Umbrella) and Section IV (Government Agencies) can provide more information:

Cloaca Connection, *III*
EA/TEF Child and Family Support Connection, Inc., *III*
NIH/National Institute of Child Health and Human Development, *IV*
TEF/VATER/VACTRL National Support Network, *II*
Tracheo Oesophageal Fistula Support Group, *II*

1050 VALINEMIA

Valinemia is a very rare metabolic disorder. It is characterized by elevated levels of the amino acid valine in the blood and urine caused by a deficiency of the enzyme valine transaminase. This enzyme is needed in the breakdown (metabolism) of valine. Infants with valinemia usually have a lack of appetite, vomit frequently, and fail to thrive. Low muscle tone (hypotonia) and hyperactivity also occur.

In addition to The National Organization for Rare Disorders (NORD) listed in Section III, the following organizations in Section II (Disease Specific) and in Section III (Umbrella) and Section IV (Government Agencies) can provide more information:

Metabolic Information Network, *III*
NIH/National Institute of Diabetes, Digestive & Kidney Diseases, *IV*
Research Trust for Metabolic Diseases in Children, *III*

1051 VARICELLA ZOSTER

Varicella-zoster is an infectious disease caused by a common virus known as herpes virus. During childhood, the virus causes chickenpox (varicella), while, during adulthood, it causes shingles (herpes zoster). Chickenpox is a highly contagious disease characterized by an itchy skin rash and fever. Chickenpox usually begins with mild constitutional symptoms such as a mild headache, moderate fever and discomfort followed by an eruption appearing in itchy groups of flat or elevated spots and blisters, which form crusts. Shingles is a painful localized recurrence of the skin rash during adulthood.

In addition to The National Organization for Rare Disorders (NORD) listed in Section III, the following organizations in Section II (Disease Specific) and in Section III (Umbrella) and Section IV (Government Agencies) can provide more information:

Centers for Disease Control and Prevention, *IV*
NIH/National Institute of Allergy and Infectious Diseases, *IV*
World Health Organization (WHO) Regional Office for the Americas (AMRO), *III*

1052 VASCULAR MALFORMATIONS OF THE BRAIN

Vascular Malformations of the Brain are conditions that affect the blood vessels in the brain. They may be classified into four groups: Arteriovenous Malformations (abnormal arteries and veins), Cavernous Malformations (enlarged blood-filled spaces), Venous Malformations (abnormal veins), and the Telangiectasias (enlarged capillary-sized vessels). Symptoms and progression of these disorders vary with the type and severity of the malformations.

In addition to The National Organization for Rare Disorders (NORD) listed in Section III, the following organizations in Section II (Disease Specific) and in Section III (Umbrella) and Section IV (Government Agencies) can provide more information:

NIH/National Institute of Neurological Disorders and Stroke, *IV*
National Vascular Malformations Foundation, Inc., *III*

1053 VASCULITIS

Vasculitis is inflammation of blood vessels. In individuals with vasculitis, inflammation damages the lining of affected blood vessels, causing narrowing, the formation of blood clots (thrombosis), and/or blockage. As a result, there may be restriction of oxygenated blood supply to certain tissues (ischemia), potentially resulting in pain, tissue damage, and, in some cases, malfunction of certain affected organs. Vasculitis may affect veins and arteries of any type or size; may involve a single organ or many organs and tissues of the body; and may be a primary disease process or occur due to or in association with a number of different underlying disorders. Therefore, the range and severity of symptoms and findings associated with vasculitis may vary greatly. The specific underlying cause of vasculitis is not fully understood. However, in most cases, it is thought to be due to disturbances of the bodys immune system.

In addition to The National Organization for Rare Disorders (NORD) listed in Section III, the following organizations in Section II (Disease Specific) and in Section III (Umbrella) and Section IV (Government Agencies) can provide more information:
American Autoimmune Related Diseases Association, Inc., *III*
NIH/National Heart, Lung and Blood Institute Information Center, *IV*

1054 VASCULITIS, CUTANEOUS NECROTIZING

Cutaneous Necrotizing Vasculitis is characterized by inflammation and tissue damage (necrosis) of blood vessel walls and associated skin (cutaneous) lesions. Cutaneous Necrotizing Vasculitis may be a primary disease process or occur due to or in association with a number of different underlying disorders (e.g., certain infections, certain autoimmune disorders) or other factors (e.g., allergic reaction or hypersensitivity to certain medications, toxins, or inhaled environmental irritants).

In addition to The National Organization for Rare Disorders (NORD) listed in Section III, the following organizations in Section II (Disease Specific) and in Section III (Umbrella) and Section IV (Government Agencies) can provide more information:
American Autoimmune Related Diseases Association, Inc., *III*
NIH/National Heart, Lung and Blood Institute Information Center, *IV*

1055 VELOCARDIOFACIAL SYNDROME

Velocardiofacial Syndrome, a rare genetic disorder, is characterized by abnormalities of the head and facial (craniofacial) area, heart defects that are present at birth (congenital heart defects), diminished muscle tone (hyptonia), mild small stature, mental retardation, slight delays in the acquisition of skills requiring the coordination of mental and muscular activities (psychomotor retardation), and/or learning disabilities. Craniofacial malformations often associated with the disorder may include incomplete closure of the roof of the mouth (cleft palate); an unusually small head (microcephaly); abnormally narrow, "almond-shaped" eyelid folds (palpebral fissues); a prominent nose with a large, rounded (bulbous) tip; abnormally flattened cheek (malar) bones; and/or a small open mouth. The most common heart defect associated with Velocardiofacial Syndrome is an abnormal opening in the fibrous partition (septum) that separates the heart's two lower chambers (ventricular septal defect). Additional symptoms and findings often associated with the disorder may include eye (ocular) defects such as clouding of the lenses of the eyes (cataracts) and/or abnormalities of blood vessels in the nerve-rich membranes lining the eyes (tortuous retinal vessels); abnormally thin fingers and hands; an underdeveloped or absent thymus; and/or other abnormalities. (The thymus is a gland in the upper portion of the chest that plays a role in the bodys immune response until puberty.) The range and severity of symptoms may vary greatly from case to case. Velocardiofacial Syndrome is inherited as an autosomal dominant genetic trait.

In addition to The National Organization for Rare Disorders (NORD) listed in Section III, the following organizations in Section II (Disease Specific) and in Section III (Umbrella) and Section IV (Government Agencies) can provide more information:
22q and You, *II*
American Heart Association, *III*
FACES: The National Craniofacial Association, *III*
NIH/National Institute of Child Health and Human Development, *IV*
NIH/National Oral Health Information Clearinghouse, *IV*
National Foundation for Facial Reconstruction, *III*
Velo-Cardio-Facial Syndrome Educational Foundation, *II*

1056 VENTRICULAR SEPTAL DEFECTS

Ventricular septal defects are heart defects that are present at birth (congenital). The normal heart has four chambers. The two upper chambers, known as atria, are separated from each other by a fibrous partition known as the atrial septum. The two lower chambers are known as ventricles and are separated from each other by the ventricular septum. Valves connect the atria (left and right) to their respective ventricles. The aorta, the main vessel of arterial circulation, carries blood from the left ventricle and away from the heart.

Ventricular septal defects can occur in any portion of the ventricular septum. The size and location of the defect determine the severity of the symptoms. Small ventricular septal defects can close on their own (spontaneously) or become less significant as the child matures and grows. Moderately-sized defects can cause congestive heart failure, which is characterized by an abnormally rapid rate of breathing (tachypnea), wheezing, unusually fast heartbeat (tachycardia), enlarged liver (hepatomegaly), and/or failure to thrive. Large ventricular septal defects can cause life-threatening complications during infancy. Persistent elevation of the pressure within the artery that carries blood away from the heart and to the lungs (pulmonary artery) can cause permanent damage to the lungs. The exact cause of ventricular septal defects is not fully understood.

In addition to The National Organization for Rare Disorders (NORD) listed in Section III, the following organizations in Section II (Disease Specific) and in Section III (Umbrella) and Section IV (Government Agencies) can provide more information:
American Heart Association, *III*
Congenital Heart Anomalies, Support, Education, & Resources, *III*
NIH/National Heart, Lung and Blood Institute Information Center, *IV*

1057 VITAMIN B12 DEFICIENCY

Vitamin B12 Deficiency is characterized by an abnormally low level of this vitamin in the blood. The disorder can be caused by a poor diet, inadequate absorption or utilization of B12 such as following stomach and intestinal surgery and increase in certain intestinal organisms. The deficiency causes changes in the blood and the central nervous system. Injection of this vitamin usually cures the disorder if the underlying cause can be corrected.

In addition to The National Organization for Rare Disorders (NORD) listed in Section III, the following organizations in Section II (Disease Specific) and in Section III (Umbrella) and Section IV (Government Agencies) can provide more information:
American Autoimmune Related Diseases Association, Inc., *III*
Cobalamin Network, *III*
NIH/National Digestive Diseases Information Clearinghouse, *IV*
NIH/National Heart, Lung and Blood Institute, *IV*

1058 VITAMIN E DEFICIENCY

Vitamin E Deficiency is extremely rare, except in people who have a disease that causes vitamin malabsorption. It is characterized by an abnormally low level of this vitamin in the blood. Vitamin E Deficiency may lead to a rare, progressive neuromuscular disease that is characterized by loss of reflexes (areflexia), loss of balance and impaired sensations. This disorder occurs most often in infants who have an impairment of their bile flow due to a disease.

In addition to The National Organization for Rare Disorders (NORD) listed in Section III, the following organizations in Section II (Disease Specific) and in Section III (Umbrella) and Section IV (Government Agencies) can provide more information:
American Liver Foundation, *III*
NIH/National Digestive Diseases Information Clearinghouse, *IV*
United Liver Association, *III*

1059 VITILIGO

Vitiligo is a dermatological condition that is characterized by an absence of melanocytes (pigment-producing cells), causing decreased pigmentation in the skin. Associated dermatological findings may vary from one or two spots to generalized depigmentation of the entire body.

In addition to The National Organization for Rare Disorders (NORD) listed in Section III, the following organizations in Section II (Disease Specific) and in Section III (Umbrella) and Section IV (Government Agencies) can provide more information:
NIH/National Institute of Arthritis and Musculoskeletal and Skin Diseases, *IV*
National Foundation for Vitiligo and Pigment Disorders, *III*
National Vitiligo Foundation, Inc., *II*

1060 VOGT KOYANAGI HARADA SYNDROME

Vogt-Koyanagi-Harada Syndrome is a rare disease of unknown origin that affects many body systems such as the eyes, ears, skin, and the covering of the brain and spinal cord (the meninges). The most noticeable symptom is a rapid loss of vision. There may also be neurological signs such as severe headache, vertigo, nausea, and drowsiness. Loss of hearing, and loss of hair (alopecia) and skin color may occur along with whitening of the hair and eyelashes (poliosis).

In addition to The National Organization for Rare Disorders (NORD) listed in Section III, the following organizations in Section II (Disease Specific) and in Section III (Umbrella) and Section IV (Government Agencies) can provide more information:
American Autoimmune Related Diseases Association, Inc., *III*
NIH/National Eye Institute, *IV*
NIH/National Institute of Neurological Disorders and

Stroke, *IV*
National Association for Visually Handicapped, *III*

1061 VON GIERKE DISEASE

Von Gierke Disease is a glycogen storage disease. This hereditary metabolic disorder is caused by an inborn lack of the enzyme glucose-6-phosphatase. This enzyme is needed to convert the main carbohydrate storage material (glycogen) into sugar (glucose), which the body uses for its energy needs. A deficiency causes deposits of excess glycogen in the liver and kidney cells.

In addition to The National Organization for Rare Disorders (NORD) listed in Section III, the following organizations in Section II (Disease Specific) and in Section III (Umbrella) and Section IV (Government Agencies) can provide more information:
Association for Glycogen Storage Disease, *III*
Metabolic Information Network, *III*
NIH/National Institute of Diabetes, Digestive & Kidney Diseases, *IV*
Research Trust for Metabolic Diseases in Children, *III*

1062 VON HIPPEL LINDAU DISEASE

Von Hippel-Lindau Disease is a rare inherited multi-system disorder characterized by the abnormal growth of blood vessels in certain parts of the body (angiomatosis). Very small blood vessels (capillaries) "knot" together to form benign growths known as angiomas. These may develop in the retinas of the eyes (retinoangioma) or in the brain (cerebellar hemangioblastoma). Benign growths may also occur in other parts of the brain, spinal cord, the adrenal glands (pheochromocytoma), and other parts of the body. The symptoms of von Hippel-Lindau Disease vary greatly and depend on the size and location of the growths. People with von Hippel-Lindau Disease are also genetically predisposed to certain types of malignant tumors (i.e., renal cell carcinoma).

In addition to The National Organization for Rare Disorders (NORD) listed in Section III, the following organizations in Section II (Disease Specific) and in Section III (Umbrella) and Section IV (Government Agencies) can provide more information:
NIH/National Eye Institute, *IV*
NIH/National Institute of Neurological Disorders and Stroke, *IV*
NIH/Patient Referral Services Unit, *IV*
VHL Family Alliance, *II*

1063 VON WILLEBRAND DISEASE

Von Willebrand Disease is a hereditary blood clotting disorder characterized by prolonged bleeding. Blood clotting is slowed due to a deficiency of the Von Willebrand factor protein and factor VIII protein (the factor VIII complex). Also, platelets do not stick normally causing excessively slow clotting time. Increased risk of excessive bleeding following surgery, dental procedures or injury occurs in individuals with this disorder. The tendency to prolonged bleeding usually decreases with age.

In addition to The National Organization for Rare Disorders (NORD) listed in Section III, the following organizations in Section II (Disease Specific) and in Section III (Umbrella) and Section IV (Government Agencies) can provide more information:
NIH/National Heart, Lung and Blood Institute Information Center, *IV*
National Hemophilia Foundation, *II*

1064 VULVOVAGINITIS

Vulvovaginitis is a common bacterial infection characterized by the simultaneous inflammation of the external parts of the female genital organs (vulva) and the canal that leads from the uterus to the external opening (vagina). It is one of the most frequent causes of genital symptoms in women. When only the vagina is inflamed, the disorder is called vaginitis. The symptoms and treatments of Vulvovaginitis depend on the specific bacteria that caused the disorder.

The most common types of vulvovaginitis are Genital Candidiasis (also called Yeast Infection), Trichomoniasis, and Nonspecific Vaginitis (also called Haemophilus Vaginalis Vaginitis, Bacterial Vaginitis or Gardnerella Vaginalis Vaginitis). Some types of vulvovaginitis are rarer than others.

Vulvovaginitis occurs when the normal acid/alkaline balance of the vagina is disturbed. Yeast, fungi and other harmful organisms that are normally present may grow in excessive amounts causing infection of the vaginal walls.

In addition to The National Organization for Rare Disorders (NORD) listed in Section III, the following organizations in Section II (Disease Specific) and in Section III (Umbrella) and Section IV (Government Agencies) can provide more information:
Centers for Disease Control and Prevention, *IV*
NIH/National Institute of Allergy and Infectious Diseases, *IV*
National Vulvodynia Association, *III*

1065 WAGR SYNDROME

WAGR Syndrome is a rare genetic syndrome in which there is a predisposition to several distinct disorders. The acronym WAGR stands for (W)ilms' Tumor, (A)niridia, (G)onadoblastoma, and Mental (R)etardation. A combination of two or more of these symptoms must be present for an individual to be diagnosed with WAGR Syndrome. The clinical picture varies, depending upon the combination of symptoms present. The only feature that has been present in all documented cases of WAGR Syndrome, with only one known exception, is the partial or complete absence of the colored portion of the eye or iris (Aniridia). Mental retardation, Wilms' Tumor (the most common form of kidney cancer in children), and/or cancer of the cells that form the testes in males or the ovaries in females (Gonadoblastoma) may or may not be present in affected individuals.

WAGR Syndrome is most often caused by a spontaneous genetic change during early embryonic development (de novo) that occurs for unknown reasons (sporadic). In a small number of cases, chromosomal abnormalities may be present in the parents of children with WAGR Syndrome. In these very rare cases, the syndrome may have been inherited as an autosomal dominant genetic trait.

In addition to The National Organization for Rare Disorders (NORD) listed in Section III, the following organizations in Section II (Disease Specific) and in Section III (Umbrella) and Section IV (Government Agencies) can provide more information:

Ambiguous Genitalia Support Network, *III*
American Cancer Society, Inc., *III*
American Kidney Fund, Inc., *III*
Candlelighters Childhood Cancer Foundation, *III*
Glaucoma Research Foundation, *II*
NIH/National Eye Institute, *IV*
NIH/National Institute of Child Health and Human Development, *IV*
National Eye Research Foundation, *III*
National Kidney Foundation, *III*
Vision Foundation, Inc., *III*

1066 WAARDENBURG SYNDROME

Waardenburg Syndrome is a hereditary disorder characterized by facial abnormalities. The inner folds of the eyelids or the tear duct may be displaced, congenital nerve deafness may occur, and often abnormal pigmentation of the iris of the eye, the skin, and/or the hair may be present.

Type I of this disorder is characterized by displacement of the fold of the eyelid, while type II does not include this feature. However, the frequency of deafness is higher in type II of the disorder.

In addition to The National Organization for Rare Disorders (NORD) listed in Section III, the following organizations in Section II (Disease Specific) and in Section III (Umbrella) and Section IV (Government Agencies) can provide more information:

Alexander Graham Bell Association for the Deaf, Inc., *III*
American Council of the Blind, Inc., *III*
American Foundation for the Blind, *III*
Council of Families with Visual Impairment, *III*
FACES: The National Craniofacial Association, *III*
NIH/National Eye Institute, *IV*
NIH/National Oral Health Information Clearinghouse, *IV*
National Association for Visually Handicapped, *III*
National Association of the Deaf, *III*
National Federation of the Blind, *III*
National Information Center on Deafness, *III*
National Organization for Albinism and Hypopigmentation, *III*
National Vitiligo Foundation, Inc., *II*

1067 WALDENSTROM'S MACROGLOBULINEMIA

Waldenstrom's Macroglobulinemia is a malignant lymph and blood cell disorder. Large quantities of homogeneous immunoglobulin-M (IgM) protein molecules are present in the blood. The disorder tends to run in families, occurring mainly among older males. An enlarged spleen and liver with abnormalities of the peripheral lymph glands are the most frequent symptoms. Weakness, anemia, fatigue and excessive bleeding, especially from the nose and mouth, also occur.

In addition to The National Organization for Rare Disorders (NORD) listed in Section III, the following organizations in Section II (Disease Specific) and in Section III (Umbrella) and Section IV (Government Agencies) can provide more information:

American Cancer Society, Inc., *III*
NIH/National Heart, Lung and Blood Institute, *IV*
NIH/Patient Referral Services Unit, *IV*
Waldenstrom's Macroglobulinemia Support Group, *II*

1068 WALDMANN DISEASE

Waldmann Disease is a rare digestive disorder characterized by the abnormal increase in the diameter (dilatation) of vessels that carry lymphatic fluid to the connective tissue under the mucous membranes of the intestines (lamina propria). The main symptoms are abdominal discomfort and swelling of the limbs. The disorder may be present at birth (congenital) or acquired.

In addition to The National Organization for Rare Disorders (NORD) listed in Section III, the following organizations in Section II (Disease Specific) and in Section III (Umbrella) and Section IV (Government Agencies) can provide more information:
March of Dimes Birth Defects Foundation, *III*
NIH/National Digestive Diseases Information Clearinghouse, *IV*
National Lymphatic and Venous Diseases Foundation, Inc., *III*

1069 WALKER WARBURG SYNDROME

Walker-Warburg Syndrome is a rare disorder that is inherited as an autosomal recessive genetic trait. Walker-Warburg Syndrome is also known as HARD +/-E Syndrome, which is an acronym for (H)ydrocephalus, (A)gyria, (R)etinal (D)ysplasia and, in some cases, (E)ncephalocele. The most consistent features of this disorder are a lack of normal folds of the brain (lissencephaly), malformations of the back portion of the brain (cerebellum), abnormalities of the retina of the eye, and progressive degeneration and weakness of the voluntary muscles (congenital muscular dystrophy).

In addition to The National Organization for Rare Disorders (NORD) listed in Section III, the following organizations in Section II (Disease Specific) and in Section III (Umbrella) and Section IV (Government Agencies) can provide more information:
Guardians of Hydrocephalus Research Foundation, *II*
Hydrocephalus Association, *II*
Lissencephaly Network, Inc., *II*
Muscular Dystrophy Association, *III*
NIH/National Institute of Neurological Disorders and Stroke, *IV*
National Hydrocephalus Foundation, *II*

1070 WANDERING SPLEEN

Congenital Wandering Spleen is a very rare birth defect characterized by the absence or underdevelopment of one or all of the ligaments that hold the spleen in its normal position in the upper left abdomen. The spleen may "wander" in the lower abdomen or pelvis and be mistaken for an unidentified abdominal mass. The symptoms of Wandering Spleen are typically related to abnormal enlargement of the spleen (splenomegaly) or the abnormal position of the spleen in the abdomen. Enlargement may be due to the twisting (torsion) of the splenic arteries and veins or a blood clot (infarct) in the spleen. Symptoms of Wandering Spleen may include abdominal pain and discomfort, nausea, vomiting, fatigue, frequent urination, and/or menstrual abnormalities. "Acquired" Wandering Spleen may occur during adulthood due to accidents or other underlying conditions that may weaken the ligaments that hold the spleen in its normal position (e.g., connective tissue disease or pregnancy).

In addition to The National Organization for Rare Disorders (NORD) listed in Section III, the following organizations in Section II (Disease Specific) and in Section III (Umbrella) and Section IV (Government Agencies) can provide more information:
NIH/National Institute of Child Health and Human Development, *IV*

1071 WEAVER SYNDROME

Weaver Syndrome is characterized by rapid growth. Usually starting before birth (prenatal onset), physical growth and bone development (maturation) can occur more quickly than average. Other symptoms can include increased muscle tone (hypertonia) with exaggerated reflexes (spasticity), slow development of voluntary movements (psychomotor retardation), specific physical characteristics, and/or foot deformities. Babies with this syndrome have a hoarse low-pitched cry.

In addition to The National Organization for Rare Disorders (NORD) listed in Section III, the following organizations in Section II (Disease Specific) and in Section III (Umbrella) and Section IV (Government Agencies) can provide more information:
Human Growth Foundation, *III*
Little People of America, *III*
Little People's Research Fund, Inc., *III*
MAGIC Foundation for Children's Growth, *III*
NIH/National Institute of Child Health and Human Development, *IV*
Support for Families with Children Having Weaver Syndrome, *II*

1072 WEGENER'S GRANULOMATOSIS

Wegener's Granulomatosis is an uncommon collagen vascular disorder that usually begins as a localized inflammation of the upper and lower respiratory tract mucosa, and usually progresses into generalized inflammation of the blood vessels (vasculitis) and kidney (glomerulonephritis). Other symptoms may include ulcerations of the mucous membranes in the nose with secondary bacterial infection, middle ear infection (otitis media) with hearing loss, cough, expectoration of blood (hemoptysis), and inflammation of the thin membrane lining the outside of the lungs and the inside of the chest cavity (pleuritis). The exact cause of Wegener's Granulomatosis is not known.

In addition to The National Organization for Rare Disorders (NORD) listed in Section III, the following organizations in Section II (Disease Specific) and in Section III (Umbrella) and Section IV (Government Agencies) can provide more information:
American Kidney Fund, Inc., *III*
American Lung Association, *III*
NIH/National Heart, Lung and Blood Institute Information Center, *IV*
National Kidney Foundation, *III*
Wegener's Foundation, *II*
Wegener's Granulomatosis Support Group, Inc. (International), *II*

1073 WEIL SYNDROME

Weil Syndrome, a rare infectious disorder, is a severe form of bacterial infection caused by Leptospira bacteria (Leptospirosis). Weil Syndrome is characterized by dysfunction of the kidneys and liver, abnormal enlargement of the liver (hepatomegaly), persistent yellowing of the skin, mucous membranes, and whites of the eyes (jaundice), and/or alterations in consciousness. In most cases, Weil Syndrome occurs among individuals who are exposed to affected animals.

In addition to The National Organization for Rare Disorders (NORD) listed in Section III, the following organizations in Section II (Disease Specific) and in Section III (Umbrella) and Section IV (Government Agencies) can provide more information:
Centers for Disease Control and Prevention, *IV*
NIH/National Institute of Allergy and Infectious Diseases, *IV*
World Health Organization (WHO) Regional Office for the Americas (AMRO), *III*

1074 WEILL MARCHESANI SYNDROME

Weill-Marchesani Syndrome is a rare genetic disorder inherited as an autosomal recessive trait. The major features of this disorder are short stature and a congenital vision defect in which the lens of the eye is unusually rounded and may dislocate.

In addition to The National Organization for Rare Disorders (NORD) listed in Section III, the following organizations in Section II (Disease Specific) and in Section III (Umbrella) and Section IV (Government Agencies) can provide more information:
Human Growth Foundation, *III*
Little People of America, *III*
Little People's Research Fund, Inc., *III*
MAGIC Foundation for Children's Growth, *III*
NIH/National Eye Institute, *IV*
NIH/National Institute of Child Health and Human Development, *IV*
National Association for Visually Handicapped, *III*

1075 WEISMANN NETTER STUHL SYNDROME

Weismann-Netter-Stuhl Syndrome is an extremely rare inherited skeletal disorder characterized by the abnormal development of bone (osseous dysplasia). Affected individuals exhibit bowing of the long portions (shafts) of the shin bone (tibia) and the outer, smaller bone of the leg below the knee (fibula). In some individuals, other bones may also be affected, such as the ribs, pelvis, spinal column, and/or bones in the arms. The primary characteristic of Weismann-Netter-Stuhl Syndrome is short stature (dwarfism). In most cases, this disorder is thought to be inherited as an autosomal dominant genetic trait.

In addition to The National Organization for Rare Disorders (NORD) listed in Section III, the following organizations in Section II (Disease Specific) and in Section III (Umbrella) and Section IV (Government Agencies) can provide more information:
Human Growth Foundation, *III*
Little People of America, *III*
Little People's Research Fund, Inc., *III*
NIH/National Institute of Child Health and Human Development, *IV*
Short Stature Foundation, *III*

1076 WELLS SYNDROME

Wells Syndrome is a rare skin disorder. It is characterized by raised, red, swollen, and warm areas of skin in a flame-shaped pattern with associated pain. The exact cause of the disease is unknown. However, bites of spiders, bees, mites, fleas, or ticks (arthropods) are often associated with this skin condition.

In addition to The National Organization for Rare Disorders (NORD) listed in Section III, the following organizations in Section II (Disease Specific) and in Section III (Umbrella) and Section IV (Government Agencies) can provide more information:
American Autoimmune Related Diseases Association, Inc., *III*
Centers for Disease Control and Prevention, *IV*
NIH/National Institute of Allergy and Infectious Diseases, *IV*

1077 WERDNIG HOFFMAN DISEASE

Werdnig-Hoffmann Disease is a rare inherited neuromuscular disorder of children. It is characterized by degenerative changes in the spinal cord (the ventral horn cells). This results in generalized muscle weakness and the progressive wasting away (atrophy) of the muscles of the trunk and extremities.

In addition to The National Organization for Rare Disorders (NORD) listed in Section III, the following organizations in Section II (Disease Specific) and in Section III (Umbrella) and Section IV (Government Agencies) can provide more information:

Alliance of Genetic Support Groups, *III*
Families of Spinal Muscular Atrophy, *III*
Jennifer Trust for Spinal Muscular Atrophy, *II*
March of Dimes Birth Defects Foundation, *III*
Muscular Dystrophy Association, *III*
Muscular Dystrophy Group of Great Britain and Northern Ireland, *III*
NIH/National Institute of Neurological Disorders and Stroke, *IV*

1078 WERNER SYNDROME

Werner Syndrome is a form of premature aging (progeria) that begins in adolescence or early adulthood and results in the appearance of old age by 30 to 40 years of age. Physical characteristics associated with the disorder may include short stature, prematurely aged appearance of the skin, premature balding, clouding of the lenses of the eyes (cataracts), and/or other abnormalities. Werner Syndrome is thought to be inherited as an autosomal recessive genetic trait.

In addition to The National Organization for Rare Disorders (NORD) listed in Section III, the following organizations in Section II (Disease Specific) and in Section III (Umbrella) and Section IV (Government Agencies) can provide more information:

International Progeria Registry, *III*
International Registry of Werner Syndrome, *II*
March of Dimes Birth Defects Foundation, *III*
NIH/National Institute on Aging, *IV*

1079 WEST SYNDROME

West Syndrome is a rare form of infantile spasm that occurs very early in the development of an infant. Unusual brain wave patterns occur (hypsarrhythmia) and possibly mental retardation. The spasms that occur may range from violent jackknife or "salaam" movements where the whole body bends in half, or they may be no more than a mild twitching of the nose or mouth. These spasms usually begin in the early months after birth and can often be helped with medication. There may be many different causes for the spasms. Neurological testing will be helpful in determining the cause.

In addition to The National Organization for Rare Disorders (NORD) listed in Section III, the following organizations in Section II (Disease Specific) and in Section III (Umbrella) and Section IV (Government Agencies) can provide more information:

Epilepsy Foundation of America, *III*
NIH/National Institute of Neurological Disorders and Stroke, *IV*
THRESHOLD (for uncontrolled seizure disorders), *III*

1080 WHIPPLE'S DISEASE

Whipple's Disease is a rare infectious disease that causes an abnormality in the metabolism and/or usage of fats (lipodystrophy) in the small intestine (localized) characterized by impairment of the ability to properly absorb nutrients (malabsorption), anemia, and joint pain. This disorder may also affect other organs of the body including the heart, lungs, brain, and eyes.

In addition to The National Organization for Rare Disorders (NORD) listed in Section III, the following organizations in Section II (Disease Specific) and in Section III (Umbrella) and Section IV (Government Agencies) can provide more information:

Association for Neuro-Metabolic Disorders, *III*
Centers for Disease Control and Prevention, *IV*
NIH/National Digestive Diseases Information Clearinghouse, *IV*

1081 WIEACKER SYNDROME

Wieacker Syndrome is a rare genetic disorder characterized by deformities of the feet (contracture), muscle atrophy, mild mental retardation and an impaired ability to move certain muscles of the eyes, face and tongue. Wieacker Syndrome is inherited as an X-linked recessive trait.

In addition to The National Organization for Rare Disorders (NORD) listed in Section III, the following organizations in Section II (Disease Specific) and in Section III (Umbrella) and Section IV (Government Agencies) can provide more information:

NIH/National Institute of Arthritis and Musculoskeletal and Skin Diseases, *IV*
NIH/National Institute of Neurological Disorders and Stroke, *IV*

1082 WIEDEMANN RAUTENSTRAUCH SYNDROME

Wiedemann-Rautenstrauch Syndrome (also known as Neonatal Progeroid Syndrome) is an extremely rare genetic disorder characterized by an aged appearance at birth (neonatal progeroid appearance); growth delays before and after birth (prenatal and postnatal growth retardation); and deficiency or absence of the layer of fat under the skin (subcutaneous lipoatrophy), causing the skin to appear abnormally thin, fragile, and wrinkled. In addition, for reasons that are not understood, abnormal deposits of fat may accumulate around the buttocks, the areas around the genitals and the anus (anogenital area), and the area between the ribs and the hips (flanks). Affected infants and children also have distinctive malformations of the head and facial (craniofacial) area including an unusually prominent forehead (frontal bossing) and sides of the skull (parietal bossing), causing the head to appear abnormally large (pseudohydrocephalus); unusually small, underdeveloped (hypoplastic) bones of the face and abnormally small facial features; a small "beak-shaped" nose that becomes more pronounced with advancing age; and/or sparse scalp hair, eyebrows, and/or eyelashes. Most infants and children with Wiedemann-Rautenstrauch Syndrome al so have unusually thin arms and legs; abnormally large hands and feet; progressive neurological and neuromuscular abnormalities; varying degrees of mental retardation; and severe delays in the acquisition of skills requiring the coordination of mental and muscular activities (psychomotor retardation). In addition, in many cases, affected infants and children are prone to repeated respiratory infections that may result in life-threatening complications. Wiedemann-Rautenstrauch Syndrome is inherited as an autosomal recessive genetic trait.

In addition to The National Organization for Rare Disorders (NORD) listed in Section III, the following organizations in Section II (Disease Specific) and in Section III (Umbrella) and Section IV (Government Agencies) can provide more information:

International Progeria Registry, *III*
NIH/National Institute of Child Health and Human Development, *IV*
NIH/National Institute of Neurological Disorders and Stroke, *IV*
United Leukodystrophy Foundation, *III*

1083 WILDERVANCK SYNDROME

Wildervanck Syndrome is a rare, congenital disorder characterized by hearing loss in which there is distortion of sound (sensorineural deafness) and fusion of certain bones of the spinal column within the neck (cervical vertebrae) and, in some cases, the upper back (thoracic vertebrae), resulting in limited motion of the neck or upper spine (Klippel-Feil Syndrome). There may also be limited movement of the eye causing difficulty in focusing (Duane Syndrome).

In addition to The National Organization for Rare Disorders (NORD) listed in Section III, the following organizations in Section II (Disease Specific) and in Section III (Umbrella) and Section IV (Government Agencies) can provide more information:

Alexander Graham Bell Association for the Deaf, Inc., *III*
American Society for Deaf Children, *III*
Deafness Research Foundation, *III*
NIH/National Arthritis and Musculoskeletal and Skin Diseases Information Clearinghouse, *IV*
NIH/National Eye Institute, *IV*
National Information Center on Deafness, *III*

1084 WILLIAMS SYNDROME

Williams Syndrome is a rare congenital disorder characterized by characteristic "elfin-like" facial features, exceptionally sensitive hearing, developmental delays, short stature, and/or an impulsive, outgoing personality. Congenital Heart Defects and/or abnormally high levels of calcium in the blood (infantile hypercalcemia) are often present in infants with Williams Syndrome. Some cases of this disorder occur for no apparent reason. Other cases are thought to be inherited as an autosomal dominant genetic trait.

In addition to The National Organization for Rare Disorders (NORD) listed in Section III, the following organizations in Section II (Disease Specific) and in Section III (Umbrella) and Section IV (Government Agencies) can provide more information:

Alliance of Genetic Support Groups, *III*
Canadian Association for Williams Syndrome, *II*
NIH/National Institute of Child Health and Human Development, *IV*
NIH/Patient Referral Services Unit, *IV*
The Arc (a national organization on mental retardation), *III*
Williams Syndrome Association, *II*

1085 WILMS' TUMOR

Wilms' Tumor is the most common form of kidney cancer in children, accounting for six to eight percent of all childhood cancers. The exact cause is not known, although it is thought to be inherited in some cases. An abdominal swelling is the most common symptom usually leading to early detection of the disease. Wilms' Tumor can often be treated successfully depending on the stage of the tumor at detection and the age and general health of the child.

In addition to The National Organization for Rare Disorders (NORD) listed in Section III, the following organizations in Section II (Disease Specific) and in Section III (Umbrella) and Section IV (Government Agencies) can provide more information:

American Cancer Society, Inc., *III*
American Kidney Fund, Inc., *III*
Candlelighters Childhood Cancer Foundation, *III*
Candlelighters Childhood Cancer Foundation Canada, *III*
National Kidney Foundation, *III*
The Arc (a national organization on mental retardation), *III*

1086 WILSON'S DISEASE

Wilson's Disease is a rare genetic disorder characterized by excess copper stored in various body tissues, particularly the liver, brain, and corneas of the eyes. Later developments include liver (hepatic) disease and central nervous system dysfunction. Early diagnosis and treatment may prevent serious long-term disability.

In addition to The National Organization for Rare Disorders (NORD) listed in Section III, the following organizations in Section II (Disease Specific) and in Section III (Umbrella) and Section IV (Government Agencies) can provide more information:
Alliance of Genetic Support Groups, *III*
American Liver Foundation, *III*
Children's Liver Alliance, *III*
March of Dimes Birth Defects Foundation, *III*
NIH/National Institute of Neurological Disorders and Stroke, *IV*
United Liver Association, *III*
WE MOVE, *III*
Wilson's Disease Association, *II*

1087 WINCHESTER SYNDROME

Winchester Syndrome is a very rare disorder believed by some scientists to be closely related to the mucopolysaccharidoses, which is a group of hereditary lysosomal storage disorders. Major symptoms of Winchester Syndrome may include short stature, arthritis-like symptoms, and eye and skin abnormalities.

In addition to The National Organization for Rare Disorders (NORD) listed in Section III, the following organizations in Section II (Disease Specific) and in Section III (Umbrella) and Section IV (Government Agencies) can provide more information:
NIH/National Arthritis and Musculoskeletal and Skin Diseases Information Clearinghouse, *IV*

1088 WISKOTT ALDRICH SYNDROME

Wiskott-Aldrich Syndrome (WAS) is a rare inherited disorder that may be characterized by recurrent infections due to defects in the immune system (i.e., partial defects in T lymphocyte and B lymphocyte systems [combined immunodeficiency]); abnormal bleeding caused by a deficiency in circulating blood platelets (thrombocytopenia); a high incidence of "autoimmune-like" symptoms; and the presence of scaling, itchy skin rashes (eczema) that may be mild in some affected individuals and severe in others. The range and severity of symptoms and physical features associated with the disorder may vary greatly from case to case. Because Wiskott-Aldrich Syndrome is inherited as an X-linked recessive genetic trait, only males are affected with the disease.

In addition to The National Organization for Rare Disorders (NORD) listed in Section III, the following organizations in Section II (Disease Specific) and in Section III (Umbrella) and Section IV (Government Agencies) can provide more information:
Immune Deficiency Foundation, *III*
International Bone Marrow Transplant Registry, *III*
International Patient Organization for Primary Immunodeficiencies, *III*
Jeffrey Modell Foundation, *III*
March of Dimes Birth Defects Foundation, *III*
NIH/National Arthritis and Musculoskeletal and Skin Diseases Information Clearinghouse, *IV*
NIH/National Heart, Lung and Blood Institute Information Center, *IV*
NIH/National Institute of Allergy and Infectious Diseases, *IV*
National Bone Marrow Transplant Link, *III*

1089 WOLF HIRSCHHORN SYNDROME

Wolf-Hirschhorn Syndrome is an extremely rare chromosomal disorder caused by a partial deletion (monosomy) of the short arm ("p") of chromosome 4. Major symptoms may include extremely wide-set eyes (ocular hypertelorism) with a broad or beaked nose, a small head (microcephaly), low-set malformed ears, mental and growth deficiency, heart (cardiac) defects, and seizures.

In addition to The National Organization for Rare Disorders (NORD) listed in Section III, the following organizations in Section II (Disease Specific) and in Section III (Umbrella) and Section IV (Government Agencies) can provide more information:
Chromosome Deletion Outreach, *III*
NIH/National Institute of Child Health and Human Development, *IV*
Wolf-Hirschhorn (4P-) Parent Contact Group, *II*
Wolf-Hirschhorn Syndrome (4p-) Support Group and Newsletter, *II*
Wolf-Hirschhorn Syndrome Support Group, *II*
World Health Organization (WHO) Regional Office for the Americas (AMRO), *III*

1090 WOLFF PARKINSON WHITE SYNDROME

Wolff-Parkinson-White Syndrome is a rare disorder involving irregularities in the heartbeat (cardiac arrhythmia). Patients have an extra conduction pathway in the heart, called the Bundle of Kent, which excessively stimulates the ventricles. Palpitations (sensation of rapid or irregular beating of the heart), weakness, and shortness of breath may occur.

In addition to The National Organization for Rare Disorders (NORD) listed in Section III, the following organizations in Section II (Disease Specific) and in Section III (Umbrella) and Section IV (Government Agencies) can provide more information:

American Heart Association, *III*
Cardiomyopathy Association, *II*
NIH/National Heart, Lung and Blood Institute Information Center, *IV*

1091 WOLFRAM SYNDROME

Wolfram Syndrome is a rare, congenital, multisystem disorder believed to be caused by both mitochondrial and nuclear gene dysfunction. Diabetes insipidus, diabetes mellitus, and vision and hearing defects are the main symptoms associated with this syndrome. Disorders of the urinary tract are also often present. Wolfram Syndrome affects males and females equally and may be inherited as a autosomal recessive trait.

In addition to The National Organization for Rare Disorders (NORD) listed in Section III, the following organizations in Section II (Disease Specific) and in Section III (Umbrella) and Section IV (Government Agencies) can provide more information:

Diabetes Insipidus Foundation, Inc., *III*
Juvenile Diabetes Foundation International, *II*
NIH/National Diabetes Information Clearinghouse, *IV*
NIH/National Eye Institute, *IV*
NIH/National Heart, Lung and Blood Institute Information Center, *IV*
National Association for Parents of the Visually Impaired, *III*
National Association for Visually Handicapped, *III*
United Mitochondrial Disease Foundation, *III*
Vision Foundation, Inc., *III*

1092 WYBURN MASON SYNDROME

Wyburn-Mason Syndrome is a rare genetic disorder that usually affects the brain, eyes and skin. Major symptoms may include discolored patches on the skin, and ballooned areas in the arteries (aneurysms) of the brain and eyes.

In addition to The National Organization for Rare Disorders (NORD) listed in Section III, the following organizations in Section II (Disease Specific) and in Section III (Umbrella) and Section IV (Government Agencies) can provide more information:

NIH/National Eye Institute, *IV*
NIH/National Institute of Neurological Disorders and Stroke, *IV*
National Aphasia Association, *II*

1093 X LINKED LYMPHOPROLIFERATIVE SYNDROME

X-linked Lymphoproliferative Syndrome (XLP) is an extremely rare inherited (primary) immunodeficiency disorder characterized by a defective immune system response to infection with the Epstein-Barr virus (EBV). This herpes virus is common among the general population and causes infectious mononucleosis (IM), usually with no long-lasting effects. However, in individuals with X-Linked Lymphoproliferative Syndrome, exposure to EBV may result in severe, life-threatening infectious mononucleosis; abnormally low levels of antibodies in the blood and body secretions (hypogammaglobulinemia), resulting in increased susceptibility to various infections; malignancies of certain types of lymphoid tissue (B-cell lymphomas); and/or other abnormalities. The range of symptoms and findings associated with XLP may vary from case to case. In addition, the range of effects may change in an affected individual over time. In most cases, individuals with XLP experience an onset of symptoms anytime from approximately six months to 10 years of age.

Approximately half of individuals with X-linked Lymphoproliferative Syndrome experience severe, life-threatening mononucleosis characterized by fever, inflammation and soreness of the throat (pharyngitis), swollen lymph glands, enlargement of the spleen (splenomegaly), enlargement of the liver (hepatomegaly), and/or abnormal functioning of the liver, resulting in yellowing of the skin, mucous membranes, and whites of the eyes (jaundice or icterus). In some cases, individuals who experience life-threatening mononucleosis infection may subsequently have an abnormal increase (i.e., proliferation) of certain white blood cells (lymphocytes and histiocytes) in particular organs, severe liver damage and/or failure, damage to the blood-cell generating bone marrow (hematopoietic marrow cells) that may result in aplastic anemia, and/or other symptoms that may result in life-threatening complications in affected children or adults. Aplastic anemia is characterized by a marked deficiency of all types of blood cells (pancytopenia) including low levels of red blood cells, certain white blood cells, and platelets (the blood cells that function to assist appropriate blood clotting). In individuals with XLP, a decrease in platelets (thrombocytopenia) results in increased susceptibility to bruising and excessive bleeding (hemorrhaging). Because X-linked Lymphoproliferative Syndrome is inherited as an X-linked recessive genetic trait, only males are affected with the disorder.

In addition to The National Organization for Rare Disorders (NORD) listed in Section III, the following organizations in Section II (Disease Specific) and in Section III (Umbrella) and Section IV (Government Agencies) can provide more information:
Alliance of Genetic Support Groups, *III*
Aplastic Anemia Foundation of America, Inc., *II*
Immune Deficiency Foundation, *III*
International Bone Marrow Transplant Registry, *III*
International Patient Organization for Primary Immunodeficiencies, *III*
Jeffrey Modell Foundation, *III*
March of Dimes Birth Defects Foundation, *III*
NIH/Hematology Branch, National Heart, Lung and Blood Institute (NHLBI), *IV*
NIH/National Cancer Institute, *IV*
NIH/National Institute of Allergy and Infectious Diseases, *IV*
National Bone Marrow Transplant Link, *III*
OncoLink: The University of Pennsylvania Cancer Center Resource, *III*

1094 X-LINKED JUVENILE RETINOSCHISIS

X-linked Juvenile Retinoschisis (RS) is a genetic disorder affecting males. Major symptoms may include poor eyesight and degeneration of the retina. The retina consists of membrane layers in the eye that receive visual images. It is composed of supportive and protective structures, nervous system components and layers including "rods" and "cones." RS is due to splitting of the retina, which, in turn, causes slow, progressive loss of parts of the fields of vision corresponding to the areas of the retina that have become split. Often, RS is associated with the development of cysts (sac-like blisters) in the retina.

In addition to The National Organization for Rare Disorders (NORD) listed in Section III, the following organizations in Section II (Disease Specific) and in Section III (Umbrella) and Section IV (Government Agencies) can provide more information:
Association for Macular Diseases, Inc., *III*
NIH/National Eye Institute, *IV*
National Association for Visually Handicapped, *III*

1095 XYY SYNDROME

XYY Syndrome is a rare chromosomal disorder that affects males. It is caused by the presence of an extra Y chromosome. Males normally have one X and one Y chromosome. Men with XYY Syndrome are usually very tall and thin. Many have severe acne during adolescence. Other symptoms may include lower than average intelligence and antisocial or behavioral problems.

In addition to The National Organization for Rare Disorders (NORD) listed in Section III, the following organizations in Section II (Disease Specific) and in Section III (Umbrella) and Section IV (Government Agencies) can provide more information:
NIH/National Institute of Mental Health, *IV*
National Alliance for the Mentally Ill, *III*
National Mental Health Association, *III*
National Mental Health Consumer Self-Help Clearinghouse, *III*
UNIQUE - Rare Chromosome Disorder Support Group, *III*

1096 XERODERMA PIGMENTOSUM

Xeroderma Pigmentosum (XP) is a group of rare inherited skin disorders that is characterized by a heightened reaction to sunlight (photosensitivity) with skin blistering occurring after exposure to the sun. In some cases, pain and blistering may occur immediately after contact with sunlight. Acute sunburn and persistent redness or inflammation of the skin (erythema) are also early symptoms of Xeroderma Pigmentosum. In most cases, these symptoms may be apparent immediately after birth or occur within the next three years. In some rare cases, symptoms may not be apparent until later in childhood. Other symptoms of Xeroderma Pigmentosum may include discolorations of the skin, weak and fragile skin, and/or scarring of the skin.

Xeroderma Pigmentosum affects the eyes as well as the skin, has been associated with several forms of cancer, and may occur along with dwarfism, mental retardation, and/or delayed development.

There are several types of Xeroderma Pigmentosum. Each type is categorized according to the capacity of the body to repair the DNA damaged by ultraviolet light. Any of the symptoms of the classic form of Xeroderma Pigmentosum may occur in any of these subdivisions. These types are: XP, Type A (XPA-Classical); XP, Type B (XPB); XP,

Type C (XPC); XP, Type D (XPD); XP, Type E (XPE); XP, Type F (XPF); XP, Type G (XPG); and XP, Dominant Type. In most cases, Xeroderma Pigmentosum is inherited as an autosomal recessive genetic trait.

In addition to The National Organization for Rare Disorders (NORD) listed in Section III, the following organizations in Section II (Disease Specific) and in Section III (Umbrella) and Section IV (Government Agencies) can provide more information:

Alliance of Genetic Support Groups, *III*
NIH/National Arthritis and Musculoskeletal and Skin Diseases Information Clearinghouse, *IV*
Skin Cancer Foundation, *III*
The Arc (a national organization on mental retardation), *III*
XP (Xeroderma Pigmentosum) Society, Inc., *II*

1097 YAWS

Yaws is an infectious tropical disease caused by the bacterium Treponema pertenue. Yaws has 3 stages of symptoms. Stage 1 Yaws is characterized by the eruption of sores on the skin. The symptoms of Stage 2 and Stage 3 Yaws may involve the bones, joints, and/or skin. Stage 2 Yaws is also known as Gangosa Syndrome (Ogo, or Rhinopharyngitis Mutilans); Stage 3 Yaws is also called Goundou Syndrome (Henpue, Henpuye, Gundo, or Anakhre). Yaws is prevalent in tropical areas of the world but rare in the United States.

In addition to The National Organization for Rare Disorders (NORD) listed in Section III, the following organizations in Section II (Disease Specific) and in Section III (Umbrella) and Section IV (Government Agencies) can provide more information:

Centers for Disease Control and Prevention, *IV*
NIH/National Institute of Allergy and Infectious Diseases, *IV*
World Health Organization (WHO) Regional Office for the Americas (AMRO), *III*

1098 YELLOW FEVER

Yellow Fever is a viral infection that causes damage to the liver, kidney, heart and gastrointestinal tract. Major symptoms may include sudden onset of fever, yellowing of the skin (jaundice) and hemorrhage. It occurs predominately in South America, the Caribbean Islands and Africa. The disease is spread through bites of infected mosquitos. Incidence of the disease tends to increase in the summer as the mosquito population increases, and it occurs year round in tropical climates.

Yellow Fever has two cycles: the sylvan cycle in which mosquitos primarily spread the disease among forest-dwelling primates, and the urban cycle in which the infection is spread from human to human.

In addition to The National Organization for Rare Disorders (NORD) listed in Section III, the following organizations in Section II (Disease Specific) and in Section III (Umbrella) and Section IV (Government Agencies) can provide more information:

Centers for Disease Control and Prevention, *IV*
NIH/National Institute of Allergy and Infectious Diseases, *IV*
World Health Organization (WHO) Regional Office for the Americas (AMRO), *III*

1099 YELLOW NAIL SYNDROME

Yellow Nail Syndrome is characterized by yellow, thickened and curved nails with almost complete stoppage of nail growth. A loss of cuticles may also be associated with this syndrome. Loosening of the nails (onycholysis) may cause loss of some of the nails. Yellow Nail Syndrome is often associated with respiratory diseases and edema (fluid in the tissue causing swelling).

In addition to The National Organization for Rare Disorders (NORD) listed in Section III, the following organizations in Section II (Disease Specific) and in Section III (Umbrella) and Section IV (Government Agencies) can provide more information:

American Lung Association, *III*
NIH/National Arthritis and Musculoskeletal and Skin Diseases Information Clearinghouse, *IV*
NIH/National Heart, Lung and Blood Institute Information Center, *IV*

1100 YUNIS VARON SYNDROME

Yunis-Varon Syndrome is an extremely rare inherited multisystem disorder with defects affecting the skeletal; ectodermal tissue (i.e., nails, hair, and teeth); and cardiorespiratory (i.e., heart and lungs) systems. It is characterized by growth retardation prior to and after birth; defective growth of the bones of the skull along with complete or partial absence of the shoulder blades (cleidocranial dysplasia); characteristic facial features; and/or abnormalities of the fingers and/or toes. Characteristic facial features may include an extremely small jaw (micrognathia), thin lips, sparse or absent eyebrows and/or eyelashes, and/or an unusually short vertical groove (philtrum) in the upper lip. Abnormalities of the fingers and toes may include absence (aplasia) or underdevelopment (hypoplasia) of the thumbs and/or the bones at the ends of the fingers and the great toes (distal phalanges). In most cases, infants with this disorder experience severe feeding problems and respiratory difficulties due, in part, to the absence or underdevelopment of the collar bones (clavicles). In addition, affected infants may have heart defects (e.g., abnormal enlargement of the heart muscle [hypertrophic cardiomyopathy]). In some cases, feeding problems, respiratory difficulties, and/or heart defects may result in life-threatening complications during infancy. Yunis-Varon Syndrome is thought to be inherited as an autosomal recessive genetic trait.

In addition to The National Organization for Rare Disorders (NORD) listed in Section III, the following organizations in Section II (Disease Specific) and in Section III (Umbrella) and Section IV (Government Agencies) can provide more information:
NIH/National Heart, Lung and Blood Institute Information Center, *IV*
NIH/National Institute of Child Health and Human Development, *IV*

1101 ZELLWEGER SYNDROME

Zellweger Syndrome is a rare hereditary disorder affecting infants. It is characterized by reduction or absence of peroxisomes in the cells of the liver, kidneys, and brain. Unusual problems in prenatal development, an enlarged liver, high levels of iron and copper in the blood, and vision disturbances are among the major manifestations of Zellweger Syndrome.

In addition to The National Organization for Rare Disorders (NORD) listed in Section III, the following organizations in Section II (Disease Specific) and in Section III (Umbrella) and Section IV (Government Agencies) can provide more information:
NIH/National Institute of Neurological Disorders and Stroke, *IV*
The Arc (a national organization on mental retardation), *III*
United Leukodystrophy Foundation, *III*

1102 ZOLLINGER ELLISON SYNDROME

Zollinger-Ellison Syndrome is an unusual ulcerative condition characterized by small tumors (usually of the pancreas) that secrete a hormone that produces excess amounts of stomach (gastric) juices. These tumors can also appear in the lower stomach wall, spleen or lymph nodes close to the stomach. Large amounts of gastric acid can be found in lower stomach areas where ulcers can form. Ulcers can appear suddenly even in areas where they are rarely found, may persist following treatment, and can be accompanied by diarrhea. Prompt medical treatment of these ulcers is necessary to prevent complications such as bleeding and perforation.

In addition to The National Organization for Rare Disorders (NORD) listed in Section III, the following organizations in Section II (Disease Specific) and in Section III (Umbrella) and Section IV (Government Agencies) can provide more information:
NIH/National Institute of Diabetes, Digestive and Kidney Diseases, *IV*

1103 **11Q RESEARCH AND RESOURCE GROUP**

6123 A Duncan Road
Petersburg, VA 23803 804-863-2114
Fax: 804-828-5343
E-mail: mspace@vcu.edu
www.ucsu.colorado.edu/~biasca/11q.html

The 11q Research and Resource Group is a not-for-profit organization dedicated to providing information, assistance, and support to parents, other family members, and health care professionals caring for children with structural abnormalities of chromosome 11, particularly abnormalities of 11q (the "long arm" of chromosome 11). The Group primarily provides information and support concerning Jacobsen Syndrome, a rare chromosomal disorder also known as "partial deletion" or "partial monosomy" of chromosome 11q. This rare chromosomal disorder may be characterized by a variety of symptoms and physical features including abnormally slow growth before and after birth, delayed psychomotor development, mental retardation, distinctive malformations of the head and facial area, abnormalities of the eyes, malformations of the hands and/or feet, defects of the heart, and/or other physical abnormalities. Established in 1996 and consisting of about 100 members, the 11q Research and Resource Group engages in patient advocacy, promotes research, and offers a variety of services including networking opportunities. In addition, the Group offers referrals, has a web site on the Internet, and provides a variety of educational materials including brochures and a regular newsletter.

President: Melanie Shopshear Pace (1996 to Present).
Year Established: 1996
Organization Members: 90

Concerned with the following diseases or disorders:
Chromosome 11, Partial Monosomy 11q

1104 **49XXXXY**

10001 NE 74th Street
Vancouver, WA 98662-3801 360-892-7547

49XXXXY is a not-for-profit self-help organization dedicated to providing mutual support to families of those affected by 49XXXXY Syndrome. 49XXXXY Syndrome is a rare chromosomal disorder that affects males and may be characterized by growth retardation, hypogonadism, craniofacial and other bone abnormalities, cardiac malformations, varying degrees of mental retardation, delayed language development, and/or behavioral problems. While males normally have one X and one Y chromosome, males with 49XXXXY Syndrome have four X chromosomes and one Y chromosome. 49XXXXY Syndrome is considered an extremely rare variant of Klinefelter Syndrome. Established in 1990, 49XXXXY enables affected families to exchange information, support, and resources through its networking program. The organization supports a pen pal program, makes appropriate referrals, and offers phone support to affected families. 49XXXXY also provides a variety of educational and support materials including a regular newsletter and brochures.

President: Kimberly Jungel (1990-Present)
Year Established: 1990

Concerned with the following diseases or disorders:
Klinefelter Syndrome

1105 **5P- SOCIETY**

7108 Katella Avenue #502
Stanton, CA 90680 714-901-1544
888-970-0777
Fax: 714-890-9112
E-mail: fivepminus@aol.com
http://www.fivepminus.org

The 5p- Society is a voluntary not-for-profit organization that is dedicated to providing information and support to individuals with a deletion of the short arm (p) of chromosome 5 and their families. The 5p- Society promotes patient advocacy, engages in patient and professional education, and provides a variety of educational and support materials, including a regular newsletter and brochures.

President: Todd Piepergerdes
Executive Director: Laura Castillo
Year Established: 1985
Organization Members: 450

Concerned with the following diseases or disorders:
Cri du Chat Syndrome

1106 **8P DUPLICATION SUPPORT GROUP**

The Genetics Center
1 Children's Plaza
The Childrens Medical Center
Dayton, OH 45404 937-226-8408
Fax: 937-463-5325

The 8p Duplication Support Group is a support organization based at The Genetics Center, Childrens Medical Center, Dayton, Ohio. Established in 1994, the Support Group is dedicated to matching families of children with chromosome 8p duplication disorders to promote the exchange of information, resources, and mutual support. Chromosome 8p duplication disorders are extremely rare chromosomal disorders in which all or a portion of the short arm ("p") of chromosome 8 appears three times rather than twice in cells of the body. These rare chromosomal disorders, known as 8p "duplications" or "trisomies" (or "inverted duplications," if the chromosomal material is also inverted) may be characterized by a variety of symptoms and physical features depending upon the exact length and location of the duplicated material on chromosome 8p. Such symptoms and physical features may include abnormally decreased muscle tone, growth delays during childhood, mental retardation, distinctive malformations of the head and facial area, abnormalities of the fingers and/or nails, cardiac defects, and/or other physical abnormalities. In addition to providing networking services, the 8p Duplication Support Group engages in patient education and provides referrals including to genetic counseling.

Executive Director: Faith Callif-Daley, M.S., C.G.C. (Contact Person)
Year Established: 1994
Organization Members: 15

1107 ABIL INC. (AGORAPHOBICS BUILDING INDEPENDENT LIVES) (ABIL, INC.)

3805 Cutshaw Avenue
Suite 415
Richmond, VA 23230 804-266-9409
Fax: 804-266-6514
E-mail: abil1996@aol.com

Agoraphobics Building Independent Lives (ABIL, Inc.) is a nonprofit "grassroots volunteer organization" dedicated to providing hope, support, and advocacy to people affected by panic attacks, phobias, and/or agoraphobia. By establishing nationwide self-help groups and providing public education, ABIL has worked since 1986 to improve treatment and awareness, both medical and social, of people with panic disorders. ABIL publishes a quarterly newsletter and brochures, establishes telephone and pen pal connections, conducts lectures, makes appropriate referrals, and maintains a database of information for the general public. If there is no local ABIL support group available, ABIL also offers guidelines, materials, and support for those interested in creating support groups in their communities. Memberships are available at a yearly rate.

President: William Harp, M.D.
Executive Director: Yolande L. Fallen, M.S.W. (Administrator)
Year Established: 1986
Organization Chapters: 30
Organization Members: 2,500

Publishes the following materials:
ABIL Handbook ~ *Handbook*
I Was Afraid to Drive My Car ~ *Brochure*
ABIL Newsletter ~ *Newsletter*

1108 ADHD CHALLENGE, INC.

P.O. Box 2277
West Peabody, MA 01910-7277
800-233-2322
TDD: 508-535-3276

ADHD Challenge, Inc. is a national not-for-profit organization dedicated to providing information and support for individuals and families affected by Attention Deficit Hyperactivity Disorder (ADHD). Attention Deficit Hyperactivity Disorder is a behavioral disorder characterized by short attention span, excessive impulsiveness, and inappropriate hyperactivity. Established in 1987 and comprised of over 2,000 members, ADHD Challenge disseminates updated information on ADHD including new research and current legislation. Educational materials include "The Challenge Newsletter," which includes interviews with experts in the ADHD field, summaries of articles from medical journals, questions and comments from readers, and news from support groups. The organization provides referrals to support groups and, when possible, to professionals and physicians; assists the scientific community in contacting patients for ADHD research; offers a networking system; and provides access to an informational database. ADHD Challenge also offers a discount prescription card to all of its members, at no cost.

Executive Director: Ralph M. Koplowitz (Editor)
Year Established: 1987
Organization Members: 2,000

Publishes the following materials:
Meet the CHALLENGE of Attention Deficit Disorder ~ *Brochure*
Thank You For Your Inquiry About Challenge ~ *Subscription Order Form*

Challenge ~ *Newsletter*
The Challenge (January/February 1997) ~ *Newsletter*
The Challenge (March/April 1997) ~ *Newsletter*
Challenge (May/June 1991) ~ *Newsletter*
Challenge (Sept/Oct 1992) ~ *Newsletter*
Challenge (March/April 1995) ~ *Newsletter*
Challenge (July/August 1996) ~ *Newsletter*
Challenge. The Proactive Teacher and the Student with an Attention Deficit ~ *Fact Sheet*
The Challenge ~ *Fact Sheet*

Concerned with the following diseases or disorders:
Attention Deficit Hyperactivity Disorder

1109 AVENUES—A NATIONAL SUPPORT GROUP FOR ARTHROGRYPOSIS MULTIPLEX CONGENITA (AVENUES)

P.O. Box 5192
Sonora, CA 95370 209-928-3688
E-mail: avenues@sonnet.com
http://www.sonnet.com/avenues

AVENUES—A National Support Group for Arthrogryposis Multiplex Congenita, a voluntary not-for-profit organization, is a national support group for people with Arthrogryposis Multiplex Congenita, a rare congenital disease characterized by the presence of multiple joint contractures. Established in 1980, AVENUES is dedicated to providing information to affected individuals, their families, and health care professionals interested in Arthrogryposis. The organization provides a variety of educational and support materials including a directory of families interested in corresponding with other affected families, a directory of medical professionals with a special interest in Arthrogryposis, a pen pal list for young correspondents, an annotated bibliography on Arthrogryposis, a regular newsletter, pamphlets, brochures, and a lecture series on audiotape.

President: Mary Anne and James Schmidt
Executive Director: Mary Anne and James Schmidt
Year Established: 1980
Organization Members: 1,200

Publishes the following materials:
What Is Arthrogryposis? ~ *Brochure*
AVENUES ~ *Newsletter*
ARTHROGRYPOSIS Information, Ontario Office, December 1993 ~ *Resource List*
Genetic Aspects of Arthrogryposis ~ *Reprint*
The Arthrogryposis Group Research Programme ~ *Reprint*
Physical Activity and Arthrogryposis ~ *Reprint*
EMG and Needle Muscle Biospy Studies in Arthrogryposis Multiplex Congenita ~ *Reprint*

Concerned with the following diseases or disorders:
Gordon Syndrome

1110 AARSKOG SYNDROME PARENTS SUPPORT GROUP

62 Robin Hill Lane
Levittown, PA 19055-1411 215-943-7131

The Aarskog Syndrome Parents Support Group is a not-for-profit self-help organization dedicated to providing information and support to parents of children with Aarskog Syndrome. This is a rare genetic disorder characterized by distinctive facial abnormalities, unusually small hands, genital abnormalities, and mild mental retardation. Established in 1993, the Aarskog Syndrome Parents Support Group offers phone and letter support; enables parents to exchange information, support, and resources through its parent-to-parent matching program; engages in patient advocacy; and supports and promotes ongoing medical research. The Aarskog Syndrome Parents Support Group also offers a variety of educational and support materials, including fact sheets, article reprints, case study information, and a regular newsletter.

Executive Director: Shannon Caranci
Year Established: 1993
Organization Members: 50

Publishes the following materials:
A Summary of Medical and Psychoeducational Aspects of Aarskog Syndrome ~ *Report*
Aarskog News Spring 1995 ~ *Newsletter*

Concerned with the following diseases or disorders:
Aarskog Syndrome

1111 ABOUTFACE INTERNATIONAL

99 Crowns Lane, 4th Floor
Toronto
Ontario, M5R 3P4
Canada 416-944-3223
800-665-3223
Fax: 416-944-2488
E-mail: aface@io.org
http://www.io.org/~aface/aface/html

AboutFace International (AFI) is a nonprofit organization dedicated to providing individual and family support to those who have facial differences. AboutFace promotes public education through school presentations and media awareness. The organization seeks to emphasize the value of the person behind every face, encouraging a greater societal acceptance of those with facial differences. Founded in 1985, AboutFace offers an international network of members for sharing information and support, community services such as hospital visits, outreach to new members and school programs, training and support to volunteers in local AboutFace chapters as well as a program to help establish a chapter in your area, and an international newsletter entitled "AboutFace," which focuses on common experiences and provides current information and resources. Educational materials include videos, booklets, and brochures entitled "My Newborn Has a Facial Difference," "You, Your Child, and the Craniofacial Team," and "Making the Difference: An Orientation Booklet on Caring for the Newborn with a Facial Difference."

President: Richard Ten Cate, M.D. (Chairperson) (1997 - present).
Executive Director: Anna Pileggi
Organization Language: Spanish (written/spoken). Portugese (spoken).
Year Established: 1985
Organization Chapters: 70
Organization Members: 5,500

Publishes the following materials:
AboutFace ~ *Mission Statement*
My Newborn has a Facial Difference ~ *Brochure*
Look at the possibilities ~ *Brochure*
You, Your Child and the Craniofacial Team ~ *Brochure*
AboutFace (Winter 1996/1997) ~ *Newsletter*
AboutFace Publications ~ *Order Form*
Making The Difference ~ *Booklet*

1112 ACHROMATOPSIA NETWORK

P.O. Box 214
Berkeley, CA 94701-0214 510-540-4700
Fax: 510-540-4767
E-mail: futterman@achromat.org
http://www.achromat.org

The Achromatopsia Network is a nonprofit organization for individuals concerned with achromatopsia. Congenital Achromatopsia is a hereditary eye defect characterized by minimal or absent function of the cone cells of the retina leading to visual impairment. Founded in 1993, the Achromatopsia Network is committed to sharing information about achromatopsia and providing resources to meet the special needs of those affected by this eye condition; helping individuals and families concerned with Achromatopsia to connect with one another; and promoting awareness and education regarding Achromatopsia with a special emphasis on accomplishing this goal among those who provide services to the visually impaired. Educational materials include a monthly newsletter and a guide written for eye care professionals entitled "Congenital Achromatopsia...A Guide for Professionals."

President: Frances Futterman (Facilitator)
Year Established: 1993
Organization Members: 300

Publishes the following materials:
The Achromatopsia Network Publications ~ *Order Form*
The Achromatopsia Network ~ *Fact Sheet*
Congenital Achromatopsia - A Guide for Professionals ~ *Booklet*

1113 ACID MALTASE DEFICIENCY ASSOCIATION, INC. (AMDA)

P.O. Box 700248
San Antonio, TX 78270-0248 210-490-7161
Fax: 210-497-3810
E-mail: tianrama@aol.com
members.aol.com/amdapage/index.htm

The Acid Maltase Deficiency Association, Inc. is a nonprofit organization directed toward the advancement of research in Acid Maltase Deficiency (also known as Pompe's Disease, Types A, B, and C). Pompe's Disease, a glycogen storage disease with onset during infancy, childhood, or adulthood, is inherited as an autosomal recessive genetic trait. Symptoms develop due to deficiency of the enzyme Alpha-1,4 glucosidase. Founded in 1995 and consisting of 70 members, the Association publishes brochures and informational literature; sponsors an annual conference for the scientific community to discuss crucial issues related to Pompe's Disease; and maintains a patient/family registry. This registry is used to disseminate information to affected families about current scientific breakthroughs, dietary information, and other issues vital to daily living.

President: Randall House (1995 - Present)
Executive Director: Marylyn House (Patient Coordinator)
Year Established: 1995
Organization Members: 70

Publishes the following materials:
AMDA. Acid Maltase Deficiency Patient Questionnaire ~ *Leaflet*
Acid Maltase Deficiency Association ~ *Brochure*
AMDA ~ *Newsletter*
Acid Maltase Deficiency Association, Inc. ~ *Brochure*

Concerned with the following diseases or disorders:
Pompe Disease

1114 ACOUSTIC NEUROMA ASSOCIATION (ANA)

P.O. Box 12402
Atlanta, GA 30355 404-237-8023
Fax: 404-237-2704
E-mail: anausa@aol.com
http://www.anausa.org

The Acoustic Neuroma Association (ANA) is a not-for-profit organization dedicated to providing information and support to individuals with an acoustic neuroma or another benign condition affecting the cranial nerves. An acoustic neuroma is a benign tumor of the eighth (auditory) cranial nerve. Established in 1981, the Acoustic Neuroma Association is also committed to disseminating information on patient rehabilitation to physicians and health care personnel and promoting and supporting research on acoustic neuroma and its effects. The Association seeks to educate the public regarding symptoms suggestive of acoustic neuroma in order to promote early diagnosis and successful treatment. In addition, the Acoustic Neuroma Association provides referrals to support groups and offers a variety of educational and support materials through its database, regular newsletter, brochures, and audiovisual aids.

President: Sallye H. Anderson (1994-Present)
Executive Director: Lois V. Lowery
Year Established: 1981
Organization Chapters: 42
Organization Members: 5,000

Concerned with the following diseases or disorders:
Acoustic Neuroma; Neurofibromatosis Type 2 (NF-2)

1115 ACOUSTIC NEUROMA ASSOCIATION OF CANADA (ANAC)

Box 369
Edmonton
Alberta, T5J 2J6
Canada
403-428-3384
TDD: 403-428-3383
E-mail: anac@compusmart.ab.ca

The Acoustic Neuroma Association of Canada (ANAC) is a not-for-profit, self-help organization dedicated to providing a comfortable environment for people who have or are facing the removal of acoustic neuromas and other tumors involving the cranial nerves. Acoustic neuromas are benign (noncancerous) tumors affecting the eighth cranial nerve, which is located in the auditory canal of the ear. Established in 1984, ANAC provides support; furnishes information on patient rehabilitation to physicians and health care personnel interested in the treatment of benign tumors and the alleviation of post surgical problems; and promotes and supports research on the cause, development, and treatment of acoustic neuromas. ANAC consists of 500 members and produces educational materials including a quarterly newsletter entitled "The Connection," a pamphlet on Acoustic Neuroma, and a brochure entitled "The Hope is Recognition and Treatment." Program activities include regular support group meetings, patient advocacy, patient networking, and patient education.

President: Shirley Entis (1994 to Present)
Executive Director: Linda Gray (Program Manager)
Organization Language: French (written/spoken)
Year Established: 1984
Organization Members: 500

Publishes the following materials:
What is the Acoustic Neuroma Association? ~ *Mission Statement*
Find it! Treat it! Beat it! ~ *Bookmark*
"The Hope Is Recognition And Treatment" ~ *Brochure*
Acoustic Neuroma ~ *Booklet*
The Connection ~ *Newsletter March 1997*

Concerned with the following diseases or disorders:
Acoustic Neuroma; Neurofibromatosis Type 2 (NF-2)

1116 ADAMS OLIVER SYNDROME SUPPORT GROUP

16 Kirton Close
Radyr Way
Llandaff
Cardiff
South Glamorean, CF5 2NB
Wales, United Kingdom

Founded in 1993, the Adams Oliver Syndrome Support Group is an organization that works to inform and create public awareness about Adams Oliver Syndrome, a rare genetic disorder characterized by distinctive malformations of the scalp and abnormalities of the fingers, toes, arms, and/or legs. The group provides an information packet on this inherited disorder and is working to build a network of people who can discuss common problems and concerns that arise for affected individuals, families, friends, and caregivers.

President: Sandra Ivins
Year Established: 1993
Organization Members: 9

Publishes the following materials:
Adams-Oliver Syndrome ~ *Disease Report*

Concerned with the following diseases or disorders:
Adams Oliver Syndrome

1117 **AGENESIS OF CORPUS CALLOSUM (ACC) NETWORK (ACC NETWORK)**

5749 Merrill Hall
Room 18
University of Maine
Orono, ME 04469-5749 207-581-3119
Fax: 207-581-3120
E-mail: um-acc@maine.maine.edu

The Agenesis of Corpus Callosum (ACC) Network is a not-for-profit self-help organization dedicated to providing information and support to families of children with Agenesis of the Corpus Callosum. This is a rare condition characterized by absence of the thick band of nerve fibers that connects the two cerebral hemispheres. Established in 1990, the Agenesis of Corpus Callosum Network also provides support to families of children with other disorders or conditions that are similar to ACC. The Agenesis of Corpus Callosum Network enables affected families to exchange information, support, and resources through its networking programs.

Executive Director: Kathy Schilmoeller
Year Established: 1990
Organization Members: 500

Concerned with the following diseases or disorders:
Agenesis of Corpus Callosum; Oculocerebrocutaneous Syndrome

1118 **AICARDI SYNDROME AWARENESS AND SUPPORT GROUP (ASASG)**

29 Delavan Avenue
Toronto
Ontario, M5P 1T2
Canada 416-481-4095

The Aicardi Syndrome Awareness and Support Group (ASASG) is a national self-help organization dedicated to providing information and support to Canadian families affected by Aicardi Syndrome and acting as an information gathering and sharing resource for health care professionals. Aicardi Syndrome, an extremely rare genetic disorder that affects only females, is characterized by absence of the thick band of nerve fibers that connects the left and right hemispheres of the brain (agenesis of the corpus callosum), seizures and spasms, characteristic retinal lesions, mental retardation, and/or other abnormalities. ASASG was established in the late 1980s in coordination with the Aicardi Syndrome Newsletter, Inc., a not-for-profit voluntary organization incorporated in the United States. ASASG is committed to providing a network of information, communication, and support to families of children with Aicardi Syndrome; strengthening and empowering families in becoming advocates for their affected children; gathering current research articles and findings regarding Aicardi Syndrome and other related topics for distribution to member families; providing information about Aicardi Syndrome to the public; and serving as a reference and resource contact for medical, educational, and professional organizations.

President: Nancy Hately
Year Established: 1987
Organization Members: Non-Membership

Publishes the following materials:
Aicardi Syndrome Newsletter ~ *Brochure*
Interview with Dr. J. Aicardi ~ *Pamphlet*
Aicardi Syndrome Bibliography ~ *Bibliography*

Concerned with the following diseases or disorders:
Aicardi Syndrome

1119 **AICARDI SYNDROME NEWSLETTER, INC. (ASN)**

PO Box 398
404 Cherry Lane
Fletcher, OH 45326 937-368-2137
Fax: 937-368-2137
E-mail: AICNews@aol.com
http://www.aicardi.com

Aicardi Syndrome Newsletter, Inc. is a voluntary not-for-profit organization dedicated to providing a network of information and support to families with children who have Aicardi Syndrome and strengthening and empowering families in becoming advocates for their children. Aicardi Syndrome, an extremely rare genetic disorder that affects only females, is characterized by absence of the thick band of nerve fibers that connects the left and right hemispheres of the brain (agenesis of the corpus callosum), seizures and spasms, characteristic retinal lesions, mental retardation, and/or other abnormalities. The organization gathers current research, articles, and findings regarding Aicardi Syndrome and other related topics for distribution to member families. In addition, the group distributes information about Aicardi Syndrome to the public and serves as a reference and resource contact for medical, education, and professional organizations. Established in 1984, the organization provides appropriate referrals for affected individuals and promotes patient advocacy, research, and legislation that benefits individuals with Aicardi

Syndrome. Aicardi Syndrome Newsletter, Inc. provides several educational materials including its monthly publication "ASN BRIEF," reports, brochures, and a bibliography of published journal articles.

President: Denise M. Park
Year Established: 1984
Organization Members: 160

Publishes the following materials:
A Medical Survey ~ *Pamphlet*
Interview with Dr. J. Aicardi, Miami Children's Hospital ~ *Pamphlet*
Aicardi Syndrome Bibliography (Limited) ~ *Bibliography*
Dear Parent ~ *Pamphlet*
A.S.N. Brief ~ *Newsletter*
Aicardi Syndrome Newsletter, A Source for Families and Professionals ~ *Brochure*

Concerned with the following diseases or disorders:
Aicardi Syndrome

1120 ALAGILLE SYNDROME ALLIANCE

10630 SW Garden Park Place
Tigard, OR 97223 503-639-6217
E-mail: cchahn@worldnet.att.net
www.athenet.net/~luxhoj/Alagillesyndrome.ht

The Alagille Syndrome Alliance is a not-for-profit voluntary organization that functions as a support network for people affected by Alagille Syndrome, an inherited chronic liver disorder. Established in 1993, the Alagille Syndrome Alliance is dedicated to providing support to children with this disorder, their family members, and health care professionals who care for people with Alagille Syndrome. The Alliance advocates for continuing medical research into the cause, prevention, and treatment of Alagille Syndrome and serves as a central location for resources related to the diagnosis and treatment of this rare disorder. The Alagille Syndrome Alliance offers a matching service to interested families as well as advice and consultation through specialists on its Scientific Advisory Board. The Alagille Syndrome Alliance provides a variety of educational and support materials including brochures, pamphlets, fact sheets, and its quarterly newsletter entitled "LiverLink."

President: Cindy L. Hahn (1993-Present)
Executive Director: Cindy L. Hahn
Year Established: 1993
Organization Members: 105

Publishes the following materials:
The Alagille Syndrome Alliance ~ *Brochure*
LiverLink ~ *Newsletter*
Alagille Syndrome: A Fact Sheet ~ *Fact Sheet*

Concerned with the following diseases or disorders:
Alagille Syndrome

1121 ALBINO FELLOWSHIP

9 Burnley Road
Hapton
Near Burnley
Lancashire, BB11 5QR
United Kingdom

The Albino Fellowship is a nonprofit organization dedicated to providing support to individuals affected by albinism, parents, families, physicians, teachers, and other interested professionals. Albinism is a group of rare inherited congenital syndromes characterized by partial or complete absence of the pigment melanin, which gives color to the eyes, skin, and hair. Established in 1979, the Albino Fellowship consists of approximately 400 members. The Fellowship has a telephone support system, conducts regional meetings, promotes research, engages in patient advocacy, and offers networking services. The Fellowship also offers a variety of materials including a regular newsletter, reports, and a complete listing of publications available for purchase.

President: Jack Campbell
Executive Director: Mark Sanderson (Honorary Secretary)
Year Established: 1979
Organization Members: 400

Publishes the following materials:
Albino Fellowship Publications List ~ *Publications List*

Concerned with the following diseases or disorders:
Albinism

1122 ALPHA-1-ANTITRYPSIN DEFICIENCY NATIONAL ASSOCIATION (A1NA)

4220 Old Shakopee Road, Suite 101
Minneapolis, MN 55437-2974 612-703-9979
800-425-7421
Fax: 612-885-0133
E-mail: brandley@Alpha1.org
http://www.alpha1.org

The Alpha-1-Antitrypsin Deficiency National Association is a not-for-profit voluntary health organization that was formed to provide information and support to people affected by Alpha-1-Antitrypsin Deficiency and their families. Alpha-1-Antitrypsin Deficiency is a rare hereditary metabolic disease characterized by low levels of the enzyme Alpha-1-Antitrypsin and progressive degenerative and destructive changes in the lungs. Founded in 1991, the organization functions as a clearinghouse for information to assist health care professionals and affected individuals. In addition, the Association engages in patient advocacy and aids in the support of medical research into the control and cure of Alpha-1-Antitrypsin Deficiency. Educational materials produced by the Association include brochures, newsletters, and videos.

President: Greg Hules (1993-Present)
Executive Director: Sandra K. Brandley
Year Established: 1991
Organization Chapters: 47
Organization Members: 900

Publishes the following materials:
Alpha 1-Antitrypsin Deficiency ~ *Brochure*
Alpha 1-Antitrypsin Deficiency. Information for Patients ~ *Pamphlet*
Facts about A1AD Related Emphysema ~ *Pamphlet*
Alpha 1-Antitrypsin Deficiency News ~ *Newsletter*

Concerned with the following diseases or disorders:
Alpha-1-Antitrypsin Deficiency

1123 **ALPORT SYNDROME—HEREDITARY NEPHRITIS STUDY**

Alport Study Department of Physiology
#156
410 Chipeta Way
Salt Lake City, UT 84108-1297 801-581-5479
Fax: 801-585-3232
E-mail: david.f.barker@m.cc.utah.edu
www.cc.utah.edu/~cla6202/ASHP.htm

The Alport Syndrome—Hereditary Nephritis Study at the University of Utah aims to discover the genetic, biochemical, and histological abnormalities that cause various kinds of hereditary nephritis including Alport Syndrome. In addition, the Study aims to devise better forms of medical management and treatments for Alport Syndrome and other types of hereditary nephritis. The ultimate goal of the study is to find a cure for these diseases. Materials produced by the Study include a bibliography of the University of Utah Study (1973-1997), an introductory letter for study participants, and reprints from medical textbooks.

President: David E. Barker, Ph.D., Principal Investigator
Executive Director: Joyce Denison (Contact Person)
Year Established: 1973

Concerned with the following diseases or disorders:
Alport Syndrome

1124 **ALZHEIMER'S ASSOCIATION (ADRDA)**

911 North Michigan Avenue
Suite 1000
Chicago, IL 60611-1676 312-335-8700
800-272-3900
Fax: 312-335-1110
E-mail: info@alz.org
http://www.alz.org

The Alzheimer's Association is a national not-for-profit voluntary organization dedicated to promoting and supporting research into the causes, cure, and prevention of Alzheimer's Disease and to providing education and support services to people with Alzheimer's Disease, their families, and caregivers. Established in 1980, the Association works through a network of more than 220 local chapters, more than 2,000 support groups, and 35,000 volunteers nationwide. The goals of the Alzheimer's Association include education, chapter formation, advocacy for improved public policy and needed legislation, and patient and family services to aid present and future patients and caregivers. Activities of the Association include the promotion of fund-raising for research through its Medical and Scientific Advisory Board; publication of the quarterly "Alzheimer's Association Newsletter"; and promotion of public awareness by publicizing such national annual events as Memory Walk and the national education conference. In addition, the Association operates a 24-hour telephone hotline to assist people with Alzheimer's Disease and their families.

President: Edward Truschke
Executive Director: Edward Truschke
Organization Language: Spanish.
Year Established: 1980
Organization Chapters: 220

Concerned with the following diseases or disorders:
Alzheimer's Disease; Binswanger's Disease; Creutzfeldt Jakob Disease; Kluver Bucy Syndrome; Pick's Disease

1125 **ALZHEIMER'S DISEASE EDUCATION AND REFERRAL CENTER (ADEAR)**

P.O. Box 8250
Silver Spring, MD 20907-8250 301-495-3311
800-438-4380
Fax: 301-495-3334
E-mail: adear@alzheimers.org
http://www.alzheimers.org/adear

The Alzheimer's Disease Education and Referral (ADEAR) Center, a nationwide service of the National Institute on Aging (NIA) and National Institutes of Health, is dedicated to translating research advances into improved care and diagnosis for individuals with Alzheimer's Disease, while focusing on the program's long-term goal: to find a way to cure and possibly prevent Alzheimer's Disease. Established in 1990, ADEAR seeks to investigate the basic mechanisms of Alzheimer's Disease, manage the symptoms, and help families cope with the effects of the disease. The organization maintains an online bibliographic database of Alzheimer's Disease education materials and resources. This database is available to the public as the "Alzheimer's Disease Subfile" of the Combined Health Information Database (CHID) and is a valuable resource for health professionals, administrators, social service workers, and caregivers. CHID contains information on patient brochures, fact sheets, books, journals, audiovisuals, directories, posters, teaching manuals, government reports and documents, and more.

Executive Director: Emily Johnson, Project Director
Year Established: 1990

Publishes the following materials:
Progress Report on Alzheimer's Disease 1994 ~ *Booklet*
Alzheimer's Disease ~ *Fact Sheet*
Alzheimer's Disease Centers Program Directory ~ *Directory*
Alzheimer's Disease Subfile of the Combined Health Information Database ~ *Fact Sheet*
Alzheimer's Disease and Its Impact: A Slide Program for General Audiences ~ *Information Sheet*
Educational Videotapes on Alzheimer's Disease Designed to Reach the African-American Community ~ *Information Sheet*
Alzheimer's Association: Fact Sheet ~ *Fact Sheet*
Multi-Infarct Dementia ~ *Fact Sheet*
Caring and Sharing ~ *Catalog*
For help...For hope...For those who care ~ *Brochure*
National Alzheimer's Library and Resource Center ~ *Mission Statement*
Alzheimer's Association Materials ~ *Catalog*
Alzheimer's Disease - A Guide to Federal Programs ~ *Book*

Concerned with the following diseases or disorders:
Alzheimer's Disease; Binswanger's Disease; Creutzfeldt Jakob Disease; Kluver Bucy Syndrome; Pick's Disease

1126 AMFAR—AMERICAN FOUNDATION FOR AIDS RESEARCH (AMFAR)

733 Third Avenue
New York, NY 10017-3204 212-682-7440
Fax: 212-682-9812
E-mail: user@amfar.org
http://www.amfar.org

AmFar—the American Foundation for AIDS Research is a nonprofit organization dedicated to the support of AIDS research (both basic biomedical and clinical), education for AIDS prevention, and sound AIDS-related public policy development. Established in 1985, AmFAR has been instrumental in educating the United States and the international community about issues germane to AIDS prevention, treatment, and public policy, with an emphasis on the global nature of the epidemic. AmFAR seeks to be a healing force in society: It is concerned about the rights of all people and strives to be a catalyst for an overall attitudinal change toward people who have, are perceived to have, or are threatened by HIV and AIDS. AmFAR funds AIDS programs, basic research, and clinical research and runs a public policy program. Educational materials include special bulletins, the "AIDS/HIV Treatment Directory," a newsletter entitled "The AmFAR Newsletter," and the "AmFAR Report." The organization maintains a web site at [http://www.amfar.org].

President: Arthur J. Ammann
Executive Director: Jerome Radwin
Organization Language: Spanish (written).
Year Established: 1985
Organization Members: Non-Membership

Publishes the following materials:
AIDS/HIV Treatment Directory ~ *Booklet*
Foundation Profile. AmFAR ~ *Mission Statement*
AmFAR. Special Bulletin (October 1995) ~ *Reprint*
AmFAR. Special Bulletin (June 1995) ~ *Reprint*
AmFAR. Special Bulletin (August 1996) ~ *Reprint*
Special Excerpt from The AmFAR Newsletter ~ *Reprint*
The AmFAR Report ~ *Newsletter Fall 1993*
The AmFAR Report ~ *Newsletter Spring 1993*
The AmFAR Report ~ *Newsletter Fall 1993*
The AmFar Report ~ *Newsletter April 1996*

Concerned with the following diseases or disorders:
AIDS (Acquired Immune Deficiency Syndrome); AIDS Dysmorphic Syndrome

1127 **AMERICAN BEHCET'S DISEASE ASSOCIATION (ABDA)**

P.O. Box 6663
Minneapolis, MN 55406 612-722-9554
800-723-4238
Fax: 612-722-2218
http://www.behcets.com

The American Behcet's Disease Association is a voluntary not-for-profit self-help organization dedicated to providing support and informational materials to people with Behcet's Disease and involved physicians. Behcet's Syndrome is a rare chronic relapsing inflammatory disorder characterized by recurrent mouth ulcers, inflammation of the eyes, genital ulcers, rashes, and/or other symptoms. The American Behcet's Disease Association produces a quarterly newsletter and conducts patient conferences and family counseling sessions. In addition, the Association distributes informational literature, makes physician referrals, and encourages patient-to-patient networking. Translations of some materials are available in both Spanish and Italian. The American Behcet's Disease Association serves the entire United States. Regional support groups are located in Sacramento CA, San Francisco CA, Phoenix AZ, Oklahoma City OK, St. Louis MO, Huntsville AL, Atlanta GA, Virginia, New York City and upstate New York, New Jersey, New England and other locations. The American Behcet's Disease Association also maintains a database of scientific research into Behcet's Disease.

President: Susan Sternfels
Organization Language: Spanish (written translation). Italian (written translation).
Year Established: 1985
Organization Members: 850

Concerned with the following diseases or disorders:
Behcet's Syndrome

1128 **AMERICAN CELIAC SOCIETY-DIETARY SUPPORT COALITION (ACS/DSC)**

58 Musano Court
West Orange, NJ 07052 201-325-8837
Fax: 201-669-8808
E-mail: bentleac@umdnj.edu

The American Celiac Society-Dietary Support Coalition is a nonprofit self-help organization that provides support, education, and encouragement for people with Celiac Sprue and other dietary disorders and food allergies, including Dermatitis Herpetiformis, Crohn's Disease, Lactose Intolerance, and Wheat Intolerance. Through patient and general education, nationwide support groups, networking, referrals, and research, ACS/DCS works to increase the awareness of dietary disorders and to identify food products that may contain gluten-gliaden, lactose, corn or soya. ACS/DCS also publishes a newsletter, patient packets, brochures, and offers audio-visual aids for its members. The society offers some Spanish language materials, and has limited Spanish and Italian speaking resources.

President: Annette Bentley
Organization Language: Spanish. Italian.

Publishes the following materials:
Whoo's Report ~ *Newsletter*
Dietary Information ~ *Factsheet*
Education, Research and Mutual Support ~ *Factsheet*

Concerned with the following diseases or disorders:
Celiac Sprue

1129 **AMERICAN COUNCIL FOR HEADACHE EDUCATION (ACHE)**

875 Kings Highway
Suite 200
Woodbury, NJ 08096 609-384-8760
800-255-2243
Fax: 609-384-5811
E-mail: headquarters@ache.smarthub.com
http://www.achenet.org

The American Council for Headache Education (ACHE) is a national voluntary nonprofit organization dedicated to advancing the treatment and management of headache and to raising the public awareness of headache as a valid, biologically based illness. Established in 1989 and consisting of approximately 35,000 members, ACHE's educational mission reaches out to health career policy makers, employers, and opinion leaders as well as to affected individuals and their families. ACHE's goal is to help affected individuals gain more control over all aspects of their lives—medical, social, and economical. The organization offers a national network of Headache Support Groups; online networking opportunities and information via Prodigy, America Online, CompuServe, and the Internet; referrals; advocacy services; and a variety of materials including local support group listings, brochures, booklets, and a regular newsletter entitled "Headache." ACHE's web site on the Internet is located at [http://www.achenet.org].

President: Fred D. Sheftell, M.D. (1995 to Present)
Executive Director: Linda McGillicuddy
Year Established: 1989
Organization Members: 35,000

Publishes the following materials:
Headache: Your Guide to Understanding Headache ~ *Brochure*
Headache: You Are Not Alone ~ *Brochure*
Headache: What Can Be Done About Headache ~ *Booklet*
Headache: Why Does My Head Hurt? ~ *Booklet*
Headache: Journal of Head and Face Pain ~ *Journal*
Migraine: The Complete Guide ~ *Order Form*
"Relief from Migraine" Video ~ *Order Form*
AASH Membership ~ *Membership Application*
Headache: Rate Card No. 17 ~ *Flyer*
Migraine: The Complete Guide ~ *Book*
Headache ~ *Newsletter*
Headache. Yor are not alone ~ *Brochure*
Headache. Why does my head hurt? ~ *Booklet*
Headache. What can be done about headache? ~ *Booklet*
Headache ~ *Newsletter*

Concerned with the following diseases or disorders:
Headache, Cluster

1130 AMERICAN HYPERLEXIA ASSOCIATION (AHA)

479 Spring Road
Elmhurst, IL 60126 630-415-2212
Fax: 630-530-5909
E-mail: info@hyperlexia.org
http://www.hyperlexia.org

The American Hyperlexia Association (AHA) is a voluntary not-for-profit organization dedicated to advancing the education and general welfare of children with Hyperlexia; promoting the social policy issues and conditions that further the full growth and potential of affected children; assisting families in accessing appropriate services; and promoting and supporting research related to Hyperlexia. Hyperlexia is a condition characterized by difficulty in understanding verbal language, inappropriate interaction with people, and a precocious ability to read words or a fascination with letters or numbers. Established in 1990, the American Hyperlexia Association is comprised of parents and relatives of children with Hyperlexia, speech and language professionals, education professionals, and other concerned individuals. The common goal is to identify Hyperlexia, promote and facilitate effective teaching techniques, and educate the public concerning Hyperlexia. The American Hyperlexia Association also provides a networking program for parents and professionals and offers a variety of educational materials including information mailings, a quarterly newsletter, announcements of AHA-sponsored events, a membership directory, a catalog for the Center for Speech and Language Disorders, fact sheets, and brochures.

President: Patti Tebbe
Year Established: 1990
Organization Members: 800

Publishes the following materials:
Center for Speech and Language Disorders Catalogue ~ *Catalogue*
Hyperlexia ~ *Brochure*
What is Hyperlexia? ~ *Report*
The Syndrome of Hyperlexia: Remediation Techniques ~ *Report*
Hyperlexia - He Reads too Soon ~ *Article*
Center for Speech and Language Disorders - Who We Are ~ *Brochure*
AHA! ~ *Newsletter*
American Hyperlexia Association ~ *Letter*

1131 AMERICAN JUVENILE ARTHRITIS ORGANIZATION (AJAO)

1330 West Peachtree Street
Atlanta, GA 30309 404-872-7100
Fax: 404-872-0457
E-mail: help@arthritis.org
http://www.arthritis.org

The American Juvenile Arthritis Organization (AJAO), a not-for-profit organization, is a Council of the Arthritis Foundation devoted to serving the needs of children, teens, and young adults with childhood rheumatic diseases and their families. These diseases include Juvenile Rheumatoid Arthritis, Lupus (Systemic Lupus Erythematosis), and Ankylosing Spondylitis. Juvenile Arthritis is medically different from the adult form of arthritis and may be far more severe in some cases. The American Juvenile Arthritis Organization was founded in 1981 to help serve the special needs of affected individuals and families, friends, and health care professionals. The Organization enables members to exchange ideas and support and serves as a clearinghouse of information for the public on topics from medications to educational rights to social services. It sponsors an annual conference; monitors and promotes legislation that benefits individuals with Juvenile Arthritis; provides appropriate referrals; and sponsors research concerning potential causes, improved treatments, preventive measures, and possible cures. The American Juvenile Arthritis Organization provides a variety of educational materials including a quarterly newsletter, pamphlets, fact sheets, self-help manuals, and a video lending library.

President: Linda Wilson (1994-Present)
Executive Director: Patricia Harrington
Year Established: 1981
Organization Members: 1,100

Publishes the following materials:
American Juvenile Arthritis Organization ~ *Factsheet*
AJAO Newsletter ~ *Newsletter*
The American Juvenile Arthritis Organization ~ *Factsheet*
Informacion la Artritis ~ *Brochure*
When Your Student Has Arthritis - A Guide for Teachers ~ *Brochure*
Remember the Arthritis Foundation in Your Will ~ *Brochure*
Arthritis Information - Pseudoxanthoma Elasticum ~ *Brochure*
Arthritis Information - Arthritis in Children ~ *Brochure*
Keys To Independence ~ *Resource Catalogue*

Concerned with the following diseases or disorders:
Ankylosing Spondylitis; Arthritis, Juvenile; Lupus

1132 AMERICAN LARYNGEAL PAPILLOMA FOUNDATION (ALPF)

P.O. Box 6108
Spring Hill, FL 34611-6108 352-686-8583
Fax: 352-686-8583
http://www.alpf.org

The American Laryngeal Papilloma Foundation is a national nonprofit voluntary health organization that was formed to promote the health and welfare of people with Laryngeal Papillomatosis and to create public awareness of the disease. Laryngeal Papilloma is a rare viral disease characterized by multiple benign growths (papillomas) in the middle and lower respiratory tract. Established in 1991, the American Laryngeal Papilloma Foundation seeks to provide funding to organizations that are engaged in medical research into the prevention and cure of Laryngeal Papillomatosis and to assist affected individuals with financial aid, TDD equipment, moral support, and counseling. Educational materials include brochures and newsletters. For patients only, there is a toll-free number in New Jersey at (800) 649-4841 (access code 17). Again, please note that this number is for affected individuals and families only.

President: William Lazar
Executive Director: Gregory Nelson Delgado
Organization Language: Spanish.
Year Established: 1991
Organization Chapters: 4
Organization Members: 70

Publishes the following materials:
National Newsletter ~ *Newsletter*
Mission Statement ~ *Mission Statement*
Please Help Them Breathe!!! ~ *Brochure*

Concerned with the following diseases or disorders:
Recurrent Respiratory Papillomatosis

1133 AMERICAN LEPROSY MISSIONS

1 ALM Way
Greenville, SC 29601 864-271-7040
800-537-7679
Fax: 864-271-7062
E-mail: amlep@leprosy.org
http://www.leprosy.org

Established in 1906, the American Leprosy Missions is a not-for-profit service organization devoted to the care of people with Leprosy and to the eventual cure of this disorder. Leprosy, also known as Hansen's Disease, is a progressive, chronic infectious disease caused by the bacteria, Mycobacterium leprae. The disorder affects nerves outside the central nervous system (peripheral nerves), particularly in the facial area and the limbs. In severe cases, loss of sensation, disfigurement, and/or blindness may occur. The Missions, a fund-raising organization, helps people with Leprosy through programs of "partner projects" in about 30 countries. The project dispenses multi-drug therapies to cure Leprosy; engages in rehabilitation; and offers vocational and other support programs. In addition, the organization mails monthly appeals and newsletters to its donors; provides educational materials to train health care workers; and manages subscriptions for the "International Journal of Leprosy." In addition, the Missions trains health care workers, surgeons, and paramedics on the appropriate treatment of affected individuals.

President: Christopher J. Doyle
Year Established: 1906

Concerned with the following diseases or disorders:
Leprosy

1134 AMERICAN LYME DISEASE FOUNDATION, INC. (ALDF)

Mill Pond Offices
293 Route 100
Somers, NY 10589 914-277-6970
800-876-5963
Fax: 914-277-6974
E-mail: alds@computer.net
http://www.w2.com/docs2/d5/lyme.html

The American Lyme Disease Foundation, Inc. (ALDF) is a nonprofit organization that is dedicated to advancing treatment, research, prevention, and public awareness of Lyme disease and other tickborne illnesses. Lyme disease is an infectious tick-transmitted disorder characterized by an early skin lesion and, subsequently, a growing red area on the skin (i.e., "bull's eye" rash). In some cases, later symptoms may include joint, neurological, and/or heart problems. Established in 1990, the Foundation's work focuses on four major field, basic, laboratory, and clinical research, and public and professional education. ALDF publishes a biannual newsletter and several brochures including "A Homeowner's Guide to the Ecology and Environmental Management of Lyme Disease," "A Quick Guide to Lyme Disease," and "Lyme Disease: Clinical Updates for Physicians." Other educational materials include reports, videos, a journal, and a selection of audiovisual aids. The Foundation also provides a toll-free informational number, a national physician referral system, and numerous support groups for affected individuals and their families.

Executive Director: David L. Weld (1991 to Present)
Year Established: 1990

Publishes the following materials:
A Homeowner's Guide to Ecology and Environmental Mnagement oif Lyme Disease ~ *Brochure*
A Quick Guide to Lyme Disease ~ *Brochure*
American Lyme Disese Foundation, Inc. Newsletter ~ *Newsletter*
Lyme Disease ~ *Reprint*
Lyme Disease: Clinical Update for Physicians ~ *Pamphlet*
National Clinical Conference on Lyme Disease ~ *Journal*
Lyme Disease: The Case of the Great Imitator ~ *Video Tape (no longer availab*
Tick Talk ~ *Video Tape (no longer availab*
The American Journal of Medicine ~ *Reprinted Journal*
A Quick Guide to Lyme disease ~ *Brochure*
American Lyme Disease Foundation, Inc. Quick Facts ~ *Fact Sheet*
Facts On Lyme Disease ~ *Fact Sheet*
ALDF's Highlights of 1996 and a Look Forward ~ *Fact Sheet*
Tick, Tick, Tick...It's Time to Pay Attention to the Dangers of Lyme Disease ~ *Reprint*
Lyme Disease: Clinical Update For Physicians ~ *Pamphlet*

Concerned with the following diseases or disorders:
Human Granulocytic Ehrlichiosis (HGE); Lyme Disease

1135 AMERICAN SLEEP APNEA ASSOCIATION (ASAA)

2025 Pennsylvania Avenue NW
Suite 905
Washington, DC 20006 202-293-3650
Fax: 202-293-3656
E-mail: assa@nicom.com
http://asaa.nicom.com

The American Sleep Apnea Association (ASAA) is a not-for-profit, health service organization dedicated to reducing injuries, disabilities, and potentially life-threatening complications that may be caused by sleep apnea, a condition characterized by breathing difficulties while sleeping. Sleep apnea may occur during childhood and/or adulthood, may be genetic, and/or may occur due to or in association with a number of different underlying disorders. Established in 1990, the Association works to improve the well-being of affected individuals and family members; promotes early diagnosis and appropriate treatment of sleep apnea through innovative efforts to educate the general public and health care professionals; and supports basic research into the causes and treatments of the disorder. The Association also fosters the nationwide ASAA A.W.A.K.E. Network, a network of self-help groups that provide additional information and support to individuals affected by sleep apnea. The American Sleep Apnea Association provides educational materials including a videotape, brochures, a regular newsletter, and guidelines to help individuals start local support groups.

President: Richard Waldhorn, M.D.
Executive Director: Christin L. Engelhardt
Year Established: 1990
Organization Members: 2,962

Concerned with the following diseases or disorders:
Apnea, Infantile; Apnea, Sleep

1136 AMERICAN SOCIETY OF ADULTS WITH PSEUDO-OBSTRUCTION, INC. (ASAP)

19 Carroll Road
Woburn, MA 01801-6161 781-935-9776
Fax: 781-933-4151
E-mail: asapgi@sprynet.com

The American Society of Adults with Pseudo-obstruction (ASAP) is an international not-for-profit organization that functions as an information resource center for people affected by Chronic Intestinal Pseudo-obstruction (CIP) and other digestive and motility disorders, their families, and physicians. Intestinal Pseudo-obstruction is a digestive disorder characterized by vomiting, constipation, and pain without evidence of obstruction. Established in 1991, the organization also provides information on other digestive motility disorders and conditions common to people with CIP. In addition, the Society offers networking services such as a young adult networking line for affected individuals from 12 to 25 years of age and distributes a list of physicians who have experience with the diagnosis and treatment of Intestinal Pseudo-obstruction. The organization also periodically distributes questionnaires to members for the purpose of collecting information. This information is then compiled and later published. The organization also offers additional educational materials including booklets, pamphlets, videos, and the "ASAP Digest," a bulletin that updates members about society activities or new medical developments in the field of motility disorders.

President: Mary-Angela De Grazia-DiTucci
Executive Director: Mary-Angela De Grazia-DiTucci
Year Established: 1991
Organization Members: 500

Publishes the following materials:
American Society of Adults with Pseudo-Obstruction, Inc. ~ *Brochure*
The ASAP Forum ~ *Newsletter*
ASAP Digest ~ *Newsletter Update*
Pain Management and Chronic Intestinal Pseudo-Obstruction ~ *Fact Sheet*
What is Chronic Intestinal Pseudo-Obstruction ~ *Fact Sheet*
Chronic Intestinal Pseudo-Obstruction ~ *Fact Sheet*
ASAP, Inc. Publication List ~ *Publication List*

Concerned with the following diseases or disorders:
Muscular Dystrophy, Oculo-Gastrointestinal

1137 AMERICAN SUDDEN INFANT DEATH SYNDROME INSTITUTE (AMERICAN SIDS INSTITUTE)

6065 Roswell Road
Suite 876
Atlanta, GA 30328 404-843-1030
800-232-7437
Fax: 404-843-0577
E-mail: prevent@sids.org
http://www.sids.org

The American Sudden Infant Death Syndrome Institute is a not-for-profit organization dedicated to preventing Sudden Infant Death Syndrome (SIDS) and to ensuring that the medical and corporate communities, government agencies, and general public share the sense of urgency in preventing SIDS. Sudden Infant Death Syndrome is characterized by the sudden death of any infant or young child that is unexpected by history and for which no adequate cause of death can be found. The Institution was founded to develop a comprehensive national program of research, clinical care, and education and to focus national attention and resources on the problem of SIDS. Most importantly, the Institute searches aggressively and with a strong sense of urgency for the means to eliminate this disorder. Established in 1983, the organization provides support groups, promotes research, engages in patient and professional education, and offers clinical services. Educational materials include a newsletter entitled "The Promise," brochures, and pamphlets.

President: Alfred Steinschneider, M.D.
Organization Language: Spanish (written/spoken).
Year Established: 1983

Publishes the following materials:
SIDS: Toward An Understanding ~ *Leaflet*
American Sudden Infant Death Syndrome Institute ~ *Brochure*
Raising Funds to Fight Sudden Infant Death Syndrome ~ *Mission Statement*
SIDS: Toward Prevention And Improved Infant Health ~ *Brochure*

Concerned with the following diseases or disorders:
Sudden Infant Death Syndrome

1138 AMERICAN SYRINGOMYELIA ALLIANCE PROJECT, INC. (ASAP)

P.O. Box 1586
300 Green Street, Suite 206
Longview, TX 75606-1586 903-236-7079
800-272-7282
Fax: 903-757-7456
E-mail: 102563.3507@compuserve.com
http://www.dataprompt.com/syringo/

The American Syringomyelia Alliance Project (ASAP), which was established in 1988, is a national nonprofit organization that functions as a clearinghouse for information on syringomyelia, a rare progressive condition characterized by the presence of abnormal, fluid-filled cavities within the spinal cord. The organization provides information to people with syringomyelia and seeks to increase public awareness of the disorder. The Project also encourages medical research and seeks to raise funds for the investigation into the possible causes of and the development of new treatments for the disorder. The American Syringomyelia Alliance Project publishes a newsletter and produces informational materials and videotapes of lectures on syringomyelia by prominent neurosurgeons. The Project also holds an annual conference to bring people with syringomyelia together and has a self-help network project.

President: H.D. White (1990-Present)
Executive Director: Patricia Williams
Year Established: 1988
Organization Members: 1,700

Publishes the following materials:
Syringomyelia - What is it? How Can You Help? ~ *Brochure*
Syringomyelia ~ *Factsheet*

Concerned with the following diseases or disorders:
Syringobulbia; Syringomyelia

1139 **AMERICAN TINNITUS ASSOCIATION (ATA)**

P.O. Box 5
Portland, OR 97207 503-248-9985
800-634-8978
Fax: 503-248-0024
E-mail: tinnitus@ata.org
http://www.ata.org

The American Tinnitus Association is a national not-for-profit self-help organization dedicated to helping people with tinnitus and their physicians. Tinnitus is a condition characterized by sensation of sound for which there is no external source. Such perceived sounds are often described as a buzzing, ringing, whistling, or clicking sensation. The Association's activities include production and distribution of public awareness materials; educational programs for the professional and lay communities; establishment of and guidance for self-help groups and their leaders; and promotion of community hearing protection programs. Founded in 1979, the organization maintains a bibliographic service and publishes a variety of informational brochures and a quarterly journal entitled "Tinnitus Today."

President: Philip O. Morton (1992-Present)
Executive Director: Gloria E. Reich, Ph.D.
Year Established: 1979
Organization Members: 16,000

Publishes the following materials:
Noise its Effects on Hearing & Tinnitus ~ *Pamphlet*
Tinnitus Family Information ~ *Brochure*
Coping with the Stress of Tinnitus ~ *Brochure*
The American Tinnitus Association ~ *Brochure*
Information About Tinnitus ~ *Brochure*
Tinnitus Today ~ *Newsletter*

Concerned with the following diseases or disorders:
Acoustic Neuroma; Meniere Disease; Tinnitus

1140 **AMYOTROPHIC LATERAL SCLEROSIS ASSOCIATION (ALSA)**

21021 Ventura Boulevard
#321
Woodland Hills, CA 91364-2206 818-340-7500
800-782-4747
Fax: 818-340-2060
TDD: 818-593-3540
E-mail: eajc27b@prodigy.com
http://www.alsa.org

The Amyotrophic Lateral Sclerosis Association (ALSA) is a national not-for-profit voluntary health organization dedicated to the fight against Amyotrophic Lateral Sclerosis (ALS). Amyotrophic Lateral Sclerosis, also known as "Lou Gehrig's Disease," is a rapidly progressive neuromuscular disease characterized by degeneration of the motor neurons responsible for transmitting electrical impulses from the brain to the voluntary muscles throughout the body. ALSA consists of a growing network of over 135 local volunteer chapters and support groups across the United States. The Association seeks to encourage, identify, fund, and monitor cutting-edge research into the cause, prevention, and possible cure of ALS. The organization also offers support on how to cope with the disease, provides referrals, and serves as the national information resource on ALS for medical professionals, affected individuals, and family members. The Information Center provides basic information about ALS and answers specific questions about the disease. ALSA also makes referrals to physicians, clinics, extended care facilities, home health agencies, visiting nurse agencies, transportation assistance, and medical equipment supplies. In addition, ALSA has a patient registry of individuals with the disease and distributes information on the latest research and clinical trials regarding ALS.

President: Steve Ross (Chairman)
Executive Director: Michael Havlicek (President & CEO)
Year Established: 1985
Organization Chapters: 135

Publishes the following materials:
Facts about ALS and The ALS Association ~ *Brochure*
ALS and The ALS Association ~ *Brochure*
Basic Home Care for ALS Patients ~ *Booklet*
Maintaining good nutrition with ALS ~ *Booklet*
ALSA Scientific Briefing ~ *Newsletter*
Caring for the Caregiver ~ *Video Order Form*
Video on Ventilator Decision ~ *Video Order Form*
LINK ~ *Newsletter*
Publications Order Form ~ *Order Form*
Certified ALS Centers ~ *Facility List*
What Is ALS ~ *Video Tape*
Managing ALS Manuals ~ *Resource List*

Concerned with the following diseases or disorders:
Amyotrophic Lateral Sclerosis; Brown Sequard Syndrome; Motor Neuron Disease; Polyglucosan Body Disease, Adult; Primary Lateral Sclerosis

1141 AMYOTROPHIC LATERAL SCLEROSIS SOCIETY OF CANADA (ALS SOCIETY OF CANADA)

6 Adelaide Street East
Suite 220
Toronto
Ontario, M5C 1H6
Canada 416-362-0269
800-267-4257
Fax: 416-362-0414
E-mail: alssoc@inforamp.net
http://www.als.ca

The Amyotrophic Lateral Sclerosis (ALS) Society of Canada is a national not-for-profit organization dedicated to providing information and support to individuals and family members affected by ALS and to promoting research to find a cure for the disorder. Amyotrophic Lateral Sclerosis (ALS), also known as "Lou Gehrig's Disease," is a rapidly progressive neuromuscular disease characterized by degeneration of the motor neurons responsible for transmitting electrical impulses from the brain to the voluntary muscles throughout the body. Established in 1977, the ALS Society, which operates in many locations across Canada, provides support and counseling for people with ALS, their families, and caregivers; raises funds to support research into the cause of and a potential cure for ALS; engages in patient advocacy; offers networking services; and provides equipment such as wheelchairs. The Society's educational materials include pamphlets, brochures, and a regular newsletter. The ALS Society of Canada also has a web site on the Internet at [http://www.als.ca].

President: Jonathan Harris (1996 to Present)
Executive Director: Suzanne Lawson
Organization Language: French (written). Spanish (written/spoken). Greek (written/spoken).
Year Established: 1977
Organization Members: Non-Membership

Publishes the following materials:
Amykotrophic Lateral Sclerosis Society of Canada "To provide care and find a cure for ALS" ~ *Brochure*

Concerned with the following diseases or disorders:
Amyotrophic Lateral Sclerosis

1142 ANENCEPHALY SUPPORT FOUNDATION (ASF)

30827 Sifton
Spring, TX 77386 281-364-9222
888-206-7526
E-mail: asf@asfhelp.com
http://www.asfhelp.com

The Anencephaly Support Foundation is a national not-for-profit organization dedicated to providing support, information, and assistance to parents and professionals who are dealing with Anencephaly. The Foundation collects medical articles dealing with causation and prevention; provides phone and mail support; provides other necessary resources; offers lectures to the medical community about issues concerning Anencephaly; and is involved in ongoing legislation designed to initiate national birth defect monitoring. Established in 1992, the Foundation provides additional education materials including support group information and personal testimonies.

President: David Andis (1992 to Present)
Executive Director: Anne Andis
Year Established: 1992
Organization Chapters: 4
Organization Members: 400

Concerned with the following diseases or disorders:
Anencephaly

1143 ANGELMAN SYNDROME FOUNDATION, INC. (ASF)

P.O. Box 12437
Gainesville, FL 32604 904-332-3303
800-432-6435
E-mail: rjbatman@aol.com

The Angelman Syndrome Foundation, Inc. (ASF) is a not-for-profit organization dedicated to educating concerned families, the medical and educational communities, interested organizations, and the general public on the diagnosis, treatment, management, and prevention of Angelman Syndrome. Angelman Syndrome is a rare genetic disorder characterized by mental and motor retardation, absence of speech, muscular abnormalities, unprovoked laughter, and characteristic facial abnormalities. Established in 1992, the Angelman Syndrome Foundation promotes patient advocacy; offers national, regional, and local support systems for affected individuals and their families; and gathers and disseminates information on genetic counseling, medical management, family counseling, behavioral management, coping methods, and educational and communication programs. The Foundation also promotes and supports research on the diagnosis, treatment, management, and prevention of Angelman Syndrome. The Angelman Syndrome Foundation offers a variety of educational and support materials through its database, regular newsletter, article reprints, brochures, pamphlets, and audiovisual materials.

President: Robert A. McCormick (1993-Present)
Year Established: 1992
Organization Members: 1,000

Publishes the following materials:
By-Laws of Angelman Syndrome Foundation, Inc. ~ *By-Laws*
Angelman Syndrome ~ *Brochure*
Facts About Angelman Syndrome ~ *Reprint*

Concerned with the following diseases or disorders:
Angelman Syndrome

1144 ANGELMAN SYNDROME SUPPORT GROUP (ASSG)

15 Place Crescent
Waterlooville
Hampshire, PO7 5UR
United Kingdom 0170 526 4224
Fax: 0170 524 1977

The Angelman Syndrome Support Group (ASSG) is an international nonprofit organization dedicated to providing information and support to families and caregivers of individuals who have Angelman Syndrome. Angelman Syndrome is a rare genetic disorder characterized by congenital mental retardation, the absence of speech, unprovoked laughter, unusual facial features, and muscular abnormalities. Established in 1986 and consisting of 450 members, ASSG maintains a patient registry and raises funds for education of affected individuals and for ongoing research into the causes, treatment, and prevention of this disorder. ASSG also offers a variety of educational materials including brochures and a regional newsletter.

President: Sheila Woolven (1986 to Present)
Organization Language: Italian (written/spoken). French (written). Spanish (written).
Year Established: 1986
Organization Members: 450

Publishes the following materials:
Facts About Angelman Syndrome ~ *Pamphlet*
What is Angelman Syndrome? ~ *Booklet*

Concerned with the following diseases or disorders:
Angelman Syndrome

1145 ANORCHIDISM SUPPORT GROUP (ASG)

P.O. Box 3025
Romford, RM3 8GX
England 01708 372597
Fax: 01708 372597

The Anorchidism Support Group (ASG) is a voluntary organization that promotes research and provides educational materials and support to individuals who are affected by Anorchia, a condition characterized by absence of one or both testes at birth. Established in 1995, ASG provides support groups for affected individuals and their families, patient networking, and educational materials including brochures and regular newsletters. The organization also provides updates concerning research into this condition.

President: Lorraine Bookless (1995 to Present)
Executive Director: David Bookless
Year Established: 1995
Organization Members: 10

Publishes the following materials:
Who Are We? And What Is Anorchidism? ~ *Brochure*
Anorchidism Support Group (April 1997) ~ *Newsletter*

1146 ANTIEPILEPTIC DRUG PREGNANCY REGISTRY (AED PREGNANCY REGISTRY)

149 CNY-MGH East
Room 5022A
Charlestown, MA 02129-2000 617-726-7739
888-233-2334
Fax: 617-724-8307
E-mail: aedregistry@helix.mgh.harvard.edu
neuro-www2.mgh.harvard.edu/aed/registry.nc
i

The Antiepileptic Drug Pregnancy Registry is a national not-for-profit research organization that was established to study the safety of antiepileptic drugs (AEDs) during pregnancy. This organization was established at the Massachusetts General Hospital with funds provided by six manufacturers of antiepileptic drugs. The Registry seeks to determine whether the frequency of birth defects is increased among infants exposed to any AEDs during pregnancy. The Registry works toward this goal through collecting and analyzing data from women in the United States and Canada during pregnancy and post delivery. The Registry hopes to enroll women during pregnancy and before any prenatal testing in order to avoid any selection bias. The Antiepileptic Drug Pregnancy Registry supplies fact sheets, flyers, general information about the potential affects of antiepileptic drugs, and slides for presentations. In addition, the Registry is working to provide assistance to Spanish speaking individuals. Pregnant women with epilepsy and their health care providers may call a toll-free number (888)

233-2334 for enrollment information. The Registry also maintains a web site.

President: Lewis B. Holmes, M.D. (Director)
Executive Director: Triptaa Surve, M.P.H. (Coordinator)
Organization Language: Spanish (spoken).
Year Established: 1996

Publishes the following materials:
AED (Antiepileptic Drug) Pregnancy Registry ~ *Mission Statement*
Massachusetts General Hospital Midical Research Consent Form ~ *Pamphlet*
AED Pregnancy Registry: Baseline Interview ~ *Pamphlet*
AED Pregnancy Registry: Patient Seventh Month Interview ~ *Pamphlet*
AED Pregnancy Registry: Postpartum Interview ~ *Pamphlet*

Concerned with the following diseases or disorders:
Epilepsy

1147 APERT SUPPORT AND INFORMATION NETWORK

P.O. Box 1184
Fair Oaks, CA 95628 916-961-1092
Fax: 916-961-1092
E-mail: apertnet@ix.netcom.com
http://www.apert.org

The Apert Support and Information Network is a voluntary not-for-profit organization dedicated to providing information, assistance, and support to parents of children with Apert Syndrome. Also known as Acrocephalosyndactyly Type 1, Apert Syndrome is a rare genetic disorder characterized by premature closure of the fibrous joints between certain bones of the skull (craniosynostosis), causing the head to appear abnormally long and narrow (acrocephaly). Additional abnormalities may typically include a prominent forehead; protruding, widely spaced eyes; and/or webbing or fusion of the fingers and/or toes (syndactyly). Established in 1995 and consisting of approximately 180 members, the Apert Support and Information Network provides networking services for affected families; engages in patient and professional education; and offers a variety of materials including a regular newsletter entitled "APERT NEWS."

President: Christine Clark (Director)
Year Established: 1995
Organization Members: 180

Publishes the following materials:
Apert Support and Information Network ~ *Mission Statement*

Concerned with the following diseases or disorders:
Apert Syndrome

1148 APERT SYNDROME PEN PALS

P.O. Box 115
Providence, RI 02901 401-421-9076

Apert Syndrome Pen Pals is a national voluntary support group dedicated to networking individuals and families who are affected by Apert Syndrome. Apert Syndrome is a rare genetic disorder characterized by premature closure of the fibrous joints between certain bones of the skull (craniosynostosis), causing the head to appear abnormally long and thin (acrocephaly). Other features include fusion or webbing (syndactyly) of the fingers and/or toes and unusual facial features. The organization enables individuals affected by Apert Syndrome and their family members to communicate with other affected families by letter.

Year Established: N/A

Concerned with the following diseases or disorders:
Apert Syndrome

1149 APERT SYNDROME SUPPORT GROUP

8708 Kathy
St. Louis, MO 63126 314-965-3356

The Apert Syndrome Support Group is a voluntary not-for-profit self-help organization dedicated to providing information and support to families of children with Apert Syndrome. Apert Syndrome is a rare genetic disorder characterized by premature closure of the fibrous joints between certain bones of the skull, fusion or webbing of the fingers and/or toes, and unusual facial features. Established in 1983, the Apert Syndrome Support Group enables affected families to exchange information, support, and resources through its networking program.

President: Beth Burns, Co-Chair, (1983-Present)
Executive Director: Daniel Burns (Co-Chair)
Year Established: 1983
Organization Members: 20

Concerned with the following diseases or disorders:
Apert Syndrome

1150 **APLASTIC ANEMIA ASSOCIATION OF CANADA**

22 Aikenhead Road
Etobicoke
Ontario, M9R 2Z3
Canada 416-235-0468
888-840-0039
Fax: 416-235-1756
E-mail: aplastic@enterprise.ca

The Aplastic Anemia Association of Canada is a voluntary, not-for-profit organization founded in 1987 that is dedicated to the support of individuals with aplastic anemia or myelodysplasia and their family members. Aplastic anemia is a rare form of anemia in which there are abnormally low levels of red blood cells, white blood cells, and platelets in the blood. Myelodysplastic syndromes are a group of related bone marrow disorders. The Association disseminates information in understandable lay terminology and has a network of volunteers with personal experience with these conditions who are able to give guidance and support during times of need. In addition, the Association informs the public about aplastic anemia and myelodysplasia, supports the Canadian Red Cross blood programs and the Unrelated Bone Marrow Registry, and raises funds for medical research.

President: Caroline Laughlin (Chairperson) (1997 to 1999)
Year Established: 1987
Organization Chapters: 4
Organization Members: 450

Publishes the following materials:
Understanding Aplastic Anemia and Myelodysplasia ~ *Brochure*

Concerned with the following diseases or disorders:
Anemia, Aplastic

1151 **APLASTIC ANEMIA FOUNDATION OF AMERICA, INC. (AAFA)**

P.O. Box 613
Annapolis, MD 21404
800-747-2820
Fax: 410-867-0240
E-mail: aafacenter@aol.com
http://www.teleport.com/nonprofit/aafa

The Aplastic Anemia Foundation of America (AAFA) is a national voluntary health organization dedicated to serving as a resource for assistance and emotional support for people with aplastic anemia, their families, and health care professionals. Aplastic anemia is a rare form of anemia in which there are abnormally low levels of red blood cells, white blood cells, and platelets in the blood. Founded in 1983, the Foundation seeks to provide updated educational materials and medical information on aplastic anemia and to support funding for ongoing medical research into the prevention, treatment, and cure of the disease. The Foundation supports the Ivan Fisher Research Study, which is a comprehensive prospective of the epidemiology and therapy of aplastic anemia. AAFA also publishes a quarterly newsletter containing stories of how others are coping with this disease and information on new medical treatments. In addition, the Foundation offers several brochures including "Communicating Patient Needs to the Medical Care Team," "Aplastic Anemia Answer Book," and "Families Coping with Hospital Life." The Aplastic Anemia Foundation has chapters across the United States and serves Canada and locations worldwide.

President: Michael I. Greenberg, M.D.
Executive Director: Marilyn M. Baker
Organization Language: Spanish. Japanese.
Year Established: 1983
Organization Chapters: 30
Organization Members: 6,000

Publishes the following materials:
ABOUT THE APLASTIC ANEMIA FOUNDATION OF AMERICA ~ *Factsheet*
APLASTIC ANEMIA ANSWER BOOK ~ *Brochure*
COMMUNICATING PATIENT AND FAMILY NEEDS TO THE MEDICAL TEAM ~ *Brochure*
Aplastic Anemia and Other Blood Disorders. Families Coping with Hospital Life. ~ *Brochure*
Aplastic Anemia Foundation of America, Inc. Newsletter ~ *Newsletter*
A BOOK FOR YOU ~ *Brochure*

Concerned with the following diseases or disorders:
Anemia, Aplastic; Anemia, Blackfan Diamond; Anemia, Fanconi's; Pure Red Cell Aplasia, Acquired

1152 **ARACHNOIDITIS INFORMATION AND SUPPORT NETWORK**

P.O. Box 1166
Ballwin, MO 63021
Fax: 314-394-5741

The Arachnoiditis Information and Support Network is a self-help organization formed in 1991. The purposes of the organization are to provide information, support, and outreach services to people affected by Arachnoiditis and to encourage research into the development of effective treatment for this disorder. Arachnoiditis is a rare disorder characterized by chronic inflammation of one of the membranes (arachnoid) that surrounds the brain and spinal cord. Symptoms may include a burning pain in the back; urinary frequency; spasms of the bladder, bowel, and/or legs; and/or unexplained skin rashes. The Network publishes a triennial newsletter, "Arachnoiditis Information and Support Network News"; provides assistance to people who wish to form local support groups; and coordinates the identification of physicians who are familiar with the treatment of this disease.

Concerned with the following diseases or disorders:
Arachnoiditis

1153 ARRHYTHMOGENIC RIGHT VENTRICULAR DYSPLASIA REGISTRY OF THE UNITED STATES (ARVD REGISTRY)

Box 245037
Tucson, AZ 85724-5037 520-626-6262
800-483-2662
Fax: 520-626-4333
E-mail: kgear@ccit.arizona.edu
http://www2.huskynet.com/ccg/rvd.html

The Arrhythmogenic Right Ventricular Dysplasia (ARVD) Registry is a not-for-profit registry that was established to identify cases of ARVD. Through long-term follow-up of enrolled patients, the Registry hopes to prevent cardiac arrest in this group of affected individuals and their families; to assess individualized therapies to prevent recurrence of irregular heart rhythms (arrythmias); to determine how initial findings predict long-term prognosis; and to evaluate the criteria for diagnosis of ARVD. The standardized diagnostic criteria for ARVD are based on the presence of major and minor criteria including structural, histological, electrocardiographic, arrhythmic, and genetic factors. The Registry provides brochures and reprints of pertinent peer-reviewed medical articles.

President: Frank I. Marcus, M.D. (Co-Director) (1996 to Present).
Executive Director: Kathleen Gear, R.N. (Registry Coordinator)
Year Established: 1996

Publishes the following materials:
ARVD Arrhythmogenic Right Ventricular Dysplasia Registry of the United States ~ *Brochure*
Arrhythmogenic Right Ventricular Dysplasia/Cardiomyopathy: A Review ~ *Reprint*
ARVD Chat (June 1997) ~ *Request Form*

1154 ARTHRITIS SOCIETY

393 University Avenue
Suite 1700
Toronto
Ontario, M4G IE6
Canada 416-967-1414
Fax: 416-967-7171
E-mail: jkonecny@arthritis.ca
http://www.arthritis.ca

The Arthritis Society is a not-for-profit organization in Canada dedicated to funding and promoting arthritis research, patient care, and public education. Arthritis, an inflammatory condition of the joints that may result in swelling and pain, is a joint disease that may be due to a number of different underlying causes. Established in 1948, the Arthritis Society, which serves 10 provincial divisions of Canada, also engages in patient advocacy; promotes patient and professional education; provides networking services for affected individuals and family members; and offers appropriate referrals. The Society also provides a variety of educational materials including a regular newsletter, brochures, and pamphlets. A toll-free number (800-321-1433) is maintained by the organization for use in Canada only.

President: Denis Morrice (Chairperson).
Executive Director: Bill Woloshyn
Organization Language: French (written).
Year Established: 1948
Organization Chapters: 10
Organization Members: Non-Membership

Publishes the following materials:
Public Education ~ *Publishers List*
Professional Information ~ *Publishers List*

Concerned with the following diseases or disorders:
Arthritis, Infectious; Arthritis, Juvenile; Arthritis, Psoriatic

1155 ARTHROGRYPOSIS GROUP (TAG)

1 The Oaks
Gillingham
Dorset, SP8 4SW
United Kingdom 01747822655
Fax: 01747822655

The Arthrogryposis Group is a not-for-profit voluntary health organization dedicated to offering contact, information, and support to people with Arthrogryposis and their families. Arthrogryposis is a non-progressive condition that limits range of movement in the joints and is accompanied by muscle weakness. Established in 1984, the organization provides information to professionals and other interested parties, encourages public awareness, and furthers research in the field. In addition, the organization sponsors regional events, activity camps, and annual conferences for all families, Group members, and other interested individuals. Educational materials produced and distributed by the organization include a quarterly newsletter, a documentary video, brochures, and an authoritative booklet.

President: Micky Macartney (1996-Present).
Executive Director: Diana Piercy
Year Established: 1984
Organization Members: 400

Concerned with the following diseases or disorders:
Arthrogryposis Multiplex Congenita

1156 ASSOCIATION STRUMPELL-LORRAIN (ASL)

9 bis rue Fabre
Besancon, F-25000
France 110381502391
Fax: 110381502391
www.infobiogen.fr/agora/associations/ASL/AS

Located in France, the Association Strumpell-Lorrain is an international voluntary organization dedicated to identifying individuals affected by familial spastic paraplegia, hereditary spasmodic paraparesis, spinocerebellar ataxia, and/or Maladie de Strumpell-Lorrain. Spastic paraplegia, a rare inherited condition, was first described by Strumpell in 1880 and is characterized by degeneration of certain parts of the brain and spinal cord (e.g., corticospinal tracts, columns of Golgi, etc.). Symptoms may include impaired ability to coordinate voluntary movements (ataxia) and uncontrolled jerky muscle movements. The Association Strumpell-Lorrain offers support and information to individuals affected by these neurological disorders. In addition, the Association publishes a regular newsletter (in French) and produces educational materials such as a brochure on familial spastic paraplegia. Reprints of medical articles are also distributed by the Association.

President: Philippe Grammont (1992 to Present)
Executive Director: Catherine Barrazza
Organization Language: French (written/spoken). Spanish (spoken). German (spoken).
Year Established: 1992
Organization Chapters: 10
Organization Members: 350

Publishes the following materials:
Vaincre Les Paraplegies Spastiques Familiales De Strumpell-Lorrain ~ *Brochure*
Fiche Technique De L'Association ~ *Mission Statement*
Compte-Rendus ~ *Summary*
ASL-Ete 95 ~ *Newsletter*
ASL (French) ~ *Brochure*
Phenotype of autosomal dominant spastic paraplegia linked to chromosome 2 ~ *Pamphlet*

Concerned with the following diseases or disorders:
Paraplegia, Hereditary Spastic

1157 ASSOCIATION FOR CHILDREN WITH DOWN SYNDROME, INC. (ACDS)

2616 Martin Avenue
Bellmore, NY 11710 516-221-4700
Fax: 516-221-5867

The Association for Children with Down Syndrome, Inc. (ACDS) is an international not-for-profit voluntary organization dedicated to providing information and support to individuals affected by Down Syndrome, their families, and health care professionals. Down Syndrome is a congenital disorder resulting from abnormalities affecting chromosome 21. In most individuals with the disorder, portions of chromosome 21 appear three times (trisomy) rather than twice in all or some (mosaicism) of the cells of the body (Trisomy 21); however, in rare cases, the disorder may result from translocations involving chromosome 21 and another chromosome. Individuals with Down Syndrome may have a variety of symptoms and physical abnormalities including characteristic malformations of the head and facial area; a short neck; malformations of the fingers, hands, and toes; short stature; congenital heart defects in some cases; and/or mental retardation. Established in 1966, the Association for Children with Down Syndrome offers a wide variety of programs and services. Its "5 Plus Program" provides recreational and social services for individuals with Down Syndrome from five years of age through adulthood and their families. The 5 Plus Program also offers support groups for adolescents, adults, and parents; workshops; referral services; health-related services; and medical information workshops. In addition, the ACDS's association with the Child Development Center/Genetics Program at North Shore University Hospital-Cornell University Medical College helps make many essential services available to ACDS families, such as pediatric cardiology, psychology, and gastroenterology services. The ACDS also promotes research, sharing results through liaisons with hospitals and universities as well as at national and regional conferences; provides families with home and hospital visitations through its Family Services Department; and has a trained parent counselor to reach out to families of newborns with Down Syndrome. Additional programs and services include parent advocacy training and assistance; regular conferences and workshops for parents and professionals; and a special library that offers up-to-date toys, books, and videos. The Association also offers additional materials including brochures, articles, manuals, bibliographies of helpful resources on certain topics (e.g., regarding genetics, legal issues and advocacy, medical/health, mental health, recreation, employment, etc.), and a regular newsletter.

President: Stuart H. Schoenfeld (1996 to Present)
Executive Director: Sam Nussbaum, C.S.W.
Organization Language: Spanish (written).
Year Established: 1966
Organization Members: 120

Publishes the following materials:
The Association For Children With Down Syndrome, Inc. 5 Plus Program ~ *Brochure*
Association For Children With Down Syndrome, Inc. ~ *Brochure*
Accent on ACDS ~ *Newsletter February 1997*

Concerned with the following diseases or disorders:
Down Syndrome

1158 ATAXIA-TELANGIECTASIA CHILDREN'S PROJECT (A-TCP)

1 West Camino Real, Suite 212
Boca Raton, FL 33432-5966 561-395-2621
800-543-5728
Fax: 561-395-2640
E-mail: bradmargus@delphi.com
http://www.med.jhu.edu/ataxia/

The Ataxia-Telangiectasia (AT) Children's Project is a national not-for-profit organization that was established in 1993. Ataxia-Telangiectasia is a rare inherited progressive disorder characterized by an impaired ability to control voluntary movement (ataxia); rapid, involuntary eye movements (nystagmus); permanent dilation of certain small blood vessels, resulting in small red lesions on the skin and other areas (telangiectasia); and immune deficiency, causing an increased predisposition to certain bacterial infections and malignancies. The purpose of the Project is to raise funds to accelerate scientific research aimed at finding a cure or a therapy that would improve the lives of children affected by Ataxia-Telangiectasia. The specific goals of the Project include finding a cure or therapy for Ataxia-Telangiectasia; increasing awareness of the disorder to help accurately diagnose affected individuals; and encouraging and funding scientific research directed at specific treatments for AT. The Project's activities also include the establishment and maintenance of a cell-bank for unlimited access by research scientists. The Ataxia-Telangiectasia Children's Project has established a National AT Clinical Center at Johns Hopkins Hospital, Baltimore, MD. It is the first of its kind in the nation and offers expert comprehensive clinical care to all children with a diagnosis of Ataxia-Telangiectasia.

President: Brad A. Margus (1993-Present)
Executive Director: Rosa M. Fernandez
Organization Language: Spanish.
Year Established: 1993

Publishes the following materials:
AT Children's Project ~ *Booklet*

Concerned with the following diseases or disorders:
Ataxia Telangiectasia

1159 ATTIA RESEARCH TRUST INTO ALD (ART INTO ALD)

36 Baker Street
London, W1M 1DG
United Kingdom 01712247112
Fax: 01712240681

The Attia Research Trust Into ALD (ARD into ALD) is a not-for-profit organization dedicated to furthering medical research into Adrenoleukodystrophy (ALD); providing grants and allowances for the purposes of medical treatment and care of children with ALD; and educating the public about ALD. Adrenoleukodystrophy is a rare inherited metabolic disorder characterized by the loss of the protective fatty sheath around nerve fibers within the brain (cerebral demyelination) and progressive degeneration of the adrenal gland (adrenal atrophy), causing progressive mental deterioration, neuromuscular abnormalities, loss of the ability to speak, blindness, and life-threatening complications. Established in 1993 and consisting of approximately 30 members, the Trust also has a support group and provides networking opportunities to parents. Educational materials include pamphlets and a regular newsletter.

President: B. J. Attia (1994 to Present)
Organization Language: Arabic (written/spoken).
Year Established: 1993
Organization Members: 30

Publishes the following materials:
Attia Research Trust into ALD ~ *Brochure*

Concerned with the following diseases or disorders:
Adrenoleukodystrophy

1160 AUTISM NETWORK INTERNATIONAL (ANI)

P.O. Box 448
Syracuse, NY 13210-0448 315-476-2462
Fax: 315-425-1978
E-mail: jisincla@mailbox.syr.edu

The Autism Network International (ANI) is a self-help and advocacy organization dedicated to supporting individuals with autism and helping them to compensate, navigate, and function in the world. Autism is a non-progressive neurological disorder characterized by language and communication deficits, withdrawal from social contacts, and extreme reactions to changes in the immediate environment. Established in 1992 and consisting of approximately 340 members, ANI is an organization run by individuals with autism who believe that the best advocates for autistic people are autistic people themselves. The Network provides a forum for people with autism to share information, peer support, and tips for coping and problem solving. In addition to promoting self-advocacy for high-functioning autistic adults, ANI also works to improve the lives of people with autism who, whether because they are young or because they do not have adequate communication skills, are unable to advocate for themselves. The Autism Network International assists people with autism who are unable to participate directly by providing information and referrals to parents and teachers. ANI's educational materials include a regular newsletter entitled "Our Voice" as well as brochures and audiovisual aids.

Executive Director: Jim Sinclair
Year Established: 1992
Organization Members: 340

Publishes the following materials:
Autism Network International "Our Voice" ~ *Newsletter*
Don't Mourn For Us ~ *Reprint*

Concerned with the following diseases or disorders:
Autism

1161 AUTISM NETWORK FOR HEARING AND VISUALLY IMPAIRED PERSONS

7510 Ocean Front Avenue
Virginia Beach, VA 23451 757-428-9036
Fax: 757-428-0019

The Autism Network for Hearing and Visually Impaired Persons is a voluntary organization that was founded to serve the needs of people with Autism who also have a hearing or visual impairment. Established in 1992, the Network was adopted as a formal committee of the Autism Society of America. The goals of the organization include the creation and maintenance of a database of people with Autism combined with a sensory disability in order to establish a network for communication, education, research, and advocacy. The Network also seeks to develop centers to diagnose and evaluate individuals with these disorders. In addition, the organization works to educate physicians within the community and present educational sessions at the Autism Society of America National Annual Conference.

President: Dolores and Alan Bartel (Contact Persons)
Year Established: 1992
Organization Members: 750

Publishes the following materials:
Composition of the Autism & Sensory Network ~ *Letter*
Autism & Sensory Impairments Network ~ *Fact Sheet*

Concerned with the following diseases or disorders:
Autism

1162 AUTISM SOCIETY OF AMERICA (ASA)

7910 Woodmont Avenue
Suite 650
Bethesda, MD 20814-3015 301-657-0881
800-328-8476
Fax: 301-657-0869

The Autism Society of America, a national not-for-profit advocacy organization established in 1965, is dedicated to providing information, assistance, support, and advocacy services to individuals with autism and their families. Autism is a nonprogressive neurological disorder characterized by language and communication deficits, withdrawal from social contacts, and extreme reactions to changes in the immediate environment. The Society supports ongoing medical research into the causes, prevention, and treatment of autism; promotes public awareness; and provides information and advocacy services to help affected individuals become fully participating members of their communities. In addition, the Society makes referrals to appropriate sources of support and treatment. The Society's educational materials include newsletters, brochures, and Spanish language materials.

President: Jacquelyn Rosen (1993-Present)
Executive Director: Veronica Zyst
Organization Language: Spanish.
Year Established: 1965
Organization Chapters: 215
Organization Members: 17,000

Concerned with the following diseases or disorders:
Autism

1163 AWAKENINGS (PARKINSON'S DISEASE INFORMATION AND NEWS)

E-mail: editor@parkinsonsdisease.com
http://www.parkinsonsdisease.com

The Awakenings web site is an open forum on the Internet concerning Parkinson's Disease (PD). This web site aims to be a reliable, current, and comprehensive resource and dialogue forum for all associated with Parkinson's Disease (PD) including affected individuals, family members, primary care physicians, specialists, researchers, caregivers, and support groups. Parkinson's Disease is a progressive neurologic disorder characterized by muscle tremor, muscular stiffness or inflexibility (rigidity), slowness of movement, and difficulty performing voluntary movements due to degeneration of or damage to certain nerve cells of the brain. The Awakenings web site provides specific information on PD and a variety of services directed toward two major audiences: that is, patients/family members and primary care physicians/specialists. Information and services provided within the site include understandable information concerning all aspects of PD, its treatment, and living with the disorder; literature updates; a FAQ (frequently asked questions) area; information concerning Parkinson's Disease associations and support groups; a case histories area for physicians; therapy updates; national and international research funding opportunities for researchers; and a "group talk" area where research teams may share information and research updates. In addition, the site includes dynamic linkage to several additional sources of information on the Internet.

Year Established: 1997

Concerned with the following diseases or disorders:
Parkinson's Disease

1164 BATTEN DISEASE SUPPORT AND RESEARCH ASSOCIATION (BDSRA)

2600 Parsons Avenue
Columbus, OH 43207-2972 614-445-4161
800-448-4570
http://bdsra.org

The Batten Disease Support and Research Association (BDSRA) is a voluntary not-for-profit organization dedicated to promoting the civil and human rights of people with Batten Disease. Batten Disease, an extremely rare inherited disorder, is a progressive degenerative neurometabolic disease characterized by gradual intellectual deterioration, seizure episodes, progressive movement (motor) impairment, and progressive visual impairment. Symptoms begin to occur at approximately five to 13 years of age. The Association seeks to maximize the opportunities of affected individuals through medical, educational, vocational, rehabilitative, and financial means and to educate lay persons and professionals concerning the special needs of people with the disease. Established in 1987, the Batten Disease Support and Research Association provides referral services to help affected families secure benefits available by law and maintains a database of individuals with Batten Disease on state, national, and international levels. The Batten Disease Support and Research Association functions as a national registry for researchers throughout the world who are studying Batten Disease. The Association also has a parent and sibling communication network that provides technical assistance and emotional support to families of affected individuals; promotes ongoing medical research on Batten Disease and makes the research results available to members; and conducts an annual conference. The Association also offers a variety of educational and support materials including a quarterly newsletter called the "Iluminator," reprints of medical journal articles, fact sheets, brochures, pamphlets, and a lending library of books and videos.

President: Larry Killen
Executive Director: Lance W. Johnston
Year Established: 1987
Organization Chapters: 10
Organization Members: 750

Publishes the following materials:
A Light in a World of Darkness ~ *Brochure*
The Illuminator ~ *Newsletter*
Battens Disease Support and Research Association Library ~ *Library List*
Article II - Purpose ~ *Fact Sheet*

Concerned with the following diseases or disorders:
Batten Disease; Santavuori Disease

1165 BECKWITH WIEDEMANN SUPPORT NETWORK (BWSN)

3206 Braeburn Circle
Ann Arbor, MI 48108
313-973-0263
800-837-2976
Fax: 313-973-9721
E-mail: a800bwsn@aol.com

The Beckwith-Wiedemann Support Network (BWSN) is a voluntary not-for-profit organization dedicated to providing peer support and information to individuals and families affected by Beckwith-Wiedemann Syndrome (BWS). Beckwith-Wiedemann Syndrome (BWS), also known as Exomphalos-Macroglossia-Gigantism Syndrome, is a rare genetic disorder characterized by a wide range of growth abnormalities including an abnormally enlarged tongue (macroglossia); excessive size and height (gigantism); and/or protrusion of portions of the intestines through an abnormal opening in the abdominal wall where the umbilical cord joined the fetal abdomen (exomphalos or omphalocele). Additional features may include abnormal enlargement of abdominal organs (visceromegaly) such as the liver and spleen; enlargement of cells within the outer layer of the adrenal glands (adrenocortical cytomegaly); improper development of the innermost tissues within the kidneys (renal medullary dysplasia); advanced bone age; and/or an increased predisposition to certain childhood cancers. Established in 1990, the Network is committed to increasing public and professional awareness of Beckwith-Wiedemann Syndrome; facilitating the flow of information among affected families and health care professionals; and promoting and supporting research into the causes, early detection, and treatment of BWS. The Beckwith-Wiedemann Support Network shares information with other BWS groups around the world and maintains a listing of appropriate referrals. The Network also maintains a toll-free help line for parents and enables affected families to exchange information, assistance, and resources through its networking program. In addition, the Network provides educational and support materials through its database, family directory, article reference list, regular newsletter, audiovisual aids, and brochures.

President: Susan Fettes (1989-Present)
Executive Director: Susan Fettes
Year Established: 1990
Organization Members: 320

Concerned with the following diseases or disorders:
Beckwith Wiedemann Syndrome; Simpson Dysmorphia Syndrome

1166 BELL'S PALSY WEB SITE AND ONLINE SUPPORT GROUP

c/o Annette Lemke
65 Calle El Avion
Camarillo, CA 93010
E-mail: Seabee86@aol.com
http://members.aol.com/seabee86/index.html

The Bell's Palsy Web Site and Online Support Group is dedicated to providing information, support, and online networking opportunities to individuals who have been diagnosed with Bell's Palsy and their family members. Bell's Palsy is characterized by paralysis of the facial nerve due to inflammation and/or compression of the nerve. The condition, which usually comes on suddenly, typically affects one side of the face and is usually temporary. The Bell's Palsy site provides a variety of online networking opportunities including corresponding with other online support group members via e-mail and engaging in regularly scheduled chats on issues that are important to individuals and family members affected by Bell's Palsy. This web site also includes understandable information on the symptoms, potential causes, and treatment of Bell's Palsy; citations from the peer-reviewed medical literature; glossaries of commonly used medical terms; information concerning how to cope with Bell's Palsy; links to additional sources of information on Bell's Palsy on the Internet; FAQs (frequently asked questions) on Bell's Palsy with answers prepared by physicians in the field; and more.

Concerned with the following diseases or disorders:
Bell's Palsy

1167 BENIGN ESSENTIAL BLEPHAROSPASM RESEARCH FOUNDATION, INC. (BEBRF)

3155 Stagg Drive
P.O. Box 12468, Suite 110
Beaumont, TX 77726-2468 409-832-0788
Fax: 409-832-0890
E-mail: bebrf@ih2000.net
http://www.blepharospasm.org/~bebrf/

The Benign Essential Blepharospasm Research Foundation is a national voluntary health organization that was formed to promote research into the cause, treatment, and potential cure of Benign Essential Blepharospasm and other disorders of the facial musculature. Benign Essential Blepharospasm is characterized by intermittent, involuntary contractions or spasms of the muscles around the eyes. In some cases, an inability to open the eyelids due to involuntary muscle spasms may result in functional blindness. Established in 1981, the Foundation provides encouragement to affected individuals and their families. To this end, the Foundation provides support through state coordinators and local support groups. District Directors coordinate activities in their regions and direct affected individuals to medical centers where these conditions are treated. The Foundation also acts as a clearinghouse for information on these disorders and distributes materials including printed brochures, bimonthly newsletters, and fact sheets.

President: Mary Lou Thompson
Executive Director: Mattie Lou Koster
Year Established: 1981
Organization Members: 6,000

Publishes the following materials:
Benign Essential Blepharospasm Research Foundation, Inc. ~ *Brochure*
Medical Information Handbook ~ *Handbook*
Benign Essential Blepharospasm Meige and Other Related Disorders ~ *Brochure*
Fact Sheet on Benign Essential Blepharospasm and Other Related Disorders ~ *Factsheet*
Blepharospasm - Patient's Perspective ~ *Brochure*
Begnign Essential Blepharospasm: Origin of Foundation, Purpose, and Implementation of Goals ~ *Brochure*
Hemifacial Spasm ~ *Factsheet*
Meige's Syndrome. Historical Aspects ~ *Factsheet*
Treatment of Blepharospasm with Botulinum Toxin ~ *Pamphlet*
Benign Essential Blepharospasm Newsletter ~ *Newsletter*

Concerned with the following diseases or disorders:
Blepharospasm, Benign Essential; Meige Syndrome

1168 BLEPHAROPHIMOSIS, PTOSIS, EPICANTHUS INVERSUS FAMILY NETWORK (BPEI FAMILY NETWORK)

SE 820 Meadow Vale Drive
Pullman, WA 99163 509-332-6628
E-mail: lschauble@wsu.edu
http://www.wsu.edu.8080/~i0144069

The Blepharophimosis, Ptosis, Epicanthus Inversus Family Network is a voluntary self-help organization dedicated to gathering and disseminating information regarding Blepharophimosis, Ptosis, Epicanthus Inversus Syndrome (BPES). BPES is a rare genetic disorder characterized by abnormal narrowness of the eyelids in a horizontal direction (blepharophimosis), drooping of the upper eyelids (ptosis), vertical eyelid folds on either side of the nose (epicanthus inversus), and/or other abnormalities. The group provides a support network to affected individuals and their families and works with medical specialists and health care professionals to help provide the best possible care for affected individuals. Established in 1994, the organization also distributes a variety of educational and support materials through its computer database, regular newsletter, reprinted journal articles, and pamphlets. The Network also conducts an annual conference for affected individuals, families, members of the medical community, research professionals, and other interested individuals.

President: Lynn Schauble (1994 to present).
Year Established: 1994
Organization Members: 50

Concerned with the following diseases or disorders:
Blepharophimosis, Ptosis, Epicanthus Inversus Syndrome

1169 BLOOM'S SYNDROME REGISTRY

NY Blood Center
310 East 67th Street
New York, NY 10021 212-570-3075
Fax: 212-570-3195

The Bloom's Syndrome Registry is a research effort dedicated to collecting clinical and genetic information about Bloom's Syndrome, a rare inherited disorder characterized by short stature; a sun-sensitive redness in a "butterfly pattern" on the face; and susceptibility to infections and proness to develop cancer of many types. Established in 1960, the Bloom's Syndrome Registry meets with affected individuals and their families, compiles information concerning their pedigree history, and collects and preserves DNA and biological specimens. In addition, the Registry maintains copies of affected individuals' medical records and updates these records with new clinical findings and medical progress. The Registry conducts ongoing research using registry data and speciment and publishes regular reports and reviews in medical journals.

Executive Director: James L. German III, M.D. (Investigator)
Year Established: 1960
Organization Members: 166

Concerned with the following diseases or disorders:
Bloom Syndrome

1170 BRACHIAL PLEXUS INJURY (ERB'S PALSY SUPPORT & INFORMATION NETWORK)

P.O. Box 533
Menasha, WI 54952 920-836-3843

The Brachial Plexus Injury (Erb's Palsy Support and Information Network) is a voluntary not-for-profit self-help organization dedicated to providing information and support to affected families, health care professionals, and social service agencies; increasing public awareness of Brachial Plexus Injury and Erb's Palsy; and discovering new ways to improve function for affected individuals. Erb's Palsy is characterized by paralysis of the shoulder and upper extremity due to injury of one or more of the nerves that control shoulder and upper extremity muscles (upper brachial plexus). Erb's Palsy usually occurs in newborns due to birth injury. Established in 1995, the Brachial Plexus Injury (Erb's Palsy Support and Information Network) engages in patient advocacy; provides appropriate referrals; and enables affected families to exchange information, support, and resources. The Network produces a wide variety of educational and support materials including a directory, a regular newsletter, journal article reprints, and brochures.

President: Brenda Moore (Chairperson 1995-Present)
Year Established: 1995

Concerned with the following diseases or disorders:
Erb's Palsy

1171 BRACHIAL PLEXUS PALSY FOUNDATION (BPPF)

210 Spring Haven Circle
Royersford, PA 19468 610-792-0974
Fax: 610-792-0974
E-mail: brachial@aol.com
http://www.membdone.com/bpp

The Brachial Plexus Palsy Foundation (BPPF) is a nonprofit organization dedicated to raising funds for support of families who have children with brachial plexus injuries. Affected children may have paralysis of the shoulder and upper extremity due to injury of one or more of the nerves that control shoulder and upper extremity muscles (upper brachial plexus). Such injuries, which may be called Erb's Palsy or Upper Brachial Paralysis, usually occur in newborns due to birth injury. The organization supports medical facilities that research and treat such injuries, holds fund-raising events to support further research, has support groups, and produces educational materials including a newsletter entitled "Outreach" and brochures.

President: Thomas J. Cirino
Executive Director: Michael F. Cirino
Organization Members: 10

Publishes the following materials:
Outreach ~ *Newsletter*
The BPP Foundation ~ *Booklet*

Concerned with the following diseases or disorders:
Erb's Palsy

1172 CDC BUSINESS RESPONDS TO AIDS AND LABOR RESPONDS TO AIDS (BRTA/LRTA)

800-458-5231
TDD: 800-243-7012
E-mail: blrs@cdcnac.org
http://www.brta-lrta.org

The Centers for Disease Control and Prevention's (CDC's) "Business Responds to AIDS and Labor Responds to AIDS (BRTA/LRTA) web site helps large and small businesses and labor organizations meet the challenges of HIV/AIDS in the workplace and the community. The web site gives an overview of BRTA/LRTA programs as well as information on where to get help setting up workplace programs. The web site also includes details about the BRTA Manager's Kit and LRTA Labor Leader's Kit and a variety of other resources for employers and employees. It offers timely information on issues related to HIV/AIDS and presents statements from business, labor, and community leaders about successful programs. The home page's headings including BRTA/LRTA; Manager's Kit and Labor Leader's Kit; Leaders Address AIDS; Current News; TV PSA; and Additional Resources (which includes dynamic links to other sources of information).

Concerned with the following diseases or disorders:
AIDS (Acquired Immune Deficiency Syndrome)

1173 CDG SOCIETY (SWEDEN)

E-mail: Rolf.Odselius@emu.lu.se
http://www.emu.lu.se/cdg/indexeng.html

The CDG Society (Sweden) provides this World Wide Web site for health care professionals, researchers, and families with children diagnosed with Carbohydrate-Deficient Glycoprotein (CDG) Syndromes. CDG Syndromes are a group of newly discovered, extremely rare inherited metabolic disorders. Although four variants of the disorder have been identified, it is suspected that more variants exist. These disorders affect most systems of the body, particularly the function of the central nervous system (i.e., the brain and spinal cord) and the peripheral nervous system (i.e., motor and sensory nerves outside the central nervous system). The most common form of CDG Syndrome is Carbohydrate-Deficient Glycoprotein Syndrome Type I (CDG1). Although symptoms may vary from case to case, individuals with CDG1 may exhibit impaired coordination and balance (cerebellar ataxia) due to underdevelopment (hypoplasia) of certain portions of the brain (e.g., cerebellum); severe muscle thinning and weakness in the legs (peripheral neuropathy); skeletal malformations; visual and/or hearing impairment; mild to severe mental retardation; and severe delays in the acquisition of skills that require the coordination of mental and muscular activity (psychomotor retardation). The purpose of this home page is to provide current information on CDGS; offer specialist resources in Sweden; provide international parent contacts through e-mail; and offer links to other patient organizations, specialist laboratories, and clinics; etc.

Organization Language: Swedish. German.

Concerned with the following diseases or disorders:
Carbohydrate deficient Glycoprotein Syndrome Type I

1174 CDGS FAMILY NETWORK

603-434-3064
E-mail: cdgforum@ultranet.com
http://www.cdgs.com

The CDGS Family Network provides this web site on the Internet for parents of children diagnosed with Carbohydrate-Deficient Glycoprotein (CDG) Syndromes. CDG Syndromes are a group of extremely rare inherited metabolic disorders. Although four variants of the disorder have been identified, it is suspected that more variants exist. These disorders affect most systems of the body, particularly the function of the central nervous system (i.e., the brain and spinal cord) and the peripheral nervous system (i.e., motor and sensory nerves outside the central nervous system). The most common form of CDG Syndrome is Carbohydrate-Deficient Glycoprotein Syndrome Type I (CDG1). The purpose of this home page is to help parents of children with CDGS assist one another in their search for information; to enable them to share experiences, support, and resources; and to provide them with understandable material on this complex group of disorders.

President: Donna Yunes

Concerned with the following diseases or disorders:
Carbohydrate deficient Glycoprotein Syndrome Type I

1175 CHARGE SYNDROME FOUNDATION, INC.

2004 Parkade
Columbia, MO 65202-3121 573-499-4694
800-442-7604
Fax: 573-499-4694
E-mail: mnorbury@mail.coin.missouri.edu

The CHARGE Syndrome Foundation is a national not-for-profit voluntary agency that was established in 1993. The mission of the Foundation is to establish, maintain, and distribute information about CHARGE Syndrome and provide support to affected families. The Foundation supports the development of information about CHARGE Syndrome, its causes, and effects on individuals, their families, and health care professionals.

In addition, the Foundation supports research into the cause and treatments of CHARGE Syndrome and works in conjunction with other organizations and institutions to accomplish its mission. Educational materials produced by the Foundation include "CHARGE Syndrome: A Booklet for Families" and a newsletter entitled "CHARGE Accounts." A bibliography, questionnaire, and a CHARGE Syndrome brochure are also available from the organization. In addition, the CHARGE Syndrome Foundation conducts a biennial conference for affected individuals, families, physicians, and other professionals such as educators and therapists.

President: Donna Lacey (1997 - Present).
Executive Director: Marion A. Norbury (Secretary/Treasurer)
Year Established: 1993
Organization Members: 300

Publishes the following materials:
CHARGE Association Related Terms ~ *Information Sheet*
2nd International CHARGE Syndrome Conference ~ *Pamphlet*
CHARGE Accounts ~ *Newsletter*
CHARGE Syndrome Parent Questionnaire ~ *Questionnaire*
CHARGE Bibliography ~ *Bibliography*
CHARGE Syndrome - A Booklet for Families ~ *Booklet*
CHARGE Syndrome - What is it? ~ *Brochure*

Concerned with the following diseases or disorders:
CHARGE Syndrome

1176 CANADIAN ANGELMAN SYNDROME SOCIETY (CASS)

P.O. Box 37
Priddis
Alberta, T0L 1W0
Canada 403-931-2415
Fax: 403-931-2415
E-mail: cass@cadvision.com

The Canadian Angelman Syndrome Society (CASS) was incorporated in 1993 as a nonprofit charity and established to educate concerned families, the medical and educational communities, and the general public on the diagnosis, treatment, and prevention of Angelman Syndrome. Angelman Syndrome is a rare genetic disorder characterized by mental and motor retardation, absence of speech, muscular abnormalities, unprovoked laughter, and characteristic facial abnormalities. CASS consists of approximately 150 members who are dedicated to educating parents and professionals about Angelman Syndrome and disseminating information on this disorder. CASS provides a regular newsletter, offers networking services for affected parents, and conducts a yearly conference.

President: Diane News
Executive Director: Jane Carscallen (Newsletter Editor)
Organization Language: French (written).
Year Established: 1993
Organization Chapters: 3
Organization Members: 150

Publishes the following materials:
Some Facts About Angelman Syndrome ~ *Brochure*

Concerned with the following diseases or disorders:
Angelman Syndrome

1177 CANADIAN ASSOCIATION FOR WILLIAMS SYNDROME (CAWS)

P.O. Box 2115
Vancouver
British Columbia, V6B 3T5
Canada 604-852-2662
Fax: 604-853-0032
www.sos.on.ca/~pmackay/williams/html

The Canadian Association for Williams Syndrome (CAWS) is a voluntary nonprofit organization dedicated to providing support and assistance to families with children affected by Williams Syndrome; maintaining a network for adults with Williams Syndrome; and supporting research into educational, behavioral, social, and medical aspects of this syndrome. Williams Syndrome is a rare congenital disorder characterized by heart and blood vessel abnormalities, high blood calcium levels, developmental delays, characteristic facial features, and/or additional abnormalities. Established in 1984 as a parent support group, the Association currently consists of 10 chapters and 360 members. CAWS is committed to locating affected families who are unaware of the Association; becoming a visible group in the medical, scientific, educational, and professional communities in order to facilitate referrals of newly diagnosed individuals; and providing a variety of educational materials to affected individuals, family members, and health care professionals. CAWS publishes a regular newsletter and maintains a web site [http://www.sos.on.ca/~pmackay/williams/html].

President: Frankie Samulski (1994 to Present)
Organization Language: French (written).
Year Established: 1984
Organization Chapters: 10
Organization Members: 360

Publishes the following materials:
Williams Syndrome. Facts ~ *Brochure*
Canadian Association for Williams Syndrome ~ *Newsletter Winter 1996*

Concerned with the following diseases or disorders:
Williams Syndrome

1178 CANADIAN CYSTIC FIBROSIS FOUNDATION (CCFF)

2221 Yonge Street
Suite 601
Toronto
Ontario, M4S 2B4
Canada 416-485-9149
800-378-2233
Fax: 416-485-0960
E-mail: postmaster@ccff.ca
http://www.ccff.ca/~cfwww/index.html

The Canadian Cystic Fibrosis Foundation (CCFF) is a national not-for-profit organization dedicated to helping individuals with cystic fibrosis (CF) and their family members. Cystic fibrosis is a rare inherited disorder that affects many exocrine ("outward-secreting") glands of the body including the sweat glands, salivary glands, and those within the pancreas and respiratory system. Due to unusually thick secretions of mucus that clog and obstruct air passages of the lungs, affected individuals experience chronic coughing and an increased susceptibility to repeated lung infections. Individuals with CF also exhibit an inability to break down food and absorb fats and nutrients properly; have abnormally salty sweat containing elevated levels of chloride and sodium; and/or may demonstrate other abnormalities. Established in 1959, the Canadian Cystic Fibrosis Foundation is committed to conducting research into improved care and treatment for CF, seeking a cure or control for the disorder, and promoting public awareness. In addition, the Foundation offers support groups, engages in patient advocacy, provides referrals, and promotes patient, professional, and general education. The Canadian Cystic Fibrosis Foundation also offers a variety of materials including brochures, guides and manuals, reports, and several newsletters. The Foundation's web site on the Internet is located at [http://www.ccff.ca/~cfwww/index.html].

President: M. Denis Mouton (1997 to Present)
Executive Director: Cathleen Morrison
Organization Language: French (written/spoken).
Year Established: 1959
Organization Chapters: 50

Publishes the following materials:
You Were Asking ~ *Brochure*
Canadian Cystic Fibrosis Foundation Annual Report 1996 ~ *Booklet*
Candid Facts (English/French) ~ *Newsletter 1997*

Concerned with the following diseases or disorders:
Cystic Fibrosis

1179 CANADIAN FANCONI ANEMIA RESEARCH FUND (CFARF)

2635 Dartmouth Drive
Penticton
British Columbia, V2A 733
Canada 250-493-2910
Fax: 250-493-2986

The Canadian Fanconi Anemia Research Fund (CFARF) is a not-for-profit voluntary organization dedicated to raising awareness of the disease in the public arena. Fanconi's Anemia is an inherited condition that leads to a deficiency of certain blood cells that are produced by the bone marrow. Established in 1994, CFARF promotes and supports research on Fanconi's Anemia, provides information and support to affected Canadian families, and gathers information regarding Fanconi's Anemia, bone marrow failure, cancer treatment, and new medications that may assist individuals with the disorder.

President: Tami Dunston-Adams (1994 to Present)
Year Established: 1994
Organization Members: 30

Concerned with the following diseases or disorders:
Anemia, Fanconi's

1180 CANADIAN HYPERLEXIA ASSOCIATION (CHA)

300 John Street
Box 87673
Thornhill
Ontario, L3T 7R3
Canada 905-886-8364
Fax: 905-886-4624
E-mail: cha@ican.net
http://home.ican.net/~cha

The Canadian Hyperlexia Association (CHA) is a not-for-profit organization dedicated to fostering awareness of hyperlexia in Canada; providing information relating to the observable characteristics of this condition; collecting, disseminating, and sharing information, practical strategies, and resources; providing networking opportunities for parents, children, and professionals; and acknowledging the value of appropriate, early, ongoing intervention. Hyperlexia is a condition that interferes with speech, language, and social interaction. From as early as 18 months to before the age of five, affected children experience an intense fascination with letters, numbers, patterns, logos, etc. and have a precocious ability to read, spell, write, and/or compute. Established in 1995 and consisting of 100 members and three chapters, CHA offers telephone support to parents, teachers, speech-language pathologists, physicians, and psychologists. The Association's educational materials include a newsletter entitled "The Reader," brochures, and audiovisual aids.

President: Robin Leszner (1995 to present).
Year Established: 1995
Organization Chapters: 3
Organization Members: 100

Publishes the following materials:
What is Hyperlexia? ~ *Fact Sheet*
Developing Language is The Key to Unlocking the Child with Hyperlexia ~ *Fact Sheet*
Selected Strategies for Helping Children with Hyperlexia ~ *Fact Sheet*
The Reader ~ *Newsletter Spring 1997*

1181 CANADIAN MARFAN ASSOCIATION

Central Plaza Postal Outlet
128 Queen Street South
P.O. Box 42257
Mississauga
Ontario, L5M 4Z0 905-826-3223
Fax: 905-826-2125
E-mail: marfan@istar.ca

The Canadian Marfan Association is an international nonprofit organization dedicated to preventing disabling symptoms and life-threatening complications of Marfan Syndrome and improving the quality of life for people affected by this disorder through comprehensive programs of education, support, and research. Marfan Syndrome is a rare inherited connective tissue disorder characterized by abnormalities of the heart and blood vessels (cardiovascular system), skeleton, and eyes. Affected individuals may be unusually tall and thin, have abnormally large hands and feet, have malformations of the chest and spine, and experience weakness of the joints, ligaments, and tendons. The Canadian Marfan Association is dedicated to increasing public awareness of Marfan Syndrome in Canada by holding public information meetings, community support group meetings, and media interviews; to providing accurate, timely information about the disorder to affected individuals, families, and physicians; to assisting people with Marfan Syndrome and their families with quality of life issues and helping them form self-help groups; and to acting as a communication liaison for people with Marfan Syndrome and the community. The Association also seeks to support and foster ongoing research in the area of connective tissue diseases. Educational materials distributed by the Association include a regular newsletter entitled "News Links" and a variety of brochures (e.g., "The Marfan Syndrome," "Chromosome 15," "The Marfan Syndrome: A Booklet for Teachers," "A Special Mouse," and "Marfan Syndrome: A Booklet for Teenagers").

Executive Director: Laura Libralesso
Organization Language: French (written/spoken).
Year Established: 1986
Organization Chapters: 9
Organization Members: 500

Publishes the following materials:
Charter by Letters Patent of the Canadian Marfan Association ~ *Mission Statement*
News Links ~ *Newsletter Winter 1997*
Marfan Syndrome. A Time Bomb ~ *Poster*
The Marfan Syndrome. Chromosome 15 ~ *Booklet*
Marfan Syndrome: A Booklet for Teenagers ~ *Booklet*
A Very Special Mouse ~ *Booklet*
A Booklet for Teachers ~ *Booklet*
Canadian Marfan Association ~ *Brochure*

Concerned with the following diseases or disorders:
Marfan Syndrome

1182 CANADIAN MULTIPLE ENDOCRINE NEOPLASIA TYPE 1, LTD.

Box 100
Meota
Saskatchewan, SOM 1XO
Canada 306-892-2080
Fax: 306-892-2080

Canadian Multiple Endocrine Neoplasia Type 1, Ltd. is an international nonprofit organization dedicated to helping others with Multiple Endocrine Neoplasia Type 1 and assisting their family members. Familial Multiple Endocrine Neoplasia Type 1 (FMEN1) is a rare genetic disorder characterized by overactivity of certain endocrine glands (e.g., pituitary, parathyroid gland, and pancreatic islet cells) and excessive production of certain hormones. A variety of symptoms and physical findings may result such as abnormally increased levels of calcium in the blood (hypercalcemia), generalized fatigue, weakness, muscle and/or bone pain, constipation and/or other digestive abnormalities, and/or additional symptoms. Established in 1996, the organization, which is affiliated with Voice of the Handicapped, is committed to collecting and distributing current information on the disease; educating the medical community about FMEN1; and providing networking services that enable affected individuals to exchange information, resources, and support.

President: Shirley Stevens (1955 to Present)
Executive Director: Cathy Fitch
Year Established: 1996
Organization Members: 18

Publishes the following materials:
Familial Multiple Endocrine Neoplasia Type 1 ~ *Fact Sheet*

1183 CANADIAN OSTEOGENESIS IMPERFECTA SOCIETY (COIS)

128 Thornhill Cres.
Chatham
Ontario, N7L 4M3
Canada 519-436-0025
Fax: 519-351-4043
E-mail: marylouk@usa.net

The Canadian Osteogenesis Imperfecta Society (COIS) is an international, nonprofit, charitable organization dedicated to assisting individuals affected by Osteogenesis Imperfecta (OI). Osteogenesis Imperfecta is a genetic disorder characterized by abnormally fragile, brittle bones. Established in 1983, the Society aims to provide emotional support on a personal level for parents and people with Osteogenesis Imperfecta; encourage and foster Canadian medical research into the underlying causes of OI; acquaint medical personnel, hospitals, educational institutions, and social agencies with all facets of Osteogenesis Imperfecta; maintain and up-to-date library of literature both medical and general pertaining to OI; promote and understand awareness of brittle bones by the public; and solicit and receive funds to carry out the aims of the Canadian Osteogenesis Imperfecta Society. The Society has approximately 400 members and can be reached by e-mail at [marylouk@usa.net].

President: Mary Lou Kearney (1993 to Present).
Year Established: 1983
Organization Members: 400

Concerned with the following diseases or disorders:
Osteogenesis Imperfecta

1184 CANADIAN PORPHYRIA FOUNDATION, INC. (CPF)

P.O. Box 1206
Neepawa
Manitoba, ROF 1HO
Canada 204-476-2800

The Canadian Porphyria Foundation Inc. (CPF) is a voluntary organization dedicated to improving the quality of life for Canadians affected by porphyria through programs of awareness, education, service, advocacy, and research. Porphyria is a group of rare genetic disorders characterized by disturbances of porphyrin metabolism. Established in 1988 and consisting of approximately 900 members, CPF is committed to promoting public and professional awareness; assembling, printing, and distributing up-to-date educational materials to physicians, health care personnel, members, and others affected by porphyria; and offering support programs to affected individuals and their families. The goals of the organization are to promote the family social welfare of affected individuals; to educate and inform physicians and others in health care about the porphyrias so that early diagnosis and proper treatment will be realized; and to promote and provide financial assistance for research into the porphyrias. The organization is also committed to encouraging, supporting, and serving physicians and researchers in their efforts to find more effective treatments for the porphyrias and to increasing physician, patient, and community awareness of the porphyrias and thereby cultivating support for research. The organization also has support groups, engages in patient advocacy, and has confidential registry. CPF's educational materials include booklets, brochures, fact sheets on the differentforms of porphyria, and a regular newsletter.

President: Lois J. Aitken (1988 to Present)
Organization Language: French (written).
Year Established: 1988
Organization Members: 900

Publishes the following materials:
Porphyria (English/French) ~ *Brochure*
A Guide To Porphyria ~ *Booklet*
Porphyria Cutanea Tarda ~ *Leaflet*
Acute Intermittent Porphyria ~ *Leaflet*

Erythropoietic Protoporphyria ~ *Leaflet*
Hereditary Coproporphyria ~ *Leaflet*
Canadian Porphyria Foundation ~ *Newsletter*

Concerned with the following diseases or disorders:
Erythropoietic Protoporphyria (EPP); Porphyria; Porphyria Cutanea Tarda; Porphyria, ALA-D; Porphyria, Acute Intermittent; Porphyria, Congenital Erythropoietic; Porphyria, Hereditary Coproporphyria; Porphyria, Variegate

1185 CANADIAN RETT SYNDROME ASSOCIATION AND RESOURCE CENTRE (CRSA)

1375 Weber Street East
P.O. Box 25058
Kitchener
Ontario, N2A 3A5
Canada 519-893-1169
Fax: 519-893-1169
E-mail: canrettres@cyberus.ca

The Canadian Rett Syndrome Association and Resource Centre (CRSA) is a not-for-profit voluntary organization dedicated to providing parents and caregivers current information, assistance, and support to ensure the best quality of life for all girls and women with Rett Syndrome. Rett Syndrome, a rare congenital neurological disorder that affects only females, is characterized by progressive degeneration of certain tissues of the brain, resulting in loss of previously acquired mental and motor skills, impaired control of voluntary movements (ataxia), episodes of uncontrolled electrical disturbances of the brain (seizures), autistic behavior, and/or other abnormalities and physical features. Established in 1985 and consisting of five provincial associations, CRSA is dedicated to providing the most current information on Rett Syndrome to affected families and health care professionals to assist in the diagnosis and treatment of the disorder; ensuring that families and caregivers understand what services are available to them in their respective provinces; offering networking services; and putting affected families and health care professionals in contact with one another. The Resource Centre provides a variety of educational materials including medical journal articles, books, videos, and a quarterly newsletter.

President: Eugene Bradley (1992 to Present)
Executive Director: Terry Boyd (Director)
Organization Language: French (written/spoken).
Year Established: 1985
Organization Chapters: 5
Organization Members: 250

Publishes the following materials:
What is RETT Syndrome ~ *Brochure*
Canadian Rett Syndrome Association ~ *Mission Statement*
Canadian Rett Syndrome Association ~ *Mission Statement*

Concerned with the following diseases or disorders:
Rett Syndrome

1186 CANADIAN SICKLE CELL SOCIETY

6999 Cote-des-Neiges
Suite 33
Montreal
Quebec, H3S 2B8
Canada 514-735-5109
Fax: 514-735-5100

The Canadian Sickle Cell Society is a not-for-profit organization dedicated to educating the at-risk population, recruiting and training volunteers, providing effective lobbying for improvement of services, and identifying individuals with sickle cell disease or traits and providing them with individual and family counseling. Sickle cell disease is a rare inherited blood disorder characterized by the presence of sickle or crescent-shaped red blood cells (erythrocytes) in the blood. The Canadian Sickle Cell Society was established in 1976 by affected family members with the assistance of medical and health professionals and community members. Program activities include volunteer training, lobbying, advocacy, counseling, support groups, and screening for sickle cell disease. The Society produces a variety of educational materials including pamphlets and brochures.

President: Horace Laryea, M.D.
Executive Director: Rosetta Cadogan
Organization Language: French (written/spoken).
Year Established: 1976

Publishes the following materials:
Sickle Cell Anemia: who-when-how? ~ *Fact Sheet*
Facts on Sickle Cell Anemia and Sickle Cell Irait ~ *Fact Sheet*

Concerned with the following diseases or disorders:
Sickle Cell Disease

1187 CANADIAN SYRINGOMYELIA NETWORK (CSN)

69 Penny Crescent
Markham
Ontario, L3P 5X7
Canada 905-471-8278
Fax: 905-882-8367
E-mail: csn@passport.ca
http://www.passport.ca/~csn

The Canadian Syringomyelia Network (CSN) is a nonprofit organization dedicated to serving as a support network for people with syringomyelia, a rare progressive condition characterized by the presence of abnormal, fluid-filled cavities within the spinal cord. Established in 1992, CSN acts as an information and referral network; builds awareness among the community; assists those who wish to establish support groups; compiles a database of people in Canada who have shown an interest in CSN and its mission; and produces a newsletter for its members and those interested in CSN's activities. The Canadian Syringomyelia Network also organizes periodic meetings and conferences, offers patient networking services, provides referrals, and produces educational materials including brochures, reports, and a regular newsletter.

President: Barbara Forrestall (1992 to Present)
Year Established: 1992
Organization Members: 230

Publishes the following materials:
Canadian Syringomyelia Network ~ *Brochure*

Concerned with the following diseases or disorders:
Arachnoiditis; Arnold Chiari Syndrome; Syringomyelia

1188 CANINE COMPANIONS FOR INDEPENDENCE (CCI)

2965 Dutton Avenue
P.O. Box 446
Santa Rosa, CA 95402-0446 707-577-1700
800-572-2275
Fax: 707-577-1711
TDD: 707-577-1756
E-mail: info@caninecompanions.org
http://www.caninecompanions.org/

The Canine Companions for Independence (CCI) is a nonprofit organization dedicated to serving the needs of people with disabilities by providing trained service, hearing, and social dogs and by providing continuing support to ensure the success of the working team. Established in 1975, CCI has been training dogs to assist people with disabilities other than blindness. The dogs at Canine Companions for Independence, trained to respond to more than 50 specialized commands, become the physical extensions of their disabled partners by performing a variety of basic tasks. The organization has four types of Assistance Dogs: Service Dogs, which increase independence by performing practical tasks for a person with a disability; Hearing Dogs, which are trained to alert people who are hearing impaired to important sounds such as a telephone, alarm clock, smoke alarm, and a baby's cry; Social Dogs, which are trained in a variety of surroundings and circumstances to enhance the quality of life for people with disabilities; and Facility Dogs, which enhance the quality of life for people through pet facilitated therapy and interactions. Consisting of 200 chapters, CCI's educational materials include a newsletter entitled "The Courier," a brochure entitled "Canine Companions for Independence," numerous fact sheets, and audio-visual aids. Program activities include the Puppy Raising Program, which provides a unique opportunity for volunteers to help create a meaningful change in someone's life. CCI puppies are raised in private homes from eight weeks of age until they are approximately 13 to 18 months old. The puppy raisers play an active role in modeling young, curious pups into enthusiastic, responsive, and confident dogs that are ready to meet the challenges of becoming service, hearing, or social dogs. Other program activities are research and education. CCI can be reached at its e-mail address at [info@caninecompanions.org] or its web site at http://www.caninecompanions.org/].

President: Jean F. Schulz (1995 to Present)
Executive Director: Corey Hudson
Year Established: 1975
Organization Chapters: 200
Organization Members: Non-Membership

Publishes the following materials:
"Heart of a Hero" ~ *Video Tape*
Lions Project for Canine Companions for Independence ~ *Brochure*
Changing Lives ~ *Brochure*
Canine Companions for Independence ~ *Brochure*
Powerful Partnerships ~ *Brochure*
Applying ~ *Brochure*
Puppy Raising Program ~ *Brochure*

1189 CARDIO-FACIAL-CUTANEOUS SYNDROME SUPPORT NETWORK

157 Alder Avenue
Egg Harbor Twnshp, NJ 08234 609-646-5606
E-mail: Redsifer@aol.com

The Cardio-Facial-Cutaneous Syndrome Support Network is a not-for-profit organization dedicated to providing information and support to affected individuals and family members. Cardio-Facial-Cutaneous Syndrome is a rare genetic disorder characterized by distinctive abnormalities of the head and facial (craniofacial) area; sparse, curly hair; skin abnormalities; cardiac defects; growth delays; psychomotor retardation; and mild to severe mental retardation. Established in 1991, the Cardio-Facial-Cutaneous Syndrome Network produces a newsletter entitled "C.F.C. Syndrome Support Newsletter." Articles from medical journals are often included with the newsletter.

President: NA
Executive Director: John and Nancy Carlson
Year Established: 1991
Organization Members: 18

Publishes the following materials:
C.F.C. Syndrome Support Newsletter ~ *Newsletter*

Concerned with the following diseases or disorders:
Cardio Facio Cutaneous Syndrome

1190 CARDIOMYOPATHY ASSOCIATION (CMA)

40 The Metro Centre
Tapits Lane
Watford
Hertfordshire, WD1 8SB
United Kingdom 01441923249977
Fax: 01441923249987

The Cardiomyopathy Association is an international not-for-profit self-help organization dedicated to providing information and support to individuals affected by cardiomyopathy, their family members, and medical professionals. Cardiomyopathy is a general diagnostic term indicating a primary noninflammatory disease of the heart muscle (myocardium) that is often due to unknown causes. Established in 1989 and consisting of 1,000 members throughout the world, the Cardiomyopathy Association publishes informational brochures on different types of cardiomyopathy. Titles include "Dilated Cardiomyopathy," "Hypertrophic Cardiomyopathy," and "Arrhythmogenic Right Ventricular Cardiomyopathy." The Association also offers videotapes on these topics. In addition to disseminating information, the Association also provides counseling to affected individuals and their family members and endeavors to open the lines of communication between affected individuals and families through an international networking program.

President: Carolyn Biro (Chairperson) (1989 to Present)
Executive Director: Gordon Rae
Year Established: 1989
Organization Members: 1,000

Publishes the following materials:
Hypertrophic Cardiomyopathy ~ *Booklet*
Dilated Cardiomyopathy ~ *Booklet*
A Booklet for Teachers on Hypertrophic Cardiomyopathy ~ *Booklet*
Cardiomyopathy Association ~ *Mission Statement*
Sudden cardiac death in the young ~ *Reprint*
Review Article. Medical Progress ~ *Leaflet*
Evidence from family studies for autoimmunity in dilated cardiomyopathy ~ *Pamphlet*
Diagnostic criteria for Arrhythmogenic Right Ventricular Cardiomyopathy ~ *Pamphlet*

Concerned with the following diseases or disorders:
Wolff Parkinson White Syndrome

1191 CELIAC SPRUE ASSOCIATION/USA, INC. (CSA/USA)

P.O. Box 31700
Omaha, NE 68131-0700 402-558-0600
Fax: 402-558-1347
http://www.csaceliacs.org

Celiac Sprue Association/USA, Inc. is a voluntary not-for-profit self-help organization that serves as a resource information center for individuals with Celiac Sprue. Celiac Sprue is a chronic hereditary intestinal malabsorption disorder caused by intolerance to gluten. Affected individuals may experience no symptoms or many symptoms. Those individuals who have symptoms may experience weight loss, chronic diarrhea, abdominal cramping, intestinal gas, weakness, fatigue, and/or a variety of other symptoms. Some may experience Dermatitis Herpetiformis, which is characterized by small itchy blisters appearing on the skin surface, most commonly on body pressure points, such as elbows, knees, and feet. The Celiac Sprue Association/USA, Inc. provides referrals to support groups and other services, engages in patient advocacy, and provides a variety of educational and support materials. These include a regular newsletter, brochures, and diet and cooking information.

Executive Director: Leon H. Rottmann
Year Established: 1979
Organization Chapters: 76
Organization Members: 7,000

Concerned with the following diseases or disorders:
Celiac Sprue; Schmidt Syndrome

1192 CENTER FOR MENTAL RETARDATION (CMR)

1621 Euclid Avenue
Keith Building
Suite 514
Cleveland, OH 44115 216-621-5858
800-899-3039
Fax: 216-621-0221

The Center for Mental Retardation (Edward I. and Fannie L. Baker International Resource Center for Down Syndrome) is an international not-for-profit organization dedicated to improving the quality of life for individuals with Down Syndrome and increasing their role as valued, contributing members of society through the implementation and promotion of services, educational programs, and research. Down Syndrome is a congenital chromosomal disorder characterized by varying degrees of mental retardation, characteristic abnormalities of the head and facial area, malformations of the hands and/or feet, congenital heart defects in approximately 25 percent of affected individuals, and/or other abnormalities. In most individuals with Down Syndrome, all or a portion of chromosome 21 appears three times rather than twice in cells of the body; however, in rare cases, the disorder may occur due to a chromosomal translocation involving chromosome 21 and another chromosome. Established in 1963, the Center for Mental Retardation offers a variety of services and programs including patient advocacy services, parent counseling and support, referral services, and patient and professional education. The Center's educational materials include brochures, pamphlets, and a regular newsletter.

President: Michael Zimmerman
Executive Director: David Pfriem
Organization Language: Spanish (written).
Year Established: 1963
Organization Members: 300

1193 CHARCOT-MARIE-TOOTH ASSOCIATION (CMTA)

601 Upland Avenue
Upland, PA 19015 610-499-7486
800-606-2682
Fax: 610-499-7487
E-mail: CMTAssoc@aol.com
http://www.charcot-marie-tooth.org

The Charcot-Marie-Tooth Association is a national voluntary health organization that functions as an educational resource for people with Charcot-Marie-Tooth Disease, their families, medical professionals, the educational community, and the general public. Charcot-Marie-Tooth Disease is a genetic neurological disorder characterized by weakness and atrophy of muscles first in the legs and, later, in the arms and hands. Founded in 1983, the Association acts as an advocate for people with Charcot-Marie-Tooth Disease by raising awareness and encouraging public and private agencies and private industry to fund and support medical research. The Association acts as a liaison between the research community and people with this disorder. It also organizes and encourages the formation of local chapters and support groups. The organization produces educational materials including brochures, a newsletter, and transcripts of medical conferences. Videotapes are also available including "Neurology & CMT," "Orthopedic Surgery Options," and "Genetics/CMOUNT."

President: Diane M. Freaney
Executive Director: Paul R. Flynn
Year Established: 1983
Organization Chapters: 15
Organization Members: 10,000

Publishes the following materials:
Charcot-Marie-Tooth Disorders ~ *Brochure*
The CMTA Report ~ *Newsletter*
CMT Facts I ~ *Newsletter*
CMT Facts II ~ *Newsletter*
Charcot-Marie-Tooth Conference ~ *Pamphlet*

Concerned with the following diseases or disorders:
Charcot Marie Tooth Disease; Roussy Levy Syndrome

1194 CHARCOT-MARIE-TOOTH INTERNATIONAL (CMT INTERNATIONAL)

1 Springbank Drive
St. Catharines
Ontario, L2S 2KI
Canada 905-687-3630
Fax: 905-687-8753
E-mail: cmtint@vaxxine.com
http://www.cmtint.org

The Charcot-Marie-Tooth International is a not-for-profit organization dedicated to helping affected individuals locate information on and medical assistance for Charcot-Marie-Tooth Disease (CMT) and related disorders. CMT is a genetic neurological disorder characterized by weakness and atrophy of muscles first in the legs and, later, in the arms and hands. Established in 1984, the CMT International engages in patient advocacy; promotes and supports research; engages in patient and professional education; and provides various forms of support to affected individuals. In addition, CMT International makes referrals to genetic counseling and other support services. CMT International also publishes a bimonthly newsletter that is distributed to more than 2,000 families in over 40 countries. A medical advisory committee informs the organization of the latest updates and findings concerning CMT and related disorders. In addition, the organization also publishes a variety of informational brochures and provides a free introductory kit to those interested in becoming members.

President: Linda Crabtree, C.M. (1984-Present)
Executive Director: Linda Crabtree
Year Established: 1984
Organization Members: 2,000

Publishes the following materials:
Charcot-Marie-Tooth Disease ~ *Brochure*
CMT Newsletter ~ *Newsletter*
Charcot-Marie-Tooth Disease/Peroneal Muscular Atrophy International Association, INC. ~ *Fact Sheet*

Concerned with the following diseases or disorders:
Charcot Marie Tooth Disease

1195 CHILDHOOD DISINTEGRATIVE DISORDER NETWORK (CDD NETWORK)

c/o Madeline Catalano
1172 Four Mile Road
Alleghany, NY 14706
E-mail: cdd@inter.com.au

The Childhood Disintegrative Disorder Network is a voluntary, nonprofit support organization consisting of families of children with Childhood Disintegrative Disorder (CDD), also known as Heller Syndrome. This condition is characterized by a significant loss of previously acquired skills such as expressive language, adaptive behavior, bladder control, etc. Established in 1995, the group's mission is to share information relating to CDD, its causes, and treatments, and to provide support and encouragement to affected families. The CDD Network works to increase its membership to encompass a larger group of affected children whose case histories may assist researchers with an interest in CDD. The network also works to promote awareness of CDD in the public and the medical establishment.

President: Madeline Catalano
Executive Director: Jenny Fairthorne
Organization Language: Japanese (written/spoken).
Year Established: 1995

Publishes the following materials:
Childhood Disintegrative Disorder Network ~ *Fact Sheet*
Childhood Disintegrative Disorder ~ *Brochure*

1196 CHILDREN AND ADULTS WITH ATTENTION DEFICIT DISORDER (CHADD)

499 NW 70th Avenue
Suite 101
Plantation, FL 33317 954-587-3700
800-233-4050
Fax: 954-587-4599
E-mail: sharon_graham@chadd.org
http://www.chadd.org

Children and Adults with Attention Deficit Disorder (C.H.A.D.D.) is a not-for-profit self-help organization dedicated to helping affected individuals of all ages achieve success. Attention Deficit Disorder (ADD) is a neurobiological disorder that is characterized by short attention span, excessive impulsiveness, and, in some cases, hyperactivity. Established in 1987 by a small group of parents and professionals, CH.A.D.D. currently has over 35,000 members and over 600 local chapters nationwide. Local chapters sponsor parent support groups, conduct meetings featuring expert speakers, work with local school systems to ensure appropriate educational services for children with ADD, and publish local newsletters. C.H.A.D.D. is developing state ADD councils to advocate for education, training, program development, health care access, employment, and other services for persons with ADD. The national office of C.H.A.D.D. provides information on the latest developments in ADD related issues, such as research and treatment, through various publications. In addition, CH.A.D.D. lobbies legislators concerning areas of importance to affected individuals, works with all forms of media to increase public awareness of ADD, provides appropriate referrals, and conducts an annual conference. C.H.A.D.D. also serves as an information resource to health care professionals working with affected individuals and offers educational materials including newsletters, a magazine, fact sheets, and brochures.

Executive Director: Sharon Graham (Director of Field Services)
Organization Language: Spanish.
Year Established: 1987
Organization Chapters: 600
Organization Members: 35,000

Publishes the following materials:
Join Forces with Chadd ~ *Brochure*
Children and Adults with Attention Deficit Disorders ~ *Fact Sheet*

Concerned with the following diseases or disorders:
Attention Deficit Hyperactivity Disorder

1197 CHILDREN'S BRAIN DISEASES FOUNDATION (CBDF)

350 Parnassus Avenue
Suite 900
San Francisco, CA 94117 415-566-5402
Fax: 415-863-3452

The Children's Brain Diseases Foundation is a national not-for-profit organization that raises funds for medical research into the causes and treatments of Batten Disease. Batten Disease, also known as Spielmeyer-Vogt Disease or Neuronal Ceroid Lipofuscinosis, Juvenile Type, is a rare progressive degenerative neurometabolic disorder characterized by gradual intellectual deterioration, seizure episodes, progressive motor impairment, and progressive visual impairment. Symptoms typically begin to occur at approximately five to 13 years of age. Founded in 1968, the Foundation provides information on Batten Disease to affected families and their physicians and promotes public understanding of the disease. Research funds are provided to investigators to help maintain the momentum of research on Batten Disease; pursue new scientific opportunities in this area of study; and promote early diagnosis, effective treatment, and prevention of Batten Disease. The Foundation produces educational brochures including "Help To Keep the Color In a Child's Life: Erase Batten Disease."

President: J. Alfred Rider, M.D., PhD
Executive Director: J. Alfred Rider, M.D., Ph.D
Year Established: 1968

Publishes the following materials:
Help to Keep the Color in a Child's Life - Erase Batten Disease ~ *Brochure*

Concerned with the following diseases or disorders:
Alexander's Disease; Batten Disease; Hydranencephaly; Joubert Syndrome; Kufs Disease; Leigh's Disease; Santavuori Disease

1198 CHILDREN'S PKU NETWORK (CPN)

1520 State Street, Suite 240
San Diego, CA 92101 619-233-3202
Fax: 619-233-0838
E-mail: pkunetwork@aol.com

The Children's PKU Network (CPN) is a not-for-profit organization dedicated to providing support and services to children with Phenylketonuria (PKU), their families, and all those involved in the treatment of this disorder. PKU is a metabolic disorder characterized by severe mental retardation, seizures, and/or other abnormalities that may be prevented through early restriction of dietary phenylalanine. The Network serves as a central operational base to assist in the gathering and dissemination of information on PKU and other related disorders, operates a national network hotline to provide PKU families with information about PKU clinics and support groups in their area, seeks to educate legislators concerning the needs of PKU families, and establishes programs for college scholarships, crisis intervention, and research. The Children's PKU Network also provides a variety of educational and support materials through its informational database, regular newsletter, reprints of medical journal articles, pamphlets, booklets, brochures, videos, and materials specifically for affected children.

President: Holly Wolf (1991-Present)
Executive Director: Suzanne Bowlby
Year Established: 1991

Publishes the following materials:
Children's PKU Network - Did You Know ~ *Brochure*
Children's PKU Network - A Non Profit Organization ~ *Brochure*
Children's PKU Network Update ~ *Brochure*
Publications Available Through Children's PKU Network ~ *Publication List*

Concerned with the following diseases or disorders:
Phenylketonuria

1199 **CHRONIC GRANULOMATOUS DISEASE ASSOCIATION, INC. (CGDA)**

2616 Monterey Road
San Marino, CA 91108 818-441-4118
E-mail: amhurley@pacificnet.net

The Chronic Granulomatous Disease Association is an international not-for-profit organization founded in 1982. The Association provides information on current treatments and medical research related to Chronic Granulomatous Disease (CGD), an X-linked or autosomal recessive immunodeficiency disorder characterized by frequent prolonged fungal and bacterial infections affecting the skin, lungs, genitourinary tract, and mucous membranes of the mouth and intestines. The organization provides emotional support to people with CGD, their families, physicians, and other organizations; provides networking services; has a physician referral service; and maintains a medical library containing medical articles about CGD and patient treatment funding information. The organization also distributes a variety of materials including booklets, guides, the "CDG Resource Directory," a patient questionnaire, a referral guide to medical articles on CGD, and a quarterly newsletter.

President: Mary Hurley (1982-Present)
Organization Language: Spanish.
Year Established: 1982
Organization Members: 600

Publishes the following materials:
Chronic Granulomatous Disease Association ~ *Questionnaire*
Chronic Granulomatous Disease Association, Inc. Fact Sheet ~ *Fact Sheet*
Chronic Granulomatous Disease Association Newsletter ~ *Newsletter*
Chronic Granulomatous Disease Reference Guide to Medical Articles ~ *Article Listing*
Chronic Granulomatous Disease - A Guide for CGD Patients and Their Famiies ~ *Booklet*

Concerned with the following diseases or disorders:
Granulomatous Disease, Chronic

1200 **CHURG-STRAUSS SYNDROME INTERNATIONAL SUPPORT GROUP (CSSISG)**

2 Saint Andrews Court
St. Augustine, FL 32084 904-824-1083
E-mail: robbins@aug.com

The Churg-Strauss Syndrome International Support Group (CSSISG) is a voluntary organization dedicated to providing information and support to families of individuals affected by Churg-Strauss Syndrome. Churg-Strauss Syndrome is a lung disorder often occurring as a complication of other disorders. Allergic blood vessel inflammation (angiitis or vasculitis) is accompanied by many inflammatory nodular lesions (granulomatosis) that may be small or granular, and are made up of compactly grouped cells. The age of onset varies from 15 to 70 years of age. The organization facilitates a support network for individuals affected by Churg-Strauss Syndrome and their caregivers. The organization's educational materials include reprints of medical journal articles. CSSISG also works to promote awareness of this disorder among medical professionals with the hope that awareness will lead to increased efforts in determining the cause, treatment, and eventual cure of Churg-Strauss Syndrome.

President: Rima Robbins
Year Established: 1997

Concerned with the following diseases or disorders:
Churg Strauss Syndrome

1201 **COFFIN-LOWRY SYNDROME FOUNDATION (CLSF)**

13827 196th Avenue, SE
Renton, WA 98059 425-204-9176
E-mail: M_C_Hoffman@msn.com

The Coffin-Lowry Syndrome Foundation is a national not-for-profit self-help organization that functions as a clearinghouse for information on Coffin-Lowry Syndrome and as a general forum for exchanging experiences, advice, and information with other families affected by this rare disorder. Coffin-Lowry Syndrome is a genetic disorder characterized by mental deficiency, an inability to speak, and musculoskeletal abnormalities. Founded in 1991, the Coffin-Lowry Syndrome Foundation seeks to become a visible group in the medical, scientific, educational, and professional communities to facilitate referrals of newly diagnosed individuals and to encourage medical and behavioral research aimed at finding the cause of Coffin-Lowry Syndrome. The organization also seeks to improve methods of social integration of people with this disorder. The Coffin-Lowry Syndrome Foundation also maintains an informational database on children with the disorder, has a mailing list of families affected by Coffin-Lowry Syndrome, provides medical journal articles, and has a quarterly newsletter.

President: Mary Hoffman
Year Established: 1991
Organization Members: 80

Publishes the following materials:
Facts About Coffin-Lowry Syndrome ~ *Brochure*
CLSF News ~ *Newsletter*

Concerned with the following diseases or disorders:
Coffin Lowry Syndrome

1202 COGAN'S CONTACT NETWORK (CCN)

P.O. Box 713
Garfield, NJ 07026-0713
Fax: 973-471-3690
TDD: 973-471-3690
E-mail: uscogans@aol.com

The Cogan's Contact Network is a national nonprofit organization formed by and for individuals who are affected by Cogan's Syndrome as a means of sharing medical information and encouraging research efforts. Cogan's Syndrome is a rare disease that is characterized by hearing impairment; dysfunction of that portion of the ear that helps to regulate balance; abnormal ringing sensations (tinnitus); and possible eye problems (e.g., interstitial keratitis). In addition to providing brochures explaining Cogan's Syndrome, the Network also disseminates copies of current medical literature and publishes a periodic newsletter. The Network also encourages ongoing medical research into the prevention and treatment of Cogan's Syndrome.

President: Anthony Yuppa (1989 to Present)
Year Established: 1989
Organization Members: 25

Publishes the following materials:
Cogan's Syndrome. Sudden Hearing Loss, Vertigo, Tinnitus, Eye Problems, Inflammatory Bowel Disease, Systemic Vascu ~ *Brochure*
Cogan's Syndrome. Information provided by Cogan's Contacts ~ *Brochure*

1203 COHEN SYNDROME SUPPORT GROUP (CSSG)

7 Woods Court
Brackley
Northants, NN13 6HP
United Kingdom 012-807-0 45

The Cohen Syndrome Support Group (CSSG) is an international nonprofit organization dedicated to providing parent to parent contact for families affected by Cohen Syndrome. Cohen Syndrome is a rare genetic disorder characterized by multiple facial, oral, and eye abnormalities, muscle weakness, obesity, and mental retardation. Children with Cohen Syndrome usually have a low birthweight, delayed growth, and obesity of the trunk that occurs during mid-childhood. Other characteristics of this disorder may include an unusually small head (microcephaly), large ears, a high nasal bridge, an abnormally short groove in the middle of the upper lip (philtrum), and prominent lips and upper central incisors. Established in 1994, CSSG publishes a quarterly newsletter and an informational brochure entitled "Cohen Syndrome, A Guide For Parents." Comprised of 29 members, the organization is dedicated to providing international networking opportunities for affected families.

President: Frances M. Osborn (1994 to Present) (Contact Person)
Organization Language: Dutch (spoken). French (spoken). German (spoken). Spanish (spoken). Italian (spoken). Norwergian (spoken). Russian (spoken). Finnish (spoken).
Year Established: 1994
Organization Members: 29

Publishes the following materials:
Cohen Syndrome. A Guide For Parents ~ *Booklet*
Cohen Syndrome ~ *Brochure*

Concerned with the following diseases or disorders:
Cohen Syndrome

1204 CONGENITAL CENTRAL HYPOVENTILATION SYNDROME (CCHS) FAMILY SUPPORT NETWORK

71 Maple Street
Oneonta, NY 13820 607-432-8872
E-mail: VanderlaanM@Hartwick.Edu

The Congenital Central Hypoventilation Syndrome (CCHS) Family Support Network is voluntary not-for-profit self-help organization dedicated to providing support and information to families with children affected by Congenital Central Hypoventilation Syndrome (CCHS). Congenital Central Hypoventilation Syndrome is a rare neurological disorder of infancy and childhood characterized by a decrease in respiratory function during sleep. Established in 1989, the CCHS Family Support Network consists of families in the United States, Canada, and across the world who have children with CCHS. The Network seeks to promote ongoing medical research into the cause, course, and treatment of CCHS; promotes the continuing education of the medical community about CCHS and affected individuals' special needs; provides appropriate referrals; promotes patient advocacy; and provides members with a phone directory of affected families. The Network also produces a regular newsletter.

President: Mary B. Vanderlaan (1989-Present)
Executive Director: Mary B. Vanderlaan
Year Established: 1989
Organization Members: 135

Publishes the following materials:
CCHS Family Newsletter ~ *Newsletter*

Concerned with the following diseases or disorders:
Central Hypoventilation Syndrome, Congenital

1205 CONJOINED TWINS INTERNATIONAL (CTI)

P.O. Box 10895
Prescott, AZ 86304-0895 520-445-0572
Fax: 520-445-8043

Conjoined Twins International (CTI) is a voluntary organization dedicated to providing moral and personal support to families of conjoined twins. Established in 1996 and consisting of 30 family members, CTI has support groups, provides networking services, promotes research, and offers referrals to physicians and hospitals with expertise in working with conjoined twins. The organization also offers educational and supportive materials through its database, reports, and regular newsletter.

Executive Director: Will L. Degeraty
Year Established: 1996
Organization Chapters: 1
Organization Members: 30

1206 CONVOMANIA, A WEB SITE FOR CHILDREN WITH CHRONIC OR SERIOUS ILLNESSES OR DISABILITIES

E-mail: mania@apple.com
http://www.mania.apple.com

Convomania is a web site on the Internet for children with serious or chronic illnesses or disabilities. Sponsored by the Worldwide Disability Solutions Group at Apple Computer in association with several partner sites including leading children's hospitals, cancer camps, and disability advocacy organizations, Convomania was created to provide kids with serious illnesses a place on the Internet where they can openly share their thoughts, concerns, and common experiences in a "cyber-community setting." The web site has several main areas designed to help children express themselves and offer support to one another: "Say It," a place where kids participate in online chats; "Stick It," a digital magnetic poetry game that helps facilitate expression; "Share It," a message board for kids to share ideas 24 hours a day; "Solve It," a place to ask questions and receive answers about living with chronic illness; "Sketch It," a digital art gallery focusing on illness-related themes; "Show It," a forum for children to express themselves using theater arts skills; and "See It," a yearbook of "Convomania" community members from around the country. Convomania is located at [http://www.mania.apple.com].

1207 COOLEY'S ANEMIA FOUNDATION, INC. (CAF)

129-09 26th Avenue
Suite 203
Flushing, NY 11354-1131 718-321-2873
800-522-7222
Fax: 718-321-3340
E-mail: NCAF@aol.com
http://www.thalassemia.org

The Cooley's Anemia Foundation, Inc. is a national not-for-profit organization dedicated to advancing the treatment and cure of Cooley's Anemia, an inherited blood disorder. Established in 1940, the Foundation conducts national programs that promote medical research and provides a variety of patient services and educational programs. The Foundation has more than 15 chapters throughout the United States and supports the Thalassemia Action Group (TAG), a support group for affected individuals and their families. The Cooley's Anemia Foundation provides information, referrals to local medical sources, medical supplies to people in need, and listings of informational materials available from the Foundation including video tapes, brochures, and regular newsletters.

President: Peter Chieco (1994-Present)
Executive Director: Gina Cioffi
Organization Language: Italian. Chinese. Greek. Spanish. Arabic.
Year Established: 1940
Organization Chapters: 16
Organization Members: 5,000

Publishes the following materials:
The Wish ~ *Video Tape*

"Tag Your It" ~ *Videotape*
The Fight Against Thalassemia ~ *Brochure*
The Cooley's Anemia Foundation, Inc. ~ *Brochure*
Cooley's Anemia Fact Sheet ~ *Fact Sheet*
Thalassemia It's Your Choice ~ *Brochure*
What is Cooley's Anemia? ~ *Booklet*
1992 Management Protocol for the Treatment of Thalassemia Patients ~ *Booklet*
Cooley's Anemia Foundation, Inc. Informational Material ~ *Material List*
Precious Time...A Gift of Life ~ *Brochure*
Lifeline ~ *Newsletter*
Investing in a fight against childhood killer ~ *Article Reprint*
Being an Italian-American Isn't Always a Wonderful Thing ~ *Flier*
Thalassemia Action Group ~ *Brochure*
TAG Newsletter ~ *Newsletter*
"T.A.G. ALONG" ~ *Flier*
My Coloring Book on Thalassemia ~ *Book*
What is Cooley's Anemia? ~ *Booklet*
The Cooley's Anemia Foundation, Inc. ~ *Brochure*
All You Need to Know About Being a Carrier of Cooley's Anemia ~ *Leaflet*
A Parent's Experience ~ *Brochure*
Cooley's Anemia Fact Sheet ~ *Fact Sheet*

Concerned with the following diseases or disorders:
Sickle Cell Disease; Thalassemia Major; Thalassemia Minor

1208 CORNELIA DE LANGE SYNDROME FOUNDATION, INC. (CDLS)

302 West Main Street
#100
Avon, CT 06001 860-676-8166
800-223-8355
Fax: 860-676-8337
E-mail: cdlsintl@iconn.net
http://cdlsoutreach.org

The Cornelia de Lange Syndrome Foundation, Inc. is an international nonprofit family support group. Cornelia de Lange Syndrome is a rare genetic disorder characterized by severe mental retardation, short stature, and characteristic craniofacial abnormalities including an abnormally short, wide head, bushy eyebrows that meet above the nose, a depressed nasal bridge, low-set ears, and other abnormalities. Established in 1981, the Foundation's mission is to ensure early and accurate diagnosis of Cornelia de Lange Syndrome and to enable families, friends, and medical professionals to make informed decisions regarding treatment options for individuals with this rare disorder. For information and support purposes, the Cornelia de Lange Syndrome Foundation publishes a number of educational materials including a bimonthly newsletter entitled "Reaching Out," a photographic and descriptive Album, a booklet entitled "Facing the Challenge: A Book for Families," and a brochure about Cornelia de Lange Syndrome. The organization also offers a toll-free informational number, holds an annual conference for parents and professionals, and promotes research into the cause and symptoms of this disorder.

President: Roy Gonella (1996 - Present).
Executive Director: Julie A. Mairano, M.S.
Year Established: 1981

Publishes the following materials:
Facts about Cornelia de Lange Syndrome ~ *Brochure*
Facing the Challenges: A Family's Guide to Cornelia de Lange Syndrome ~ *Booklet*
Reaching Out ~ *Newsletter*
Album 1993-1994 ~ *Book*
Attention All Professionals "CdLS Link" ~ *Application*
CdLS Video Library ~ *Order Form*

Concerned with the following diseases or disorders:
Cornelia de Lange Syndrome

1209 CREUTZFELDT-JAKOB DISEASE FOUNDATION, INC. (CJD FOUNDATION)

P.O. Box 611625
Miami, FL 33261-1625 305-891-7579
E-mail: crjakob@aol.com
http://members.aol.com/crjakob

The Creutzfeldt-Jakob Disease (CJD) Foundation, Inc., a national voluntary not-for-profit organization, is dedicated to promoting research into CJD, increasing awareness of the disorder, and reaching out to families with loved ones affected by CJD. Creutzfeldt-Jakob Disease is an extremely rare degenerative brain disorder (i.e., spongiform encephalopathy) characterized by the sudden onset of rapidly progressive neurological and neuromuscular symptoms. Such symptoms, which may include lack of coordination, muscle weakness, impairment of vision, dementia, repeated shock-like muscle spasms (myoclonus), coma, and susceptibility to repeated respiratory infections, may result in life-threatening complications less than a year after the disorder becomes apparent. Established in 1993, the CJD Foundation collects and disseminates information on CJD, provides referrals, and offers general information on other human prion diseases such as Gerstmann-Straussler-Scheinker Disease, Kuru, and Fatal Familial Insomnia as well as suspected prion disorders in animals (such as Bovine Spongiform Encephalopathy, also known as "Mad Cow Disease," scrapie, etc.). The CJD Foundation also has a web site on the Internet that provides understandable information on Creutzfeldt-Jakob Disease; enables family members of affected individuals to exchange information, support, and resources; and provides a bibliographic listing of additional references on prion disorders including government, scientific, and medical publications. The site also provides links to indepth articles from the peer-reviewed medical literature concerning these disorders and offers dynamic links to other helpful sources of information on the Internet. The CJD Foundation's web site is located at [http://members.aol.com/crjakob].

President: Mayra R. Lichter (1993 to Present)
Executive Director: Cecile L. Sardo (Secretary)
Organization Language: Spanish (written/spoken).
Year Established: 1993

Publishes the following materials:
Creutzfeldt-Jakob Disease Foundation, Inc. ~ *Leaflet*
Reprints ~ *Pamphlet*
Creutzfeldt-Jakob Disease Foundation, Inc. ~ *Leaflet*

Concerned with the following diseases or disorders:
Creutzfeldt Jakob Disease

1210 CRI DU CHAT SYNDROME SUPPORT GROUP

7 Penny Lane
Barwell
Leicester, LE9 8HJ
United Kingdom 01455 841680
E-mail: jeff@cridchat-u-net.com
http://www.personal.u-net.com/~cridchat

The Cri Du Chat Syndrome Support Group is an international nonprofit organization located in the United Kingdom. Established in 1991 and consisting of 180 families, the Group exists primarily to support parents and caregivers of individuals with Cri Du Chat Syndrome and to provide appropriate information on this disorder. Cri Du Chat, a rare chromosomal disorder caused by a partial deletion of chromosomal material from the short arm of chromosome 5 (5p deletion), is characterized by a distinctive catlike cry during infancy, mild to severe mental retardation, and craniofacial abnormalities including widely spaced eyes, a broad nasal bridge, an abnormally small head (microcephaly), and round face. The Cri Du Chat Syndrome Support Group is committed to providing support for families and caregivers through a network of area families; raising awareness of Cri Du Chat Syndrome among medical professionals, parents, caregivers, and the general public; raising funds to promote and support ongoing research into the treatment of this disorder; distributing information; and organizing an annual conference and family meeting for affected families and health care professionals. The Support Group publishes a regular newsletter, distributes informational brochures on the disorder, and maintains a web site at [http://www.personal.u-net.com/~cridchat].

President: Angela Stokes (Coordinator) (1994 to Present)
Executive Director: Ray Clarke (Chairman)
Year Established: 1991
Organization Members: 180

Publishes the following materials:
Providing Support and Friendship for Families and Carers ~ *Brochure*
Cri Du Chat Syndrome Support Group ~ *Brochure*
Cri Du Chat Syndrome Support Group Newsletter (Winter 96/97) ~ *Newsletter*

Concerned with the following diseases or disorders:
Cri du Chat Syndrome

1211 CUSHING SUPPORT AND RESEARCH FOUNDATION, INC. (CSRF)

65 East India Row
#22B
Boston, MA 02110 617-723-3674
Fax: 617-723-3674
http://world.std.com/~CSRF/

The Cushing Support and Research Foundation, Inc. is a not-for-profit organization dedicated to providing information and support to individuals and family members affected by Cushing's Disease and Cushing's Syndrome. Cushing's Syndrome is a rare endocrine disorder caused by abnormally increased secretion of adrenocortical hormones due to tumors of the adrenal cortex or part of the pituitary gland or prolonged intake of glucocorticoids. When symptoms are due to increased levels of adrenocortical hormones resulting from excessive pituitary secretion, the disorder is called Cushing's Disease. Established in 1995, the Cushing Support and Research Foundation is committed to increasing public awareness of these two disorders; serving as a source of information and support for health care professionals; and raising and distributing funds for Cushing's Disease and Cushing's Syndrome research. The Foundation also enables affected individuals to exchange information, resources, and support through its networking program; provides appropriate referrals (e.g., to support groups); and offers a variety of educational materials including a newsletter, fact sheets, and brochures.

President: Louise Pace
Executive Director: Mary Brim
Year Established: 1995
Organization Members: 300

Publishes the following materials:
Cushing Syndrome ~ *Factsheet*
The Cushing's Newsleter ~ *Newsletter*

Concerned with the following diseases or disorders:
Cushing Syndrome

1212 CUTANEOUS LYMPHOMA NETWORK

234 Goodman Street
Pavilion A-3
Cincinnati, OH 45267-0523

The Cutaneous Lymphoma Network, which is associated with the University of Cincinnati's Department of Dermatology, is a not-for-profit organization dedicated to providing educational and supportive resources to individuals who have Cutaneous T-Cell Lymphoma, a group of lymphomas or neoplasms of lymphoid tissue characterized by malignant infiltration of the skin. Established in 1989, the group publishes a quarterly newsletter entitled "Cutaneous Lymphoma Network" for affected individuals, family members, and health care professionals. The newsletter includes medical articles on Cutaneous T-Cell Lymphoma (CTCL), excerpts from symposia on CTCL, reprints of articles, and subscriber letters. It also has listings of resources for information and support, a medical question-and-answer column, and listings of books, videos, and other materials of interest. A form to register for the Network's pen pal service, which enables affected individuals to communicate directly with one another, is also included in the newsletter.

President: Judi Van Horn, RN, Editor
Executive Director: Debra Breneman, MD
Year Established: 1989
Organization Members: 1,500

Publishes the following materials:
Cutaneous Lymphoma Network ~ *Newsletter*

Concerned with the following diseases or disorders:
Mycosis Fungoides

1213 CYCLIC VOMITING SYNDROME ASSOCIATION (CVSA)

13180 Caroline Court
Elm Grove, WI 53122 414-784-6842
Fax: 414-821-5494
E-mail: kadams@post.its.mcw.edu
http://www.beaker.iupui.edu/cvsa/

The Cyclic Vomiting Syndrome Association (CVSA) is a voluntary not-for-profit self-help organization dedicated to giving affected individuals, families, and health care professionals the opportunity to offer and receive support and share knowledge about Cyclic Vomiting Syndrome (CVS). The organization also promotes ongoing medical research into CVS; increases worldwide public and professional awareness of the syndrome; and serves as a resource center for information on CVS. Established in 1993 by parents of children with CVS and health care professionals, the Cyclic Vomiting Syndrome Association provides appropriate referrals, promotes patient advocacy, and enables affected families to network nationally and internationally to exchange information and provide mutual support. In addition, the Cyclic Vomiting Syndrome Association offers a variety of educational materials to parents, health care professionals, and the general public through its computer database, regional directory, regular newsletter, reports, brochures, and videos.

President: Kathleen Adams (1993-Present)
Organization Language: Spanish. German. French. Russian. Greek.
Year Established: 1993
Organization Chapters: 11
Organization Members: 600

Publishes the following materials:
Cyclic Vomiting Syndrome Association ~ *Bibliography*
Cyclic Vomiting Syndrome A Fact Sheet ~ *Fact Sheet*
Do You Know A Child Who Vomits For Prolonged Periods? ~ *Brochure*
Educational Video Order Form ~ *Order Form*
CVSA Materials List ~ *Materials List*
CVSA News ~ *Newsletter*

Concerned with the following diseases or disorders:
Cyclic Vomiting Syndrome

1214 CYSTIC FIBROSIS FOUNDATION (CFF)

6931 Arlington Rd.
Bethesda, MD 20814 301-951-4422
800-344-4823
Fax: 301-951-6378

The Cystic Fibrosis Foundation (CFF) is a voluntary not-for-profit organization dedicated to raising funds for research to find a cure for cystic fibrosis (CF) and improving the quality of life for individuals with the disease. Cystic fibrosis is a rare inherited disorder that affects many exocrine ("outward-secreting") glands of the body including the sweat glands, salivary glands, and those within the pancreas and respiratory system. Established in 1955 and currently consisting of more than 70 chapters and branch offices across the country, the Cystic Fibrosis Foundation funds its own network of CF research centers at leading universities and medical schools throughout North America. It provides a variety of grants to scientists to fund CF research and finances over 100 CF care centers nationwide. The organization supports clinical trials at its care centers to test new drug therapies for CF and works closely with Congress, the Food and Drug Administration, and pharmaceutical companies to speed the development of new drugs to treat CF. The Foundation offers affected individuals, family members, health care professionals, and the public a variety of informational materials including research updates, regular newsletters, and brochures on several topics such as health insurance and financial assistance programs.

President: Robert J. Beall, PhD
Executive Director: C. Richard Mattingly
Year Established: 1955
Organization Chapters: 70

Publishes the following materials:
Make a Difference in the Life of a Child ~ *Factsheet*
Foundation Facts ~ *Factsheet*
Facts About CF ~ *Factsheet*
Gene Therapy and CF ~ *Factsheet*
Homeline ~ *Factsheet*
Commitment ~ *Newsletter*

Concerned with the following diseases or disorders:
Cystic Fibrosis

1215 CYSTINOSIS FOUNDATION, INC.

2516 Stockbridge Drive
Oakland, CA 94611
800-392-8458
Fax: 510-482-8119
E-mail: jdzhotz@qnis.net
www-cystinosisfoundation.ucsd.edu

The Cystinosis Foundation is a not-for-profit self-help organization dedicated to providing information and support to individuals affected by Cystinosis, a rare inherited lysosomal disorder characterized by the abnormal accumulation of cystine crystals in tissues throughout the body, which may cause certain organs to malfunction. Three main forms of Cystinosis are recognized: Infantile Nephropathic Cystinosis, Adolescent Cystinosis (also called Intermediate or Juvenile Cystinosis), and Adult Cystinosis (also known as Benign Cystinosis). Established in 1983, the Cystinosis Foundation is committed to raising awareness of the disorder in the medical and research communities and the public. The Foundation offers support to affected individuals and their families; provides appropriate referrals; engages in patient, family, and professional education; and promotes and supports research. The Cystinosis Foundation provides a directory and a regular newsletter, which includes medical updates, editorials, member feedback, and listings of literature concerning Cystinosis.

President: Jean Hobbs Hote (1983-Present)
Year Established: 1983
Organization Members: 150

Concerned with the following diseases or disorders:
Cystinosis

1216 CYSTINURIA SUPPORT NETWORK (CSN)

21001 NE 36th Street
Redmond, WA 98053 425-868-2996
E-mail: cystinuria@aol.com

The Cystinuria Support Network is a national self-help organization that functions as a mutual aid and support network for people with Cystinuria and their caregivers. Cystinuria is a rare genetic disorder characterized by excessive urinary excretion of the amino acid cystine and other amino acids, and the formation of urinary cystine kidney stones (calculi). The Network was developed to provide a central resource for networking affected individuals for the purpose of mutual support and practical advice. The organization allows people to come together with their own unique strengths, hopes, and concerns to offer support and understanding to one another. Established in 1994, the Cystinuria Support Network publishes a periodic newsletter with input from group participants and medical professionals.

President: Jann P. Ledbetter (1994-Present)
Executive Director: Jann P. Ledbetter
Year Established: 1994
Organization Members: 100

Publishes the following materials:
Cystinuria Support Network News ~ *Newsletter*

Concerned with the following diseases or disorders:
Cystinuria

1217 **DES ACTION**
1615 Broadway
Suite 510
Oakland, CA 94612 510-465-4011
800-337-9288
Fax: 510-465-4815
E-mail: desact@well.com
http://www.desaction.org

DES Action is a nonprofit organization that offers medical information, physician referrals, special publications, and quarterly newsletters to help those exposed in-utero to the estrogen hormone DES (Diethylstilbestrol). DES was given to patients under the mistaken belief that it would prevent miscarriages. Unfortunately, it causes serious side effects resulting in birth defects in affected newborns. Founded in 1979, DES Action offers a toll-free hotline for affected individuals and their families, promotes research, has educational programs, engages in patient advocacy, and works for appropriate government legislation in the area of DES. DES Action also offers reports, a newsletter entitled "Voice," and brochures entitled "DES Daughters," "DES Sons," and "Talking About DES: A Guide for Families." Many of the publications are available in Spanish. Consisting of 3,500 members, DES Action is able to serve affected individuals and families worldwide through its sister groups in Australia, Belgium, Canada, France, the Netherlands, Ireland, Italy, and England.

President: Amanda Sherman (1995 to Present).
Executive Director: Nora Cody
Organization Language: Spanish (written).
Year Established: 1979
Organization Chapters: 22
Organization Members: 3500

Publishes the following materials:
Find Out About DES Exposure ~ *Brochure*
DES. Could You Be A DES Son? ~ *Brochure*
Were You Born Between 1938 and 1971 Or Pregnant Then? If So, You Could Be Exposed To DES ~ *Booklet*
Talking About DES. A Family Guide for DES-Exposed Mothers, Daughters, and Sons ~ *Booklet*
DES Daughters. Women Born Between 1938 and 1971 Who Were Exposed to DES Before Birth ~ *Booklet*
Facts About DES ~ *Fact Sheet*
Women Who Took DES. A guide for Women Who Took DES During Pregnancy From 1938 to 1971 ~ *Booklet*
Find Out About DES Exposure. If you were born between 1938 and 1971 ~ *Brochure*
Could You Be A DES Son? ~ *Brochure*
DES Daughters. ~ *Booklet*

1218 **DANCING EYE SYNDROME SUPPORT TRUST (DES SUPPORT TRUST)**
78 Quantock Road
Worthing
West Sussex, BN13 2HQ
United Kingdom 01903 532383
Fax: 01903 532383
E-mail: rasr@mistral.co.uk

Dancing Eye Syndrome Support Trust is an international voluntary organization based in the United Kingdom that is dedicated to providing information and support to individuals affected by Dancing Eye Syndrome and their families. Dancing Eye Syndrome (also known as Kinsbourne Syndrome or Opsoclonus Myoclonus) is a rare neurological disorder of unknown cause that typically becomes apparent between the ages of one to three years, although, in rare cases, it may occur at any time during childhood or early adolescence. The disorder is characterized by an unsteady gait; rhythmic, involuntary motions of certain areas during voluntary movements (intention tremor); brief, shock-like muscle spasms of the arms, legs, or entire body (myoclonus); and irregular, rapid, horizontal and vertical eye movements (opsoclonus). Formed in 1988 as a support group in the United Kingdom, the Dancing Eye Syndrome Support Trust became a trust in 1997. The Trust is committed to enabling parents of affected children to exchange information, support, and resources. In addition, the Dancing Eye Syndrome Support Trust holds regular meetings for members, promotes research, and offers a variety of materials including pamphlets and a regular newsletter.

President: Jane Stanton-Roberts (Secretary) (1994 to Present)
Year Established: 1997
Organization Members: 48

Publishes the following materials:
Dancing Eye Syndrome Support Trust ~ *Brochure*

Concerned with the following diseases or disorders:
Kinsbourne Syndrome

1219 **DANDY-WALKER SYNDROME NETWORK (DWSN)**
5030 142nd Path West
Apple Valley, MN 55124 612-423-4008

The Dandy-Walker Syndrome Network (DWSN) is a nonprofit organization that provides information and support to individuals and family members affected by Dandy-

Walker Syndrome and the physicians who treat them. Dandy-Walker Syndrome is a rare malformation of the brain that is present at birth. Established in 1996, DWSN offers family networking services and a variety of materials including studies that explain the effects of Dandy Walker Syndrome.

President: Desiree Fleming
Year Established: 1996

Concerned with the following diseases or disorders:
Dandy Walker Malformation

1220 DANISH APERT SYNDROME ASSOCIATION (DANMARKS APERTFORENING)

Dronningeengen 17
Vedbaek, DK-2950
Denmark 45 4589 0300
Fax: 45 4589 0300

The Danish Apert Syndrome Association (Danmarks Apertforening) is an international voluntary not-for-profit organization dedicated to providing information and support to individuals and family members affected by Apert Syndrome. Also known as Acrocephalosyndactyly Type I, Apert Syndrome is a rare genetic disorder characterized by premature closure of the fibrous joints between certain bones of the skull (craniosynostosis), causing the head to appear abnormally long and narrow (acrocephaly). Additional abnormalities may typically include a prominent forehead; protruding, widely spaced eyes; and/or webbing or fusion of the fingers and/or toes (syndactyly). Established in 1991, the Association is committed to establishing and supporting contacts between individuals and families affected by Apert Syndrome; increasing awareness of the disorder; ensuring appropriate, effective treatments; and advocating on behalf of affected individuals with health care institutions and professionals. The Association also promotes and supports research; establishes and maintains contacts with other international not-for-profit organizations; has support groups; and offers family networking services. The Association's materials include a regular newsletter.

President: Soeren Lildal (1991 to Present)
Organization Language: Danish (written/spoken).
Year Established: 1991
Organization Members: 15

Concerned with the following diseases or disorders:
Apert Syndrome

1221 DAVID G. JAGELMAN INHERITED COLORECTAL CANCER REGISTRIES

Dept. of Colorectal Cancer Registry
A-111 Cleveland Clinic Found
9500 Euclid Ave.
Cleveland, OH 44195 216-444-6470
800-998-4785
Fax: 216-445-6343

Established in 1978, the David G. Jagelman Inherited Colorectal Cancer Registries is a not-for-profit academic medical center recognized as a National Referral Center and an international resource for diseases of the colon and rectum. Dedicated to identifying, educating, and serving affected individuals, the organization has an educational division, a research institute, and a hospital and outpatient clinic. The organization offers risk assessments and appropriate screening tests; maintains computerized registries of affected individuals and those who may be at risk (e.g., for Familial Adenomatous Polyposis, Hereditary Nonpolyposis Colorectal Cancer, and Familial Colon Cancer). It suggests surveillance protocols and reviews surgical options for affected individuals. David G. Jagelman Inherited Colorectal Cancer Registries also provides a variety of educational and support materials including brochures, pamphlets, articles, and a newsletter called "Family Matters."

President: Dr. James Church (Director)
Executive Director: Ellen McGannon (Coordinator)
Year Established: 1978
Organization Members: 5,000

Publishes the following materials:
Inherited Colorectal Cancer Screening Program - What is Your Risk? ~ *Brochure*
Familial Adenomatous Polyposis-A Guide for People at Risk ~ *Pamphlet*
Familial Adenomatous Polyposis - A Guide for Parents ~ *Booklet*
Family Matters ~ *Newsletter*

1222 DERCUM'S CONNECTION (TDC)

712 Lincoln Avenue
Leesburg, FL 34748 352-728-4367

The Dercum's Connection is an international not-for-profit organization dedicated to serving as a liaison between affected individuals, physicians, and researchers; gathering and disseminating information and documentation concerning Dercum's Disease; and fostering research into the treatment and possible cure of the disorder. Dercum's Disease, also known as Adiposis Dolorosa, is characterized by painful, localized swelling and weakness in certain areas of the body due to pressure on particular nerves from abnormal fatty deposits. The disorder, which is of unknown cause, affects primarily women. Established in 1996, the Dercum's Connection has a registry of individuals with the disorder, offers patient networking services, engages in patient advocacy, promotes research, engages in patient and professional education, and has a database of information concerning Dercum's Disease.

President: Linda R. Robinson (1996 to Present)
Year Established: 1996
Organization Members: 4

Concerned with the following diseases or disorders:
Dercum Disease

1223 DIAMOND BLACKFAN ANEMIA REGISTRY (DBAR)

Mount Sinai School of Medicine
Pediatric Hematology/Oncology
One Gustave Levy Place
Box 1208
New York, NY 10029 212-241-6031
Fax: 212-360-6921
E-mail: avlachos@smtplink.mssm.ed
None.

The Diamond Blackfan Anemia Registry (DBAR), associated with the Department of Pediatric Hematology/Oncology at Mount Sinai School of Medicine, is a research organization dedicated to acquiring, analyzing, and disseminating information on Diamond Blackfan Anemia to affected individuals, their families, and medical professionals. Diamond Blackfan Anemia (DBA) is a rare genetic disorder characterized by moderate to severe deficiency of red blood cells. Blood cell abnormalities may be accompanied by an unusual physical appearance, paleness, weakness, and lethargy. The Registry was established in 1993 to better understand the cause(s) in order to develop treatment alternatives and, ultimately, find a cure for DBA. Affected individuals and/or their families enroll in the Registry by completing a registration form. This is followed by a detailed questionnaire which is completed by the affected individual, his or her family, and physician(s). Families can choose to have their name released to a family support group and they also receive a regular

Executive Director: Adrianna Vlachos, M.D.
Organization Language: Spanish (spoken). French (spoken). Greek (spoken).
Year Established: 1993
Organization Members: 250

Concerned with the following diseases or disorders:
Anemia, Blackfan Diamond

1224 DYSAUTONOMIA FOUNDATION, INC. (FD)

20 East 46th Street
Room 302
New York, NY 10017 212-949-6644
Fax: 212-682-7625
http://www.med.nyu.edu/fd/fdcenter.html

The Dysautonomia Foundation is a national nonprofit organization founded in 1951 by parents of children with Familial Dysautonomia, a rare genetic disorder characterized by dysfunction of the autonomic nervous system (ANS). Symptoms and findings may include absence of pain sensation, defective secretion and discharge of tears (lacrimation), unusual fluctuations of body temperature, unstable blood pressure, skin blotching, impaired coordination, abnormally decreased reflex responses (hyporeflexia), and/or other abnormalities. The Foundation has chapters located throughout the United States, Canada, the United Kingdom, and Israel. The Foundation supports ongoing medical research and the clinical care of children with this disorder by maintaining the Familial Dysautonomia Treatment and Evaluation Center at New York University Medical Center, New York, New York and the Israeli Familial Dysautonomia Center at Hadassah Hospital in Jerusalem, Israel. In addition, the Foundation is dedicated to funding basic medical research studies, particularly studies related to identification of the Familial Dysautonomia gene. The Foundation also provides updated informational materials to members, parents, medical professionals, and other interested individuals. Such materials include a regular newsletter, brochures, and pamphlets.

President: Gerald Adler (1993-Present)
Executive Director: Lenore F. Roseman
Year Established: 1951
Organization Chapters: 16
Organization Members: 8,500

Publishes the following materials:
Are You The One? ~ *Brochure*
Dysautonomia Treatment & Evaluation Center ~ *Brochure*

Dysautonomia ~ *Brochure*
Dys/course ~ *Newsletter*

Concerned with the following diseases or disorders:
Dysautonomia, Familial

1225 DYSTROPHIC EPIDERMOLYSIS BULLOSA RESEARCH ASSOCIATION-UNITED KINGDOM (DEBRA (UK))

DEBRA House
13 Wellington Business Park
Dukes Ride
Crowthorne
Berkshire, RG45 6LS
United Kingdom 44 1344771961
E-mail: debra.uk@btinternet.com
http://www.debra.org.uk

The Dystrophic Epidermolysis Bullosa Research Association (DEBRA)—United Kingdom is a nonprofit voluntary organization dedicated to offering information, assistance, and support to people whose lives are affected by Epidermolysis Bullosa (EB). EB is a group of genetic disorders in which there is a defect causing the skin layers to separate and blister either spontaneously or at the slightest friction. Symptoms usually are apparent at or shortly after birth. Established in 1978 by a group of parents with children affected by EB, DEBRA is committed to funding international research into the causes of and possible cures for EB; providing specialist nursing and paramedical staff to support families and professionals; and publishing an extensive range of informational materials for the medical community and the general public. DEBRA is also committed to providing specialist equipment or financial support in cases of special need; organizing, where appropriate, holidays for individuals with EB and their families; coordinating and assisting in the development of EB support groups worldwide; and encouraging the development of local treatment in the regions throughout the United Kingdom. DEBRA provides referrals including to genetic counseling, engages in patient advocacy and lobbying, offers networking services, and engages in patient and professional education. The organization offers a wide range of educational materials including fact sheets, brochures, pamphlets, bookletson all aspects of EB for professionals and affected families, bibliographies of medical journal articles published on EB, and videos. DEBRA also has a web site on the Internet at [http://www.debra.org.uk].

President: Philip Evans
Executive Director: John Dart
Year Established: 1978
Organization Members: 700

Publishes the following materials:
More Than Skin Deep. How DEBRA is helping people with the genetic skin blistering condition EB ~ *Video Tape*
Coping With Epidermolysis Bullosa. A Guide for Affected Adults ~ *Booklet*
Diet For Epidermolysis Bullosa ~ *Booklet*
DEBRA. Guidelines for parents on the play and development of the child with Epidermolysis Bullosa ~ *Booklet*
A Guideline To Physiotherapy For Parents Of Children With Dystrophic Epidermolysis Bullosa ~ *Booklet*
Dental Care for your child ~ *Booklet*
Nutrition For Babies With Dystrophic Epidermolysis Bullosa ~ *Booklet*
Epidermolysis Bullosa: A Guide For Parents, Schools And Playgroups ~ *Booklet*
Care And Management Of Children With Dystrophic Epidermolysis Bullosa ~ *Booklet*
A Bibliography of Epidermolysis Bullosa ~ *Bibliography*
Supplementum 133. A bibliography of Epidermolysis Bullosa ~ *Bibliography*
DEBRA. More than Skin Deep ~ *Brochure*
Can I Go It Alone ~ *Booklet*
DEBRA. Epidermolysis Bullosa ~ *Booklet*
EB Simplex ~ *Fact Sheet*
DEBRA News ~ *Newsletter*
Annual Report 1997 ~ *Booklet*

Concerned with the following diseases or disorders:
Epidermolysis Bullosa

1226 EARL J. GOLDBERG APLASTIC ANEMIA FOUNDATION (EJGAAF)

P.O. Box 2231
Glenview, IL 60025 847-559-0688

The Earl J. Goldberg Aplastic Anemia Foundation is a nonprofit volunteer organization that functions as the Chicago area chapter of the Aplastic Anemia Foundation of America. Aplastic Anemia is a rare form of anemia in which there are abnormally low levels of red blood cells, white blood cells, and platelets in the blood. Founded in 1979, the organization provides patient and family support, supports medical research into Aplastic Anemia, and promotes public awareness and education. Educational materials include an "Answer Book," local chapter information brochures, and newsletters.

President: Caryl Kaufman
Year Established: 1979
Organization Chapters: 8
Organization Members: 130

Publishes the following materials:
EJGAAF Newsletter ~ *Newsletter*
Aplastic Anemia the "Not Enough" Disease ~ *Brochure*
Aplastic Anemia Answer Book ~ *Pamphlet*

1227 **EHLERS-DANLOS SYNDROME SUPPORT GROUP UK**

1 Chandler Close
Richmond
North Yorkshire, DL10 5QQ
United Kingdom 01748 823867
Fax: 01748 823867
E-mail: EDS_UK@compuserve.com
ourworld.compuserve.com/homepages/EDS_UK/

The Ehlers-Danlos Syndrome Support Group UK is an international not-for-profit self-help organization dedicated to informing, encouraging, and assisting those with Ehlers-Danlos Syndrome (EDS) and their family members. Ehlers-Danlos Syndrome (EDS) is a group of rare inherited connective tissue disorders characterized by abnormalities of the skin, ligaments, and internal organs. Although symptoms and physical features may vary greatly depending upon the specific form of EDS present, many affected individuals may have thin, fragile, hyperextensible skin that may bruise easily; abnormally loose joints that are prone to repeated dislocations; widespread tissue fragility with bleeding and poor healing of wounds; and/or other abnormalities. Established in 1992, the Ehlers-Danlos Syndrome Support Group UK is committed to raising awareness of EDS among the medical and professional communities; supporting research into the causes, treatment, and cure of EDS; and enabling members of the organization to exchange information, support, and resources. The Group also maintains a listing of medical specialists who have experience with EDS; holds a biennial National Conference; produces booklets, information sheets, and other materials on all aspects of EDS; offers a "Key Facts Medical Card" that is available in several languages to help affected individuals alert medical professionals to key aspects concerning EDS; and has a regular newsletter entitled "Fragile Links."

President: Valerie Burrows (1985 to Present)
Executive Director: M. Moffat
Year Established: 1992
Organization Members: 492

Publishes the following materials:
Ehlers-Danlos Syndrome ~ *Booklet*
A Guide for Teachers ~ *Booklet*
Pregnancy and Childbirth in Ehlers-Danlos Syndrome ~ *Booklet*
Ehlers-Danlos Syndrome ~ *Information Sheet*
Booklets, Ehlers-Danlos-Syndrome ~ *Order Form*
Information Sheets Available ~ *Order Form*
NO Maybe It Is EDS ~ *Factsheet*
A Guide For Teachers ~ *Booklet*
Ehlers-Danlos Syndrome ~ *Booklet*
Pregnancy and Childbirth in Ehlers-Danlos Synddrome ~ *Booklet*
Ehlers-Danlos Support Group ~ *Information Sheet*

Concerned with the following diseases or disorders:
Ehlers Danlos Syndrome

1228 **EOSINOPHILIC FASCIITIS (SHULMAN'S SYNDROME) HOME PAGE**

E-mail: thrasher@freenet.edmonton.ab.ca
www.freenet.edmonton.ab.ca/~thrasher/

The Eosinophilic Fasciitis (Shulman's Syndrome) Home Page is a web site on the Internet dedicated to providing information and support to individuals with Eosinophilic Fasciitis, family members, health care professionals, and other interested individuals. Eosinophilic Fasciitis is a disorder of unknown cause characterized by symmetric and painful inflammation, swelling, and loss of elasticity of the tissues of the hands, arms, legs, and feet. This web site provides general information on the disorder including diagnostic and treatment information and a Frequently Asked Questions (FAQ) area; personal stories; a bibliography; linkage to sources of information concerning clinical trials; dynamic linkage to additional Internet resources; and more.

Concerned with the following diseases or disorders:
Eosinophilic Fasciitis

1229 **EPILEPSY CANADA (EC)**

1470 Peel Street
Suite 745
Montreal
Quebec, H3A 1T1
Canada 514-845-7855
800-860-5499
Fax: 514-845-7866
E-mail: epilepsy@epilepsy.ca
http://www.epilepsy.ca

Epilepsy Canada (EC) is a not-for-profit organization dedicated to enhancing the quality of life for persons affected by epilepsy. Epilepsy is a group of disorders of the central nervous system characterized by repeated uncontrolled electrical disturbances in the brain. Established in 1966, EC is committed to establishing understanding and acceptance of epilepsy through the promotion of research, facilitation of education, and the implementation of awareness initiatives. Consisting of 21 members, the organization produces educational materials including a newsletter entitled "Lumina," a pamphlet entitled "Your Medication for Epilepsy," and a brochure entitled "Answers to Your Questions, Epilepsy." EC maintains a web site at [http://www.epilepsy.ca].

President: James LaMartina
Executive Director: Denise Crepin
Organization Language: French (written/spoken).
Year Established: 1966
Organization Members: 21

Publishes the following materials:
"The cure for epilepsy is in your pocket" ~ *Brochure*
Answers to your questions ~ *Brochure*
What parents need to know ~ *Brochure*
Seniors and seizures ~ *Brochure*
Your Medication for Epilepsy ~ *Brochure*
Lumina (English/French) ~ *Booklet*

Concerned with the following diseases or disorders:
Epilepsy; Epilepsy, Myoclonic Progressive Familial; Myoclonus, General; Perisylvian Syndrome, Congenital Bilateral

1230 **ERB'S PALSY GROUP**
22 Glenview Road
Hemel Hempstead
Hertfordshire, HP1 1TE
United Kingdom 1442 212422
Fax: 1442 212422

The Erb's Palsy Group is an international nonprofit self-help organization dedicated to providing support and information to families in England and North and South Ireland who are affected by Erb's Palsy. Erb's Palsy is a paralysis of the shoulder and upper extremity that is most commonly seen in newborns. This disorder is characterized by an abnormal positioning (adduction) and internal turning of the shoulder with a rotation of the forearm. This type of nerve injury may be caused by abnormal stretching of the shoulder during a difficult labor, a delivery where the buttocks present first (breech), or excessive sideways movement of the neck during delivery. Founded in 1992, the Erb's Palsy Group publishes a self-titled newsletter and distributes several informational brochures and fact sheets. Titles include "Obstetrical Erb's Palsy," "Nerve Grafts," and "Shoulder Release." A series of brochures geared to educators is also available. The Group also provides guidelines for starting and maintaining local support groups.

President: Debbie Clark (1996 to Present)
Executive Director: Karen Hillyer
Year Established: 1992
Organization Members: 510

Publishes the following materials:
Obstetrical Erb's Palsy (Brachial Plexus Paralysis) ~ *Fact Sheet 1*
Nerve Grafts ~ *Fact Sheet 2*
Shoulder Release (Subscapularis Release) ~ *Fact Sheet 3*
Erb's Palsy/Brachial Plexus Paralysis ~ *Fact Sheet*
Information Sheet for Schools. Number One for Primary, Nursery and Playgroups ~ *Pamphlet*
Information Sheet Tips for Pre-School Parents ~ *Pamphlet*
Tips for Hosting Coffee Mornings ~ *Pamphlet*
Information Sheets for Schools. Number Two for Middle and Upper Schools ~ *Pamphlet*
Erb's Palsy Group ~ *Newsletter May 1977*

Concerned with the following diseases or disorders:
Erb's Palsy

1231 **ERYTHROPOIETIC PROTOPORPHYRIA RESEARCH AND EDUCATION FUND (EPPREF)**
Channing Laboratory
Harvard Medical School
Brigham & Women's Hospital
181 Longwood Avenue
Boston, MA 02115-5804 617-525-2249
Fax: 617-731-1541
E-mail: mmmathroth@bics.bwh.harvard.edu

The Erythropoietic Protoporphyria Research and Education Fund (EPPREF) is a not-for-profit organization dedicated to disseminating knowledge about Erythropoietic Protoporphyria (EPP) to affected individuals, physicians, and the general public; operating and maintaining a referral service for individuals with EPP; and assisting physicians in any way necessary to bring about optimal care for affected individuals. Erythropoietic Protoporphyria is a rare inherited metabolic disorder characterized by a deficiency of the enzyme ferrochelatase (FECH). Due to abnormally low levels of FECH, excessive amounts of protoporphyrin accumulate in the plasma, red blood cells, and the liver. Symptoms may include hypersensitivity of the skin to sunlight and some types of artificial light (photosensitivity); itchiness and redness of the skin and/or a burning sensation after exposure to light, particularly on the skin of the hands, arms, and face; and/or, in rare cases, complications related to liver and gallbladder function. Established in 1978, the EPPREF, which is based at Channing Laboratory, Harvard Medical School, Brigham & Women's Hospital, offers diagnostic services to physicians, maintains a registry, and plans to publish articles concerning EPP within the peer-reviewed medical literature. The EPPREF, which currently has approximately 250 members, also publishes a regular newsletter, entitled "EP-PREF News," that contains items of interest to affected individuals and physicians.

President: Micheline M. Mathews-Roth, M.D.
Organization Language: French (written/spoken).
Year Established: 1978
Organization Members: 250

Publishes the following materials:
EPPREF NBEWS ~ *Newsletter*
EPP Questionaire - 1993 ~ *Questionairre*

Concerned with the following diseases or disorders:
Erythropoietic Protoporphyria (EPP)

1232 EUROPEAN CHROMOSOME 11Q NETWORK

Else Mauhsstraat 7
Wageningen, 6708 NJ
Netherlands 0317423345
E-mail: avbetuw@wxs.nl
http://home.wxs.nl/~avbetuw/home.htm

The European Chromosome 11q Network is an international self-help organization dedicated to providing information, assistance, and support to parents of children with abnormalities of the long arm of chromosome 11 (11q). Such 11q chromosome disorders include Jacobsen Syndrome, a rare chromosomal disorder also known as "partial deletion" or "partial monosomy" of chromosome 11q; duplication (or "trisomy") of chromosomal material on 11q; or other chromosomal abnormalities. Associated symptoms and physical features depend upon the exact length, location, and nature of the specific 11q chromosomal abnormality in question. Established in 1996, the European Chromosome 11q Network is dedicated to networking parents of affected children, collecting and disseminating information concerning 11q chromosomal disorders, following the latest scientific developments, promoting research, and organizing international conferences on 11q disorders for affected families. The European Chromosome 11q Network provides a regular newsletter and has a web site on the Internet at [http://www.worldaccess.nl/~avbe].

President: Annet van Betuw (1996 - Present).
Organization Language: Dutch (written/spoken). German (written/spoken). French (written/spoken). Spanish (written/spoken). Portuguese (written/spoken).
Year Established: 1996
Organization Members: 30

Concerned with the following diseases or disorders:
Chromosome 11, Partial Monosomy 11q; Chromosome 11, Partial Trisomy 11q

1233 EUROPEAN MARFAN SUPPORT NETWORK (EMSN)

70 Greenways
Courtmoor
Fleet
Hampshire, GU13 9XD
United Kingdom 01252 810472
Fax: 01252 810473
E-mail: marfan@thenet.co.uk
http://www.thenet.co.uk/~marfan

The European Marfan Support Network is a not-for-profit organization dedicated to serving as a liaison with Marfan Syndrome Parent Organizations across Europe. Marfan Syndrome is a rare inherited connective tissue disorder characterized by abnormalities of the heart and blood vessels (cardiovascular system), skeleton, and eyes. Affected individuals may be unusually tall and thin, have abnormally large hands and feet, have malformations of the chest and spine, and experience weakness of the joints, ligaments, and tendons. Established in 1990, the Network is committed to ensuring the availability of current medical information for affected individuals, family members, physicians, and other health care professionals; encouraging effective medical management; and promoting research towards a cure for the disorder. The organization also engages in patient advocacy, offers patient networking services, has support groups, produces an annual magazine entitled "In Touch," and offers written materials in several languages including Spanish, French, German, Italian, and Russian. The European Marfan Support Network also has a web site on the Internet at [http://www.thenet.co.uk/~marfan].

President: Diane Rust (Coordinator/Founder) (1990 to Present)
Organization Language: Flemish (written). French (written). Dutch (written). Finnish (written). Danish (written). Norwegian (written). German (written). Greek (written). Italian (written). Russian (written). Swedi
Year Established: 1990
Organization Members: 13

Concerned with the following diseases or disorders:
Marfan Syndrome

1234 **EVANS SYNDROME SUPPORT AND RESEARCH GROUP**
5630 Devon Street
Port Orange, FL 32127 904-760-3031
Fax: 904-760-5583
E-mail: 73142.1315@compuserve.com

The Evans Syndrome Support and Research Group is a not-for-profit self-help organization dedicated to providing information and support to individuals with Evans Syndrome. This is a disorder characterized by acquired hemolytic anemia, the chronic premature destruction of red blood cells and thrombocytopenia, abnormally low levels of circulating blood platelets. Established in 1992, the Group provides appropriate referrals, offers various forms of support, and provides educational materials to affected individuals, family members, and health care professionals.

President: Lou Addington (1992-Present)
Organization Language: French.
Year Established: 1992
Organization Members: 25

1235 **FD FAMILIAL DYSAUTONOMIA FOUNDATION (FD FOUNDATION)**
343 Clark Avenue West
Thornhill
Ontario, L4J 7K5
Canada 905-764-5335
Fax: 905-764-7752

The FD Familial Dysautonomia Foundation is an international, voluntary, not-for-profit organization dedicated to supporting clinical treatment, laboratory research, genetic testing and counseling, and parent and family support groups for children and adults with Familial Dysautonomia. Familial Dysautonomia, also know as Riley-Day Syndrome, is a rare genetic disorder of the autonomic nervous system (ANS) characterized by diminished sensitivity to pain, lack of overflow tearing in the eyes, a decrease in the number of knob-like projections that cover the tongue (fungiform papillae), unusual fluctuations of body temperature, and unstable blood pressure. Founded in 1982, the Foundation provides educational materials including reports, brochures, and a newsletter. The Foundation consists of approximately 2,300 members in Canada and the United States.

President: Gilda Israeli & Dena Weiman (1994 to Present)
Year Established: 1982
Organization Chapters: 20
Organization Members: 2,300

1236 **FEL (FAMILIAL ERYTHROPHAGOCYTIC LYMPHOHISTIOCYTOSIS) NETWORK (FELN)**
2519 West Twonig
San Angelo, TX 76901 915-949-4228

The FEL Network, which is affiliated with the Histiocytosis X Association of America, is a national not-for-profit self-help organization that is dedicated to providing information and support to individuals with Familial Erythrophagocytic Lymphohistiocytosis (FEL), their families, and physicians. FEL, a rare inherited systemic disorder that typically becomes apparent from early infancy to five years of age, may be characterized by recurrent fevers, recurrent infections, irritability, failure to grow and gain weight at the expected rate (failure to thrive), anemia, intermittently low levels of certain white blood cells (granulocytopenia) and/or platelets (thrombocytopenia) in the blood, and/or other findings. Established in 1990, the FEL Network is committed to offering networking services for the purposes of mutual support and information exchange; supplying affected individuals, family members, and health care professionals with information from the peer-reviewed medical literature; and conducting family conferences.

Executive Director: Kay Wojtek
Year Established: 1990

1237 **FRAXA RESEARCH FOUNDATION, INC. (FRAXA)**
P.O. Box 935
West Newbury, MA 01985-0935 978-462-1866
Fax: 978-463-9985
E-mail: fraxa@seacoast.com
http://www.fraxa.org

The FRAXA Research Foundation is a voluntary not-for-profit organization dedicated to providing support for individuals affected by Fragile X Syndrome, an X-linked disorder characterized by metal retardation, a large jaw, a high forehead, enlarged testes, and/or other abnormalities in affected males and, in some cases, mild mental retardation in females (heterozygotes). The Foundation is also committed to aiding the research efforts of concerned medical professionals throughout the United States. Founded in 1994 by parents of children with Fragile X Syndrome, the FRAXA Research Foundation is dedicated to educating public officials and the general population about Fragile X and to supporting ongoing medical research. The Foundation works toward these goals by awarding research grants to physicians whose purpose is to find treatments for Fragile X Syndrome and by encouraging the publication of articles to increase awareness of Fragile X Syndrome. In addition, the FRAXA Research Foundation puts families with affected children in touch with one another and welcomes questions about this disorder from concerned individuals. The FRAXA Research Foundation produces educational and support materials including brochures, newsletters, and pamphlets. Individual chapters hold dances, golf tournaments, and other functions.

President: Katherine N. Clapp (1994-Present)
Executive Director: Kathrine N. Clapp
Year Established: 1994
Organization Chapters: 27
Organization Members: 800

Publishes the following materials:
Supporting Research for the Treatment of Fragile X Syndrome ~ *Brochure*
Fraxa Research Foundation, Inc. Newsletter ~ *Newsletter*

Concerned with the following diseases or disorders:
Fragile X Syndrome

1238 FROST: FRIENDS OF THE OSTEOPETROSIS SUPPORT TRUST (FROST)

37 Reade Road
Holbrook
Ipswich, IPG 202
United Kingdom 01473328083

FROST: Friends of the Osteopetrosis Support Trust is a voluntary not-for-profit organization dedicated to supporting families with children who have Osteopetrosis, a rare genetic disorder characterized by increased bone density and brittle bones. Established in 1994, the Trust has members throughout the United States, the United Kingdom, Canada, and across the world. FROST offers financial assistance and helps provide special equipment to affected children. It also promotes and supports ongoing medical research and provides referrals to genetic counseling, support groups, and other services. FROST produces and distributes a variety of educational materials including information leaflets, medical fact sheets, and a newsletter.

President: Sylvia McLean (1994-Present)
Executive Director: Margaret Wright
Year Established: 1994
Organization Members: 20

Publishes the following materials:
O.S.T. Osteopetrosis Support Trust ~ *Fact Sheet*
FROST ~ *Newsletter*
Osteopetrosis ~ *Fact Sheet*

Concerned with the following diseases or disorders:
Osteopetrosis

1239 FABRY DISEASE HOME PAGE

E-mail: fabry@scisun.sci.ccny.cuny.edu
http://www.sci.ccny.cuny.edu/~fabry/

The Fabry Disease Home Page is a web site offered by The City College of New York. The home page provides information on Fabry Disease in lay terminology for patients and family members as well as clinical and biochemical information in medical terminology. Fabry Disease is a rare inherited disorder of lipid metabolism characterized by the abnormal accumulation of certain fatty substances (i.e., glycolipids such as glycosphingolipid) in various organs in the body. The purpose of the Fabry Disease Home Page is to educate affected individuals and family members about the disease, to provide a worldwide communication network, and to alert physicians and patients to new therapeutic approaches. Affected individuals, family members, and health care professionals with Fabry Disease patients may provide their e-mail addresses to this site to receive forwarded information about the disease as it becomes available. This home page also provides dynamic linkage to other appropriate web sites and provides listings of relevant article citations on Fabry Disease.

Concerned with the following diseases or disorders:
Fabry Disease

1240 **FABRY SUPPORT & INFORMATION GROUP (FSIG)**

P.O. Box 569
Concordia, MO 64020-0569 816-463-1382
Fax: 816-463-1356
E-mail: jcjohnson@vax1.rainis.net
jjohnson@cpgnet.com
http://www.cpgnet.com/fsig.nsf

The Fabry Support and Information Group is a national not-for-profit self-help organization dedicated to providing emotional support and disseminating information to individuals with Fabry Disease and their families. Fabry Disease is a rare inherited disorder of lipid metabolism characterized by the abnormal accumulation of certain fatty substances (i.e., glycolipids such as glycosphingolipid) in various organs of the body. Symptoms may include clusters of wart-like discolorations on the skin (angiokeratomas), abdominal pain, and/or visual impairment. Established in 1996, the organization, which has approximately 70 members, is committed to offering support to affected families, increasing the understanding of Fabry Disease, and offering networking services for affected individuals, their friends, and their families. The organization offers a variety of educational materials including a regular newsletter.

President: Jack C. Johnson
Year Established: 1996
Organization Members: 70

Publishes the following materials:
Fabry Support & Information Group (April 1997) ~ *Newsletter*

Concerned with the following diseases or disorders:
Fabry Disease

1241 **FACIO-SCAPULO-HUMERAL SOCIETY, INC. (FSH SOCIETY, INC.)**

3 Westwood Road
Lexington, MA 02173 781-860-0501
Fax: 781-860-0599
E-mail: carol.perez@fshsociety.org
http://disability.ucdavis.edu

Facio-Scapulo-Humeral Society, Inc. (FSH Society) is a voluntary not-for-profit organization created to address issues and needs specifically related to Facio-Scapulo-Humeral Muscular Dystrophy (FSHD), a rare inherited neuromuscular disorder. Established in 1989, the Facio-Scapulo-Humeral Society is dedicated to encouraging and promoting ongoing scientific and clinical research and development into the nature of Facio-Scapulo-Humeral Syndrome through solicitation of grants and contributions from private foundations, the pharmaceutical industry, and others. The Society also seeks to develop educational programs aimed at the medical community, government bodies, and the public. The Society accumulates and disseminates timely information about FSHD and actively cooperates with related organizations to foster communication among all interested parties. In addition, Facio-Scapulo-Humeral Society promotes professional education; provides appropriate referrals including to support groups; and promotes patient advocacy and legislation beneficial to individuals with FSHD. The Society offers a variety of educational and support materials including brochures, fact sheets, and a newsletter.

President: Daniel Paul Perez (1992-Present)
Executive Director: Carol A. Perez
Year Established: 1989
Organization Chapters: 3
Organization Members: 600

Publishes the following materials:
FSH Society, Inc. ~ *Fact Sheet*
Board of Directors ~ *Directors Listing*
Scientific Advisory Board ~ *Advisor Listing*
FSH Watch ~ *Newsletter*

Concerned with the following diseases or disorders:
Muscular Dystrophy, Landouzy Dejerine

1242 **FAMILIES WITH MOYAMOYA SUPPORT NETWORK**

4900 McGowan Street SE
Cedar Rapids, IA 52403
800-261-6692

Families with Moyamoya Support Network is a not-for-profit voluntary health organization composed of families who are affected by Moyamoya Disease. Moyamoya Disease is a progressive disease that affects the blood vessels in the brain (cerebrovascular). The disorder is characterized by narrowing and/or closing of the main artery to the brain (carotid). This lack of blood may cause paralysis of the feet, legs, or upper extremities. Headaches, various vision problems, mental retardation, and psychiatric problems may also occur. The Network seeks to share information and support to help affected individuals and families cope with the impact of this rare disease. Established in 1992, the organization provides a forum through which members can receive emotional support and learn about Moyamoya Disease, treatment options, and sources of treatment. Educational materials produced by the organization include a bibliographic list of medical journal articles about Moyamoya Disease and brochures.

President: Dawn Gruettner (1992-Present)
Year Established: 1992
Organization Members: 60

Concerned with the following diseases or disorders:
Moyamoya Disease; Valinemia

1243 **FAMILY EMPOWERMENT NETWORK: SUPPORTING FAMILIES AFFECTED BY FAS/FAE (FEN)**
519 Lowell Hall
610 Langdon Street
Madison, WI 53703 608-262-8971
800-462-5254
Fax: 608-265-3352
E-mail: fen@mail.des.wisc.edu

The Family Empowerment Network: Support For Families Affected by FAS/FAE (Fetal Alcohol Syndrome and Fetal Alcohol Effects) is a voluntary organization established to empower families affected by Fetal Alcohol Syndrome and Fetal Alcohol Effects through programs of education and support. The goals of the Network are to provide support, education, and training to families affected by FAS/FAE and provide information and training to professionals involved with families affected by FAS/FAE. The organization networks families with support groups and professionals on a national level; conducts an annual family retreat; maintains a toll-free family information line; conducts an annual conference; and offers ongoing technical assistance. The Network also provides a variety of materials including the quarterly newsletter "FEN Pen."

Executive Director: Raymond Kessel, PhD
Year Established: 1992
Organization Members: 500

Publishes the following materials:
FEN ~ *Brochure*
FEN Pen ~ *Newsletter*

Concerned with the following diseases or disorders:
Fetal Alcohol Syndrome

1244 **FANCONI ANEMIA RESEARCH FUND, INC. (FARF)**
1902 Jefferson Street
Suite 2
Eugene, OR 97405 541-687-4658
800-828-4891
Fax: 541-687-0548
E-mail: fafund@rio.com
http://www.rio.com/~fafund

The Fanconi Anemia Research Fund is a national voluntary organization that raises funds for medical research into Fanconi's Anemia, an inherited condition that leads to a deficiency of certain blood cells that are produced by the bone marrow. This disorder occurs mainly in children and is characterized by abnormalities of the heart, kidneys, and skeleton. Established in 1989, the organization supports numerous investigators who are working on various approaches to gene identification and therapy. The Fanconi Anemia Research Fund sponsors an annual international Fanconi Anemia Research Symposium to stimulate scientific progress and collaborative research among the different scientific disciplines. In addition, the Fund develops and maintains a communication network that supplies information and mutual support to parents of affected children and their physicians. Educational materials include the "FA Handbook," "FA Family Newsletter," "Scientific Supplement," and the "Bulletin."

President: Joyce Owen (1994-Present)
Executive Director: Linda DeSpain
Organization Language: Spanish.
Year Established: 1989
Organization Members: 3,000

Publishes the following materials:
Mark Your Calendars! ~ *Information Sheet*
We're Fighting For Life - One Step at a Time ~ *Brochure*
A Handbook for Families & Their Physicians ~ *Handbook*
International Fanconi Anemia Family Directory ~ *Directory*
FA family newsletter ~ *Newsletter*
Scientific Supplement ~ *Newsletter*
Fanconi Anemia Research Fund, Inc. ~ *Fact Sheet*
Family Education and Support Network ~ *Member Information Form*

Concerned with the following diseases or disorders:
Anemia, Fanconi's

1245 **FETAL ALCOHOL EDUCATION PROGRAM (FAEP)**
7 Kent Street
Brookline, MA 02146 617-739-1424
Fax: 617-566-4019

The Fetal Alcohol Education Program is a professional, not-for-profit organization that seeks to prevent Fetal Alcohol Syndrome (FAS) and Fetal Alcohol Effects (FAE) and to treat the conditions that result from alcohol consumption during pregnancy. Established in 1974, the Fetal Alcohol Education Program works to educate the professional and lay communities about the various risks and aspects of Fetal Alcohol Syndrome and Fetal Alcohol Effects. To accomplish this goal, the Fetal Alcohol Education Program produces teaching materials about FAS and FAE and conducts nationwide workshops to disseminate this information. In addition, the Fetal Alcohol Education Program conducts research into FAS/FAE, offers referrals, conducts phone consultations, and provides a variety of educational materials including pamphlets, brochures, article reprints, and audiovisual aids.

Executive Director: Barbara A. Morse, PhD
Year Established: 1974

Publishes the following materials:
Alcohol, Drugs & The Fetus: A Teaching Package ~ *Brochure*
FAS: Parent and Child ~ *Price Card*
Alcohol, Drugs and the Fetus ~ *Manual List*
Here's to Healthy Babies! ~ *Book Information Sheet*
Order Form for Fetal Alcohol Education Program ~ *Order Form*
Reprints - Fetal Alcohol Education Program ~ *Price List*
Identification, Prevention and Treatment of FAS An Intensive Seminar ~ *Registration Form*

Concerned with the following diseases or disorders:
Fetal Alcohol Syndrome

1246 FIBROMYALGIA ALLIANCE OF AMERICA, INC. (FMAA)

P.O. Box 21990
Columbus, OH 43221-0990 614-457-4222
Fax: 614-457-2729
E-mail: Masaathoff@aol.com

The Fibromyalgia Alliance of America, Inc. is a professional self-help not-for-profit organization dedicated to improving the lives of people affected by Fibromyalgia. Established in 1986, the Alliance provides state-of-the-art knowledge concerning Fibromyalgia to the medical community; supports research into the causes of Fibromyalgia and effective treatments for Fibromyalgia; educates the public and private sector about Fibromyalgia; and provides information and support to affected individuals, their families, and others. The Fibromyalgia Alliance produces educational and support materials including a quarterly newsletter, brochures, pamphlets, audio and vidieo tapes, and books on Fibromyalgia and chronic illness. The Alliance also sponsors national patient conferences.

President: Mary Anne Saathoff, RN, BSN (1992-Present)
Executive Director: Mary Anne Saathoff, RN, BSN
Year Established: 1986
Organization Members: 5,000

Concerned with the following diseases or disorders:
Fibromyalgia

1247 FOUNDATION FOR PULMONARY HYPERTENSION, INC. (FPH)

P.O. Box 61540
New Orleans, LA 70161 504-533-5888
Fax: 504-533-2447

The Foundation for Pulmonary Hypertension is a national not-for-profit research organization that was established in 1984. Pulmonary Hypertension is a condition characterized by abnormally high blood pressure in the arteries that supply the lungs. Pulmonary Hypertension may be an isolated condition that may occur for unknown reasons (Primary Pulmonary Hypertension) or may occur due to or in association with other underlying disorders or conditions (Secondary Pulmonary Hypertension). The mission of the Foundation is to provide "seed money" for pioneering research into the causes and treatments of Pulmonary Hypertension. The Foundation supports the development of clinical treatments for people with Primary and Secondary Pulmonary Hypertension and informs and educates affected individuals about their conditions. In some cases, the group make appropriate referrals for further evaluation and possible treatment. Educational materials distributed by the Foundation include a regular newsletter and fact sheets.

President: Stephen A. Hansel (1984-Present)
Executive Director: Dr. Alfred P. Fishman
Year Established: 1984
Organization Chapters: 1
Organization Members: 175

Publishes the following materials:
The Foundation for Pulmonary Hypertension, Inc. December 20, 1994 ~ *Fact Sheet*
Update of Transplantation Developments Related to Pulmonary Problems ~ *Fact Sheet*
Primary Pulmonary Hypertension ~ *Fact Sheet*
Jacksonville Foundation Funds Research into Rare Disease ~ *Article Reprint*

Concerned with the following diseases or disorders:
Pulmonary Hypertension, Primary; Pulmonary Hypertension, Secondary

1248 FREEMAN-SHELDON PARENT SUPPORT GROUP (FSPSG)

509 East Northmont Way
Salt Lake City, UT 84103 801-364-7060
Fax: 801-585-7395
E-mail: FSPSG@aol.com
http://members.aol.com/fspsg

Established in 1982, the Freeman-Sheldon Parent Support Group is an international voluntary organization that acts as a clearinghouse for information and as a support group for families and individuals affected by Freeman-Sheldon Syndrome. Freeman-Sheldon Syndrome is a rare genetic disorder characterized by distinctive abnormalities of the head and facial area including an abnormally small mouth that has a "whistling" appearance; a flat, expressionless face; and/or deeply set, widely spaced eyes. In many cases, additional abnormalities may also be present including malformations of the fingers and/or the feet. The Group seeks to provide emotional support, shared experiences, and current medical findings to affected individuals and families and serves as a resource for health care providers, educators, and the general public. The Freeman-Sheldon Parent Support Group actively encourages and participates in medical research studies regarding the cause and treatment of this disease. The Group also produces educational materials including brochures, a newsletter, a members-only directory, and a bibliography of current medical literature.

Executive Director: Joyce Dolcourt
Year Established: 1982
Organization Members: 69

Publishes the following materials:
Bibliography of the Medical Literature for Freeman-Sheldon Syndrome - December 1994 ~ *Bibliography*
FSPSG Newsletter ~ *Newsletter*
Freeman-Sheldon Syndrome ~ *Brochure*

Concerned with the following diseases or disorders:
Freeman Sheldon Syndrome

1249 GALACTOSAEMIA SUPPORT GROUP (GSG)

31 Cotysmore
Sutton Coldfield
West Midlands, B75 6BJ
United Kingdom

The Galactosaemia Support Group (GSG) is a self-help organization that establishes contact and fosters support between patients of all ages with Galactosaemia, a genetic disorder resulting from defective metabolism of galactose. GSG also offers guidance on foods that are lactose-free, promotes public and professional awareness about Galactosaemia, and raises funds to support Galactosaemia research. GSG publishes a newsletter and informational leaflets. Although it is based in the United Kingdom, the Group will assist those who contact them from other countries.

President: Sue Benington
Organization Members: 90

Publishes the following materials:
Galactosaemia - What's That? ~ *Brochure*

Concerned with the following diseases or disorders:
Galactosemia

1250 GAUCHERS ASSOCIATION

25 West Cottages
London, NW6 1R5
United Kingdom 171-433-1121
E-mail: gaucher@wisebuy.co.uk
http://www.gaucher.org.uk

The Gauchers Association is a nonprofit international support network whose mission is to provide information and support to families in Europe and elsewhere whose lives have been affected by Gaucher's Disease. Gaucher's Disease is the most common type of lipid storage disease (which includes Tay-Sachs, Fabry's, and Neimann-Pick diseases) and is characterized by anemia, fatigue, easy bruising, and a tendency to bleed more easily than normal. Established in 1991 and currently consisting of 150 members, the Gauchers Association provides information to the general public and medical professionals about Gaucher's Disease, maintains a registry of individuals affected by the disease that may help to assess the prevalence and distribution of affected families, and actively encourages ongoing medical research. The group maintains a web site that is also available in French; portions are available in German.

President: Susan Lewis (Honorary Secretary) (1991 - Present)
Organization Language: French (written). German (written)
Year Established: 1991
Organization Members: 150

Concerned with the following diseases or disorders:
Gaucher Disease

1251 **GIANT CELL MYOCARDITIS REGISTRY**

Mayo Clinic
ATTN: Leslie T. Cooper, M.D.
200 First Street SW
Rochester, MN 55905 507-284-3680
Fax: 507-266-1617
E-mail: cooper.leslie@mayo.edu
www.mayo.edu/cv/wwwpg_cv/research/cv_trial.

The Giant Cell Myocarditis Study Group was established in 1994 to gather a multicenter database on Idiopathic Giant Cell Myocarditis and the related disorder Cardiac Sarcoidosis. Giant Cell Myocarditis (GCM), a rare disorder that presents with inflammation of the heart muscle, often affects young, previously healthy individuals. GCM is characterized by the progressive inability of the heart to pump blood effectively to the lungs and the rest of the body (progressive congestive heart failure) and irregularities in the rhythm of the heartbeat (arrhythmias) originating in the lower chambers of the heart (ventricular arrhythmia), resulting in potentially life-threatening complications. Cardiac Sarcoidosis, which is frequently confused with GCM due to similar symptoms and clinical findings, is chararacterized by involvement of the heart in Sarcoidosis. Sarcoidosis, a rare multisystem disorder of unknown cause, is characterized by the formation of rounded, granular, inflammatory nodules (tubercles) consisting of cells resembling those that line internal and external surfaces of the body (epithelioid tissue). The Giant Cell Myocarditis Registry conducts several clinical observational studies to better define the natural history, demographics, and effect of treatment on Giant Cell Myocarditis and Cardiac Sarcoidosis. In addition to the efforts to define the clinical spectrum of these disorders, the Registry seeks to better define the causes of Giant Cell Myocarditis in an effort to produce more effective treatments. The Registry also enables interested registry participants to network with one another, promoting understanding of the disorder and enabling affected individuals and family members to better cope with GCM. In addition, the Registry provides reprints from the peer-reviewed medical literature and bibliographies of medical journal article citations concerning Giant Cell Myocarditis and Cardiac Sarcoidosis.

President: Leslie T. Cooper, M.D.
Year Established: 1994

1252 **GLAUCOMA RESEARCH FOUNDATION (GRF)**

490 Post Street
Suite 830
San Francisco, CA 94102 415-986-3162
800-826-6693
Fax: 415-986-3763
E-mail: info@glaucoma.org
http://www.glaucoma.org

The Glaucoma Research Foundation is a national voluntary organization dedicated to protecting and preserving the sight and independence of people with glaucoma through research and education. Glaucoma is a condition characterized by abnormally increased pressure of the fluid of the eye, potentially resulting in partial or complete loss of vision without appropriate treatment. Established in 1978, the Glaucoma Research Foundation provides information and support concerning the various forms of glaucoma including normal tension, pigmentary, congenital, childhood, open-angle, closed-angle, exfoliative, pseudoexfoliative, and secondary glaucoma. The Foundation engages in patient and professional education; has a national, telephone-based Glaucoma Support Network; and conducts and supports various glaucoma research efforts including the Glaucoma Family History Project, the Glaucoma Research Eye Donor Network, and the Normal Tension Glaucoma Study. The Foundation's educational materials include a reference booklet in English and Spanish entitled "Understanding and Living with Glaucoma"; a booklet on childhood glaucoma; brochures; information packets; glaucoma fact sheets; videos; and a quarterly newsletter entitled "GLEAMS." The Glaucoma Research Foundation also has a web site on the Internet at [http://www.glaucoma.org].

President: Lars Vistnes, M.D. (1996 to Present).
Executive Director: Tara Steele
Organization Language: Spanish (written).
Year Established: 1978
Organization Members: Non-Membership

Concerned with the following diseases or disorders:
Aniridia Cerebellar Ataxia Mental Deficiency; Cogan Reese Syndrome; Essential Iris Atrophy; Megalocornea Mental Retardation Syndrome; WAGR Syndrome

1253 **GLUTEN INTOLERANCE GROUP OF NORTH AMERICA (GIG)**
P.O. Box 23053
Seattle, WA 98102-0353 206-325-6980
Fax: 206-850-2394

The Gluten Intolerance Group of North America is a not-for-profit self-help organization dedicated to providing information and support to individuals with Celiac Sprue and/or Dermatitis Herpetiformis, their families, and health care professionals. Celiac Sprue is a chronic, hereditary, intestinal malabsorption disorder caused by intolerance to gluten. Affected individuals may experience no, few, or many symptoms. Those who do have symptoms may experience weight loss, chronic diarrhea, abdominal cramping, intestinal gas, weakness, fatigue, and/or other symptoms. Some may experience Dermatitis Herpetiformis, which is characterized by small itchy blisters on the skin surface, most commonly on body pressure points, such as elbows, knees, and feet. The organization enables members to exchange information, support, and resources through its networking program; has staffed phone lines to answer inquiries; and offers a variety of educational and support materials. Such materials include a patient resource guide, cookbooks, book reviews, research reports, information on specific drug therapies, brochures, videotapes for purchase or rental, and a quarterly newsletter.

President: Dr. Elaine Hartsook (1974-Present)
Executive Director: Elaine Hartsook, M.D.
Organization Language: Spanish.
Year Established: 1974
Organization Members: 2,000

Concerned with the following diseases or disorders:
Celiac Sprue; Duhring Disease

1254 **GROUP B STREP ASSOCIATION (GBSA)**
P.O. Box 16515
Chapel Hill, NC 27516 919-932-5344
Fax: 919-932-3657
http://www.groupbstrep.org

The Group B Strep Association (GBSA) is a voluntary not-for-profit organization dedicated to educating the public about Group B Streptococcus (GBS) bacterial infections during pregnancies. Established in 1990 by parents whose babies were affected by GBS infections, the Group B Strep Association works closely with its Medical Advisory Board of researchers and physicians to help bring about guidelines for testing and treatment of GBS. The organization promotes routine screening of pregnant women for GBS and generates continuing support for vaccine research. The Group B Strep Association promotes patient advocacy, public awareness, and beneficial legislation and provides a variety of educational and support materials to patients, family members, health care professionals, and the general public. These include a biannual newsletter, and brochures.

President: Gina Burns (1990-Present)
Executive Director: Gina Burns
Year Established: 1990
Organization Members: 2,000

Publishes the following materials:
Awareness of Group B Streptococcus Infection During Pregnancy ~ *Brochure*
Update ~ *Newsletter*
Group B Strep Association Medical Advisory Board 1995 ~ *Medical Advisory List*

Concerned with the following diseases or disorders:
Streptococcus, Group B

1255 **GUARDIANS OF HYDROCEPHALUS RESEARCH FOUNDATION (GHRF)**
2618 Avenue Z
Brooklyn, NY 11235 718-743-4473
800-458-8655
Fax: 718-743-1171

The Guardians of Hydrocephalus Research Foundation is a national voluntary health organization dedicated to aiding and assisting children with Hydrocephalus and their families. Hydrocephalus is an abnormal accumulation of cerebrospinal fluid, causing a build-up of pressure inside the head. The efforts of the Foundation are directed at disseminating information to the general public so that a better understanding of Hydrocephalus will be established. The Foundation supports research into the causes, prevention, and cure of Hydrocephalus. For example, the Foundation conducts a research program at the New York University Medical Center, interacts with physicians and medical centers across the United States and Canada including the Universities of California at San Francisco and San Diego, the Texas Medical Center, and Sick Children's Hospital in Toronto, Canada. The Foundation also offers networking services to parents and supports the development of Satellite Information Centers, which are designed to form a network of information, assistance, and support. The Foundation's materials include pamphlets, reprints, fact sheets, and booklets.

President: Michael Fischetti Sr.
Year Established: 1977
Organization Chapters: 12
Organization Members: 5,000

Publishes the following materials:
Guardians of Hydrocephalus Research Foundation ~ *Pamphlet*
What is Hydrocephalus? ~ *Brochure*
An Introduction to Hydrocephalus ~ *Booklet*
About Hydrocephalus - A Book for Parents ~ *Booklet*
For Parents of Children with Hydrocephalus ~ *Brochure*

Concerned with the following diseases or disorders:
Acrocallosal Syndrome, Schinzel Type; Agenesis of Corpus Callosum; Craniosynostosis, Primary; Dandy Walker Malformation; Diencephalic Syndrome; Encephalocele; Hydranencephaly; Hydrocephalus; MASA Syndrome; Walker Warburg Syndrome

1256 GUILLAIN-BARRE SYNDROME FOUNDATION INTERNATIONAL (GBS)

P.O. Box 262
Wynnewood, PA 19096 610-667-0131
Fax: 610-667-7036
E-mail: GBINT@ix.netcom.com
http://www.webmast.com/gbs/

The Guillain-Barre Syndrome Foundation, which was established in 1980, provides emotional support and assistance to people affected by this rare disease of the peripheral nervous system. The Foundation currently consists of approximately 18,000 members in 160 chapters. The Foundation arranges personal visits to affected individuals in hospitals and rehabilitation centers, when possible; fosters research into the cause, treatment, and other aspects of the disorder; and directs affected individuals with long-term disabilities to resources for vocational, financial, and other forms of assistance. The Foundation's Medical Advisory Board includes neurologists who are active in Guillain-Barre research, physicians in rehabilitation medicine, and physicians who have had Guillain-Barre Syndrome. The Guillain-Barre Syndrome Foundation also supplies informational materials such as a directory, newsletters, and other literature about the disorder, including a comprehensive 55 page booklet entitled "An Overview for the Layperson."

President: Robert Benson (1980-Present)
Executive Director: Estelle Benson
Organization Language: Spanish. French. German. Dutch.
Year Established: 1980
Organization Chapters: 160
Organization Members: 18,000

Publishes the following materials:
A Brief Description of the Support Group ~ *Factsheet*
An Overview for the Layperson ~ *Brochure*
Acute Idiopathic Polyneuritis ~ *Brochure*
Chapter Directory ~ *Directory*
The Communicator ~ *Newsletter*
Support, Education, and Research Offer ~ *Flyer*

Concerned with the following diseases or disorders:
Guillain Barre Syndrome

1257 HME CONTACT GROUP

3 Linn Drive
Netherlee
Glasgow, G44 3PT
Scotland 0141 633 2617

The HME Contact Group is an international voluntary not-for-profit organization dedicated to providing support to individuals with Hemimegalencephaly (HME) and their families and friends and to providing educational services to affected individuals and their families. Hemimegalencephaly is a rare brain disorder characterized by abnormal enlargement of one half of the cerebral hemisphere. Founded in 1991, the HME Contact Group has approximately 40 members. The HME Contact group organizes family meetings, offers networking services, provides up-to-date publications on HME, and publishes an annual newsletter. The HME Contact Group also offers information on Epidermal Nevus Syndrome (Linear Nevus Sebaceous Syndrome), Proteus Syndrome, and Hemispherectomy. Epidermal Nevus Syndrome is characterized by the association of distinctive birth marks (nevus) on the skin in association with other abnormalities, particularly those of the central nervous system and skeleton. Proteus Syndrome is a rare disorder characterized by multiple lesions of the lymph vessels (lipolymphohemangiomas), overgrowth of one side of the body (hemihypertrophy), an abnormally large head (macrocephaly), partial gigantism of the feet, and abnormal coffee-colored (cafe-au-lait) spots on the skin. Hemispherectomy is a surgical procedure in which part or all of a cerebral hemisphere is removed.

President: Dagmar and David Kerr (Contact Persons) (1991 to Present)
Organization Language: German (spoken).
Year Established: 1991
Organization Members: 40

Publishes the following materials:
A specialist has diagnosed Hemimegalencephaly in your child ~ *Fact Sheet*
HME Contact Group ~ *Newsletter No. 4 1996*
Vision in Hemimegalencephaly ~ *Fact Sheet*
Hemimegalencephaly ~ *Fact Sheet*
Hemispherectomy ~ *Fact Sheet*

Concerned with the following diseases or disorders:
Epidermal Nevus Syndrome; Proteus Syndrome

1258 HEMANGIOMA SUPPORT SYSTEM

c/o Cynthia Schumerth
1215 Monterey Terrace
DePere, WI 54115 920-336-9399

The Hemangioma Support System is a national self-help organization dedicated to providing moral support to families affected by hemangiomas. Hemangiomas are benign tumors that are caused by abnormal distribution of blood vessels. Such tumors most commonly occur in infancy or childhood. The organization provides information on Capillary and Cavernous Hemangiomas and offers networking services to affected families, enabling them to exchange information, support, and resources.

President: Cynthia Schumerth
Executive Director: Leslie Andrisiak

Concerned with the following diseases or disorders:
Cavernous Hemangioma; Hemangioma Thrombocytopenia Syndrome

1259 HEMOCHROMATOSIS FOUNDATION, INC. (HF)

P.O. Box 8569
Albany, NY 12208 518-489-0972
Fax: 518-489-0227
http://Branch.com/hemo/hemo.html

The Hemochromatosis Foundation is a national not-for-profit organization dedicated to finding a cure for Hemochromatosis. Hereditary Hemochromatosis (HH) is a metabolic disorder characterized by increased absorption of dietary iron. Without appropriate treatment, excessive iron may accumulate in the liver, heart, pancreas, and other organs, causing organ dysfunction and tissue damage. Established in 1971, the Foundation is committed to fostering understanding of the disease by supporting activities that encourage research; advising legislative and regulatory bodies at the local and federal levels; increasing general awareness of Hemochromatosis to help ensure early diagnosis and prompt treatment; and improving the quality of life for affected individuals and family members. The Foundation also establishes local chapters; sponsors discussion groups where people share their experiences; and provides physician referrals, general information, and local contacts. Educational materials produced by the Foundation include a brochure series.

President: NA
Executive Director: Tim Casey
Year Established: 1971
Organization Chapters: 1
Organization Members: 6,000

Publishes the following materials:
Hereditary (Genetic or Idiopathic) Hemochromatosis ~ *Brochure*
What you don't know about IRON can kill you ~ *Brochure*
The Hemochromatosis Foundation, Inc. ~ *Mission Statement*

1260 HEREDITARY HEMORRHAGIC TELANGIECTASIA (HHT) FOUNDATION INTERNATIONAL, INC.

P.O. Box 8087
New Haven, CT 06530 313-561-2537
800-448-6389
Fax: 313-561-4585
E-mail: hhtinfo@hht.org
http://www.hht.org

The HHT Foundation International is a not-for-profit self-help organization dedicated to increasing public and professional awareness and understanding of Hereditary Hemorrhagic Telangiectasia (HHT). This disorder, also known as Osler Weber Rendu Syndrome, is a rare inherited blood vessel malformation characterized by the dilation of small vessels under the skin, leading to skin lesions and bleeding under the skin. The organization also supports ongoing medical research into the causes, prevention, and treatment of HHT; has support groups; offers referrals through a toll-free number; and offers a variety of materials including informational brochures and a quarterly newsletter.

President: Rita Van Bergijk
Organization Language: Dutch.
Year Established: 1990
Organization Chapters: 3
Organization Members: 402

Publishes the following materials:
A Rare Genetic Blood Vessel Disorder ~ *Brochure*

Concerned with the following diseases or disorders:
Hemorrhagic Telangiectasia, Hereditary

1261 HEREDITARY SPASTIC PARAPLEGIA (HSP)/FAMILIAL SPASTIC PARAPARESIS (FSP) PAGE

E-mail: FIssues@aol.com
http://www.geocities.com/HotSprings/Spa/2847/

The Hereditary Spastic Paraplegia (HSP)/Familial Spastic Paraparesis (FSP) Page is a web site on the Internet dedicated to providing information, assistance, and support to individuals and family members affected by the hereditary neuromuscular disease known as Hereditary Spastic Paraplegia or Familial Spastic Paraparesis. HSP is an inherited neurological condition characterized by progressive muscle weakness, stiffness, and muscle spasms that first develop in the legs and may later spread to other parts of the body. The HSP/FSP Page provides understandable information on the condition, treatment, and current investigational studies. In addition, the site conducts surveys concerning FSP/HSP, offers dynamic linkage to other helpful sources of information and support on the Internet, and provides a variety of online networking opportunities including an e-mail discussion list and online support group (the "HSP-L ListServ E-Mail List") and the HSP/FSP Bulletin Board.

Concerned with the following diseases or disorders:
Paraplegia, Hereditary Spastic

1262 HERMANSKY-PUDLAK SYNDROME NETWORK, INC.

One South Road
Oyster Bay, NY 11771-1905 516-922-3440
800-789-9477
Fax: 516-922-4022
E-mail: appell@theonramp.net
http://www.medhelp.org/web/hpsn.htm

The Hermansky-Pudlak Syndrome (HPS) Network, a special interest group of the National Organization of Albinism and Hypopigmentation, is a voluntary not-for-profit support group for people and families affected by Hermansky-Pudlak Syndrome. This is an inherited form of albinism that is characterized by lack of pigmentation in the skin, hair, and eyes; visual abnormalities; poor blood clotting due to platelet abnormalities; and abnormal storage of a wax-like material, called ceroid, in certain organs of the body. Established in 1992, the HPS Network is dedicated to networking individuals, families, and physicians for the purposes of education and research. The HPS Network is in frequent communication with researchers and communicates information concerning developments to its members. In addition, the Hermansky-Pudlak Syndrome Network provides a variety of educational and support materials through its database, reports, brochures, pamphlets, and regular newsletter. Please note that individuals who wish to communicate with the organization via fax should notify the Network before initiating transmission.

President: Donna Jean Appell, RN (1992-Present)
Year Established: 1992
Organization Members: 600

Publishes the following materials:
HPS Network Hermansky-Pudlak Syndrome Network ~ *Pamphlet*

Concerned with the following diseases or disorders:
Hermansky Pudlak Syndrome

1263 HIDRADENITIS SUPPORT GROUP

E-mail: annastesia1475@geocities.com
http://www.cyberhighway.net/~stesia

The Hidradenitis Support Group is a web site dedicated to providing information, assistance, support, and networking opportunities to men and women affected by this disorder. Hidradenitis Suppurativa is a chronic condition characterized by obstruction and painful inflammation of certain sweat glands, particularly the aprocrine glands; secondary bacterial infection; swelling; rupture; and progressive scarring due to recurrences. The site provides understandable information on the disorder, debunks common myths about the disease, and offers links to other sources of helpful information on the Internet. The site also enables affected individuals to subscribe to the support group's mailing list (listserv) to correspond with others around the world who are also affected by the disorder. To subscribe, send an e-mail message to [hidradenitis-request@UserHome.com] and leave the subject field of the message blank. In the body of the message, type subscribe and you will then be added to the group's mailing list.

Concerned with the following diseases or disorders:
Hidradenitis Suppurativa

1264 **HOLT-ORAM SYNDROME SUPPORT GROUP (HOSSG)**

21 Forth Road, Rivers Estate
Redcar
Cleveland, TS10 1PN
United Kingdom 164-248-5379
E-mail: 106524.33@compuserve.com

The Holt-Oram Syndrome Support Group is a voluntary not-for-profit self-help organization that is dedicated to providing information and support to individuals affected by Holt-Oram Syndrome, their families, and medical professionals. Holt-Oram Syndrome is a rare hereditary disorder characterized by heart defects and skeletal malformations affecting the thumbs and forearms. Established in 1994 and currently consisting of approximately 100 members, the Group provides networking services to affected families; offers support to all members of affected families; and promotes awareness of the syndrome among professional organizations and other interested parties. In addition, the organization provides educational materials including brochures and newsletters.

President: Andrew D. Sigsworth
Year Established: 1994
Organization Members: 100

Publishes the following materials:
Helping Those Who Have To Cope ~ *Brochure*
HOSSG News ~ *Newsletter*
Helping Those Who Have To Cope ~ *Brochure*
What is the Holt-Oram syndrome? ~ *Factsheet*
Aims of the Holt-Oram Syndrome Support Group ~ *Factsheet*
Cardiac Problems ~ *Factsheet*
Skeletal Defects ~ *Factsheet*

Concerned with the following diseases or disorders:
Holt Oram Syndrome

1265 **HUNTINGTON SOCIETY OF CANADA (HSC)**

13 Water Street North
P.O. Box 1269
Cambridge
Ontario, N1R 7G6
Canada 519-622-1002
800-998-7398
Fax: 519-622-7370
E-mail: hsc@wat.hookup.net

The Huntington Society of Canada is a national not-for-profit network of volunteers and professionals dedicated to finding a cure and treatment for Huntington's Disease and improving the quality of life for affected individuals and family members. Huntington's Disease (HD) is an inherited degenerative brain disorder characterized by irregular, involuntary movements (chorea); abnormal gait; slurred speech; and progressive disorientation and loss of intellectual function (dementia). Founded in 1973 to fight Huntington's Disease through research, service, and education, the Society now includes over 50 volunteer chapters and area representatives in all areas of Canada; an expanding network of professional counselors and caregivers; an international team of scientists and physicians; the National Office in Cambridge, Ontario; the Huntington Society of Quebec; and several sister organizations in other countries, forming the International Huntington Association. The Huntington Society of Canada funds basic and clinical research into the cause, cure, and treatment of HD (including partial funding of the research that located the disease gene for HD in 1993); supports the Canadian HD DNA Bank for testing and research; provides information to affected families and professionals; and raises awareness of HD across Canada. The Society also sponsors summer holiday and day activity programs for affected individuals; runs local support groups; offers crisis counseling and referral services; and provides a variety of materials on HD including a videotape and manual series concerning techniques of care, several booklets on all aspects of the disorder, and a national quarterly newsletter entitled "Horizon."

Executive Director: Isla Horvath (Director of Communications)
Organization Language: French (written/spoken).
Year Established: 1973
Organization Chapters: 60
Organization Members: 10,000

Publishes the following materials:
What is a Champion? ~ *Brochure*
Understanding Huntington's Disease. A Resource for Families ~ *Booklet*
Huntington Society of Canada (Summer 1997) ~ *Newsletter*

Concerned with the following diseases or disorders:
Huntington's Disease

1266 **HUNTINGTON'S DISEASE SOCIETY OF AMERICA (HDSA)**

140 West 22nd Street
Sixth Floor
New York, NY 10011-2420 212-242-1968
800-345-4372
Fax: 212-243-2443
E-mail: curehd@hdsa.ttisms.com
http://hdsa.mgh.harvard.edu

The Huntington's Disease Society of America (HDSA) is a national voluntary health organization dedicated to improving the lives of people with Huntington's Disease (HD) and to finding a cure for this disease. Huntington's Disease is an inherited degenerative brain disorder characterized by irregular, involuntary movements (chorea); abnormal gait; slurred speech; and progressive disorientation and loss of intellectual function (dementia). Established in 1986 and currently consisting of 40,000 members and 31 chapters across the United States, the Society supports medical research into the causes and treatment of Huntington's Disease, maintains a national network of services and referrals to assist affected individuals and families and offers a variety of materials through its brochures, newsletters, reports, audiovisual aids, and directory.

President: Mikal Kitchens
Executive Director: Barbara Boyle
Year Established: 1986
Organization Chapters: 32
Organization Members: 40,000

Publishes the following materials:
1993 Annual Report ~ *Brochure*
The Marker ~ *Newsletter*
A Disease of Both Mind and Body ~ *Brochure*
So You Got the News ~ *Brochure*
A Neurologist Speaks About Huntington's Disease ~ *Booklet*
Publications ~ *Pamphlet*
Guidelines for Genetic Testing for Huntington's Disease ~ *Pamphlet*
Neurology ~ *Brochure*
Basic Information Materials Order Form ~ *Order Form*
A Neurologist Speaks About Huntington's Disease ~ *Booklet*
A Family Member Speaks About Huntington's Disease ~ *Booklet*
Care of the Patient and Family with Huntington's Disease: A Guide for Clinicians ~ *Booklet*

Concerned with the following diseases or disorders:
Huntington's Disease

1267 **HYDROCEPHALUS ASSOCIATION**

870 Market Street
Suite 955
San Francisco, CA 94102 415-732-7040
Fax: 415-732-7044
E-mail: hydroassoc@aol.com
http://neurosurgery.mgh.harvard.edu/ha/

The Hydrocephalus Association is a national not-for-profit voluntary organization that provides support, education, and advocacy for families affected by hydrocephalus. Hydrocephalus is a condition characterized by inhibition of the normal flow of cerebrospinal fluid (CSF) and abnormal widening (dilatation) of the cerebral spaces of the brain (ventricles), causing accumulation of CSF in the skull and potentially increased pressure on brain tissue. The goals of the Association are to ensure that affected families and individuals receive personal support, comprehensive educational materials, and ongoing quality medical care. Established in 1983, the organization provides a variety of services including an OutReach Program that provides one-to-one personal support for families and individuals; educational meetings in the San Francisco area; social gatherings; networking with other support groups and organizations nationwide; and an annual scholarship awarded to young adults with hydrocephalus. Educational materials include books, resource guides, a directory, and a quarterly newsletter.

President: Emily S. Fudge (1994-Present)
Executive Director: Emily S. Fudge
Year Established: 1983
Organization Members: 2,000

Publishes the following materials:
Sobre Hidrocefalia Un Libro para los Padres ~ *Book*
Hydrocephalus Association ~ *Fact Sheet*
Hydrocephalus Fact Sheet ~ *Fact Sheet*
Hydrocephalus Adult Onset ~ *Fact Sheet*
Information Sheet - Primary Care Needs of Children with Hydrocephalus ~ *Fact Sheet*
Information Sheet - Learning Disabilities in Children with Hydrocephalus and Spina Bifida ~ *Fact Sheet*
Information Sheet - Eye Problems Associated with Hydrocephalus ~ *Fact Sheet*
Information Sheet - Survival Skills for the Family Unit ~ *Fact Sheet*
Information Sheet - Individualized Education Program Communication Skills for Parents ~ *Fact Sheet*
Information Sheet - Pediatric Pain Assessment ~ *Fact Sheet*
Information Sheet - How to be an Assertive Parent on the Treatment Team ~ *Fact Sheet*
Information Sheet - Preparing Your Child for Surgery ~ *Fact Sheet*
Information Sheet - Tax Considerations for Parents of Disabled Children ~ *Fact Sheet*
Information Sheet - Social Skills Development in Children with Hydrocephalus ~ *Fact Sheet*

Hydrocephalus Association Resource Guide Additions ~ *Resource Guide*
Hydrocephalus Association Resource Guide ~ *Resource Listing*
National Directory of Hydrocephalus Support Groups ~ *Directory*
Hydrocephalus Association Directory of Pediatric Neurosurgeons ~ *Directory*

Concerned with the following diseases or disorders:
Acrocallosal Syndrome, Schinzel Type; Agenesis of Corpus Callosum; Arnold Chiari Syndrome; Craniosynostosis, Primary; Dandy Walker Malformation; Diencephalic Syndrome; Encephalocele; Hydranencephaly; Hydrocephalus; MASA Syndrome; Mulibrey Nanism Syndrome (Perheentupa Syndrome); Pallister Hall Syndrome; Walker Warburg Syndrome

1268 HYDROCEPHALUS RESEARCH FOUNDATION, INC.

1670 Green Oak Circle
Lawrenceville, GA 30243 770-995-9570
Fax: 770-995-8982
E-mail: ann_liakos@atlmug.org

The Hydrocephalus Research Foundation, Inc. is an international voluntary organization dedicated to improving treatments and outcomes for individuals with hydrocephalus and closely related conditions, disorders, and diseases of the central nervous system. Hydrocephalus is a condition characterized by inhibition of the normal flow of cerebrospinal fluid (CSF) and abnormal widening (dilatation) of the cerebral spaces of the brain (ventricles), causing accumulation of CSF in the skull and potentially increased pressure on brain tissue. Established in 1980, the Hydrocephalus Research Foundation engages in patient advocacy and lobbying efforts, offers family networking services, promotes research, makes referrals, and provides a variety of educational materials. Such materials include brochures, pamphlets, videos, and a regular newsletter.

President: Ann Marie Liakos
Year Established: 1980
Organization Members: Non-Membership

Concerned with the following diseases or disorders:
Arnold Chiari Syndrome; Hydrocephalus; Mulibrey Nanism Syndrome (Perheentupa Syndrome); Pallister Hall Syndrome

1269 HYDROCEPHALUS SUPPORT GROUP, INC. (HSG)

P.O. Box 4236
Chesterfield, MO 63006-4236 314-532-8228
Fax: 314-995-4108
E-mail: hydro@inlink.com

The Hydrocephalus Support Group, Inc. (HSG) is an international nonprofit self-help organization dedicated to providing information, assistance, and support to individuals affected by hydrocephalus and their family members. Hydrocephalus is a condition characterized by inhibition of the normal flow of cerebrospinal fluid (CSF) and abnormal widening (dilatation) of the cerebral spaces of the brain (ventricles), causing accumulation of CSF in the skull and potentially increased pressure on brain tissue. Founded in 1986 and currently consisting of 1,000 members, HSG provides patient referrals, engages in patient advocacy, offers networking services, promotes research, and conducts meetings with speakers who discuss all aspects of hydrocephalus and related conditions. HSG also has a library of over 150 articles and tapes concerning hydrocephalus and provides pamphlets, brochures, and a quarterly newsletter.

President: Debby Buffa
Year Established: 1986
Organization Members: 1,000

Publishes the following materials:
Hydrocephalus Support Group, Inc. ~ *Brochure*

Concerned with the following diseases or disorders:
Arnold Chiari Syndrome; Dandy Walker Malformation; Hydrocephalus; Mulibrey Nanism Syndrome (Perheentupa Syndrome); Pallister Hall Syndrome

1270 HYPERACUSIS NETWORK

444 Edgewood Drive
Green Bay, WI 54302 414-468-4663
Fax: 414-432-3321
E-mail: dmalcore@aol.com

The Hyperacusis Network is an international self-help organization for individuals affected by hyperacusis, a condition characterized by intolerance and painful sensitivity to normal environmental sound. Established in 1991, the network provides information on hyperacusis, tinnitus, recruitment, vertigo, and Meniere's Disease. Consisting of 700 members, the organization shares ways to cope with hyperacusis; provides ongoing support; offers information and assistance in securing disability benefits; and reports on current research and treatment options through a monthly newsletter.

President: Dan Malcore (Indefinite)
Year Established: 1991
Organization Chapters: 1
Organization Members: 700

Publishes the following materials:
Hyperacusis ~ *Newsletter*
The Hyperacusis Network. Hyperacusis and Recruitment ~ *Brochure*
Hyperacusis Network. Supplement ~ *Pamphlet*
Hyperacusis Network ~ *Mission Statement*

1271 HYPERTROPHIC CARDIOMYOPATHY ASSOCIATION OF AMERICA (HCAA)

PO Box 306
Hibernia, NJ 07842 973-983-7429
E-mail: lfas1282@aol.com
http://www.hcma-heart.com

The Hypertrophic Cardiomyopathy Association of America is a national self-help organization dedicated to providing information and support to individuals with Hypertrophic Cardiomyopathy (HCM) and family members. HCM is a primary noninflammatory disease of the heart muscle characterized by enlargement of the lower left chamber of the heart (left ventricle) and the fibrous partition dividing the two ventricles (interventricular septum), causing obstruction of ventricular outflow and reduced cardiac output. The organization provides information to the medical community, acts as a referral service for affected individuals and family members, offers networking services, and promotes and supports research.

President: Lisa Salberg
Executive Director: unknown
Year Established: 1996
Organization Members: 50

1272 HYPOGLYCEMIA ASSOCIATION, INC. (HAI)

P.O. Box 165
Ashton, MD 20861-0165 202-544-4044

The Hypoglycemia Association, Inc. (HAI) is a nonprofit self-help organization dedicated to educating the public about hypoglycemia. Hypoglycemia is a common condition characterized by abnormally low blood sugar (glucose) level. Established in 1967, the organization publishes educational materials include a booklet entitled "A Diet For Living With Hypoglycemia," a self-titled pamphlet, and many other information sheets. The organization promotes patient, professional, and general education.

President: Dorothy Schultz
Executive Director: Marge Smith
Year Established: 1967
Organization Members: Non-Membership

Publishes the following materials:
A Diet For Living With Hypoglycemia ~ *Booklet*
Feeding Yourself In All Sorts Of Circumstances ~ *Pamphlet*
Hypoglycemia Association, Inc. ~ *Mission Statement*
Case Histories, Book Reviews and the Internet ~ *Leaflet*
Announcements ~ *Fact Sheet*
Available Literature List ~ *Bibliography*
Get Under The Health Umbrella with HAI ~ *Brochure*
Medical Heroes ~ *Pamphlet*

Concerned with the following diseases or disorders:
Hypoglycemia

1273 HYPOKALEMIC PERIODIC PARALYSIS RESOURCE PAGE

E-mail: editor@calexplorer.com
http://www.calexplorer.com/ushkpp.html

The Hypokalemic Periodic Paralysis Resource Page is a web site on the Internet dedicated to helping individuals who have been diagnosed with Primary Hypokalemic Periodic Paralysis (HKPP). HKPP is a metabolic disorder characterized by recurring episodes of progressively flaccid paralysis or weakness. During such episodes of muscle weakness, levels of potassium in the blood are abnormally low. In most cases, the disorder is inherited as an autosomal dominant genetic trait; however, in some cases, HKPP may occur sporadically. The Hypokalemic Periodic Paralysis Resource Page provides understandable information on HKPP; provides dynamic linkage to several additional sources of helpful information on the Internet; and offers several online networking opportunities including the ability to subscribe to its HKPP listserv, enabling affected individuals and family members to exchange histories, experiences, coping techiques, support, and research resources. The Hypokalemic Periodic Paralysis Resource Page is located at [http://www.calexplorer.com/ushkpp.html].

1274 HYPOPARATHYROIDISM NEWSLETTER

2835 Salmon Street
Idaho Falls, ID 83406 208-524-3857
E-mail: jesand@ida.net

The Hypoparathyroidism Newsletter is a self-help group that publishes a newsletter for the purpose of providing a support system for people with Hypoparathyroidism and their families. Hypoparathyroidism is a condition characterized by abnormally decreased levels of calcium in the blood due to insufficient production of parathyroid hormones. Symptoms may include weakness; muscle cramps; abnormal sensations such as tingling, burning, and numbness (paresthesia) of the hands; excessive nervousness; uncontrollable cramping spasms of certain muscles; and/or other symptoms. Established in 1994, the group also seeks to inform health care professionals about this rare condition. The Hypoparathyroidism Newsletter allows affected individuals to share experiences and offer information of mutual interest.

President: James E. Sanders
Year Established: 1994

Publishes the following materials:
Hypoparathyroidism Newsletter ~ *Newsletter*

Concerned with the following diseases or disorders:
Hypoparathyroidism; Kenny Caffe Syndrome

1275 IP SUPPORT NETWORK

34929 Elm
Wayne, MI 48148 313-729-7912

The IP Support Network is a national voluntary self-help organization dedicated to providing information and support to individuals and families affected by Incontinentia Pigmenti (IP); promoting knowledge of the disorder in the medical community; and increasing public awareness. Incontinentia Pigmenti is a hereditary disorder characterized by discolorations and lesions of the skin, often occurring in association with abnormalities of the eyes, hair, nails, teeth, and/or central nervous system. Established in 1992, the IP Support Network enables affected individuals to exchange mutual support, information, and resources through its networking program. The IP Support Network also publishes a quarterly newsletter entitled "The IP Party Line," which includes personal accounts written by individuals with IP and their families as well as a directory of members. In addition, the IP Support Network provides reprints of medical journal articles on Incontinentia Pigmenti.

President: Colleen Kidder
Executive Director: Colleen Kidder
Year Established: 1992
Organization Members: 50

Publishes the following materials:
Party Line ~ *Newsletter*
Incontinentia Pigmenti ~ *Reprint*

Concerned with the following diseases or disorders:
Incontinentia Pigmenti

1276 ITP ASSOCIATION

45/8 Avraham Keren Street
Kfar Saba, 44208
Israel 972 9 7657950
Fax: 972 9 7410784
E-mail: aliuneh@tamam.iai.co.il

The ITP (Idiopathic Thrombocytopenic Purpura) Association was established in 1997 in Israel as a support group for individuals with ITP, a condition characterized by deficiency of circulating blood platelets resulting in bleeding into the skin and other organs. The Association is committed to providing its members with current information concerning ITP research and its treatment, conducting periodic meetings with guest speakers from all medical and para-medical fields, promoting and supporting ITP research programs all over the world, and continually working to locate ITP specialists who will support such research. The ITP Association exchanges information with the ITP Society in New York and the Association in England; supports the Hebrew language in written and spoken forms; supports the French language in written form only; and distributes educational materials to its members. Such materials include leaflets and a regular newsletter. The Association welcomes all those with an interest in ITP and can be reached at its e-mail address at [aliuneh@tamam.iai.co.il].

President: Evi Hamany
Executive Director: Yvonne Weiss
Organization Language: Hebrew (written/spoken). French (written).
Year Established: 1997
Organization Members: 30

Concerned with the following diseases or disorders:
Purpura, Idiopathic Thrombocytopenic

1277 ITP PEOPLE PLACE

E-mail: ITPpeople1.aol.com
http://www.itppeople.com

ITP People Place is a web site on the Internet dedicated to providing information, support, resources, and online networking opportunities to individuals with Idiopathic Thrombocytopenia Purpura (ITP). ITP is characterized by abnormally low levels of circulating blood platelets (thrombocytopenia) without a readily apparent cause or underlying disease (idiopathic). The disorder may be characterized by small areas of abnormal bleeding (minor hemorrhages) within skin (dermal) layers or layers below the mucous membranes (submucosal), causing the appearance of small purplish spots on the skin (petechia); bleeding from mucous membranes that may be manifested by nose bleeds, for example; increased susceptibility to bruising; and/or other symptoms. In some cases, affected individuals may exhibit fever, slight enlargement of the spleen (splenomegaly), and/or other characteristics. The ITP People Place site offers understandable information about the potential underlying causes of ITP, symptoms and findings associated with the disorder, current treatments, and research conducted on ITP. The site also provides listings of peer-reviewed medical journal articles in several categories (including ITP in Children, ITP and Pregnancy, ITP in Adults, Gammaglobulin, Splenectomy, Methylprednisone, and Other Treatments); offers dynamic linkage to other helpful sources of information on the Internet; and offers online visitors the opportunity to participate in several surveys (such as a general ITP survey and a children's survey) whose results are then shared on the site. ITP People Place also offers several online networking opportunities including a Message Board where visitors can read and post messages, questions, and comments and a Mailing List that enables subscribers to receive a listing of others who would like to communicate with one another via e-mail.

Concerned with the following diseases or disorders:
Purpura, Idiopathic Thrombocytopenic

1278 ITP SOCIETY

Children's Blood Foundation
333 East 38th Street
New York, NY 10016 212-297-4340
800-487-7010

The ITP Society is a not-for-profit organization dedicated to promoting the welfare of and addressing the issues that affect people with Immune or Idiopathic Thrombocytopenic Purpura (ITP), a condition characterized by deficiency of circulating blood platelets resulting in bleeding into the skin and other organs. The ITP Society was founded in 1994 under the auspices of The Children's Blood Foundation. The Society's goals are to provide patient support and give appropriate referrals; support ongoing medical research to advance the knowledge and treatment of ITP; and educate the public and medical communities about the disorder. The ITP Society provides educational and support materials including fact sheets, brochures, and a booklet entitled "What's It Called Again?"

President: Mela Stevens
Executive Director: Debra Ressler, M.D.
Year Established: 1994

Publishes the following materials:
What's It Called Again? ~ *Brochure*

Concerned with the following diseases or disorders:
Purpura, Idiopathic Thrombocytopenic

1279 IVH PARENTS

P.O. Box 56-1111
Miami, FL 33256-1111 305-232-0381
Fax: 305-232-9890
E-mail: 72167.633@compuserve.com

IVH Parents is a voluntary not-for-profit self-help organization dedicated to sharing information concerning intraventricular hemorrhages (IVHs) of the brain, providing support to affected individuals and their families, and conducting ongoing follow-up. Established in 1984, the group consists of parents as well as professionals who work with affected children including physicians from several specialties, therapists, nurses, researchers, and teachers. Intraventricular hemorrhage of the brain, or bleeding into the brain's cerebrum, can occur after a premature birth or due to a traumatic full-term birth. Intraventricular hemorrhage may result in cerebral palsy, hydrocephalus, sensory loss, seizures, mental retardation, or multiple disabilities. IVH Parents enables families with affected children to network with one another in order to exchange information and mutual support. The organization also has a registry of children with IVH, provides a directory of members, and publishes a regular newsletter for parents and professionals.

President: Ronnie Londner
Executive Director: Ronnie Londner
Organization Language: Spanish. German.
Year Established: 1984
Organization Members: 350

Publishes the following materials:
IVH Parents Fact Sheet ~ *Fact Sheet*

1280 IDIOPATHIC VENTRICULAR FIBRILLATION REGISTRY OF THE UNITED STATES (IVF REGISTRY)

P.O. Box 245037
Tucson, AZ 85724-5037 520-626-6262
800-483-2662
Fax: 520-626-4333
E-mail: ivfreg@ccit.arizona.edu

The Idiopathic Ventricular Fibrillation (IVF) Registry is a not-for-profit registry that was established to identify cases of IVF. Through long-term follow-up of enrolled patients, the Registry hopes to identify cardiovascular and biobehavioral predictors of the recurrence of Ventricular Fibrillation. The rate of recurrence is currently estimated to be 25 percent within two years. Previously unidentified risk factors may be applicable to individuals at risk for sudden death due to organic heart disease. The Registry is the counterpart to a similar registry in Europe called UCARE (Unexplained Cardiac Arrest Registry of Europe). The IVF Registry will ultimately pool its data with UCARE. This will identify a large group of patients and allow data to be determined with sufficient numbers to answer questions of natural history, recurrence rate, relative efficacy of device treatments (e.g., pacemakers) versus pharmacotherapy, and risk factors predictive of recurrence. The Registry provides reprints of pertinent medical articles.

President: Frank I. Marcus, M.D. (1996 to Present)
Executive Director: Kathleen Gear, R.N. (Coordinator)
Year Established: 1996

Publishes the following materials:
Idiopathic Ventricular Fibrillation Registry of the United States ~ *Brochure*
Current Perspectives. Consensus Statement of the Joint Steering Committees of the Unexplained Cardiac Arrest Regis ~ *Pamphlet*

1281 IGA NEPHROPATHY SUPPORT NETWORK

964 Brown Avenue
Huntington Valley, PA 19006 215-663-0536

The IgA Nephropathy Support Network is a national voluntary organization dedicated to helping people with IgA Nephropathy and their families. IgA Nephropathy is a kidney disorder characterized by chronic inflammation of the kidney, blood in the urine (hematuria), abnormally increased levels of protein in the urine (proteinuria), deposits of IgA immunoglobulin in certain areas of the kidney, and other symptoms and physical findings. The primary goal of the IgA Nephropathy Support Network is to function as a clearinghouse for information on IgA Nephropathy. To further this goal, the Network has prepared pamphlets on the disease and maintains an extensive database of current medical literature related to IgA Nephropathy. Patient concerns and the latest medical research are covered in the organization's biannual newsletter entitled "Network News." The IgA Nephropathy Support Network also promotes research into the causes, treatments, and possible cures of IgA Nepropathy.

President: Dale M. Hellegers (1992-Present)
Year Established: 1993
Organization Chapters: 1

Publishes the following materials:
IgA Nephropathy Support Network ~ *Fact Sheet*
IgA Nephropathy: Questions & Answers A Guide For Parents ~ *Pamphlet*
Network News ~ *Newsletter*

Concerned with the following diseases or disorders:
IGA Nephropathy

1282 INDEPENDENT HOLOPROSENCEPHALY SUPPORT SITE

E-mail: Tim.Smith@gashead.demon.co.uk
http://www.team17.com/~tsmith/HPE/

The Independent Holoprosencephaly Support Site is a web site on the Internet dedicated to enabling families of children with Holoprosencephaly (HPE) to share information, support, common experiences, and resources. Holoprosencephaly is a condition that results from failure of the prosencephalon section of the forebrain to divide into hemispheres during embryonic development. Associated abnormalities, which may vary greatly in range and severity, may include midline facial defects such as closely set eyes (hypotelorism), absence of certain front teeth (incisors), an abnormally small head (microcephaly), cleft lip and/or cleft palate, incomplete development or absence of the nose, and/or, in severe cases, cyclopia. Affected individuals may also experience psychomotor delays, mental retardation, seizures, and/or other abnormalities. The Independent Holoprosencephaly Support Site provides referrals to holoprosencephaly organizations, describes the various forms of holoprosencephaly in understandable terminology, offers a glossary of commonly used medical terms, and discusses research that has identified the gene responsible for HPE on chromosome 7. The Support Site also enables online visitors to subscribe to the HPE e-mail list, enabling affected families to regularly communicate with one another to exchange information and resources via e-mail. In addition, the site provides an "Update" area where online visitors can read postings from other affected families. The HPE site also provides dynamic linkage to other helpful web sites on the Internet in several categories such as "Chromosomes and Gene Resources," "Hydracephaly Specific," "Neurology Resources," "Friends and Families," "General Disability," "Mailing Lists," and "Pediatric Resources." The Independent Holoprosencephaly Support Site is located at [http://www.team17.com/~tsmith/HPE/].

Concerned with the following diseases or disorders:
Holoprosencephaly

1283 INTERNATIONAL 11;22 TRANSLOCATION NETWORK

232 Kent Avenue
Timmins
Ontario, P4N 3C3
Canada 705-268-3099
Fax: 705-268-3099
E-mail: stpierre@ntl.sympatico.ca
http://www.nt.net/~stpierre/index.html

Established in 1996, the International 11;22 Translocation Network is an international voluntary health organization dedicated to bringing families together who have children with chromosomal abnormalities due to Chromosome 11;22 Translocations. Chromosome 11;22 balanced translocations usually do not result in associated symptoms or abnormalities in carriers. (A translocation is said to be "balanced" if pieces of two or more chromosomes break off and trade places, creating an altered but balanced set of chromosomes.) However, because they may result in reproductive cells (eggs in females or sperm cells in males) with "unbalanced" sets of chromosomes, carriers have an increased risk of having offspring with an unbalanced translocation (i.e., an altered set of chromosomes resulting in extra and/or missing chromosomal material in certain chromosomal locations). In such cases, affected infants and children may exhibit low muscle tone, cleft palate, genital abnormalities, heart defects, hip dislocation, kidney malfunction, and/or other abnormalities. Symptoms and physical findings may vary in range and severity from case to case depending upon the exact length, location, and nature of the resulting chromosomal abnormality. The Network participates in ongoing clinical research at Children's Hospital in Philadelphia, PA; brings together affected families for the purposes of mutual support and information exchange; and publishes brochures and a regular newsletter entitled "Together." The organization also maintains a web site at [http://www.nt.net/~stpierre/index.html].

President: Stephanie St-Pierre (Founder).
Organization Language: French (written/spoken). German (written). Dutch (written). Spanish (written).
Year Established: 1996
Organization Chapters: 1
Organization Members: 40

Publishes the following materials:
International 11;22 Translocation Network ~ *Brochure*
Together! ~ *Newsletter May 1997*
Site-Specific Reciprocal Translocation,t(11;22) (q23;q11), in Several Unrelated Families With 3:1 Meiotic Disjuncti ~ *Reprint Pamphlet*
International 11;22 Translocation Network (Dutch) ~ *Fact Sheet*
International 11;22 Translocation Network (Spanish) ~ *Fact Sheet*
International 11;22 Translocation Network (French) ~ *Fact Sheet*
International 11;22 Translocation Network (German) ~ *Fact Sheet*

1284 INTERNATIONAL CENTER FOR FABRY DISEASE

Human Genetics
Mt. Sinai Fifth Avenue at 100th Street
Box 1203
New York, NY 10029 212-241-6944
Fax: 212-348-5811
http://www.mssm.edu/crc/fabry/

The International Center for Fabry Disease is a voluntary not-for-profit organization dedicated to aiding in the diagnosis, treatment, and management of Fabry Disease, a rare inherited disorder of lipid metabolism characterized by the abnormal accumulation of certain fatty substances in various organs of the body. Symptoms may include clusters of discolorations on the skin (angiokeratomas), abdominal pain, and/or visual impairment. Later in the course of the disease, kidney failure, heart problems, and/or neurological symptoms may cause serious complications. Established in 1974, the International Center for Fabry Disease promotes and supports ongoing research on Fabry Disease and engages in patient and professional education. The Center also makes appropriate referrals and provides educational and support information to affected individuals, family members, health care professionals, and the general public through its database, reports, and brochures. The Center maintains a web site at [http://www.mssm.edu/crc/fabry/].

President: Robert Desnick
Executive Director: Christine Eng, M.D.
Organization Language: Spanish.
Year Established: 1974
Organization Members: 600

Concerned with the following diseases or disorders:
Fabry Disease

1285 INTERNATIONAL DYSLEXIA ASSOCIATION (IDA)

Chester Building
Suite 382
8600 LaSalle Road
Baltimore, MD 21286-2044 410-296-0232
800-222-3123
Fax: 410-321-5069
E-mail: info@interdys.org
http://www.interdys.org

The International Dyslexia Association (IDA) is a voluntary not-for-profit international organization concerned with the complex issues of dyslexia. IDA membership consists of a variety of professionals in partnership with people with dyslexia and their families. Established in 1949, IDA is committed to helping affected individuals achieve their personal potential, strengthening their learning abilities, and removing educational, social, and cultural barriers to language acquisition and use. In addition, the IDA actively promotes effective teaching approaches and related clinical educational intervention strategies for affected people. The Association supports and encourages interdisciplinary study and research; facilitates the exploration of causes and early identification of dyslexia; and is committed to the wide dissemination of research-based knowledge on the condition. IDA provides a bibliography of published materials on dyslexia and a variety of educational brochures and referral services.

President: Gordon F. Sherman, Ph.D.
Executive Director: J. Thomas Viall
Year Established: 1949
Organization Chapters: 46
Organization Members: 12,000

Publishes the following materials:
What is Dyslexia? ~ *Brochure*

Concerned with the following diseases or disorders:
Dyslexia

1286 INTERNATIONAL FIBRODYSPLASIA OSSIFICANS PROGRESSIVA ASSOCIATION (IFOPA)

P.O. Box 3578
Winter Springs, FL 32708 407-365-4194
Fax: 407-365-4194
E-mail: ifopa@vol.com
http://www.med.upenn.edu/ortho/fop

The International Fibrodysplasia Ossificans Progressiva (FOP) Association is a voluntary not-for-profit organization for men, women, and children with FOP, an extremely rare connective tissue disorder in which the body produces bone in abnormal locations. Established in 1988, the Association is dedicated to promoting and funding research on FOP and making medical resources available to affected individuals. The organization assists individuals with FOP in any manner reasonably related to their medical concerns including making adaptive equipment and transportation available. The Association seeks to educate affected individuals, family members, health care and other professionals, and the public about this disorder and foster relationships and the sharing of information between people with FOP. The organization also engages in patient advocacy, provides appropriate referrals, and offers a variety of educational materials including a quarterly newsletter, reports, brochures, and a directory of articles and videos.

President: Jeannie L. Peeper (1988-Present)
Executive Director: Jeannie L. Peeper
Year Established: 1988
Organization Members: 109

Publishes the following materials:
IFOPA ~ *Brochure*
THE F.O.P. CONNECTION ~ *Newsletter*
International FOP Association Resource Center Guide ~ *Pamphlet*

Concerned with the following diseases or disorders:
Fibrodysplasia Ossificans Progressiva (FOP)

1287 **INTERNATIONAL FOUNDATION FOR ALTERNATING HEMIPLEGIA OF CHILDHOOD (IFAHC)**

239 Nevada Street
Redwood City, CA 94062 650-365-5436
Fax: 650-365-5798
E-mail: laegan@aol.com
http://www.phoenix.net/~ifahc

The International Foundation for Alternating Hemiplegia of Childhood (IFAHC) is a voluntary not-for-profit organization dedicated to promoting professional and public awareness of Alternating Hemiplegia of Childhood (AHC) and providing current information to affected individuals and their families. AHC is a rare neurological disorder characterized by frequent, temporary episodes of paralysis on one side of the body (hemiplegia); temporary paralysis of the muscles that control eye movement (transient ocular palsies); sudden, involuntary movements of limbs and facial muscles (choreoathetosis); and/or excessive sweating with changes in skin color and body temperature (autonomic nervous system dysfunction). Symptoms usually become apparent before the age of 18 months. Founded in 1993 by two families who have children affected by this disorder, the organization supports ongoing medical research into the cause, treatment, and potential cure of AHC. For example, the Foundation raises funds for research at the Children's Hospital of Detroit. The Foundation also disseminates information about this disorder to promote proper diagnosis; maintains a registry of families, affected children, and physicians who are familiar with AHC; has a medical advisory board; and produces brochures and a regular newsletter.

President: L. Neil Jackson (1997 to Present)
Executive Director: Lynn Egan (Contact Person)
Year Established: 1993
Organization Members: 125

Publishes the following materials:
Alternating Hemiplegia of Childhood ~ *Brochure*
Caring for a $1 Million Baby ~ *Reprint*
International Foundation for Alternating Hemiplegia of Childhood ~ *Newsletter*

Concerned with the following diseases or disorders:
Alternating Hemiplegia of Childhood

1288 **INTERNATIONAL JOSEPH DISEASES FOUNDATION, INC. (IJDF)**

P.O. Box 2550
4047 First Street
Suite 107
Livermore, CA 94551-2550 510-371-1287
Fax: 510-371-1288

International Joseph Diseases Foundation, Inc. is a not-for-profit voluntary organization that was established in 1977. The Foundation is dedicated to assisting individuals who are affected by or may be at risk for Joseph's Disease by providing information on the disorder, supporting and promoting clinical research, and helping affected individuals locate medical, social, and genetic counseling services. Joseph's Disease is a rare inherited disorder of the central nervous system characterized by the slow degeneration of certain areas of the brain. The Foundation also engages in public and professional education and offers a variety of materials including fact sheets, a flier on the history of the disease, and a bibliography.

President: Merton Murray (1993-Present)
Executive Director: Rose Marie Silva
Organization Language: Portuguese.
Year Established: 1977
Organization Members: 3,000

Publishes the following materials:
Machado-Joseph Disease Bibliography ~ *Bibliography*
Fact Sheet - Joseph Disease ~ *Brochure*
International Joseph Diseases Foundation ~ *Brochure*

Concerned with the following diseases or disorders:
Joseph's Disease

1289 **INTERNATIONAL LESCH-NYHAN DISEASE ASSOCIATION**

11402 Ferndale Street
Philadelphia, PA 19116 215-677-4206

The International Lesch-Nyhan Disease Association is a not-for-profit, self-help organization dedicated to providing information and support to families of children diagnosed with Lesch-Nyhan Disease. Lesch-Nyhan Disease is a rare inborn error of purine metabolism characterized by the absence of the enzyme HPRT. Symptoms include impaired kidney function, joint pain, muscle weakness, neurological impairment, and self-mutilating behavior such as lip and finger biting and/or head banging. Established in 1994, the International Lesch-Nyhan Disease Association promotes awareness of the disease among health care professionals and the general public and engages in patient advocacy. It also enables affected families to exchange information, support, and resources and offers a variety of informational and support information through its database, directory, article reprints, and brochures.

President: Leslie Cornely (1994-Present)
Year Established: 1994
Organization Members: 85

Concerned with the following diseases or disorders:
Lesch Nyhan Syndrome

1290 INTERNATIONAL LONG QT SYNDROME REGISTRY

P.O. Box 653
University of Rochester Medical Center
Rochester, NY 14642-8653 716-275-5391
Fax: 716-473-2751

The International Long QT Syndrome Registry is a research organization that maintains an international database on Long QT Syndrome. The aim of the Registry, which has been helpful in providing information on many aspects of Long QT Syndrome, is to improve understanding of the genetics and natural history of this rare heart disorder. It also seeks to improve treatments for affected individuals. Efforts toward improved treatments are aided by families with the disorder and physicians who participate in this worldwide registry program. The Registry also produces an informational pamphlet for affected families and publishes in the peer-reviewed medical literature.

Executive Director: Jennifer Robinson, MS
Year Established: 1975

Publishes the following materials:
LONG QT SYNDROME An Information Pamphlet for Families ~ *Pamphlet*

Concerned with the following diseases or disorders:
Cardio Auditory Syndrome; Romano Ward Syndrome

1291 INTERNATIONAL MYELOMA FOUNDATION (IMF)

2120 Stanley Hills Drive
Los Angeles, CA 90046 213-654-3023
800-452-2873
Fax: 213-656-1182
E-mail: TheIMF@aol.com
http://myeloma.org/

The International Myeloma Foundation (IMF)) is a not-for-profit voluntary health organization dedicated to improving the quality of life for people affected by myelomas, tumors of the bone marrow. Established in 1990, the Foundation is committed to promoting research into the prevention, treatment, and cure of myelomas. The Foundation also offers nationwide support groups, engages in patient advocacy, offers referrals, and engages in patient and professional education. In addition, the Foundation offers a variety of informational brochures, audiovisual aids, and a regular newsletter.

President: Susan Lavitt Novis
Executive Director: Brian G.M. Durie, M.D. (Chairman of the Board)
Year Established: 1990
Organization Members: 17,600

Publishes the following materials:
Myeloma Today ~ *Newsletter*
Multiple Myeloma Patient Handbook ~ *Handbook*

Concerned with the following diseases or disorders:
Myeloma, Multiple

1292 INTERNATIONAL OPITZ FRIAS SYNDROME ASSOCIATION

116 June Avenue
Nanaimo
BC, V9S 4R7
Canada 604-754-7088
Fax: 604-754-7088

The International Opitz Frias Syndrome Association is a not-for-profit voluntary organization consisting of families and medical professionals who are committed to enhancing the quality of life for people affected by Opitz Frias/G/BBB Syndrome. This is a rare inherited disorder characterized by widely set eyes (hypertelorism), undescended testicles (cryptorchidism) and abnormal placement of the urinary opening (meatus) on the underside of the penis in males (hypospadias), incomplete closure of the roof of the mouth (cleft palate), an abnormal groove in the upper lip (cleft lip), swallowing difficulties (choking, aspiration), and/or other abnormalities. Established in 1994, the Association offers support services, engages in patient advocacy, and compiles and disseminates information concerning Opitz Frias/G/BBB Syndrome.

President: Celine Towstego (1994-Present)
Executive Director: Lon Towstego
Year Established: 1994
Organization Members: 7

Publishes the following materials:
Helping One Another ~ *Brochure*

Concerned with the following diseases or disorders:
Opitz Syndrome

1293 **INTERNATIONAL POLIO NETWORK**

4207 Lindell Boulevard
#110
St. Louis, MO 63108-2915 314-534-0475
Fax: 314-534-5070
TDD: 800-735-2966
E-mail: gini_intl@msn.com

Established in 1960, the International Polio Network is a not-for-profit voluntary organization dedicated to supporting the independent living, self direction, and personal achievement of people with disabilities worldwide. The Network is committed to ongoing educational and advocacy efforts related to poliomyelitis and its late effects (also known as Post Polio Syndrome). Post Polio Syndrome is characterized by a history of polio at least 10 years previously and partial recovery of function after initial infection followed by progressive weakness in previously affected muscles for which there is no other definitive cause. In addition to continuing its work with respiratory polio survivors, the International Polio Network has expanded its role to include other ventilator users through the International Ventilator Users Network (IVUN). The International Polio Network promotes patient and professional education, has a network of support groups, conducts workshops and conferences, and offers a networking program. The Network also provides a variety of materials including directories, newsletters, booklets, and brochures.

President: Martin B. Wice, M.D. (1993-Present)
Executive Director: Joan L. Headley
Year Established: 1960

Concerned with the following diseases or disorders:
Post Polio Syndrome

1294 **INTERNATIONAL REGISTRY OF WERNER SYNDROME (IRWS)**

University of Washington
Department of Pathology
Box 357470
Health Science Building K543
Seattle, WA 98195 206-543-5088
Fax: 206-685-8356
E-mail: gmmartin@u.washington.edu

The International Registry of Werner Syndrome (IRWS), associated with the Department of Pathology of the University of Washington, is a not-for-profit research organization dedicated to providing clinical and genetic information on Werner Syndrome to health care professionals and researchers. Werner Syndrome, a rare autosomal recessive disorder, is characterized by abnormally short stature in childhood and premature aging beginning in adolescence or early adulthood. Established in 1986, IRWS works to ascertain and genotype individuals with Werner Syndrome from around the world and to establish and cryopreserve cell lines from affected individuals.

President: George M. Martin, M.D. (Principal Investigator) (1986 to Present)
Executive Director: Junko Oshima, M.D., Ph.D.
Organization Language: Japanese (written/spoken).
Year Established: 1986
Organization Members: Non-Membership

Publishes the following materials:
International Registry of Werner Syndrome ~ *Mission Statement*
Registry Form. Donor Consent Form ~ *Pamphlet*

Concerned with the following diseases or disorders:
Werner Syndrome

1295 **INTERNATIONAL RETT SYNDROME ASSOCIATION (IRSA)**

9121 Piscataway Road
Suite 2-B
Clinton, MD 20735 301-856-3334
800-818-7388
Fax: 301-856-3336
E-mail: irsa@paltech.com
http://www2.paltech.com/irsa/irsa.htm

Established in 1984, the International Rett Syndrome Association is a not-for-profit voluntary organization dedicated to serving as an information and referral center for physicians and families of children with Rett Syndrome. Rett Syndrome, a rare congenital neurological disorder that affects only females, is characterized by progressive degeneration of certain tissues of the brain, resulting in loss of previously acquired mental and motor skills, impaired control of voluntary movements (ataxia), episodes of uncontrolled electrical disturbances of the brain (seizures), autistic behavior, and/or other abnormalities and physical features. The Association's mission includes supporting and promoting research into the prevention, control, and cure of the disorder; increasing public awareness; and providing emotional support for affected families. The International Rett Syndrome Association engages in patient advocacy; promotes family and professional education; provides referrals to support groups, genetic counseling, and other services; and promotes legislation beneficial to affected individuals and families. The Association also provides a variety of educational and support information through its directory, quarterly newsletter, books, audiovisual materials, brochures, and fliers.

President: Kathy Hunter (1984-Present)
Executive Director: Kathy Hunter
Year Established: 1984
Organization Members: 2,000

Publishes the following materials:
Bridges A Book of Hope and Inspiration for Families ~ *Book*
Educational and Therapeutic Intervention in Rett Syndrome ~ *Book*
Parent Idea Book ~ *Booklet*
Epilepsy and Rett Syndrome ~ *Booklet*
Orthopaedic Problems in Rett Syndrome ~ *Booklet*
What is Rett Syndrome ~ *Brochure*
Rett Syndrome: A Therapeutic Approach ~ *Videotape*
Rett Syndrome: A Physician's Approach ~ *Videotape*
Rett Syndrome: A Conversation With Families ~ *Videotape*
Rett Syndrome: A Closer Look ~ *Videotape*

Concerned with the following diseases or disorders:
Rett Syndrome

1296 INTERNATIONAL WALDENSTROM'S MACROGLOBULINEMIA FOUNDATION (WMSG)

5080 Timberchase Way
Sarasota, FL 34238 941-927-4963
Fax: 941-927-7037
E-mail: asmokler@bigfoot.com
http://www.iwmf.com

The Waldenstrom's Macroglobulinemia Support Group (WMSG) is a nonprofit support and information organization for individuals with Waldenstrom's Macroglobulinemia (WM), a malignant lymph and blood cell disorder characterized by abnormal enlargement of the liver and spleen (hepatosplenomegaly), weakness, anemia, fatigue, and excessive bleeding. Established in 1994, WMSG publishes a monthly newsletter that provides information on current therapies and clinical evaluations. Comprised of nearly 1,000 members throughout the world, the organization also offers a telephone support networking service and provides support and understanding to individuals and families affected by WM. WMSG also maintains a database containing information regarding WM, medications that may be used to treat the disorder, and updates on ongoing clinical research studies. The organization maintains a web site at [http://www.erols.com/asmokler/wmsg.htm] and sponsors an Internet discussion group.

President: Arnold Smokler (Chairman) (1994 to Present)
Year Established: 1994
Organization Chapters: 4
Organization Members: 972

Publishes the following materials:
WM Newsletter ~ *Newsletter*
WMSG Newsletter (May-June 1997) ~ *Newsletter*
WMSG Newsletter (January 1997) ~ *Newsletter*
Waldenstrom's Macroglobulinemia. What It Is! ~ *Reprint*
The Waldenstrom's Macroglobulinemia Support Group ~ *Brochure*
The Waldenstrom's Macroglobulinemia Support Group. Clinical Information (Section I) ~ *Pamphlet*
The Waldenstrom's Macroglobulinemia Support Group. Clinical Information (Section II) ~ *Pamphlet*

Concerned with the following diseases or disorders:
Waldenstrom Macroglobulinemia

1297 INTERSTITIAL CYSTITIS ASSOCIATION OF AMERICA, INC. (ICA)

P.O. Box 1553
Madison Square Station
New York, NY 10159-1553 212-979-6057
800-435-7422
Fax: 212-677-6139
E-mail: icainfo@aol.com
http://www.ichelp.com

The Interstitial Cystitis Association of America (ICA) is a voluntary not-for-profit organization working on behalf of all individuals with Interstitial Cystitis (IC), an inflammatory disease of the bladder in which chronic inflammation of the lining of the bladder and swelling of the bladder's interior walls result in pressure and pain above the pubic area and frequency and urgency of urination. Established in 1984 by individuals with Interstitial Cystitis, the Association is dedicated to providing affected individuals with the most current information on the disease; offering a support network to affected individuals and their families; increasing awareness of the disease among the medical community and the general public; and establishing a National Database to compile and study data concerning Interstitial Cystitis and promote research to find an effective treatment and cure for IC. The Interstitial Cystitis Association of America also promotes patient advocacy; testifies before Congress to support legislation beneficial to people with IC; funds several research projects for Interstitial Cystitis including its own Pilot Research Project Program; and conducts ICA national meetings and scientific workshops for Interstitial Cystitis researchers. The Association offers a variety of materials to affected individuals and the medical community including a regular newsletter entitled "Update," reports, journal article reprints, transcripts of workshops, brochures, videos, andaudiotapes.

President: Vicki Ratner, M.D. (1984-Present)
Executive Director: Debra Slade
Year Established: 1984
Organization Members: 15,000

Publishes the following materials:
ICA ~ *Brochure*
Interstitial Cystitis Association Self-Help ~ *Brochure*
Interstitial Cystitis Association - IC and Diet ~ *Brochure*
Interstitial Cystitis Association - IC and Sex ~ *Brochure*
Interstitial Cystitis Foundation - IC and Pregnancy ~ *Brochure*
ICA Resource Materials ~ *Resource List*

Concerned with the following diseases or disorders:
Interstitial Cystitis

1298 INTERSTITIAL CYSTITIS INFORMATION CENTER (ICIC)

5000 King Richard Drive
Annandale, VA 22003 703-323-7066
Fax: 703-323-7066

The Interstitial Cystitis Information Center is a not-for-profit organization dedicated to providing information, assistance, and support to individuals with Interstitial Cystitis (IC). IC is a slowly progressive inflammatory disease of the bladder characterized by pressure and pain above the pubic area as well as abnormal frequency and urgency of urination. Symptoms associated with the disorder occur due to chronic inflammation of the lining of the bladder and swelling of the bladder's interior walls. Established in 1995, the Interstitial Cystitis Information Center advocates on behalf of affected individuals and family members, maintains a database of information, promotes professional and public education on IC, and provides an informational resource listing at minimal cost to inquirers regarding all facets of IC.

Executive Director: Kay H. Benton, B.S., M.A.
Year Established: 1995
Organization Members: Non-Membership

Publishes the following materials:
Interstitial Cystitis Information Center ~ *IC Information Listings*

Concerned with the following diseases or disorders:
Interstitial Cystitis

1299 IVEMARK SYNDROME ASSOCIATION

52 Keward Avenue
Wells
Somerset, BA5 1TS
United Kingdom 174-967-2603

The Ivemark Syndrome Association is a voluntary not-for-profit organization dedicated to providing information and support to families affected by Ivemark Syndrome. Ivemark Syndrome, a rare disorder that is usually apparent at birth, is characterized by absence of the spleen, malformations of the cardiovascular system, and abnormal displacement of the abdomen and intestines. Founded in 1996, the Association aims to offer support to other familes affected by Ivemark Syndrome; to raise awareness of the disorder within the medical community and among other interested individuals; and to network families in similar situations. Educational materials include a regular newsletter.

President: Liz Fisher
Executive Director: Ingrid Gladki
Year Established: 1996

Publishes the following materials:
Ivemark Syndrome Association ~ *Brochure*

Concerned with the following diseases or disorders:
Ivemark Syndrome

1300 JAMA MIGRAINE INFORMATION CENTER

E-mail: migraine@ama-assn.org
www.ama-assn.org/special/migraine/migraine
.

The JAMA Migraine Information Center, a web site on the Internet, is a collection of peer-reviewed resources for physicians, other health care professionals, affected individuals, family members, and the general public. The site is produced and maintained by editors and staff of the "Journal of the American Medical Association" (JAMA) under the direction of an editorial review board of leading migraine authorities. The site includes a Treatment Center section containing clinical guidelines and related resources and a Library containing reviews of major migraine articles published in the medical literature as well as article selections from American Medical Association (AMA) journals and other publishers. The site also has an Education and Support Center that includes patient education material as well as information concerning support and information groups; a Newsline section containing updates from Reuters Health Information Services, summaries from major professional meetings, and reports on the science that underlies migraines; and a Best of the Net section containing a collection of additional web links selected by the site's editorial reviewers.

Concerned with the following diseases or disorders:
Headache, Cluster

1301 JDF THE DIABETES RESEARCH FOUNDATION (JDF)

89 Granton Avenue
Richmond Hill
Ontario, L4B 2N5
Canada
905-889-4171
800-668-0274
Fax: 905-889-4209
http://www.jdfc.ca

JDF The Diabetes Research Foundation is an international not-for-profit organization in Canada dedicated to raising funds to support and promote diabetes research. Diabetes is a chronic metabolic disorder that affects the body's ability to properly manufacture or utilize insulin, a hormone necessary for the body to transport food glucose into cells for energy. There are several types of diabetes including Insulin-Dependent Diabetes Mellitus, IDDM (also known as Juvenile Diabetes); Non-Insulin Dependent (Type II, also known as Adult-Onset Diabetes); and Gestational Diabetes. Established in 1974 and consisting of 14 chapters, JDF supports research advances in therapies to reduce the risk of diabetes-caused blindness, decrease the number of amputations due to diabetes, and control high blood pressure associated with diabetes; disease management practices that help maintain tight control of glucose levels to prevent or delay complications of diabetes; and practices that afford women with diabetes the opportunity for safe pregnancies and healthy children. JDF also supports advancements in methods to detect the earliest signs of diabetes; therapeutic treatments to prevent or delay the disease's onset; experimental techniques for programming cells from outside the pancreas to produce insulin; and research that has contributed to the increased understanding of transplantation immunology, which has helped to make transplantation of pancreatic tissue a reality. JDF publishes a quarterly magazine entitled "Countdown Canada," regularly produces "Research News Updates," and has a web site on the Internet at [http://www.jdfc.ca].

President: Mike Hopkins
Executive Director: Kate MacDonald
Year Established: 1974
Organization Chapters: 14
Organization Members: Non-Membership

Publishes the following materials:
Research News Summer 1997 ~ *Newsletter*
Countdown Canada ~ *Magazine*

Concerned with the following diseases or disorders:
Diabetes, Insulin Dependent

1302 JENNIFER TRUST FOR SPINAL MUSCULAR ATROPHY (JTSMA)

296 Avon House
New Broad Street
Stratford-Upon-Avon
Warwick, CV37 6HW
United Kingdom
01789 267520
Fax: 01789 268371
E-mail: anita@jtsma.demon.co.uk
http://www.jtsma.demon.co.uk

The Jennifer Trust for Spinal Muscular Atrophy (JTSMA) is a support group run by parents of children with spinal muscular atrophy (SMA) and adults who have SMA. Spinal muscular atrophy is the name given to a group of inherited disorders that result in the progressive deterioration of the spinal nerves controlling voluntary movement. The main purpose of the group is to provide support, information, understanding, and friendship to those whose lives are affected by SMA. Established in 1985 and currently consisting of 1,500 members, JTSMA conducts an annual weekend conference, has an area contact network of people who provide local support to affected individuals and family members, and offers a variety of educational materials including informational leaflets, booklets, a JTSMA Library Book List, a JTSMA Toy List, and a regular newsletter entitled Holding Hands. JTSMA also maintains a web site at [http://www.jtsma.demon.co.uk].

President: Craig Hamilton (1994 to Present).
Executive Director: Anita Macaulay
Year Established: 1985
Organization Members: 1,500

Publishes the following materials:
Severe (Type I) Spinal Muscular Atrophy ~ *Booket*
Intermediate (Type II) Spinal Muscular Atrophy ~ *Brochure*

Concerned with the following diseases or disorders:
Kugelberg Welander Syndrome; Werdnig Hoffman Disease

1303 JOUBERT SYNDROME PARENTS-IN-TOUCH NETWORK

6931 South Carlinda Avenue
Columbia, MD 21046 410-997-8084
Fax: 410-992-9184
E-mail: Joubert@erols.com

The Joubert Syndrome Parents-In-Touch Network is an international network of parents who share emotional support, knowledge, and experiences about Joubert Syndrome, a rare genetic disorder characterized by partial or complete absence of a certain area of the brain (cerebellar vermis), diminished muscle tone (hypotonia), mental retardation, psychomotor retardation, abnormal eye movements, and respiratory abnormalities including episodes of abnormally rapid breathing. Established in 1992, the organization maintains a networking list, produces a regular newsletter, conducts biannual conferences, promotes public awareness, and seeks to educate physicians and their support teams about this rare disorder.

President: Cheryl Duquette (1994-Present)
Year Established: 1992
Organization Members: 85

Publishes the following materials:
Parents-In-Touch Network ~ *Brochure*
Parents-In-Touch ~ *Newsletter*
1994 Conference Video ~ *Order Form*

Concerned with the following diseases or disorders:
Joubert Syndrome

1304 JUVENILE DIABETES FOUNDATION INTERNATIONAL (JDF)

432 Park Ave South
New York, NY 10016 212-889-7575
800-533-2873
Fax: 212-532-8791
E-mail: JBroch@jdf.usa.com.

Juvenile Diabetes Foundation International is a national voluntary health agency dedicated to supporting and funding research into the cause, treatment, prevention, and cure of diabetes, a chronic metabolic disorder that affects the body's ability to properly manufacture or utilize insulin, a hormone necessary for the body to transport food glucose into cells for energy. Juvenile Diabetes, also known as Insulin-Dependent Diabetes or Diabetes Mellitus Type I, most commonly becomes apparent in affected individuals between the ages of 10 to 16 years. Founded in 1970, the Foundation also provides information, assistance, and support to affected individuals; promotes public awareness; provides referrals; and offers a variety of educational materials including brochures and fact sheets.

President: Stephen Leeper, DDS
Executive Director: Kenneth Farber
Organization Language: Spanish.
Year Established: 1970

Publishes the following materials:
Diabetes and Nerve Disease ~ *Pamphlet*
Living with Diabetes ~ *Brochure*
Oral Medications and Type II Diabetes ~ *Pamphlet*
Diabetes and Your Heart ~ *Pamphlet*
Diabetes and Your Eyes ~ *Pamphlet*
Diabetes and Kidney Disease ~ *Pamphlet*
Dental Care and Diabetes ~ *Pamphlet*
Foot Care and Diabetes ~ *Pamphlet*
Low Blood Sugar Emergencies ~ *Pamphlet*
Diet, Exercise and Diabetes ~ *Pamphlet*
A Child with Diabetes is in Your Care ~ *Pamphlet*
Monitoring Your Blood Sugar ~ *Pamphlet*
Pregnancy and Diabetes ~ *Pamphlet*
Information About Insulin ~ *Pamphlet*
Your Child Has Diabetes ~ *Pamphlet*
What You Should Know About Diabetes ~ *Pamphlet*
Helping Research Find A Cure ~ *Pamphlet*
JDF and You: The Search for a Cure ~ *Pamphlet*
The Following Books Are Available From The Juvenile Diabetes Foundation ~ *Order Form*
Diabetes Fact Sheet ~ *Fact Sheet*

Concerned with the following diseases or disorders:
Alstrom Syndrome; Arthritis, Juvenile; Ataxia Telangiectasia; Ataxia, Friedreich's; Diabetes, Insulin Dependent; Retinopathy, Diabetic; Schmidt Syndrome; Wolfram Syndrome

1305 KFS (KLIPPEL-FEIL SYNDROME) NETWORK ONLINE

E-mail: g.catalan@student.murdoch.edu.au
http://home1.gte.net/kfsnet/index.htm

The KFS (Klippel-Feil Syndrome) Network Online, a web site on the Internet, provides understandable information on all aspects of Klippel-Feil Syndrome; abstracts summarizing medical journal articles published on the disorder; linkage to other web sites that provide additional information, support, and resources; and international online networking opportunities for individuals with KFS and family members. In individuals with Klippel-

Feil Syndrome, certain bones (vertebrae) in the spinal column within the neck may be missing and/or fused, causing shortness of the neck, limited neck motion, and an abnormally low hairline.

President: Gale Catalan (Founder)

Concerned with the following diseases or disorders:
Klippel Feil Syndrome

1306 KAWASAKI FAMILIES' NETWORK

46-111 Nahewai Place
Kaneohe, HI 96744 808-525-8053
Fax: 808-525-8055
E-mail: machado@hawaii.edu
kawasaki@compuserve.com 1022
ourworld.compuserve.com/homepages/kawasaki

The Kawasaki Families' Network is a not-for-profit organization dedicated to providing information and support to individuals and families affected by Kawasaki Syndrome, an inflammatory disease of childhood characterized by fever, skin rash, swollen lymph nodes, and inflammation of the blood vessels. Inflammatory changes cause destructive lesions in blood vessels and may lead to complications involving the liver, gall bladder, and heart. Established in 1996 and currently consisting of approximately 70 members, the Network facilitates networking opportunities through the mail and the Internet and offers educational materials including a regular newsletter entitled "Heartlines." The Network maintains a web site at [http://ourworld.compuserve.com/homepages/kawasaki] and a listserv at [kawasaki-l@hawaii.edu].

President: Vicki Viotti Machado
Year Established: 1996
Organization Members: 70

Publishes the following materials:
Heartlines ~ *Newsletter*

Concerned with the following diseases or disorders:
Kawasaki Syndrome

1307 KLINEFELTER SYNDROME AND ASSOCIATES (KS&A)

P.O. Box 119
Roseville, CA 95678-0119 916-773-2999
Fax: 916-773-1449
E-mail: ks47xxy@ix.netcom.com
http://www.genetic.org/ks/index.shtml

Klinefelter Syndrome & Associates is a national voluntary organization dedicated to supporting individuals and families whose lives have been affected by Klinefelter Syndrome, a rare chromosomal disorder. Males normally have one X and one Y chromosome; however, those with Klinefelter's Syndrome carry at least one extra X chromosome in cells of the body (somatic). Associated symptoms and physical features may not become apparent until puberty. Such abnormalities may include abnormal smallness of the testes, infertility due to impaired function of the testes, breast enlargement (gynecomastia), unusually long legs, and/or other symptoms and physical features. Established in 1990 and currently consisting of approximately 1,500 members, the organization has national and regional support groups; offers confidential networking services; has an outreach program to the medical community to help ensure earlier diagnosis of the disorder; and offers patient pamphlets and a regular newsletter entitled "The Even Exchange."

Executive Director: Melissa Aylstock
Year Established: 1990
Organization Chapters: 5
Organization Members: 1,500

Publishes the following materials:
Meet Nick and Kent ~ *Brochure*
Klinefelter Syndrome ~ *Brochure*
Understanding Klinefelter Syndrome ~ *Booklet*
The Even Exchange ~ *Newsletter*

Concerned with the following diseases or disorders:
Klinefelter Syndrome

1308 KLIPPEL-TRENAUNAY SUPPORT GROUP

4610 Wooddale Avenue
Edina, MN 55424 612-925-2596
Fax: 612-925-4708
E-mail: vesse001@maroon.tc.umn.edu
http://www.umn.edu/nlhome/m474/vesse001/k-t.html

The Klippel-Trenaunay Support Group is a voluntary self-help organization dedicated to providing support for individuals affected with Klippel-Trenaunay Syndrome and their families. Klippel-Trenaunay Syndrome is a rare congenital disorder characterized by the presence of a port-wine stain on the skin, excessive growth of the soft tissues and/or bones, venous malformations, and lymphatic abnormalities. Established in 1986, the organization conducts biannual meetings of affected individuals and their families to enable them to exchange information, experiences, and support; makes medical advisors available during these meetings; and provides phone support to members. In addition, the Group maintains a confidential group roster so that members may correspond with one another and raises awareness of the disease among the medical community and the general public. The Klippel-Trenaunay Support Group provides a variety of educational materials including a periodic newsletter, brochures, and a list of current medical articles on K-T Syndrome.

President: Judy Vessey (1986-Present)
Year Established: 1986
Organization Members: 500

Publishes the following materials:
Klippel-Trenaunay and the K-T Support Group Informational Brochure ~ *Brochure*
Guide to Medical Terminology ~ *Brochure*

Concerned with the following diseases or disorders:
Klippel Trenaunay Syndrome

1309 KNIEST SYNDROME GROUP (KSG)

4956 Queen Avenue South
Minneapolis, MN 55410 612-922-6184
Fax: 612-922-8732
E-mail: sondrols@aol.com

The Kniest Syndrome Group (KSG) is an international voluntary organization dedicated to providing financial, educational, and emotional support to individuals and families affected by Kniest Syndrome. Kniest Syndrome is a form of dwarfism characterized by short stature and unusually short, malformed arms and legs (short-limbed dwarfism); a short, "barrel-shaped" chest; swelling and stiffness of joints; abnormal sideways curvature of the spine (scoliosis); an abnormally flat face with protruding eyes and low nasal bridge; visual and/or hearing impairment; and/or other abnormalities. Established in 1997 and consisting of approximately 50 members, the Kniest Syndrome Group is committed to providing networking services to individuals and families affected by Kniest Syndrome; financial support for medical needs (i.e., for items not covered by many insurance companies such as glasses, hearing aids, etc.); college funds for affected children; and current, complete medical information on Kniest Syndrome. The organization also engages in professional education, offers support services, and provides a variety of materials including pamphlets, brochures, reports, a directory, and a regular newsletter.

Executive Director: Cory Sondrol
Year Established: 1997
Organization Members: 50

Publishes the following materials:
Individuals and Families with Kniest Syndrome ~ *Mission Statement*

Concerned with the following diseases or disorders:
Kniest Syndrome

1310 LAM FOUNDATION

10105 Beacon Hills Drive
Cincinnati, OH 45241 513-777-6889
Fax: 513-777-4109
E-mail: lamfoundtn@juno.com
http://www.lam.uc.edu

The LAM Foundation is a national non-profit organization dedicated to finding a cure for lymphangioleiomyomatosis (LAM). Lymphangioleiomyomatosis is a very rare progressive lung disease that affects females of childbearing age. The disease is characterized by the abnormal growth of smooth muscle, leading to airway obstruction and cystic lesions (blebs) in the lungs. The symptoms of Lymphangioleiomyomatosis may include shortness of breath, coughing, and/or difficulty breathing (dyspnea), especially following periods of exercise or exertion. Affected individuals may experience repeated episodes of chest pain due to fluid accumulations around the lungs (pleural effusions), potentially resulting in collapse of a lung (pneumothorax) is also common in females with this disorder. The exact cause of Lymphangioleiomyomatosis is not known. Founded in 1995, the organization believes that the cause of the disease will be uncovered by scientific research. The LAM Foundation's main objectives are to support efforts by the scientific community to develop better methods of prevention, diagnosis, and treatment; to undertake activities that will increase the amount of funding nationwide to support research on LAM; and to serve as an information resource to women affected by LAM and their families. The Foundation publishes a periodic newsletter, a brochure entitled "A Breath of Hope," and a leaflet entitled "Facts About Lymphangioleiomyomatosis (LAM)." Also available through the Foundation is a directory of women affected by LAM that enables sharing of information and support. The Foundation supports fund-raising initiatives, conducts conferences, and encourages the formation of national chapters.

President: Sue Byrnes (1995 toPresent). (Founder)
Year Established: 1995
Organization Chapters: 2
Organization Members: Non-Membership

Publishes the following materials:
Facts about Lymphangioleiomyomatosis ~ *Pamphlet*
A Breath of Hope ~ *Brochure*

Concerned with the following diseases or disorders:
Lymphangioleiomyomatosis

1311 LANGER-GIEDION SYNDROME ASSOCIATION (LGSA)

89 Ingham Avenue
Toronto
Ontario, M4K 2W8
Canada 416-465-3029
Fax: 416-465-4963
E-mail: kinross@istar.ca
http://www.geocities.com/HotSprings1930B

The Langer-Giedion Syndrome Association (LGSA) is an international not-for-profit organization dedicated to providing information and support to individuals and family members affected by Langer-Giedion Syndrome, also known as Trichorhinophalangeal Syndrome Type II (TRPS 2). Langer-Giedion Syndrome is an extremely rare genetic, multisystem disorder that belongs to the group of diseases known as Ectodermal Dysplasias. Langer-Giedion Syndrome is characterized by fine, thin hair; unusual facial features; progressive growth retardation resulting in short stature; abnormally short fingers and toes (brachydactyly); "cone-shaped" formation of the "growing ends" of certain bones; development of multiple bony growths (exostoses) projecting outward from the surfaces of various bones of the body; and/or additional abnormalities. The Langer-Giedion Syndrome Association, established in 1997, consists of an international network of families and professionals committed to helping individuals with the disorder. The Association provides networking services and an annual members' directory, engages in patient and professional education, has a patient registry, engages in patient advocacy, and provides a variety of educational materials. These materials include its regular newsletter entitled "Links," reports, brochures, pamphlets, and information available through its web site on the Internet.

President: Raquel Rozenberg (Founder)
Executive Director: Louise Kinross
Year Established: 1997

Concerned with the following diseases or disorders:
Trichorhinophalangeal Syndrome Type II

1312 LATE ONSET TAY-SACHS FOUNDATION

1303 Paper Mill Road
Erdenheim, PA 19038 215-836-9426
800-672-2022
Fax: 215-836-5438
E-mail: mpf@bellatlantic.net
http://www.webknx.com/LOTSF/

The Late Onset Tay-Sachs Foundation is a national voluntary health organization dedicated to the education of the medical community and general public regarding the late onset form of Tay-Sachs Disease. Tay-Sachs Disease is a rare genetic disorder progressive destruction of the central nervous system. Symptoms may include hand tremors, clumsiness, speech impledments, swallowing problems, and problems with gait and balance, and muscle weakness. Established in 1994, the Foundation serves people affected by this disorder, their family members, and health care professionals. It is a source of emotional support through support group activities, patient advocacy, patient education, and genetic counseling. The Late Onset Tay-Sachs Foundation supplies audio visual aids, a newsletter entitled "The Horizon," referrals, and brochures.

President: Marc P. Fishbein (1994-Present)
Year Established: 1994
Organization Members: 300

Publishes the following materials:
Late Onset Tay-Sachs Disease ~ *Brochure*

1313 LATEX ALLERGY INFORMATION SERVICE (LAIS)

176 Roosevelt Avenue
Torrington, CT 06790 860-482-6869
Fax: 860-482-7640
E-mail: 76500.1452@compuserve.com
http://www.latexallergyhelp.com

The Latex Allergy Information Service is a national voluntary service organization that provides up-to-date information on latex allergy. The Service helps to establish regional support groups and develop educational materials used to increase latex allergy awareness among medical professionals and the public. Many people who have an allergy to latex may not be aware of how to avoid contact with latex. The Service provides lists of products that contain latex and non-latex alternatives. Hospital guidelines and protocols for the management of people with latex allergy are also available from the organization. Educational materials produced by the organization include a newsletter entitled Latex Allergy News, a fact sheet on guidelines for the management of people with this allergy, and lists of products that contain latex.

Executive Director: Debra Adkins
Year Established: 1993
Organization Chapters: 48
Organization Members: 7,000

1314 LAURENCE MOON BARDET BIEDL SYNDROME (LMBBS)

c/o The Foundation Fighting Blindness
Executive Plaza 1
11350 McCormick Road
Suite 800
Hunt Valley, MD 21031 410-785-1414
888-394-3937
Fax: 410-771-9470
TDD: 800-683-5551
http://www.blindness.org

The Laurence Moon Bardet Biedl Syndrome is a national not-for-profit voluntary organization dedicated to the support of individuals with Laurence Moon Bardet Biedl Syndrome and their families. The group publishes a newsletter twice a year that offers support and networking to members. Founded in 1975, the organization also publishes the names, addresses, and phone numbers of members for the purpose of mutual support and information sharing. The organization also produces and distributes educational brochures and pamphlets.

President: Jessica Beach (Contact Person)
Executive Director: Bob Gray
Year Established: 1973
Organization Members: 50

Concerned with the following diseases or disorders:
Bardet Biedl Syndrome; Laurence Moon Syndrome

1315 LEONARD WOOD MEMORIAL AMERICAN LEPROSY FOUNDATION (LWN OR ALM)

11600 Nebel Street
Rockville, MD 20852 301-984-1336
Fax: 301-770-0580

The Leonard Wood Memorial American Leprosy Foundation is a not-for-profit research organization that is dedicated to providing information on and conducting research into the treatment and eventual cure of leprosy. Leprosy is a progressive, chronic infectious disease caused by the bacteria, Mycobacterium leprae. This disease affects the nerves that are located outside the central nervous system and the skin, mucous membranes, and eyes. The organization seeks to conduct, maintain, and support laboratory investigations, clinical studies, and related research with the goal of eradicating the disease. The Foundation is also committed to the dissemination of information concerning the source, diagnosis, treatment, and prevention of leprosy. In addition, it seeks to voluntarily aid, establish, maintain, and support clinics, hospitals, and laboratories for the diagnosis and treatment of this disease. The Foundation, to the extent of its financial ability, hopes to leave no scientific step untaken that holds any promise of finding the ultimate solution of Hansen's Disease (leprosy). Information and reports are provided and research is being conducted on Leprosy at the Foundation's clinical facility in the Philippines.

President: Gerald P. Walsh, M.D. (Scientic Director)
Executive Director: Priscilla Reed (Admin. Director)
Year Established: 1928

Publishes the following materials:
Leonard Wood Memorial American Leprosy Foundation ~ *Annual Report 1993-1994*

1316 LES TURNER AMYOTROPHIC LATERAL SCLEROSIS FOUNDATION, LTD. (LES TURNER ALS FDT)

3325 Main Street
Skokie, IL 60076 847-679-3311
Fax: 847-679-9103
E-mail: info@LTurner-ALS.org

The Les Turner Amyotrophic Lateral Sclerosis Foundation is a voluntary health organization dedicated to raising funds for ALS research, patient services, and public awareness. Amyotrophic Lateral Sclerosis (ALS), also known as Lou Gehrig's Disease, is a progressive neurological disease that causes impaired breathing, speaking, and swallowing, as well as muscle weakness and eventually total paralysis. Intellectual function remains unaffected and there is no known cure. The Les Turner ALS Foundation was established in 1977 and provides educational materials for affected individuals and family members, health care professionals, and the general public. Program services include referrals and counseling; audio-visual aids and periodic newsletters entitled "ALS Dialogue" and "ALS Today." Consisting of over 971 members, the organization offers support groups and patient networking to affected individuals, family members, and caregivers. Annual events include a one and five mile family hike and a "Music and Record Sale," in which musical and electronic items are donated and sold to raise money to benefit the Foundation and ALS research.

President: Harvey Gaffen (1979 to Present)
Executive Director: Wendy Abrams
Year Established: 1977
Organization Members: 971

Publishes the following materials:
Questions and Answers About ALS ~ *Pamphlet*
ALS Q and A. Information about Amyotrophic Lateral Sclerosis and the Les Turner ALS Foundation ~ *Brochure*
Serving the Amyotrophic Lateral Sclerosis Patient ~ *Brochure*
A Legacy of Caring ~ *Brochure*
We're Going To Get This Gene ~ *Reprint*
Teepu Siddique, M.D. (Director) Neuromuscular Disorders Program Nortwestern University Medical School ~ *Fact Sheet*
From Harvard Medical School. Harvard Health Letter ~ *Reprint*
ALS Patient/Family/Caregiver Reading List ~ *Pamphlet*
Ventilation: "The Decision Making Process" ~ *Video Tape*
ALS Resource Guide ~ *Resource Binder*
Medlife ~ *Reprint*
Rilutek. Some Specifics ~ *Fact Sheet*
Scientists hail discovery of gene that triggers ALS ~ *Reprint*
Opening the lines of communication ~ *Reprint*
Altered-gene mice a boon to science ~ *Reprint*
ALS Dialogue ~ *Newsletter*
Als Today ~ *Newsletter*
Critical Support Services ~ *Pamphlet*
Drug Development Update ~ *Pamphlet*

Concerned with the following diseases or disorders:
Amyotrophic Lateral Sclerosis

1317 LEUKEMIA SOCIETY OF AMERICA, INC. (LSA)

600 Third Avenue
4th Floor
New York, NY 10016
212-573-8484
800-955-4572
Fax: 212-856-9686
E-mail: infocenter@leukemia.org
http://www.leukemia.org

The Leukemia Society of America, Inc. is a national not-for-profit voluntary health agency dedicated to curing leukemia and its related cancers such as lymphoma, multiple myeloma, and Hodgkin's Disease and to improving the quality of life of affected individuals and their families. The Society, which was established in 1949 and has 57 chapters across the country, sponsors research, patient aid, public and professional education, and community service programs. The Leukemia Society of America's educational resources include a toll-free public education resource phone line, a newsletter, brochures, fact sheets, booklets, and videos.

President: Dwayne Howell
Year Established: 1949
Organization Chapters: 57

Publishes the following materials:
Free Public Educational Materials ~ *Materials List*

Concerned with the following diseases or disorders:
Anemia, Sideroblastic; Leukemia, Chronic Lymphocytic; Leukemia, Chronic Myelogenous; Leukemia, Hairy Cell; Lymphoma, Gastric, Non-Hodgkins Type; Myeloma, Multiple; Radiation Syndromes

1318 LI-FRAUMENI SYNDROME INTERNATIONAL REGISTRY

Cancer Institute
CE&C
44 Binney Street
Suite 201
Boston, MA 02115
617-632-3158
800-828-6622
Fax: 617-632-3161
http://www.dfci.harvard.edu

The Li-Fraumeni Syndrome International Registry is a not-for-profit health organization dedicated to compiling data concerning families with Li-Fraumeni Syndrome and providing them with information regarding surveillance and intervention options. Li-Fraumeni Syndrome is a familial disorder consisting of the appearance of early breast cancer. Established in 1969, the Registry provides referrals to genetic counseling and other services and works to educate affected families and health care professionals. It provides a variety of educational and support materials, including a regular newsletter, videotapes concerning genetic testing, brochures, and fliers.

President: David Nathan
Executive Director: Fred Li
Organization Language: Interpreters.
Year Established: 1969
Organization Chapters: 1
Organization Members: 300

1319 **LIPOMYELOMENINGOCELE FAMILY SUPPORT NETWORK (LFSN)**

321 Hopewell Street
Birdsboro, PA 19508 610-582-5937
E-mail: gmcafee@postoffice.ptd.net
http://develop.mainquad.com/web/chrisMc/support.ht

The Lipomyelomeningocele Family Support Network (LFSN) is a self-help organization dedicated to supporting families affected by lipomyelomeningocele/tethered cord syndrome. Lipomyelomeningocele is a soft tissue mass including fat and fibrous elements that extends into the spinal canal through a defect in the spine. Tethered cord syndrome is a disorder characterized by progressive neurological deterioration due to unnatural stretching of the spinal cord caused by adhesions in the spinal cords or nerves. Established in 1997, LFSN consists of 70 members. Educational materials include a self-titled brochure, a newsletter entitled "LFSN NEWS," and pamphlets. Program activities include a support group, family matching, pen pal list, online mailing list, and a chat room.

Executive Director: Chris McAfee
Year Established: 1997
Organization Members: 70

Publishes the following materials:
Lipomyelomeningocele Family Support Network. A Support Network for Families Affected by Lipomyelomeningocele/Tethe ~ *Brochure*
LFSN News ~ *Newsletter*
CLASS Notes ~ *Newsletter*

Concerned with the following diseases or disorders:
Tethered Spinal Cord Syndrome

1320 **LISSENCEPHALY CONTACT GROUP**

12 Didsbury Park
Didsbury
Manchester, M20 5LJ
United Kingdom 0161 445 3539

The Lissencephaly Contact Group is an international self-help organization in the United Kingdom dedicated to networking affected families and promoting awareness of Lissencephaly and other rare, related brain conditions. Lissencephaly is a rare birth defect in which the folds of the brain are incompletely formed; as a result, the brain has a smooth surface instead of the normal folds and grooves. In some cases, affected individuals may exhibit additional abnormalities, such as a small head (microcephaly), episodes of uncontrolled electrical disturbances in the brain (seizures), and/or other physical abnormalities. Severe mental retardation may also be present. Lissencephaly may be due to a spontaneous (de novo) genetic change that occurs for unknown reasons (sporadic), be inherited as an autosomal recessive genetic trait, or occur in association with various underlying disorders. Beginning in 1988 as a few families with children affected by Lissencephaly, the Lissencephaly Contact Group was officially established the following year. The Contact Group is committed to enabling affected families to share information and experiences; helping interested families meet and/or correspond; and obtaining and disseminating current information on Lissencephaly for the benefit of affected families and interested professionals. The Contact Group also provides referrals and offers a variety of educational materials including brochures, pamphlets, and a regular newsletter.

President: Kathleen Wood (Contact Person)
Year Established: 1988
Organization Members: 80

Publishes the following materials:
Lissencephaly. Can We Help ~ *Brochure*

Concerned with the following diseases or disorders:
Lissencephaly

1321 **LISSENCEPHALY NETWORK, INC.**

716 Autumn Ridge Lane
Fort Wayne, IN 46804 219-432-4310
Fax: 219-432-4310
http://www.lissencephaly.org/

The Lissencephaly Network is a non-profit organization that serves children with Lissencephaly and their families throughout the United States, Canada, and Mexico. Lissencephaly is a rare birth defect in which the folds of the brain are incompletely formed; as a result, the brain has a smooth surface instead of the normal folds and grooves. In some cases, affected individuals may exhibit additional abnormalities, such as a small head (microcephaly), episodes of uncontrolled electrical disturbances in the brain (seizures), and/or other physical abnormalities. Established in 1991, the Lissencephaly Network offers updated and accurate medical information, referrals to genetic counseling, equipment sharing, and parent-to-parent talks. The Lissencephaly Network publishes a newsletter three times a year and has a directory that lists members. A comprehensive database is maintained on medical and developmental histories of affected children. A variety of informational materials is produced and distributed by the Lissencephaly Network including Update for Physicians, articles, and reprints of medical journal articles.

President: Dianne Fitzgerald (1991-Present)
Executive Director: Dianna Fitzgerald
Year Established: 1991
Organization Members: 285

Publishes the following materials:
The Lissencephaly Network, Inc. ~ *Fact Sheet*
Lissencephaly Information for Parents ~ *Article*
Update for Physicians ~ *Pamphlet*

Concerned with the following diseases or disorders:
Lissencephaly; Perisylvian Syndrome, Congenital Bilateral; Walker Warburg Syndrome

1322 LONG QT SYNDROME EUROPEAN INFORMATION CENTER (LQTS-EIC)

Ronnerweg 2
Nidau, 2560
Switzerland 041323315835
Fax: 041323448335
E-mail: jmettler@bielnews.ch
www.bielstar.ch/customers/jmettler/qt.html

The Long QT Syndrome (LQTS) European Information Center is a web site on the Internet created by an individual with LQTS from Switzerland. There are two forms of Long QT Syndrome, one without deafness (Romano Ward Syndrome) and one with deafness (Jervell and Lange-Nielsen Syndrome). Long QT Syndrome is characterized by an abnormality in the heart's electrical system. In the lower chambers (ventricles) of the heart, the normal duration of one phase of electrical activity is referred to as the Q-T interval. In Long QT Syndrome, there are abnormally prolonged intervals of electrical activity in the ventricles (prolonged Q-T), resulting in seizures and a fast, uneven heartbeat (ventricular fibrillation). The main goal of the web site is to provide information about Long QT Syndrome to affected individuals, their families, medical professionals, and interested individuals worldwide. The site also provides information on diagnostic criteria and potential therapies and has dynamic linkage to sites with further information. The web site is supported by Prof. Dr. Peter J. Schwartz, Chairman of Cardiology at the University of Pavia, Italy.

President: Jon Mettler
Organization Language: German (written/spoken).
Year Established: 1997
Organization Members: Non-Membership

Concerned with the following diseases or disorders:
Cardio Auditory Syndrome; Romano Ward Syndrome

1323 LOWE SYNDROME ASSOCIATION (LSA)

222 Lincoln Street
West Lafayette, IN 47906 765-743-3634
E-mail: kayeuulsa@aol.com
http://www.medhelp.org/lowesyndrome

The Lowe Syndrome Association is an international voluntary health organization composed of parents, health care professionals, and other interested individuals. It was formed to provide information to parents of children with Lowe Syndrome. Established in 1983, the organization fosters communication and networking among affected families for the purpose of mutual support and information exchange. The Lowe Syndrome Association also seeks to support medical research leading to prevention and more effective treatments for Lowe Syndrome. Educational publications are designed to provide accurate and timely information to parents, teachers, and physicians all over the world. These publications include brochures, a planned publications list, and a booklet entitled "Living with Lowe Syndrome."

President: Candy Smith (1993-Present)
Year Established: 1983
Organization Members: 300

Publishes the following materials:
Lowe's Syndrome: Questions & Answers ~ *Fact Sheet*
Care Today ... Cure Tomorrow ~ *Brochure*
On The Beam ~ *Newsletter*

Concerned with the following diseases or disorders:
Lowe's Syndrome

1324 LUPUS CANADA

P.O. Box 64034
5512 - 4 Street NW
Calgary
Alberta, T2K 6J1
Canada 403-274-5599
800-661-1468
Fax: 403-274-5596
E-mail: lupuscan@cadvision.com
http://www.lupuscanada.org

Lupus Canada is a national association of regional lupus support groups and their various branches. These groups of volunteers are dedicated to providing support and information to people who have lupus, their families, and friends. Lupus is a chronic autoimmune disorder that can affect any organ of the body. In lupus, the body's immune system that defends against invading or "foreign" organisms (e.g., viruses, bacteria, germs) begins to malfunction and fails to distinguish between the body's own tissues and these foreign invaders. As a result, the body's natural defenses (antibodies) begin to attack the body's own tissue. Established in 1987, Lupus Canada produces educational materials including a pamphlet entitled "Introduction to Lupus," a booklet entitled "Lupus: The disease with 1000 faces," and a video entitled "Lupus: Disease in Disguise." Interested individuals can contact Lupus Canada at its e-mail address [lupuscan@cadvision.com] or on the world wide web at [http://www.lupuscanada.org].

President: Mae Boa (1996 to Present)
Executive Director: P.K. O'Brien
Organization Language: French (written).
Year Established: 1987
Organization Chapters: 121
Organization Members: 12

Publishes the following materials:
"Lupus" Disease in Disguise ~ *Video Tape*
An Introduction To Lupus ~ *Brochure*
SLE and the Related Connective Tissue Diseases: Clinical and Laboratory Diagnosis ~ *Brochure*
The disease with 1000 faces (French) ~ *Booklet*
The disease with 1000 faces ~ *Booklet*

Concerned with the following diseases or disorders:
Lupus

1325 LUPUS FOUNDATION OF AMERICA, INC. (LFA)

1300 Piccard Drive
Suite 200
Rockville, MD 20850 301-670-9292
800-558-0121
Fax: 301-670-9486
http://www.lupus.org/lupus

The Lupus Foundation of America is a national not-for-profit organization that was established in 1977. The primary purposes of the Foundation are the eradication of Lupus through research, the early detection of undiagnosed cases through awareness promotion, and the alleviation of suffering through patient support programs. The Lupus Foundation has more than 90 local chapters serving hundreds of thousands of people throughout the United States and 73 International Associated Groups in 37 countries worldwide. The Services provided by the Foundation and its chapters include informational materials, referrals, patient educational meetings and seminars, support groups, hospital visits, grants, and bequests. The Foundation functions as an advocate for people with Lupus and seeks to raise awareness and understanding of the disorder among elected and appointed government officials. To this end, the Foundation participates in coalitions with other health agencies to make its mission known to decision and policy makers. A wide variety of educational materials are produced by the organization including brochures, pamphlets, and a newsletter entitled "Lupus News." Some materials are available in Spanish.

President: V. Terry Bell (1996-Present)
Organization Language: Spanish.
Year Established: 1977
Organization Chapters: 98
Organization Members: 46,000

Publishes the following materials:
Brochures ~ *Publications List*
Brochure and Fact Sheets ~ *Publications List*
Organizational Fact Sheet ~ *Fact Sheet*
List of Publications ~ *Publications List*
Lupus News ~ *Newsletter*
Lupus 1993 Annual Report ~ *Report*
Que Es Lupus? ~ *Brochure*
Vivir Bien Con Lupus ~ *Brochure*
La Enfermedad Renal Y Lupus ~ *Brochure*
Enfermedad Cardiopulmonar Y Lupus ~ *Brochure*
Depresion Y Lupus ~ *Brochure*
Enfermedad Neurologica Y Lupus ~ *Brochure*
Vasculitis Y Lupus ~ *Brochure*
El Lupus, Las Infecciones, Y Las Immunizaciones ~ *Brochure*
Examenes De Laboratorio Y El Diagnostico Del Lupus ~ *Brochure*
Lupus Y Los Hombres ~ *Brochure*
Dolor De Los Musculos Y Las Articulaciones En El Lupus ~ *Brochure*
Desordenes De La Sangre En Les ~ *Brochure*
What is Lupus? ~ *Brochure*
Living Well With Lupus ~ *Brochure*
Laboratory Tests Used in the Diagnosis of Lupus ~ *Brochure*
Medications ~ *Brochure*

Concerned with the following diseases or disorders:
Antiphospholipid Syndrome; Lupus; Mixed Connective Tissue Disease (MCTD)

1326 LYME DISEASE FOUNDATION (LDF)

1 Financial Plaza 18th Floor
Hartford, CT 06103 860-525-2000
800-886-5963
Fax: 860-525-8425
E-mail: lymefnd@aol.com
http://www.lyme.org

The Lyme Disease Foundation, Inc. (LDF) is a voluntary not-for-profit organization dedicated to finding the solutions to Lyme Disease and other tick-borne disorders. Established in 1988, the Lyme Disease Foundation funds research on Lyme Disease (LD), conducts international scientific conferences, and publishes a peer-reviewed scientific journal. It has successfully lobbied Congress for federal funds dedicated to Lyme Disease education and research. In addition, the Lyme Disease Foundation provides appropriate referrals, promotes patient advocacy, and supports the development of educational programs for affected individuals, family members, the medical and scientific communities, and the public. The Lyme Disease Foundation's many educational and support materials include a monthly self-help newsletter and a Lyme Disease Awareness Pack. A Lyme Disease Scientific Pack includes reprints of medical articles, scientific slide show information, and guidelines for establishing and conducting a self-help group. In addition, the Foundation distributes educational program materials for students, workplace and community education program materials, poster sets, brochures, and videotapes.

President: Karen Vanderhoof-Forschner (1988-Present)
Executive Director: Thomas E. Forschner
Year Established: 1988
Organization Members: 90,000

Publishes the following materials:
LDF Educational Material - Tick Alert Card ~ *Fact Sheet*
LDF Educational Material - Self-Help ~ *Fact Sheet*

1327 LYME DISEASE RESOURCE CENTER

P.O. Box 1423
Ukiah, CA 95482 707-468-8460
E-mail: pcm@pacific.net

The Lyme Disease Resource Center is a voluntary not-for-profit education and communication center dedicated to supporting people affected by Lyme Disease, the public, physicians, and any others interested in this disorder. Established in 1990, the Lyme Disease Resource Center educates the public about Lyme Disease, its risks, and preventive measures. It provides a forum for physicians and other health care professionals to exchange ideas and information concerning symptoms, diagnosis, and treatments for Lyme Disease and functions as a communication center for individuals and groups who assist people with Lyme Disease. The Center also has a network of Lyme Disease support groups; engages in patient advocacy; and provides referrals to medical professionals or support groups. The Resource Center offers a variety of educational and support materials through its directory, audio visual aids, brochures, Spanish language brochure, and regular newsletter.

President: Phyllis Mervine
Year Established: 1990
Organization Members: 4,000

Concerned with the following diseases or disorders:
Lyme Disease

1328 MAAP SERVICES, INC. (MAAP)

P.O. Box 524
Crown Point, IN 46307 219-662-1311
Fax: 219-662-0638
E-mail: chart@netnitco.net

The MAAP Services, Inc. is a nonprofit organization dedicated to assisting family members of more advanced individuals with autism by offering information and advice on autism, and by providing the opportunity to network with others in similar circumstances. In addition, MAAP Services works to inform professionals and the general public about more advanced individuals with autism and how to meet their needs. Autism is a syndrome; individuals with this syndrome experience difficulty in verbal and/or nonverbal communications, which ranges in extremes from not speaking at all to being unable to interpret body language or participate comfortably in two-way conversation. Established in 1984, MAAP Services, Inc. supports professionals and families of individuals with autism by responding to phone calls and letters from family members, professionals, and individuals with autism who need support and advice. Consisting of 2,000 members, the organization produces educational materials including "The MAAP," a quarterly newsletter that allows subscribers to exchange information, learn about issues related to autism, and share with others who face similar challenges; disseminates specific print materials relevant to high-functioning individuals with autism; and distributes a pamphlet entitled "MAAP Services, Inc." The organization conducts conferences, workshops, and meetings of parent groups; supports education; and provides appropriate referrals. MAAP can be reached at its e-mailaddress at [chart@netnitco.net].

President: Susan J. Moreno (1991 to Present)
Organization Language: Spanish (written).
Year Established: 1984
Organization Members: 2,000

Publishes the following materials:
What is MAAP Services, Inc.? ~ *Brochure*
The Maap ~ *Newsletter*
Tips For Teaching High-Functioning People With Autism ~ *Reprint*

Concerned with the following diseases or disorders:
Autism

1329 MCAD (MEDIUM CHAIN ACYL-COA DEHYDROGENASE DEFICIENCY) FAMILY SUPPORT GROUP

805 Montrose Drive
Greensboro, NC 27410 336-547-8682
E-mail: goulddan@aol.com
http://www.cinternet.net/FOD

The MCAD (Medium-Chain Acyl-CoA Dehydrogenase Deficiency) Family Support Group is a self-help organization devoted to the nationwide networking of families affected by this disorder. MCAD Deficiency is a very rare inherited metabolic disorder characterized by a deficiency of the enzyme medium chain acyl-CoA dehydrogenase. This enzyme is found to be most active in the liver, certain white blood cells (leukocytes), and certain connective tissue cells (fibroblasts) and is necessary for the breakdown (oxidation) of certain fats (medium chain fatty acids). Failure to break down these fats can lead to the abnormal accumulation of fatty acids in the liver and the brain. In infants with MCAD Deficiency, symptoms may include recurrent episodes of unusually low levels of a certain sugar (glucose) in the blood (hypoglycemia), lack of energy (lethargy), vomiting, and/or liver malfunction. Because MCAD Deficiency is a rare genetic metabolic deficiency that may be unfamiliar to many physicians, many affected families feel that they have not received the information and support that they require. The MCAD Family Support Group was established in 1991 to help fulfill MCAD families' special needs by providing them with practical information, support, and regular updates on medical research and pharmaceutical news that concerns MCAD. The MCAD Family Support Group produces and distributes information and support through periodic newsletters, letters, and phone calls. A Family List enables members to contact other families affected by MCAD.

President: Deb Lee Gould, MEd. (1991-Present)
Executive Director: Deb Lee Gould, MEd.
Year Established: 1991
Organization Members: 450

Publishes the following materials:
MCAD Communications Network "All In This Together" ~ *Newsletter*
1995 MCAD Family List ~ *Directory*

Concerned with the following diseases or disorders:
Medium Chain Acyl CoA Dehydrogenase Deficiency

1330 MHE (MULTIPLE HEREDITARY EXOSTOSES) FAMILY SUPPORT GROUP (MHE)

1727 Ironwood Drive
Idaho Falls, ID 83402 208-523-6459
http://www.radix.net/~hogue/mhe

The MHE (Multiple Hereditary Exostoses) Family Support Group is a national organization dedicated to providing counseling, medical information, and a forum for individuals and families affected by MHE. MHE is a rare disorder in which bony growths or bumps (exostoses) form on the bones of affected individuals. These growths vary in size, location, and number depending upon the individual. Established in 1993, MHE consists of 40 members. Educational materials include a brochure entitled "Multiple Hereditary Exostoses, What Is It?" Program activities include a support group, genetic counseling referrals, advocacy, and education.

President: Penny Flake
Executive Director: Evelyn Hogue
Year Established: 1993
Organization Members: 40

Publishes the following materials:
Mulitple Hereditary Exostoses. What is it? ~ *Brochure*
The Natural History of Hereditary Multiple Exostoses ~ *Reprint*
MHE Family Support Group. Dear Friends: ~ *Letter*
MHE Family Support Group ~ *Mission Statement*

Concerned with the following diseases or disorders:
Exostoses, Multiple

1331 ML 4 (MUCOLIPIDOSIS TYPE IV FOUNDATION) (ML4 FOUNDATION)

719 East 17th Street
Brooklyn, NY 11230 718-434-5067
Fax: 718-859-7371
E-mail: ML4www@aol.com
http://www.ML4.org

The Mucolipidosis Type IV Foundation is a not-for-profit voluntary organization of parents and professionals committed to raising funds for medical research into the cause and possible treatments for Mucolipidosis Type IV. Established in 1983, the Foundation uses all donations to fund scientific research. Areas of medical research that the Foundation supports include the definition of the exact biochemical mechanism of the disorder; improvement of diagnostic measures; development of a carrier screening test; development of treatments; and discovery of a cure. In addition, the Foundation is a major support system for families affected by Mucolipidosis Type IV. The Foundation has recently awarded grants to Dr. Roscoe Brady (National Institutes of Health), Dr. Edwin Kolodny (New York University Medical Center), and Dr. Gideon Bach (Hadassah Hospital Genetics Team). Educational materials produced by the Foundation include a brochure and fact sheet.

President: Randy Yudenfriend Glaser
Executive Director: Steve Schottenfeld
Year Established: 1983
Organization Chapters: 2

Publishes the following materials:
What Is Mucolipidosis IV? ~ *Fact Sheet*
ML4 Mucolipidosis IV Foundation ~ *Brochure*
Mucolipidosis Type IV: Clinical Spectrum and Natural History ~ *Reprint*

Concerned with the following diseases or disorders:
Ganglioside Sialidase Deficiency

1332 MSL (MULTIPLE SYMMETRICAL LIPOMATOSIS) HELP (MSL HELP)

P.O. Box 2426
Stamford, CT 06906 203-359-4822

MSL (Multiple Symmetrical Lipomatosis) Help is a self-help organization dedicated to identifying persons with this condition in order to form a network of mutual information sharing and support. MSL, also known as Madelung's Disease or Lanois-Bensaude Syndrome, is a disorder of fat metabolism (lipid storage) that results in an unusual accumulation of fat deposits around the neck and shoulders. Established in 1996, MSL Help works toward its objectives including information sharing and resources; providing encouragement; and helping to educate other people and the medical community. The organization produces educational materials including a brochure entitled "Multiple Symmetrical Lipomatosis." Program activities include networking and education.

President: Sister Mary Ellen Boyle, Esq. (Contact Person)
Year Established: 1996
Organization Members: 12

Publishes the following materials:
Multiple Symmetrical Lipomatosis ~ *Brochure*

1333 MALIGNANT HYPERTHERMIA ASSOCIATION (MHA)

Toronto General Hospital
200 Elizabeth Street
CCRW-2, Room 834
Toronto
Ontario, M5G 2C4
Canada 416-340-3238
Fax: 416-340-4960
http://www.advantage.com

The Malignant Hyperthermia Association (MHA) is a registered charitable organization dedicated to reducing complications associated with Malignant Hyperthermia. Malignant Hyperthermia is a hereditary disorder in which a person does not react appropriately to certain drugs (e.g., anesthetics) due to a genetic abnormality. Founded in 1976, the MHA has three main objectives: education, communication, and research. It provides financial support to current test standardization and genetic and lymphocyte research. In addition, the organization also produces educational materials including a periodic newsletter entitled "Hotline," and other literature of interest to the general public and medical professionals.

President: Morris Altman, M.D. (1996 to Present)
Executive Director: Elysse Clamen
Organization Language: French.
Year Established: 1979
Organization Members: 1,000

Publishes the following materials:
Malignant Hyperthema ~ *Fact Poster*
Notification Letter to MH Family Members ~ *Fact Sheet*
Campers/Daycare Advice ~ *Fact Sheet*
Malignant Hyperthermia Association. Medical Bibliography ~ *Pamphlet*
MHA Drug List (Revised, 1989) ~ *Pamphlet*
A Guide to Malignant Hyperthermia ~ *Booklet*
Preparations for Elective Surgery ~ *Reprint*
Genetics and Malignant Hyperthermia ~ *Reprint*
Phosphorus Nuclear Magnetic Resonance Spectroscopy: A possible test for MH? ~ *Reprint*
Heat Stroke and Malignant Hyperthermia ~ *Reprint*
Stress and Pain Control for MH Patients ~ *Reprint*

Concerned with the following diseases or disorders:
Malignant Hyperthermia

1334 MALIGNANT HYPERTHERMIA ASSOCIATION OF THE UNITED STATES (MHAUS)

32 South Main Street
Sherburne, NY 13460-1069 607-674-7901
800-986-4287
Fax: 607-674-7910
E-mail: mhaus@norwich.net
http://www.mhaus.org

The Malignant Hyperthermia Association of the United States is a national not-for-profit voluntary organization dedicated to reducing morbidity and mortality related to Malignant Hyperthermia. Founded in 1981, the Malignant Hyperthermia Association of the United States seeks to improve the medical care of people with Malignant Hyperthermia and provide support information for people with this rare disorder and their families. It seeks to improve scientific understanding of Malignant Hyperthermia and promote ongoing medical research related to Malignant Hyperthermia and other related syndromes. Educational materials produced by the organization include numerous brochures about the disorder, a booklet entitled "Understanding Malignant Hyperthermia," a newsletter, and a directory of United States Malignant Hyperthermia Muscle Biopsy Test Centers.

President: Dallas D. Pennington (1994-Present)
Executive Director: Richard A. Hillman
Year Established: 1981
Organization Members: 2,700

Publishes the following materials:
Emergency Therapy for Malignant Hyperthermia ~ *Poster*
Directory - US Malignant Hyperthermia Muscle Biopsy Centers ~ *Directory Listing*
The Communicator (MHAUS) ~ *Newsletter*
Understanding Malignant Hyperthermia ~ *Booklet*
What is Mhaus? ~ *Brochure*
Clinical Update 1994 - Managing Malignant Hyperthermia ~ *Brochure*
Dantrolene Sodium - The Specific Treatment for Malignant Hyperthermia ~ *Brochure*
Preventing Malignant Hyperthermia - An Anesthesia Protocol ~ *Brochure*
Managing Malignant Hyperthermia - Drugs and Equipment ~ *Brochure*
Testing for Susceptibility to Malignant Hyperthermia ~ *Brochure*
The Job's Not Done Yet...1993/94 Annual Report ~ *Report*

Concerned with the following diseases or disorders:
Central Core Disease; Malignant Hyperthermia; Myotonia Congenita; Neuroleptic Malignant Syndrome; Pseudocholinesterase Deficiency; Schwartz Jampel Syndrome

1335 MAPLE SYRUP URINE DISEASE FAMILY SUPPORT GROUP (MSUD)

24806 SR 119
Goshen, IN 46526 219-862-2992
Fax: 219-862-2012
E-mail: msud@hsonline.net
http://www.msud-support.org/

The Maple Syrup Urine Disease Family Support Group (MSUD) is a non-profit organization dedicated to providing opportunities for support to affected individuals and their families, encouraging research, and disseminating educational materials. Maple Syrup Urine Disease is a rare inherited matabolic disorder that, if left untreated, can result in mental retardation, physical disabilities, and life-threatening complications. In infants with MSUD, three branched chain amino acids (leucine, iosleucine, and valine) abnormally accumulate in the blood causing harmful effects that interfere with brain functions. Established in 1982, MSUD publishes a periodic newsletter entitled "Magic." The support group conducts an annual national education conference; produces and distributes educational materials such as brochures on Maple Syrup Urine Disease; and organizes a symposium held every two years. The organization maintains a site on the World Wide Web at [http://www.msud-support.org].

President: Wayne Brubacher (1990 to Present).
Executive Director: Dawn Marie Hahn
Year Established: 1982
Organization Members: 430

Publishes the following materials:
Maple Syrup Urine Disease ~ *Brochure*
Maple Syrup Urine Disease ~ *Brochure*
Maple Syrup Urine Disease Newsletter ~ *Newsletter*

Concerned with the following diseases or disorders:
Maple Syrup Urine Disease

1336 MARFAN ASSOCIATION UK

Rochester House
5 Aldershot Road
Fleet
Hampshire, GU13 9NG
United Kingdom 01252 810472
Fax: 01252 810473
E-mail: marfan@thenet.co.uk
http://www.thenet.co.uk/~marfan

The Marfan Association UK is a service, research, and advocacy organization dedicated to supporting, educating, and researching Marfan Syndrome. Marfan Syndrome is an inherited disorder that affects the connective tissues of the heart and blood vessels (cardiovascular system). Established in 1984, the Marfan Association works with affected individuals, family members, specialists, researchers, general practitioners, and other medical specialists in the support role. Consisting of 1,200 members and 70 support groups, the organization produces educational materials including a self-titled newsletter, reports, brochures, fact sheets, and a directory. Program activities sponsored by the organization include awareness meetings, which are underway nationally on a continuing basis (a Marfan text is provided as appropriate) and support meetings which are planned in its offices. The organization works to improve the effectiveness of the Marfan Support Network and provides translations of its materials in Spanish, Italian, Greek, Russian, Norwegian, Dutch, French, Danish, and several other languages. Marfan Association UK can be reached at its e-mail address at [marfan@thenet.co.uk] or its web site at [http://www.thenet.co.uk/~marfan].

President: Diane Rust (Chairman/Support Coordinator) (1984 to present).
Organization Language: Spanish (written). Italian (written). Greek (written). Russian (written). Norwegian (written). Dutch (written). French (written). Danish (written).
Year Established: 1984
Organization Chapters: 70
Organization Members: 1,200 Families

Publishes the following materials:
Marfan Association UK (February 1997) ~ *Newsletter*
Marfan 'In Touch' Magazine ~ *Magazine*

Concerned with the following diseases or disorders:
Marfan Syndrome

1337 MASTOCYTOSIS SOCIETY, INC.

11208 Vienna Drive
Denton, MD 21629 410-479-1808
Fax: 410-479-1808
E-mail: masto@dmv.com
http://www.gil.com.au/comm/mast/

The Mastocytosis Society is a voluntary not-for-profit self-help organization dedicated to providing information and support to individuals with Mastocytosis and their caregivers. Mastocytosis is the name given to a group of rare disorders that are caused by a proliferation of mast cells. Established in 1994, the Mastocytosis Society produces a periodic newsletter entitled "The Mastocytosis Chronicles" that is distributed to more than 200 subscribers across the United States and throughout the world. The newsletter includes editorials, a letter forum, reprints of physicians' case studies, bibliographies listing recent medical journal articles on Mastocytosis and helpful hints. A Kid's Corner is reserved for children with Mastocytosis. The newsletter also provides an "Ask the Chemist" column in which a pharmacist who also has Mastocytosis answers questions from affected individuals concerning medications and their use for the treatment of Mastocytosis.

Publishes the following materials:
The Mastocytosis Chronicles ~ *Newsletter*
The Mastocytosis Chronicles (Welcome Edition) ~ *Newsletter*

Concerned with the following diseases or disorders:
Mastocytosis

1338 MATHEWS FOUNDATION FOR PROSTATE CANCER RESEARCH

817 Commons Drive
Sacramento, CA 95825-6655 916-567-1400
800-234-6284
Fax: 916-927-5218
E-mail: mathews@sna.com
http://www.mathews.org

The Mathews Foundation for Prostate Cancer Research is a nonprofit health organization dedicated to providing information and support to individuals affected by prostate cancer and their families. Prostate cancer is characterized by malignant cell development arising in the prostate gland. Symptoms may include increased frequency of urination, poor flow of urine, and difficulties beginning urination due to enlargement of the prostate. Established in 1988, the Mathews Foundation provides affected individuals and their families with information pertinent to prostate cancer so that they can make informed treatment choices. The Foundation also works to raise funds for research into the cause(s), treatment, and ultimate cure of prostate cancer. Educational materials produced by the organization include a regular newsletter entitled "BreakThrough," brochures, pamphlets, and reprints of pertinent medical literature.

President: Mary Lou Wright (1989 to present).
Organization Language: Spanish (written).
Year Established: 1988
Organization Members: Non-membership.

Concerned with the following diseases or disorders:
Cancer, Prostate

1339 MELNICK-NEEDLES SYNDROME SUPPORT GROUP

4 Kivner Lane
Bexhill-On-Sea
East Suffex, TN40 2ST
United Kingdom 01424217790

The Melnick-Needles Syndrome Support Group is a voluntary self-help organization dedicated to helping families of children with Melnick-Needles Syndrome (MNS). This is a rare hereditary disorder characterized by abnormal bone development and characteristic abnormalities of the head and face (craniofacial) area. Established in 1994 as an affiliate of Contact a Family, the Melnick-Needles Syndrome Support Group is committed to providing information, assistance, and moral support to member families as well as those whose children have just been diagnosed. The Support Group also works to raise awareness among professionals and disseminates information concerning treatment options. It enables affected families to share their experiences and resources with one another and works to make contact with other affected families. The Melnick-Needles Support Group provides members with fact sheets on MNS.

President: G. Carter
Executive Director: G. Carter
Year Established: 1994
Organization Members: 2

Concerned with the following diseases or disorders:
Melnick Needles Syndrome

1340 MENIERE'S AUSTRALIA, INC. (MA INC.)

P.O. Box 202
Moonah
Tasmania, 7009
Australia 01161362341494
Fax: 0116136234194
http://www.tassie.net.au/~meniere

The Meniere's Australia, Inc. (MA Inc.) is a not-for-profit organization dedicated to promoting and advancing the interests of people with Meniere's Disease, so as to help them improve the quality of their lives, and to have the community become more aware of the disease. Meniere's Disease is a disorder characterized by recurrent prostrating dizziness (vertigo), possible hearing loss, and ringing sounds (tinnitus). Established in 1981, MA Inc. assists people with Meniere's Disease adjust to the daily routine of life through counseling and advice gained from the experiences of members and other people whose expertise is considered to be of assistance. It also assists the families of affected individuals to understand their special needs. The organization works to collect and disseminate information to increase community awareness and knowledge about Meniere's Disease. MA Inc. consists of 600 members and 11 chapters and produces educational materials including leaflets on various aspects of Meniere's Disease, a newsletter, a publications list, and an order form. Program activities include a support group, patient advocacy, research, patient and professional education, and referrals.

President: Vincent Cockburn (Senior Executive Officer) (1993 to Present)
Executive Director: Gordon Hancock (Officer)
Year Established: 1981
Organization Chapters: 12
Organization Members: 3,000

Publishes the following materials:
Meniere's Disease ~ *Fact Sheet*
Meniere's Disease - An Information Book for People with Meniere's Disease ~ *Book*
Meniere's Australia, Inc. Rules of the Association ~ *Leaflet*
People with Meniere's Disease don't just have one disability ~ *Fact Sheet*
Vertigo ~ *Fact Sheet*
Meniere's Tears in the Ears ~ *Fact Sheet*
Some hints on reducing salt in your diet ~ *Fact Sheet*
Meniere's Disease ~ *Brochure*
Meniere's Disease ~ *Fact Sheet*
Impaired Hearing ~ *Fact Sheet*

Concerned with the following diseases or disorders:
Meniere Disease

1341 MENIERE'S DISEASE AND DIZZINESS SUPPORT GROUP

511 Ellen Avenue
Royal Oak, MI 48073-3359 248-585-8519
Fax: 248-585-8519
TDD: 810-585-8519
E-mail: 72724.2263@Compuserve.Com

The Meniere's Disease and Dizziness Support Group is a not-for-profit self-help organization dedicated to helping individuals affected by Meniere's Disease to cope in society, family, and employment. Meniere's Disease is characterized by recurrent dizziness (vertigo), possible hearing loss, and ringing sounds (tinnitus). Established in 1989, the organization provides educational materials and maintains support groups for affected individuals and their families. Monthly meetings include professional speakers such as a specialist in the medical treatment and surgery of the ear (otologist); a specialist in the diagnosis and treatment of neurological disorders (neurologist); ear, nose, and throat specialist; physical therapist; and nutritionist. In addition, the Group helps affected individuals to help themselves to prevent an episode of symptoms.

President: Marie Key
Executive Director: Marie Key
Year Established: 1989
Organization Members: 102

Publishes the following materials:
Meniere's Disease vs. Meniere's Syndrome ~ *Reprint*
Steady (The Quarterly Newsletter of The Meniere's Network) ~ *Reprint*
Dizziness (Vertigo) ~ *Reprint*
News Release ~ *Reprint*
Aging hearing cells produce annoying ringing of the ears ~ *Reprint*
Symptomatology and Dcfinition of Mcnicrc's Discasc - *Reprint*
Benign Paroxysmal Positional Vertigo ~ *Reprint*
Tinnitus in Burnt-Out Meniere's Disease ~ *Reprint*
Neruotology ~ *Reprint*
Medi-News ~ *Reprint*
Better than Dramamine ~ *Reprint*

Concerned with the following diseases or disorders:
Meniere Disease

1342 MENIERE'S NETWORK

1817 Patterson Street
Nashville, TN 37203 615-329-7807
800-545-4327
Fax: 615-329-7935
TDD: 615-239-7849
E-mail: FYIEAR@aol.com
http://www.theearfound.com

The Meniere's Network, a national network of patient support groups, is administered by the EAR (Education and Auditory Research) Foundation, a not-for-profit organization dedicated to integrating persons who have hearing impairments into the mainstream of society through public awareness and medical education. Meniere's Disease is a disorder of the inner ear characterized by episodic vertigo, nausea, ringing or roaring in the ear, and hearing loss. The Meniere's Network is dedicated to providing networking and support services that enable affected individuals to share common experiences, mutual support, information, resources, and coping strategies. The Network has members in all states throughout the United States, has over 35 support groups across the country, offers an international pen pal service, and has a "telephone buddy" service. The Meniere's Network also educates health care professionals and the public about Meniere's Disease. The Network offers a variety of educational materials including a quarterly newsletter entitled "STEADY" and a 28-page booklet entitled "An Introduction to Meniere's Disease."

President: C. Gary Jackson, M.D. (1997-Present)
Executive Director: Edward Thompson
Year Established: 1971
Organization Chapters: 1

Publishes the following materials:
Steady ~ *Newsletter*

Concerned with the following diseases or disorders:
Meniere Disease; Tinnitus

1343 MERALGIA PARESTHETICA FOUNDATION (MPF)

414 Erie Street SE
Apt. 2
Minneapolis, MN 55414 612-627-9415
E-mail: macew001@gold.tc.umn.edu
http://www.angelfire.com/mn/meralgia

The Meralgia Paresthetica Foundation is a general service organization dedicated to providing information, assistance, and support to individuals with Meralgia Paresthetica (MP) and their families. Also known as Lateral Femoral Cutaneous Neuropathy (LFCN), Meralgia Paresthetica is an uncommon condition in which direct mechanical pressure or traction on the lateral femoral cutaneous nerve of the thigh may cause burning, tingling, and numbness toward the front, side (anterolateral) area of the thigh (entrapment neuropathy). Such mechanical pressure or traction on the nerve may result from a number of factors such as obesity, swelling of the abdomen due to abnormal accumulation of fluid in the abdominal cavity (ascites), or pregnancy; in addition, tight garments (e.g., belts, jeans, backpack straps), prolonged standing, and/or other factors may exacerbate symptoms. Although the course of MP tends to be benign in most cases, symptoms may continue periodically for several years. Established in 1995, the Meralgia Paresthetica Foundation promotes research, offers understandable information on MP, and has a web site on the Internet. Its web site includes an indepth "A to Z" listing of medical journal article citations published from the peer-reviewed medical literature on Meralgia Paresthetica. The Foundation's web site is located at [http://www.angelfire.com/mn/meralgia].

President: Karen E. MacEwan (1995 to Present).
Year Established: 1995
Organization Members: 1

Publishes the following materials:
Meralgia Paresthetica Foundation. Reference Pages ~ *Pamphlet*

1344 METATROPIC DYSPLASIA DWARF REGISTRY

3393 Geneva Drive
Santa Clara, CA 95051 408-244-6354
Fax: 408-296-6317
E-mail: figone@netgate.net

The Metatropic Dysplasia Dwarf Registry is a group comprised of parents and adults with Metatropic Dwarfism who have united to form a self-help group for the purpose of mutual support. The Registry collects and exchanges information about metatropic dwarfism, which is a very rare form of dwarfism. The Registry seeks to gather information that will help affected individuals, their families, and physicians. Established in 1980, the Metatropic Dysplasia Dwarf Registry was formed to collect data and case histories from families with metatropic dwarfism. To this end, the Registry distributes a detailed registry questionnaire for the purposes of gathering information, networking, and mutual support. A list of physicians who are specialists in care and treatment of people with dwarfism is also available from the Registry.

President: Shirley Figone (1980-Present)
Year Established: 1980
Organization Members: 29

Publishes the following materials:
Voluntary Metatrophic Dwarf Registry ~ *Information/Registration Packe*
Metatrophic Dyplasia ~ *Fact Sheet*
Physicians with Expertise in Dwarfism National Medical Advisory Board ~ *Advisory Board Listing*

Concerned with the following diseases or disorders:
Metatropic Dysplasia I

1345 MICRO & ANOPHTHALMIC CHILDREN'S SOCIETY (MACS)

Publishes the following materials:
MACS Newsletter ~ *Newsletter*
MACS Patron: Anne Diamond ~ *Brochured*

Concerned with the following diseases or disorders:
Aicardi Syndrome; Chromosome 13, Partial Monosomy 13q; Chromosome 5, Trisomy 5p; Lenz Microphthalmia Syndrome; Oculocerebrocutaneous Syndrome; Phocomelia Syndrome; Schwartz Jampel Syndrome; Trisomy 13 Syndrome; Velocardiofacial Syndrome; Walker Warburg Syndrome

1346 MOEBIUS SYNDROME FOUNDATION

P.O. Box 993
Larchmont, NY 10538 914-834-6008

The Moebius Syndrome Foundation is a national not-for-profit voluntary organization that was founded in 1994. The mission of the Foundation is to help individuals with Moebius Syndrome, their families, and physicians. Moebius Syndrome is a rare disorder characterized by paralysis of the 6th and 7th cranial nerves, resulting in a lack of facial expression, lack of lateral eye movement, and lack of blinking. In some cases, other cranial nerves may be involved. The Foundation provides a network of information and communication to affected individuals and their families and seeks to educate the medical community and general public about this disorder. In addition, the Foundation promotes funding for ongoing medical research. Funds are used to support scientific research into the development of new diagnostic tests, treatments, and a cure for this disorder. Educational materials produced by the Foundation include a brochure entitled "Life Without a Smile" and a newsletter called "Moebius Syndrome Foundation."

President: Kathryn Kim Campbell
Year Established: 1994
Organization Members: 250

Publishes the following materials:
Life without a smile ~ *Brochure*

Concerned with the following diseases or disorders:
Moebius Syndrome

1347 MOEBIUS SYNDROME SUPPORT GROUP

39521 Rowan Court
Palmdale, CA 93551 805-267-2570
Fax: 310-477-8640
http://www.ciaccess.com/moebius

The Moebius Syndrome Support Group is a non-profit voluntary health organization that provides information, support, and networking to people with Moebius Syndrome and their families. Moebius Syndrome is a rare disorder characterized by paralysis of the 6th and 7th cranial nerves, resulting in a lack of facial expression, lack of lateral eye movement, and lack of blinking. In some cases, other cranial nerves may be involved. Established in 1990, the Group also provides referrals and telephone support. Video tapes of the 1994 Moebius Syndrome Conference are available from the Group. Educational materials produced by the Group include pamphlets, newsletters, a directory of people with Moebius Syndrome, and a bibliography of journal articles about this disorder.

President: Lori Thomas (1991-Present)
Executive Director: Vicki McCarrell
Year Established: 1991
Organization Chapters: 3
Organization Members: 285

Publishes the following materials:
Moebius Syndrome Support Network ~ *Brochure*
Moebius Syndrome News ~ *Newsletter*

Concerned with the following diseases or disorders:
Moebius Syndrome

1348 MONTGOMERY HEART FOUNDATION FOR CARDIOMYOPATHY

6205 Pilgrim Road
Baltimore, MD 21214 410-254-6370
Fax: 410-254-6379
E-mail: rmonty@welchlink.welch.jhu.edu
http://www.med.jhu.edu/cardiomyopathy

The Montgomery Heart Foundation for Cardiomyopathy is a not-for-profit organization dedicated to providing private funding to support genetic research for familial cardiomyopathy and raising awareness of the disease to help promote the advancement of a cure. Cardiomyopathy is a term used to describe a heterogeneous group of disorders causing primary heart muscle dysfunction in both men and women, often leading to heart failure or life-threatening complications. Established in 1993, the Foundation provides direct financial support for research studies focusing on the cause and treatment of cardiomyopathies; creates a constituency for cardiomyopathy and makes the needs and interests of this known to researchers, clinicians, and the general public; facilitates the flow of information between researchers, clinicians, and affected individuals about new developments and breakthroughs; informs the general public about this disease; and offers up-to-date information to affected individuals and their families and helps them to understand what it means to have this disease.

President: Robert A. Montgomery, M.D., Ph.D. (1993 to Present)
Executive Director: Meg Friske Montgomery (Administrator)
Year Established: 1993
Organization Members: Non-Membership

Publishes the following materials:
Striving to Stop the Cycle of Inherited Heart Disease ~ *Brochure*

1349 MORBUS FABRY HOMEPAGE GERMANY

E-mail: Korzilius@t-online.de
home.t-online.de/home/026232710-0001/fabrye.htm

Morbus Fabry Homepage Germany is a web site on the Internet that was created by three individuals with Fabry Disease. Provided in an English and a German version, this site is dedicated to providing information on Fabry Disease to affected individuals, family members, health care professionals, and others. Fabry Disease is a rare inherited disorder of lipid metabolism characterized by the abnormal accumulation of certain fatty substances (i.e., glycolipids such as glycosphingolipid) in various organs of the body. Symptoms may include clusters of wart-like discolorations on the skin (angiokeratomas), abdominal pain, and/or visual impairment. In addition to providing information concerning Fabry Disease, this site also provides dynamic links to several additional home pages on the Web, many of which are specifically dedicated to providing information, services, support, and resources to individuals affected by the disorder. For example, links are provided to such sites as the International Fabry Disease Homepage, Fabry Support & Information Group (USA), Fabry Disease Support Group (GB), and the National Institutes of Health's (NIH's) Fabry Disease Homepage.

Organization Language: German.

Concerned with the following diseases or disorders:
Fabry Disease

1350 MYASTHENIA GRAVIS FOUNDATION OF AMERICA (MGFA)

222 South Riverside Plaza
Suite 1540
Chicago, IL 60606 312-258-0522
800-541-5454
Fax: 312-258-0461
E-mail: MGFA@aol.com
http://www.med.unc.edu/mgfa/

The Myasthenia Gravis Foundation of America is national not-for-profit agency dedicated to assisting people with Myasthenia Gravis through programs of research, education, information, and patient services. The Foundation supports funding for medical research and promotes public awareness of Myasthenia Gravis. Myasthenia Gravis is a rare autoimmune disease affecting the neuromuscular junction and producing weakness of voluntary muscles. The Foundation also disseminates educational materials to those affected by this disease, their families, medical professionals, and the interested public. Organizational activities conducted by the Foundation include support groups and patient advocacy. The Myasthenia Gravis Foundation produces national and chapter newsletters, numerous brochures and pamphlets, a Survival Guide, health alert cards, and manuals for nurses and physicians. Founded in 1952, the Myasthenia Gravis Foundation has grown to more than 37 chapters and 100 support groups.

President: Raina M. Ernstoff, M.D.
Executive Director: Edward S. Trainer
Year Established: 1952
Organization Chapters: 35
Organization Members: 23,000

Publishes the following materials:
A PRACTICAL GUIDE TO MYASTHENIA GRAVIS ~ *Brochure*
Emergency Management of Myasthenia Gravis ~ *Brochure*
IMURAN ~ *Brochure*
PLASMAPHERESIS ~ *Brochure*
MYASTHENIA GRAVIS FOUNDATION ~ *Brochure*
PREDNISONE ~ *Brochure*
FACTS ABOUT MYASTHENIA GRAVIS FOR PATIENTS AND FAMILIES ~ *Brochure*
MYASTHENIA GRAVIS FOUNDATION NATIONAL NEWSLETTER ~ *Newsletter*
MESTINON ~ *Brochure*
MYASTHENIA GRAVIS Survival Guide ~ *Brochure*
MYASTHENIA GRAVIS Physician's Manual ~ *Brochure*

Concerned with the following diseases or disorders:
Eaton Lambert Syndrome; Myasthenia Gravis; Schmidt Syndrome

1351 MYASTHENIA GRAVIS LINKS

E-mail: PKHL45B@prodigy.com
http://pages.prodigy.com/myasthenia/

Myasthenia Gravis Links, a web site on the Internet, contains information on Myasthenia Gravis for affected individuals, family members, physicians, health care professionals, researchers, and the general public. Myasthenia Gravis is a rare autoimmune disease affecting the neuromuscular junction and producing weakness of voluntary muscles. This web site provides information on Myasthenia Gravis in understandable terminology, more detailed and technical medical information covering every aspect of the disorder (e.g., diagnosis, causes, treatments, etc.), a variety of online networking opportunities (including listservs, chat rooms, newsgroups, bulletin boards, etc.), and links to additional organizations within the United States and across the world that provide information and support for those affected by Myasthenia Gravis. This comprehensive site also includes dynamic links to information on research and researchers around the world who are investigating the causes and potential treatments for Myasthenia Gravis, links to other helpful online resources (including to web sites with non-English Myasthenia Gravis information), listings of newsletters that provide information on the disorder, and more.

Concerned with the following diseases or disorders:
Myasthenia Gravis

1352 MYOTUBULAR MYOPATHY RESOURCE GROUP

2602 Quaker Drive
Texas City, TX 77590 409-945-8569
Fax: 409-945-2162
E-mail: gscoggin@aol.com
http://members.aol.com/xmtm/homepage.htm

Established in 1993, the Myotubular Myopathy Resource Group is a not-for-profit voluntary organization dedicated to enabling affected families to exchange support, resources, and information about this rare disorder. X-linked Myotubular Myopathy is a rare disorder characterized by weakness of the respiratory muscles causing respiratory distress. In addition, infants with this form of myotubular myopathy are generally weak and have a loss of muscle tone causing poor sucking and an inability to swallow. Weakness of the jaw, tongue, lips, cheeks, mouth, throat, and neck muscles may also be present. The Resource Group is also committed to identifying affected families, educating the medical community about the disorder, working with several researchers who are attempting to locate the responsible gene, and offering educational materials, including fact sheets, reports, and a regular newsletter.

President: Gary Scoggin
Executive Director: Pamela Scoggin
Year Established: 1993
Organization Members: 120

Publishes the following materials:
X-Linked Myotubular Myopathy Resource Group ~ *Fact Sheet*
Myotubular Myopathy Families ~ *Newsletter*

Concerned with the following diseases or disorders:
Myopathy, Myotubular

1353 NAEVUS SUPPORT GROUP (NSG)

58 Necton Road
Wheathampstead
Herts, AL4 8AU
United Kingdom

The Naevus Support Group is voluntary self-help group dedicated to providing support and information to individuals affected by various types of birthmarks. Established in 1985, the Naevus Support Group works toward its various goals: to provide information on various types of birthmarks; to introduce parents of children with similar birthmarks to each other; to provide support by existing members to newcomers; to deal with every inquiry on a personal basis; not to impose any charges for the services offered until the expenditure is so great that gifts will not cover expenses; to be voluntary and independent; to produce two newsletters per year; and to hold two informal get-togethers per year. The organization provides educational materials including a newsletter, brochures, booklets, and fact sheets.

President: John Renate O'Neill, Founder
Year Established: 1985
Organization Members: 600

Concerned with the following diseases or disorders:
Blue Rubber Bleb Nevus; Dysplastic Nevus Syndrome; Epidermal Nevus Syndrome

1354 NAIL-PATELLA SYNDROME (NPS) WEB SITE

E-mail: PACALI@aol.com
http://members.aol.com/PACALI/index.html

The Nail-Patella Syndrome Web Site is a site on the Internet created by Carol Ferensak, an individual with Nail-Patella Syndrome who has traced the disorder back three generations in her family. Nail-Patella Syndrome (NPS), an extremely rare inherited disorder, may be characterized by improper development of the fingernails and/or toenails; absence and/or underdevelopment of the knee caps (patellae); underdevelopment of certain bones and/or webbing of skin at the bend of the elbow(s); abnormal projections of bone from the upper portion of both sides of the hipbone (bilateral iliac horns); and/or, in some cases, eye abnormalities. Approximately 30 to 40 percent of affected individuals may also experience abnormalities in kidney function (nephropathy) that may be apparent during childhood or later in life. The NPS Web Site is dedicated to providing information on the disorder as well as enabling affected individuals and family members to locate one another, share their stories, and exchange information, support, mutual concerns, and resources. The site provides indepth, understandable information on NPS; includes information on ongoing research and enables affected individuals and family members to contact researchers via e-mail for more details; has dynamic linkage to additional sources of information on NPS on the Internet; and provides a variety of online networking opportunities. For example, the site enables affected individuals and family members to post their personal stories to a message board area, read the many stories already posted in this area, and send direct e-mail to those who posted such stories; offers regular live chats; and more.

President: Carol Ferensak (site creator)

Concerned with the following diseases or disorders:
Nail Patella Syndrome

1355 NAIL-PATELLA SYNDROME (NPS) WEB SITE (UNITED KINGDOM)

E-mail: alan@reck-bates.demon.co.uk
www.reck-bates.demon.co.uk/nps/nps.html

The Nail-Patella Syndrome (NPS) Web Site is a site on the Internet created by Alan Bates, an individual with Nail-Patella Syndrome in the United Kingdom. Nail-Patella Syndrome (NPS), an extremely rare inherited disorder, may be characterized by improper development of the fingernails and/or toenails; absence and/or underdevelopment of the knee caps (patellae); underdevelopment of certain bones and/or webbing of skin at the bend of the elbow(s); abnormal projections of bone from the upper portion of both sides of the hipbone (bilateral iliac horns); and/or, in some cases, eye abnormalities. Approximately 30 to 40 percent of affected individuals may also experience abnormalities in kidney function (nephropathy) that may be apparent during childhood or later in life. The NPS Web Site is dedicated to providing information on the disorder, enabling affected individuals and family members to locate one another, providing online visitors with linkage to additional sources of information, and offering support resources to individuals who live in the United Kingdom. (Although support resources are specific to the U.K., the majority of the information within this site is helpful for all individuals and family members affected by NPS.) The NPS Web site provides indepth, understandable information on the disorder; offers information concerning ongoing research in the U.K. and the United States and the ability to e-mail researchers for additional information; provides dynamic linkage to additional sources of information; and offers several online networking opportunities by enabling affected individuals and family members to post their personal stories, read those stories already posted to the area, and send direct e-mail to those who posted such stories.

President: Alan Bates (site creator)

Concerned with the following diseases or disorders:
Nail Patella Syndrome

1356 NAIL-PATELLA SYNDROME WEB SITE

Johns Hopkins University School of Medicine
Baltimore, MD 21287-4922
E-mail: imcintos@welchlink.welch.jhu.edu
http://www.med.jhu.edu/nps/index.html

The Nail-Patella Syndrome Web Site, a site on the Internet, consists of information provided by Dr. Iain McIntosh of Johns Hopkins University School of Medicine, Baltimore, MD. Dr. McIntosh is the principal investigator of the research team that narrowed the location of the gene responsible for Nail-Patella Syndrome to a small interval on chromosome 9 (9q34). His team is continuing its research to identify the specific gene responsible for the disorder. Nail-Patella Syndrome (NPS), an extremely rare inherited disorder, may be characterized by improper development of the fingernails and/or toenails; absence and/or underdevelopment of the knee caps (patellae); underdevelopment of certain bones and/or webbing of skin at the bend of the elbow(s); abnormal projections of bone from the upper portion of both sides of the hipbone (bilateral iliac horns); and/or, in some cases, eye abnormalities. Approximately 30 to 40 percent of affected individuals may also experience abnormalities in kidney function (nephropathy) that may be apparent during childhood or later in life. The Nail-Patella Syndrome Web Site provides understandable information on the disorder; includes an introduction to basic genetics and an explanation of how NPS may be inherited; describes Dr. McIntosh's ongoing studies to locate the NPS gene; enables affected individuals or family members to request additional information concerning such research and potential participation; contains a bibliography of citationsfrom the peer-reviewed medical literature concerning NPS; and offers dynamic linkage to additional sources of helpful information on the Internet.

President: Dr. Iain McIntosh (principal investigator, site creator)

Concerned with the following diseases or disorders:
Nail Patella Syndrome

1357 NARCOLEPSY NETWORK, INC. (NN)

277 Fairfield Avenue
Suite 310B
Fairfield, NJ 07004 973-276-0115
Fax: 973-227-8224
E-mail: narnet@aol.com
http://www.websciences.org/narnet

The Narcolepsy Network is a national voluntary organization that was formed to serve the needs of people with narcolepsy. It is composed of people with narcolepsy, their families, friends, health care professionals, and other interested individuals. The Network is dedicated to improving the quality of life for people with narcolepsy and finding a cure for this disorder. To this end, the organization maintains a network of local support groups and chapters. The organization promotes programs of communication, advocacy, research, support, and education. A booklet entitled "Narcolepsy: A Guide to Understanding" provides information on narcolepsy. Topics covered within the booklet include the symptoms, causes, diagnosis of the disorder, associated sleep apnea, treatments, and social implications. The organization also distributes a reading list, bibliography, and an educational materials order form.

President: Robert L. Cloud, Esq.
Executive Director: Howard Wolfe
Year Established: 1986
Organization Chapters: 40

Publishes the following materials:
Narcolepsy - A Funny Disorder That's No Laughing Matter ~ *Book*
Narcolepsy - A Guide to Understanding ~ *Booklet*
Narcolepsy - Questions and Answers ~ *Brochure*

Concerned with the following diseases or disorders:
Apnea, Sleep; Narcolepsy

1358 NATIONAL ALLIANCE OF BREAST CANCER ORGANIZATIONS (NABCO)

9 East 37th Street
10th Floor
New York, NY 10016 212-889-0606
888-806-2226
Fax: 212-689-1213
E-mail: nabcoinfo@aol.com
http://www.nabco.org

The National Alliance of Breast Cancer Organizations (NABCO) is a not-for-profit network of breast cancer organizations dedicated to providing information, education, assistance and referrals to anyone with questions about breast cancer. It acts as a voice for the interests and concerns of breast cancer survivors and women at risk. Breast Cancer is one of the most common forms of cancer. Established in 1986, NABCO has information specialists who can answer questions about breast cancer; provide referrals to experts, support, practical resources, and how to get a second opinion; and provide background reading about risk, detection, diagnosis, and treatment. These services are available free of charge by telephone, mail, or on the Internet. Aside from its role as a source of up-to-date, accurate information for media, medical organizations, professionals, patients and their families, NABCO advocates for regulatory change and legislation that benefits individuals with breast cancer locally, on the state level, and in Washington D.C. Consisting of 350 members, the organization produces educational materials including a quarterly publication entitled "NABCO News," a guide to more than 2,000 publications entitled "NABCO Breast Cancer Resource List," and a brochure entitled "Take Charge of Your Breast Health." Programs include patient advocacy, government legislation, and education. NABCO can be reached at its e-mail address at [nabcoinfo@aol.com] or its web site address at[http://www.nabco.org].

Executive Director: Amy Langer
Year Established: 1986
Organization Members: 350

Publishes the following materials:
Network Publications. Promoting communication in the field of learning disabilities ~ *Brochure*
Network Outreach ~ *Brochure*
The Learning Disabilities Network ~ *Brochure*
The National Alliance of Breast Cancer Organizations ~ *Mission Statement*
Questions about Breast Cancer? NABCO Has the Answers ~ *Brochure*
Take Charge of Your Breast Health ~ *Brochure*
Myth or Fact? ~ *Brochure*
NABCO News ~ *Newsletter*
Breast Cancer Resource List (1996/97 Edition) ~ *Booklet*
National Alliance of Breast Cancer Organizations. The First Ten Years ~ *Booklet*
NABCO. Questions and Answers about Breast Cancer and Young Women ~ *Pamphlet*
How to Get A Low-Cost Mammogram ~ *Fact Sheet*
Getting the Best Mammogram ~ *Fact Sheet*
Myths and Facts about the Detection of Breast Cancer ~ *Fact Sheet*
Myths and Facts about the Risk of Developing Breast Cancer ~ *Fact Sheet*
Myths and Facts about the Treatment of Breast Cancer ~ *Fact Sheet*
Myths and Facts about Breast Cancer Follow-Up Care and Survival ~ *Fact Sheet*
Facts About Breast Cancer in the USA ~ *Fact Sheet*
National Breast Cancer Organizations ~ *Mission Statement*

1359 NATIONAL ALOPECIA AREATA FOUNDATION (NAAF)

710 C Street
Suite 11
San Rafael, CA 94901 415-456-4644
Fax: 415-456-4274
E-mail: NAAF@compuserve.com

The National Alopecia Areata Foundation is a voluntary health organization and the main source of funding for research on basic hair biology and Alopecia Areata. Established in 1981, the Foundation leads medical research efforts by raising private funds and awarding grants to qualified investigators at university centers in the United States, Canada, and Europe. It also seeks to inform government officials about Alopecia Areata in an effort to obtain federal funding for research studies on this disorder. The Foundation conducts ongoing public awareness programs to increase the public's understanding of this disorder. As a worldwide center for educational materials, the Foundation supplies a wide variety of information, support, and resources for people with Alopecia Areata and their physicians. Numerous brochures, a handbook, a Foundation report, newsletters, a novel entitled "Herman," and a video called "This Weird Thing That Makes My Hair Fall Out" are available from the Foundation.

President: Vera H. Price, M.D. (1992-Present)
Executive Director: Vicki Kalabokes
Organization Language: Spanish. Greek.
Year Established: 1981
Organization Chapters: 58

Publishes the following materials:
Ayudese A Si Mismo ~ *Brochure*
Alopecia Areata ~ *Brochure*
Alopecia Areata: A Children's Perspective ~ *Brochure*
Helping You Cope with ALOPECIA AREATA ~ *Brochure*
Parents Talking to Parents About Alopecia Areata ~ *Brochure*
HELP YOURSELF ~ *Brochure*
What You Should Know About Alopecia Areata ~ *Brochure*
Coping with Alopecia Areata ~ *Brochure*
Summary of the Second International Research Workshop on Alopecia Areata ~ *Brochure*
BASH FOR BALDNESS ~ *Brochure*
National Alopecia Areata Foundation Newsletter ~ *Newsletter*
HERMAN ~ *Book*
"This Weird Thing That Makes My Hair Fall Out" ~ *Videotape*
A Decade of Progress ~ *Brochure*
Newsletter of the National Alopecia Areata Foundation ~ *Newsletter*

Concerned with the following diseases or disorders:
Alopecia Areata

1360 NATIONAL APHASIA ASSOCIATION

P.O. Box 1887
Murray Hill Station
New York, NY 10156-0611
800-922-4622
Fax: 212-989-7777

The National Aphasia Association is a not-for-profit organization that is dedicated to increasing public awareness of aphasia and other communication disorders. Aphasia is a neurological condition in which communication and/or language skills are impaired. Established in 1987, the Association's activities include sponsoring support groups, promoting advocacy and legislative programs, supporting ongoing medical research, and maintaining an informational database. The National Aphasia Association publishes a quarterly newsletter and distributes educational brochures. A Young People's Network matches young people together for the purpose of peer support and information exchange.

President: Martha Taylor Sarnd, M.D. (1987-Present)
Executive Director: Karen Klein
Year Established: 1987

Concerned with the following diseases or disorders:
Apraxia; Landau Kleffner Syndrome; MASA Syndrome; Wyburn Mason Syndrome

1361 NATIONAL ASSOCIATION FOR PSEUDOXANTHOMA ELASTICUM (NAPE)

1420 Odgen Street
Denver, CO 80218-1910 303-832-5055
Fax: 303-832-3765
E-mail: pxenape@estreet.com
http://www.ttuhsc.edu/pages/NAPE/

The National Association for Pseudoxanthoma Elasticum (NAPE) is a voluntary not-for-profit organization dedicated to disseminating information on Pseudoxanthoma Elasticum (PXE). PXE is a rare connective tissue disease that is inherited and progressive and affects the elastic tissues of the body; abnormal accumulations of calcium salts (calcifications) develop within elastic fibers of the skin, eyes, and cardiovascular system (i.e., heart and blood vessels). The Association promotes and supports ongoing medical research into possible new treatments, prevention, and eventual cure for PXE. Established in 1988, the National Association for Pseudoxanthoma Elasticum promotes patient advocacy and provides referrals to support groups, genetic counseling, and other services. The National Association for Pseudoxanthoma Elasticum produces and distributes a variety of educational materials to affected individuals, families, health care professionals, and the general public. These educational services include a computerized database, member directory, newsletters, reports, journal articles, brochures, and audio tapes.

President: Claudia McCallister
Executive Director: Joyce Kohn (Office Manager)
Year Established: 1988
Organization Chapters: 1
Organization Members: 300

Publishes the following materials:
Pseudoxanthoma Elasticum ~ *Publications List*
Greetings from Denver ~ *Fact Sheet*
A Pyramid of Hope ~ *Article*
From East to West Coast ~ *Article*
Pseudoxanthoma Elasticum (PXE) Summary ~ *Fact Sheet*
Treatment Recommendations for PXE ~ *Fact Sheet*
Reader's Info Exchange ~ *Letter*
Q & A's - Medical Corner ~ *Information Sheet*

PXE Awareness ~ *Newsletter*
PXE Awareness - Special Edition ~ *Newsletter*

Concerned with the following diseases or disorders:
Pseudoxanthoma Elasticum (PXE)

1362 NATIONAL ATTENTION DEFICIT DISORDER ASSOCIATION (ADDA)

9930 Johnnycake Ridge Road
Suite 3E
Mentor, OH 44060
440-350-9595
800-487-2282
Fax: 440-350-0223
E-mail: NATLADDA@aol.com
http://www.add.org

The National Attention Deficit Disorders Association is a not-for-profit organization that was founded in 1989. The mission of the organization is to educate the public about Attention Deficit Disorder and to serve the information needs of affected individuals. The Association provides referrals to local support groups and physicians; resource materials on medications; coping strategies; and advocacy programs. Educational materials produced by the organization include a bimonthly newsletter and a variety of brochures directed at children, adolescents, and adults with Attention Deficit Disorders.

President: Nancy Eisenberg
Executive Director: Diana Vvicich, Office Coordinator
Year Established: 1989
Organization Members: 2000

Publishes the following materials:
ADDAlog ~ *Catalog*
The 1st Annual ADDA Adult ADD Conference ~ *Announcement*

Concerned with the following diseases or disorders:
Attention Deficit Hyperactivity Disorder

1363 NATIONAL AUTISTIC SOCIETY (NAS)

276 Willesden Lane
London, NW2 5RB
United Kingdom
01814511114
Fax: 01814515865

The National Autistic Society (NAS) is an international non-profit support organization dedicated to providing support and information to individuals affected by autism and their families and to act as an advocate for these individuals to ensure that they are provided equal opportunities in all aspects of life. Founded in 1962 and comprised of 3,500 members, NAS offers a national diagnostic and assessment service; supports ongoing clinical research; maintains a directory of affected individuals; owns and manages full-time schools and adult residential facilities; coordinates conferences for parents, caregivers, and practitioners; runs an information service for people with autism and related disorders; and provides appropriate referrals. NAS also publishes a newsletter entitled "Connection," reports, a journal, and brochures. The Society is a member of many other societies and organizations, including the National Council for Voluntary Organizations and Autism Europe. Memberships are available.

Executive Director: Geraldine Peacock (Chief Executive)
Year Established: 1962
Organization Members: 3,500

Publishes the following materials:
In Your Working Life You Can Expect to Meet Several People with Autism ~ *Brochure*
What is Asperger Syndrome? ~ *Brochure*
Publications 1995 - National Autistic Society ~ *Publications List*
Could this be Autism? ~ *Booklet*
Fact Sheet - National Autistis Society ~ *Mission Statement*
Connection ~ *Newsletter*

Concerned with the following diseases or disorders:
Asperger's Syndrome; Autism

1364 NATIONAL BREAST CANCER COALITION (NBCC)

1707 L Street North West
Suite 1060
Washington, DC 20036
202-296-7477
Fax: 202-265-6854
E-mail: pgoddard@natlbcc.org
http://www.natlbcc.org

The National Breast Cancer Coalition (NBCC) is a not-for-profit voluntary organization dedicated to working to eradicate breast cancer, the most common form of cancer among females in the United States. The Coalition achieves its goals by focusing national attention on breast cancer and involving all those concerned about this disease as advocates for action, advances, and change. The Coalition informs, supports, and directs affected individuals and concerned others in knowledgeable and effective advocacy efforts. Nationwide, members are bringing about meaningful progress in breast cancer policy through legislative and regulatory input, promotion of media coverage, and participation in activities such as marches and campaigns. Established in 1991, the Coalition has grown to more than 350 organizations, representing several million affected individuals, professionals, families, and friends. Coalition members include cancer support, information, and service groups, as well as women's, consumer health, and provider organizations. Thousands of individuals are members of the Coalition's National Action Network. The goals of the National Breast Cancer Coalition are to promote research into the cause of, optimal treatments and cure for breast cancer through increased funding, recruitment, and training of scientists and improved coordination and distribution of research funds; to improve access to high-quality breast cancer screening, diagnosis, treatment, and care for all women, particularly the underserved and uninsured, through legislation and change in the regulation and delivery of breast health care; and to increase the involvement and influence of those living with breast cancer in the areas of legislation, regulatory process, and all aspects of clinical trial design, including access to clinical trials. Consisting of 400 organizational members and 50,000 individual members, the organization produces educational materials including a pamphlet entitled "National Breast Cancer Coalition: Research, Access, and Influence," a booklet entitled "Leadership, Education and Advocacy Development," and an essay entitled "The Face of Breast Cancer." Program activities include an annual conference, patient advocacy, networking, and research. The NBCC can be reached at its web site at [http://www.natlbcc.org].

President: Fran Visco (1991 to Present)
Executive Director: Jane Reese-Coulbourne (Vice President)
Organization Language: Spanish (written/spoken).
Year Established: 1991
Organization Chapters: 400
Organization Members: 50,000

Publishes the following materials:
The National Breast Cancer Coalition ~ *Mission Statement*
Leadership, Education and Advocacy Development ~ *Leaflet*
End The Breast Cancer Epidemic ~ *Brochure*

Concerned with the following diseases or disorders:
Cancer, Breast

1365 NATIONAL CARCINOID SUPPORT GROUP, INC. (NCSG)

P.O. Box 44233
Madison, WI 53744-4233 608-271-0487
E-mail: jean@mick.com
http://members.aol.com/thencsg

The National Carcinoid Support Group, Inc. (NCSG) is an international not-for-profit self-help organization dedicated to supporting those with rare carcinoid tumors through peer-to-peer networking and networking with health care professionals who have experience with carcinoid tumors; acting as a clearinghouse of information on carcinoid tumors; and providing support to affected individuals and family members through online and telephone conferences. Carcinoid tumors are rare tumors that primarily arise in the gastrointestinal tract or the lung, although they may occur in several other organs, such as the appendix, pancreas, ovaries, testicles, or other locations. The symptoms associated with carcinoid tumors depend upon their location and other factors. In some cases, affected individuals may experience "Carcinoid Syndrome" if the tumor secretes serotonin or other biologically active substances, causing episodes of flushing of the skin of the face and neck, wheezing, diarrhea, and/or other symptoms. Established in 1994 and consisting of approximately 360 members, the National Carcinoid Support Group provides a variety of services including patient networking, support groups, and referrals. The organization also provides a variety of educational materials including reports on all aspects of carcinoid tumors, brochures, pamphlets, and a regular newsletter. NCSG also maintains a web site on the Internet at [http://members.aol.com/thencsg].

President: Ruth E. Ray (1997 to Present).
Executive Director: Jean Mickelson Michaux
Year Established: 1994
Organization Members: 360

Publishes the following materials:
Hope Lines. Knowledge is Power! ~ *Newsletter*
Hope Lines. Liver Embolization ~ *Newsletter*
The National Carcinoid Support Group Inc. ~ *Pamphlet*
The National Carcinoid Support Group Inc. ~ *Pamphlet*
What is Carcinoid? ~ *Fact Sheet*
Is Carcinoid Cancer Hereditary? ~ *Fact Sheet*
What is Cryosurgery ~ *Fact Sheet*
Surgery ~ *Fact Sheet*
Radioisotopes ~ *Fact Sheet*
Angiogenesis ~ *Fact Sheet*
Can Sandostatin Help Fight The Tumors? ~ *Fact Sheet*
What is Octreotide? ~ *Fact Sheet*
What Causes Carcinioid Cancer? ~ *Fact Sheet*

Concerned with the following diseases or disorders:
Carcinoid Syndrome

1366 **NATIONAL CHRONIC FATIGUE SYNDROME & FIBROMYALGIA ASSOCIATION (NCFSFA)**

P.O. Box 18 426
Kansas City, MO 64133 816-313-2000
Fax: 816-524-6782
E-mail: KEAL55A@prodigy.com

The National Chronic Fatigue Syndrome & Fibromyalgia Association is a voluntary health organization that was incorporated in 1988. The Association was formed to educate and inform the public about the nature and impact of Chronic Fatigue Syndrome and related disorders. In 1993, Fibromyalgia was added to the organization's educational efforts. The primary focus of The National Chronic Fatigue Syndrome & Fibromyalgia Association is to offer scientifically accurate information to people with Chronic Fatigue Syndrome and Fibromyalgia. Brochures, booklets, and videos are available from the organization. A periodic newsletter and fact sheet are also produced and distributed by the organization.

President: Orvalene Prewitt (1988 to Present)
Executive Director: Orvalene Prewitt
Year Established: 1988
Organization Chapters: 2
Organization Members: 3,000

Publishes the following materials:
The Thief of Vitality ~ *Brochure*
Chronic Fatigue Syndrome in Men ~ *Brochure*
Social Security Disability Benefits Information ~ *Brochure*
A School's Guide for Students with CFS ~ *Brochure*
CFS In the Workplace ~ *Brochure*
Chronic Fatigue Syndrome (CFS) and School Success ~ *Brochure*
CFS and Employment ~ *Brochure*
Neuropsychological Rehabilitation ~ *Brochure*
Coping Skills: How to Maintain Your Equilibrium in the CFS Balancing Act ~ *Brochure*
Understanding the Emotions Surrounding Chronic Fatigue Syndrome ~ *Brochure*
A Guide for Physicians ~ *Brochure*
Chronic Fatigue Syndrome - A Pamphlet for Physicians ~ *Pamphlet*
Arthritis Information Fibromyalgia ~ *Brochure*
The Facts About Chronic Fatigue Syndrome ~ *Brochure*
Chronic Fatigue Syndrome Awareness Month ~ *Brochure*
General Information Packet ~ *Newsletter*
CFS: Addressing the Realities of a Chronic Illness ~ *Video Tape*
Fact Sheet ~ *Factsheet*
Heart of America Newsletter ~ *Newsletter*
Multidisciplinary Innovations in Research, Theory & Clinical Practice ~ *Journal*

Concerned with the following diseases or disorders:
Chronic Fatigue Syndrome; Fibromyalgia

1367 **NATIONAL CONGENITAL CMV DISEASE REGISTRY**

6621 Fannin Street
MC 3-2371
Houston, TX 77030-2399 713-770-4330
Fax: 713-770-4347
E-mail: cmv@bcm.tmc.edu

The National Congenital CMV Disease Registry, based at Baylor College of Medicine in Houston, Texas, collects information on infants born after 1990 with Congenital Cytomegalovirus (CMV). The Registry is committed to identifying disease patterns over time; describing factors that may increase a mother's risk of delivering an infant with congenital cytomegalovirus infection; and providing the foundation for future intervention programs and collaborative research. All newborns with a confirmed diagnosis of Congenital CMV are eligible to be registered. In addition to these activities, the Congenital CMV Disease Registry functions as a national clearinghouse for information about congenital CMV. It distributes reprints of medical articles on human cytomegalovirus infection, publishes a newsletter entitled "CMV Updates," and maintains a CMV Parent-To-Parent Support Network.

President: Gail Demmler, Prinicipal Investigator
Year Established: N/A

Publishes the following materials:
CMV Updates ~ *Newsletter*
CMV Infection in Young Women ~ *Reprint*
Clinical Advancements in the Treatment of Infections ~ *Reprint*

Concerned with the following diseases or disorders:
Cytomegalovirus Infection

1368 **NATIONAL CONGENITAL PULMONARY LYMPHANGIECTASIS FOUNDATION**

119 Marge Lane
Somerset, PA 15501 814-445-3686
Fax: 814-445-8565
E-mail: vbrf@twd.net

The National Congenital Pulmonary Lymphangiectasis Foundation (NCPLF) is a not-for-profit self-help organization dedicated to educating the public on CPL and promoting awareness as well as research. CPL is a rare disease that usually affects infants. CPL causes respiratory distress due to rigidity of the lungs and is also linked to severe problems with the cardiovascular system. Established in 1995, the Foundation conducts programs such as local support groups and patient/family networking. NCPLF serves information resource for affected families to receive support and appropriate referrals. Educational materials available from the Foundation include audiovisual aids and brochures. In addition, a patient registry is maintained. Consisting of an active membership of 25 to 30 people, the Foundation offers program activities including support group meetings. The ultimate mission of the NCPLF is to find a cure for CPL through research.

Year Established: 1995
Organization Members: 25 to 50

1369 NATIONAL DEPRESSIVE AND MANIC-DEPRESSIVE ASSOCIATION (NATIONAL DMDA)

730 North Franklin Street
Suite 501
Chicago, IL 60610-3526
800-826-3632
Fax: 312-642-7243
http://www.ndmda.org

The National Depressive and Manic-Depressive Association (National DMDA) is a nonprofit self-help organization dedicated to educating patients, families, professionals, and the public concerning the nature of depressive and manic-depressive illnesses as medical diseases; to foster self-help for patients and families; to eliminate discrimination and stigma frequently associated with these diseases; to improve access to appropriate medical care; and to advocate for research toward the elimination of these illnesses. Depression (also known as unipolar disorder) and manic-depressive illness (also known as bipolar disorder) are mood disorders characterized by medical illnesses involving disruptions in brain functions. Established in 1986, the National DMDA has a single goal: to help people improve the quality of their lives. The Association accomplishes this by responding to requests for information, supporting research, combating the stigma associated with these diseases, and educating the public and those with depressive illnesses. Consisting of 275 chapters, the organization publishes educational materials including a self-titled pamphlet, a booklet entitled "Depressive Illness: The Medical Facts, The Human Challenge," and a newsletter entitled "Outreach." The organization's activities include support groups, patient advocacy, and educational programs. The National DMDA can be reached at its web site on the Internet at [http://www.ndmda.org].

President: Mark Gottlieb (1997 to 1998)
Executive Director: Lydia Lewis
Year Established: 1986
Organization Chapters: 275
Organization Members: Non-Membership

Publishes the following materials:
National DMDA ~ *Newsletter*
Expert Consensus Treatment Guidelines for Bipolar Disorder: A guide for Patients and Families ~ *Leaflet*
National Depressive and Manic-Depressive Association ~ *Booklet*
Bookstore Catalog ~ *Bibliography*
Diagnosis, Treatment and Support ~ *Booklet*
Chapter Directory (1997) ~ *Booklet*
Just a Mood....Or Real Depresion? ~ *Leaflet*
Suicide and Depressive Illness ~ *Booklet*
Depressive Illness: The Medical Facts The Human Challenge ~ *Booklet*
In Bipolar Illness: Rapid Cycling & It's Treatment ~ *Leaflet*
When Treatments Fail ~ *Booklet*

Concerned with the following diseases or disorders:
Manic Depression, Bipolar

1370 NATIONAL DOWN SYNDROME CONGRESS (NDSC)

1605 Chantilly Drive
Suite 250
Atlanta, GA 30324-3269
404-633-1555
800-232-6372
Fax: 404-633-2817
E-mail: ndsc@charitiesusa.com
http://members.carol.net/ndsc

The National Down Syndrome Congress (NDSC), a not-for-profit organization established in 1971, is committed to building a sense of community among all those concerned with Down Syndrome. The Congress provides leadership in the formation of public policy and encourages ethically responsible research in all aspects of Down Syndrome. The organization seeks to educate professionals, parents, and the community about Down Syndrome and fosters self-advocacy, rights, and full participation in all aspects of community life. The National Down Syndrome Congress is also dedicated to developing position statements on major issues; providing a network that links state and local groups and affiliates; and enhancing relationships within the organizations' communities and the broader disability community. The National Down Syndrome Congress provides a telephone hotline offering information on any subject related to Down Syndrome. It conducts an annual convention, provides appropriate referrals, and coordinators a local parent group network and maintains directory of such groups to promote parent-to-parent and parent-to-professional networking. The National Down Syndrome Congress provides a variety of educational and support materials through its regular journal "Down Syndrome News," reports, brochures, and bibliographies of relevant materials.

President: Maureen Babula (1993-Present)
Executive Director: Frank Murphy
Year Established: 1971
Organization Chapters: 600
Organization Members: 10,000

Publishes the following materials:
National Down Syndrome Congress - Facts About Down Dyndrome ~ *Fact Sheet*
Down Syndrome ~ *Pamphlet*
The National Organization of Parents and Professionals ~ *Brochure*

Concerned with the following diseases or disorders:
Down Syndrome; Trisomy

1371 NATIONAL DOWN SYNDROME SOCIETY (NDSS)

666 Broadway
8th Floor
New York, NY 10012-2317 212-460-9330
800-221-4602
Fax: 212-979-2873
E-mail: info@ndss.org
http://www.ndss.org/

The National Down Syndrome Society is a national voluntary not-for-profit organization dedicated to providing support to people affected by Down Syndrome and increasing public awareness. The National Down Syndrome Society's goals are to promote better understanding of Down Syndrome and help affected individuals reach their personal potential; support research about this genetic disorder; and disseminate accurate and up-to-date information on Down Syndrome to parents, professionals, and other interested individuals. Established in 1979, the Society also supports several pilot demonstration programs to address specific areas of concern among families affected by Down Syndrome. It confers scholar awards and two-year grants to promising young scientific students and conducts a biannual research symposium. The Society also provides referrals to medical professionals and support groups and holds conferences to update research advances. The National Down Syndrome Society has an extensive supply of educational and support materials including a series of fact sheets, a bibliography of reading materials, brochures, pamphlets, booklets, fliers, and videos. A magazine entitled "News N Views" and a quarterly newsletter entitled "The National Down Syndrome Society Update" are also available from the Society.

President: Elizabeth F. Goodwin (1979-Present)
Executive Director: Myra Madnick
Year Established: 1979
Organization Chapters: 34
Organization Members: 52,000

Publishes the following materials:
Background - NDSS ~ *Mission Statement*
Fact Sheet - NDSS ~ *Fact Sheet*
Questions and Answers About Down Syndrome ~ *Information Sheet*
NDSS Down Syndrome Research Program ~ *Information Sheet*
Suggested List of Readings and Viewings ~ *Reading List*
Increase Awareness and Understanding of Down Syndrome ~ *Video List*
Order Form - NDSS ~ *Publications List*
Can You Use Exceptional Parent ~ *Article Reprint*
Down Syndrome - Advances in Medical Care ~ *Publications List*
National Down Syndrome Society UPDATE ~ *Newsletter*
Living and Learning in the Community ~ *Publications List*
Brick by Brick ~ *Brochure*
This Baby Needs You Even More ~ *Brochure*
NEWS VIEWS ~ *Magazine*
National Down Syndrome Society Educational Materials ~ *Order Form*
Down Syndrome: Myths and Truths ~ *Fact Sheet*

Concerned with the following diseases or disorders:
Down Syndrome

1372 NATIONAL ECZEMA ASSOCIATION FOR SCIENCE AND EDUCATION (NEA OR NEASE)

1221 South West Yamhill
Suite 303
Portland, OR 97205 503-228-4430
800-818-7546
Fax: 503-273-8778

The National Eczema Association for Science and Education (NEA) is a nonprofit organization dedicated to informing, educating, and providing resources for individuals affected by eczema; increase public awareness of the disease; support research to discover the cause, treatment, and cure of atopic dermatitis-eczema; and represent individuals with eczema in order to help improve their quality of life. Atopic Dermatitis-Eczema is a disease that causes itchy, inflamed skin that most typically affects the insides of the elbows, backs of the knees and the face, but can cover most of the body. NEA was established in 1988 in Portland, Oregon by a group of affected individuals, nurses, doctors, and others concerned with the enormous social, medical, and economic consequences of this disease. NEA is governed by a Board of Directors. The Association is guided by a Scientific Advisory Committee comprised of physicians and scientists who donate their time and expertise. Consisting of 3,000 members and eight chapters, the Association produces educational materials including a brochure entitled "All About Atopic Dermatitis," a video entitled "Suffering in Silence," and a newsletter entitled "The Advocate." Programs and activities include a support group, patient advocacy, patient networking, education, and the support of research.

Executive Director: Contact Office.
Organization Language: Spanish (written).
Year Established: 1989
Organization Chapters: 8
Organization Members: 3,000

Publishes the following materials:
National Eczema Association for Science and Education ~ *Brochure*

Concerned with the following diseases or disorders:
Dermatitis, Contact; Ichthyosis Congenita

1373 NATIONAL ECZEMA SOCIETY

163 Eversholt Street
London, NW1 1BU
United Kingdom 0171 388 4097
Fax: 0171 388 5882

The National Eczema Society is a self-help organization dedicated to improving the quality of life for people with eczema, other skin diseases, related conditions, and their carers. Established in 1975, the Society works primarily to empower people with eczema to receive the quality of treatment and care that they have a right to expect. The Society also works to identify and seek to resolve issues that affect the interests of affected interests; raise awareness about the rights and needs of affected individuals; and campaign actively on behalf of affected individuals. In addition, the Society will help to develop and fund patient-centered training programs aimed at health professionals to improve their knowledge and understanding of eczema's treatment and management and a systematic and comprehensive program of research into the causes of, and cure for, eczema. The Association produces educational materials including a quarterly journal entitled "Exchange," brochures, fact sheets, and booklets.

President: Peter Longland, Chairperson
Executive Director: Christina Funnell, Chief Executive
Year Established: 1975
Organization Members: 13,000

Publishes the following materials:
A Practical Guide to the Management of Eczema...Community Healthcare Nurses ~ *Booklet*
A Practical Guide to the Management of Eczema...Pharmacists ~ *Booklet*
A Practical Guide for Employers...Eczema At Work ~ *Booklet*
NES Informs...Eczema and Diet ~ *Booklet*
National Eczema Society Publications ~ *Order Form*
Chinese Medicinal Plants for Atopic Eczema ~ *Information Sheet*
Cyclosporin A New Treatment for Atopic Eczema ~ *Information Sheet*
Hand Eczema and Dermatitis ~ *Information Sheet*
Nickel Allergy ~ *Information Sheet*
Seborrhoeic Eczema in Adults ~ *Information Sheet*
Cradle Cap & Seborrhoeic Eczema in Infants ~ *Information Sheet*
Working with Eczema ~ *Information Sheet*
Questions Need Answers ~ *ILnformation Sheet*
Varicose Eczema ~ *Information Sheet*
Urticaria ~ *Information Sheet*
Exchange ~ *Quarterly Journal*
The Management and Treatment of Eczema ~ *Book*
Your Baby and Child with Eczema ~ *Book*
Eczema. Dermatitis and Sensitive Skin ~ *Brochure*
National Eczema Society. Annual Report and Accounts (1996 Summary) ~ *Booklet*

1374 NATIONAL FOUNDATION FOR ECTODERMAL DYSPLASIAS (NFED)

219 East Main Street
P.O. Box 114
Mascoutah, IL 62258-0114 618-566-2020
Fax: 618-566-4718
E-mail: nfed1@aol.com and nfed2@aol.com
http://www.nfed.org

The National Foundation for Ectodermal Dysplasia (NFED), which was established in 1981, is a not-for-profit service organization committed to assisting people with Ectodermal Dysplasia (ED) to live not only normal life spans, but normal life styles. Ectodermal Dysplasias (EDs) are a group of rare inherited multisystem disorders that typically affect the hair, teeth, nails, and/or skin. The Foundation provides informational materials and support for families affected by Ectodermal Dysplasia in the United States and around the world. It also assists medical and dental professionals with useful information on early diagnosis and treatment options. NFED maintains a database of health care professionals who have experience in treating people with Ectodermal

Dysplasia and conducts educational meetings for families and health care providers. The Foundation provides financial assistance to qualified families for medically necessary care and publishes educational materials for all interested individuals. Other services include a scholarship program and dental implant program. Current research projects include studies to identify the genes responsible for the various types of Ectodermal Dysplasia, the mechanisms by which these genes cause the features of ED, and the treatment of ED.

President: Frank C. Hazzard (1990-Present)
Executive Director: Mary Kaye Richter
Year Established: 1981

Publishes the following materials:
Lifting Hopes for the Future ~ *Brochure*
The Educator ~ *Newsletter*
Charley's Story ~ *Pamphlet*
The Ectodermal Dysplasias ~ *Brochure*
A Dental Guide to Ectodermal Dysplasias ~ *Brochure*
A Family Guide to the Ectodermal Dysplasias ~ *Brochure*
A Guide to the Skin, Hair, and Nails in the Ectodermal Dysplasias ~ *Brochure*
An EENT* Guide to the Ectodermal Dysplasias ~ *Brochure*
Evan's New Teeth ~ *Brochure*

Concerned with the following diseases or disorders:
APECED Syndrome; Amelogenesis Imperfecta; Anodontia; Dentin Dysplasia, Coronal; Dentin Dysplasia, Radicular; Dentinogenesis Imperfecta Type III; Dyskeratosis Congenita; Ectodermal Dysplasias; Ectrodactyly Ectodermal Dysplasia Cleft Lip/Palate; Focal Dermal Hypoplasia; Hay Well's Syndrome; Oculo Dento Digital Dysplasia; Rapp Hodgkins Syndrome; Rieger Syndrome; Setleis Syndrome; Tooth and Nail Syndrome; Tricho Dento Osseous Syndrome; Trichorhinophalangeal Syndrome Type I; Trichorhinophalangeal Syndrome Type II; Trichorhinophalangeal Syndrome Type III

1375 NATIONAL FRAGILE X FOUNDATION (NFXF)

1441 York Street
Suite 303
Denver, CO 80206 303-333-6155
800-688-8765
Fax: 303-333-6155
E-mail: natlfx@sprintmail.com
http://www.medhelp.org/www/fragilex

The National Fragile X Foundation is a not-for-profit organization dedicated to promoting educational awareness and supporting research into the nature of Fragile X Syndrome. Fragile X Syndrome is an inherited defect of the X chromosome that causes mental retardation. Established in 1985, the National Fragile X Foundation produces a variety of educational and support materials. These materials include handbooks, brochures, a newsletter, pamphlets, and numerous audio-visual aids, such as "Educational Strategies & Issues for Children with Fragile X Syndrome" and "Fragile X Syndrome: Medical and Educational Approaches to Intervention."

President: Jeffrey S. Cohen
Executive Director: Stephen Holloway
Year Established: 1984
Organization Chapters: 40
Organization Members: 8000

Concerned with the following diseases or disorders:
Fragile X Syndrome

1376 NATIONAL GRAVES' DISEASE FOUNDATION (NGDF)

2 Tsitsi Court
Brevard, NC 28712 704-877-5251
E-mail: jake@support-group.com
http://www.ngdf.org/

The National Graves' Disease Foundation (NGDF) is a national voluntary not-for-profit organization dedicated to providing resources, referrals, and current medical information to people with Graves' Disease. Information provided by the Foundation incorporates a multidisciplinary approach to the treatment of Graves' Disease. The Foundation also promotes professional education through lectures and forums and public education through the distribution of literature, lectures, and presentations in the media and the community. Established in 1990, the National Graves' Disease Foundation offers a one-on-one individual support network and assists in the development of locally based support groups. It establishes liaison relationships with major hospitals and research institutions, both nationally and internationally. The National Graves' Disease Foundation's Medical and Advisory Board consists of representatives from a variety of disciplines who play essential roles in the treatment and support of individuals with Graves' Disease (e.g., endocrinology, surgery, ophthalmology, pharmacology, internal medicine, and family practice). The National Graves' Disease Foundation offers a variety of educational materials to patients, their families, health care professionals, and the general public through its computer database, bulletins, brochures, newsletters, videos, and audio tapes.

President: Nancy Hord Patterson (1990-Present)
Executive Director: Nancy Hord Patterson
Year Established: 1990

Publishes the following materials:
The National Graves' Disease Foundation Presents The Third Annual Family-Patient Conference in Pittsburgh ~ *Conference Brochure*
An Invitation to Join the National Graves' Disease Foundation ~ *Brochure*
Commonly Asked Questions About Graves' Disease ~ *Brochure*
Bulletin Order Form ~ *Order Form*
National Graves' Disease Foundation ~ *Resource List/Order Form*
NDGF News ~ *Newsletter*
Invitation to Join the National Graves' Disease Foundation/Bulletin Order Form ~ *Membership Application/Order F*
Living With Graves' Disease ~ *Bulletin*
Graves' Disease - Eye Interventions ~ *Bulletin*
Graves' Disease - Rehabilitative Surgery ~ *Bulletin*
Graves' Disease - Eyelid Surgery ~ *Bulletin*
Graves' Disease ~ *Bulletin*
Eye Changes with Graves' Disease - Continuing Concepts ~ *Bulletin*
Thyroid Eye Disease - Double Vision and Loss of Vision ~ *Bulletin*
Graves' Ophthalmopathy & Radiation Therapy ~ *Bulletin*
Me, Bush and Graves' Disease ~ *Bulletin*
Dry Eyes ~ *Bulletin*
A Letter from Your Eye Doctor ~ *Bulletin*
Anatomical Pictures of Normal vs Graves' Eye Muscles ~ *Bulletin*
Treatment of Graves' Disease by the "Atomic Cocktail" ~ *Bulletin*
Graves' Disease and Pregnancy ~ *Bulletin*
Signs & Symptoms of Thyroid Disease ~ *Bulletin*

Concerned with the following diseases or disorders:
Graves' Disease

1377 NATIONAL HEMOPHILIA FOUNDATION (NHF)

110 Greene Street
Suite 303
New York, NY 10012 212-219-8180
800-424-2634
Fax: 212-966-9247
E-mail: nhfofnyc@aol.com
http://www.hemophilia.org

Founded in 1948, the National Hemophilia Foundation is a national not-for-profit organization dedicated to the treatment and cure of hemophilia, related bleeding disorders, and complications of those disorders, including HIV infection. Estalished in 1948, the Foundation also strives to support people with hemophilia, their families, and physicians; increase public awareness of hemophilia; and advocate on behalf of affected individuals. The Foundation is also committed to disseminating current information on hemophilia and other clotting disorders; raising funds for medical research; and promoting legislation beneficial to affected individuals and family members. The Foundation produces a variety of educational materials include regular newsletters, brochures, and audio-visual aids.

President: Ray Stanhope
Executive Director: Stephen E. Bajardi
Organization Language: Spanish.
Year Established: 1948
Organization Chapters: 46
Organization Members: 20,000

Concerned with the following diseases or disorders:
Afibrinogenemia, Congenital; Factor IX Deficiency; Factor XIII Deficiency; Hageman Factor Deficiency; Hemophilia; Von Willebrand Disease

1378 NATIONAL HYPERTENSION ASSOCIATION, INC. (NHA)

324 East 30th Street
New York, NY 10016 212-889-3557
Fax: 212-447-7032

The National Hypertension Association, Inc. (NHA) is a not-for-profit organization dedicated to combating the chronic health problem of high blood pressure (hypertension) by developing, directing, and implementing effective programs to promote research, educate the public, and ensure prompt detection and effective treatment of hypertension. The NHA is committed to researching the causes of essential hypertension and enhancing the understanding of certain secondary types of hypertension through basic laboratory research studies, thereby improving treatment of these conditions; educating and alerting the public to the severe, life-threatening dangers of hypertension and informing physicians as well as medical students of the most current advances in its causes, diagnosis, treatment, and prevention; and detecting hypertension wherever it exists in the most economical and effective way and urging treatment if indicated. Established in 1977 by a group of concerned scientists, doctors, and philanthropists, NHA offers charitable blood pressure screening, provides work-site detection programs, and has a well-defined program of basic and clinical research to gain better insight into the causes of hypertension. Materials include brochures, pamphlets, a regular newsletter, reports, and information packets.

President: William M. Manger, M.D., Ph.D. (1977 to Present)
Executive Director: Francine R. Rowley
Year Established: 1977
Organization Members: Non-Membership

Publishes the following materials:
National Hypertension Association, Inc. Annual Report 1996 ~ *Booklet*
Hypertension and You. What you need to know ~ *Brochure*
News Report ~ *Newsletter*

Concerned with the following diseases or disorders:
Conn Syndrome; Polycystic Kidney Diseases

1379 NATIONAL INCONTINENTIA PIGMENTI FOUNDATION (NIPF)

30 East 72nd Street
New York, NY 10021 212-452-1231
Fax: 212-452-1406
E-mail: nipf@pipeline.com
http://www.medhelp.org/www/nipf.htm

The National Incontinentia Pigmenti Foundation is a national non-profit organization that was founded in 1995. Guided by a Scientific Advisory Council, the Foundation is comprised of affected individuals, physicians, educators, parents, relatives, and volunteers — all of whom are interested in taking a leadership role in supporting research, education, and funding for Incontinentia Pigmenti (IP). IP is a rare genetic disorder affecting the skin, hair, and teeth. The most prominent feature of Incontinentia Pigmenti is a progressive skin rash, which typically has four stages of development. Symptoms may vary greatly in severity from person to person, even within the same family. Although most affected individuals have normal function of the nervous system, in some cases, neurological complications, including seizures and/or mental retardation, can occur as a consequence of IP. The mission of the National Incontinentia Pigmenti Foundation is to encourage and support research on IP and to provide family support and education. Research goals include support of ongoing genetic studies to map and identify the IP gene; creation of an accurate and safe prenatal diagnostic test for IP; development of a database to accurately assess clinical variations, natural history, and prognostic indicators; and the development of transgenic mouse models. Family support is offered by the Foundation. To this end, the organization publishes a self-titled periodic newsletter; maintains a national database of health professionals who are experienced with IP; directs people to appropriate medical resources and consultants; offers emotional support and the sharing of resources. In addition, the Foundation seeks to provide the medical care community with relevant medical information on IP; create awareness of IP on a worldwide basis; and collect and catalogue medical articles on IP. The National Incontinentia Pigmenti Foundation maintains a site on the World Wide Web at [http://www.medhelp.org/www/nipf.htm].

President: Susanne Bross Emmerich (1995 to Present)
Organization Language: German (spoken).
Year Established: 1995
Organization Members: 400

Publishes the following materials:
National Incontinentia Pigmenti Foundation ~ *Newsletter*
Incontinentia Pigmenti ~ *Pamphlet*
Eye Examination of Children Affected with IP ~ *Reprint*
National Incontinentia Pigmenti Foundation ~ *Newsletter*
Incontinentia Pigmenti Bibliography ~ *Bibliography*

Concerned with the following diseases or disorders:
Incontinentia Pigmenti

1380 NATIONAL KERATOCONUS FOUNDATION (NKCF)

Cedars-Sinai Medical Center
8700 Beverly Boulevard
Davis Research Building, #5069
Los Angeles, CA 90048 310-855-6455
800-521-2524
Fax: 310-652-8411
E-mail: nkcf@csmc.edu
http://www.csmc.edu/nkcf/

The National Keratoconus Foundation (NKCF) is a non-profit, tax exempt organization founded to disseminate educational materials to individuals affected by Keratoconus (KC) and their families, as well as to eye care professionals. Keratoconus is characterized by the slow progressive enlargement of the curved transparent outer layer of fibrous tissue covering the eyeball. The disease leads to visual impairment. Established in 1985, NKCF supports research into keratoconus and its causes, treatments, and eventual cure. Informational materials include a reference guide entitled "What Is Keratoconus?" brochures, and a quarterly newsletter. Program activities include communication channels for affected individuals and their families through an outreach program and an information "WARMLINE." Consisting of 500 members, the NKCF maintains a registry of individuals affected by keratoconus and eye care providers who have a special interest and expertise in treating people with keratoconus.

President: Jon Pynoos, Ph.D.
Executive Director: Catherine Warren
Organization Language: French (written). Spanish (written). Hindi (written). Hebrew (written).
Year Established: 1985
Organization Members: 500

Publishes the following materials:
National Keratoconus Foundation ~ *Brochure*
What is Keratoconus - A Reference Guide for Patients & Their Families ~ *Booklet*
NKCF ~ *Newsletter*

Concerned with the following diseases or disorders:
Keratoconus

1381 NATIONAL KIDNEY CANCER ASSOCIATION (NKCA)

1234 Sherman Avenue
Suite 203
Evanston, IL 60202-1375 847-332-1051
800-850-9132
Fax: 847-332-2978
E-mail: office@nkca.com
http://www.ncka.org

The National Kidney Cancer Association is a national non-profit organization comprised of people who have been affected by kidney cancer, their families and friends, physicians, and researchers. The Association is dedicated to improving the quality of care and increasing survival of individuals affected by kidney cancer. Established in 1990, the Association works toward three primary goals: to provide information to affected individuals and physicians; to sponsor and conduct research on kidney cancer; and to act as an advocate on a federal level and with insurance companies and employers on behalf of affected individuals and their families. Comprised of 4,000 members and 17 chapters, the organization publishes "Kidney Cancer News," a quarterly newsletter, as well as several informational brochures including "We Have Kidney Cancer," "Interleukin-2 Therapy: What You Should Know," and "Kidney Cancer: Emotional vs. Rational." The Association holds support group meetings several times a year in various cities so that individuals who have kidney cancer can learn how others have dealt with their disease. In addition, the Association conducts a yearly national convention that brings individuals together with leading physicians and researchers in the field of kidney cancer.

President: Eugene P. Schonfeld
Executive Director: Carl F. Dixon
Year Established: 1990
Organization Chapters: 17
Organization Members: 4,000

Publishes the following materials:
Kidney Cancer News ~ *Newsletter*
Kidney Cancer - Emotional vs. Rational ~ *Brochure*
"We Have Kidney Cancer" ~ *Booklet*
Kidney Cancer News Special Edition to be Saved ~ *Newsletter*
What You Should Know ~ *Booklet*
Kidney Cancer News (Febuary 1997) ~ *Newsletter*
Reflections. A Guide to End of Life Issues for You and Your Family ~ *Booklet*
Interleukin-2 and Biologic Therapy ~ *Booklet*
Kidney Cancer News (May 1997) ~ *Newsletter*
13 Steps to World Class Cancer Care ~ *Brochure*
Access to Cancer Drugs World Wide ~ *Brochure*
A Prescription For Physicians Suffering From Advocacy Deficit ~ *Brochure*

1382 NATIONAL LEUKEMIA RESEARCH ASSOCIATION, INC. (NLRA)

585 Stewart Avenue
Suite 536
Garden City, NY 11530 516-222-1944
Fax: 516-222-0457

The National Leukemia Research Association, Inc. (NLRA) was founded in 1965 as a not-for-profit voluntary organization dedicated to raising funds to support research efforts into the causes and cure of leukemia and to provide patient aid to those families in need while meeting the expense incurred in leukemia treatment. Leukemia is any of several types of cancer in which there is usually an abnormal accumulation of white blood cells within the bone marrow often resulting in decreased production of red blood cells, platelets, and normal white blood cells. Other organs such as the liver, lymph nodes, and brain may fail to function properly as they are infiltrated by leukemia cells. As part of its Patient Aid Services Program, NLRA requests families seeking aid submit an application to the Patient Aid director. All claims are investigated by the Patient Aid committee and money is allocated to the affected families covering drugs, lab fees, and other valid claims after review by committee; unusual and extraordinary expenses will also be considered based upon need and availability of funds. As part of its Scientific Investigation Program, a Medical Advisory Committee consisting of prominent internationally known and respected specialists in the field of blood disorders (hematologists) reviews research grants submitted yearly for consideration of funding.

The objectives of this committee are to direct the funds of the NLRA into the most promising projects and where funding would not duplicate other funding sources. The objectives of NLRA are to find the causes and cure for leukemia.

President: Gilbert A. Schwab
Executive Director: Allan D. Weinberg
Year Established: 1965
Organization Members: Non-Membership

Publishes the following materials:
National Leukemia Research Association, Inc. ~ *Brochure*

Concerned with the following diseases or disorders:
Leukemia, Chronic Lymphocytic; Leukemia, Chronic Myelogenous; Leukemia, Hairy Cell

1383 NATIONAL MARFAN FOUNDATION (NMF)

382 Main Street
Port Washington, NY 11050 516-883-8712
800-862-7326
Fax: 516-883-8040
E-mail: staff@marfan.org
http://www.marfan.org

The National Marfan Foundation is a voluntary not-for-profit organization dedicated to the support and education of people affected by Marfan Syndrome. The Foundation was established in 1981 by families and individuals affected by Marfan Syndrome, an inherited disorder of the connective tissue that may affect the skeleton, lungs, eyes, heart, blood vessels, and/or other areas of the body. The National Marfan Foundation has a three-fold purpose: to support and promote research; disseminate accurate and timely information about this condition to affected individuals, family members, and physicians; and provide means for affected individuals and relatives to share experiences, support one another, and improve their medical care. To help meet these goals, the Foundation sponsors research grants to investigators studying any or all disciplines involved in Marfan Syndrome and conducts annual conferences. It has a network of chapters, support groups, and contacts across the country and provides a variety of educational and support materials for affected individuals, family members, health care professionals, teachers, and other professionals. These materials include a newsletter called "Connective Issues," an annual research supplement, booklets, and a listing of thousands of articles and books on Marfan Syndrome. Other informational materials include brochures, fact sheets, videos, and a guide for physical educators, coaches, and physicians outlining physical activities for affected individuals.

President: Priscilla Ciccariello, Chair (1984-Present)
Executive Director: Carolyn Leuering
Year Established: 1981
Organization Chapters: 65
Organization Members: 14.500

Publishes the following materials:
NMF The National Marfan Foundation 1994 Request for Research Proposals ~ *Brochure*
Connective Issues ~ *Newsletter*
1993-1994 Research Achievements ~ *Fact Sheet*
The Marfan Syndrome ~ *Fact Sheet*
Marfan Syndrome - A Guide for Eye Care Professionals ~ *Brochure*
Publications and Videos about the Marfan Syndrome ~ *Brochure*
The Marfan Syndrome: A Booklet for Teenagers ~ *Booklet*
The Marfan Syndrome: A Booklet for Teachers ~ *Booklet*
How John Was Unique ~ *Booklet*
Physical Activity Guidelines for Physical Educators, Coaches, and Physicians ~ *Booklet*
What could be wrong with a casual game of basketball? Plenty. ~ *Poster*
Medical Panel Update ~ *Videotape*

Concerned with the following diseases or disorders:
Marfan Syndrome; Mixed Connective Tissue Disease (MCTD)

1384 NATIONAL MULTIPLE SCLEROSIS SOCIETY (NMSS)

733 Third Avenue
New York, NY 10017 212-986-3240
800-344-4867
Fax: 212-986-7981
E-mail: info@nmss.org
http://www.nmss.org

The National Multiple Sclerosis Society is a voluntary not-for-profit advocacy organization dedicated to advancing the cure, prevention, and treatment of Multiple Sclerosis and improving the lives of affected individuals. Multiple Sclerosis (MS) is a chronic disorder of the central nervous system that causes the destruction of the covering (myelin sheath) over nerve cells. Established in 1946, the National Multiple Sclerosis Society, which has over 140 chapters throughout the United States, seeks to provide services, further education, and promote public policy development on behalf of individuals with Multiple Sclerosis. The Society promotes and supports research; engages in patient, professional, and community education; advocates on behalf of people with MS; and promotes legislation beneficial to affected individuals. The National Multiple Sclerosis Society produces a wide variety of educational and support materials including a regular newsletter, brochures, pamphlets, and video aids.

President: Gen. Michael Dugan
Executive Director: Gen. Michael Dugan
Year Established: N/A
Organization Chapters: 142

Publishes the following materials:
MS 1993 Annual Report ~ *Brochure*
National Multiple Sclerosis Society ~ *Fact Sheet*

Concerned with the following diseases or disorders:
Multiple Sclerosis

1385 NATIONAL NARCOLEPSY REGISTRY (NNR)

729 15th Street NW
4th Floor
Washington, DC 20005 202-347-3471
Fax: 202-347-3472
E-mail: natsleep@erols.com
http://www.sleepfoundation.org

The National Narcolepsy Registry (NNR) is a not-for-profit research organization dedicated to providing researchers with information to advance research, diagnosis, and treatment of narcolepsy; to finding the gene(s) that may cause or contribute to narcolepsy; and to developing better treatments, a better quality of life for affected individuals and their families; and progressing toward a cure. Narcolepsy is a rare disorder characterized by abnormal drowsiness during the day, sudden extreme muscle weakness (cataplexy), hallucinations, paralysis while sleeping, and disrupted sleep during the night. Established in 1996, NNR is a confidential database of genetic information provided by individuals with narcolepsy. It is used for the sole purpose of promoting further research on narcolepsy. The first registry of its kind, the NNR is part of the National Sleep Foundation's (NSF) "Towards the Cause of Narcolepsy" program. The NSF urges individuals who have been diagnosed with narcolepsy and their family members to use the registry as an opportunity to contribute to narcolepsy research. Consisting of 500 members, the NNR produces educational materials including a brochure entitled "National Narcolepsy Registry." NNR can be reached at its e-mail address at [natsleep@erols.com] or its web site at [http://www.sleepfoundation.org].

President: Michael Thorpy, M.D. (Director)
Executive Director: Kate Lynch (Coordinator)
Year Established: 1996
Organization Members: 500

Publishes the following materials:
National Narcolepsy Registry ~ *Brochure*
National Narcolepsy Registry ~ *Brochure*

Concerned with the following diseases or disorders:
Narcolepsy

1386 NATIONAL NEUROFIBROMATOSIS FOUNDATION, INC. (NNFF)

95 Pine Street
16th Floor
New York, NY 10005 212-344-6633
800-323-7938
Fax: 212-747-0004
TDD: 212-344-6633
E-mail: nnff@aol.com
http://www.nf.org

The National Neurofibromatosis Foundation (NNFF), Inc. is a not-for-profit voluntary organization dedicated to improving the well-being of pat individuals and families affected by Neurofibromatosis Type I (NF1) and Type II (NF2). NF1 is a rare inherited disorder characterized by the development of multiple benign tumors on the covering of nerve fibers and the appearance of brown spots and freckles on the skin. NF2 is a rare inherited disorder characterized by the development of benign tumors on both auditory nerves and in other areas of the body. Established in 1978, the Foundation is dedicated to sponsoring scientific research aimed at finding the causes and cures for the neurofibromatoses, promoting the development of clinical activities, creating public awareness, and providing patient support services. In addition, NNFF promotes education of health care professionals, offers patient advocacy, and provides referrals to genetic counseling and support groups. The National Neurofibromatosis Foundation offers educational and supportive information through its directory, database, pamphlets, newsletters, handbooks, and audio-visual aids. The Foundation supports several languages including English, Spanish, French, Italian, Vietnamese, Turkish, Arabic, Greek, and Chinese. The National Neurofibromatosis Foundation's home page can be reached on the World Wide Web at http://neurofibromatosis.org or http://nf.org.

President: Peter Bellermann (1986-Present)
Organization Language: Spanish. French. Italian. Vietnamese.
Year Established: 1978
Organization Chapters: 26
Organization Members: 33,000

Publishes the following materials:
Questions & Answers ~ *Brochure*
Neurofibromatosis. Information for Patients and Families ~ *Pamphlet*
Neurofibromatosis Type 2: Information for Patients and Families ~ *Pamphlet*
Facing Neurofibromatosis: A Guide for Teens ~ *Pamphlet*
The Child with Neurofibromatosis I ~ *Pamphlet*
Achieving in Spite of... A Booklet on Learning Disabilities ~ *Booklet*

Concerned with the following diseases or disorders:
Acoustic Neuroma; Neurofibromatosis Type 1 (NF-1); Neurofibromatosis Type 2 (NF-2)

1387 NATIONAL NEUTROPENIA NETWORK (NNN)

P.O. Box 205
6348 North Milwaukee Avenue
Chicago, IL 60646
800-638-8768
E-mail: Bolyard@U.Washington.EDU

The National Neutropenia Network is a not-for-profit professional self-help organization dedicated to providing a support system for affected individuals and their families, coordinating nationwide efforts to promote awareness of neutropenia, and distributing educational materials. Neutropenia is an abnormal decrease in the number of circulating white blood cells (neutrophils) in the blood. Established in 1994, the Network supports general and clinical research related to neutropenia; provides information to families, the medical community, and the general public concerning the needs of affected individuals; and collects and distributes the latest medical data on neutropenia. The Network is also committed to helping affected individuals and family members work with hospitals, physicians, nurses, and other health care professionals and identifying people and families whose lives are affected by neutropenia. The Network also seeks to identify the psychological effects of dealing with chronic illness and encouraging families to seek appropriate support.

President: Beth Jacobs (1994-Present)
Executive Director: Beth Jacobs
Year Established: 1994
Organization Members: 300

Concerned with the following diseases or disorders:
Hyper IgM Syndrome; Neutropenia, Chronic; Neutropenia, Cyclic; Shwachman Syndrome

1388 NATIONAL NIEMANN-PICK DISEASE FOUNDATION, INC. (NNPDF)

3734 East Olive Avenue
Gilbert, AZ 85234-3117
602-497-6638
Fax: 602-497-6346
E-mail: stevekenyon@netwrx.net
http://www.nnpdf.org/

The National Niemann-Pick Disease Foundation, Inc. is an international voluntary not-for-profit organization made up of parents, medical professionals, friends, relatives, and others who are committed to finding a cure for Niemann-Pick Disease (NPD). Niemann-Pick is a group of rare inherited diseases in which excessive amounts of a fatty substance called sphingomyelin and/or cholesterol accumulate in many organs of the body. Established in 1984, the National Niemann-Pick Disease Foundation is dedicated to promoting medical research into the cause and cure of Niemann-Pick Disease; providing medical and educational information to assist in the correct diagnosis and referral of children with Niemann-Pick Disease; and providing support to families of affected children. The Foundation is also committed to facilitating genetic counseling for parents who are known carriers of Niemann-Pick Disease; encouraging the sharing of research information among scientists; and supporting legislation that is beneficial to affected individuals and family members. The National Niemann-Pick Disease Foundation also conducts a national conference that gives families the opportunity to network with one another and meet with medical professionals and researchers. The Foundation provides a variety of educational and support materials through its database, directory, reports, regular newsletter, and brochures.

President: Stephen J. Kenyon
Year Established: 1991
Organization Members: 2,000

Publishes the following materials:
For the Children ~ *Brochure*
Niemann-Pick Newsletter ~ *Newsletter*
NPD Background ~ *Fact Sheet*

What is Niemann-Pick, type C? ~ *Fact Sheet*
Membership Application ~ *Application Form*
A Clinical Staging Classification for type C Niemann-Pick Disease ~ *Report*
General Information on the Educational Management of Young People with Niemann-Pick Disease Type C ~ *Fact Sheet*
National Niemann-Pick Disease Foundation Inc. ~ *Poster*

Concerned with the following diseases or disorders:
Niemann Pick Disease

1389 NATIONAL ORGANIZATION ON FETAL ALCOHOL SYNDROME (NOFAS)

1819 H Street NW
Suite 750
Washington, D.C. 20006 202-785-4585
800-666-6327
Fax: 202-466-6456
E-mail: nofas@erols.com
http://www.nofas.org

The National Organization on Fetal Alcohol Syndrome is a voluntary not-for-profit service agency dedicated to eliminating birth defects caused by alcohol consumption during pregnancy and improving the quality of life for all those affected by Fetal Alcohol Syndrome. Established in 1990, the organization is committed to increasing public awareness of Fetal Alcohol Syndrome (FAS) and Fetal Alcohol Effects (FAE); assisting in community empowerment and the promotion of preventive education through media campaigns; and training health care professionals, educators, and community members in addressing the specialized needs of affected children. The organization is also committed to serving as a national clearinghouse for local, regional, and state Fetal Alcohol Syndrome organizations to ensure the effective exchange of information and resources. In addition, the National Organization on Fetal Alcohol Syndrome engages in patient advocacy; promotes and supports research; provides appropriate referrals; and offers educational and supportive information through its database, directory, regular newsletter, reports, and brochures. Materials are available in English and Spanish.

President: Lance Friedsam
Year Established: 1990
Organization Members: 14,000

Publishes the following materials:
National Organization on Fetal Alcohol Syndrome ~ *Brochure*
Unas pocas bebidas, un posible dano eterno ~ *Brochure*
Fetal Alcohol Syndrome Fact Sheet ~ *Factsheet*
NOFAS Materials ~ *Order Form*

Concerned with the following diseases or disorders:
Fetal Alcohol Syndrome

1390 NATIONAL PKU FOUNDATION

6301 Tejas Drive
Pasadena, TX 77503 281-487-4802
Fax: 281-487-2089

The National PKU Foundation is a voluntary not-for-profit organization dedicated to promoting awareness of Phenylketonuria (PKU). This is a rare metabolic disorder of infancy caused by a deficiency of the liver enzyme phenylalanine hydroxylase. Impairment in the metabolism of the amino acid phenylalanine results in excess accumulation of phenylalanine. Phenylketonuria is a severe progressive disorder that can produce mental retardation if it is not treated early. The National PKU Foundation provides parents of affected children with information and support, engages in patient advocacy, and promotes and supports research.

President: Polly Kollman
Year Established: 1989
Organization Members: 300

Concerned with the following diseases or disorders:
Phenylketonuria

1391 NATIONAL PKU NEWS

6869 Woodlawn Avenue NE #116
Seattle, WA 98115-5469 206-525-8140
Fax: 206-525-5023
E-mail: schuett@pkunews.org
http://pkunews.org

National PKU News is a not-for-profit organization devoted to providing news and information to all persons involved in the treatment of Phenylketonuria (PKU). This is a rare metabolic disorder caused by a deficiency of the liver enzyme phenylalanine hydroxylase. Impairment in the metabolism of the amino acid phenylalanine results in excess accumulation of phenylalanine. Phenylketonuria is a severe progressive disorder that, if not treated early, can produce mental retardation. Founded in 1989, National PKU News publishes a newsletter three times a year and has approximately 2,000 subscribers from the United States, Canada, and 30 foreign countries. National PKU News also publishes educational materials regarding treatment of PKU. Food lists and cookbooks are also distributed by the organization.

President: Virginia E. Schuett
Executive Director: Virginia E. Schuett
Year Established: 1989
Organization Members: 2,000

Publishes the following materials:
National PKU News ~ *Newsletter*
Special Pre-Publication Announcement ~ *Order Form*
Low Protein Cookery for PKU ~ *Order Form*
Nutrient Content of Recipes from Low Protein Cookery for PKU ~ *Order Form*
Low Protein Bread Machine Baking for PKU ~ *Order Form*
National PKU News: News and Information About Phenylketonuria ~ *Order Form*

Concerned with the following diseases or disorders:
Phenylketonuria

1392 NATIONAL PEDIATRIC MYOCLONUS CENTER (NPMC)

1828 L Street North West
Suite 402
Washington, DC 20036 202-861-5823
Fax: 202-785-4188
E-mail: pranz@aol.com

The National Pediatric Myoclonus Center (NPMC) is a nonprofit organization dedicated to providing the best care possible for children with myoclonus, a neurological movement disorder characterized by sudden, involuntary contractions of skeletal muscles. Such care includes making the correct diagnosis, searching for all reversible (curable) causes, making the best drug treatments available, providing information about myoclonus, obtaining psychological and emotional support for the children and their families, and bringing them together with other similar families. Established in 1990, NPMC also wishes to establish the scope of the problem and increase awareness among federal, private, and pharmaceutical agencies. To accomplish this goal, it has assembled experts in dozens of disciplines. Those experts may perform electrical brain wave studies (EEG and EP), IQ and other tests of mental function (neuropsychological testing), blood tests for rare disorders, eye examinations (neuro-opthalmology), analysis of the chemicals in spinal fluid (neurochemistry), measurement of movement (videotaping), determination of the source of myoclonus (back-averaging), x-ray studies of brain structure (MRI or CT scan), and advanced studies of brain function (PET scan). Consisting of 200 members, the organization provides educational materials including pamphlets entitled "What is Myoclonus?," "What is Progressive Myoclonus Epilepsy?," and "What is the Treatment for Myoclonus?" Program activities include patient advocacy, research, education, and referrals. NPMC can be reached at its e-mail address at [pranz@aol.com].

President: Michael R. Pranzatelli, M.D. (Director)
Executive Director: Elizabeth D. Tate, F.N.P., C., M.N. (Manager)
Year Established: 1990
Organization Members: 200

Publishes the following materials:
What is Myoclonus? ~ *Pamphlet*
What is Progressive Myoclonus Epilepsy? ~ *Pamphlet*
What is the Opsoclonus Myoclonus Syndrome? ~ *Pamphlet*
What is the Treatment for Myoclonus? ~ *Pamphlet*
What is the National Pediatric Myoclonus Center? ~ *Mission Statement*
Advances in the Treatment of Pediatriac Movement Disorders ~ *Repritn*
Myoclonic Disorders ~ *Reprint*
The Immunopharmacology of the Opsoclonus-Myoclonus Syndrome ~ *Reprint*
The Neurobiology of the Opsoclonus-Myoclonus Syndrome ~ *Reprint*

Concerned with the following diseases or disorders:
Batten Disease; Epilepsy, Myoclonic Progressive Familial; Kinsbourne Syndrome; Myoclonus, General

1393 NATIONAL PEDICULOSIS ASSOCIATION (NPA)

P.O. Box 610189
Newton, MA 02161 617-449-6487
Fax: 617-449-8129
http://www.headlice.org

The National Pediculosis Association is a not-for-profit health agency dedicated to promoting public education about Pediculosis and the prevention and treatment of lice and scabies. Pediculosis is the medical term for any type of louse infestation. Incorporated in 1983, the National Pediculosis Association has worked to build awareness about head lice prevention and has helped to standardize head lice control policies nationwide. In addition, the National Pediculosis Association seeks to protect children from the misuse of potentially harmful lice and scabies pesticidal treatments. The National Pediculosis Association produces several educational materials including catalogs, brochures, pamphlets, guides for pharmacists and child care providers, and a quarterly newsletter entitled "Progress." The Association offers many products through its catalogs including t-shirts, coloring books, stickers, and aprons.

President: Deborah Z. Altschuler (1990-Present)
Executive Director: Linda Menditto (Operations)
Year Established: 1983

Publishes the following materials:
I've got you under my skin... ~ *Brochure*

You ought to Have Your Head Examined ~ *Brochure*
Not just another lousy catalog ~ *Catalog*
Keep your wits not your nits ~ *Booklet*
The Latest Greatest Coloring Book About Lice ~ *Coloring Book*
Pharmacist's Guide to Controlling Head Lice ~ *Brochure*
Child Care Provider's Guide To Controlling Head Lice ~ *Brochure*
Dear Parent: National Pediculosis Association ~ *Letter*
Questions & Answers: Moving Toward More Effective Pediculosis Prevention In Schools ~ *Fact Sheet*
The National Pediculosis Association's Progress ~ *Newsletter*

1394 NATIONAL PEMPHIGUS VULGARIS FOUNDATION (NATIONAL PV FOUNDATION)

1098 Euclid Avenue
Berkeley, CA 94708 510-527-4970
Fax: 510-527-8497
E-mail: PVnews@aol.com

The National Pemphigus Vulgaris Foundation is a non-profit, voluntary organization formed to increase awareness of Pemphigus Vulgaris (PV) among the general public and the medical community and to function as an information clearinghouse on PV. Pemphigus is a group of rare autoimmune skin disorders characterized by the development of blisters in the outer layer of the skin and on mucous membranes that line the mouth, eyes, and rectum. Founded in 1994, the Foundation seeks to provide emotional and informational support to individuals who have been diagnosed with Pemphigus Vulgaris, their families, and friends. A quarterly newsletter entitled "The PV Foundation News" disseminates information on the disease and current treatments to all interested parties. With the assistance of medical specialists and researchers from Johns Hopkins Medical Center and New York University Medical Center, the Foundation works toward one of its principal goals: to raise funds for more extensive research into finding a cure for this disease. The Foundation also gathers information on PV from sources worldwide and plans to form chapters and support groups.

President: Janet S. Lehne (1994 to Present)
Year Established: 1994
Organization Chapters: 3

Publishes the following materials:
The PV Foundation News ~ *Newsletter*
The National Pemphigus Vulgaris Foundation ~ *Brochure*

Concerned with the following diseases or disorders:
Pemphigus

1395 NATIONAL PRUNE BELLY SYNDROME NETWORK

100 UCLA Medical Plaza
Suite 690
Los Angeles, CA 90095 310-825-6865
Fax: 310-794-9962

The National Prune Belly Syndrome Network is a self-help organization dedicated to providing support and information concerning Prune Belly Syndrome, a rare disorder in which partial absence of certain abdominal muscles occurs in association with intestinal, renal, and urogenital abnormalities. Established in 1986, the organization promotes the education of affected individuals, their families, and health care and other professionals by providing reprints of medical journal articles concerning all aspects of Prune Belly Syndrome.

President: Richard Ehrlich, M.D.
Year Established: 1986

Concerned with the following diseases or disorders:
Prune Belly Syndrome

1396 NATIONAL PSORIASIS FOUNDATION (NPF)

6600 SW 92nd Avenue
Suite 300
Portland, OR 97223-7195 503-244-7404
800-723-9166
Fax: 503-245-0626
E-mail: getinfor@NPFUSA.org
http://www.psoriasis.org/

The National Psoriasis Foundation is a voluntary not-for-profit organization dedicated to providing support to and improving the quality of life for individuals with psoriasis, a chronic skin disorder; educating the public; and promoting and supporting research for psoriasis. Established in 1968 by affected individuals, physicians, and researchers, the National Psoriasis Foundation is committed to publishing the most current information on psoriasis and providing a forum for affected individuals to speak out. The organization promotes funding for psoriasis research and seeks to establish an alliance between affected people, the medical and scientific communities, and the pharmaceutical industry. The National Psoriasis Foundation promotes patient advocacy and legislation beneficial to affected individuals; provides appropriate referrals (e.g., to support groups); and offers a variety of educational materials. These materials include a regular newsletter and reports.

Executive Director: Gail M. Zimmerman
Year Established: 1968
Organization Members: 38,000

Publishes the following materials:
Overview of Psoriasis Treatments ~ *Brochure*
A Guide to Understanding Psoriasis ~ *Brochure*

Concerned with the following diseases or disorders:
Arthritis, Psoriatic; Psoriasis

1397 NATIONAL RESOURCE CENTER FOR SPECIAL NEEDS ADOPTION

16250 Northland Drive
Suite 120
Southfield, MI 48075 248-443-7080
Fax: 248-443-7099

The National Resource Center for Special Needs Adoption is not-for-profit organization dedicated to the children and professionals involved in special needs adoption. Established in 1985, the organization works toward its goal of improving the effectiveness and quality of adoption and post adoption services for children with special needs nationwide. Such children include those who are older; of minority heritage; have medical, developmental, or emotional challenges; and/or are members of sibling groups who need one family to adopt them. The Center seeks to further its goals through providing a forum for adoption practitioners, policy makers, and advocates to enable them to contribute and share their knowledge and experiences; providing ongoing technical assistance; and developing and distributing educational materials to enhance the practices related to the adoption of children with special needs. The Center also provides training to interested individuals through conferences, workshops, and other various presentations. Training is divided into the Special Needs Adoption Curriculum, post-legal adoption services curriculum, Cultural Competence in Child Welfare curriculum, and parent orientation curriculum. Educational materials produced by the National Resource Center for Special Needs Adoption include a newsletter entitled "Roundtable" and numerous videotapes and books.

President: Judith K. McKenzie, M.S.W. (Executive Director)
Executive Director: Drenda Lakin, M.S.W., A.C.S.W. (Center Director)
Year Established: 1985
Organization Members: Non-Membership

Publishes the following materials:
National Resource Center For Special Needs Adoption ~ *Mission Statement*
The Center Source. Child Welfare Resources (1997) ~ *Leaflet*

1398 NATIONAL RETINOBLASTOMA PARENT GROUP

110 Allen Road
Bow, NH 03304 603-224-4085

The National Retinoblastoma Parent Group is a not-for-profit self-help organization dedicated to providing information and support to parents of children with Retinoblastoma, a malignant tumor appearing in one or both eyes. Established in the late 1980s, the National Retinoblastoma Parent Group provides a variety of educational and support materials including a regular newsletter and medical journal article reprints concerning Retinoblastoma.

President: Susan Laventure
Organization Language: Spanish.
Year Established: 1990
Organization Members: 500

Concerned with the following diseases or disorders:
Chromosome 13, Partial Monosomy 13q; Retinoblastoma

1399 NATIONAL REYE'S SYNDROME FOUNDATION, INC. (NRSF)

426 North Lewis Street
P.O. Box 829
Bryan, OH 43506-0829 419-636-2679
800-233-7393
Fax: 419-636-3366
E-mail: reyessyn@mail.bright.net
http://www.bright.net/~reyessyn

The National Reye's Syndrome Foundation, Inc. is a voluntary not-for-profit service organization dedicated to providing funding for basic research, awareness programs for the general public and the medical community, and emotional support and guidance for individuals with Reye's Syndrome and their families. Reye's Syndrome is a rare childhood disease that usually follows a viral infection, such as influenza or chicken pox, and is strongly associated with the use of salicylates (e.g., aspirin). The syndrome may be characterized by liver failure, low levels of glucose in the blood, and brain damage. Established in 1974, the National Reye's Syndrome Foundation promotes patient and family advocacy; provides appropriate referrals (e.g., to support groups); and offers a variety of educational and supportive information through its database, bulletins, fact sheets, brochures, audiovisual aids, and regular newsletter. Languages supported by the Foundation include English, Spanish, Laotian, Cambodian, and Vietnamese.

President: John E. Freudenberger
Executive Director: Sandra K. Nelson
Year Established: 1974
Organization Chapters: 140
Organization Members: 10,000

Publishes the following materials:
Language, Learning and Behavior ~ *Pamphlet*
National Reye's Syndrome Foundation ~ *Brochure*
Because You Need to Know ~ *Brochure*
Reye's Syndrome ~ *Report*
The New York Times - October 23, 1992 ~ *Reprint*
Reye's Syndrome: Review and Update ~ *Report*
Here Come the Bugs ~ *Report*
Preparations Containing Aspirin and Aspirin-Like Compounds ~ *Products List*
Public Health Service Study of Reye's Syndrome and Medications ~ *Report*
Reye's Syndrome - Health Education Unit 10 ~ *Report*
Reye's Syndrome: A Medical Mystery ~ *Report*
Consequences of Reye Syndrome ~ *Report*
Intellectual and emotional sequelae of Reye's Syndrome ~ *Report*
Neuropsychologic Consequences of Reye Syndrome ~ *Report*
IN THE NEWS ~ *Newsletter*

Concerned with the following diseases or disorders:
Reye Syndrome

1400 NATIONAL ROSACEA SOCIETY

800 S. Northwest Highway
Suite 200
Barrington, IL 60010 847-382-8971
888-662-5874
Fax: 847-382-5567
E-mail: rosaceas@aol.com
http://www.rosacea.org

The National Rosacea Society is a national not-for-profit voluntary organization dedicated to offering information and support to people with Acne Rosacea, a rare skin disorder characterized by flushing and skin eruptions on the face. The organization publishes a quarterly newsletter entitled "Rosacea Review," which provides affected individuals with tips on proper care, new information on the disease and a forum for sharing experiences and insights. Other educational materials produced and disseminated by the Society include "Rosacea: What You Should Know," a public service booklet on rosacea; "Rosacea Tripwires," a chart of lifestyle factors that can trigger flare-ups in various individuals; a patient diary checklist to be used to help identify and avoid lifestyle factors that affect individual cases; a bibliography of books and articles on rosacea; articles on specific aspects of the disease; facts sheets; news realeases; and brochures. The Society has instituted a physician referral service, which provides lists, by local zip code, of dermatologists who have informed the Society that they treat rosacea and are willing to accept new patients.

Executive Director: Sam Huff (Director)
Year Established: 1990
Organization Chapters: 1

Concerned with the following diseases or disorders:
Acne Rosacea

1401 NATIONAL SARCOIDOSIS RESOURCE CENTER

P.O. Box 1593
Piscataway, NJ 08855-1593 908-699-0733
Fax: 908-699-0882
E-mail: nsrc@microfone.net
http://www.microfone.net/nsrc/

The National Sarcoidosis Resource Center is an international not-for-profit organization dedicated to providing support and information to individuals affected by sarcoidosis, their families, and any interested individuals. Sarcoidosis, a rare disorder of unknown cause, is characterized by the formation of small rounded nodules (tubercles) of tissue consisting of cells resembling those that line internal and external surfaces of the body (epithelioid tissue). Almost any organ or tissue may be affected, including the eyes, skin, lungs, spleen, liver, and lymph nodes. Acute Sarcoidosis may be characterized by fever, generalized muscle aches, breathlessness, arthritis, enlarged lymph nodes, and other symptoms. Chronic, progressive, systemic Sarcoidosis may cause a wide variety of symptoms that may include fever, arthritis, numbness, appearance of a purplish rash on the face, bloodshot eyes, and additional abnormalities. Established in 1992 by an individual with sarcoidosis, the Center provides information to people throughout the United States, Canada, and Europe. The Center maintains a registry of more than 15,000 affected individuals; provides referrals to physicians; assists in the formation of self-help groups; coordinates a networking program; and holds an annual "Sarcoidosis Awareness Day Celebration." In addition, the Center conducts on ongoing study of the symptoms and demographics of individuals with sarcoidosis.

President: Sandra Conroy
Year Established: 1992

Concerned with the following diseases or disorders:
Sarcoidosis

1402 NATIONAL SCOLIOSIS FOUNDATION (NSF)

72 Mount Auburn Street
Watertown, MA 02172
E-mail: scoliosis@aol.com

The National Scoliosis Foundation is a not-for-profit organization dedicated to promoting and assisting screening programs for scoliosis (a sideways curvature of the spine) and kyphosis (a front-to-back curvature of the spine) and creating and promoting cooperating networks of educational, health care, and social services professionals from public and private institutions. It acts as a clearinghouse of information about scoliosis and kyphosis and serves as a resource to people working for enactment of postural screening acts by state legislatures and Departments of Education. The National Scoliosis Foundation offers a variety of educational and support materials through its computer database; information packets for parents, affected young people and adults, and health care professionals; and educational multimedia units for teachers. The Foundation also offers videos, fact sheets, medical updates, books, educational posters, brochures, pamphlets, reprints of magazine and medical journal articles, screening information for the detection of scoliosis and kyphosis, and a biannual newsletter, The Spinal Connection.

President: Joseph O'Brien
Year Established: 1976
Organization Members: 1,600

Concerned with the following diseases or disorders:
Ataxia, Friedreich's; Marinesco Sjogren Syndrome; Stenosis, Spinal

1403 NATIONAL SJOGREN'S SYNDROME ASSOCIATION (NSSA)

P.O. Box 42207
Phoenix, AZ 85080-2207 602-516-0787
800-395-6772
Fax: 602-516-0111
E-mail: NSSA@aol.com
http://www.sjogrens.org/

The National Sjogren's Syndrome Association is a voluntary not-for-profit self-help organization dedicated to the identification, control, and cure of Sjogren's Syndrome. Sjogren's Syndrome, a disorder of unknown cause, is characterized by deficient moisture production of the mucous-secreting glands, particularly the tear ducts of the eyes (lacrimal) and the salivary glands of the mouth. Associated symptoms and physical abnormalities may include abnomal dryness, itching, and burning of the eyes (keratoconjunctivitis sicca); abnormal dryness of the mouth, resulting in cavities, other dental disorders, and loss of odor and taste sensations; and, when the lungs are affected, increased susceptibility to repeated respiratory infections. Many affected individuals also experience rheumatoid arthritis. Sjogren's Syndrome, which primarily affects middle-aged women, is thought to be due to an abnormal autoimmune response. Founded in 1990, the organization provides support to affected individuals and health care professionals world-wide; acts as a resource to those seeking informational materials about the syndrome; promotes and supports research; and sponsors support groups throughout the United States. In addition, the National Sjogren's Syndrome Association engages in patient advocacy; makes appropriate referrals; and conducts regional and national conferences. The Association offers a variety of educational and supportive information through its database, patient guide, member newsletter entitled "Sjogren's Digest," and quarterly publications known as the Patient Education Series.

President: Dr. Ari Askari
Executive Director: Barbara Henry
Year Established: 1990
Organization Members: 10,000

Publishes the following materials:
If ~ *Brochure*
Learning to Live With Sjogren's Syndrome ~ *Brochure*
What is Sjogren's Syndrome ~ *Factsheet*
The Many Faces of Sjogren's Syndrome ~ *Factsheet*
Patient Education Series ~ *Pamphlet*
Sjogren's Digest ~ *Brochure*
Sjogren's Syndrome: A Guide For The Patient ~ *Pamphlet*

Concerned with the following diseases or disorders:
Mikulicz Syndrome; Sjogren Syndrome

1404 NATIONAL SPASMODIC DYSPHONIA ASSOCIATION (NSDA)

One E. Wacker Drive
Suite 2430
Chicago, IL 60601-1905 312-755-0198
800-795-6732
Fax: 312-803-0138
E-mail: nsda@aol.com
http://www.geocities.com/hotsprings/5914/

The National Spasmodic Dysphonia Association is a voluntary not-for-profit organization devoted to the interests of individuals with Spasmodic Dysphonia and the physicians, speech pathologists, medical schools, and voice treatment centers that serve them. Spasmodic Dysphonia is a neurological disorder affecting the muscles of the larynx; it is characterized by abnormal, involuntary movement of the vocal cords, resulting in difficult, strained speech and/or intermittent breathlessness. Established in 1990, the National Spasmodic Dysphonia Association is committed to increasing the quality of life for affected individuals; ensuring increased access to information and resources for affected individuals and family members; and promoting awareness of Spasmodic Dysphonia in the medical community and the general public. The Association is also committed to promoting research into the causes and treatment of Spasmodic Dysphonia and encouraging and assisting in the formation of local support groups. In addition, the National Spasmodic Dysphonia Association engages in patient advocacy; promotes legislation beneficial to affected individuals; and provides appropriate referrals. The organization offers a variety of informational materials including a regular newsletter, brochures, audio-visual aids, and listings of treatment centers and support groups.

President: John Hunsinger (1996 to Present)
Executive Director: Valerie Levitan
Year Established: 1990
Organization Members: 5,000

Publishes the following materials:
Dear Friends ~ *Letter*
What is the National Spasmodic Dysphonia Association ~ *Factsheet*
Spasmodic Dysphonia Support Groups ~ *Address List*
Spasmodic Dysphonia Videotapes ~ *Factsheet*
Medical Centers Providing Botox for Spasmodic Dysphonia ~ *Address List*

Concerned with the following diseases or disorders:
Dysphonia, Chronic Spasmodic

1405 **NATIONAL SPASMODIC TORTICOLLIS ASSOCIATION (NSTA)**
PO Box 5849
Orange, CA 92863-5849 714-516-1824
800-487-8385
Fax: 714-516-1824
http://www.bluheronweb.com/nsta/nsta.htm

The National Spasmodic Torticollis Association is a self-help not-for-profit international organization dedicated to increasing awareness of Spasmodic Torticollis; providing support for affected individuals and family members; and promoting and supporting research on the disorder. Spasmodic Torticollis is a neurological disorder that affects the muscles of the neck, causing the head to turn or pull toward the shoulder. Established in 1980, the National Spasmodic Torticollis Association's main purpose is providing an extensive support network to affected individuals. The Association is also committed to helping affected individuals locate physicians with knowledge of Spasmodic Torticollis; engaging in patient advocacy; and supporting and promoting research into effective treatments for Spasmodic Torticollis. The National Spasmodic Torticollis Association also conducts an annual symposium and offers a variety of educational materials including a quarterly newsletter, brochures, pamphlets, and videos.

President: Janet Richter
Executive Director: Patricia L. Murray
Year Established: 1980
Organization Chapters: 37
Organization Members: 3,200

Publishes the following materials:
Remember...You are not alone ~ *Brochure*
For Just a Little $ ~ *Brochure*
NSTA Newsletter ~ *Newsletter*

Concerned with the following diseases or disorders:
Spasmodic Torticollis

1406 **NATIONAL STROKE ASSOCIATION (NSA)**
96 Inverness Drive East
Suite 1
Englewood, CO 80112-5112 303-649-9299
800-787-6537
Fax: 303-649-1328
E-mail: info@stroke.org
http://www.stroke.org

The National Stroke Association (NSA) is an international not-for-profit voluntary health organization dedicated to reducing the incidence and severity of stroke through prevention, medical treatment, rehabilitation, family support, and research. During a stroke, interruption of oxygenated blood supply to the brain or leakage of blood outside of blood vessel walls may cause damage to a portion of the brain. Depending upon the exact location and duration of lack of oxygenated blood supply to brain tissue (ischemia), affected individuals may experience a variety of symptoms such as weakness, paralysis, speech impairment, sensory abnormalities, and/or life-threatening complications. Established in 1984, the National Stroke Association promotes patient, physician, and public education; engages in patient advocacy efforts; and promotes research into improved stroke prevention, treatment, and rehabilitation. The organization, which currently has six chapters and approximately 8,775 members, offers networking services that enable affected individuals and family members to exchange information, assistance, and support; maintains a registry; offers support groups; and makes appropriate referrals. In addition, the NSA offers a stroke information hotline and provides a variety of materials including reports, brochures, pamphlets, videos, audiovisual aids, and a quarterly newsletter.

President: Harold Todd (1995 to present).
Executive Director: Karen Iannella (Vice President)
Organization Language: Spanish (written).
Year Established: 1984
Organization Chapters: 6
Organization Members: 8,775

Publishes the following materials:
Joining NSA ~ *Brochure*
Recurrent Stroke ~ *Brochure*
Reducing Risk and Recognizing Symptoms ~ *Brochure*
Know the Warning Sings of Stroke ~ *Brochure*
The Brain at Risk - Understanding and Preventing Stroke ~ *Booklet*
Stroke Prevention Screening Program ~ *Brochure*
Publications, Products and Programs ~ *Brochure*
To Order NSA Stroke Education Materials ~ *Order Form*
NSA Membership Application ~ *Membership Application*
Stroke Education Materials ~ *Order Form*
The Road Ahead: A Stroke Recovery Guide ~ *Order Form*
Family Caregivers Guide ~ *Order Form*
Ted's Stroke ~ *Order Form*
The Caregiver Survival Series ~ *Order Form*
Be Stroke Smart ~ *Newsletter*
Journal of Stroke and Cerebrovascular Diseases ~ *Order Form*
Stroke Clinical Updates ~ *Reprint*

Concerned with the following diseases or disorders:
Antiphospholipid Syndrome; Sneddon Syndrome

1407 NATIONAL STUTTERING PROJECT

5100 East La Palma Avenue
Suite 208
Anaheim Hills, CA 92807 714-693-7480
800-364-1677
Fax: 714-693-7554
E-mail: NSPmail@aol.com

National Stuttering Project (NSP) is a not-for-profit organization dedicated to people affected by stuttering. Established in 1977, NSP provides education, support, and empowerment tools to children and adults who stutter. In addition the organization serves their families and the speech-language pathologists who work with affected individuals. Consisting of 46 chapters and 5,000 members, the NSP also serves as an advocate and raises the consciousness of the general public about stuttering. Educational materials produced by the organization include a monthly newsletter entitled "Letting Go," audio-visual aids, and informational brochures such as "A Guide for Parents of Children Who Stutter" in English and Spanish. A networking support system, including local support groups, seeks to provide emotional support and information. The Project also operates a toll-free national support hotline.

President: Michael Sugarman (1977 to present)
Year Established: 1977
Organization Chapters: 64
Organization Members: 4,600

Publishes the following materials:
National Stuttering Project ~ *Brochure*
A Guide for Parents of Children Who Stutter ~ *Booklet*
Support Yourself and the NSP! ~ *Order Form*

1408 NATIONAL SUBACUTE SCLEROSING PANENCEPHALITIS REGISTRY

University of South Alabama
P.O. Box 70191
2451 Fillingim Street
Mobile, AL 36615 334-471-7834
Fax: 334-476-8277

The National Subacute Sclerosing Panencephalitis (SSP) Registry is a formal registry for people with SSP. Based at the Department of Neurology, University of South Alabama, the organization maintains an international registry of people with Subacute Sclerosing Panencephalitis. Subacute Sclerosing Panencephalitis is a rare inflammatory disease of the brain that usually affects children and is characterized by the progressive loss of previously acquired motor and mental skills.

President: John Rothrock, M.D.
Year Established: N/A

Concerned with the following diseases or disorders:
Subacute Sclerosing Panencephalitis

1409 NATIONAL SUDDEN INFANT DEATH SYNDROME RESOURCE CENTER (NSCR)

8201 Greensboro Drive
#600
McLean, VA 22102 703-821-8955
Fax: 703-821-2098
http://www.circsol.com/sids

The National Sudden Infant Death Syndrome (SIDS) Resource Center is a professional for profit health organization that provides information services and technical assistance concerning SIDS and related topics in order to promote understanding of SIDS and to comfort those affected by a SIDS loss. Established in 1981, the Resource Center assists the National Center of Education's Maternal and Child Health Bureau (MCHB) by providing its services to State MCHB-supported projects and State SIDS programs funded through the Maternal and Child Health Block Grant. The Resource Center also offers its services to parents, family members, care providers, counselors, medical and legal professionals, researchers, program planners, policymakers, and the general public. The Resource Center maintains automated databases of SIDS technical literature, public awareness materials, MCHB materials, and organizations concerned with SIDS. The Center also develops and distributes bibliographies of materials on SIDS, fact sheets, and other educational materials, including its "Information Exchange" newsletter; tracks information and resources on current developments related to SIDS; conducts customized database searches; and refers those making inquiries to State SIDS programs and other regional and national organizations, as appropriate.

Executive Director: Olivia Cowdrill
Year Established: 1981

Concerned with the following diseases or disorders:
Sudden Infant Death Syndrome

1410 NATIONAL TUBEROUS SCLEROSIS ASSOCIATION (NTSA)

8181 Professional Place
Suite 110
Landover, MD 20785 301-459-9888
800-225-6872
Fax: 301-459-0394
E-mail: ntsa@ntsa.org
http://www.ntsa.org

The National Tuberous Sclerosis Association is a voluntary not-for-profit organization dedicated to improving the quality of life of individuals and families affected by Tuberous Sclerosis. Tuberous Sclerosis is a hereditary disorder characterized by benign, tumor-like nodules of the brain and/or retinas, skin lesions, seizures, and/or mental retardation. Established in 1974, the Association is committed to promoting and sponsoring medical research studies into the diagnosis, cause, management, and cure of Tuberous Sclerosis and ensuring that affected individuals and families have access to appropriate medical services, support services, and resource information. The organization is involved in the development of public and professional educational programs aimed at increasing awareness of Tuberous Sclerosis and prompting early diagnosis and effective treatment. The National Tuberous Sclerosis Association also provides referrals to genetic counseling, support groups, and other services; promotes patient advocacy and legislation beneficial to affected individuals; and conducts international symposia on Tuberous Sclerosis. The Association provides a variety of educational and supportive information through its database, directory, regular newsletter, reports, audio-visual materials, and brochures.

President: Barbara K. Witten
Year Established: 1974
Organization Members: 1,700

Publishes the following materials:
Tuberous Sclerosis ~ *Brochure*
Medical Education Conference Series ~ *Brochure*
Tuberous Sclerosis - An Awareness for Teachers ~ *Brochure*
My Child Has Tuberous Sclerosis ~ *Brochure*
Clinical Manifestations Of Tuberous Sclerosis ~ *Brochure*
NTSA 20Th Anniversary International Symposium ~ *Brochure*
Understanding Your Brother or Sister With Tuberous Sclerosis ~ *Pamphlet*
Resources ~ *Brochure*
NTSA 1994 Annual Report ~ *Brochure*

Concerned with the following diseases or disorders:
Tuberous Sclerosis

1411 NATIONAL VITILIGO FOUNDATION, INC. (NVFI)

305 South Broadway
Suite 403
Tyler, TX 75702 903-531-0074
Fax: 903-531-9767
E-mail: 73071.33@compuserve.com
http://pegasus.uthct.edu/vitiligo/index.html

The National Vitiligo Foundation, Inc. is a voluntary not-for-profit self-help organization dedicated to providing information and support to individuals with vitiligo, a skin disorder in which pigment cells are destroyed, resulting in irregularly shaped white patches on the skin. Established in 1985, the Foundation is committed to locating, informing, and counseling affected individuals and family members; increasing public awareness and concern for affected individuals; and promoting and funding scientific and clinical research into the cause, treatment, and cure of vitiligo. The Foundation is interested in broadening the concern for people with vitiligo within the medical community and establishing a central vitiligo center and local treatment facilities across the country. In addition, the National Vitiligo Foundation promotes patient advocacy and legislation beneficial to affected individuals and engages in patient, professional, and community education. The Foundation provides a variety of informational materials including a quarterly newsletter, guidelines for physicians concerning the treatment of patients with vitiligo, fact sheets, pamphlets, and handbooks for patients, physicians, and schools.

President: Allen L. Locklin (1985-Present)
Executive Director: Jerri Bossley
Year Established: 1985
Organization Chapters: 11
Organization Members: 8,000

Publishes the following materials:
Vitiligo A Manual for Physicians ~ *Brochure*
Vitiligo A Handbook for Schools ~ *Brochure*
Vitiligo A Handbook for Patients ~ *Brochure*
Vitiligo ~ *Brochure*
Vitiligo Newsletter ~ *Newsletter*
This is Vitiligo ~ *Fact Sheet*
Guidelines for the Treatment of Patients with Vitiligo ~ *Fact Sheet*
Dear Vitiligo Friend, ~ *Letter*

Concerned with the following diseases or disorders:
Vitiligo; Waardenburg Syndrome

1412 **NEMALINE MYOPATHY NEWSLETTER**
c/o Jane Lionberger
722 Langwood Drive
Houston, TX 77079-4405 281-493-0860

The Nemaline Myopathy Newsletter is a not-for-profit self-help organization dedicated to sharing information on Namaline Myopathy. Nemaline Myopathy is a rare inherited neuromuscular disease that is usually apparent at birth (congenital) and characterized by extreme muscle weakness (hypotonia). Established in 1991, the Nemaline Myopathy Newsletter consists of 37 members. Educational materials include a newsletter, reports, and a directory. Program activities include a support group, networking, referrals, and phone support.

President: Jane Lionberger (Contact Person) (1991 to Present)
Year Established: 1991
Organization Members: 37

Concerned with the following diseases or disorders:
Nemaline Myopathy

1413 **NEPHROGENIC DIABETES INSIPIDUS PARENT SUPPORT GROUP OF CHOP (NDI PARENT SUPPORT GROUP)**
c/o Mary Evans-Lee
201 Jay Street A-8 S
Stowe, PA 19464 610-326-7955
Fax: 215-590-3705

The Nephrogenic Diabetes Insipidus Parent Support Group is a self-help organization dedicated to providing information and support to individuals and families affected by Diabetes Insipidus. Diabetes Insipidus is a rare metabolic disease that is characterized by a deficiency of the hormone vasopressin (antidiuretic hormone [ADH]), which is produced in the posterior lobe of the pituitary gland. Excessive thirst and urination are the major symptoms of this disorder. The NDI Parent Support Group's mission is to let affected families know that there are others with this condition. Established in 1995 and consisting of 20 members and one chapter, the group publishes two newsletters each year and expects to publish a pamphlet directed toward caregivers and schools. The organization maintains coordinates an active networking program and telephone support system.

President: Mary Evans-Lee (Contact Person)
Year Established: 1995
Organization Chapters: 1
Organization Members: 20

Concerned with the following diseases or disorders:
Diabetes Insipidus

1414 **NEUROBLASTOMA CHILDREN'S CANCER SOCIETY**
P.O. Box 957672
Hoffman Estates, IL 60195 847-490-0700
800-532-5162
Fax: 847-490-0705
http://www.granitewebworks.com/nccs.htm

The Neuroblastoma Children's Cancer Society is a not-for-profit voluntary organization dedicated to significantly accelerating potential cures for neuroblastoma and its related children's cancers and to improve the quality of life of affected individuals and their families. The organization is an advocate for children and their families and is dedicated to providing support in the following ways: promoting research by highly trained medical professionals; providing research grant awards to medical specialists locally and nationwide; educating health care professionals on early detection and the latest advances in treatments and diagnosis; maintaining updated information on current treatment and diagnosis; maintains updated information on current treatments; providing moral, practical, and emotional support for affected individuals and their families through newsletters, Internet interaction, toll-free telephone support, etc.; and providing a resource booklet that lists non-profit organizations and other resources that offer support for affected families. Consisting of 500 members, the Society produces educational materials including a resource handbook and a newsletter entitled "HOPE for Families and Friends of Children With Neuroblastoma."

President: Jim Sexton (1994 to Present)
Executive Director: Dori Sexton
Year Established: 1994
Organization Members: 500

Publishes the following materials:
HOPE for more tomorrow's for children with Neuroblastoma ~ *Brochure*
HOPE for families and friends of children with Neuroblastoma ~ *Newsletter*

Concerned with the following diseases or disorders:
Beckwith Wiedemann Syndrome

1415 NEUROFIBROMATOSIS, INC. (NF)

8855 Annapolis Road
Suite 110
Lanham, MD 20706-2924 301-577-8984
800-942-6825
Fax: 301-577-0016
TDD: 410-461-5213
E-mail: nfinc1@aol.com
http://members.aol.com/NFInc1/index.htm

Neurofibromatosis, Inc. is a national voluntary not-for-profit organization dedicated to providing information, support, and advocacy to individuals and family members affected by Neurofibromatosis Type I (NF1) and Type II (NF2). NF1 is a rare inherited disorder characterized by the development of multiple benign tumors on the covering of nerve fibers and the appearance of brown spots and freckles on the skin. NF2 is a rare inherited disorder characterized by the development of benign tumors on both auditory nerves and in other areas of the body. Established in 1988, Neurofibromatosis, Inc. services the needs of affected individuals through coordinated educational, support, and clinical and research programs. The organization provides information about NF1 and NF2 to affected individuals, family members, health care and other professionals, and the general public; provides referrals to local medical resources; and assists in identifying community support services. Neurofibromatosis, Inc. also encourages and supports medical, clinical, educational, and sociological research into the prevention, treatment, cure, and/or effects of the Neurofibromatoses. It educates federal, state, and local governments concerning the needs of affected families and promotes greater awareness and understanding of the Neurofibromatoses among medical providers, educators, employers, and the general public. In addition, Neurofibromatosis, Inc. sponsors local and national conferences for NF families and providers of care; networks with other voluntary health organizations; and offers educational and supportive information through its regular newsletter, booklets, audio-visual aids, pamphlets, and brochures. Neurofibromatosis, Inc. also provides listings of medical resources and patient support groups throughout the United States and Canada. Languages supported by the organization include English, Spanish, and American Sign Language.

President: Michael Elamingo (1994-Present)
Executive Director: Mary Ann Wilson
Year Established: 1988
Organization Chapters: 9
Organization Members: 12,000

Publishes the following materials:
Acoustic Neuroma Consensus Statement ~ *Booklet*
Medical Resources for the Treatment of NF and Patient Support Groups ~ *Resource Booklet*
Understanding Neurofibromatosis ~ *Booklet*
Is There a Place for Me? New NF Video ~ *Flier*
Neurofibromatosis ~ *Consensus Reprint*
Neurofibromatosis Ink ~ *Newsletter*
NF ~ *Brochure*
NF, Inc. Serving NF Families ~ *Brochure*

Concerned with the following diseases or disorders:
Neurofibromatosis Type 1 (NF-1); Neurofibromatosis Type 2 (NF-2)

1416 **NEUROPATHY ASSOCATION**

P.O. Box 2055
Lenox Hill Station
New York, NY 10021 212-692-0662
800-247-6968
Fax: 212-692-0668
E-mail: info@neuropathy.org
http://www.neuropathy.org/neuropathy

The Neuropathy Association is a national not-for-profit organization established to help people with disorders that affect the peripheral nerves. The organization is dedicated to providing patient support and education to individuals affected by peripheral neuropathy; advocating for patients' interests and promoting research into the cause and cure of peripheral neuropathy. The objectives of the Association are to provide support through education and sharing information and experiences related to peripheral neuropathy; enhance physician awareness through education to help identify, evaluate, and treat peripheral neuropathy; increase public awareness of the nature and extent of peripheral neuropathy and the need for early intervention and research; encourage pharmaceutical and biotechnology companies to develop new therapies and devices for treatment of neuropathy; and encourage government support for research into the causes and treatments of neuropathy and the need for special accommodations and facilities for people with neuropathy. The organization publishes several brochures and a periodic newsletter entitled "Neuropathy News."

Concerned with the following diseases or disorders:
Neuropathy, Peripheral

1417 **NEUTROPENIA SUPPORT ASSOCIATION, INC. (NSAI)**

P.O. Box 243
905 Corydon Avenue
Winnepeg
Manitoba, R3M 3S7
Canada 204-489-8454
800-663-8876
E-mail: stevensl@neutropenia.ca
http://www.neutropenia.ca

The Neutropenia Support Association, Inc. (NSAI) is a voluntary charity dedicated to increasing the awareness and understanding of neutropenia. Cyclic Neutropenia is a rare blood disorder characterized by episodes of abnormally low levels of certain white blood cells called neutrophils; recurrent infections with fever usually occur as a result of this finding. Chronic Neutropenia is a blood disorder in which bone marrow does not produce sufficient numbers of neutrophils; affected individuals are typically more susceptible to recurring infections from fungus and bacteria. Chronic Neutropenia may last for months or years and it can affect both children and adults. NSAI was founded in Canada in 1989, and has since expanded to become the only organization of its kind in the world, with a "National Neutropenia Network" forming in the United States and communication and collaborations between NSAI and other rare disorder, cancer, and health organizations continually growing stronger. The Association's services are geared for affected individuals, families, and the medical community, and include genetic counseling from medical advisors, support groups, public and professional education, an international disease registry, networking opportunities, and advocating for patient/family rights and more legislation in this area. NSAI also maintains an "Information Library," operates a toll-free hotline, produces audio-visual aids and publishes a periodic newsletter and informationalbrochures; at present, published materials are available in both English and French. Brochures include "Neutropenia: Causes, Consequences, and Care" and "Chemotherapy and Neutropenia."

President: Lorna Stevens (1989 to Present) (Founder).
Executive Director: Jim & Janis Benzelock (Volunteers).
Organization Language: French (written/spoken).
Year Established: 1989
Organization Members: Non-Membership

Publishes the following materials:
La Neutropenie - Causes, consequences et conduit a tenir ~ *Booklet*
Neutropenia - Causes, Consequences, and Care ~ *Booklet*
Chimiotherapie et Neutropenie ~ *Booklet*
Chemotherapy and Neutropenia ~ *Booklet*
Neutropenia Support Assoc. Inc. ~ *Newsletter*
Our Mandate Is: ~ *Mission Statement*
A Patient's Guide to Therapy with Neupogen ~ *Booklet*
Neutropenia Support Association, Inc. ~ *Financial Reoport*
Severe Chronic Neutropenia Chemo Therapy Induced ~ *Videotape*
Focusing On The Future ~ *International Registry Informa*
Sammy Syringe...Sammy's Special Stuff ~ *Booklet*
Marvin's Marvelous Medicine ~ *Booklet*
Your Body and G-CSF ~ *Booklet*

Concerned with the following diseases or disorders:
Hyper IgM Syndrome; Neutropenia, Chronic; Neutropenia, Cyclic

1418 **NEVOID BASAL CELL CARCINOMA SYNDROME (NBCCS) SUPPORT NETWORK**

162 Clover Hill Street
Marlboro, MA 01752 508-485-4873
800-815-4447
Fax: 301-847-2012
E-mail: souldansur@aol.com

The NBCCS (Nevoid Basal Cell Carcinoma Syndrome) Support Network is a not-for-profit organization that was established in 1994. The Network was formed to address the medical and psychosocial concerns of people with Nevoid Basal Cell Carcinoma Syndrome. NBCCS is a rare inherited syndrome characterized by the appearance of multiple basal cell cancers of the skin at an early age, occurring in association with skeletal anomalies, palmar and plantar depressions or "pits," and other abnormalities. Founded by two long-term survivors, the Network grew out of a desire to provide support, education, treatment information, resources, and advocacy to others diagnosed with NBCCS, their families, and friends. The Network also seeks to provide information to physicians and other interested health care providers in order to raise their awareness of this disorder and its treatments. The NBCCS Network is committed to reaching as many people as possible with this disorder and providing them with a multitude of services. The organization offers appropriate referrals; provides an opportunity to network with other affected individuals, family members, and health care professionals; and offers educational and supportive information through its directory, regular newsletter, reports, and brochures.

President: Penni Fischer (1994-Present)
Executive Director: Susan A. Charron
Year Established: 1994
Organization Members: 320

Publishes the following materials:
NBCCS NETWORK SUPPORT ~ *Brochure*
NBCCS Support Network Newsletter ~ *Newsletter*

Concerned with the following diseases or disorders:
Nevoid Basal Cell Carcinoma Syndrome

1419 **NEVUS NETWORK (NN)**

The Congenital Nevus Support Group
P.O. Box 1981
Woodbridge, VA 22193 703-492-0253
E-mail: nevusnet@bigfoot.com
http://www.nevusnetwork.org

The Nevus Network is a voluntary not-for-profit self-help organization dedicated to providing support and information to individuals with congenital nevi (birthmarks or moles) and other rare nevus syndromes. Established in 1983, the organization provides a network of support through letters, phone calls, and personal meetings; engages in patient advocacy; and provides referrals to support groups. In addition, the Nevus Network offers educational and supportive information through its directory, information sheets, and brochures. The organization also publishes a regular newsletter that includes research updates, letters from readers, and information concerning nevus support groups. Languages supported by the Nevus Network include English, French, and Spanish.

President: Bari J. Bett
Organization Language: French. Spanish.
Year Established: 1983
Organization Chapters: 10
Organization Members: 336

Publishes the following materials:
Nevus Network ~ *Newsletter*
Congenital Nevi (Moles) Basic Information ~ *Factsheet*
The Nevus Network offers: Educational Material ~ *Information List*

Concerned with the following diseases or disorders:
Blue Rubber Bleb Nevus; Cutis Marmorata Telangiectatica Congenita; Dysplastic Nevus Syndrome; Epidermal Nevus Syndrome; Klippel Trenaunay Syndrome; Sturge Weber Syndrome

1420 **NEVUS OUTREACH, INC. (NOI)**

1616 Alpha Street
Lansing, MI 48910 517-487-2306
E-mail: info@nevus.org
http://www.nevus.org

Nevus Outreach, Inc. (NOI) is a voluntary health organization formed in 1997 by a group of parents dedicated to improving medical knowledge and treatment for individuals with Giant Congenital Nevi and related disorders such as Neurocutaneous Melanosis. Giant Congenital Nevi is characterized by the presence of large, darkly pigmented moles or birthmarks (nevi) at birth. Although such nevi may vary in size and shape and may cover any area of the body, they are often present on the chest, the shoulders, the upper back, the area covered by bathing trunks, the lower arms and legs, and/or various areas on the face and/or scalp. Individuals with giant nevi have an abnormally increased risk of developing malignant melanoma, a form of skin cancer. In addition, the nevus cells that appear on the skin may form in the central nervous system in some cases (Neurocutaneous Melanosis), which may cause neurological abnormalities and potentially life-threatening complications. The Nevus Outreach is committed to providing information, assistance, and support to affected individuals and family members; promoting additional research; and increasing awareness of these conditions among dermatologists and other health care professionals. NOI provides understandable information on these disorders; publishes a biannual newsletter entitled "Nevus News"; provides periodic updates on important events and announcements; and sponsors an annual conference to enable affected individuals and family members to network with one another and to interact with medical specialists in the field. The Nevus Outreach also acts as an advocate for affected families, helps make travel assistance arrangements for treatment, and provides referrals to other relevant organizations. In addition, the NOI has a web site on the Internet that provides information on nevi disorders, online networking opportunities, and dynamic links to other helpful sources of information and support on the Internet.

President: Kevin Williams
Organization Language: French. Spanish. Dutch.
Year Established: 1997

Concerned with the following diseases or disorders:
Blue Rubber Bleb Nevus; Dysplastic Nevus Syndrome; Epidermal Nevus Syndrome; Sturge Weber Syndrome

1421 NEW ONSET JUVENILE DERMATOMYOSITIS (JDMS) REGISTRY

Children's Memorial Medical Center
2300 Children's Plaza Center
Chicago, IL 60614 773-880-3333
Fax: 773-880-4179
E-mail: e-mendez@nwu.edu

The New Onset Juvenile Dermatomyositis (JDMS) Registry is a five-year project that has been funded by the National Institutes of Health's (NIH's) National Institute of Arthritis and Musculoskeletal and Skin Diseases (NIAMS) since 1994. Dermatomyositis is a progressive connective tissue disorder characterized by inflammatory and degenerative changes of the muscles and of the skin. Muscle abnormalities may include muscle weakness, stiffness, and degeneration (atrophy), while skin abnormalities may include a reddish-purple rash on the upper eyelids (Heliotrope rash); reddish-purple, horn-like growths on the surface of the knuckles, elbows, and/or knees (Gottron's sign); and/or a red rash (erythema) affecting the skin of the face, neck, and/or upper torso. Although the symptoms of Juvenile (Childhood) Dermatomyositis (JDMS) are similar to those associated with the adult form of the disorder, onset is usually more sudden. In addition, abnormal accumulations of calcium deposits (calcifications) in muscle and skin tissues, as well as involvement of the digestive (gastrointestinal) tract are more common in the childhood form of Dermatomyositis. The purpose of the JDMS Registry is to help determine the prevalence and incidence of Juvenile Dermatomyositis, the circumstances surrounding the onset of JDMS, and the influences that ethnic background may have on the disease's course. The goals of the Registry include learning the possible causes of the disorder, increasing recognition of JDMS and facilitating diagnosis, determining better treatments based upon the outcomes affected children have experienced with medical and physical therapy, and facilitating JDMS research by physicians and scientists across the United States. In addition, the Registry provides a regular newsletter entitled "New Onset Juvenile Dermatomyositis Registry Newsletter" to participating children and families as well as physicians and other health care providers who give their time and support to the Registry. Physicians with pediatric patients that have been diagnosed within the last six months are encouraged to contact the JDMS Registry for more information.

President: Lauren M. Pachman, M.D. (Principal Investigator)
Organization Language: Spanish (written).
Year Established: 1994

Concerned with the following diseases or disorders:
Dermatomyositis

1422 NON-KETOTIC HYPERGLYCINEMIA (NKH) PARENT NETWORK (NKH PARENT NETWORK)

c/o Karen Carter
2236 Birchbark Trail
Clearwater, FL 34623 813-799-4977
Fax: 813-441-4942
E-mail: Ketchcar@aol.com

The Non-Ketotic Hyperglycinemia (N.K.H.) Parent Network is an international voluntary organization dedicated to providing information and support to parents with children affected by Non-Ketotic Hyperglycinemia. A rare inherited metabolic disorder that affects infants soon after birth, Non-Ketotic Hyperglycinemia is caused by an impairment in the breakdown of the amino acid glycine. As a result, affected infants exhibit an abnormal accumulation of glycine in body fluids, primarily the blood, cerebrospinal fluid, and urine. Symptoms and physical features may include failure to gain weight and grow at the expected rate; abnormally low muscle tone; drowsiness; episodes of uncontrolled electrical disturbances in the brain; repeated, brief, shock-like muscle spasms of the arms, legs, or entire body; and mild to severe mental retardation. Established in 1995, the Non-Ketotic Hyperglycinemia Parent Network provides networking services that enable parents and family members to exchange information, support, and resources. The N.K.H. Parent Network, which has approximately 60 members, also has a registry, provides referrals, and offers educational materials including a regular newsletter entitled the "N.K.H. Parent Network Newsletter."

President: Karen Carter (1995 to Present)
Year Established: 1995
Organization Members: 60

Publishes the following materials:
NKH Parent Network Newsletter ~ *Newsletter*
Children With Non-Ketotic Hyperglycinemia. List of Members ~ *Pamphlet*

Concerned with the following diseases or disorders:
Non-Ketotic Hyperglycinemia

1423 NOONAN SYNDROME SUPPORT GROUP, INC. (TNSSG)

P.O. Box 145
Upperco, MD 21155 410-374-5245
888-686-2224
E-mail: wandar@bellatlantic.net
http://noonansyndrome.org

The Noonan Syndrome Support Group (TNSSG) is a national non-profit organization that is dedicated to the sharing of information and encouragement among individuals whose lives have been affected by Noonan Syndrome. Noonan Syndrome is a genetic disorder characterized by a lack of sexual development; short stature; possible mental retardation; a webbed neck; skeletal and/or heart defects; and various other malformations. Persons with Noonan Syndrome have normal chromosomes (karyotype is normal), while their physical appearance is different from their peers. Persons with Noonan Syndrome have widely varying symptoms. Established in 1996 and composed of 225 members, the organization publishes a quarterly newsletter entitled "The Noonan Connection." TNSSG maintains a Resource Center that gives its members access to the most recent medical journal articles and studies. Support group meetings are held for those who live near other network members. Affected individuals, their families, and friends from all over the world are able to receive encouragement and information via TNSSG's Web Site. The organization also offers forums where physicians and other professionals can provide information on living with the daily challenges of Noonan Syndrome. TNSSG works to enhance public awareness and fight misconceptions about Noonan Syndrome by providing information to the media, medical community, and schools.

President: Wanda H. Robinson (Founder)
Year Established: 1996
Organization Members: 225

Publishes the following materials:
The Noonan Syndrome ~ *Fact Sheet*
Noonan Connection (Volume 1.2 Winter 96/97) ~ *Newsletter*
The Noonan Syndrome (Spring 1997) ~ *Newsletter*
The Noonan Syndrome Support Group ~ *Brochure*
List of NS Characteristics/Symptoms ~ *Fact Sheet*
The Noonan Syndrome Support Group ~ *Brochure*
The Noonan Syndrome Support Group, Inc. Available Articles ~ *List*
What Do I Do Once I Am Told My Child Has Noonan Syndrome? ~ *Reprint*
Noonan Syndrome: A clinical description emphasizing the cardiac findings ~ *Pamphlet*

Concerned with the following diseases or disorders:
Noonan Syndrome

1424 NORRIE DISEASE ASSOCIATION (NDA)

Massachusetts General Hospital
E. #6217
149 13th Street
Charlestown, MA 02129 617-726-5718
Fax: 617-724-9620
E-mail: sims@helix.mgh.harvard.edu
http://neuro-www.mgh.harvard.edu/medbie.html

The Norrie Disease Association is a voluntary not-for-profit service organization dedicated to providing support and information to people with Norrie Disease and their families. Norrie Disease is a rare inherited disorder characterized by blindness in both eyes at birth; some affected children may later develop mild to profound hearing loss and varying degrees of mental retardation. Established in 1994, the Norrie Disease Association compiles and disseminates educational and research information on the disorder; maintains a patient registry; and provides referrals to medical and/or genetic services. The Association also provides educational and supportive information through its database, directory, and flyers.

Executive Director: Katherine B. Sims, M.D.
Year Established: 1994
Organization Members: 30

Concerned with the following diseases or disorders:
Norrie Syndrome

1425 NORTH AMERICAN MALIGNANT HYPERTHERMIA REGISTRY

Penn State University
Dept. of Anesthesiology
P.O. Box 850
Hershey, PA 17033-0850 717-531-6936
Fax: 717-531-6221

The North American Malignant Hyperthermia Registry is a not-for-profit research organization that is dedicated to acquiring, analyzing, and disseminating patient-specific clinical and laboratory information concerning susceptibility to malignant hyperthermia (MH). Malignant Hyperthermia is an inherited condition characterized by a rapid rise in body temperature and other serious symptoms after an affected individual has been given general anesthesia. Established in 1987, the North American Malignant Hyperthermia Registry maintains a central database of individuals with MH susceptibility and similar syndromes. It provides physicians with current medical information concerning MH susceptibility status of affected individuals who consent to be registered. The Registry also provides database services to participating MH diagnostic testing referral centers for standardization and validation of MH diagnostic testing procedures. In addition, the Registry coordinates storage of blood and tissue samples at each MH diagnostic referral center as part of the North American MH research repository. It investigates the epidemiology of MH to improve diagnosis, treatment, and prevention of MH episodes and gives registered affected individuals the security of knowing that any physician will be able to obtain specific information on their MH susceptibility status.

President: Dennis Landers, M.D., Ph.D.
Executive Director: Marilyn Green Larach, M.D.
Year Established: 1987

Publishes the following materials:
Malignant Hyperthermia Registry ~ *Brochure*
AMRA Report Adverse Metabolic Reaction to Anesthesia ~ *Report*
Already Known As ~ *Report*

Concerned with the following diseases or disorders:
Central Core Disease; Malignant Hyperthermia; Neuroleptic Malignant Syndrome; Pseudocholinesterase Deficiency

1426 NORTH AMERICAN RIDING FOR THE HANDICAPPED ASSOCIATION (NARHA)

P.O. Box 33150
Denver, CO 80233 303-452-1212
800-369-7433
Fax: 303-252-4610
E-mail: narha@frii.com
http://www.narha.org

The North American Riding for the Handicapped Association (NARHA) is a national nonprofit equestrian organization dedicated to serving individuals with disabilities by giving disabled individuals the opportunity to ride horses. NARHA establishes safety standards, provides continuing education, and offers networking opportunities for both its individuals and operating center members. Riders are encouraged to expand the limits of their abilities in environments that promote success. Established in 1969, NARHA is headquartered in Denver, CO with a membership of approximately 3,200 and 450 operating centers. The organizations produces educational materials including fact sheets, brochures, booklets, a newsletter entitled "NARHA," audio-visual tapes, and a directory. Significant NARHA programs include the Operating Center Accreditation and the Instructor Certification. Both programs help insure the high quality and safe instruction offered by local operating centers. NARHA also provides many educational opportunities through regional workshops, an annual conference, and regional and state networks. In addition, the NARHA offers the American Hippotherapy Association (AHA), a special interest section of the NARHA. The AHA is dedicated to promoting research, education, and communication among physical and occupational therapists, and others utilizing the horse in a treatment approach based on principles of classic hippotherapy.

Executive Director: William Scebbi
Year Established: 1969
Organization Chapters: 1
Organization Members: 3,200

Publishes the following materials:
You can make a difference ~ *Brochure*

1427 OBSESSIVE-COMPULSIVE FOUNDATION, INC. (OCF)

P.O. Box 70
Milford, CT 06460-0070 203-878-5669
Fax: 203-874-2826
E-mail: jphs28a@prodigy.com
http://pages.prodigy.com.alwillen/ocf.html

The Obsessive-Compulsive Foundation is a national not-for-profit organization dedicated to giving support to individuals with Obsessive-Compulsive Disorder, their families and friends, medical professionals, and other concerned individuals. Obsessive-Compulsive Disorder is an anxiety disorder characterized by recurrent obsessive or compulsive thoughts that may interfere with the affected individual's normal routine, occupational functioning, social activities, and personal relationships. Established in 1986, the Obsessive-Compulsive Foundation raises funds for research; compiles and disseminates the latest treatment information; and engages in patient advocacy. The Foundation also provides appropriate referrals, including to support groups and engages in patient, professional, and community education. Informational and supportive materials include a bimonthly newsletter, semi-annual children's newsletter, quarterly newsletter for support group leaders, booklets, and brochures.

President: Susan Duffy
Executive Director: James W. Broatch, MSW
Organization Language: Spanish.
Year Established: 1986
Organization Chapters: 8
Organization Members: 10,000

Publishes the following materials:
Obsessive Compulsive Disorder - Questions and Answers ~ *Brochure*
Check It Out ~ *Newsletter*
Learning to Live With OCD ~ *Brochure*
School Personnel: A Critical Link ~ *Brochure*
OCD Newsletter ~ *Newsletter*
Kidscope "The OCD Kids Newsletter" ~ *Newsletter*

Concerned with the following diseases or disorders:
Obsessive Compulsive Disorder; Trichotillomania

1428 OLLIER/MAFFUCCI SELF-HELP GROUP

1824 Millwood Road
Sumter, SC 29150 803-775-1757
E-mail: Olliers@aol.com
http://uhsweb.edu/olliers/olliers.htm

The Ollier/Maffucci Self-Help Group, a national not-for-profit self-help organization, is a support group for individuals and families affected by Ollier's Disease, a rare disorder of bone development usually beginning during childhood and Maffucci Syndrome, a rare congenital disorder characterized by multiple benign skin and bone lesions which in some cases, may be progressive. Established in 1987, the Group is dedicated to providing support to affected individuals and family members, gathering and disseminating information about Ollier's Disease and Maffucci Syndrome, and spreading awareness among health care professionals and the general public. The Group's goals are to establish means of communication for persons with the disease, and to inform the world at large about those people's problems; help people with the disease cope with the physical and psychological burden; provide a forum for individuals with Ollier's Disease and Maffucci Syndrome so they can communicate with each other; collect information on these diseases and/or on research in related fields; and raise awareness of the Group's existence, activities, and the services it provides. In addition, the Group enables members to network with one another and works with physicians and other organizations to increase awareness and understanding of Ollier's Disease and Maffucci Syndrome. The Group provides educational materials including reports and a regular newsletter entitled "Ollier's News," which is published four times a year and discusses medical information and current research studies. The Ollier/Maffucci Self-Help Group also maintains close contact with its members; updates members list and case histories; improves and periodically updates its web site; periodically updates the Ollier/Maffucci/Ilizarov libraries; and create a database of experienced doctors and hospitals.

President: Bonnie M. Schmid (1988-Present)
Year Established: 1987
Organization Members: 92

Publishes the following materials:
Ollier's Disease Self-Help Group ~ *Newsletter*
Parents Searching for Answers ~ *Flyer*

Concerned with the following diseases or disorders:
Maffucci Syndrome; Ollier Disease

1429 ONGWANADA FRAGILE X RESOURCE CENTRE

191 Portsmouth Avenue
Kingston
Ontario, K7L 1L2
Canada
613-548-4417
Fax: 613-548-1743

The Ongwanada Fragile X Resource Center is a voluntary organization that is dedicated to providing support and information concerning Fragile X Syndrome. Fragile X Syndrome is an inherited defect of the X chromosome that causes mental retardation. Established in 1948, the Center provides information on genetic counseling; genetic testing; parent and family support; networking options for parents; research opportunities; a registry; and educational materials. These materials include a newsletter, Spanish language materials, and pamphlets such as "Fragile X Syndrome" or "Alcohol and Pregnancy." Fragile X Syndrome is also known as Martin-Bell Syndrome, FRAXA, X-linked Mental Retardation and Macroorchidism, and Marker X Syndrome.

President: Pat Frost (Contact Person)
Organization Language: French (spoken). Spanish (written/spoken).
Year Established: 1948
Organization Members: 100

1430 ONTARIO FEDERATION FOR CEREBRAL PALSY (OFCP)

1630 Lawrence Avenue West
Suite 104
Toronto
Ontario, M6L 1C5
Canada
416-244-9686
Fax: 416-244-6543
E-mail: ofcp@the.connection.com
http://www.connection.com/ofcp/

The Ontario Federation for Cerebral Palsy (OFCP), a voluntary, non-profit, charitable organization is dedicated to working with and for people with cerebral palsy and other disabilities. The Federation is also committed to initiating programs, personal attendant care services, and facilities; promoting public and professional awareness and education; offering family support groups; and promoting and supporting research. Cerebral palsy, a nonprogressive motor disorder thought to be due to a prenatal brain defect or brain injury during birth, is characterized by spastic paralysis, impaired control of voluntary movements (ataxia), seizures, and/or mental retardation. Established in 1947 and consisting of 50 member groups, OFCP offers a variety of programs and services including several annual conferences, workshops and seminars, consumer peer support, and publication and distribution of printed and audiovisual materials on cerebral palsy and related issues. The Federation also developed the International Cerebral Palsy Registry to help parents of affected children as well as adults with cerebral palsy make direct contact with others to support one another and share information and strategies in their pursuit to become empowered and self-directed. OFCP also offers information packets developed for parents, grandparents, adolescents, young adults, teachers, and other professionals; provides a reference library for parents and professionals; and assists in the development ofregional member groups and community support programs. In addition, OFCP has developed a "Service Information Database for People With Disabilities Program" (SIDD), offering current comprehensive disability-specific information on a variety of service needs in a user-friendly computer format for people of all ages with all types of physical and developmental disabilities. The Federation offers a variety of educational materials including booklets, pamphlets, videos, self-help guides, information packets, and a regular newsletter entitled "Participaper." OFCP also has a web site on the Internet at [http://www.connection.com/ofcp/].

President: Gloria Neamtu
Executive Director: Clarence Meyers
Year Established: 1947
Organization Chapters: 50

Publishes the following materials:
Participating Families Program ~ *Brochure*
A Guide to Cerebral Palsy ~ *Booklet*
The Ontario Federation for Cerebral Palsy. Video Library ~ *Catalogue*
Important Facts About The OFCP Household Pickup Service ~ *Brochure*
Ontario Federation for Cerebral Palsy. Prevention ~ *Brochure*
OFCP Disability Myths ~ *Brochure*

What is Cerebral Palsy? ~ *Brochure*
The Ontario Federation for Cerebral Palsy ~ *Brochure*
Participaper ~ *Newsletter*

1431 **ONTARIO FIBROMYALGIA ASSOCIATION**
393 University Avenue
Suite 1700
Toronto
Ontario, M5G 1E6
Canada 416-979-7228
800-321-1433
Fax: 416-979-8366
http://www.arthritis.ca

The Ontario Fibromyalgia Association, one of five specific disease associations of The Arthritis Society of Canada, is a not-for-profit organization dedicated to promoting and supporting research on fibromyalgia and providing information and support to affected individuals, family members, and health care professionals. Fibromyalgia is a chronic disorder characterized by pain throughout much of the body. Established in 1986, the Ontario Fibromyalgia Association has several chapters and offers more than 40 support groups in Ontario for affected individuals, family members, and friends. The Association also promotes patient advocacy and offers a variety of materials to affected individuals, family members, health care professionals, and the general public. These materials include a quarterly newsletter entitled "Tender Points," reports, guides, booklets, brochures, pamphlets, videos, and assistive devices.

President: Lois R. Whittaker
Executive Director: Joanne Wright (Director of Support Services)
Year Established: 1986
Organization Chapters: 11
Organization Members: 3,000

Publishes the following materials:
The 1995 Fibromyalgia Research Campaign ~ *Announcement*
OFA Membership Questionaire ~ *Questionaire*
Arthritis News ~ *Subscription Form*
Arthritis Information - Coping With Pain ~ *Brochure*
OFA Tender Points ~ *Newsletter*
Lifelines ~ *Article*
Tender Points ~ *Newsletter*
Pain and Tender Points: Fibrositis/Fibromyalgia and Related Syndromes ~ *Reprint*
The Arthritis Society Fibromyalgia (Fibrositis) Syndrome ~ *Brochure*
Ontario Fibromyalgia Association - An Introduction ~ *Brochure*
Literature and Assistive Devices for Fibromyalgia Patients ~ *Resource Listing*
Benefits of O.F.A. Membership ~ *Membership Fact Sheet*
The Ontario Fibromyalgia Association Patient Videos ~ *Fact Sheet*
Graded Sit-ups for Abdominal Muscle Power ~ *Flier*

Concerned with the following diseases or disorders:
Fibromyalgia

1432 **OPITZ FAMILY NETWORK**
P.O. Box 516
Grand Lake, CO 80447 970-627-8935
Fax: 970-627-8935
E-mail: opitznet@rkymtnhi.com
http://rkymtnhi.com/opitz/

The Opitz Family Network is a voluntary not-for-profit self-help organization dedicated to providing support to individuals and family members affected by Opitz Syndrome. Opitz Syndrome is a rare hereditary disorder characterized by widely set eyes, hernias, undescended testicles and abnormal placement of the urinary opening on the underside of the penis in males, partial or total absence of the thick band of nerve fibers that connects the left and right hemispheres of the brain (hypoplasia or agenesis of the corpus callosum), swallowing difficulties, and/or additional abnormalities. Established in 1994, the Opitz Family Network provides phone support; promotes the sharing of information, resources, and support among affected families; engages in patient advocacy; and offers appropriate referrals. The Network also maintains a database of members, engages in professional education, and offers a variety of educational and support materials including a regular newsletter and brochures.

President: Janet Wharton
Executive Director: Janet Wharton
Year Established: 1994
Organization Members: 30

Concerned with the following diseases or disorders:
Opitz Syndrome

1433 **OPSOCLONUS-MYOCLONUS SUPPORT NETWORK, INC. (OMS-PARENT TALK)**
724 North Street
Jim Thorpe, PA 18229 717-325-3302
E-mail: clquinn@ptdprolog.net
http://www.geocities.com/hotsprings/spa/2190

Opsoclonus-Myoclonus Syndrome Parent Talk is a not-for-profit organization dedicated to providing information and support to parents of children with Opsoclonus-Myoclonus Syndrome. Myoclonus is a neurological movement disorder characterized by sudden, involuntary contractions of a muscle or groups of muscles. Opsoclonus is a condition in which there are nonrhythmic vertical and horizontal movements of the eyes. Established in 1994, Opsoclonus-Myoclonus Syndrome Parent Talk enables parents to network with other affected families whose children are in a similar age group. This networking program gives affected families the opportunity to exchange information, support, and resources. Opsoclonus-Myoclonus Syndrome Parent Talk also publishes a quarterly newsletter.

President: Connie Quinn (Contact Person)
Executive Director: Connie Quinn
Year Established: 1994
Organization Members: 28

Concerned with the following diseases or disorders:
Kinsbourne Syndrome; Myoclonus, General

1434 OSTEOGENESIS IMPERFECTA FOUNDATION, INC. (OIF)

804 West Diamond Avenue
Suite 210
Gaithersburg, MD 20878 301-947-0083
800-981-2663
Fax: 301-947-0456
E-mail: bonelink@aol.com
http://www.oif.org

The Osteogenesis Imperfecta Foundation, Inc. is a voluntary organization dedicated to improving the quality of life for individuals affected by Osteogenesis Imperfecta through research, education, awareness, and mutual support. Osteogenesis Imperfecta (OI) is a genetic disorder characterized by abnormally fragile bones. Established in 1970, the Osteogenesis Imperfecta Foundation offers information and support to affected individuals and family members. It promotes public and professional education, encourages and supports research for OI, and promotes health care legislation benefiting affected individuals. In addition, the Foundation provides appropriate referrals, conducts local and regional meetings for members, holds biennial national conferences on OI, provides a peer contact network, and promotes patient advocacy. The Osteogenesis Imperfecta Foundation offers a variety of educational and support materials through its computer database, directory, regular newsletter, resource list, brochures, booklets, and videos.

President: Joseph Antolini
Year Established: 1970
Organization Chapters: 1

Publishes the following materials:
Resources Form OIF ~ *Resource List/Order Form*
OIF Needs You Please, Become a Member Today ~ *Brochure*
Osteogenesis Imperfecta OIF Foundation ~ *Brochure*
We're Growing Stronger ~ *Brochure*
The Care of a Baby and Child with Osteogenesis Imperfecta ~ *Brochure*
El cuidado del bebe y del nino con Osteogenesis Imperfecta ~ *Brochure*

Concerned with the following diseases or disorders:
Osteogenesis Imperfecta

1435 PKR (POLYCYSTIC KIDNEY RESEARCH) FOUNDATION

4901 Main St.
#200
Kansas City, MO 64112-2634 816-931-2600
800-753-2873
Fax: 816-931-8655
E-mail: pkdcure@pkrfoundation.org
http://www.kumc.edu/pkrf

The PKR (Polycystic Kidney Research) Foundation is an international not-for-profit voluntary organization that was established in 1982. The Foundation is committed to providing emotional support and educational materials to people with Polycystic Kidney Disease and their families. The Foundation seeks to promote public awareness of polycystic kidney disease and raise funds that will support ongoing medical research into the causes, treatment, and prevention of this disease. The PKR Foundation conducts informational seminars and conferences; provides phone support for newly diagnosed affected individuals and publishes a quarterly newsletter. It assists in the formation and maintenance of new support groups and makes appropriate referrals to physicians who are familiar with this disorder.

President: Dan Larson (1994-Present)
Year Established: 1982
Organization Chapters: 45

Concerned with the following diseases or disorders:
Polycystic Kidney Diseases

1436 PRISMS (PARENTS & RESEARCHERS INTERESTED IN SMITH-MAGENIS SYNDROME) (PRISMS)

11875 Fawn Ridge Lane
Reston, VA 22094 703-709-0568
Fax: 703-709-0568
E-mail: acmsmith@nhgri.mh.gov

PRISMS (Parents & Researchers Interested in Smith-Magenis Syndrome) is a national not-for-profit organization that was established in 1993. The primary goals of the group are to serve as a national network of support for families with individuals who have Smith-Magenis Syndrome (SMS) and provide centralized communication between families and researchers interested in the treatment of Smith-Magenis Syndrome. PRISMS seeks to increase public and professional awareness of this disorder and serve as a national clearinghouse for information about SMS. In addition, the group fosters the development of new programs that benefit people with Smith-Magenis Syndrome and their families and supports research into the causes, management, and treatment of this rare disorder. Smith-Magenis Syndrome is a rare chromosomal disorder characterized by a specific pattern of physical, behavioral, and developmental features. SMS is caused by the absence of genetic material (deletion) from a certain region on chromosome 17. Educational materials produced by PRISMS include a brochure entitled "What is Smith-Magenis Syndrome?" and a newsletter entitled "Spectrum."

President: Margaret Miller (1993-Present)
Executive Director: Ann C.M. Smith
Year Established: 1993
Organization Members: 90

Publishes the following materials:
What is Smith-Magenis Syndrome? ~ *Brochure*
Spectrum ~ *Newsletter*

Concerned with the following diseases or disorders:
Smith Magenis Syndrome

1437 PXE INTERNATIONAL, INC. (PXE, INT.)

23 Mountain Street
Sharon, MA 02067 781-784-3817
Fax: 781-784-3817
E-mail: pxeinter@aol.com or pxe@tiac.net
http://www.med.harvard.edu/programs/PXE

PXE International, Inc. is a voluntary organization established in 1995 for the purpose of disseminating information on Pseudoxanthoma Elasticum (PXE) to affected individuals, families, and doctors. PXE is a rare connective tissue disease that is inherited and progressive and affects the elastic tissues of the body; abnormal accumulations of calcium salts (calcifications) develop within elastic fibers of the skin, eyes, and cardiovascular system (i.e., heart and blood vessels). The goals of PXE International include dissemination of information to affected individuals, families, and physicians; support of research; review of the literature; and establishment of a patient support network. Educational materials are written both for lay people and medical specialists, in as many languages as possible and include "MemberGram," the organization's newsletter. Composed of 800 members, the organization maintains an international registry of affected individuals, families, and helpful medical specialists. It networks throughout the world, providing written, telephone, e-mail, and meeting connections. A blood and tissue bank has been created so that patient information and tissue samples can be anonymously available to approved ongoing research projects concerning PXE. In addition, the organization conducts an annual international conference.

President: Sharon F. Terry (1995 to present)
Organization Language: French, German, Spanish (written/spoken). Italian (written).
Year Established: 1995
Organization Chapters: 21
Organization Members: 800

Publishes the following materials:
Patient Information ~ *Brochure*
Paeudoxanthoma Elasticum (PXE) and Skin ~ *Reprint*
PXE and the Eye ~ *Reprint*
A Review of Pseudoxanthoma Elasticum for Pediatricians and Family Practitioners ~ *Pamphlet*
PXE and the Dermatologist ~ *Factsheet*
Angioid Streaks ~ *Reprint*
PXE and the Primary Care Practitioner ~ *Reprint*
PXE and Dentistry ~ *Reprint*
Coalition of Patient Advocates for Skin Disease Research ~ *Brochure*
PXE International, Inc. Patient Information ~ *Brochure*
PXE and the Eye ~ *Reprint*
Pseudoxanthoma elasticum (PXE) and Skin ~ *Reprint*
Your Child and PXE ~ *Reprint*
PXE and the Primary Care Practitioner ~ *Reprint*
PXE and Pregnancy ~ *Reprint*
Angioid Streaks ~ *Reprint*
PXe and the Dermatologist ~ *Reprint*
PXE and Dentistry ~ *Reprint*
Pseudoxanthoma Elasticum and the Pediatricians ~ *Reprint*
PXE International MemberGram Fall/Winter 1996 ~ *Newsletter*
PXE International MemberGram Spring 1997 ~ *Newsletter*

Concerned with the following diseases or disorders:
Pseudoxanthoma Elasticum (PXE)

1438 PALLISTER-HALL FOUNDATION

RFD Box 3000
Fairground Road
Bradford, VT 05033

The Pallister-Hall Foundation is a voluntary not-for-profit organization dedicated to serving individuals and families affected by Pallister-Hall Syndrome. This is a rare disorder characterized by a benign tumor in a certain area of the brain (hypothalamic hamartoblastoma), extra fingers and/or toes, an absent or extremely small anal opening, and decreased pituitary function. Established in 1994 by concerned parents and health care professionals, the Foundation provides referrals to physicians and genetic professionals, offers access to research on Pallister-Hall Syndrome, and promotes the exchange of information, support, and resources through networking with other families. The Foundation also promotes awareness of Pallister-Hall Syndrome among the health care community and the general public. The Pallister-Hall Foundation plans to offer educational and support materials through fact sheets and a regular newsletter.

President: Felicia Johnson (1994-Present)
Executive Director: Debra Messer
Year Established: 1994
Organization Members: 10

Concerned with the following diseases or disorders:
Pallister Hall Syndrome

1439 PALLISTER-KILLIAN FAMILY SUPPORT GROUP

3700 Wyndale Court
Fort Worth, TX 76109 817-927-8854
Fax: 817-927-2073

The Pallister-Killian Family Support Group is a voluntary not-for-profit organization dedicated to facilitating and promoting networking between families who have loved ones with Pallister-Killian Syndrome. Pallister-Killian Syndrome is a rare chromosomal disorder characterized by distinctive facial abnormalities, mental retardation, lack of muscle tone, and streaks of skin lacking color. Established in 1991, the Pallister-Killian Family Support Group is affiliated with the Alliance of Genetic Support Groups. The Pallister-Killian Family Support Group sends individual personalized letters to those requesting information. The group has received communications from families in the United States as well as many other countries around the world.

President: Susan Garnett, MSW, Coordinator
Year Established: 1991

Concerned with the following diseases or disorders:
Pallister Killian Mosaic Syndrome

1440 PARENT PROJECT FOR DUCHENNE MUSCULAR DYSTROPHY RESEARCH

125 Marymont Court
Middletown, OH 45042 513-424-7452
800-714-5437
Fax: 513-425-9907
E-mail: santolo@soho.ios.com
http://www.parentdmd.org

The Parent Project for Duchenne Muscular Dystrophy Research is a not-for-profit national health organization dedicated to funding ongoing medical research to find a cure for Duchenne Muscular Dystrophy. Duchenne Muscular Dystrophy is a chronic, progressive, inherited form of muscular dystrophy usually beginning in early childhood; it is characterized by enlargement of muscles, weakness in the pelvis and shoulders, muscular atrophy, and additional symptoms. Established in 1994, the organization has a scientific review board in place to channel funding to those areas currently lacking in research funding. The Parent Project provides current information on Duchenne Muscular Dystrophy and related disorders such as Becker Muscular Dystrophy through brochures and audio-visual materials.

President: Patricia A. Furlong (1994-Present).
Executive Director: Carol D. Henderson (Chairman)
Year Established: 1994
Organization Chapters: 4
Organization Members: 3,000

Publishes the following materials:
Do you remember....childhood memories. ~ *Brochure*

1441 PARENTS OF GALACTOSEMIC CHILDREN, INC. (PGC)

2871 Stage Coach Drive
Valley Springs, CA 95252 209-772-2449
E-mail: gayled3@aol.com or baure@cy-net.net
http://www.galactosemia.org

Parents of Galactosemic Children, Inc. is a non-profit voluntary health organization dedicated to maximizing the potential for the development of individuals with galactosemia, which is a rare genetic metabolic disorder. Galactosemia is characterized by the inability of the body to break down (metabolize) galactose, which is a normal byproduct of lactose (e.g., milk) metabolism. The affected individual is missing the enzyme that converts galactose to glucose. Serious complications can occur including abnormal enlargement of the liver, kidney failure, cataracts, and/or brain damage. The objectives of the organization are to provide support and educational information to families affected by galactosemia and interested health care professionals; facilitate communication between professionals and families with galactosemia; and support professionals in the research of the treatment of galactosemia. Parents of Galactosemic Children, Inc. provides support to parents of affected children; publishes a self-titled periodic newsletter; seeks to stimulate ongoing clinical research; distributes educational materials on galactosemia (e.g., a brochure entitled "Parents of Galactosemic Children"); operates a parent help line; and distributes appropriate dietary information on the disease. Established in 1985 and consisting of 400 members, the organization also operates a web site at [http://www.galactosemia.org].

President: Gayle Dennis (1988 to Present)
Year Established: 1985
Organization Members: 1,200

Publishes the following materials:
Parents of Galactosemic Children, Inc. ~ *Brochure*
Parents of Galactosemic Children, Inc. (Fall 1996) ~ *Newsletter*

Concerned with the following diseases or disorders:
Galactosemia

1442 PARKINSON'S DISEASE FOUNDATION, INC. (PDF)

710 West 168th Street
New York, NY 10032 212-923-4700
800-457-6676
Fax: 212-923-4778
E-mail: pdfepmc@aol.com
http://www.parkinsons-foundation.@org

Parkinson's Disease Foundation, Inc. is a national not-for-profit organization dedicated to funding medical research to investigate the cause and cure of Parkinson's Disease and related disorders. Established in 1957, the Foundation has a post-doctoral training program, offers extramural research grants, and makes referrals to physicians who treat Parkinson's Disease. The Foundation strives to provide individuals with Parkinson's Disease a better quality of life and, ultimately, find the cause and a cure. Other activities of the organization include counseling, supporting advocacy efforts, and providing referrals to self-help groups. In addition, the Foundation has a Research Advisory Board composed of internationally known neurological scientists. The Parkinson's Disease Foundation conducts symposia and distributes a variety of educational materials including brochures, booklets, a manual for health care professionals, and a regular newsletter.

President: Lewis P. Rowland, M.D.
Executive Director: Robin Elliott
Year Established: 1957
Organization Members: 91,000

Publishes the following materials:
Parkinson's Disease Foundation ~ *Annual Report*
Exercises for the Parkinson Patient with Hints for Daily Living ~ *Pamphlet*
Progress, Promise and Hope! ~ *Pamphlet*
The Parkinson Patient at Home ~ *Pamphlet*
Parkison's Disease Foundation ~ *Brochure*
Parkinson's Disease Foundation Newsletter ~ *Newsletter*

Concerned with the following diseases or disorders:
Parkinson's Disease

1443 PEDIATRIC/ADOLESCENT GASTROESOPHAGEAL REFLUX ASSOCIATION, INC. (PAGER)

P.O. Box 1153
Germantown, MD 20875-1153 301-601-9541
E-mail: gergroup@aol.com
http://www.reflux.org

The Pediatric/Adolescent Gastroesophageal Reflux Association, Inc. (PAGER) is a non-profit, parent-led organization dedicated to offering support and information to parents of children with gastroesophageal reflux and related disorders. Gastroesophageal reflux is the inappropriate backward flow of stomach contents into the esophagus. A diagnosis of gastroesophageal reflux (GER) is given only when the "backwashing" is causing problems. A child is said to have Gastroesophageal Reflux Disease (GERD) if the backwashing has caused damage, such as failure to gain weight; respiratory symptoms including asthma, choking, and repeated infections due to aspiration; and/or esophageal irritation and scarring. Founded in 1992, PAGER disseminates information on pediatric gastroesophageal reflux and related disorders; provides support and education to individuals and families affected by GER; and promotes public awareness of the condition. Consisting of 300 members, PAGER publishes a monthly newsletter containing stories from families, research updates, practical ideas for affected individuals and families, and a list of new members. Also available is medical literature on GER and related disorders with descriptions of tests, procedures, medications, and parent-tested home care techniques. Program activities include monthly support and information meetings.

President: Beth Anderson (1992 to Present) (Founder).
Year Established: 1992
Organization Chapters: 1
Organization Members: 300

Publishes the following materials:
What is the Pediatric/Adolescent Gastroesophageal Reflux Association? ~ *Brochure*
Pediatric/Adolescent Gastroesophageal Reflux Association, Inc. (PAGER) ~ *Newsletter*

Concerned with the following diseases or disorders:
Gastroesophageal Reflux

1444 PERIODIC PARALYSES RESOURCE CENTER

E-mail: paragon@pe.net
http://www.pe.net/~paragon/PPMSD.html

The Periodic Paralyses Resource Center is a Web site on the Internet dedicated to providing information, assistance, and support to individuals with disorders characterized by loss of motion or sensation at irregular intervals (periodic paralysis). Such disorders include Hyperkalemic Periodic Paralysis, Hypokalemic Periodic Paralysis, Normokalemic Periodic Paralysis, Anderson Cardiodysrhythmic Periodic Paralysis, Thyrotoxic Periodic Paralysis, various myotonias and myopathies, and periodic paralyses related to sleep disorders. The Periodic Paralyses Resource Center site is also committed to providing information and assistance to family members of affected individuals, physicians, other health care professionals, and researchers. The site provides patient information on periodic paralysis disorders; links to online discussion groups on specific disorders for affected individuals, family members, and/or health care professionals; an online newsletter; notes on research; information concerning diagnosis; information on certain medications and pharmacology; and dynamic links to other helpful resources on the Internet in categories such as cell biology and anatomy, important sites and associations, periodic paralyses sources, researchers, references and bibliographies, sleep disorder sources, and more. The site also provides a preliminary summary of a periodic paralysis survey to provide information that may be helpful for potential research subjects and to gather information that may assist affected individuals and those assisting them with the control and management of periodic paralysis. The Periodic Paralyses Resource Center also includes a case study section that will present stories, in the patients' own words, describing the natural history of their disease, their search for diagnosis, treatment, etc.

1445 PHENYLALANINE HYDROXYLASE LOCUS DATABASE (PAHDB) HOME PAGE

E-mail: pahdb@www.debelle.mcgill.ca
http://www.mcgill.ca/pahdb/

The objectives of the Phenylalanine Hydroxylase Locus Database (PAHdb) web site are twofold. First, the site provides affected individuals, family members, health care professionals, and others with understandable information concerning phenylketonuria (PKU), an inborn error of metabolism characterized by progressive severe mental retardation, episodes of uncontrolled electrical disturbances of the brain (seizures), and/or other abnormalities that may be prevented through early restriction of dietary phenylalanine. The site posts the indepth booklet entitled the "Montreal Children's Hospital's Hyperphenylalaninemia Resource Booklet for Families" and offers dynamic linkage to additional sources of information and support. The web site is also dedicated to providing researchers, physicians, and other interested individuals with access to current information concerning mutations of the phenylalanine hydroxylase (PAH) gene. The majority of such mutations result in deficient activity of the liver enzyme phenylalanine hydroxylase and abnormal accumulation and excretion of dietary phenylalanine (hyperphenylalaninemia). The most severe manifestation may be PKU, while, in other cases, affected individuals may have benign conditions that cause few or no apparent symptoms. PAH mutation data within the database is collated from both published articles as well as communications from approximately 90 investigators across the world who are members of the PAH Mutation Analysis Consortium. The database provides online users several searchable fields including mutation name, population, geographic location, gene region, mutation type, phenotype, author's name, etc. The complete information provided for each mutation is regularly updated from both published data and personal communications from consortium members.

Concerned with the following diseases or disorders:
Phenylketonuria

1446 PHOENIX SOCIETY FOR BURN SURVIVIORS, INC.

11 Rust Hill Road
Levittown, PA 19056-2311 215-946-2876
800-888-2876
Fax: 215-946-4788
E-mail: info@burns-phoenix-society.org
http://www.burns-phoenix-society.org

The Phoenix Society for Burn Survivors, Inc. is an international non-profit self-help organization dedicated to helping burn survivors and their families return to happy and productive lives following injury. The Society's major goal is to ease the psychosocial adjustment of severely burned individuals during and after hospitalization so they may resume full and productive lives within their communities. This is achieved through a series of support programs including peer counseling, family group meetings, and re-entry programs. The Phoenix Society works mainly through volunteer Area Coordinators who are burn survivors themselves or parents of burned children. They provide peer support and counseling to affected individuals and their families under the guidance and approval of medical professionals. Established in 1977 and consisting of 350 chapters, the Society publishes a quarterly newsletter entitled "The Icarus File" which contains information about Society activities and developments in the field of burns (treatment, prevention, etc.). Other program activities include a pen pal program and "Operation Magic Carpet," in which the Society arranges to bring survivors of severe burns from third world countries for reconstructive surgery at no charge. The Society arranges transportation, housing, interpreters, and other needs. The Society also works with the American Red Cross in providing counseling and other support services in the event of burn disaster and provides referrals for paramedical cosmetologists, manufacturers of artificial devices (prosthetics), and specialized legal assistance. The organization offers verbal and written support for individuals who speak Spanish.

President: George Pessotti (1995 to Present)
Executive Director: Alan J. Breslau
Organization Language: Spanish (written/spoken).
Year Established: 1977
Organization Chapters: 350
Organization Members: 9,500

Publishes the following materials:
The Phoenix Society For Burn Survivors, Inc. ~ *Brochure*
Burn Scars ~ *Brochure*
Hidden Burns ~ *Brochure*
Humor and the Burn Patient ~ *Brochure*
Itching. What Helps? ~ *Brochure*
How We Select Our Volunteers ~ *Brochure*
The Icarus File ~ *Newsletter*

1447 POLIO CONNECTION OF AMERICA

P.O. Box 182
Howards Beach, NY 11414 718-835-5536
Fax: 718-738-1946

Polio Connection of America, also known as the New York Post-Polio Support Group, is a voluntary not-for-profit organization dedicated to locating polio survivors and providing them with information concerning Post-Polio Syndrome. The syndrome, which is characterized by gradual deterioration of muscle function, can occur from 10 to more than 30 years after the onset of polio. Established in 1980, the organization is committed to locating, informing, and supporting polio survivors affected with Post-Polio Syndrome to help them receive appropriate treatment. Polio Connection of America provides appropriate referrals as well as a variety of educational materials including a regular newsletter, brochures, and booklets.

President: Eleanor Berk
Executive Director: Walter Berk
Year Established: 1980
Organization Chapters: 2150
Organization Members: 40,000

1448 POLIO SOCIETY

4200 Wisconsin Avenue
Suite 106273
Washington, DC 20016 301-897-8180
Fax: 202-466-1911

The Polio Society is a national not-for-profit voluntary organization that was established in 1984. The Society was created to provide educational resources and support group services to people who had polio and are now experiencing the late effects of polio. Governed by a Board of Directors composed primarily of polio survivors and their family members, the Society's programs and services are funded by membership dues, gifts, and private contributions. Activities of the organization include the maintenance of a national membership database of polio survivors and health care professionals; sponsorship of major national UPDATE conferences about post-polio issues; and the publication of "OPTIONS," a quarterly newsletter that contains information on current medical research, available resources, support activities, and first-hand accounts from the polio community. In addition, the Society provides state-of-the-art medical and psychosocial information about the late effects of polio, including audio and video tapes of conference presentations, current scientific and lay articles, and polio-related publications. The organization also promotes public awareness of the late effects of polio through poster campaigns, local and national newspapers, radio, and network television.

President: Ed Grebenstein
Executive Director: Jessica Scheer, Ph.D
Year Established: 1984

Concerned with the following diseases or disorders:
Post Polio Syndrome

1449 POLYCYSTIC OVARIAN SYNDROME ASSOCIATION (PCO SUPPORT)

PO Box 360878
Strongsville, OH 44136 216-846-0895
E-mail: info@pcosupport.org
http://www.pcosupport.org

The Polycystic Ovarian Syndrome Association is a voluntary organization dedicated to promoting research, understanding, and communicating the most up-to-date information concerning polycystic ovarian syndrome (PCOS) among its membership body. PCOS is a disorder characterized by the absence of menstruation or irregular and abnormal menstruation, excessive amounts of body hair, excessive body weight, and infertility. Established in 1997, the Polycystic Ovarian Syndrome Association seeks to fulfill the following objectives: to provide a central resource of information for women with PCOS; to support research on medical and/or surgical protocols to further understand the cause of PCOS and treat its associated symptoms; to promote awareness of PCOS to the public; to educate physicians and other healthcare professionals to recognize and more fully understand PCOS and the nature of its treatment; to provide a social support network for women with PCOS and their families; to bring about an understanding of the short term and long term complications of PCOS; and to encourage approval by government health organizations of drugs and procedures that have been identified as being beneficial to women with PCOS. Consisting of 88 members, the Association produces educational materials including a periodic newsletter, brochures, a directory, and a database. Program activities include a support group, patient advocacy programs, networking, research and educational programs, and appropriate referrals. The Polycystic Ovarian Syndrome Association can be reached at its web site on the Internet at [http://www.pcosupport.org].

Executive Director: Christine Gray (Acting Director & Contact Person)
Year Established: 1997
Organization Members: 88

1450 POSTPARTUM SUPPORT INTERNATIONAL (PSI)

927 North Kellogg Avenue
Santa Barbara, CA 93111 805-967-7636
Fax: 805-967-0608
E-mail: thonikman@compuserve.com
http://www.iup.edu/an/postpartum/

Postpartum Support International (PSI) is a not-for-profit voluntary organization dedicated to increasing awareness among public and professional communities about the emotional changes women often experience during pregnancy and after the birth of a baby. Established in 1987, PSI is an international network that focuses on postpartum mental health and social support. PSI's objectives are to provide current information to members on the diagnosis and treatment of postpartum mood and anxiety disorders; to advocate research into the cause (etiology), diagnosis, and treatment of postpartum mood and anxiety disorders; to provide education about mental health issues of childbearing; to address legal and insurance coverage issues; to encourage collaboration with related organizations, to encourage health care professional participation in PSI; to encourage the formation of new groups; and to sponsor an annual PSI conference to review progress on achieving these objectives. Consisting of 300 members, PSI produces educational materials including a self-titled brochure, audio visual aids, and a regular newsletter. Program activities include a support group, patient advocacy, networking, education, and referrals. PSI also maintains a web site on the Internet at [http://www.iup.edu/an/postpartum/].

President: Ann Dunnewold, Ph.D. (1996 to Present)
Executive Director: Jane Honikman, M.S.
Organization Language: Spanish (written).
Year Established: 1987
Organization Members: 300

Publishes the following materials:
Postpartum Support International ~ *Brochure*
PSI. Member Organizations' Resources and Other Publications ~ *Bibliography*

1451 PRADER-WILLI CONNECTION

40 Holly Lane
Roslyn Heights, NY 11577 516-621-2445
800-358-0682
Fax: 516-484-7154
E-mail: info@pwsyndrome.com
http://www.pwsyndrome.com

The Prader-Willi Connection is a for-profit organization founded in 1933. With more than 6,000 members, it is the largest Prader-Willi membership organization in the world. There is no charge for membership. Participants receive newsletters, brochures, and access to a 24-hour fax hot-line and the Information Forum on the Internet. Educational materials include a newsletter entitled "Prader-Willi Perspectives" and brochures entitled "Children with P.W.S. - Information for School Staff" and "Physical Therapy Intervention."

President: Sheldon L. Tarakan
Executive Director: Jacqueline Kelly
Year Established: 1993
Organization Members: 6,600

Concerned with the following diseases or disorders:
Prader Willi Syndrome

1452 PRADER-WILLI FOUNDATION, INC.

223 Main Street
Port Washington, NY 11050 516-944-8136
800-253-7993
Fax: 516-944-3173
E-mail: foundation@prader-willi.inter.net
http://www.prader-willi.org

The Prader-Willi Foundation, Inc., is a national, not-for-profit public charity that, under the direction of a national Board of Directors made up of parents and professionals in many fields, carries out its mission of funding projects for the betterment of individuals with Prader-Willi Syndrome (PWS) and their families. Prader Willi Syndrome is a complex multisystem disorder characterized by muscular weakness during infancy (infantile hypotonia); failure to thrive; a decrease in the efficiency of the testes or ovaries (hypogonadism); short stature and impaired intellectual and behavioral functioning. Eating excessive amounts of food (hyperphagia) leads to severe obesity in early childhood and adolescence. According to its Bylaws, the major purposes of The Foundation are the publication and dissemination of information in printed and electronic media; the provision of information and referral, advocacy, and support services to individuals with PWS and their families; the support of residential living programs and projects; the financial support of organizations, from national organizations to local support groups, dedicated to serving individuals with PWS and their families; the direct support of crisis intervention services for individuals with PWS and their families; as well as other services, programs and activities approved by the Board of Directors that will result in an enhanced quality of life for individuals with Prader-Willi syndrome. In addition, the Foundationsupports state and regional Prader-Willi organizations throughout the nation by awarding conference grants; provides funding for families with financial need to attend national Prader-Willi conferences; provides families with partial "camperships" to help send their children to summer camp; sponsors research in many areas of concern. Currently, the Foundation is sponsoring a year-long project at the University of California at Los Angeles. The Prader-Willi Foundation also provides appropriate referrals, promotes education of professionals and the general public, and offers a variety of educational materials, including a regular newsletter and brochures.

President: Sheldon L. Tarakan (1993-Present)
Executive Director: Sheldon L. Tarakan
Year Established: 1993

1453 PRADER-WILLI SYNDROME ASSOCIATION (PWSA (UK))

2 Wheatsheaf Close
Horsell
Woking
Surrey, GU21 4BP
England 014-837-24784

The Prader Willi Syndrome Association (PWSA) is a voluntary organization located in the United Kingdom and dedicated to promoting the care, welfare, treatment, interests, education, and advancement of persons affected by Prader Willi Syndrome. These goals are achieved by contacting and supporting families concerned with the disorder; raising funds; inviting and receiving contributions by way of subscriptions and donations; establishing mutual self-help groups; and fostering and supporting ongoing research. Prader Willi Syndrome is a complex multisystem disorder characterized by muscular weakness during infancy (infantile hypotonia); failure to thrive; a decrease in the efficiency of the testes or ovaries (hypogonadism); short stature and impaired intellectual and behavioral functioning. Eating excessive amounts of food (hyperphagia) leads to severe obesity in early childhood and adolescence. Established in 1981, PWSA consists of 500 members and six chapters. The Association produces various educational materials including a periodic newsletter and brochures. In addition, the Association, conducts regular support group meetings and supports ongoing patient advocacy.

President: John Booth (Chairman) (1955 to Present)
Executive Director: Rosemary Johnson (Contact Person)
Organization Language: French (written). Spanish (written). Dutch (written).
Year Established: 1981
Organization Chapters: 6
Organization Members: 800

Publishes the following materials:
Prader-Willi Syndrome - What is It? ~ *Brochure*
PWSA (UK) Book Order Form ~ *Order Form*
Constitution of The Prader-Willi Syndrome Association (UK) ~ *Constitution*
Prader-Willi News ~ *Newsletter*
Prader-Willi Syndrome Association (UK). Services and Information ~ *Leaflet*

Concerned with the following diseases or disorders:
Prader Willi Syndrome

1454 PRADER-WILLI SYNDROME ASSOCIATION, NATIONAL HEADQUARTERS (PWSA)

5700 Midnight Pass Road
Suite 6
Sarasota, FL 34242 941-312-0400
800-926-4797
Fax: 941-312-0142
E-mail: PWSAUSA@aol.com
http://www.athenet.net/~pwsa_usa/index.html

The Prader-Willi Syndrome Association (USA) is a non-profit voluntary health organization. Founded in 1975, the Association provides parents and healthcare professionals with a national and international network of information, support sevices, and research endeavors to expressly meet the needs of children and adults with Prader-Willi Syndrome and their families. The organization comprises parents, professionals and other interested individuals who are taking active roles in improving the lives of people with Prader-Willi Syndrome. Goals include normalizing life for people with Prader-Willi Syndrome and their families, improving communication and education, and acting as a lifetime advocate for affected individuals. The Association also supports research, interdisciplinary communication, and increased professional knowledge of treatments. Educational materials include various brochures and pamphets.

President: Jerry Park
Executive Director: Janalee Heinemann
Organization Language: Spanish. French.
Year Established: 1975
Organization Chapters: 42
Organization Members: 1,600

Publishes the following materials:
Prader-Willi Syndrome Management ~ *Brochure*
Prader-Willi Syndrome Assocation U.S.A. ~ *Brochure*
My Child Has Prader-Willi Syndrome? Now What? ~ *Brochure*
The Gathered View ~ *Newsletter*
Publications of the Prader-Willi Syndrome Assocation (USA) ~ *Factsheet*
Prader-Willi Syndrome Association (USA) Membership Application ~ *Application*

Concerned with the following diseases or disorders:
Prader Willi Syndrome

1455 PREGNANCY AND INFANT LOSS CENTER (PILC)

1421 East Wayzata Boulevard
#30
Wayzata, MN 55391 612-473-9372
Fax: 612-473-8978

The Pregnancy and Infant Loss Center, a national not-for-profit service organization, was established in 1983 by parents and professionals to serve the unique needs of bereaved families and their care providers. The Center is dedicated to providing information, referrals, comfort, understanding, and resources to individuals and families who have experienced the death of an infant; encouraging and promoting healthy grieving as affected families work towards healing; helping individuals and families utilize their own support networks to the fullest; and providing information, education, and consultation services to professional caregivers and the general public in order to increase sensitivity, understanding, and awareness of miscarriage, stillbirth, and infant death. The Pregnancy and Infant Loss Center provides referrals to appropriate national and local support groups, other bereaved parents, counselors, and nationwide resources; offers educational programs for parents and professional care providers; and has volunteer opportunities that may aid in the healing process, offer individuals a chance to reach out to others, and provide educational experiences. The Center offers a variety of materials for affected parents, young siblings, and other family members as well as health care providers including booklets, handbooks, and brochures; special items; videos; and a quarterly newsletter entitled "Loving Arms."

Executive Director: Charlene Nelson (Director).
Organization Language: Spanish (written).
Year Established: 1983
Organization Members: 1,000

Publishes the following materials:
Pregnancy And Infant Loss Center ~ *Brochure*
Loving Arms ~ *Newsletter*
Resources Available Through the Pregnancy and Infant Loss Center ~ *Resource List*

1456 PRIMARY BILIARY CIRRHOSIS PATIENT SUPPORT NETWORK

R. R. 5, Highway 43
Perth
Ontario, K7H 3C7
Canada 613-267-2517
Fax: 613-267-2084
E-mail: pbc@superaje.com

The Primary Biliary Cirrhosis Patient Support Network is a not-for-profit organization established in 1981 to serve the needs of people with Primary Biliary Cirrhosis and their families. The purpose of the organization is to provide information, emotional support, and encouragement to families affected by Primary Biliary Cirrhosis. In addition, the organization seeks to educate medical professionals and the general public about liver disease, transplantation, and organ donation. Members of the Network form strong friendships and organizational meetings provide an environment of non-critical mutual support assistance. An important aspect of this group is confidentiality and anonymity. The Support Network publishes a newsletter, fact sheet, a pamphlet on Primary Biliary Cirrhosis, and a potential member informational letter.

President: Kathlene or Rod Dawson
Year Established: 1981
Organization Members: 325

Publishes the following materials:
Primary Biliary Cirrhosis PBC ~ *Brochure*
PBC Patient Support Network Philosophy ~ *Fact Sheet*
Primary Biliary Cirrhosis Patient Support Network ~ *Membership Form and Introducto*
Reprint Articles List ~ *Article List*
PBC Newsletter ~ *Newsletter*

Concerned with the following diseases or disorders:
Cirrhosis, Primary Biliary

1457 PROGRESSIVE OSSEOUS HETEROPLASIA ASSOCIATION (POHA)

33 Stonehearth Square
Indian Head Park, IL 60525 708-246-9410

The Progressive Osseous Heteroplasia Association (POHA) is a non-profit, voluntary organization dedicated to raising funds for research into finding appropriate treatment and a cure for Progressive Osseous Heteroplasia (POH). POH is an extremely rare disorder characterized by the abnormal development of bone in areas of the body where bone is not normally present (heterotopic ossification). The disorder first appears as areas of patchy bone formation (ossification) on the skin during infancy; heterotopic ossification progresses to involve superficial and deep connective tissues, areas of fat beneath the skin (subcutaneous fat), muscles, tendons, ligaments, and the bands of fibrous tissues that support muscle (fascia). In addition to serving as a patient education organization, POHA strives toward an additional goal, to raise sufficient funds to make the medical world more aware of POH. Established in 1995, the Association produces educational materials including a handbook entitled "What is POH? A Guidebook for Families," reprints of scientific and medical journal articles about POH, and a videotape of a 1995 symposium on Fibrodysplasia Ossificans Progressiva (FOP), a similar but distinct rare disorder.

President: Catherine M. Jacobs (1995 to present)
Executive Director: Fred B. Gardner (Treasurer)
Year Established: 1995
Organization Chapters: 1
Organization Members: 5

Publishes the following materials:
The Katelyn Foundation ~ *Brochure*
Observation - Progressive Osseous Heteroplasia ~ *Reprint*
The Ian Foundation ~ *Factsheet*

Concerned with the following diseases or disorders:
Progressive Osseous Heteroplasia (POH)

1458 PROTEUS SYNDROME FOUNDATION

609 South East Mount Vernon Drive
Blue Springs, MO 64014 816-229-9132
E-mail: Abscit@aol.com
http://www.kumc.edu/gec/support/proteus.html

The Proteus Syndrome Foundation is a national voluntary not-for-profit organization dedicated to providing information, assistance, and support to children with Proteus Syndrome and their families. Proteus Syndrome is a rare, extremely variable disorder of unknown cause that may be characterized by partial enlargement of the hands and/or feet; overgrowth of one side of the face, body, and/or arms and legs (hemihypertrophy); and/or an abnormally large head (macrocephaly) or asymmetry of the skull. Additional features include the development of benign fat cell tumors (lipomas) primarily beneath the skin (subcutaneous) that may, in some cases, consist of newly formed blood vessels (hemangiomas) and/or elements of the lymphatic system (lymphangiomas); distinctive birth marks (nevus) on the skin that may be raised and have a rough texture; deep lines and overgrowth of soft tissue on the soles of the feet; and/or other abnormalities. Established in 1995, the Proteus Syndrome Foundation is committed to providing networking opportunities for affected individuals and family members; compiling a family directory; and creating a database of affected families around the world to help physicians and families obtain as much information as possible before making choices concerning surgeries and therapies. The Foundation also works closely with researchers to promote clinical studies into Proteus Syndrome; communicates ongoing research efforts to affected families; provides referrals; engages in patient and professional education; and offers a variety of materials including brochures, pamphlets, and a regular newsletter entitled "The Proteus Foundation Newsletter." The Foundation also has a web site on the Internet at [http://www.kumc.edu/gec/support/proteus.html].

President: Kim Hoag (1995 to Present)
Executive Director: Barbara King
Organization Language: Spanish (written).
Year Established: 1995
Organization Chapters: 1
Organization Members: 50

Publishes the following materials:
What you need to know about Proteus Syndrome ~ *Brochure*
The Proteus Foundation Newsletter ~ *Newsletter Spring 1997*

Concerned with the following diseases or disorders:
Proteus Syndrome

1459 PSEUDOTUMOR CEREBRI SOCIETY (PTC SOCIETY)

1319 Butternut St.
Apt. 3
Syracuse, NY 13208 315-464-3937
Fax: 315-464-6663
E-mail: mtanay@aol.com

The Pseudotumor Cerebri Society (PCS) is a national, voluntary not-for-profit organization dedicated to bringing together individuals with pseudotumor cerebri (PTC) in order for them to share common experiences and other information. Pseudotumor cerebri is a condition characterized by increased pressure inside the skull, swelling of the optic disc, headaches, nausea, vomiting, and/or paralysis (palsy) of the sixth cranial nerve. Established in 1992, the Pseudotumor Cerebri Society provides information to affected individuals, family members, and health care professionals concerning pseudotumor cerebri, treatments, research advances, and ways to a better life for affected individuals. The Society conducts monthly meetings for members; provides a pen pal service; engages in patient advocacy; offers appropriate referrals; and provides assistance to those interested in starting support groups. The Pseudotumor Cerebri Society also offers a variety of educational and support materials including a regular newsletter and brochures.

President: Marina Tanay (1996 - Present).
Executive Director: Deborah Friedman, M.D.
Year Established: 1992

Concerned with the following diseases or disorders:
Pseudotumor Cerebri

1460 PSEUDOTUMOR CEREBRI SUPPORT NETWORK (PTC SUPPORT NETWORK)

6632 Kennington Square South
Pickerington, OH 43147 614-837-4301
Fax: 614-837-5913

The Pseudotumor Cerebri (PTC) Support Network is a national non-profit support organization dedicated to supporting research, treatment, and medical care of individuals who are diagnosed with pseudotumor cerebri. Pseudotumor cerebri is a syndrome of increased pressure inside the skull. It is most often seen in obese females between the ages of 20 and 50 years. Symptoms can mimic those of a brain tumor; however, no tumor is involved. Symptoms of pseudotumor cerebri include headache of varying degrees of severity (often mild), typically unrelieved by medication. A swelling of the optic disc (papilledema) with progressive visual loss occurs in a small percentage of the patients. Established in 1992, the PCT Network publishes a periodic newsletter to help keep individuals with pseudotumor cerebri informed of current treatments and ongoing research. In addition to putting individuals in touch with one another, the Network also has a volunteer support system composed of individuals diagnosed with Pseudotumor Cerebri who provide information and support by telephone on a regional basis. A spring 1997 gathering is planned for "People Living with Pseudotumor Cerebri."

President: Jennifer Duncan (Indefinite).
Year Established: 1992

Publishes the following materials:
Pseudotumor Cerebri Support Network (Summer/Fall 1996) ~ *Newsletter*
Pseudotumor Cerebri Support Network (Spring/Summer 1997) ~ *Newsletter*

1461 PSORIATIC ARTHROPATHY ALLIANCE (PAA)

P.O. Box 111
St. Albans
Hertfordshire, AL2 3JQ
United Kingdom 192-367-2837
Fax: 192-367-2837
E-mail: davidc@paalliance.org
http://www.paalliance.org

The Psoriatic Arthropathic Alliance (PAA) is a non-profit support and informational organization for individuals affected by psoriatic arthropathy (PA) and other related conditions. Psoriatic arthropathy is a rheumatoid-like arthritic condition that is associated with psoriasis of the skin or nails, and a negative rheumatoid arthritis (RA) serology laboratory test. The disorder is more common in females than males. The mission of the PAA is to provide support and information to individuals affected by PA. Established in 1993, the Alliance also monitors medical and health care services and supports research into the causes, prevention, and management of PA and related conditions. In addition, the group acts as a lobbyist for patient rights. Consisting of 1,000 members, the Alliance produces educational materials that are available to medical professionals, medical students, and the general public. PAA publishes a periodic newsletter and a journal and offers a networking service.

President: Julie and David Chandler
Year Established: 1993
Organization Members: 1,000

Publishes the following materials:
Healthy Skin for Every Body ~ *Brochure*
Psoriatic Arthropathy - When to Treat ~ *Factsheet*
Psoratic Arthropathy - Did You Know? ~ *Factsheet*
Psoriatic Arthropathy - The Feet ~ *Factsheet*
Psoriatic Arthropathy Allliance Newsletter ~ *Newsletter*
Skin & Bones Connection ~ *News Journal*
PAA ~ *Brochure*
Psoriatic Arthritis ~ *Brochure*
What is Psoriatic Arthritis? ~ *Brochure*
PAA Journal ~ *Booklet*
PAA Newsletter ~ *Newsletter*

Concerned with the following diseases or disorders:
Arthritis, Psoriatic; Psoriasis

1462 PULMONARY HYPERTENSION ASSOCIATION (PHA)

P.O. Box 24733
Speedway, IN 46224-0733 215-591-9016
800-748-7274
Fax: 215-542-5692
E-mail: 76330.751@compuserve.com
http://www.phassociation.org

The Pulmonary Hypertension Association (PHA) is a national not-for-profit voluntary organization that provides educational information and fellowship to people with Primary or Secondary Pulmonary Hypertension. Pulmonary Hypertension is a condition characterized by abnormally high blood pressure in the arteries that supply the lungs. Pulmonary

Hypertension may be an isolated condition that may occur for unknown reasons (Primary Pulmonary Hypertension) or may occur due to or in association with other underlying disorders or conditions (Secondary Pulmonary Hypertension). Established in 1992, the organization addresses issues pertinent to people with these disorders such as current research, early detection, orphan drug designations, organ donor awareness, and organ transplantation. The Association's activities include conducting international conferences on Pulmonary Hypertension; providing a networking service to help affected individuals contact one another by phone or through the mail; offering referrals; and publishing a quarterly newsletter entitled "Pathlight." The Pulmonary Hypertension Association also offers additional educational and support materials including fact sheets, booklets, and pamphlets.

President: Bonnie Dukart (1996 - Present)
Year Established: 1992
Organization Chapters: 20
Organization Members: 1,200

Publishes the following materials:
Hearts and Hands ~ *Brochure*
United Patients' Association for Pulmonary Hypertension, Inc. ~ *Information Sheet*
Primary Pulmonary Hypertension ~ *Brochure*
UPAPH Scientific Advisory Board ~ *Board List*
General Information about PPH Family Registry ~ *Fact Sheet*
Physicians Experienced with Treating PPH Patients ~ *Address List*
Pathlight ~ *Newsletter*

Concerned with the following diseases or disorders:
Pulmonary Hypertension, Primary; Pulmonary Hypertension, Secondary

1463 RSDHOPE GROUP (RSDHOPE GROUP)

P.O. Box 875
Harrison, ME 04040-0875 207-583-4589
E-mail: rsdhope@mail.org
http://www.rsdhope.org

The RSDHope Group is a national not-for-profit organization dedicated to increasing awareness of Reflex Sympathetic Dystrophy Syndrome (RSDS) among affected individuals, their family members, health professionals, and the general public. RSDS is a rare disorder of the sympathetic nervous system that is characterized by chronic, severe pain following a simple trauma, break or fracture, sharp force injury, or surgery. The sympathetic nervous system is that part of the autonomic nervous system which regulates involuntary, bodily functions such as increasing heart rate, constricting blood vessels, and increasing blood pressure. Excessive or abnormal responses of portions of the sympathetic nervous system are thought to be responsible for the pain associated with Reflex Sympathetic Dystrophy Syndrome. The symptoms of RSDS typically begin with burning pain, especially in an arm, finger(s), palm of the hand(s), and/or shoulder(s). In some individuals, RSDS may occur in one or both legs or it may be localized to one knee or hip. Established in 1995, the RSDHope Group consists of 750 members. The organization produces educational materials including a quarterly newsletter, seminars, videotapes, information packets, and computer and postal pen pals.

President: A. Robert Orsini (Chairperson) (1995 to Present)
Executive Director: Keith R. Orsini (Contact Person)
Year Established: 1995
Organization Members: 750

Publishes the following materials:
RSDS Seminar Tape 1 ~ *Video Tape*
RSDS Seminar Tape 2 ~ *Video Tape*
Reflex Sympathetic Dystrophy Syndrome ~ *Video Tape*
RSDHope Group. Maine RSDS Group ~ *Newsletter Summer 1997*
Letter From Bob Orsini, Director (and Dad). Letter From Lynne Orsini. Treasurer (and Mom) ~ *Letter*
Reflex Sympathetic Dystrophy Syndrome (RSDS) ~ *Pamphlet*
Reflex Sympathetic Dystrophy Syndrome. Fact and Fiction ~ *Pamphlet*
RSDHope/Maine RSDS Patient Advovacy Group ~ *Fact Sheet*
Reflex Smypathetic Dystrophy Patient Guide ~ *Reprint*
RSDS Patient's Favorite Line ~ *Fact Sheet*
We Need To Teach Doctors To Care ~ *Reprint*
Neurological Associates. Dr. H. Hooshmand's RSD Puzzles ~ *Leaflet*
RSD Puzzle #1-B ~ *Pamphlet*
RSDS help is available for sufferers ~ *Reprint*
Glossary of Medical Terms ~ *Fact Sheet*

Concerned with the following diseases or disorders:
Reflex Sympathetic Dystrophy Syndrome (RSDS)

1464 RASMUSSEN'S SYNDROME AND HEMISPHERECTOMY SUPPORT NETWORK (RSHSN)

8235 Lethbridge Road
Millersville, MD 21108 410-987-5221
Fax: 410-987-5221
E-mail: rssnlynn@aol.com

The Rasmussen's Syndrome and Hemispherectomy Support Network is a national not-for-profit organization dedicated to providing information and support to individuals affected by Rasmussen's Syndrome (Rasmussen's Encephalitis) and Hemispherectomy. Rasmussen's Syndrome is a rare central nervous system disorder characterized by chronic active inflammation of the brain (encephalitis) and epileptic seizures of varying degrees of severity. Progressive symptoms including paralysis (usually of one side of the body) and mental retardation may also occur. Although the exact cause of this disorder is not known, it is thought to result from an unidentified viral infection. Hemispherectomy is a form of surgery commonly used in the treatment of Rasmussen's Syndrome. Founded in 1994 and comprised of 120 members, RSHSN publishes a periodic newsletter and disseminates reprints of medical journal articles concerning Rasmussen's Syndrome and its treatments. RSHSN also maintains a support network that provides encouragement and information to individuals affected by Rasmussen's Syndrome and their families.

President: Al and Lynn Miller (Founders)
Organization Language: Spanish (written). French (written). Spanish (written). Russian (written).
Year Established: 1994
Organization Chapters: 1
Organization Members: 120

Publishes the following materials:
My Name is Lynn Miller ~ *Information Packet*
Family History and Information ~ *Questionnaire*
Mission Statement ~ *Pamphlet*

Concerned with the following diseases or disorders:
Encephalitis, Rasmussen's

1465 RAYNAUD'S & COLD SUFFERERS NETWORK

94 Mercer Avenue
Hartsdale, NY 10530 914-682-8341
Fax: 914-946-4685
E-mail: Lwunderman@aol.com

Raynaud's and Cold Sufferers Network is a self-help organization dedicated to sharing information and help in coping with daily activities among individuals who are affected by Raynaud's Disease and Phenomenon. Raynaud's Disease is a common vascular disorder characterized by episodes of constriction of very small blood vessels in the fingers. Symptoms may include numbness, tingling, and cold sensations in the fingers. The purpose of the Network is to share information and to provide support in dealing with everyday activities, such as holding a cold glass of soda or shopping in the refrigerated section of a supermarket. Founded in 1992, the Network also works to increase public awareness of Raynaud's Disease and is active in patient recruitment for ongoing clinical trials and eventually funding for research. Consisting of approximately 280 members, the Network produces educational materials including the newsletter "Cold Cuts" and a brochure about the disease. In addition, the Network coordinates a national networking program and holds informal support group meetings in the New York metropolitan area.

President: Lynn Wunderman (1992 to Present) (Founder)
Year Established: 1992
Organization Members: 281

Publishes the following materials:
Raynaud's & Cold Sufferers Network ~ *Brochure*
Cold Cuts ~ *Newsletter*

1466 REACH OUT FOR YOUTH WITH ILEITIS AND COLITIS, INC.

15 Chemung Place
Jericho, NY 11753 516-822-8010
Fax: 516-822-8010
E-mail: spell16@ix.netcom.com

Reach Out for Youth with Ileitis and Colitis, Inc. is a non-profit support organization dedicated to assisting families whose children have Inflammatory Bowel Disease (IBD) such as Ileitis or Colitis. Ulcerative Colitis is an inflammatory disease of the large intestine and is characterized by diarrhea, abdominal pain, fever, and bleeding from the rectum. Decreased appetite and weight loss may also occur. Ileitis or Crohn's Disease, also an inflammatory bowel disorder, can affect any portion of the digestive system and has symptoms that are similar to those of Colitis. Established in 1979 and consisting of approximately 400 members, the organization has helped hundreds of families cope with the effects of IBD. The group's goals include providing educational materials and emotional support to affected individuals and their families and organizing fundraising efforts to promote research into the causes and treatment of IBD. Educational seminars and a quarterly newsletter entitled "Inner Circle" assist members by keeping them informed of current activities. A hotline offers interested individuals the opportunity to communicate on a one-to-one basis, especially when acute symptoms are present. Reach Out also continues to support the IBD clinical database established 13 years ago as a crucial research tool.

President: Richard Spellman (1995 to Present)
Executive Director: Susan Spellman
Year Established: 1979
Organization Chapters: 1
Organization Members: 400

Publishes the following materials:
The Inside Story - Your Child And Inflammatory Bowel Disease ~ *Brochure*
Inner Circle ~ *Newsletter*

Concerned with the following diseases or disorders:
Colitis, Collagenous; Colitis, Ulcerative

1467 RECURRENT RESPIRATORY PAPILLOMATOSIS FOUNDATION (RRP FOUNDATION)

PO Box 6643
Lawrenceville, NJ 08648-0643 609-530-1443
Fax: 609-530-1912
E-mail: wfs@gfdl.gov or mstern@pucc.princeton.edu
http://members.aol.com/rrpf/RRPF.html

The Recurrent Respiratory Papillomatosis Foundation is a national not-for-profit voluntary organization created to provide support and information to people with Recurrent Respiratory Papillomatosis and their families. Established in 1992, the Foundation seeks to serve as an information resource for affected individuals and their physicians, to promote public awareness, and to aid in the prevention, cure, and treatment of Recurrent Respiratory Papillomatosis. In addition, the Foundation endeavors to educate the medical community about Recurrent Papillomatosis, to facilitate early diagnosis of the disease, and to implement risk reduction measures. The nucleus of the network is the RRP Newsletter. It includes support network information, statistics, individual case histories, treatment developments, and additional information that furthers understanding and awareness of Recurrent Respiratory Papillomatosis.

President: Marlene Stern (1994-Present)
Executive Director: William Stern
Organization Language: Spanish.
Year Established: 1992
Organization Members: 400

Publishes the following materials:
Recurrent Respiratory Papillomatosis Foundation Description and Mission ~ *Factsheet*
Recurrent Respiratory Papillomatosis Newsletter ~ *Newsletter*

Concerned with the following diseases or disorders:
Recurrent Respiratory Papillomatosis

1468 REFLEX SYMPATHETIC DYSTROPHY NETWORK

E-mail: info@rsdnet.org
http://www.rsdnet.org

The Reflex Sympathetic Dystrophy Network is a web site on the Internet dedicated to providing information, support, resources, and online networking opportunities to individuals with Reflex Sympathetic Dystrophy (RSD). RSD is a rare disorder or group of disorders of the sympathetic nervous system characterized by chronic, severe pain and related sensory abnormalities, abnormal blood flow, sweating, and other symptoms following bone fracture, muscle sprain, or injury to blood vessels or nerves. The RSD Network site provides information concerning current research on RSD; a Frequently Asked Questions (FAQ) and answers area that provides understandable information on the disorder; and current medical journal references and abstracts on RSD. The site also offers a listing of suggested readings on the disorder; dynamic linkage to additional sources of information on the Internet; and the "RSDNet-L," an online discussion list (ListServ) for people with RSD, individuals who care about someone with the disorder, and health care professionals who treat those with RSD. The ListServ also offers current subscribers archives of past mailing list correspondence. (Those interested in joining the online discussion list may locate simple instructions within the RSD Network's web site.)

President: Karen Strauss (Executive Director)

Concerned with the following diseases or disorders:
Reflex Sympathetic Dystrophy Syndrome (RSDS)

1469 REFLEX SYMPATHETIC DYSTROPHY SYNDROME ASSOCIATION OF AMERICA (RSDSA)

116 Haddon Avenue
Suite D
Haddonfield, NJ 08033 609-795-8845
Fax: 609-795-8845
http://www.cyboard.com/rsds

The Reflex Sympathetic Dystrophy Syndrome Association of America (RSDSA) is a not-for-profit organization founded to promote and support research into the causes and cure of Reflex Sympathetic Dystrophy Syndrome (RSDS). The Association's mission also includes the establishment of a national data bank for coordination of research and treatment information; establishment and organization of support groups for affected individuals and their families; and promotion of awareness of Reflex Sympathetic Dystrophy Syndrome among health care professionals and the general public. Founded in 1984, the Association provides a referral service to physicians, offers a pen pal service, and promotes patient advocacy. The Reflex Sympathetic Dystrophy Syndrome Association offers a variety of educational materials and services including an information packet, a quarterly newsletter, a statistical report on Reflex Sympathetic Dystrophy Syndrome derived from member questionnaires, reference articles, brochures, booklets, and videos. The Association also provides several special services to health care professionals, including an annual professional membership directory, an annual digest of current articles on Reflex Sympathetic Dystrophy Syndrome, and educational in-service conferences.

President: Francis J. Davis
Executive Director: Rosalyn Davis
Year Established: 1984
Organization Members: 4,000

Publishes the following materials:
Help Us Stop the Pain ~ *Booklet*
RSDS. The Pain that Doesn't Stop. ~ *Brochure*
RSDSA Review ~ *Newsletter*

Concerned with the following diseases or disorders:
Reflex Sympathetic Dystrophy Syndrome (RSDS)

1470 RESEARCH FOR RETT FOUNDATION (RRF)

P.O. Box 50347
Mobile, AL 36605 334-479-8293
800-422-7388
Fax: 334-479-8293

Research for Rett Foundation is a national not-for-profit voluntary organization dedicated to raising funds for critical ongoing medical research into Rett Syndrome, hosting medical research symposia, and funding grant applications. The Foundation is also committed to expanding public awareness of and encouraging Rett Syndrome research within the National Institute of Child Health and Human Development. Rett Syndrome, a rare congenital neurological disorder that affects only females, is characterized by progressive degeneration of certain tissues of the brain, resulting in loss of previously acquired mental and motor skills, impaired control of voluntary movements (ataxia), episodes of uncontrolled electrical disturbances of the brain (seizures), autistic behavior, and/or other abnormalities and physical features. The Foundation provides a variety of educational materials including brochures and fact sheets.

President: Patty Cofer
Executive Director: Anna Luce
Year Established: 1988

Publishes the following materials:
Rett Syndrome - What Is It? ~ *Videotape*
Battling Rett Syndrome ~ *Article*
Connections ~ *Article*
RETT Girls ~ *Article*
Rett Syndrome: One Mothers Story ~ *Article*
Rett Syndrome - What is it? Know the Facts. ~ *Brochure*
Fact Sheet - The Research for Rett Foundation, Inc. ~ *Fact Sheet*
Rett Syndrome - Alan K Percy ~ *Reprint*

Concerned with the following diseases or disorders:
Rett Syndrome

1471 RESTLESS LEGS SYNDROME FOUNDATION, INC. (RLFS)

4410 19th Street NW
Rochester, MN 55901-6624 507-287-6465
Fax: 507-287-6312
E-mail: rlsf@millcomm.com
http://www.rls.org

The Restless Legs Syndrome Foundation is a national nonprofit organization dedicated to providing educational materials on Restless Legs Syndrome and related sleep disorders to people affected by these disorders, physicians, and other health care professionals. The goals of the Foundation include the development, production, and distribution of medically approved materials for educational purposes and the expansion of awareness of Restless Legs Syndrome by using mass media to inform the general public about this disorder. In addition, the Foundation provides networking services for people with Restless Legs Syndrome, their families, and health professionals within their communities to share information, assistance, and support. In addition, the Restless Legs Syndrome Foundation supports medical research studies and encourages medical and nursing schools to include Restless Legs Syndrome in their curricula. The Foundation produces educational materials including brochures, bulletins, a mission or vision statement, and newsletters.

President: Sheila Connolly (Chair)
Year Established: 1993
Organization Chapters: 96
Organization Members: 5,100

Publishes the following materials:
The Restless Legs Syndrome Foundation, Inc. Mission Statement ~ *Pamphlet*
History of RLS Foundation and Previous Accomplishments ~ *Factsheet*
You Are Not Alone ~ *Brochure*
The Night Walkers Newsletter ~ *Newsletter*
RLS Information Bulletin ~ *Bulletin*

Concerned with the following diseases or disorders:
Restless Legs Syndrome

1472 RETINITIS PIGMENTOSA INTERNATIONAL (RPI)

23241 Ventura Blvd. #117
Woodland Hills, CA 91364 818-992-0500
800-344-4877
Fax: 818-992-3265

Retinitis Pigmentosa International (RPI) is a not-for-profit organization dedicated to promoting and supporting research to find effective treatments and cures for Retinitis Pigmentosa, Macular Degeneration, and other degenerative eye diseases. The organization promotes the education of family members, friends, physicians, and educators about the special needs of people who are visually impaired. It maintains an ongoing public awareness campaign and supports its human service programs, including its school for the blind, audiovision talking greeting cards, and TheatreVision (accessible movies for blind individuals). Established in 1972, Retinitis Pigmentosa International offers facilities that demonstrate visual aids for people who are partially-sighted and provides personal counseling, psychological counseling, and mobility training. The organization provides referrals to genetic counselors and support groups and offers a variety of educational materials including a regular newsletter and brochures.

President: Helen Harris (1972-Present)
Executive Director: Helen Harris
Year Established: 1972
Organization Chapters: 50
Organization Members: 35,000

Publishes the following materials:
Fighting Blindness ~ *Brochure*

Concerned with the following diseases or disorders:
Acanthocytosis; Alstrom Syndrome; Bardet Biedl Syndrome; Coats' Disease; Cone Dystrophy; Leber's Congenital Amaurosis; Loken Senior Syndrome; Norrie Syndrome; Refsum Syndrome; Retinitis Pigmentosa; Retinoschisis; Usher's Syndrome

1473 ROBINOW SYNDROME FOUNDATION

15955 Uplander Street NW
Andover, MN 55304-2501 612-434-1152
Fax: 612-788-2331

The Robinow Syndrome Foundation is a not-for-profit, self help organization dedicated to providing information and support to individuals and family members affected by Robinow Syndrome. Robinow Syndrome is an extremely rare inherited disorder characterized by mild to moderate short stature (dwarfism) due to growth delays after birth; distinctive abnormalities of the head and facial (craniofacial) area; additional skeletal malformations; and/or genital abnormalities. The disorder may be inherited as an autosomal dominant or recessive genetic trait. Established in 1991, the Foundation engages in patient and professional education, provides referrals, has yearly conventions for members, and maintains a database. The Foundation is also committed to collecting data from original case studies and including new and recent information. The Robinow Syndrome Foundation offers a variety of educational materials including brochures, pamphlets, reports, audiovisuals, and a regular newsletter.

President: Karla M. Kruger (1991 to Present)
Year Established: 1991
Organization Members: 31

Concerned with the following diseases or disorders:
Robinow Syndrome

1474 RUBINSTEIN-TAYBI PARENT GROUP (RTS PARENT GROUP)

P.O. Box 146
Smith Center, KS 66967-0146 785-697-2984
Fax: 785-697-2985
E-mail: lbaxter@ruraltel.net
http://www.tucson.com/rts/

The Rubinstein-Taybi Parent Group is a voluntary not-for-profit self-help organization that is dedicated to providing information, assistance, and support to parents, health care professionals, and others who care for children with Rubinstein-Taybi Syndrome (RTS). Established in 1984, the Rubinstein-Taybi Parent Group provides a list of families affected by this disorder for the purpose of mutual support and information exchange. In addition, the Group works with individuals, families, and various organizations around the world to help them start RTS support groups; and promotes and supports research on RTS.

The organization provides a variety of educational and support materials, including a directory, a periodic newsletter, brochures, and pamphlets. The Group also informs members about research being conducted on Rubinstein-Taybi Syndrome and timely journal articles published in the peer-evaluated medical literature.

President: Lorrie Baxter (1984-Present)
Executive Director: Lorrie Baxter (Coordinator)
Year Established: 1984
Organization Members: 318

Publishes the following materials:
Rubinstein-Taybi Syndrome ~ *Brochure*

Concerned with the following diseases or disorders:
Rubinstein Taybi Syndrome

1475 SIDS ALLIANCE (SIDS ALLIANCE)

1314 Bedford Avenue
Suite 210
Baltimore, MD 21208 410-653-8226
800-221-7437
Fax: 410-653-8709
E-mail: sidshq@charm.net

The SIDS Alliance is a tax exempt charitable organization whose mission is to help parents whose lives have been touched by Sudden Infant Death Syndrome (SIDS); to educate the community about SIDS; and to support SIDS research. Sudden Infant Death Syndrome (SIDS) is the sudden death of any infant or young child that is unexpected by history and in which no adequate cause for death can be found. The SIDS Alliance was established in an effort to unite parents and friends affected by SIDS with medical, business, and civic groups concerned about the health of infants. With 77 local affiliates, the SIDS Alliance strives to achieve increased public participation and support for programs about SIDS. The Alliance is engaged in ongoing efforts to expand its scientific programs, strengthen services for families, and provide public education and advocacy opportunities. An important goal is to improve community understanding and elevate SIDS to the level of societal concern appropriate to one of the major causes of infant mortality. The SIDS Alliance assists parents to organize local chapters and provides services to them. Established in 1987, it publishes a periodic newsletter; distributes literature such as an informational brochure entitled "Facts About SIDS"; and disseminates information to community agencies and medical groups about SIDS. The Alliance advocates programs of professional counseling.

President: Judith S. Jacobson, EVP (1996 to Present)
Year Established: 1987
Organization Chapters: 77
Organization Members: 77

Publishes the following materials:
What Every New Parent Should Know: Facts About Sudden Infant Death Syndrome & Reducing the Risks for SIDS ~ *Brochure*
Facts About SIDS ~ *Brochure*

1476 SIDS EDUCATIONAL SERVICES, INC. (SIDS-ES)

2905 64th Avenue
Cheverly, MD 20785 301-773-9671
Fax: 301-322-2620

SIDS Educational Services, Inc. (SIDS-ES) is a voluntary self-help organization that assists those who have lost children to Sudden Infant Death Syndrome (SIDS) to deal with their grief. Sudden Infant Death Syndrome (SIDS) is the sudden death of any infant or young child that is unexpected by history and in which no adequate cause for death can be found. The organization publishes a 290 page book entitled "The SIDS Survival Guide" that is written by parents who have been affected by SIDS and experts for bereaved families and professionals. Also available is a brochure "Empathetic Support to Newly-Bereaved Families and Those Who Care About Them." SIDS-ES provides free peer contact assistance to newly bereaved families and has a book sponsorship program whereby companies, individuals, and groups donate books to newly bereaved families (often via SIDS support groups) as well as to public libraries, hospitals, doctors, police officials, and emergency responders.

President: Kee Schuth Marshall (1995 to Present).
Executive Director: Joani Nelson Horchler
Year Established: 1994

Publishes the following materials:
Empathetic Support to Newly-Bereaved SIDS Families and Those Who Care About Them ~ *Brochure*
The SIDS Survival Guide ~ *Book*

1477 SARCOID NETWORKING ASSOCIATION (SNA)

13925 80th Street East
Puyallup, WA 98372-3614 253-845-3108
Fax: 253-845-3108
E-mail: VBLR29A@Prodigy.com

The Sarcoid Networking Association (SNA) is a national not-for-profit self-help organization dedicated to providing information and support to individuals and family members affected by Sarcoidosis. Sarcoidosis, a rare disorder of unknown cause, is characterized by the formation of small rounded nodules (tubercles) of tissue consisting of cells resembling those that line internal and external surfaces of the body (epithelioid tissue). Almost any organ or tissue may be affected, including the eyes, skin, lungs, spleen, liver, and lymph nodes. Acute Sarcoidosis may be characterized by fever, generalized muscle aches, breathlessness, arthritis, enlarged lymph nodes, and other symptoms. Chronic, progressive, systemic Sarcoidosis may cause a wide variety of symptoms that may include fever, arthritis, numbness, appearance of a purplish rash on the face, bloodshot eyes, and additional abnormalities. Established in 1992, the SNA promotes research, works to increase professional and public awareness of Sarcoidosis, and provides networking services that enable affected individuals and family members to exchange information, support, and resources. The Association also engages in patient advocacy, has a directory, makes appropriate referrals, and offers a variety of materials including pamphlets, brochures, audiovisual aids, and a regular newsletter entitled "Sarcoidosis Networking."

President: Dolores O'Leary
Executive Director: Joe Ornowski
Year Established: 1992
Organization Members: Non-Membership

Publishes the following materials:
Sarcoidosis Networking (May/June 1997) ~ *Newsletter*
Sarcoidosis Networking (May/June 1996) ~ *Newsletter*
Sarcoidosis Networking (January/February 1997) ~ *Newsletter*

Concerned with the following diseases or disorders:
Sarcoidosis

1478 SARCOIDOSIS NETWORK FOUNDATION, INC. (REACH)

7475 La Palma Avenue
Buena Park, CA 90620 714-739-1398
888-638-9692
Fax: 714-739-2325

The Sarcoidosis Network Foundation, Inc. is a non-profit organization dedicated to supporting research to discover a cause, cure, and prevention of Sarcoidosis; promoting education and awareness; and improving the quality of life for those affected by Sarcoidosis. Sarcoidosis is a disorder that affects many body systems and is characterized by small round lesions of granulated tissue. Symptoms vary depending on the severity of the disease and the specific areas of the body that are affected. Fever, weight loss, and joint pain (arthralgia) may be initial symptoms of Sarcoidosis. Persistent fever is especially common with liver (hepatic) involvement. Abnormal enlargement of certain lymph nodes (peripheral lymphadenopathy) is also common and usually asymptomatic. Both enlarged and normal-sized lymph nodes may contain the characteristic sarcoid tubercles. Established in 1992, the Foundation provides educational materials about Sarcoidosis. Monthly support groups are available for affected individuals and their family members and caregivers as well as the general public. A quarterly newsletter entitled "R.E.A.C.H" is available along with referral services for physicians, and counseling and disability referrals. Patient networking has been established to give affected individuals and family members an opportunity to share their experiences with others. In addition, the Foundation provides charitable assistance to Sarcoidosis research program to help discover a cure and prevention for Sarcoidosis.

President: Earl Jacobs, Jr. (1989 to Present)
Year Established: 1992

Publishes the following materials:
Mission Statement ~ *Mission Statement*
Statement of Services and Activities ~ *Fact Sheet*
REACH (April-May-June 1997) ~ *Newsletter*
Sarcoidosis Network ~ *Brochure*
What Is Sarcoidosis? Where Is It Found? ~ *Pamphlet*
What is Sarcoidosis? ~ *Fact Sheet*
Body Map ~ *Body Map*
Are You Between The Ages Of 20 - 45? ~ *Fact Sheet*

Concerned with the following diseases or disorders:
Sarcoidosis

1479 SARCOIDOSIS RESEARCH INSTITUTE (SRI)

3475 Central Avenue
Memphis, TN 38111 901-774-7294
Fax: 901-766-6951
http://www.netten.net/~soskelnt/

The Sarcoidosis Research Institute is a national not-for-profit organization established in 1991. The Institute is dedicated to providing up-to-date information to individuals with Sarcoidosis and conducting forums for affected individuals and their families. Sarcoidosis, a rare disorder of unknown cause, is characterized by the formation of small rounded nodules (tubercles) of tissue consisting of cells resembling those that line internal and external surfaces of the body (epithelioid tissue). Almost any organ or tissue may be affected, including the eyes, skin, lungs, spleen, liver, and lymph nodes. Acute Sarcoidosis may be characterized by fever, generalized muscle aches, breathlessness, arthritis, enlarged lymph nodes, and other symptoms. Chronic, progressive, systemic Sarcoidosis may cause a wide variety of symptoms that may include fever, arthritis, numbness, appearance of a purplish rash on the face, bloodshot eyes, and additional abnormalities. The Institute also seeks to increase public awareness of Sarcoidosis and channel appropriate information to the medical community. Educational materials produced by the Sarcoidosis Research Institute include a brochure entitled "Answer's to Your Questions about Sarcoidosis" and a video called "Sarcoidosis: An Overview."

President: Paula Yette Polite (1994-Present)
Year Established: 1991
Organization Chapters: 2

Publishes the following materials:
Answers to Your Questions About... Sarcoidosis ~ *Brochure*

Concerned with the following diseases or disorders:
Sarcoidosis

1480 SCAPULOPERONEAL DISEASE ASSOCIATION (SPDA)

610 Navesink Avenue
Ocean Gate, NJ 08740 908-269-0357
Fax: 908-269-0357

The Scapuloperoneal Disease Association (SPDA) is an international self-help and research organization dedicated to providing information, assistance, and support to individuals and family members affected by Scapuloperoneal Muscular Dystrophy. Scapuloperoneal Muscular Dystrophy, a rare inherited muscular dystrophy that may become apparent early in life, is characterized by slowly progressive muscle weakness of the upper arms and shoulder blade area (scapula) as well as certain leg muscle groups below the knee (peroneal). Established in 1994, the SPDA provides networking services that enable affected individuals and family members to exchange information, support and resources; promotes basic and clinical research development; fosters communication among related organizations; serves to represent individuals and family members affected by Scapuloperoneal Muscular Dystrophy; and accumulates and disseminates information and materials concerning this disorder.

President: Michael S. Curivan (1994 to Present).
Executive Director: Patricia A. Curivan
Year Established: 1994
Organization Members: 65

Concerned with the following diseases or disorders:
Myopathy, Scapuloperoneal

1481 SCHIZ KIDZ BUDDIES ONLINE SUPPORT GROUP FOR SCHIZENCEPHALY

E-mail: wrights@televar.com
www.geocities.com/Heartland/Meadows/7384/

Schiz Kidz Buddies Online Support Group for Schizencephaly is a web site on the Internet for parents, other family members, physicians, therapists, and friends of children born with Schizencephaly. Schizencephaly is a rare brain malformation due to improper development of the cerebral hemispheres of the brain during embryonic growth (neuronal dysmigration). Affected infants and children may have variable symptoms that may include seizure disorders, developmental delays, mental retardation, visual impairment, eating difficulties, and/or other symptoms. The Schizencephaly Online Support Group's web site provides general information on the condition, a variety of online networking opportunities, and dynamic links to additional sources of helpful information on the Internet. Online networking opportunities include the Group's daily "E-mail Loop," which offers affected family members the opportunity to share experiences, ask questions, and gain invaluable support from others who "have been there." The web site also will include more indepth information concerning schizencephaly written by pediatricians and pediatric neurologists and will enable parents and other family members to share questions with such specialists. The online support group also offers a special birthday club that provides affected children with stuffed animals, birthday cards, and balloons on their special days. The Schiz Kidz Online Support Group for Schizencephaly Web site is located at [http://www.geocities.com/Heartland/Meadows/7384/].

President: Judi Wright and Lynn Niedzwiecki (Co-founders)
Year Established: 1997
Organization Members: 45

1482 SCLERODERMA FEDERATION, INC.

Peabody Office Building
1 Newbury Street
Peabody, MA 01960 508-535-6600
800-422-1113
Fax: 508-535-6696
E-mail: sclerofed@aol.com
http://www.scleroderma.org

Scleroderma Federation, Inc. is an international voluntary not-for-profit federation of scleroderma support groups. Established in 1982, the Federation is dedicated to promoting the welfare of people with Scleroderma and their families by providing educational and emotional support; enhancing public and professional awareness of the disease; and promoting and supporting medical research designed to identify causes, prevention methods, improved treatments, and a potential cure. The Federation's member organizations function locally and regionally to assist affected individuals and their families. These member organizations provide telephone helplines, conduct educational meetings and workshops led by health care professionals; supply medical referrals; arrange networking among individuals with scleroderma; and offer other support services. At the national and international levels, the Scleroderma Federation serves as an advocate for funding and support of Scleroderma research as well as legislation benefiting people with the disease. The Federation also serves as a clearinghouse for information on Scleroderma and offers a variety of educational and support materials including a quarterly newsletter, brochures, pamphlets, booklets, and audio-visual aids.

President: Peter Meyer (1994-Present)
Executive Director: Jacqueline Magoon
Year Established: 1982
Organization Chapters: 13
Organization Members: 15,000

Publishes the following materials:
Understanding and Managing Scleroderma ~ *Brochure*
Helpful Hints ~ *Brochure*
Medication Update ~ *Brochure*
About Scleroderma ~ *Brochure*
Localized Scleroderma ~ *Brochure*
The Beacon ~ *Newsletter*

Concerned with the following diseases or disorders:
Eosinophilia Myalgia; Eosinophilic Fasciitis; Peyronie Disease; Scleroderma

1483 SCLERODERMA INFO EXCHANGE, INC. (SDINFO)

150 Hines Farm Road
Cranston, RI 02921 401-943-3909
Fax: 401-946-5666
E-mail: hshinc.@yahoo.com

The Scleroderma Info Exchange, Inc. (SDInfo) is a not-for-profit organization dedicated to collecting and disseminating information concerning Scleroderma, a rare connective tissue disorder of the skin. Established in 1981, the Exchange engages in patient education, promotes patient advocacy, and provides both educational and support information to affected individuals, family members, health care professionals, and the public. One of the goals of the Scleroderma Info Exchange is locating a site on Internet to store Worldwide Web documents concerning Scleroderma.

President: Nancy D. Hersey (1981-Present)
Year Established: 1981

Concerned with the following diseases or disorders:
Chromosome 21 Ring; Mixed Connective Tissue Disease (MCTD); Peyronie Disease; Raynaud's Disease and Phenomenon; Scleroderma

1484 SCLERODERMA RESEARCH FOUNDATION (SRF)

2320 Bath Street
Suite 315
Santa Barbara, CA 93105 805-563-9133
800-441-2873
Fax: 805-563-2402
E-mail: srfcure@srfcure.org
http://www.srfcure.org

The Scleroderma Research Foundation is a voluntary research non-profit organization dedicated to finding a cure for Scleroderma by funding and facilitating ongoing medical research. The Foundation also seeks to increase public awareness and understanding of this disorder. Established in 1987, the Scleroderma Research Foundation created a team of scientific and biomedical advisors to identify and address key issues that may lead to a cure. The efforts of the Foundation and its advisory team have led to the opening of the Bay Area Scleroderma Research Center in San Francisco and the East Coast Scleroderma

Research Center in Baltimore, both cross-institutional, multi-disciplinary research facilities. With participation of the National Institutes of Health (NIH) and several institutes and universities, the Foundation has also assisted in the creation of clinical laboratory tests that provide for the early diagnosis of several forms of Scleroderma. Moreover, with the assistance of the Foundation, significant progress has been achieved in the development of animal models for Scleroderma that may be a step toward development and evaluation of potential therapies. The Scleroderma Research Foundation has also been involved in the establishment of the importance of key cells that serve as catalysts in Scleroderma's onset. The Scleroderma Research Foundation provides a variety of educational materials to affected individuals, family members, health care and research professionals, and the general public through its computer database, newsletters, articles, and video documentaries.

President: Sharon Monsky (Board Chairman)
Executive Director: Kevin C. Looper (Executive Vice President)
Year Established: 1987

Publishes the following materials:
The Mission of the Scleroderma Research Foundation ~ *Fact Sheet*
Scleroderma Research Foundation ~ *Newsletter*
A Fast-Tracker on a Life-or-Death Mission ~ *Article Reprint*
The Power of Two ~ *Videotape*

Concerned with the following diseases or disorders:
Mixed Connective Tissue Disease (MCTD);
Scleroderma

1485 SCOTTISH SOCIETY FOR AUTISTIC CHILDREN (SSAC)

Hilton House
Alloa Business Park
Whins Road
Alloa, FK10 3SA
Scotland 01259 720044
Fax: 01259 720051

The Scottish Society for Autistic Children (SSAC) is a not-for-profit voluntary organization dedicated to providing the best possible care, support, and education for people of all ages with autism throughout Scotland. SSAC also works to raise the awareness of autism among the general public and professionals working in this field. Autism is a genetic disorder characterized by difficulties in relating to, or understanding, other people and social situations; difficulties in acquiring any form of communication; and a lack of imaginative ability, often substituted by obsessive, repetitive behavior and a strong resistance to change. Established in 1976, SSAC has programs that provide residential and day services for people with autism from all over Scotland. Staff aim to identify the strengths and needs of the service-users and devise strategies that maximize their potential. This is carried out in a caring environment in which affected individuals receive the necessary support and guidance to maintain a satisfying and enjoyable lifestyle. Consisting of 500 members and 15 chapters, the organizations produces educational materials including a booklet entitled "The Scottish Society for Autistic Children Information Pack" and a magazine entitled "In Touch."

President: Andrew Lester (1993 to Present)
Executive Director: Donald Liddell
Year Established: 1976
Organization Chapters: 15
Organization Members: 500

Publishes the following materials:
The Scottish Society for Autistic Children. Information Pact ~ *Booklet*
In Touch ~ *Members Magazine*

1486 SELECTIVE MUTISM FOUNDATION, INC. (SMF, INC.)

P.O. Box 450632
Sunrise, FL 33345-0632 954-748-7714
Fax: 954-748-7714

Selective Mutism Foundation, Inc. is a national non-profit voluntary health organization dedicated to developing and disseminating educational materials on selective mutism (SM) to affected individuals, families, professionals, and the general public; increasing the knowledge and sensitivity of professionals who treat individuals experiencing selective mutism; finding the cause and cure for this condition; improving treatments and medications for selective mutism; and developing and implementing interventions in public schools. In addition, the Foundation promotes ongoing research and develops educational testing materials. Selective mutism (SM), formerly known as Elective Mutism, is a psychiatric disorder most commonly found in children. It is characterized by a persistent failure (for more than one month) to speak in select settings. Affected children understand spoken language and have the ability to speak. In most cases, affected children speak to their parents and a few selected others. In some cases, they do not speak to certain individuals in their household. The exact cause of this disorder is not known. Established in 1991 and consisting of 600 members, the organization produces a quarterly newsletter and brochures that address the needs of families affected by SM. In addition, the Foundation networks affected families for the purposes of mutual support and information exchange.

President: Sue Newman (Co-Founder/Director) (1991 to Present)
Executive Director: Carolyn Miller (Co-Founder/Director)
Year Established: 1991
Organization Members: 600

Publishes the following materials:
Understanding Selective Mutism. A silent cry for help! ~ *Brochure*

Concerned with the following diseases or disorders:
Mutism, Selective

1487 SELECTIVE MUTISM GROUP WEB SITE

E-mail: rotkh@flinet.com
http://www.flinet.com/~diverse/smg/

The Selective Mutism Group Web Site was begun by a parent of a child with Selective Mutism who was unable to find the answers to his questions. Selective Mutism is a rare psychiatric condition occurring primarily during childhood. Although affected individuals understand language use and have the ability to speak, they demonstrate a persistent failure to speak in particular settings over a period of time. For example, in many cases, although affected children may speak to their parents and a few select others, they may not speak in school or in other social situations. Most affected children function normally in other ways and learn age appropriate skills; however, some may have additional disabilities. The Selective Mutism Group Web Site is dedicated to furthering research and offering information and support to affected individuals, family members, and educators who work with affected children. The site provides an interactive location for all those affected by Selective Mutism to enable them to ask questions and find answers, keep up with current research, and locate dynamic links to additional sources of information and support on the Internet. The site's CAAP Question and Answer Page, which is offered in collaboration with the UCLA Neuropsychiatric Institute's Child and Adolescent Anxiety Program (CAAP), a clinical research program, enables affected individuals, family members, and educators to receive answers to their questions from qualified professionals whoare currently researching Selective Mutism. The site also features parents' stories, additional information to assist teachers of affected children, a forum area where online users can ask questions and reply to posted messages, and a pen pal area where affected individuals and family members can leave their names and e-mail addresses so that others may correspond with them and provide more personal support.

1488 SEVERE CHRONIC NEUTROPENIA INTERNATIONAL REGISTRY (SCN INTERNATIONAL REGISTY)

Puget Sound Plaza
Suite 620
1325 4th Avenue
Seattle, WA 98101-2509
206-543-9749
800-726-4463
Fax: 206-543-3668
E-mail: Registry@u.washington.edu
http://scnir.medicine.washington.edu

Established in March of 1994, the Severe Chronic Neutropenia International Registry is a research organization supported by Amgen, Inc. and directed by an advisory board of physicians who treat individuals with Severe Chronic Neutropenia (SCN). Chronic Neutropenia is a blood disorder in which the bone marrow produces a decreased number of certain white blood cells known as neutrophils. Abnormally low levels of neutrophils can cause affected individuals to become more susceptible to certain bacterial infections. The mission of the Registry is to establish a worldwide database of treatment and disease related outcomes for individuals diagnosed with SCN. It is hoped that the information collected will lead to improved medical care and a focus for future medical research. The Registry, which serves the entire United States, Canada, nine European countries, Australia and Israel, works with two data coordinating centers and seven regional referral centers. The Registry provides information to affected individuals and health care professionals in the form of reports.

President: Dale C. Dale, M.D. (Co-Director)
Executive Director: Professor Karl Welte (Co-Director)
Year Established: 1994
Organization Chapters: 9
Organization Members: 526

Publishes the following materials:
Focusing on the Future ~ *Brochure*

Concerned with the following diseases or disorders:
Neutropenia, Chronic; Neutropenia, Cyclic

1489 SEVERE CHRONIC NEUTROPENIA INTERNATIONAL REGISTRY AUSTRALIA (SCNIRAU)

2nd Floor Marian House
St. John of God Hospital
1002 Mair Street
Ballarat, 3350
Australia 61 3 5333 4811
Fax: 61 3 5333 4813
E-mail: scnirau@ballarat.edu.au
http://freyja.ballarat.edu.au:8080/~scnirau/

The Severe Chronic Neutropenia International Registry Australia (SCNIRAU) is the Australian division of the Severe Chronic Neutropenia International Registry. The Australian division, which registered its first patient in 1994, currently has over 30 patients registered, while over 400 patients are registered internationally. Chronic Neutropenia is a blood disorder characterized by abnormally low levels of certain white blood cells known as neutrophils that are produced by the bone marrow and play an essential role in fighting infection. Individuals with Chronic Neutropenia may be abnormally susceptible to certain bacterial infections and may experience other associated symptoms and/or findings. The International Registry is committed to documenting the clinical course of Severe Chronic Neutropenia (SCN); monitoring and assessing long-term safety of primary treatments in individuals with SCN in the United States, Canada, Europe, and Australia; and studying the incidence and outcome of certain previously identified adverse events including osteoporosis, splenomegaly, cytogenetic abnormalities, myeloplastic syndrome, and leukemia. The International Registry is also dedicated to evaluating growth and development and hematologic parameters; monitoring for clinically significant changes in primary treatment response over time; establishing a physician network to increase the understanding of SCN; and establishing a demographic database to allow for future research. The Australian division provides affected individuals and family members with several services including offering understandable information on SCN; reprints from the peer-reviewed medical literature concerning the disorder; and a web site on the Internet with information on the disorder, protocol information for those interested in becoming registry participants, and dynamic linkage to other helpful sources of information on the Internet.

Year Established: 1994

Concerned with the following diseases or disorders:
Neutropenia, Chronic; Neutropenia, Cyclic

1490 SHARE AND CARE COCKAYNE SYNDROME NETWORK

P.O. Box 552
Stanleytown, VA 24168 540-629-2369
Fax: 540-647-3739

The Share & Care Cockayne Syndrome Network is a voluntary health organization that began as a parent support group. The Network expanded to include affected families and health care professionals who are interested in the care of people with Cockayne Syndrome. Cockayne Syndrome is a rare inherited disorder characterized by growth retardation, abnormal sensitivity to light (photosensitivity), an abnormally small head (microcephaly), and a prematurely aged (progeroid) appearance. Children with this disorder may scar easily and have an increased amount of color (pigmentation) in the skin. The purpose of the Network is to provide support and information for families affected by Cockayne Syndrome. The sharing of information helps people make informed decisions regarding the care of children with this rare disorder. Established in 1993, the organization produces an informational pamphlet and a periodic newsletter.

President: Teresa Wall
Executive Director: Thaddeus E. Kelly, MD, PhD
Year Established: 1993
Organization Members: 300

Publishes the following materials:
Share & Care ~ *Newsletter*
Share & Care Cockayne Syndrome Network ~ *Brochure*

Concerned with the following diseases or disorders:
Cockayne Syndrome

1491 **SHWACHMAN SYNDROME SUPPORT INTERNATIONAL**

418 Quincy Street
St. Louis, MO 63116 314-352-1821
E-mail: 4sskids@mvp.net
http://www.xmission.com/~4sskids

The Shwachman Syndrome Support is a non-profit voluntary health organization that functions as an international support system for people with Shwachman Syndrome and their families. Shwachman Syndrome is an extremely rare inherited disorder with multiple and varied manifestations. In most cases, the disorder may be characterized by signs of insufficient absorption (malabsorption) of fats and other nutrients due to abnormal development of the pancreas (pancreatic insufficiency); abnormal bone development affecting the rib cage and/or bones in the arms and/or legs (metaphyseal dysostosis); short stature; and/or improper functioning of the bone marrow (bone marrow dysfunction), resulting in low levels of circulating blood cells (hematologic abnormalities). The organization maintains a central registry and medical profiles of individuals with this disorder. The registry also contains the names of medical professionals who have experience in treating people with Shwachman Syndrome or who have expressed a desire to treat people with this disorder. Established in 1994, the support group publishes a periodic newsletter and seeks to increase awareness of this disorder among the medical community and the public. Other goals of the Shwachman Syndrome Support are to stimulate interest in ongoing medical research, improve treatments, and develop informational brochures and pamphlets.

President: Joan Mowery (1994-Present)
Year Established: 1994
Organization Members: 300

Publishes the following materials:
help us grow...... ~ *Brochure*

Concerned with the following diseases or disorders:
Shwachman Syndrome

1492 **SHY DRAGER SYNDROME SUPPORT GROUP (SDS)**

1607 Silver Avenue SE
Albuquerque, NM 87106
800-737-4999

The Shy Drager Syndrome Support Group is a not-for-profit self-help organization that was established in 1987. Shy-Drager Syndrome is a rare neurological disorder characterized by progressive failure of the autonomic nervous system. The autonomic nervous system is the part of the nervous system that controls a variety of vital involuntary body functions. These include regulation of heart rate, blood pressure, sweating, bowel and bladder control, as well as a variety of other bodily functions. Symptoms of Shy-Drager Syndrome include unusually low blood pressure while standing upright (orthostatic hypotension), loss of bladder and bowel control, and/or lack of sweating. The mission of the Group is to insure that individuals with Shy Drager Syndrome and their caregivers will be able to locate appropriate support systems, other resources, and avenues to medical professionals who are familiar with this rare disorder. Located in Albuquerque, New Mexico, the Support Group serves the entire United States, Canada, Mexico, and Europe. The group maintains a directory and makes appropriate medical referrals.

Executive Director: Dorothy Trainor Kingsbury
Year Established: 1987
Organization Members: @400

Concerned with the following diseases or disorders:
Shy Drager Syndrome

1493 **SICKLE CELL DISEASE ASSOCIATION OF AMERICA, INC. (SCDAA)**

200 Corporate Pointe
Suite 495
Culver City, CA 90230-7633 310-216-6363
800-421-8453
Fax: 310-215-3722

The Sickle Cell Disease Association of America (SCDAA) is a voluntary service organization dedicated to educating the public and providing support to people affected by Sickle Cell Disease. The Association was founded in 1971 as the umbrella organization for community-based groups providing support and services to persons affected by sickle cell conditions. The Association seeks to educate the public about sickle cell disease and the sickle cell trait and develop educational materials on these conditions for extensive circulation. It also educates legislators on issues regarding sickle cell disease and other genetic disorders and fosters ongoing medical research to improve the well-being of those affected by sickle cell disease. In addition, the Association supports research, advocates on behalf of all individuals affected by sickle cell diseases, and provides appropriate referrals to medical professionals. The Association is the only national community-based voluntary health agency working full-time to resolve issues surrounding sickle cell conditions. The Sickle Cell Disease Association provides an extensive supply of resources. These include guidebooks, brochures, pamphlets, audio and visual tapes, fact sheets, and a periodic newsletter entitled "Sickle Cell News."

President: Dr. Kwaku Ohene-Frempong, Director.
Executive Director: Lyndra K. Anderson
Year Established: 1971
Organization Chapters: 75

Concerned with the following diseases or disorders:
Sickle Cell Disease; Thalassemia Major; Thalassemia Minor

1494 SIMON FOUNDATION FOR CONTINENCE

P.O. Box 815
Wilmette, IL 60091 847-864-3913
800-237-4666
Fax: 847-864-9758

The Simon Foundation for Continence is a not-for-profit voluntary organization dedicated to removing the social stigma of this condition and to educating both medical professionals and affected individuals about cure, treatment, and management techniques. Incontinence is a condition in which one loses bladder control. Established in 1982, the Foundation has worked to raise public awareness and educate people that incontinence can be cured or managed satisfactorily. Much of its work goes on behind the scenes by Foundation staff, attending different programs to educate physicians and nurses about the need of people affected by incontinence. The Foundation is constantly meeting with manufacturers to help develop better incontinence products at lower prices for consumers. In the last two years, spokespersons from the Foundation have appeared on over 400 television and radio talk shows, bringing awareness about continence to millions of people. Educational materials include a quarterly newsletter entitled "The Informer" and a book entitled "Managing Incontinence: A Guide to Living With the Loss of Bladder Control." The Foundation coordinates regular support group meetings, encourages constant patient advocacy, and supports patient, professional, and general education programs.

President: Cheryle B. Gartley
Executive Director: Connie Fairbanks
Year Established: 1982
Organization Members: 100,000

Publishes the following materials:
The Solution Starts With You ~ *Brochure*
I Will Manage. A Program to Promote Continence ~ *Brochure*
The Simon Foundation ~ *Mission Statement*

1495 SISTERS NETWORK, INC. (SN, INC.)

8787 Woodway Drive
Suite 4207
Houston, TX 77063 713-781-0255
Fax: 713-780-8998
http://users.aol.com/sistersnet/sis.html

Sisters Network, Inc. is a national not-for-profit organization dedicated to providing informational and emotional support to African-American women who have been affected by breast cancer and to increasing local and national attention that breast cancer has in the African-American community. Established in 1994, Sisters Network addresses the needs of African-American women facing breast cancer through its local chapters and partnerships with existing service providers. The primary services of the Network are to provide emotional and psychological support; a resource for medical research; community cancer education and awareness programs; a speakers bureau; in-home sister-to-sister support; and a self-titled periodic newsletter. Sisters Network advocates early detection as the best defense against breast cancer through monthly breast self-exams; annual breast exams by a doctor; and mammography screening starting at age 35. Sisters Network, Inc. maintains a site on the world wide web and can be reached at [http://users.aol.com/sistersnet/sis.html].

President: Karen E. Jackson (1994 to Present)
Year Established: 1994
Organization Chapters: 15
Organization Members: 500

Publishes the following materials:
Sisters Network ~ *Newsletter Jan-March 1997*
Sisters Network ~ *Newsletter Jan-March 1997*

Concerned with the following diseases or disorders:
Cancer, Breast

1496 **SJOGREN'S SYNDROME FOUNDATION, INC. (SSF)**
333 North Broadway
Jericho, NY 11573 516-933-6365
800-475-6473
Fax: 516-933-6368
http://www.sjogrens.com

The Sjogren's Syndrome Foundation is an international not-for-profit organization founded in 1983 to serve the needs of people affected by Sjogren's Syndrome. Sjogren's Syndrome, a disorder of unknown cause, is characterized by deficient moisture production of the mucous-secreting glands, particularly the tear ducts of the eyes (lacrimal) and the salivary glands of the mouth. Associated symptoms and physical abnormalities may include abnomal dryness, itching, and burning of the eyes (keratoconjunctivitis sicca); abnormal dryness of the mouth, resulting in cavities, other dental disorders, and loss of odor and taste sensations; and, when the lungs are affected, increased susceptibility to repeated respiratory infections. Many affected individuals also experience rheumatoid arthritis. Sjogren's Syndrome, which primarily affects middle-aged women, is thought to be due to an abnormal autoimmune response. The mission of the Foundation is to support and educate individuals affected by Sjogren's Syndrome and their families; educate health care professionals and the general public about the disorder; and stimulate interest in research toward improved treatments and an eventual cure. In addition, the Sjogren's Syndrome Foundation provides referrals to physicians who treat people with Sjogren's Syndrome; to local chapters; and to support groups. The Foundation offers postgraduate fellowships and student fellowships to stimulate continuing research into the cause and possible cure for Sjogren's Syndrome. The Foundation conducts comprehensive symposia on Sjogren's Syndrome. Regional chapters and support groups conduct smaller regional and local gatherings. The Sjogren's Syndrome Foundation produces an extensive array of educational and support materials. These include audio and visual tape materials, a library of medical articles, a medical referral listing, a monthly newsletter, and a handbook entitled "The Sjogren's Syndrome Handbook: An Authoritative Guide."

President: NA
Executive Director: Alexis Stegemann
Year Established: 1983
Organization Chapters: 10
Organization Members: 7,400

Publishes the following materials:
Sjogren's Syndrome Foundation Information Packet ~ *Information Packet*
An Overview: How to Recognize and Treat Sjogren's Syndrome ~ *Fact Sheet*

Concerned with the following diseases or disorders:
Mikulicz Syndrome; Mixed Connective Tissue Disease (MCTD); Sjogren Syndrome

1497 **SMITH LEMLI-OPITZ/RSH ADVOCACY AND EXCHANGE (SLO OR RSH)**
32 Ivy Lane
Glen Mills, PA 19342 610-361-9663
http://members.aol.com/slo97/index.htm

The Smith-Lemli-Opitz/RSH Advocacy & Exchange is a voluntary not-for-profit organization dedicated to educating the medical community, parents of affected children, educators, and the public about Smith-Lemli-Opitz/RSH Syndrome. Established in 1988, the organization was created by 37 families with children affected by this rare disorder. The organization's purpose is to enable members to exchange information and experiences in an atmosphere of mutual support. In addition to informal networking, the Advocacy & Exchange sponsors regular national meetings where physicians, scientists, and parents can meet to learn more from each other. The organization now includes families from the United States, Canada, and throughout the world. The Exchange is devoted to patient advocacy, an ongoing exchange of information and support, and promoting and funding research on SLO/RSH. The organization produces educational materials including brochures and a regular newsletter.

President: Barbara Hook (1988-Present)
Year Established: 1988
Organization Chapters: 2
Organization Members: 100

Publishes the following materials:
Smith-Lemli-Optiz Syndrome ~ *Brochure*

Concerned with the following diseases or disorders:
Smith Lemli Opitz Syndrome

1498 SOTOS SYNDROME SUPPORT ASSOCIATION (SSSA)

3 Danada Square East
Suite 235
Wheaton, IL 60187 630-682-8815
E-mail: ssa@well.com
http://www.well.com./user/sssa/

The Sotos Syndrome Support Association (SSSA) is a voluntary not-for-profit organization dedicated to providing information and support to individuals affected by Sotos Syndrome, their families, and health care professionals. Sotos Syndrome is a rare genetic disorder characterized by excessive growth that occurs prior to and after birth (prenatally and postnatally). At birth, affected infants have unusually increased body length that is abnormal in proportion to weight, which may also be above average; in addition, newborns typically demonstrate advanced bone growth, abnormally large hands and/or feet, and characteristic facial features. The purpose of the Association is to establish a social support environment for professionals and families of individuals affected by Sotos Syndrome so that they can meet to exchange ideas and help one another cope; enhance the understanding of Sotos Syndrome through education; coordinate an annual meeting in which to meet, organize, and discuss association business; and provide an opportunity for professionals working with individuals affected by Sotos Syndrome to collect data for research and to meet colleagues. Established in 1988, the Association produces educational materials including brochures, a 55 page booklet entitled "A Handbook for Families," and a quarterly newsletter for members to network ideas, articles, and inspirations.

President: Debra Shively (1994-Present)
Year Established: 1988
Organization Members: 250

Concerned with the following diseases or disorders:
Sotos Syndrome

1499 SPECIAL PARENTS PROJECT

5954 Van Keppel Road
Forestville, CA 95436 707-887-1011
Fax: 707-887-2154
E-mail: brucer@monitor.net

The Special Parents Project is a voluntary not-for-profit organization dedicated to providing caring outreach, training, advocacy, and support for families who are adjusting to the distress of having an infant or young child with disabilities. Established in 1994, the objective of the Special Parents Project is to give parents tools to enhance their family's quality of life and their ability to be effective advocates for their children. The organization accomplishes this through the creation of a comprehensive survival guide, parent network and support groups, community outreach, research, and multi-media materials. The broader purpose of the Special Parents Project is to build increased public understanding of the circumstances faced by these families — underserved members of our local and national community whose needs transcend ethnicity, social class, occupation, and financial status. Educational materials include reports and a database. The organization coordinates support groups, encourages networking, supports research, promotes education, and provides appropriate referrals. The Special Parents Project can be reached at its e-mail address at [brucer@monitor.net].

Executive Director: Lorna Catford
Year Established: 1994

Publishes the following materials:
The Special Parents Project ~ *Mission Statement*

1500 SPINA BIFIDA ASSOCIATION OF AMERICA (SBAA)

4590 MacArthur Boulevard NW
Suite 250
Washington, DC 20007-4226 202-944-3285
800-621-3141
Fax: 202-944-3295
E-mail: sbaa@sbaa.org
http://www.sbaa.org

The Spina Bifida Association of America (SBAA) is a not-for-profit association dedicated to promoting the rights and well-being of individuals with spina bifida. The Association supports research into the causes, treatment, and prevention of the disease and seeks to increase public awareness of spina bifida and its prevention. Educational advancement, social and vocational development, and mainstreaming of individuals with disabilities are also goals of the Association. Established in 1973 to address the specific needs of the spina bifida community, the Association's chapters comprise affected individuals, family members, health care professionals, and health institutions. The Association promotes the continuing education to health care professionals involved in the treatment of spina bifida. It maintains a toll-free information and referral service, provides direct program services for its members and chapters, conducts public awareness campaigns, and holds an annual national conference addressing spina bifida issues. The Spina Bifida Association of America publishes a bimonthly newsletter, produces and distributes publications on the entire spectrum of spina bifida issues, and provides a variety of brochures and fact sheets.

Executive Director: Larry Pencak
Year Established: 1973
Organization Chapters: 80
Organization Members: 6,000

Publishes the following materials:
SB Spina Bifida Association of America ~ *Introduction Sheet*
SBAA Class Assistance Programs ~ *Brochure*
INSIGHTS ~ *Newsletter*
SB Spina Bifida Association of America ~ *Introduction Sheet*
About the SBAA ~ *Information Sheet*
NIS Information Sheet ~ *Information Sheet*
General Information about Spina Bifida ~ *Information Sheet*
Facts about The Americans With Disabilities Act ~ *Fact Sheet*
1995 Spina Bifida Chapter List ~ *Chapter List*
Update: Latex Allergy ~ *Fact Sheet*
SBAA Publication List ~ *Publication List*
Cassette Order Form ~ *Order Form*
SB ~ *Brochure*

Concerned with the following diseases or disorders:
Fetal Valproate Syndrome; Spina Bifida; Tethered Spinal Cord Syndrome

1501 SPONDYLITIS ASSOCIATION OF AMERICA (SAA)

P.O. Box 5872
Sherman Oaks, CA 91413 818-981-1616
800-777-8189
Fax: 818-981-9826
E-mail: Information@spondylitis.org
http://www.spondylitis.org

The Spondylitis Association of America is a national voluntary self-help organization dedicated to supporting the advancement of research into Ankylosing Spondylitis; educating health care professionals; and lending support to people affected by Ankylosing Spondylitis and their families. Established in 1983, the Spondylitis Association of America seeks to help affected individuals lead more productive lives. The Association also desires to familiarize the medical community with Spondylitis and supports ongoing investigations into new advanced treatments. The Association hopes to educate medical professionals about the early symptoms of AS and to promote research into this disease and other related disorders. The Spondylitis Association of America offers services to people with Ankylosing Spondylitis, Reiter's Syndrome, Psoriatic Arthritis and Spondylitis Associated with Inflammatory Bowel Diseases. The Association produces a variety of educational materials including pamphlets, brochures, and a newsletter.

President: Laura Schafer, R.N. (1994-Present)
Executive Director: Jane Bruckel
Year Established: 1983
Organization Members: 3,000

Publishes the following materials:
Spondylitis Association of America - We're Here to Help You ~ *Brochure*
Spondylitis Association of America Order Form ~ *Order Form*
Spondylitis Plus ~ *Brochure*
Fight Back Home Exercise Video ~ *Brochure*
Spondylitis Association of America ~ *Brochure*
Juvenile Ankylosing Spondylitis ~ *Pamphlet*
A Guidebook for Patients ~ *Booklet*
Spondylitis Plus Spondylitis Association of America Quarterly ~ *Newsletter*

1502 STEVE ANTANAS STAVRO FAMILIAL GASTROINTESTINAL CANCER REGISTRY

Mt. Sinai Hospital Familial GI Cancer Registry
Pavilion A-3 Suite 1157
Toronto
Ontario, M5G 1X5
Canada 416-586-8334
Fax: 416-586-8644
E-mail: GICANREG@MSHRI.ON.CA

The Steve Antanas Stavro Familial Gastrointestinal Cancer Registry is a professional and research center dedicated to providing professional services as well as emotional support to people affected by familial gastrointestinal cancer and their families. Established in 1980, the center conducts research studies and has an investigative team focused on innovative surgical techniques related to gastrointestinal cancer. The center also has a molecular diagnostic program and offers a screening service for family members who may be at risk for the hereditary form of the disease. Along with its scientific and medical departments, the center also has a genetic counseling department that offers advice and support to affected individuals and families. The Steve Antanas Stavro Familial Gastrointestinal Cancer Registry maintains a database of affected individuals and produces educational and support materials including pamphlets, brochures, family guides, and a biannual newsletter. The Registry relays information regarding hospital and community resources through a patient library.

Executive Director: Teri Berk, Clinical Coordinator
Organization Language: French. Spanish.
Year Established: 1980
Organization Members: 350

Concerned with the following diseases or disorders:
Polyposis, Familial

1503 STEVENS JOHNSON SYNDROME SUPPORT GROUP (SJS SUPPORT GROUP)
9285 North Utica Street
Westminster, CO 80030 303-430-9559
E-mail: SJSUPPORT@aol.com
http://members.aol.com/sjsupport/index.html

The Stevens Johnson Syndrome (SJS) Support Group is a national non-profit support group dedicated to providing emotional support to individuals affected by SJS and their families. Stevens-Johnson Syndrome is a severe form of Erythema Multiforme characterized by blistery lesions on the mucous membranes of the mouth, throat, anogenital region, eyelids and corneal lining. Established in 1995, the group's mission is to provide current information on SJS, its causes and treatments, and to distribute this information through a nationwide networking system. Educational materials include reprints of current medical information on SJS.

President: Jean Farrell
Year Established: 1995
Organization Members: 7

Publishes the following materials:
SJS Support. The Julie Foundation for Allergic Drug Reactions ~ *Mission Statement*
Julie's Story ~ *Biography*

1504 STICKLER INVOLVED PEOPLE (SIP)
15 Angelina
Augusta, KS 67010 316-775-2993
E-mail: houch@southwind.net
http://geocities.com/hotsprings/9572

The Stickler Involved People (SIP) is a voluntary organization dedicated to educating and giving support to those affected by Stickler Syndrome. Stickler Syndrome is a rare genetic disorder that affects connective tissue, including the joints, eyes, palate, heart, and hearing. The disorder is characterized by possible vision problems, hearing loss, early arthritis, cleft palate, and heart murmurs. The disorder is extremely variable from case to case. Established in 1995, the organization focuses on patient networking and communication as the most effective and personal means of helping people who have this condition. In addition, the group utilizes its newsletter and on-line correspondence to continue and further develop interpatient contact. SIP publishes disease and treatment-specific informational brochures, a quarterly self-titled newsletter, and physician updates; relays past experiences, advice, and ways to cope from individuals who are willing to share their stories; and offers a networking service and a database of information for affected individuals. The group hopes to develop a "pen pal" system for patients, families, and friends.

President: Pat Houchin (Coordinator) (1995 to Present).
Year Established: 1995
Organization Members: 300

Publishes the following materials:
What You Need To Know First!! ~ *Brochure*
Stickler Involved People Newsletter (September 1996) ~ *Newsletter*
Stickler Involved People Newsletter (March 1997) ~ *Newsletter*
Stickler Incvolved People. Annual Financial Report ~ *Financial Statement*
Stickler Syndrome. Genetic Screening Information ~ *Brochure*
Stickler syndrome: A Diagnostic Aid ~ *Brochure*
Ideas. We want to Share ~ *Brochure*
Stickler Syndrome. What your Doctor Needs to Know ~ *Brochure*

Concerned with the following diseases or disorders:
Stickler Syndrome

1505 STICKLER SYNDROME SUPPORT GROUP
27 Braycourt Avenue
Walton-on-the-Thames
Surrey, KT12 2A2
United Kingdom 01932229421

The Stickler Syndrome Support Group is a voluntary health organization located in the United Kingdom. The Group is dedicated to the support of parents of children with this rare genetic disorder. Stickler Syndrome is a rare genetic disorder that affects connective tissue, including the joints, eyes, palate, heart, and hearing. The disorder is characterized by possible vision problems, hearing loss, early arthritis, cleft palate, and heart murmurs. The disorder is extremely variable from case to case. The Support Group offers parents an opportunity to contact other affected families for support, information, and advice. Through the Group's newsletter, parents can share experiences and keep abreast of new advances in medical research. The Group plans to maintain a comprehensive registry of people who have been diagnosed with this disorder. Educational materials distributed by the organization include an informational brochure and reprints of articles from medical literature.

Executive Director: Wendy Hughes
Year Established: 1990
Organization Members: 600

Concerned with the following diseases or disorders:
Stickler Syndrome

1506 STRANG-CORNELL HEREDITARY COLON CANCER PROGRAM (SCPC)

428 East 72nd Street
New York, NY 10021 212-746-5656
Fax: 212-746-8765
E-mail: mbertag@mail.med.cornell.edu
http://www.strang.org

The Strang-Cornell Hereditary Colon Cancer Program (SCPC) is a not-for-profit organization dedicated to providing individuals with Familial Adenomatous Polyposis (FAP) and Hereditary Nonpolyposis Colorectal Cancer (HNPCC) clinical and educational services, as well as to foster participation in research. Colorectal cancer is a common disease in the United States. While most cases of colorectal cancer are sporadic, up to ten percent are hereditary. Hereditary colorectal cancer includes the polyposis syndromes, of which Familial Adenomatious Polyposis is the most common, and the nonpolyposis syndromes, broadly referred to as Hereditary Nonpolyposis Colorectal Cancer. Established in 1934, this program is a collaboration between the Strang Cancer Prevention Center and the New York Hospital-Cornell Medical Center. SCPC includes three divisions: registries for FAP and HNPCC, which are maintained with the assistance of a full-time registrar; clinical and pre-clinical research, including the study of predictors of malignant potential, chemoprevention of colon cancer, gastrointestinal immune function, molecular diagnostics, and dietary intervention; and clinical services, inclusive of medical and surgical treatment, with specialists in nutrition, psychological and genetic counseling. Educational materials include two pamphlets entitled "Nutrition Consultation Program" and "Hereditary Colon Cancer Program." Program activities include a support group, genetic counseling, patientnetworking, education, and referrals. SCPC can be reached at its e-mail address at [MBERTAG@mail.med.cornell.edu] or its web site at [www.strang.org].

President: Michael B. Osborne, M.D. (1996 to Present)
Executive Director: Andrew J. Dannenburg, M.D.
Organization Language: Spanish. Chinese.
Year Established: 1934
Organization Members: Non-Membership

Publishes the following materials:
Nutrition Consultation Program ~ *Brochure*
Hereditary Colon Cancer Program ~ *Brochure*

Concerned with the following diseases or disorders:
Polyposis, Familial

1507 STURGE-WEBER FOUNDATION (SWF)

P.O. Box 418
Mt. Freedom, NJ 07970-0418 973-895-4114
800-627-5482
Fax: 973-895-4846
E-mail: SWF@pobox.com
http://www.pobox.com/~swf

The Sturge-Weber Foundation (SWF) is a not-for-profit organization for parents, professionals, and others concerned with Sturge-Weber Syndrome (SWS). A congenital disorder of unknown cause, SWS is characterized by facial discoloration and neurological abnormalities. Established in 1987, the Sturge-Weber Foundation is dedicated to acting as a clearinghouse of information on all aspects of Sturge-Weber Syndrome and offering support to all interested parties. The group seeks to educate the medical community, government agencies, and the general public about SWS; promote the funding of ongoing medical research on the disorder; and establish a registry of individuals with Sturge-Weber Syndrome. The Sturge-Weber Foundation provides appropriate referrals and offers a variety of educational and support materials. These include a resource guide, medical articles, and brochures on all aspects of Sturge-Weber Syndrome. Other educational resources available from the Foundation include booklets, physical recommendation papers, a VHS video tape, and a quarterly newsletter.

Executive Director: Karen Ball
Organization Language: Italian. Spanish. French.
Year Established: 1987

Publishes the following materials:
Research Pledge Program ~ *Brochure*

The Laymen's Guide to Sturge-Weber Medical Terminology ~ *Brochure*
A Guide For Schools ~ *Brochure*
What is Glaucoma? ~ *Fact Sheet*
A Booklet for Kids ~ *Booklet*
Laser Treatment for Port Wine Stains ~ *Booklet*
Color Me Different - Color Me The Same ~ *Coloring Book*
Branching Out ~ *Newsletter*
The Sturge-Weber Foundation Resource Guide ~ *Resource Guide*
"Branching out with Wisdom" ~ *Handbook*
Sturge-Weber Syndrome ~ *Membership Application*
SWF Education Materials ~ *Resource List*

Concerned with the following diseases or disorders:
Cavernous Hemangioma; Klippel Trenaunay Syndrome; Sturge Weber Syndrome

1508 STUTTERING FOUNDATION OF AMERICA (SFA)

PO Box 11749
3100 Walnut Grove Road #603
Memphis, TN 38111-0749 901-452-7343
800-992-9392
Fax: 901-452-3931
E-mail: stuttersfa@aol.com
http://www.stuttersfa.org

The Stuttering Foundation of America (SFA) is a not-for-profit organization dedicated to people affected by stuttering. Established in 1947, SFA is dedicated to the improved treatment and the prevention of stuttering. The Foundation publishes a periodic newsletter and numerous informational brochures including "If You Think Your Child Is Stuttering," "The Child Who Stutters at School: Notes to the Teacher," "Turning to Therapy," and "Using the Telephone, A Guide for People Who Stutter." Several publications are also directed toward medical professionals who serve the stuttering community. The Foundation maintains a toll-free Hotline on stuttering and a nationwide resource list for individuals seeking a speech-language pathologist who specializes in stuttering. In addition, the Foundation in collaboration with Northwestern University co-sponsors an annual "Workshop for Specialists: Stuttering Therapy." This is an in-depth two week training program.

President: Jane Fraser (1982 to Present)
Organization Language: Spanish (written).
Year Established: 1947
Organization Members: Non-Membership

Publishes the following materials:
Services Provided By The Stuttering Foundation Of America ~ *Fact Sheet*
Stuttering Foundation Of America ~ *Catalog*
Hot To React When Speaking With Sommeone Who Stutters ~ *Fact Sheet*
Using The Telephone A Guide for People Who Stutter ~ *Brochure*
If You Think Your Child Is Stuttering ~ *Brochure*
The Child Who Stutters at School: Notes to the Teacher ~ *Brochure*
Turning on to Therapy ~ *Brochure*
National Stuttering Awareness Week ~ *Brochure*
Stuttering Foundation of America ~ *Newsletter*
A Stutterer's Story ~ *Book*
Stuttering and Your Child: Questions and Answers ~ *Book*
Do You Stutter: A Guide for Teens ~ *Book*
Stuttering Therapy: Prevention and Intervention with Children ~ *Book*
Stuttering Therapy: Transfer and Maintenance ~ *Book*
Counseling Stutterers ~ *Book*
If Your Child Stutters ~ *Book*
Therapy For Stutterers ~ *Book*
Stuttering: An Integration of Contemporary Therapies ~ *Book*
Treating the School Age Stutterer: A Guide for Clinicians ~ *Book*
To The Stutterer ~ *Book*
Stuttering: Successes and Failures in Therapy ~ *Book*
Self-Therapy for the Stutterer ~ *Book*

1509 SUDDEN INFANT DEATH SYNDROME ALLIANCE, INC. (SIDS ALLIANCE)

1314 Bedford Avenue
Suite 210
Baltimore, MD 21208 410-653-8226
800-221-7437
Fax: 410-653-8709
E-mail: sidshq@charm.net

The Sudden Infant Death Syndrome Alliance is a national voluntary health organization uniting parents, caregivers, and researchers with government, business, and community service groups in a nationwide movement to advance the support of SIDS families and hasten the elimination of SIDS through medical research. The SIDS Alliance was created in 1987 as an umbrella organization for the many diverse national, regional, and local agencies involved in SIDS. In 1991, these organizations formally merged operations and the Sudden Infant Death Syndrome Alliance became an organization dedicated exclusively to solving the mystery of SIDS. The SIDS Alliance funds medical research and offers emotional support nationally and locally. Programs include support to families who have lost babies to SIDS. The Alliance supplies up-to-date information on SIDS to the public, particularly new and expectant parents. The organization operates a nationwide 24-hour toll-free hotline.

President: Parker K. Petit (1991-Present)
Executive Director: Judith S. Jacobson
Year Established: 1987
Organization Chapters: 53
Organization Members: 3,000

Publishes the following materials:
What Every Parent Should Know ~ *Brochure*
Facts About SIDS ~ *Brochure*
Synopsis ~ *Newsletter*

Concerned with the following diseases or disorders:
Apnea, Infantile; Sudden Infant Death Syndrome

1510 SUPPORT GROUP FOR 9P-

c/o Beverly Udell
675 North Round Table Drive
Las Vegas, NV 89110 702-453-0788
Fax: 702-453-0788

The Support Group for 9p- is a voluntary not-for-profit organization dedicated to providing information and support to parents of children with 9p- Syndrome and health care professionals who work with affected individuals. 9p- Syndrome is a rare chromosomal disorder caused by a partial deletion of the short arm (p) of chromosome 9. The disorder may be characterized by abnormalities of the head and face, a short neck, widely spaced nipples, genital abnormalities, and/or moderate mental retardation. Established in the mid-1980s, the Support Group for 9p- is dedicated to educating affected individuals and family members, professionals, and the general public. The Support Group also supports and promotes research, provides appropriate referrals, and offers a variety of educational and support materials, including reports and brochures.

President: Jonathan Storr (Co-Chairperson)
Executive Director: Beverly Udell
Year Established: 1984
Organization Members: 75

Concerned with the following diseases or disorders:
Chromosome 9, Partial Monosomy 9p

1511 SUPPORT GROUP FOR BRACHIAL PLEXUS INJURY (SGBP)

18 Staci Lane
Webster, NY 14580 716-787-0197
Fax: 716-872-6158
E-mail: JDeBryne@aol.com

The Support Group for Brachial Plexus Injury was established in 1990 to provide resources and emotional support to families impacted by Erb's Palsy and other brachial plexus injuries by advising on how best to receive and obtain insurance and treatment for this disorder. Erb's Palsy is caused by an injury to one of more of the nerves that control the muscles of the shoulder and upper extremities (upper brachial plexus) and is characterized by a paralysis of the shoulder and upper extremity. Erb's Palsy usually occurs in newborns and as a result of a difficult delivery.

President: Jeff DeBryne (1997 to present)
Year Established: 1990
Organization Members: Non-Membership

Concerned with the following diseases or disorders:
Erb's Palsy

1512 SUPPORT GROUP FOR MONOSOMY 9P

43304 Kipton Nickle Plate Road
LaGrange, OH 44050 216-775-4255
E-mail: jstorr@ix.netcom.com

The Support Group for Monosomy 9P is a national self-help organization that distributes information on monosomy 9P to interested individuals. As a forum for sharing, the organization enables parents with children with monosomy 9P to exchange their experiences for the purpose of mutual support and assistance. Medically oriented information is also available to health care professionals. Established in 1984, the Network maintains a listing of affected families and offers it to first time callers who wish to network with other affected families. The Network also seeks to foster ongoing research into the nature of monosomy 9P. The organization distributes an educational brochure on this disorder.

Executive Director: John Storr
Organization Language: Spanish. Japanese.
Year Established: 1984
Organization Members: 100

Publishes the following materials:
Support for 9P- ~ *Factsheet*
Support for 9P ~ *Brochure*
Apoyo Para 9P ~ *Factsheet*

Concerned with the following diseases or disorders:
Chromosome 9, Partial Monosomy 9p

1513 SUPPORT FOR FAMILIES WITH CHILDREN HAVING WEAVER SYNDROME

4357 153rd Avenue
SE
Belluvue, WA 98006 206-747-5382

Support for Families with Children Having Weaver Syndrome is a voluntary advocacy organization dedicated to providing support and information to families and caregivers of individuals with Weaver Syndrome. This is a rare disorder characterized by faster than normal physical growth and bone development, distinct facial abnormalities, and developmental delays. Established in 1995, Support for Families with Children Having Weaver Syndrome is a grassroots organization committed to establishing a network for affected individuals and developing comprehensive information on treatment options. Recommendations for optimal education and physical and social development are also made by the group. The organization supports ongoing medical research to determine the underlying cause of Weaver Syndrome.

President: Patty Mayer and Jane Croteau
Year Established: 1995
Organization Members: 10

Concerned with the following diseases or disorders:
Weaver Syndrome

1514 SWEDISH SJOGREN'S SYNDROME ASSOCIATION

Box 359
Malmo, 20123
Sweden 46 40 97 7955
Fax: 46 46 30 7353
E-mail: mailbox@sjogrensyndrom.se
http://www.sjogrensyndrom.se

The Swedish Sjogren's Syndrome Association is an international not-for-profit organization dedicated to providing information and support to individuals with Sjogren's Syndrome, family members, and health care professionals. Sjogren's Syndrome, a disorder of unknown cause, is characterized by deficient moisture production of the mucous-secreting glands, particularly the tear ducts of the eyes (lacrimal) and the salivary glands of the mouth. Associated symptoms and physical abnormalities may include abnomal dryness, itching, and burning of the eyes (keratoconjunctivitis sicca); abnormal dryness of the mouth, resulting in cavities, other dental disorders, and loss of odor and taste sensations; and, when the lungs are affected, increased susceptibility to repeated respiratory infections. Many affected individuals also experience rheumatoid arthritis. Sjogren's Syndrome, which primarily affects middle-aged women, is thought to be due to an abnormal autoimmune response. Established in 1989, the Swedish Sjogren's Syndrome Association provides networking opportunities that enable affected individuals and family members to exchange information, support, and resources; engages in patient education; and offers a variety of materials including reports and a regular newsletter. The Association also has a web site on the Internet in both English and Swedish that explains the history of Sjogren's Syndrome, discusses current research in Sweden and around the world, provides information concerning the disorder, and offers dynamic linkage to other helpful sources of information on the Internet.

President: Inger Siwersson
Organization Language: Swedish (written/spoken).
Year Established: 1989
Organization Members: 800

Publishes the following materials:
Torkarbladet ~ *Newsletter*
Torkarbladet Sjogrens Syndrom ~ *Newsletter*

Concerned with the following diseases or disorders:
Sjogren Syndrome

1515 TAR SYNDROME ASSOCIATION (TARSA)

212 Sherwood Drive
Linwood, NJ 08221 609-927-0418
Fax: 609-653-8639
E-mail: spp212@aol.com

The TAR Syndrome Association, also known as TARSA, is an international not-for-profit self-help organization that was established in 1981. The group functions as a support system and educational resource for families affected by Thrombocytopenia Absent Radius (TAR) Syndrome. TAR Syndrome is a rare hereditary disorder characterized by abnormally low levels of circulating blood platelets and underdevelopment or absence of the radius, one of the bones of the forearm. In some cases, symptoms may include kidney abnormalities and congenital heart disease. Educational materials produced by the TAR Syndrome Association include informational brochures and an annual newsletter.

President: Sandra Puriton (1981-Present)
Year Established: 1981
Organization Members: 100

Concerned with the following diseases or disorders:
Thrombocytopenia Absent Radius Syndrome;
Thrombocytopenia, Essential

1516 TEF/VATER/VACTRL NATIONAL SUPPORT NETWORK

15301 Grey Fox Road
Upper Marlboro, MD 20772 301-952-6837
Fax: 301-952-6837

The TEF/VATER/VACTRL National Support Network is a voluntary not-for-profit self-help organization dedicated to providing information and support to adults and families of children with narrowing of the esophageal atresia, tracheoesophageal fistula, and VATER/VACTRL Association. Esophageal atresia is a condition in which the tube that carries food from the mouth to the stomach (esophagus) ends in a pouch instead of connecting to the stomach. Tracheoesophageal fistula is an abnormal connection between the esophagus and the windpipe (trachea) that may result in food being aspirated into the lungs. VATER Association is a rare disorder that affects several organ systems of the body. VATER/VACTERL is an acronym that stands for (V)ertebral defects, (A)nal atresia/imperforate anus, (C)ardiac defects, (T)racheo(E)sophageal defects, (R)enal defects, or (R)adial (L)imbs defects. Established in 1992, the TEF/VATER/VACTRL National Support Network is committed to promoting and supporting research, engaging in patient advocacy, ensuring the appropriate treatment of affected individuals, and promoting patient and professional education. The Network also provides appropriate referrals, such as to genetic counseling; promotes legislation beneficial to affected individuals; and offers a variety of educational and support materials through its database, directory, brochures, and a regular newsletter.

Executive Director: Greg Burke, P.A.
Year Established: 1992
Organization Chapters: 8
Organization Members: 250

Concerned with the following diseases or disorders:
Esophageal Atresia and/or Tracheoesophageal Fistula; VACTERL Association

1517 TMJ ASSOCIATION, LTD.

PO Box 26770
Milwaukee, WI 53226-0770 414-259-3223
Fax: 414-259-8122
E-mail: TMJ@execpc.com

The TMJ (Temporomandibular Joint) Association, Ltd. is a national not-for-profit voluntary organization that promotes awareness of temporomandibular joint disorders and provides information and support for people with TMJ disorders and their families through the development of a national network of members. In addition, the Association promotes research into the causes of TMJ and the development of safe and effective treatments. Established in 1986, the Association has provided testimony to a special National Institute of Dental Research panel and played an instrumental role in NIH's utilization of a multi-institute approach to basic research of temporomandibular joint disorders. Additional testimony before the Senate Appropriations Committee played a vital role in the creation of an intensive educational program for medical professionals and the public and the stimulation of controlled scientific research into the nature of the disorder. In addition, the Association was instrumental in notifying the national media about the Vitek implant recall and creating a TMJ implant registry. The Association publishes a quarterly newsletter that keeps readers updated on current research and medical, legal, legislative, and insurance issues; the newsletter also provides a forum for sharing ideas and asking questions. In addition, the TMJ Association provides informational brochures and pamphlets.

President: Terrie Cowley (1991-Present)
Year Established: 1986
Organization Chapters: 28
Organization Members: 5,000

Publishes the following materials:
Lifeline ~ *Newsletter*
TMD ~ *Reprint*
TMD Temporomandibular Disorders ~ *Pamphlet*
The TMJ Association: Help and Hope ~ *Brochure*
Temporomandibular Joint Disorders ~ *Brochure*
Causes ~ *Brochure*
Diagnosis ~ *Brochure*
The TMJ Report ~ *Newsletter*

Concerned with the following diseases or disorders:
Temporomandibular Joint Dysfunction (TMJ)

1518 TARDIVE DYSKINESIA/TARDIVE DYSTONIA NATIONAL ASSOCIATION (TD/TDNA)

4424 University Way NE
P.O. Box 45732
Seattle, WA 98145-0732 206-522-3166

The Tardive Dyskinesia/Tardive Dystonia National Association (TD/TDNA) is a voluntary not-for-profit self-help organization dedicated to providing information and support to individuals with Tardive Dyskinesia or Tardive Dystonia, family members, health care professionals, and the general public. Tardive Dyskinesia is an involuntary movement disorder resulting from use of neuroleptic drugs that are prescribed to control psychiatric or gastrointestinal problems. Tardive Dystonia is a minor variant of Tardive Dyskinesia. Established in 1988, TD/TDNA is committed to encouraging research on Tardive Dyskinesia and Tardive Dystonia; enabling affected individuals to exchange information, support, and resources through its networking program; and advocating on behalf of affected individuals. TD/TDNA also engages in patient and professional education; provides appropriate referrals; and conducts national and international workshops. In addition, the Tardive Dyskinesia/Tardive Dystonia National Association offers a variety of educational materials to affected individuals, family members, health care professionals, and the general public, including reports, journal article reprints, and brochures.

President: Thomas Graham, III
Executive Director: Sonya Kjaer
Year Established: 1988
Organization Members: 3,000

Concerned with the following diseases or disorders:
Tardive Dyskinesia

1519 TOURETTE SYNDROME ASSOCIATION, INC. (TSA)

42-40 Bell Boulevard
Bayside, NY 11361-2861 718-224-2999
888-486-8738
Fax: 718-279-9596
E-mail: tourette@ix.netcom.com
http://TSA.mgh.harvard.edu/

The Tourette Syndrome Association, Inc. (TSA) is a national nonprofit organization dedicated to serving the needs of individuals affected by Tourette Syndrome and their families. Tourette Syndrome (TS) is a hereditary neurologic movement disorder characterized by repetitive motor and vocal tics. Symptoms may include involuntary movement of the extremities, shoulders, and face accompanied by uncontrollable sounds and/or inappropriate words. Symptoms tend to be variable and follow a chronic waxing and waning course. Founded in 1972 and currently consisting of 54 chapters and approximately 8,000 members, TSA's mission is to identify the cause, find a cure, and control the effects of Tourette Syndrome. To this end, TSA facilitates a research grant award program and coordinates both a volunteer national Medical Advisory Board and a Scientific Advisory Board. The Association produces a variety of educational materials including brochures, a quarterly newsletter, and videotapes. In addition, TSA maintains a crisis hotline, provides physician referral listings, and engages in patient advocacy.

President: Alfred Sklaver (1994-Present)
Executive Director: Judit Unger
Year Established: 1972
Organization Chapters: 54
Organization Members: 7,800

Publishes the following materials:
Catalog of Videos ~ *Brochure*
Questions and Answers about Tourette Syndrome ~ *Brochure*
Catalog of Publications and Films ~ *Brochure*
TSA Permanent Research Fund Recipients: 1994 ~ *Brochure*
Tourette Syndrome Association, Inc. Newsletter ~ *Newsletter*
Brain Bank Brochure ~ *Brochure*

Concerned with the following diseases or disorders:
Obsessive Compulsive Disorder; Tourette Syndrome

1520 TOURETTE SYNDROME FOUNDATION OF CANADA (TSFC)

3675 Keele Street
Suite 203
North York
Ontario, M3J 1M6
Canada 416-636-2800
800-361-3120
Fax: 416-636-1688
E-mail: tsfc.org@sympatico.ca

The Tourette Syndrome Foundation of Canada (TSFC) is a national voluntary health organization dedicated to providing support and information to Canadian families affected by Tourette Syndrome. Tourette Syndrome (TS) is a hereditary neurologic movement disorder characterized by repetitive motor and vocal tics. Symptoms may include involuntary movements of the extremities, shoulders, and face accompanied by uncontrollable sounds and/or inappropriate words. Symptoms tend to be variable and follow a chronic waxing and waning course. TSFC's mission is to help families affected by Tourette Syndrome by gathering and distributing information about the disorder; promoting local self-help and professional services; and stimulating and funding research into the cause, treatment, and potential cure of TS. Founded in 1976 and consisting of 26 chapters, TSFC organizes workshops and symposiums to increase the knowledge and sensitivity of health care professionals; provides periodic forums for scientists, clinicians, and others working in the field of Tourette Syndrome; develops and maintains lists of physicians who diagnose and treat TS; and supports the Brain Bank Program and collaborates with other agencies dealing with neurological disorders. The Foundation publishes a tri-annual newsletter entitled "The Green Leaflet" and provides brochures, pamphlets, reports, and audiovisual aids.

President: Judy Rogers (1997 to Present)
Executive Director: Rosie Wartecker
Organization Language: French (written/spoken).
Year Established: 1976
Organization Chapters: 26
Organization Members: 1,500

Publishes the following materials:
Questions and Answers on Tourette Syndrome (French) ~ *Brochure*
Questions and Answers on Tourette Syndrome ~ *Brochure*
The Green Leaflet (English/French) ~ *Newsletter*

Concerned with the following diseases or disorders:
Tourette Syndrome

1521 TRACHEO OESOPHAGEAL FISTULA SUPPORT GROUP (TOFS)

St. George's Centre
91 Victory Road
Netherfield
Nottingham, NG4 2NN
United Kingdom 0115 9400694
Fax: 0115 9400694
E-mail: dobbs@nnotts.co.uk
http://www.cityscape.co.uk/users/jw58/

The Tracheo Oesophageal Fistula Support Group (TOFSG) is an international voluntary organization dedicated to providing information and support to parents who have a child born with tracheo-esophogeal fistula (TOF). In TOF, a section of the baby's throat is abnormally joined to the windpipe (esophagus) making it difficult for food and saliva to pass into the stomach. Established in 1982, TOFSG consists of an 800 plus family membership and a national network of volunteers, all of whom are parents of children with TOF. The Support Group receives calls from affected families and professionals; maitains contact with sister organizations in other countries; and maitains a databank of information on matters such as feeding problems, tube feeding, and financial assistance. A video has been produced that explains the condition and the problems affecting children with TOF. In addition, TOFSG raises funds to support its own work, to purchase equipment for hospitals and individuals, and to finance research. Support groups for affected individuals, family members, and healthcare professionals are provided along with educational materials. In addition to educational materials, audiovisual aides entitled, "Your Life In Their Hands," "History of TOF," and "Reach," along with many others are available. A national conference for members and professionals is organized every two years. A yearly magazine entitled "Chew" and a bi-monthly newsletter are also available. Fund-raising is undertaken to assist hospitals to purchase specialized equipment. The group operates a site on the World Wide Web at [http://www.cityscape.co.uk/users/jw58/].

President: David Dobbs, M.D. (Chairman)
Executive Director: Christine Sherterd (Secretary)
Organization Language: French (written). Italian (written).
Year Established: 1982
Organization Members: 600

Publishes the following materials:
For Babies Born Unable to Swallow ~ *Brochure*
Oseophageal Atresia and Tracheo Oesophageal Fistula ~ *Pamphlet*
TOFS ~ *Mission Statement*
Tracheo Oesophageal Fistula and Oesophageal Atresia ~ *Pamphlet*
TOFS. For babies born unable to swallow ~ *Brochure*
The teacher's guide to the TOF child ~ *Brochure*
Vater Association. A basic guide ~ *Brochure*
Oesophageal Atresia and Tracheo Oesophageal Fistula. A Guide for New Parents ~ *Leaflet*
Tracheo-Oesophageal Fistula support. A registered charity for babies born unable to swallow ~ *Mission Statement*
Tracheo Oesophageal Fistula and Oesophageal Atresia ~ *Pamphlet*
The TOF Child. The Early Years ~ *Fact Sheet*
Chest Problems after Repair of Tracheo-Oesophageal Fistula and Oesophageal Atresia ~ *Reprint*
TOFS News (April 1997) ~ *Newsletter*
TOF Video Loan List ~ *List*

Concerned with the following diseases or disorders:
Gastroesophageal Reflux; VACTERL Association

1522 TRANSVERSE MYELITIS ASSOCIATION (TMA)

3548 Tahoma Place West
Tacoma, WA 98466-2142 253-565-8156
E-mail: srulyosef@aol.com
http://members.aol.com/TMAssocWA/index.html

The Transverse Myelitis Association (TMA) is a not-for-profit self-help organization dedicated to providing mutual support to families affected by transverse myelitis. Transverse myelitis is an acute spinal cord inflammation involving both sides of the spinal cord. Established in 1994, the Transverse Myelitis Association enables affected families to exchange information, support, and resources; engages in patient advocacy; provides a pen pal service; conducts group meetings; and offers phone support. The Association also offers appropriate referrals; engages in patient and professional education; and serves as a clearinghouse of information on transverse myelitis, offering a variety of reports and brochures.

President: Deanne Gilmur
Year Established: 1994

Concerned with the following diseases or disorders:
Myelitis

1523 TREACHER COLLINS FOUNDATION (TCF)

P.O. Box 683
Norwich, VT 05055-0683 802-649-3050
800-823-2055

The Treacher Collins Foundation is an organization of families, individuals, and medical professionals who are interested in developing and sharing knowledge and experiences about Treacher Collins Syndrome and related conditions. A national voluntary health organization, the Foundation seeks to support, inform, and network families and individuals with these conditions and to serve as a resource for current information about Treacher Collins Syndrome. Established in 1988, the Treacher Collins Foundation provides medical referrals, educational materials, and information on other service providers who are familiar with Treacher Collins Syndrome. Recognizing the value of mutual peer support, the Foundation cites networking as a primary goal. In addition, the Foundation promotes medical research activities aimed at improving the quality of life of people with Treacher Collins Syndrome and related disorders. Specific educational materials produced by the organization include a newsletter, booklets, bibliographies, vocabulary lists, and resources and referral lists.

President: David Drazin, Ph.D.
Executive Director: Hope Charkins M.S.W.
Year Established: 1988

Publishes the following materials:
The Treacher Collins Foundation Welcomes You ~ *Brochure*
Treacher Collins Syndrome: An Overview ~ *Brochure*
Treacher Collins Syndrome - Vocabulary List ~ *Vocabulary List*
American Resource List ~ *Pamphlet*
Treacher Collins Syndrome Bibliography ~ *Bibliography*
Newsletter ~ *Newsletter*

Concerned with the following diseases or disorders:
Treacher Collins Syndrome

1524 TRIAD SICKLE CELL ANEMIA FOUNDATION (TSCAF)

1102 East Market Street
P.O. Box 20964
Greensboro, NC 27401 910-274-1507
800-733-8297
Fax: 910-275-7984
http://www.greensboro.com/sickle/

The Triad Sickle Cell Anemia Foundation is a non-profit community health agency committed to providing a comprehensive array of services to individuals with sickle cell disease, their families, and the community. Founded in 1971 by a group of concerned citizens, the Triad Sickle Cell Anemia Foundation continues to improve the quality of life for people with sickle cell disease and their families. The Triad Sickle Cell Anemia Foundation offers a variety of educational and support services including sickle cell screening and genetic counseling; educational presentations and health fairs; case management services and home health care; sickle cell clinics; summer enrichment camps; and psychological counseling and support groups. Other unique services include daycare referrals, education and employment assistance, financial assistance, healthcare referrals, in-school counseling, medical reimbursement referrals, tutoring, transportation, and vocational rehabilitation referrals.

President: Thomas Boone (1993-Present)
Executive Director: Gladys Robinson
Year Established: 1971

Publishes the following materials:
About Sickle-Cell Trait and Anemia ~ *Booklet*
Learning About Hemoglobins ~ *Booklet*
Your Child and Sickle Cell Anemia ~ *Booklet*
Fact Sheet for Parents of Newborns who have Sickle Cell-Thalassemia Disease ~ *Fact Sheet*
Fact Sheet for Parents of Newborns who have Sickle Cell Trait ~ *Fact Sheet*
Fact Sheet for Parents of Newborns who have Sickle Cell Anemia ~ *Fact Sheet*
Fact Sheet for Parents of Newborns who have Sickle Cell-Hemoglobin C Disease ~ *Fact Sheet*
Fact Sheet on Thalassemia ~ *Fact Sheet*
Fact Sheet on Hemoglobin C ~ *Fact Sheet*
Fact Sheet for Parents of Newborns who have Hemoglobin C Trait ~ *Fact Sheet*
Fact Sheet on Sickle-Beta Thalassemia Disease ~ *Fact Sheet*
Improving the Quality of Life for Sickle Cell Disease Patients and Their Families ~ *Brochure*
Sickle Cell Disease in Newborns and Infants - A Guide for Parents ~ *Brochure*

Concerned with the following diseases or disorders:
Sickle Cell Disease

1525 TRIGEMINAL NEURALGIA ASSOCIATION (TNA)

P.O. Box 340
Barnegat Light, NJ 08006 609-361-1014
Fax: 609-361-0982
E-mail: tna@csionline.net
neurosurgery.mgh.harvard.edu/tna/#services

The Trigeminal Neuralgia Association is a national voluntary not-for-profit organization dedicated to providing information, mutual aid, support, and encouragement to people with Trigeminal Neuralgia (TN) and their families. Trigeminal Neuralgia (or Tic Douloureux) is a disorder of the trigeminal (fifth) cranial nerve that causes intense, episodic pain in areas of the face supplied by the trigeminal nerve. Founded in 1990, the Association is also committed to increasing public and professional awareness of the disorder and reducing the isolation of those affected by Trigeminal Neuralgia. The organization serves as a resource and information clearinghouse to centralize current data and medical efforts on treatment of TN and encourages medical research to determine the cause of and effective treatment for this disorder. The Association's Medical Advisory Board consists of key specialists in the medical and surgical treatment of TN, dentistry, and pain management. The Trigeminal Neuralgia Association also has a network of local support groups that enable affected individuals to share experiences, receive support and encouragement, and obtain current information on the disorder's treatment. In addition, the Association promotes patient advocacy; provides appropriate referrals; and conducts an educational outreach program to medical and dental practitioners and the general public. The Association produces and distributes a wide variety of educational materials including a quarterly newsletter and brochures.

President: Claire W. Patterson (1990-Present)
Executive Director: Claire W. Patterson
Year Established: 1990
Organization Chapters: 13
Organization Members: 2,500

Publishes the following materials:
TNA MUTUAL SUPPORT GROUPS/CONTACT PERSONS ~ *Factsheet*
Information, Support, Encouragement... ~ *Brochure*
TNAlert ~ *Newsletter*

Concerned with the following diseases or disorders:
Trigeminal Neuralgia (Tic Douloureux)

1526 TRISOMY 12P PARENT SUPPORT ORGANIZATION

105 Mill Pond Road
Roswell, GA 30076 770-993-4796

The Trisomy 12p Parent Support Organization is an international not-for-profit self-help organization dedicated to providing information, assistance, and support to families of individuals with trisomies of the short arm ("p") of chromosome 12 or other abnormalities involving the 12th chromosome. Chromosome 12, Trisomy 12p is an extremely rare chromosomal disorder in which a portion of the short arm of the 12th chromosome (12p) appears three times (trisomy) rather than twice in cells of the body. The disorder may be characterized by abnormal growth delays after birth (postnatal growth retardation); delays in the acquisition of skills requiring the coordination of mental and muscular activity (psychomotor retardation); mental retardation; abnormally diminished muscle tone (hypotonia); characteristic malformations of the head and facial (craniofacial) area; abnormally short, wide hands; and/or other abnormalities. Associated symptoms and physical findings may vary from case to case, depending upon the exact length and location of the duplicated portion of chromosome 12p. Established in 1997, the Trisomy 12p Parent Support Organization provides networking opportunities that enable affected families to exchange information, support, and helpful resources.

Executive Director: Cindy Smith
Year Established: 1997
Organization Members: 20

1527 TRISOMY 9 INTERNATIONAL PARENT SUPPORT (9-TIPS)

Children's Hospital
Div. Gen. & Met.
3901 Beaubien Boulevard
Detroit, MI 48201-2196 909-862-4470
E-mail: atoddna@sprynet.com

Trisomy 9 International Parent Support (TIPS) is a not-for-profit organization that is dedicated to assisting families who have children with Trisomy 9. Chromosomal disorders included are Trisomy 9p, Trisomy 9 Mosaic, Trisomy 9q, Partial Trisomy 9, and other complex chromosomal abnormalities involving extra chromosomal material from chromosome 9. The organization offers an international mutual support network for the purposes of information exchange and emotional support. The network also informs parents of any medical professionals who are familiar with these rare chromosomal disorders. Educational materials include biannual newsletters, a map that details the geographic distribution of cases in the United States, and a bibliography of medical articles related to Trisomy 9.

President: Alice Todd (Contact)
Year Established: N/A
Organization Members: 40

Concerned with the following diseases or disorders:
Chromosome 9, Tetrasomy 9p; Chromosome 9, Trisomy 9P (Multiple Variants); Chromosome 9, Trisomy Mosaic; Trisomy

1528 TUBEROUS SCLEROSIS ASSOCIATION (TSA)

Little Barnsley Farm
Catshill
Bromsgrove
Worcestershire, B61 0NQ
United Kingdom 0 1527 871898
Fax: 0 1527 579419
E-mail: tsassn@compuserve.com
ourworld.compuserve.com/homepages/tsassn

The Tuberous Sclerosis Association (TSA), an international self-help organization located in the United Kingdom, was established in 1977 by a group of parents and interested physicians dedicated to providing support to individuals with Tuberous Sclerosis (TS) and their families, increasing awareness of the disorder, and promoting fundraising to support research. Tuberous Sclerosis, a rare genetic disorder that affects the skin and nervous system, may be characterized by the development of white skin patches, red or brown birthmarks, and/or a characteristic facial rash across the cheeks and nose; developmental delays; episodes of uncontrolled electrical disturbances in the brain that cause convulsive seizures (epilepsy); mental retardation in some cases; and/or the development of benign tumors, particularly of the brain, retina, kidney, heart, and skin. The Tuberous Sclerosis Association has helped to establish specialist, multidisciplinary TS clinics in Leeds, Bath, Cambridge, Northern Ireland (Craigavon), and Scotland (Edinburgh) that offer advice on diagnosis, management, and genetic counseling and work closely with local medical staff involved with the individuals and family members in question. The TSA also supports and promotes research into the causes and management of TS through its Education and Research Fund; is in touch with over 1,000 affected families across the world as well as interested professionals from the medical, social support, and education fields; offers networking opportunities to affected families that enable them to exchange information, support, and resources; and provides support to affected individuals, family members, and caregivers through visits and telephone support. In addition, the Association advises on where to obtain assistance concerning social services, benefits, and educational concerns and has a Family Care Worker who engages in patient and family advocacy. The TSA also has an International TS Research Symposium every three to four years for physicians who are conducting research on all aspects of the disorder; organizes regional meetings with speakers who address local groups; holds an Annual General Meeting for members, friends, and professionals during which physicians gives presentations on Tuberous Sclerosis; and has a Family Weekend Conference when affected families spend time together and benefit from shared experiences. The Tuberous Sclerosis Assocation offers a variety of materials including brochures, leaflets, fact sheets, videos, and a regular newsletter entitled "TS Scan."

President: Janet Medcalf (1986 to Present)
Year Established: 1977
Organization Members: 1,200

Publishes the following materials:
Tuberous Sclerosis...more than just skin deep ~ *Booklet*
Tuberous Sclerosis ~ *Brochure*
What the Teacher of a TS Child Should Know ~ *Brochure*
Tuberous Sclerosis International ~ *Factsheet*
Tuberous Sclerosis Association. Support. Research. Awareness. Education ~ *Brochure*
Tuberous Sclerosis ~ *Brochure*
Tuberous Sclerosis International (French, German, English, Italian, Spanish, Dutch) ~ *Mission Statement*
What the Teacher of a TS Child Should Know ~ *Brochure*

Concerned with the following diseases or disorders:
Tuberous Sclerosis

1529 TUBEROUS SCLEROSIS CANADA (TSCST)

2443 New Wood Drive
Oakville
Ontario, L6H 5Y3
Canada 905-257-1997
800-347-0252
E-mail: jillian.dasilva@ablelink.org

Tuberous Sclerosis Canada Sclerose Tubereuse (TSCST) is a not-for-profit organization dedicated to raising public awareness of Tuberous Sclerosis Complex (TSC); encouraging mutual support between families affected by TSC; and promoting research and education. Tuberous Sclerosis, a rare genetic disorder that affects the skin and nervous system, may be characterized by the development of white skin patches, red or brown birthmarks, and/or a characteristic facial rash across the cheeks and nose; delays in reaching developmental milestones (e.g., sitting, crawling, walking); episodes of uncontrolled electrical disturbances in the brain that cause convulsive seizures (epilepsy); mental retardation in some cases; and/or the development of benign tumors, particularly of the brain, retina, kidney, heart, and skin. Established in 1990 and consisting of 130 members, TSCST facilitates a self-help network in which families affected by Tuberous Sclerosis support one another by telephone and share information about local services that may be available. Educational materials are available in French and English and include a self-titled quarterly newsletter and brochures entitled "There's More You Need to Know About Tuberous Sclerosis" and "Tuberous Sclerosis Complex — What To Expect."

President: Jillian DaSilva (1994 to Present)
Organization Language: French (written/spoken).
Year Established: 1990
Organization Members: 130

Publishes the following materials:
Tuberous Sclerosis Complex. What To Expect (Part I) ~ *Brochure*
Tuberous Sclerosis Complex. Wht To Expect (Part II) ~ *Brochure*
There's More You Need To Know about Tuberous Sclerosis ~ *Brochure*
Tuberous Sclerosis Canada Sclerose Tubereuse ~ *Newsletter Spring 1997*

Concerned with the following diseases or disorders:
Tuberous Sclerosis

1530 TURNER'S SYNDROME SOCIETY

814 Glencairn Avenue
North York
Ontario, M6B 2A3
Canada 416-781-2086
800-465-6744
Fax: 416-781-7245

The Turner's Syndrome Society is a non-profit charitable organization dedicated to improving the quality of life for individuals and families affected by Turner's Syndrome. Turner's Syndrome is a rare chromosomal disorder that affects 1 in approximately 2,500 females. Females normally have two X chromosomes. However, in those with Turner's Syndrome, one X chromosome is absent or is damaged. Affected females may exhibit short stature, webbing of the neck, absence of secondary sexual development, infertility, and/or other abnormalities. Established in 1981, the Turner's Syndrome Society provides support services for individuals with Turner's Syndrome and their families and disseminates up-to-date medical information to affected families, physicians and other health care professionals, and the general public. Educational materials include a quarterly newsletter entitled "Turner's Syndrome News," brochures and booklets such as "The X's and O's of Turner's Syndrome," "Growing Up Small," and "Tall and Small - A Book About Height," and a video documentary entitled "Very Special People." The Society also offers support groups and holds an annual conference that presents new medical findings and provides an opportunity for a free exchange of information between affected individuals and family members. The Society has approximately 500 members and 12 chapters.

President: Mary K.S. Edwards
Executive Director: Sandi Hofbauer
Organization Language: French (written).
Year Established: 1981
Organization Chapters: 12
Organization Members: 500

Publishes the following materials:
The Turner's Syndrome Society ~ *Mission Statement*
The X's and O's of Turner's Syndrome ~ *Booklet*
Turner's Syndrome News ~ *Newsletter*
Resource Order Form - Turner's Syndrome Society ~ *Order Form*

Concerned with the following diseases or disorders:
Turner Syndrome

1531 TURNER'S SYNDROME SOCIETY OF THE UNITED STATES

1313 South East 5th Street
Suite 327
Minneapolis, MN 55414 612-379-3607
800-365-9944
Fax: 612-379-3619
E-mail: tesch005@tc.umn.edu
http://www.turner-syndrome-us.org

Established in 1988, the Turner's Syndrome Society of the United States is a national not-for-profit self-help organization dedicated to increasing awareness and understanding of

Turner's Syndrome and providing an active networking program for affected individuals. Turner's Syndrome is a rare chromosomal disorder in females that is characterized by the absence or abnormalities of one X chromosome. Symptoms may include short stature, lack of sexual development at puberty, a webbed neck, heart defects, and/or other abnormalities. The Society makes referrals to appropriate support and treatment centers and promotes the continuing education of physicians and other health care professionals. In addition, the organization supports ongoing medical research and enables individuals with Turner's Syndrome to exchange information, support, and resources through its networking program. The Turner's Syndrome Society also offers a variety of educational materials including a regular newsletter, audio-visual aids, and brochures.

President: Cheryl Fourt (1995-Present)
Executive Director: Lynn Georgi Tesch
Organization Language: German. Italian.
Year Established: 1988
Organization Chapters: 36
Organization Members: 1,000

Concerned with the following diseases or disorders:
Turner Syndrome

1532 UNITED CEREBRAL PALSY ASSOCIATION (UCPA)

1660 L Street NW
Suite 700
Washington, D.C. 20036 202-776-0406
800-872-5827
Fax: 202-776-0414
TDD: 202-973-7197
E-mail: ucpanatl@ucpa.org
http://www.ucpa.org

The United Cerebral Palsy Association is a national not-for-profit self-help organization dedicated to providing information and support to individuals with Cerebral Palsy and their families. Cerebral Palsy is a neurological movement disorder characterized by lack of muscle control and impairment in the coordination of movement. Established in 1949, the United Cerebral Palsy Association supports its more than 160 local affiliates; these affiliates provide a variety of programs and services for affected families, including support groups. The United Cerebral Palsy Association offers several educational and support materials including a quarterly magazine, regular newsletters, and research reports. In addition, the Association conducts regular forums on America On-Line.

President: Michael Simonson
Executive Director: Michael W. Morris
Year Established: 1949
Organization Chapters: 162

Concerned with the following diseases or disorders:
Cerebral Palsy

1533 UNITED PARKINSON FOUNDATION (UPF)

833 West Washington Boulevard
Chicago, IL 60607 312-733-1893
Fax: 312-733-1896
E-mail: upf_itf@msn.com

The United Parkinson Foundation (UPF) is an international voluntary not-for-profit organization dedicated to patient services; education of affected individuals, family members, and health care professionals; and promotion and support of research for Parkinson's Disease and related disorders. Established in 1963, the United Parkinson Foundation offers an extensive referral service to guide affected individuals to proper diagnosis and clinical care. The organization also provides personal responses by phone or mail to members who contact the Chicago office with specific questions. The Foundation conducts an annual seminar series for affected individuals and family members with presentations by guest speakers from the United Parkinson Foundation's Medical Advisory Board. The United Parkinson Foundation also raises funds to support neurological research in the form of grants to established scientists whose primary interest is Parkinson's Disease. In addition, the United Parkinson Foundation provides referrals to genetic counseling and support groups; promotes patient advocacy; and offers a variety of educational and support materials. These materials include regular newsletters, exercise materials, fact sheets, reports, brochures, audio-visual aids, and information concerning recent advances in research.

President: Harold L. Klawans, M.D.
Executive Director: Judy Rosner
Year Established: 1962
Organization Members: 36,000

Concerned with the following diseases or disorders:
Parkinson's Disease

1534 UNITED SCLERODERMA FOUNDATION, INC. (USF)

P.O. Box 399
Watsonville, CA 95076 408-728-2202
800-722-4673
Fax: 408-728-3328
E-mail: outreach@scruznet.com
http://www.scleroderma.com

The United Scleroderma Foundation, Inc. (USF) is a not-for-profit organization dedicated to providing educational and emotional support for people with scleroderma and their families; increasing awareness of scleroderma; and supporting research to determine the disorder's cause, treatment, and cure. Established in 1975, the United Scleroderma Foundation testifies before Congress concerning the needs of people with scleroderma and works to increase public awareness through all forms of media. The organization raises research funding; institutes research grants; and conducts an annual conference. The Foundation also networks with other national health agencies on common concerns; assists people with scleroderma in securing Social Security and Disability benefits; and works with the medical community to promote better care and treatment. In addition, the United Scleroderma Foundation provides a physician referral service; a list of medical centers with specific interest in scleroderma; and a variety of educational and support materials. These materials include brochures, a regular newsletter, current medical information on scleroderma, videotapes of USF'S annual conferences, and a listing of self-help aids.

President: Jack E. Andrews (1994-Present)
Executive Director: Denise Brockerman
Year Established: 1975
Organization Chapters: 56
Organization Members: 11,935

Publishes the following materials:
United Scleroderma Foundation, Inc. Scope of Services ~ *Fact Sheet*
United Scleroderma Foundation Inc. FACT SHEET ~ *Fact Sheet*

Concerned with the following diseases or disorders:
Mixed Connective Tissue Disease (MCTD); Peyronie Disease; Scleroderma

1535 USHER FAMILY SUPPORT (UFS)

4918 42nd Avenue South
Minneapolis, MN 55417 612-724-6982
E-mail: kadbmn@aol.com

Usher Family Support (UFS) is a newsletter for individuals and family members affected by Usher's Syndrome, a rare inherited disorder characterized by congenital deafness in association with Retinitis Pigmentosa (RP). RP is characterized by degeneration of the retina leading to progressive loss of vision. The UFS Newsletter is published quarterly and contains articles, poems, pictures, and letters of interest to affected individuals and family members. All included materials are reviewed by Usher Family Support's Advisory Board.

Executive Director: Helen Anderson (Contact Person)
Year Established: 1995

Concerned with the following diseases or disorders:
Usher's Syndrome

1536 VHL FAMILY ALLIANCE (VHLFA)

171 Clinton Road
Brookline, MA 02146-5815 617-232-5946
800-767-4845
Fax: 617-734-8233
E-mail: info@vhl.org
http://www.vhl.org

The VHL Family Alliance is a voluntary not-for-profit organization dedicated to improving diagnosis, treatment, and quality of life of individuals and families affected by von Hippel-Lindau Disease (VHL). VHL is an inherited multisystem disorder characterized by the abnormal growth of blood vessels in certain areas of the body (angiomatosis) such as the retinas, the brain, the spinal cord, and/or the adrenal glands. Established in 1993, the Alliance is committed to distributing current information about VHL to affected individuals, family members, and physicians; promoting research studies and providing research grants; establishing a VHL Registry; and enabling affected individuals to exchange information, resources, and mutual support through its networking programs. The Alliance also helps establish standards for clinics that specialize in the diagnosis and treatment of VHL and provides referrals to designated clinical care centers in the United States and across the world. In addition, the Alliance offers telephone support; engages in patient and family advocacy; and assists in the development of local chapters. The organization provides a variety of educational materials including a quarterly newsletter, patient handbooks, guides, booklets, audiovisual aids, and pamphlets. The Alliance provides support materials in several languages including English, French, Spanish, Italian, Dutch, German, Portuguese, Danish, Norwegian, Polish, and Japanese.

President: Joyce Wilcox Graff/Peggy Marshall (Co-Chairs)
Executive Director: Altheada Johnson
Organization Language: Spanish. French. Italian. Dutch. German. Portuguese. Danish. Norwegian. Polish. Japanese.
Year Established: 1993
Organization Chapters: 27

Publishes the following materials:
VHL Family Alliance Annual Report 1993-1994 ~ *Brochure*
VHL Family Forum ~ *Newsletter*
El Arbol Genealogico De Su Salud ~ *Pamphlet*
Todo Lo Que Debe Saber Sobre La Enfermedad De von Hippel-Lindau (VHL) ~ *Pamphlet*
What is VHL? ~ *Brochure*
VHL...Not So Rare After All ~ *Brochure*
Help Us Put the Puzzle Together ~ *Brochure*
What You Need to Know About VHL ~ *Brochure*
Your Family Health Tree ~ *Brochure*
Que Es VHL? ~ *Brochure*
La Enfermedad De VHL No Es Tan Infrecuente, Despues De Todo ~ *Brochure*
Von Hippel-Lindau... ~ *Brochure*
VHL ~ *Brochure*
Public Service Announcement ~ *Announcement*
VHL...Not So Rare After All ~ *Brochure*

Concerned with the following diseases or disorders:
Von Hippel Lindau Disease

1537 VELO-CARDIO-FACIAL SYNDROME EDUCATIONAL FOUNDATION

110-45 Queens Boulevard
Forest Hills, NY 11375 718-261-8049
Fax: 718-261-7346

The Velo-Cardio-Facial Syndrome Educational Foundation is a national not-for-profit self-help organization dedicated to providing information and support to individuals affected by Velo-Cardio-Facial Syndrome, their families, and physicians. Velo-Cardio-Facial Syndrome, also known as Shprintzen Syndrome, is a rare inherited disorder characterized by cleft palate, malformations of the jaw, heart abnormalities, and/or learning disabilities. The Foundation is committed to offering family programs, providing parent-to-parent networking, distributing educational materials about Velo-Cardio-Facial Syndrome, publishing an informational newsletter, and distributing a questionnaire regarding the medical diagnosis and management of children with this disorder.

President: Judy Ziet
Executive Director: Joan Kerrs
Year Established: 1993

Concerned with the following diseases or disorders:
Velocardiofacial Syndrome

1538 WEGENER'S FOUNDATION

9000 Rockville Pike
Building 31
Room 1B
30W
Bethesda, MD 20892 301-496-8331

The Wegener's Foundation is a voluntary not-for-profit research organization dedicated to providing information and support to individuals with Wegener's Granulomatosis, family members, caregivers, and the medical community. Wegener's Granulomatosis is a rare multisystem disorder characterized by inflammation of the walls of blood vessels, the formation of tumor-like masses or nodules in air passages, generalized inflammation of the kidney (glomerulonephritis), and associated symptoms and findings. The policies of the Wegener's Foundation are formulated by its Board of Directors, composed of affected individuals as well as health care professionals who are working to find treatments for the disorder. Established in 1988, the Foundation is committed to providing information and support services to affected individuals and family members and promoting research into the causes and treatments of the disorder. The Foundation promotes public understanding and awareness of the disorder and disseminates timely information to health care workers in diverse medical fields. The Wegener's Foundation also provides appropriate referrals to medical assistance; engages in patient advocacy; and offers a variety of support and educational materials including pamphlets, brochures, fact sheets, and a regular newsletter.

President: Linda Baltrusch (1994-Present)
Year Established: 1988
Organization Members: 300

Publishes the following materials:
Backgrounder ~ *Fact Sheet*
The Wegener's Foundation ~ *Brochure*
Wegener's Foundation News ~ *Newsletter*

Concerned with the following diseases or disorders:
Wegener's Granulomatosis

1539 **WEGENER'S GRANULOMATOSIS SUPPORT GROUP, INC. (INTERNATIONAL) (WGSGI)**
P.O. Box 28660
Kansas City, MO 64188-8660 816-436-8211
800-277-9474
Fax: 816-436-8211
E-mail: wgjimiva@uit.net
http://www.wgsg.org/wgsg

The Wegener's Granulomatosis Support Group, Inc. (International) is a voluntary not-for-profit self-help organization dedicated to providing information on Wegener's Granulomatosis; helping affected families understand the nature of the disease; and raising public awareness. Wegener's Granulomatosis is a rare multisystem disorder characterized by inflammation of the walls of blood vessels, the formation of tumor-like masses or nodules in air passages, generalized inflammation of the kidney (glomerulonephritis), and associated symptoms and findings. Established in 1986, the Group has several chapters and approximately 3,500 members. The organization engages in patient and family advocacy; operates a toll-free hotline; conducts national seminars; and provides a variety of informational materials including a bimonthly newsletter, a clinical information packet, videotapes, and audiotapes. The Wegener's Granulomatosis Support Group, Inc. (International) also maintains a web site at [http://www.wgsg.org/wgsg].

President: Iva N. Roe
Year Established: 1986
Organization Chapters: 14
Organization Members: 3,500

Concerned with the following diseases or disorders:
Wegener's Granulomatosis

1540 **WILLIAMS SYNDROME ASSOCIATION (WSA)**
1312 North Campbell
Suite 34
Royal Oak, MI 48067 248-541-3630
Fax: 248-541-3631
E-mail: TMonkaba@aol.com
http://www.williams-syndrome.org

The Williams Syndrome Association is a national voluntary not-for-profit organization dedicated to improving the lives of individuals with Williams Syndrome, a rare congenital disorder characterized by heart and blood vessel abnormalities, high blood calcium levels, developmental delays, characteristic facial features, and/or additional abnormalities. Established in 1983, the Association is committed to locating affected individuals and their families and disseminating current medical and educational information to families, professionals, and the public. In addition, the organization seeks to increase professional awareness of and interest in Williams Syndrome and supports ongoing research into the educational, behavioral, social, and medical aspects of the disorder. The Williams Syndrome Association engages in patient and family advocacy; provides appropriate referrals including to support groups; and holds annual regional conferences, social gatherings, and biennial conventions. The Association also provides a variety of informational materials to families, health care professionals, teachers, and others through its database, directory, quarterly newsletter, reports, medical monitoring guidelines for physicians, brochures, pamphlets, and audiovisual aids.

President: Terry Monkaba (1994-Present)
Executive Director: Diane McCloskey Dueweke
Year Established: 1983
Organization Members: 6,000

Publishes the following materials:
"Heart to Heart" ~ *Newsletter*
Williams Syndrome Information For Teachers ~ *Booklet*
Key Features of Williams Syndrome ~ *Fact Sheet*
Evolving Consensus Document ~ *Fact Sheet*
Resource Order Form ~ *Order Form*
Facts About Williams Syndrome ~ *Brochure*
"Heart to Heart" ~ *Newsletter*

Concerned with the following diseases or disorders:
Williams Syndrome

1541 **WILSON'S DISEASE ASSOCIATION**
4 Navaho Dr.
Brookfield, CT 06804-3124 203-775-9666
800-399-0266
TDD: 540-743-1415
E-mail: hasellner@worldnet.att.net
http://www.medhelp.org/wda/wil.htm

The Wilson's Disease Association is a voluntary self-help not-for-profit organization dedicated to providing information and support to people with Wilson's Disease, a rare inherited disorder of copper metabolism in which copper abnormally accumulates in the liver and is slowly released into other tissues and organs of the body. As the disorder progresses, abnormal copper accumulation may cause liver disease such as inflammation of the liver (hepatitis) and cirrhosis; diminished kidney function; and abnormalities of brain function resulting in muscle rigidity, tremors, speech difficulties, and impaired memory and judgment and distinct personality changes (dementia). The Wilson's Disease Association makes referrals to physicians for appropriate diagnosis and treatment, to genetic counseling, and to support groups. The Association also engages in patient and professional education; promotes public awareness of Wilson's Disease; conducts annual conferences; and offers educational and support information through its database, directory, regular newsletter, and brochures.

President: H. Ascher Sellner, MD (1994-Present)
Year Established: N/A
Organization Chapters: 4
Organization Members: 500

Publishes the following materials:
President's Message ~ *Fact Sheet*
Wilson's Disease Update ~ *Report*
Annual Meeting - Wilson's Disease Association ~ *Bulletin*
Wilson's Disease ~ *Report*
Wilson's Disease Inheritance ~ *Report*

Concerned with the following diseases or disorders:
Wilson's Disease

1542 WOLF-HIRSCHHORN (4P-) PARENT CONTACT GROUP

2048 South 182nd Circle
Omaha, NE 68130-2749 402-330-7135
E-mail: tombecr@aol.com or 1bentley@orednet.org

The Wolf-Hirschhorn (4P-) Parent Contact Group is a voluntary not-for-profit self-help organization dedicated to educating parents about Wolf-Hirschhorn Syndrome and networking them with other parents of affected children. Wolf-Hirschhorn Syndrome, a rare chromosomal disorder caused by a partial deletion of the short arm ("p") of chromosome 4, may be characterized by widely set eyes, an abnormally small head, cleft palate, low-set ears, undescended testicles in affected males, and/or mental and/or psychomotor retardation. Established in 1985, the Wolf-Hirschhorn Parent Contact Group provides a variety of educational and support materials through its directory and regular newsletter.

President: Larry Bentley (1996-Present)
Executive Director: Becky Richardson (Contact Person)
Year Established: 1985
Organization Members: 200

Publishes the following materials:
Wolf Hirschorn Syndrome 4P "Clare" ~ *Booklet*

1543 WOLF-HIRSCHHORN SYNDROME (4P-) SUPPORT GROUP AND NEWSLETTER

c/o Brenda Grimmett
5536 Virginia Court
Amherst, OH 44001 440-282-1460
E-mail: blgrimmett@centuryinter.net
http://www.members.aol.com/lbent503/whs

The Wolf-Hirschhorn Syndrome (4P-) Support Group and Newsletter is a not-for-profit self-help organization dedicated to providing information and support to parents of children with Wolf-Hirschhorn Syndrome. Wolf-Hirschhorn Syndrome, a rare chromosomal disorder caused by a partial deletion of the short arm (p) of chromosome 4, is characterized by widely set eyes, an abnormally small head, cleft palate, low-set ears, undescended testicles in affected males, and/or mental and/or psychomotor retardation. Established in 1991, the Wolf-Hirschhorn Syndrome (4P-) Support Group and Newsletter serves as a liaison between affected families and researchers who are conducting clinical trials to study Wolf-Hirschhorn Syndrome. The organization also provides referrals to physicians and genetic counseling; engages in patient advocacy; and provides affected families with the opportunity to exchange information, support, and resources through its networking program. In addition, the Group holds gatherings of member families from across the country. The organization also offers a variety of educational and support information through its database, family directory, regular newsletter, reports, article reprints, audiotapes of family gatherings, and brochures. In addition, the organization publishes biographies that highlight the progress of member families' affected children.

President: Brenda Grimmett (1991-Present)
Year Established: 1991
Organization Members: 300

Concerned with the following diseases or disorders:
Wolf Hirschhorn Syndrome

1544 WOLF-HIRSCHHORN SYNDROME SUPPORT GROUP

2B Harvesters Close
Rainham
Kent, ME8 8PA
United Kingdom 01634372218
Fax: 01634372218

The Wolf-Hirschhorn Syndrome Support Group is a not-for-profit self-help organization in the United Kingdom dedicated to gathering and disseminating information about Wolf-Hirschhorn Syndrome and enabling parents of affected children to exchange information, support, and resources through its parent networking program. Wolf-Hirschhorn Syndrome, a rare chromosomal disorder caused by a partial deletion of the short arm (p) of chromosome 4, is characterized by widely set eyes, an abnormally small head, cleft palate, low-set ears, undescended testicles in affected males, and/or mental and/or psychomotor retardation. Established in 1986, the Group coordinates fund-raising activities; acts as a contact point for physicians and other health care professionals who are conducting research into the disorder; and provides information on the disorder to affected families, health care professionals, and other interested individuals. The Group provides a variety of educational and support materials through its database, directory, regular newsletter, reports, and brochures.

President: Christine Violet Hilder (1986-Present)
Executive Director: Christine Voilet Hilder
Year Established: 1986
Organization Members: 80

Concerned with the following diseases or disorders:
Wolf Hirschhorn Syndrome

1545 X-LINKED ALPHA THALASSEMIA FAMILY SUPPORT NETWORK

1437 Cool Springs Drive
Mesquite, TX 75181 972-222-0050
E-mail: nordtx@earthlink.net

The X-linked Alpha Thalassemia Family Support Network is a national self-help organization dedicated to providing information and support to individuals and families affected by X-Linked Alpha Thalassemia Mental Retardation Syndrome (ATR-X). ATR-X, an extremely rare disorder that is fully expressed in males only, is characterized by alpha thalassemia, severe mental retardation, severe delays in the acquisition of skills requiring coordination of mental and muscular activities (psychomotor retardation), genital abnormalities, and characteristic facial abnormalities. The Network engages in patient advocacy, promotes patient and general education and offers networking services.

President: David and Dayna Hughes (Contact Persons)
Year Established: 1996
Organization Members: Non-Membership

1546 XP (XERODERMA PIGMENTOSUM) SOCIETY, INC. (XP SOCIETY)

Box 4759
Poughkeepsie, NY 12601 914-473-4735
Fax: 914-473-4735
E-mail: xps@xps.org
http://www.xps.org

Xeroderma Pigmentosum (XP) Society, Inc. is a national not-for-profit organization dedicated to increasing public awareness of XP and related conditions; providing direct support to individuals affected by XP and their families through information exchange and financial support; and promoting increased medical research to achieve a cure for XP. Founded in 1995, the XP Society currently has approximately 2,000 members. Xeroderma Pigmentosum is a group of rare inherited skin disorders that is characterized by a heightened reaction to sunlight (photosensitivity) with skin blistering occurring after exposure to the sun. In some cases, pain and blistering may occur immediately after contact with sunlight. Acute sunburn and persistent redness or inflammation of the skin (erythema) are also early symptoms of Xeroderma Pigmentosum. In most cases, symptoms may be apparent immediately after birth or occur within the next few years. The Society publishes a quarterly newsletter entitled "XP Report," distributes "The Xeroderma Pigmentosum Handbook, A Practical Guide to Living With XP," and sponsors "Camp Sundown," a yearly family summer camp for individuals affected by XP and their families.

President: Daniel Mahar (1995 to Present)
Executive Director: Caren Mahar
Organization Language: Italian (spoken). Spanish (spoken). French (spoken). Russian (spoken). German (spoken).
Year Established: 1995
Organization Chapters: 1
Organization Members: 2,000

Publishes the following materials:
XP Report ~ *Newsletter*
Understanding Xeroderma Pigmentosum ~ *Booklet*
The Xeroderma Pigmentosum Handbook ~ *Booklet*

Concerned with the following diseases or disorders:
Xeroderma Pigmentosum

1547 Y-ME NATIONAL BREAST CANCER ORGANIZATION

212 West Van Buren
4th Floor
Chicago, IL 60607
312-986-8338
800-986-8228
Fax: 312-294-8598
E-mail: info@y-me.org
http://www.y-me.org

The Y-Me Breast Cancer Organization is a national nonprofit support organization that provides information, hotline counseling, educational programs, and self-help meetings for individuals with breast cancer, their families, and friends. Y-Me was established in 1978 and is the largest and most comprehensive breast cancer support organization in the country. Y-Me has helped thousands of women live with their diagnoses. There is strong evidence that because of this support, women are able to withstand treatment with less disruption to their daily lives. Most of all, Y-Me gives hope to women and men who fear cancer by letting them know that there are others who are leading active, fulfilling lives despite their illnesses. Y-Me activities include hotline services in which trained peer counselors who have experienced breast cancer answer questions and lend support; open door educational meetings for individuals who have had breast cancer or are concerned about it; presurgical counseling and referral services; inservice programs for health care professionals; and a wig and prosthesis bank. The Y-Me Breast Cancer Organization produces educational materials including a newsletter, brochures, Spanish language materials, and booklets. In addition, as a founding member of the National Breast Cancer Coalition, Y-Me provides information on public policy and legislative activities related to breast cancer.

President: Michelle Melin (Director of Patient Services)
Organization Language: Spanish (written).
Year Established: 1978
Organization Chapters: 19
Organization Members: 4,000

Publishes the following materials:
A Women's Guide for Breast Care ~ *Brochure*
The Teen Guide for Breast Care ~ *Brochure*
When the Woman You Love has Breast Cancer ~ *Booklet*
For Single Women with Breast Cancer ~ *Booklet*
Breast Cancer Information and Support (Spanish) ~ *Brochure*
A Woman's Guide For Breast Care (Spanish) ~ *Brochure*
Para La Mujer Que Vive Sola Y Tiene Cancer Del Seno ~ *Booklet*
Cuando La Mujer Que Tu Amas Tiene Caner Del Seno ~ *Booklet*
A Program for and about People Concerned about Breast Cancer ~ *Mission Statement*

Concerned with the following diseases or disorders:
Cancer, Breast

1548 22Q AND YOU

The Department of Clinical Genetics
The Children's Hospital of Philadelphia
One Children's Center
34th Street and Civic Center Boulevard
Philadelphia, PA 19104 215-590-2920
Fax: 215-590-3298
E-mail: lunny@email.chop.edu
cbil.humgen.upenn.edu/VCFS/index.html

22q and You, located at the Children's Hospital of Philadelphia, is a national nonprofit voluntary health organization dedicated to providing educational information and support to individuals, families, and medical professionals interested in chromosome 22q11.2 deletion. This chromosomal disorder is also known as DiGeorge Anomaly and Velocardiofacial Syndrome (VCFS). Opitz G/BBB Syndrome, Asymmetric Crying Face Syndrome, CATCH 22, and conotruncal cardiac anomaly are also included in this group of disorders. Velocardiofacial Syndrome is a rare disorder in which cleft palate, heart abnormalities, learning disabilities, and distinct physical features are all present. Other findings may include the absence or underdevelopment of the thymus, hearing loss, eye abnormalities, curvature of the spine (scoliosis), inguinal or umbilical hernia, and/or absent or unusually small tonsils and adenoids. This disorder is inherited as an autosomal dominant trait and is the most common syndrome related to cleft palate without cleft lip. Established in 1996 and consisting of 1,500 members, 22q and You publishes a quarterly newsletter entitled "22q and You." In addition, the group maintains a site on the World Wide Web at [http://cbil.humgen.upenn.edu/VCFS/index.html].

Executive Director: Donna McDonald-McGinn, M.S. (Associate Director)
Organization Language: Spanish (written).
Year Established: 1996
Organization Chapters: 5
Organization Members: 1,500

Publishes the following materials:
Color Me Healthy ~ *Leaflet*
22q And You ~ *Newsletter - Winter 1997*
22q And You ~ *Newsletter - Fall 1996*
22q And You ~ *Newsletter - Winter 1997*

Concerned with the following diseases or disorders:
DiGeorge Syndrome; Opitz Syndrome; Velocardiofacial Syndrome

1549 AMEND: AIDING MOTHERS AND FATHERS EXPERIENCING NEONATAL DEATH

4324 Berrywick Terrace
St. Louis, MO 63128 314-487-7582

AMEND: Aiding Mothers and Fathers Experiencing Neonatal Death is a not-for-profit organization dedicated to offering support and encouragement to parents who are having a normal grief reaction to the loss of their baby. Established in 1974, AMEND offers a free counseling service to parents who have experienced the loss of an infant through miscarriage, stillbirth, or neonatal death. All counselors have been trained via professional leadership and are on call 24 hours a day. All information is confidential and no names are disclosed. Counselors are available whenever grieving parents have a need to talk. Counselors do not dispense medical advice or information. It is through listening, understanding, and caring that they are able to assist in easing the pain of neonatal loss. Educational materials include a brochure entitled "AMEND, A One-on-One Peer Contact for Bereaved Parents."

President: Martha Eise (Co-ordinator)
Executive Director: Maureen Connelly (Referral Co-ordinator)
Year Established: 1974
Organization Members: 12

Publishes the following materials:
AMEND. A one-on-one peer contact for bereaved parents ~ *Brochure*

1550 ARCH NATIONAL RESOURCE CENTER FOR CRISIS AND RESPITE CARE SERVICES

800 Eastowne Drive
Suite 105
Chapel Hill, NC 27514 919-490-5577
800-473-1727
Fax: 919-490-4905
E-mail: HN4735@connectinc.com
http://chtop.com

Established in 1991, ARCH National Resource Center for Respite and Crisis Care Services, a not-for-profit consortium of several organizations, is dedicated to providing support to service providers and families through training, technical assistance, evaluation, and research. Respite, temporary relief for caregivers and families, is a service in which care is provided to children with disabilities, with chronic or terminal illnesses, and/or who are at risk of abuse or neglect.

Respite can occur in out-of-home and in-home settings for any length of time depending upon family needs and available resources. Crisis nurseries are a form of respite that focus on children who are at risk of abuse or neglect. Respite helps prevent out-of-home placements and possible abuse and neglect situations, preserves the family unit, and supports family stability. The Center's staff offers training, technical assistance, and support materials to state and local agencies to help them develop and maintain effective respite programs. The Center also conducts surveys of local programs, state level summaries, site visits, and other activities to evaluate and manage current services and improve the system of family support sevices. In addition, the Center offers informational resources to the public including acccss to electronic bulletin boards; a national registry of consultants; a database of respite options for families/caregivers; and a lending library of books, journals, and audiovisuals.

Executive Director: Linda Baker
Year Established: 1991
Organization Members: 473

Publishes the following materials:
ARCH ~ *Brochure*

1551 ABIDING HEARTS

P.O. Box 5245
Bozeman, MT 59717 406-388-8001
Fax: 406-587-7197
E-mail: hearts@imt.net
http://www.imt.net/~hearts

Abiding Hearts is a not-for-profit organization dedicated to providing support and information to parents continuing their pregnancies after prenatal testing has revealed the presence of birth defects, some of which may be life-threatening. Established in 1993, Abiding Hearts provides a network of contact parents in a growing number of areas across the United States, enabling the exchange of support, information, and resources between new members and parents who have already experienced similar circumstances. Abiding Hearts also promotes patient advocacy; provides referrals to support groups and other services; and offers a variety of educational and support materials to parents and other affected family members, health care professionals, and the general public through its directory, brochures, reports, and its regular newsletter.

President: Maria La Fond Visscher (1993-Present)
Executive Director: Kathleen Johnson
Year Established: 1993
Organization Chapters: 5
Organization Members: 20

1552 ABOUTFACE U.S.A.

P.O. Box 93
Limekiln, PA 19535 610-689-4476
800-225-3223
Fax: 610-689-4479
E-mail: abtface@aol.com
http://www.interlog.com/~abtface

AboutFace U.S.A. is a national voluntary health organization dedicated to providing individual and family support to those who have facial differences. The organization offers information, practical advice, and the opportunity to network with others who share similar concerns and experiences. AboutFace promotes public education through school presentations and media awareness. The organization seeks to emphasize the value of the person behind every face, encouraging a greater acceptance of those with facial differences in society. As part of its networking program, the organization provides a toll-free support number. AboutFace publishes pamphlets, booklets, and a newsletter six times a year. Literature is geared to families, health care professionals, and the general public. A comprehensive lending library provides books and videotapes to members. The organization develops local chapters for the purposes of support, education, and public awareness. In conjunction with the Cleft Palate Foundation, AboutFace sponsors an annual conference for families and professionals. An advocacy program helps families to access insurance coverage. To this end, volunteers in many states provide advice and information and a database of members' insurance experiences.

Executive Director: Pamela H. Onyx
Organization Language: Spanish. French.
Year Established: 1985
Organization Chapters: 25
Organization Members: 5,000

Publishes the following materials:
AboutFace - Erin, Age 7 ~ *Brochure*
My Newborn has a Facial Difference ~ *Brochure*
You, Your Child and the Craniofacial Team ~ *Brochure*

AboutFace ~ *Newsletter*
Apert, Crouzon and other Craniosynostosis Syndromes ~ *Booklet*
Making The Difference ~ *Orientation Package*
We all have different faces ~ *Brochure*
For Parents, Teachers and Young Adults ~ *Resource List*
For Children ~ *Resource List*
The Beauty Within ~ *Resource List*
AbouFace Publications Order Form ~ *Order Form*
For the Very First Time, We Knew We Were Not Alone ~ *Brochure*
My Newborn has a Facial Difference ~ *Brochure*
You, Your Child and the Craniofacial Team ~ *Brochure*
Look at the Possibilities ~ *Brochure*

Concerned with the following diseases or disorders:
Apert Syndrome; Baller Gerold Syndrome; Blepharophimosis, Ptosis, Epicanthus Inversus Syndrome; Carpenter Syndrome; Cerebro Oculo Facio Skeletal Syndrome; Chromosome 7, Monosomy 7p2; Cleft Palate and Cleft Lip; Craniofrontonasal Dysplasia; Craniometaphyseal Dysplasia; Craniosynostosis, Primary; Crouzon Disease; Encephalocele; Fraser Syndrome; Frontofacionasal Dysplasia; Frontonasal Dysplasia; Goodman Syndrome; Greig Cephalopolysyndactyly Syndrome; Hallermann Streiff Syndrome; Jackson-Weiss Syndrome; Maxillofacial Dysostosis; Maxillonasal Dysplasia, Binder Type; Moebius Syndrome; Oral Facial Digital Syndrome; Orocraniodigital Syndrome; Pallister W Syndrome; Pfeiffer Syndrome; Popliteal Pterygium Syndrome; Pyknodysostosis; Rapp Hodgkins Syndrome; Roberts Syndrome; Saethre Chotzen Syndrome; Sakati Syndrome; Seckel Syndrome; Summitt Syndrome; Telecanthus with Associated Abnormalities; Treacher Collins Syndrome; Tricho Dento Osseous Syndrome

1553 ALEXANDER GRAHAM BELL ASSOCIATION FOR THE DEAF, INC.

3417 Volta Place, NW
Washington, D.C. 20007-2778 202-337-5220
800-432-7543
Fax: 202-337-8314
E-mail: agbell2@aol.com
http://www.agbell.org

The Alexander Graham Bell Association for the Deaf, Inc. is a not-for-profit organization dedicated to helping hearing-impaired individuals by developing maximal use of residual hearing, speech reading, and speech and language skills and promoting better public understanding of hearing loss. The Association seeks to promote detection of hearing loss in early infancy as well as prompt and continued use of appropriate hearing aids and collaborates on research relating to auditory or verbal communication. Established in 1890 by Alexander Graham Bell, the organization is also committed to working for better educational opportunities for affected children; providing in-service training for teachers; and offering scholarships. In addition, the Association disseminates information on hearing impairment, its causes, and options for remedial treatment and collaborates with physicians, audiologists, speech/language specialists, and educators to promote educational, vocational, and social opportunities for affected individuals. The organization also supports legislation beneficial to affected individuals, conducts international conferences, and has one of the world's largest historical collections of information on deafness. The Association answers inquiries on all areas of hearing impairment and provides a variety of materials. These include textbooks, videotapes, and materials for parents; information on hearing aids, lip-reading, and auditory training; a magazine entitled "VOLTA VOICES"; and a journal called the "VOLTA REVIEW."

President: Nan Ellen East (1996 to Present)
Executive Director: Donna Dickman, Ph.D.
Year Established: 1890
Organization Chapters: 26
Organization Members: 5,800

Publishes the following materials:
Fall & Winter 1994-95 Publications ~ *Publications List*
Alexander Graham Bell Association for the Deaf, Inc. - Objectives ~ *Mission Statement*

Concerned with the following diseases or disorders:
Acoustic Neuroma; Bjornstad Syndrome; Usher's Syndrome; Waardenburg Syndrome; Wildervanck Syndrome

1554 ALLERGY AND ASTHMA NETWORK—MOTHERS OF ASTHMATICS, INC. (AAN-MA)

3554 Chain Bridge Road
Suite 200
Fairfax, VA 22030 703-385-4403
Fax: 703-352-4354
E-mail: aanma@aol.com
http://www.podi.com/health/aanma

The Allergy and Asthma Network—Mothers of Asthmatics, Inc. (AAN-MA) is a not-for-profit organization dedicated to helping individuals affected by asthma and allergy through education, support, and resources. Established in 1985 and currently consisting of 5,000 members, AAN-MA works to educate the general public; provide an essential communication link among the home, school, physicians, the pharmaceutical industry, and the government on allergies and asthma; offer emotional support to affected individuals and their families; and provide accurate guidance and clearly written resources on allergies and asthma. AAN-MA has a toll-free hotline and offers a variety of materials including a monthly newsletter, various publications, and videos on allergies and asthma. AAN-MA also maintains a web site at [http://www.podi.com/health/aanma].

President: Nancy Sander (1986 to Present)
Executive Director: Barbara Tomayko
Organization Language: Spanish (written).
Year Established: 1985
Organization Members: 5,000

Publishes the following materials:
Let's Fix Asthma and Allergies ~ *Brochure*
Allergy and Asthma Network Mothers of Asthmatics, Inc. ~ *Mission Statement*
The MA Report ~ *Newsletter*

1555 ALLIANCE FOR TECHNOLOGY ACCESS (ATA)

2175 East Francisco Boulevard
Suite L
San Rafael, CA 94901 415-455-4575
800-455-7970
Fax: 415-455-0654
TDD: 415-455-0491
E-mail: atainfo@ATAccess.org
http://www.ATAccess.org

The Alliance for Technology Access (ATA) is a not-for-profit organization dedicated to providing technology information to people with disabilities. ATA was established in 1987 and consists of 42 resource centers nationwide that provide direct services to help people with disabilities explore computer hardware systems, adaptive devices, telecommunication services, and software. Technology vendors who belong to the Alliance are dedicated to helping consumers obtain the most current information, best service, and quality products currently available. Materials include the ATA Resource Center list, ATA Vendor Member List, a sample application entitled "Partners in the Promise," and "Computer Resources for People With Disabilities." The Alliance has over 40 community based resource centers in 34 states and the Virgin Islands. Each center provides information on and training in the use of microcomputer technology. ATA also maintains a web site at [http://www.ATAccess.org].

President: Mary Lester (Contact Person / Associate Director)
Executive Director: Frederick A. Fiedler
Year Established: 1987
Organization Members: 42

Publishes the following materials:
Alliance for Technology Access ~ *Mission Statement*
Alliance for Technology Access - Resource Centers ~ *Resource List*
Computer Resources for People with Disabilities ~ *Order Form*
Invitation to Join. Partners in the Promise of Technology ~ *Leaflet*
Alliance for Technology Access. Resource Centers ~ *Pamphlet*

1556 ALLIANCE OF GENETIC SUPPORT GROUPS

35 Wisconsin Circle, Suite 440
Chevy Chase, MD 20815 301-652-5553
800-336-4363
Fax: 301-654-0171
E-mail: alliance@capaccess.org
http://medhelp.org/www/agsg.htm

The Alliance of Genetic Support Groups is a consortium of national voluntary organizations for individuals and families who have genetic disorders. Dedicated to fostering a partnership between genetic consumers and professionals, the Alliance provides referrals to support groups, services, and genetic counseling on its toll-free telephone line. In addition, the Alliance promotes education in the field of genetics and provides technical assistance to its member organizations. It encourages communication among support groups and provides a forum for identifying concerns and needs common to its constituency. The Alliance represents the consumer viewpoint before private and government forums and holds national conferences on topics timely and relevant to genetic consumers and professionals. The Alliance offers a variety of materials including the "Directory of National Genetic Voluntary Organizations."

Executive Director: Mary Davidson

Publishes the following materials:
Health Insurance Resource Guide ~ *Guide Book*
Publications Order Form ~ *Form*
Directory of National Genetic Voluntary Organizations and Related Resources ~ *Book*
Alliance of Genetic Support Groups ~ *Brochure*
Integrating Consumers Into The Regional Genetics Networks ~ *Pamphlet*
Informed Consent: Participation in Genetic Research Studies ~ *Pamphlet*
Media Reporting In The Genetic Age. Conference Proceedings ~ *Booklet*
Media Reporting In The Genetic Age. A Guide for Consumer Groups ~ *Booklet*

Media Reporting In The Genetic Age. Points To Consider. ~ *Booklet*
Genetic Resources To Know About ~ *Factsheets*
Bibiography: Media Coverage, Public Attitudes and Labeling of People with Disabilities ~ *Factsheet*
How to Develop Good Public Relations And Favorable Publicity ~ *Factsheets*
Unhandicapping Our Language ~ *Factsheet*

Concerned with the following diseases or disorders:
Achondroplasia; Adrenoleukodystrophy; Agammaglobulinemias, Primary; Aicardi Syndrome; Albinism; Alexander's Disease; Alkaptonuria; Alpha-1-Antitrypsin Deficiency; Amyloidosis; Anemia, Blackfan Diamond; Anemia, Fanconi's; Anencephaly; Angelman Syndrome; Apert Syndrome; Arthrogryposis Multiplex Congenita; Ataxia Telangiectasia; Ataxia, Friedreich's; Beckwith Wiedemann Syndrome; Carnitine Deficiency Syndromes; Cataract Dental Syndrome; Catel Manzke Syndrome; Chromosome 11, Partial Monosomy 11q; Chromosome 11, Partial Trisomy 11q; Chromosome 9, Trisomy 9P (Multiple Variants); Clubfoot; Crohn's Disease; Cystic Fibrosis; Cystinosis; Cystinuria; Cytochrome C Oxidase Deficiency; Dandy Walker Malformation; DiGeorge Syndrome; Diabetes Insipidus; Dysautonomia, Familial; Dystonia, Torsion; Ectodermal Dysplasias; Endocardial Fibroelastosis (EFE); Epidermolysis Bullosa; Epilepsy; Exostoses, Multiple; Factor XIII Deficiency; Focal Dermal Hypoplasia; Gaucher Disease; Glycogen Storage Disease VIII; Gottron's Syndrome; Hemochromatosis, Hereditary; Hemophilia; Huntington's Disease; Hydrocephalus; Hyper IgM Syndrome; Hypercholesterolemia; Joubert Syndrome; Kearns Sayre Syndrome (KSS); Keratoconus; Kugelberg Welander Syndrome; Laurence Moon Syndrome; Leigh's Disease; Lenz Microphthalmia Syndrome; MASA Syndrome; MELAS Syndrome; MERRF Syndrome; Malignant Hyperthermia; Marfan Syndrome; Mediterranean Fever, Familial; Megalocornea Mental Retardation Syndrome; Muscular Dystrophy, Duchenne; Myopathy, Sc apuloperoneal; Narcolepsy; Nemaline Myopathy; Neurofibromatosis Type 1 (NF-1); Nezelof's Syndrome; Non-Ketotic Hyperglycinemia; Opitz Syndrome; Osteogenesis Imperfecta; Phenylketonuria; Polyposis, Familial; Prader Willi Syndrome; Retinitis Pigmentosa; Rett Syndrome; Rubinstein Taybi Syndrome; Schinzel Syndrome; Schwartz Jampel Syndrome; Seitelberger Disease (Infantile Neuroaxonal Dystrophy); Setleis Syndrome; Severe Combined Immunodeficiency; Sickle Cell Disease; Simpson Dysmorphia Syndrome; Tay Sachs Disease; Thalassemia Major; Thalassemia Minor; Three M Syndrome; Tooth and Nail Syndrome; Tuberous Sclerosis; Velocardiofacial Syndrome; Werdnig Hoffman Disease; Wiedemann Rautenstrauch Syndrome; Williams Syndrome; Wilson's Disease; Xeroderma Pigmentosum; Yunis Varon Syndrome

1557 AMBIGUOUS GENITALIA SUPPORT NETWORK (AGSN)

P.O. Box 313
Clements, CA 95227-0313 209-727-0313
E-mail: esagsn@hotmail.com

The Ambiguous Genitalia Support Network is a voluntary health organization consisting of affected individuals, parents, other family members, and professionals. Established in 1994, the Ambiguous Genitalia Support Network is dedicated to providing information, assistance, and support to families of children diagnosed with ambiguous genitalia.

President: Cherie Sintes (1994-Present)
Year Established: 1994
Organization Chapters: 1
Organization Members: 20

Publishes the following materials:
Needs Assessment Survey ~ *Survey*

Concerned with the following diseases or disorders:
Ablepharon Macrostomia Syndrome; Adrenal Hyperplasia, Congenital (General); WAGR Syndrome

1558 AMERICAN AMPUTEE FOUNDATION (AAF)

P.O. Box 250218
Little Rock, AR 72225 501-666-2523
Fax: 501-666-8367

The American Amputee Foundation (AAF) is a not-for-profit organization dedicated to researching and gathering information on amputation including studies, product information, services, self-help publications, and hundreds of articles that have been written in this area of study. Established in 1975, AAF responds to over 5,000 inquiries for both direct and indirect assistance each year. During the past years, AAF has helped with insurance claims, justification letters to payers, testimony, and life-care planning; direct financial aid for prosthetic devices and home modifications; technical assistance in developing self-help programs; hospital visitations; and counseling services. In addition, the Foundation deals with thousands of telephone inquiries and referrals each year. AAF consists of chapters in various states around the country that are self-supporting and provide a variety of peer support programs. The Foundation also maintains a list of amputee support groups and provides the "National Resource Directory" for consumers and professionals.

Executive Director: Jack Erst
Year Established: 1975

Publishes the following materials:
What is AAF? ~ *Mission Statement*
Phantom Pain. Relief Without Medication? ~ *Fact Sheet*
Phantom Limb Pain ~ *Reprint*
Amputee Support Groups ~ *Pamphlet*
AAF National Resource Directory ~ *Booklet*

1559 AMERICAN ANOREXIA AND BULIMIA ASSOCIATION, INC. (AABA)

165 West 42nd Street
New York, NY 10036 212-575-6200
Fax: 212-778-0698

The American Anorexia and Bulimia Association, Inc. (AABA), a national not-for-profit health organization established in 1978, is dedicated to the prevention, treatment, and cure of eating disorders. As a source of public information on the growing field of eating disorders, AABA answers more than 20,000 inquiries each year from affected individuals, family members, professionals, schools, media, and the general public. The Association publishes a quarterly newsletter, brochures, and other educational materials.

President: Diane Mickley, M.D. (1990-Present)
Executive Director: Randi Wirth, Ph.D.
Year Established: 1978
Organization Chapters: 4
Organization Members: 1,000

Publishes the following materials:
American Anorexia/Bulimia Association, Inc. ~ *Brochure*
AABA Membership & Book Order Form ~ *Order Form*
Dear Friend ~ *Pamphlet*
Facts on Eating Disorders ~ *Pamphlet*
Body Politics - Why You Should Eat ~ *Pamphlet*
Questions to Ask a Potential Therapist ~ *Questionnaire*
How To Help a Friend With An Eating Disorder ~ *Report*
A Hunger for Happiness ~ *Report*
Newsletter/Winter 1995 ~ *Newsletter*

Concerned with the following diseases or disorders:
Anorexia Nervosa; Bulimia

1560 AMERICAN ASSOCIATION OF KIDNEY PATIENTS (AAKP)

100 South Ashley Drive
Suite 280
Tampa, FL 33602 813-223-7099
800-749-2257
Fax: 813-223-0001
E-mail: aakpnat@aol.com
http://www.aakp.org

The American Association of Kidney Patients (AAKP) is a not-for-profit organization committed to serving the needs of people with kidney disorders and their families. Established in 1969, the Association's programs include support for people dealing with the physical, emotional, and social impacts of kidney diseases. The Association assists affected individuals to adjust to their own particular circumstances and challenges. The organization offers a variety of educational materials including a quarterly magazine called "AAKP Renalife."

President: Joseph D. White (1995-Present)
Executive Director: Kris Robinson
Year Established: 1969
Organization Chapters: 22
Organization Members: 5,000

Publishes the following materials:
NA-K Counter ~ *Booklet*
The Importance of Having Enough Iron ~ *Brochure*
AAKP ~ *Membership Application*
Someday...Someone May Be Eternally Grateful to You ~ *Brochure*
AAKP Bulletin ~ *Newsletter*
AAKP Advisory ~ *Information Sheet*
Americans With Disabilities Act of 1990: Your Rights in the Workplace ~ *Brochure*
Renalife - The 25 Year Story... ~ *Booklet*

Concerned with the following diseases or disorders:
Hepatorenal Syndrome; Nail Patella Syndrome; Ochoa Syndrome; Renal Agenesis, Bilateral; Renal Glycosuria

1561 AMERICAN ASSOCIATION OF SUICIDOLOGY (AAS)

4201 Connecticut Avenue, NW
Suite 310
Washington, DC 20008 202-237-2280
Fax: 202-237-2282
E-mail: amyjomc@ix.netcom.com
http://www.cyberpsych.org

The American Association of Suicidology (AAS) is a not-for-profit, voluntary organization dedicated to understanding and preventing suicide. Founded in 1967, AAS promotes research, public awareness programs, and education and training for professionals and volunteers. In addition, it serves as a national clearinghouse for information on suicide. Membership of AAS includes mental health professionals, researchers, suicide prevention and crisis intervention centers, school districts, crisis center volunteers, survivors of suicide, and a variety of lay persons who have an interest in suicide prevention. A primary objective of AAS is to help suicide prevention and crisis intervention centers throughout the United States and Canada provide quality services. AAS develops public service announcements regarding suicide prevention and sponsors yearly conferences and training for clinicians as well as those who have lost someone to suicide. Educational materials produced by the organization include "Suicide and Life-Threatening Behavior," a quarterly journal entitled "Newslink," a quarterly newsletter, and a number of suicide prevention pamphlets. AAS maintains a web site at [http://www.cyberpsych.org].

President: Cheryl A. King, Ph.D. (1997-1998)
Executive Director: Alan L. Berman, Ph.D.
Year Established: 1967
Organization Members: 1,200

Publishes the following materials:
Understanding and Preventing Suicide ~ *Brochure*
Suicide Prevention and Survivors of Suicide ~ *Resource List*
News Link ~ *Newsletter*
Undrstanding and Helping the Suicidal Person ~ *Fact Sheet*
Elderly Suicide Fact Sheet ~ *Fact Sheet*
Youth Suicide Fact Sheet ~ *Fact Sheet*
USA Suicide: 1994 Official Final Data ~ *Fact Sheet*

1562 AMERICAN ASSOCIATION OF UNIVERSITY AFFILIATED PROGRAMS FOR PERSONS WITH DEVELOPMENTAL DISABILITIES (AAUAP)

6830 Fenton Street
#410
Silver Spring, MD 20910 301-588-8252
Fax: 301-588-2842
TDD: 301-588-3319
http://www.waisman.wisc.edu/aauap/

The American Association of University Affiliated Programs for Persons with Developmental Disabilities is a not-for-profit professional organization that functions as the central office for University Affiliated Programs and as their representative to the federal government. The mission of the Association is to support the independence, productivity, integration, and inclusion of individuals with developmental disabilities and their families. The group responds to the specific needs of people with developmental disabilities by preparing individuals for careers in the field of developmental disabilities. The organization provides support to affected individuals through the provision of technical assistance and community training. Another objective of the Association is to disseminate information about developmental disabilities and to contribute to the evolution of new knowledge through research and field testing of various models and the evaluation of existing practices.

President: Sheryl White-Scott (1997 - Present)
Executive Director: William Jones, Ph.D
Year Established: N/A
Organization Members: 70

1563 AMERICAN AUTOIMMUNE RELATED DISEASES ASSOCIATION, INC. (AARDA)

Michigan National Bank Building
15475 Gratiot Avenue
Detroit, MI 48205 313-371-8600
800-598-4668
Fax: 313-371-6002
E-mail: aarda@aol.com
http://www.aarda.org/

The American Autoimmune Related Diseases Association, Inc. (AARDA) is a national not-for-profit voluntary health agency dedicated to bringing a national focus to autoimmunity, a major cause of serious chronic diseases. The Association was founded for the purposes of supporting research to find a cure for autoimmune diseases and providing services to affected individuals. In addition, the Association's goals include increasing the public's awareness that autoimmunity is the cause of more than 80 serious chronic diseases; bringing national focus and collaborative effort among state and national voluntary health groups that represent autoimmune diseases; and serving as a national advocate for individuals and families affected by the physical, emotional, and financial effects of autoimmune disease. The American Autoimmune Related Diseases Association produces educational and support materials including fact sheets, brochures, pamphlets, and a newsletter entitled "In Focus."

President: Robert Meyer (1994-Present) (Chairman)
Executive Director: Virginia T. Ladd
Year Established: 1991
Organization Chapters: 14
Organization Members: 10,000

Publishes the following materials:
Coping with Autoimmunity ~ *Brochure*
American Autoimmune Diseases Association, Inc. - Lupus ~ *Article Reprint*
American Autoimmune Diseases Association, Inc. - Pemphigus Vulgaris ~ *Fact Sheet*
American Autoimmune Diseases Association, Inc. - Primary Biliary Cirrhosis ~ *Reprint*
American Autoimmune Related Diseases Association, Inc. - Chronic Inflammatory Demyelinating Polyneuropathy (CIDP) ~ *Reprint*
Chronic Active Hepatitis ~ *Fact Sheet*
Polymyositis & Dermatomyositis ~ *Fact Sheet*
Autoimmune Hemolytic Anemia ~ *Fact Sheet*
Discoid Lupus ~ *Fact Sheet*
Crohn's Disease ~ *Fact Sheet*
Mixed Connective Tissue Disease ~ *Fact Sheet*
Fibromyalgia ~ *Fact Sheet*
Cardiomyopathy ~ *Fact Sheet*
Polychrondritis ~ *Fact Sheet*
Addison's Disease ~ *Fact Sheet*
Systemic Lupus Erythematosus (SLE) ~ *Fact Sheet*

Chronic Idiopathic Thrombocytopenic Purpura (ITP) ~ *Fact Sheet*
Systemic Scleroderma ~ *Fact Sheet*
Temporal Arteritis/Giant Cell Vasculitis ~ *Fact Sheet*
Sjogren's Syndrome ~ *Fact Sheet*
Pernicious Anemia ~ *Fact Sheet*
Ulcerative Colitis ~ *Fact Sheet*

Concerned with the following diseases or disorders:
Acrodermatitis Enteropathica; Addison's Disease; Alveolitis, Fibrosing; Amenorrhea, Primary; Anemia, Hemolytic, Acquired Autoimmune; Anemia, Hemolytic, Cold Antibody; Anemia, Pernicious; Antiphospholipid Syndrome; Arteritis, Giant Cell; Arteritis, Takayasu; Balo Disease; Bullous Pemphigoid; Castleman's Disease; Cerebellar Degeneration, Subacute; Chronic Inflammatory Demyelinating Polyneuropathy; Churg Strauss Syndrome; Conjunctivitis, Ligneous; Cryoglobulinemia, Essential Mixed; Cutis Laxa; Dermatomyositis; Devic Disease; Eaton Lambert Syndrome; Eosinophilic Fasciitis; Goodpasture Syndrome; Granulomatosis, Lymphomatoid; Guillain Barre Syndrome; Hemoglobinuria, Paroxysmal Cold; Hyper IgM Syndrome; Landau Kleffner Syndrome; Lichen Sclerosus; Melkersson Rosenthal Syndrome; Mikulicz Syndrome; Mixed Connective Tissue Disease (MCTD); Mucha Habermann Disease; Neuropathy, Congenital Hypomyelination; POEMS Syndrome; Pars Planitis; Parsonage Turner Syndrome; Pemphigoid, Benign Mucosal; Pemphigus; Polyarteritis Nodosa; Posterior Uveitis; Pure Red Cell Aplasia, Acquired; Purpura, Henoch Schonlein; Pyoderma Gangrenosum; Sarcoidosis; Schmidt Syndrome; Stiff Man Syndrome; Tolosa Hunt Syndrome; Urticaria, Cold; Vasculitis; Vasculitis, Cutaneous Necrotizing; Vitamin B12 Deficiency; Vogt Koyanagi Harada Syndrome; Wells Syndrome

1564 AMERICAN BRAIN TUMOR ASSOCIATION (ABTA)

2720 River Road
Suite 146
Des Plaines, IL 60018
847-827-9910
800-886-2282
Fax: 847-827-9918
E-mail: ABTA@aol.com
neurosurgery.mgh.harvard.edu/ABTA/

The American Brain Tumor Association (ABTA) is a not-for-profit organization dedicated to eliminating brain tumors through the funding and promotion of ongoing medical research. The organization provides educational materials and objective resource information to people with brain tumors, their families, and medical professionals with treatment responsibility. The American Brain Tumor Association promotes excellence in patient care and advocates the investigation of innovative research and treatment approaches. The American Brain Tumor Association encourages networking through mutual support groups and produces a wide variety of informational materials including a newsletter known as "Message Line" and other informational brochures. It also offers a Pen Pal program, resource listings of treatment facilities, physicians' listings, and referrals to other related organizations. The American Brain Tumor Association was established in 1973 and services the United States and Canada.

President: Gail Segal (1993-Present)
Executive Director: Naomi Berkowitz
Year Established: 1973
Organization Members: 40,000

Publishes the following materials:
A Primer of Brain Tumors ~ *Booklet*
ABOUT EPENDYMOMA ~ *Brochure*
Dictionary for Brain Tumor Patients ~ *Pamphlet*
About Metastatic Tumors to the Brain and Spine ~ *Pamphlet*
ABOUT MEDULLOBLASTOMA/PNET (MEDULLOBLASTOMA) ~ *Brochure*
ABOUT GLIOBLASTOMA MULTIFORME AND ANAPLASTIC ASTROCYTOMA ~ *Brochure*
ABOUT MENINGIOMA ~ *Brochure*
Tumor del Cerebro. Compartiendo la Esperanza ~ *Brochure*
About Oligodendroglioma And Mixed Glioma ~ *Brochure*
About Pituitary Tumors ~ *Brochure*
Chemotherapy of Brain Tumors ~ *Pamphlet*
Immunotherapy of Brain Tumors ~ *Pamphlet*
Radiation Therapy of Brain Tumors Part 1: Basic Guide ~ *Brochure*
Radiation Therapy of Brain Tumors Part 2: Background and Research Guide ~ *Pamphlet*
Shunts ~ *Brochure*
Alex's Journey ~ *Booklet*
When Your Child is Ready to Return to School ~ *Brochure*
Message Line ~ *Newsletter*
Coping With A Brain Tumor Part I: From Diagnosis to Treatment ~ *Pamphlet*
Coping With A Brain Tumor Part II: During and After Treatment ~ *Pamphlet*
Organizing a Support Group ~ *Brochure*
Using a Medical Library ~ *Brochure*

Concerned with the following diseases or disorders:
Astrocytoma, Benign; Astrocytoma, Malignant; Brain Tumors, General; Gerstmann Syndrome; Glioblastoma Multiforme; Medulloblastoma; Meningioma; Pallister Hall Syndrome

1565 AMERICAN CANCER SOCIETY, INC. (ACS)

1599 Clifton Road NE
Atlanta, GA 30329
404-320-3333
800-227-2345
Fax: 404-325-2217
http://www.cancer.org

The American Cancer Society (ACS) is a nationwide community-based voluntary health organization dedicated to eliminating cancer as a major health problem by preventing cancer and diminishing problems associated with a diagnosis of cancer through programs of research, education, advocacy, and service. Founded in 1913 and consisting of two million volunteers, the Society funds ongoing medical research by scientists who are studying cancer. In addition, the media and public rely on the Society for statistical research and epidemiology data. Through the "Resources, Information, and Guidance Program," the ACS provides callers with information about cancer, ACS services, and other resources in the community that meet the practical, social, psychological, social, and other needs of individuals and families affected by cancer. The Society also publishes guidelines that assist physicians in establishing appropriate recommendations for the prevention and early treatment of the disease. In addition, the ACS actively seeks to educate policy makers at all levels of government about the history of cancer and the impact of health related legislation on the lives of people with cancer.

President: Raymond Lenhard, M.D. (1996 to Present)
Executive Director: John Seffrin, Ph.D.
Year Established: 1913
Organization Chapters: 57
Organization Members: Non-Membership

Concerned with the following diseases or disorders:
Ameloblastoma; Astrocytoma, Malignant; Ataxia Telangiectasia; Bowen's Disease; Brain Tumors, General; Cancer, Breast; Cancer, Colon; Cancer, Lung; Cancer, Prostate; Cancers, Skin, General; Carcinoid Syndrome; Carcinoma, Renal Cell; Carcinoma, Squamous Cell; Castleman's Disease; Cerebellar Degeneration, Subacute; Cystic Hygroma; Diencephalic Syndrome; Drash Syndrome; Dysplastic Nevus Syndrome; Fibromatosis, Congenital Generalized; Gardner Syndrome; Glioblastoma Multiforme; Granulomatosis, Lymphomatoid; Hodgkin's Disease; Leukemia, Chronic Lymphocytic; Leukemia, Chronic Myelogenous; Leukemia, Hairy Cell; Lymphangioma, Cavernous; Lymphoma, Gastric, Non-Hodgkins Type; Lynch Syndromes; Maffucci Syndrome; Medulloblastoma; Melanoma, Malignant; Meningioma; Mycosis Fungoides; Myelofibrosis, Idiopathic; Myeloma, Multiple; Nevoid Basal Cell Carcinoma Syndrome; Paget's Disease of the Breast; Pancreatic Islet Cell Tumor; Peutz Jeghers Syndrome; Pheochromocytoma; Polyposis, Familial; Pseudomyxoma Peritonei; Radiation Syndromes; Retinoblastoma; Sarcoma, Ewing's; Tongue Carcinoma; WAGR Syndrome; Waldenstrom Macroglobulinemia; Wilms' Tumor

1566 AMERICAN CHRONIC PAIN ASSOCIATION (ACPA)

P.O. Box 850
Rocklin, CA 95677 916-632-0922
Fax: 916-632-3208
E-mail: ACPA@Pacbel.net
members.tripod.com/~widdy/ACPA.html

The American Chronic Pain Association is a nonprofit self-help organization that provides assistance and hope to individuals with chronic pain. Established in 1980, the American Chronic Pain Association operates support groups throughout the United States and offers its members positive and constructive methods for dealing with chronic pain. Groups usually consist of approximately 10 members who learn useful techniques for pain management through discussion, mutual support, and informational exchanges. Educational materials produced by the American Chronic Pain Association include "Help & Hope" pamphlets and brochures, guidelines for the selection of a pain unit, the "American Chronic Pain Association Member Workbook," tapes, and the "American Chronic Pain Association Chronicle."

Executive Director: Penney Cowan
Year Established: 1980
Organization Chapters: 850

Publishes the following materials:
The ACPA Chronicle ~ *Newsletter*
American Chronic Pain Association: Help and Hope ~ *Brochure*
The American Chronic Pain Association Help and Hope ~ *Pamphlet*
Ten Concepts Moving from Patient to Person ~ *Fact Sheet*
Guidelines to Help Select A Pain Unit ~ *Fact Sheet*
ACPA Member Workbook, Tape, and Chronicle Order Form ~ *Order Form*

Concerned with the following diseases or disorders:
Dercum Disease; Fibromyalgia; Reflex Sympathetic Dystrophy Syndrome (RSDS)

1567 AMERICAN COUNCIL OF THE BLIND, INC. (ACB)

1155 15th Street
Suite 720
Washington, DC 20005 202-467-5081
800-424-8666
Fax: 202-467-5085
E-mail: info@acb.org
http://www.acb.org

The American Council of the Blind is a national not-for-profit advocacy organization for people who are blind or visually impaired. Established in 1961, the Council is dedicated to improving the well-being of all blind and visually impaired people. To this end, the Council serves as a representative national organization and seeks to improve the social, economic, and cultural levels of affected individuals. The Council is dedicated to improving educational and rehabilitation opportunities and cooperating with public and private institutions and organizations concerned with services for people who are blind. The Society produces a variety of publications including the "Braille Forum." Produced in Braille, large print, four track cassette, and on computer disk, the magazine contains articles on employment, legislation, sports and leisure activities, new products and services, human interest stories, and other information. The Society also supports a national toll-free information and referral service.

President: Paul Edwards
Executive Director: Oral Miller
Year Established: 1961
Organization Chapters: 70
Organization Members: 45,000

Concerned with the following diseases or disorders:
Bardet Biedl Syndrome; Choroideremia; Coats' Disease; Laurence Moon Syndrome; Leber's Congenital Amaurosis; Leber's Optic Atrophy; Macular Degeneration; Macular Degeneration, Polymorphic; Norrie Syndrome; Retinitis Pigmentosa; Retinopathy, Arteriosclerotic; Retinopathy, Hypertensive; Retinoschisis; Usher's Syndrome; Waardenburg Syndrome

1568 AMERICAN FOUNDATION FOR UROLOGIC DISEASE (AFUD)

1128 North Charles Street
Baltimore, MD 21201
800-242-2383
Fax: 410-468-1808
E-mail: admin@afud.org
http://www.access.digex.net/~afud

The American Foundation for Urologic Disease (AFUD) is a national not-for-profit health organization dedicated to the prevention and cure of urologic diseases through the expansion of medical research and the education of health care professionals and the public. Such urologic diseases include bladder cancer, urinary incontinence, urinary tract disorders, interstitial cystitis, kidney stones, benign prostatic hyperplasia, prostate cancer, prostatitis, and sexual dysfunction. Established in 1987, the Foundation sponsors a Research Scholar Program to encourage physicians to conduct research into urologic diseases, provides appropriate referrals, engages in patient advocacy, and offers networking services. AFUD also offers a variety of educational materials including brochures, pamphlets, and a quarterly magazine entitled "Family Urology." In addition, the Foundation has a web site on the Internet at [http://www.access.digex.net/~afud].

Executive Director: Thomas M. Bruckman
Organization Language: Spanish (written).
Year Established: 1987
Organization Members: Non-Membership

Concerned with the following diseases or disorders:
Alport Syndrome; Carcinoma, Renal Cell; Cystinosis; Exstrophy of the Bladder; Hematuria, Benign, Familial; Hepatorenal Syndrome; IGA Nephropathy; Interstitial Cystitis; Loken Senior Syndrome; Medullary Cystic Disease; Medullary Sponge Kidney; Nail Patella Syndrome; Peyronie Disease; Polycystic Kidney Diseases; Prostatitis; Renal Agenesis, Bilateral; Renal Glycosuria

1569 AMERICAN FOUNDATION FOR THE BLIND (AFB)

11 Penn Plaza
Suite 300
New York, NY 10001
212-502-7600
800-232-5463
Fax: 212-502-7777
TDD: 212-502-7662
E-mail: afbinfo@afb.org
http://www.afb.org

The American Foundation for the Blind (AFB) is a national not for-profit voluntary organization established in 1921 and recognized as Helen Keller's cause in the United States. AFB is the leading national resource for people who are blind or visually impaired, the organizations that serve them, and the general public. The mission of AFB is to enable people who are blind or visually impaired to achieve equality of access and opportunity that will ensure freedom of choice in their lives. AFB fulfills this mission through four primary areas of activity regarding the non-medical aspects of blindness and visual impairment. These include: the development, collection and dissemination of information on blindness and visual impairment; identification, analysis, and resolution of critical issues related to blindness and visual impairment; education of the public and policy makers as to the needs and capabilities of people who are blind or visually impaired; and the production and distribution of talking books and other audio materials. AFB records and duplicates talking books under contract to the Library of Congress and publishes books, pamphlets, videos, and periodicals about blindness for professionals and health care consumers. In addition, AFB publishes the "Journal of Visual Impairment & Blindness."

President: Carl R. Augresso
Year Established: 1921

Publishes the following materials:
Disabled Americans at Work ~ *Brochure*
Visually Impaired Professional Personnel ~ *Brochure*
Helen Keller ~ *Brochure*
Helen Keller An Annotated Bibliography ~ *Brochure*
Guide to Toys for Children who are Blind or Visually Impaired ~ *Brochure*
Referring blind & low vision patients for Rehabilitation Services ~ *Brochure*
Careers & Technology Information Bank: Student Program ~ *Brochure*
Career Choice for Blind and Visually Impaired Students: Career Planning and Placement Offices ~ *Brochure*
Don't Settle For Just A Job - Choose A Career ~ *Brochure*
Aging and Vision: Making The Most Of Impaired Vision ~ *Brochure*
A vision impairment of the later years: macular degeneration ~ *Brochure*
Getting help for a disabled child - advice from parents ~ *Brochure*
Touch the Baby ~ *Brochure*
Low Vision Questions and Answers: Definitions, Devices, Services ~ *Brochure*
Diabetes, Vision Impairment, and Blindness ~ *Brochure*
What do you do when you see a blind person? ~ *Brochure*
When You Have a Visually Handicapped Child in Your Classroom: Suggestions for Teachers ~ *Brochure*
You seem like a regular kid to me! ~ *Brochure*
Creating careers for blind people: rehabilitation and technology ~ *Brochure*
What to Do When You Meet a Deaf-Blind Person ~ *Brochure*
A Different Way of Seeing ~ *Brochure*
Braille Literacy ~ *Brochure*

Concerned with the following diseases or disorders:
Bardet Biedl Syndrome; CHARGE Syndrome; Choroideremia; Coats' Disease; Laurence Moon Syndrome; Leber's Congenital Amaurosis; Leber's Optic Atrophy; Macular Degeneration; Macular Degeneration, Polymorphic; Norrie Syndrome; Retinitis Pigmentosa; Retinopathy, Arteriosclerotic; Retinopathy, Diabetic; Retinopathy, Hypertensive; Retinoschisis; Septo Optic Dysplasia; Usher's Syndrome; Waardenburg Syndrome

1570 AMERICAN HEALTH ASSISTANCE FOUNDATION (AHAF)

15825 Shady Grove Road
Suite 140
Rockville, MD 20850 301-948-3244
800-437-2423
Fax: 301-258-9454
http://www.ahaf.org

The American Health Assistance Foundation (AHAF) is a national nonprofit health organization dedicated to raising funds for scientific research on age-related and degenerative diseases, educating the public about these diseases, and providing financial assistance to Alzheimer's Disease patients and their caregivers. Some of the age-related and degenerative diseases with which AHAF is concerned include Alzheimer's disease, glaucoma, heart disease, and stroke. AHAF is an umbrella organization comprised of four separate and distinct programs: Alzheimer's Disease Research, National Glaucoma Research, National Heart Foundation, and the Alzheimer's Family Relief Program. Currently AHAF supports 15 investigations focusing on the causes of and potential cures for Alzheimer's disease, 16 research projects studying glaucoma, and six studies of heart disease and stroke. Since its inception in 1973, AHAF has awarded more than $40 million in research grants. The Alzheimer's Family Relief Program has provided more than $1.3 million in emergency assistance grants since it began in 1988. The Foundation produces educational materials including brochures, pamphlets, booklets, and a regular newsletter. AHAF also maintains a web site on the Internet at [http://www.ahaf.org].

Executive Director: Janet R. Michaels
Year Established: 1973
Organization Members: Non-Membership

1571 AMERICAN HEARING RESEARCH FOUNDATION

55 East Washington Street
Suite 2022
Chicago, IL 60602 312-726-9670
Fax: 312-726-9695

The American Hearing Research Foundation is a voluntary organization dedicated to providing support for medical research into the causes, prevention, and cure of deafness, impaired hearing, and balance disorders and to promoting hearing health education. Established in 1966, the American Hearing Foundation consists of 30 members. The organization provides referrals and produces educational materials including a regular newsletter and pamphlets entitled "Facts and Fancies About Hearing Aids," "Care of the Ears and Hearing for Health," and "So You Have Had An Ear Operation...What Next?"

President: Wiley H. Harrison, M.D. (1988 to Present)
Executive Director: William L. Lederer
Year Established: 1966
Organization Members: 30

Publishes the following materials:
So You Have Had An Ear Operation...What Next? ~ *Leaflet*
Care of the Ears and Hearing for Health ~ *Leaflet*
Facts and Fancies about Hearing Aids ~ *Leaflet*
American Hearing Research Foundation ~ *Newsletter*

Concerned with the following diseases or disorders:
Tinnitus

1572 AMERICAN HEART ASSOCIATION (AHA)

7272 Greenville Avenue
Dallas, TX 75231-4596 214-373-6300
800-242-8721
Fax: 214-706-1341
E-mail: inquire@amhrt.org
http://www.amhrt.org

The American Heart Association (AHA), a national not-for-profit voluntary health agency funded by private contributions, is dedicated to the reduction of death and disability from cardiovascular diseases including heart diseases and stroke. The Association consists of approximately 2,000 community organizations in all states, the District of Columbia, and Puerto Rico. More than 3.7 million people volunteer with the Association to fight cardiovascular diseases, the nation's number one cause of death and leading cause of disability. Preventing heart disease and stroke is the first priority of the American Heart Association. In support of this goal, the Association has contributed more than one billion dollars to cardiovascular research since 1949. The Association also distributes a variety of educational materials and sponsors continuing medical education (CME) seminars and meetings.

President: Dr. Suzanne Oprail, M.D.
Executive Director: Thom R. Winkler
Year Established: 1949
Organization Chapters: 2,200

Concerned with the following diseases or disorders:
Apert Syndrome; Atrial Septal Defects; Atrioventricular Septal Defect; Broad Beta Disease; Cardio Auditory Syndrome; Cardio Facio Cutaneous Syndrome; Cat Eye Syndrome; Cayler Syndrome; Chromosome 8, Monosomy 8p2; Chromosome 9, Tetrasomy 9p; Cor Triatriatum; Dextrocardia with Situs Inversus; Endocardial Fibroelastosis (EFE); Endocarditis, Infective; Endomyocardial Fibrosis; Goodman Syndrome; Gorlin Chaudhry Moss Syndrome; Heart Block, Congenital; Holt Oram Syndrome; Hypercholesterolemia; Hyperlipoproteinemia Type IV; Hypoplastic Left Heart Syndrome; Kearns Sayre Syndrome (KSS); LEOPARD Syndrome; Mitral Valve Prolapse Syndrome; Mulibrey Nanism Syndrome (Perheentupa Syndrome); Myopathy, Desmin Storage; Pulmonary Hypertension, Primary; Pulmonary Hypertension, Secondary; Raynaud's Disease and Phenomenon; Retinopathy, Arteriosclerotic; Retinopathy, Hypertensive; Romano Ward Syndrome; Sakati Syndrome; Tetralogy of Fallot; Truncus Arteriosus, Persistent; Velocardiofacial Syndrome; Ventricular Septal Defects; Wolff Parkinson White Syndrome

1573 AMERICAN KIDNEY FUND, INC. (AKF)

6110 Executive Boulevard
Suite 1010
Rockville, MD 20852 301-881-3052
800-638-8299
Fax: 301-881-0898
E-mail: helpline@akfinc.org
http://www.arbon.com/kidney

The American Kidney Fund, Inc. (AKF) is a national not-for-profit health organization dedicated to providing direct financial aid to dialysis patients, transplant recipients, and donors to help cover the cost of treatment-related expenses. Grants are available to help patients afford the costs of medication, transportation, transient dialysis, and special dietary needs. Established in 1971, the American Kidney Fund promotes and supports research for kidney diseases, kidney donor development, and public and professional education. The American Kidney Fund publishes a newsletter as well as several brochures on kidney diseases, other related disorders, treatments, nutrition, and organ donation. Some selections are written specifically for children. Several brochures are also available in Spanish.

President: George A. Pocter, M.D. (1993-Present)
Executive Director: Francis J. Soldovere
Organization Language: Spanish. German.
Year Established: 1971
Organization Chapters: 3

Publishes the following materials:
Directory of American Kidney Fund Publications ~ *Resource List/Order Form*

Concerned with the following diseases or disorders:
Alport Syndrome; Arginino Succinic Aciduria; Bartter's Syndrome; Blue Diaper Syndrome; Branchio Oto Renal Syndrome; Carbamyl Phosphate Synthetase Deficiency; Citrullinemia; Cystinuria; Drash Syndrome; Fraser Syndrome; Hematuria, Benign, Familial; Hemolytic Uremic Syndrome; Hepatic Fibrosis, Congenital; Hepatorenal Syndrome; IGA Nephropathy; Loken

Senior Syndrome; Medullary Cystic Disease; Medullary Sponge Kidney; Mullerian Aplasia; Myeloma, Multiple; N-Acetyl Glutamate Synthetase Deficiency; Nail Patella Syndrome; Ochoa Syndrome; Polycystic Kidney Diseases; Purpura, Henoch Schonlein; Renal Agenesis, Bilateral; Renal Glycosuria; WAGR Syndrome; Wegener's Granulomatosis; Wilms' Tumor

1574 AMERICAN LIVER FOUNDATION (ALF)

1425 Pompton Avenue
Cedar Grove, NJ 07009-1000 973-256-2550
800-223-0179
Fax: 973-256-3214
E-mail: webmail@liverfoundation.org
http://www.liverfoundation.org

The American Liver Foundation is a national voluntary not-for-profit organization dedicated to the prevention, treatment, and cure of diseases of the liver through programs of research and education. Established in 1976, the Foundation's activities include support groups, patient advocacy, support of medical research, and patient and professional education. Educational materials include brochures on Hepatitis, Cirrhosis, Biliary Atresia, liver transplantation, gallstones, and Hereditary Hemochromatosis. Fact sheets are also available on a variety of liver diseases including Alagille Syndrome, Alpha-1-Antitrypsin Deficiency, Cancer of the Liver, Fatty Liver, Gilbert Syndrome, Primary Biliary Cirrhosis, Porphyria, and others. Videotapes produced by the Foundation include "A Healthy Liver: A Happier Life," "Foundations for Decision Making," "Hepatitis B: Patient Information," "Hepatitis C: A Guide for Primary Care Physicians," and "The Visionaries." The Foundation also offers liver wellness and substance abuse prevention programs to elementary schools and corporations.

President: John M. Vierling, M.D.
Executive Director: Alan P. Brownstein
Organization Language: Spanish.
Year Established: 1976
Organization Chapters: 23
Organization Members: 20,000

Publishes the following materials:
Your Liver Lets You Live ~ *Brochure*
Viral Hepatitis: Everybody's Problem? ~ *Brochure*
Cirrhosis: Many Causes ~ *Brochure*
Hepatitis A, B, & C ~ *Brochure*
Biliary Atresia ~ *Brochure*
Como Puedes Quererme Si No Me Conoces? ~ *Brochure*
Enfermedades hepaticas sobre las que usted debe estar informado ~ *Brochure*
Calculos y Otros Trastornos de la Vesicula Biliar: Problema Nacional de Salud ~ *Brochure*

Concerned with the following diseases or disorders:
Alagille Syndrome; Alpha-1-Antitrypsin Deficiency; Antithrombin III Deficiency; Banti's Syndrome; Biliary Atresia, Extrahepatic; Budd Chiari Syndrome; Caroli Disease; Cat Eye Syndrome; Cholangitis, Primary Sclerosing; Cholestasis; Cirrhosis, Primary Biliary; Crigler Najjar Syndrome Type I; Dubin Johnson Syndrome; Fascioliasis; Gilbert Syndrome; Hepatic Fibrosis, Congenital; Hepatitis B; Hepatitis, Neonatal; Hepatitis, Non-A, Non-B (Hepatitis C); Hepatorenal Syndrome; Kernicterus; Polycystic Liver Disease; Vitamin E Deficiency; Wilson's Disease

1575 AMERICAN LUNG ASSOCIATION (ALA)

1740 Broadway
New York, NY 10019 212-315-8700
800-586-4872
Fax: 212-265-5642
E-mail: info@lungusa.org
http://www.lungusa.org

The American Lung Association (ALA) is a national not-for-profit voluntary health organization dedicated to the prevention, cure, and control of all types of lung disease such as asthma, emphysema, tuberculosis, and lung cancer. This is accomplished through programs of community service, public health education, advocacy, and research. The ALA was established in 1904 as the National Association for the Study and Prevention of Tuberculosis. As the number of tuberculosis cases declined over the years, the association widened its focus to include other forms of lung disease and, in 1973, changed its name to the American Lung Association. The Association offers assistance through support groups, genetic counseling, patient networking, referrals, and the development and dissemination of educational materials. Such materials include reports, brochures, audiovisual aids, and Spanish language materials.

President: Donald Clark
Organization Language: Spanish (written).
Year Established: 1904
Organization Members: Non-Membership

Publishes the following materials:
American Lung Association ~ *Mission Statement*

Concerned with the following diseases or disorders:
APECED Syndrome; Alpha-1-Antitrypsin Deficiency; Alveolitis, Extrinsic Allergic; Alveolitis, Fibrosing; Atrial Septal Defects; Atrioventricular Septal Defect; Berylliosis; Bronchopulmonary Dysplasia (BPD); Churg Strauss Syndrome; Cystic Fibrosis; Dextrocardia with Situs Inversus; Dilatation of the Pulmonary Artery, Idiopathic; Emphysema, Congenital Lobar;

Goodpasture Syndrome; Granulomatosis, Lymphomatoid; Histiocytosis X; Kartagener Syndrome; Lymphangioleiomyomatosis; Pneumonia, Interstitial; Pulmonary Alveolar Proteinosis; Pulmonary Hypertension, Primary; Pulmonary Hypertension, Secondary; Respiratory Distress Syndrome, Adult; Respiratory Distress Syndrome, Infant; Sarcoidosis; Tuberculosis; Wegener's Granulomatosis; Yellow Nail Syndrome

1576 AMERICAN MEDICAL ASSOCIATION (AMA) PHYSICIAN SELECT

http://www.ama-assn.org/aps/amahg.htm

The American Medical Association (AMA) is a professional association of physicians and medical students dedicated to the health of America. The AMA's web site on the Internet includes an arca called "AMA Physician Select" or "On-line Doctor Finder" that provides information on most licensed physicians in the United States and its possessions, including more than 650,000 doctors of medicine (MD) and doctors of osteopathy or osteopathic medicine (DO). All physician credential data have been verified for accuracy and authenticated by accrediting agencies, medical schools, residency training programs, licensing and certifying boards, and other data sources. Physician Select is intended for use by the general public to allow them quick access to information on physicians. Online users can search for physicians by physician name, medical specialty, and location. Physician medical specialty categories that may be selected during a Physician Select search include allergy and immunology, anesthesiology, cardiology, dermatology, diabetes, emergency medicine, family practice/general practice, geriatrics, internal medicine, medical genetics, neurological surgery, neurology, obstetrics and gynecology, oncology, ophthalmology, orthopedics, other, otolaryngology, pathology, pediatrics, physical medicine and rehabilitation, plastic surgery, preventive medicine, psychiatry, radiology, surgery, and urology. Specific physician profiles include their location and phone numbers; primary and, if appropriate, secondary practice specialties; medical school and residency training information; major professional activities; and confirmation of board certification.

1577 AMERICAN METHADONE TREATMENT ASSOCIATION, INC.

217 Broadway
Suite 304
New York, NY 10007 212-566-5555
Fax: 212-349-2944

The American Methadone Treatment Association, Inc. was founded in 1983 to promote the growth and development of methadone treatment services. The Association currently represents over 15 states and the District of Columbia, providing treatment to more than 105,000 individuals in approximately 550 programs. Committed to enhancing the quality of patient care, the American Methadone Treatment Association, in conjunction with the American Society of Addiction Medicine, developed clinical guidelines to assist individual practitioners and policy makers in the development of effective methadone treatment services. In addition, the Association focuses on federal, state, and program specific treatment policies; advocates on behalf of affected individuals and their families; engages in professional and public education; and promotes the coordination of and communication among methadone treatment programs. The Association also convenes a national conference every 18 months for researchers, treatment personnel, and policy makers, and provides a variety of materials including fact sheets, brochures, and a quarterly newsletter entitled "News Report" that provides an analysis of leading federal and state initiatives in methadone treatment.

President: Mark W. Parrino (1984 to Present)
Year Established: 1983
Organization Chapters: 17
Organization Members: 550

Publishes the following materials:
Methadone Maintenance Treatment ~ *Fact Sheet*
American Methadone Treatment Association New Report ~ *Reprint*
Acronyms ~ *Fact Sheet*

1578 AMERICAN ORGAN TRANSPLANT ASSOCIATION (AOTA)

3335 Cartwright Road
Missouri City, TX 77459 281-261-2682
Fax: 281-499-2315
E-mail: aota@phoenix.com

The American Organ Transplant Association (AOTA) is a nonprofit organization dedicated to helping defray out-of-pocket expenses for organ transplant recipients. Founded in 1987, the Association also seeks to generate increased public awareness of organ transplantation and to provide information on the need, importance, and success of transplantation. AOTA engages in fund-raising, supplies necessary support services to affected individuals, provides referrals to appropriate agencies, and lobbies for government legislation on behalf of the transplant community. In addition, AOTA arranges air transportation for over 60 patients and family members per year to and from transplant centers for evaluation and check-ups; donations of some medications; discounted rental cars for affected individuals and hospital personnel; free transportation to hospitals for patients anywhere in the country; and free hotel accommodations for three nights for family members who accompany patients to the hospital. AOTA offers a variety of materials including brochures, a regular newsletter, and a booklet entitled "Life After Transplantation."

President: Sandi Berman Hartig (1993 to Present).
Executive Director: Ellen Gordon Woodall
Year Established: 1987
Organization Members: 200

Publishes the following materials:
Helping to Bear the Cost of Living ~ *Brochure*
AOTA Items ~ *Newsletter*
Expenses as a % of Revenues ~ *Fact Sheet*
Life After Transplantation ~ *Booklet*

1579 AMERICAN PARALYSIS ASSOCIATION (APA)

500 Morris Avenue
Springfield, NJ 07081 973-379-2690
800-225-0292
Fax: 973-912-9433
E-mail: paralysis@aol.com
http://www.apacure.com

The American Paralysis Association is a national not-for-profit research and self-help organization that was established in 1982. The mission of the Association is to encourage and support worldwide research activities designed to speed the progress toward a cure for paralysis caused by spinal cord injury and various central nervous system disorders. The Association has also provided seed money for innovative medical research studies that are largely responsible for recent breakthroughs in the prevention of spinal cord injury and its treatments. In addition, the Association sponsors international conferences on spinal injury, providing an important forum for the exchange of information among leaders in the field of spinal cord injury research. Educational materials produced by the organization include brochures, a publication called "Progress in Research," and a newsletter entitled "Walking Tomorrow."

President: Mitchell R. Stoller (1993-Present)
Executive Director: Susan P. Howley
Year Established: 1982
Organization Chapters: 5
Organization Members: 12,000

1580 AMERICAN PORPHYRIA FOUNDATION

P.O. Box 22712
Houston, TX 77227 713-266-9617
Fax: 713-871-1788
http://www.enterprise.net/apf/

The American Porphyria Foundation is a national voluntary health organization established in 1981 to enhance public awareness of and education about the porphyrias and to aid in advancing treatments of these disorders. Porphyria is a group of rare genetic disorders characterized by disturbances of porphyrin metabolism. The Foundation serves people with porphyria and physicians by serving as an information source and exchange. It also provides individuals with the opportunity to participate in research, support groups, political action programs, seminars, and fund-raising projects. The Foundation produces a variety of publications including a general brochure and several disease specific brochures. The Foundation also maintains a web site at [http://www.enterprise.net/apf/].

Executive Director: Desiree Lyon
Year Established: 1981
Organization Members: 3,000

Publishes the following materials:
When the Sun Can't Shine ~ *Brochure*
American Porphyria Foundation ~ *Brochure*
Hematin ~ *Brochure*
American Porphyria Foundation The Porphyrias An Overview ~ *Brochure*
American Porphyria Foundation Acute Intermittent Porphyria ~ *Brochure*
American Porphyria Foundation Erythropoietic Protoporphyria (EPP) ~ *Brochure*
American Porphyria Foundation Diet and Nutrition in Porphyria ~ *Brochure*
American Porphyria Foundation Porphyria Cutanea Tarda ~ *Brochure*

Concerned with the following diseases or disorders:
Erythropoietic Protoporphyria (EPP); Porphyria; Porphyria Cutanea Tarda; Porphyria, ALA-D; Porphyria, Acute Intermittent; Porphyria, Congenital Erythropoietic; Porphyria, Hereditary Coproporphyria; Porphyria, Variegate

1581 **AMERICAN PRINTING HOUSE FOR THE BLIND**

1839 Frankfort Avenue
P.O. Box 6085
Louisville, KY 40206-0085 502-895-2405
800-223-1839
Fax: 502-899-2274
E-mail: info@aph.org
http://www.aph.org

The American Printing House for the Blind is a national not-for-profit voluntary self-help organization dedicated to assisting blind individuals and their families. Established in 1858, the American Printing House for the Blind offers "Readers Digest" in Braille, "Newsweek" and "Time" magazines on cassettes, and various books on cassettes. In addition, the organization also provides a newsletter, brochures, and pamphlets. The organization also offers referrals to other appropriate organizations for further support and assistance.

President: Tuck Tinsley, III
Organization Language: Spanish (written).
Year Established: 1858
Organization Members: Non-Membership

Concerned with the following diseases or disorders:
Bardet Biedl Syndrome; Retinitis Pigmentosa

1582 **AMERICAN PSEUDO-OBSTRUCTION & HIRSCHSPRUNG'S DISEASE SOCIETY, INC. (APHS, INC.)**

158 Pleasant Street
North Andover, MA 01845 508-685-4477
800-394-2747
Fax: 508-685-4488
E-mail: aphs@mail.tiac.net
http://www.tiac.net/users/aphs

The American Pseudo-obstruction and Hirschsprung's Disease Society, Inc. is an international support organization that was established in 1988. The Society promotes public awareness of gastrointestinal motility disorders, particularly Intestinal Pseudo-obstruction and Hirschsprung's Disease. Intestinal Pseudo-obstruction, a digestive disorder that may be present at birth, is characterized by vomiting, constipation, and pain without evidence of obstruction. Hirschsprung's Disease, a condition that usually becomes apparent during early infancy or early childhood, is characterized by absense of groups of nerve fibers in the muscular wall of the colon. As a result, feces may accumulate in the colon, causing abnormal widening of the colon, continuous spasms of the colon, abdominal bloating, diarrhea, vomiting, and other symptoms. Established in 1988, the Society provides information and support to affected individuals and families through a variety of programs including parent-to-parent networking and annual educational symposia. Through various fund-raising activities and events, the Society encourages and supports ongoing medical research in the area of gastrointestinal motility disorders. The organization also provides a variety of publications including brochures, pamphlets, reports, and a regular newsletter.

President: Andrea M. Anastas (1988 to Present)
Organization Language: Spanish (written).
Year Established: 1988
Organization Members: 1,700

Publishes the following materials:
North American PEDIATRIC PSEUDO-OBSTRUCTION SOCIETY,INC. ~ *Brochure*
Hirschsprung's Disease Questions and Answers For Parents ~ *Brochure*
APHS ~ *Factsheet*
Hirschsprung's Disease ~ *Factsheet*
Chronic Intestinal Pseudo-obstruction ~ *Factsheet*
APHS Newsletter ~ *Newsletter*
Hirschsprung's Disease Chapter 133 ~ *Reprint*
Hirschsprung Disease ~ *Reprint*
What is New in Gastrointestinal Motility ~ *Reprint*
Pediatric Gastroesophageal Reflux: A Guide for the Primary Care Physician ~ *Brochure*
Gastroesophageal Reflux in Children ~ *Factsheet*
Gastroesophageal Reflux: One Reason Why Baby Won't Eat ~ *Reprint*
Chronic Intestinal Pseudo-obstruction Chapter 7 ~ *Reprint*
Chronic Intestinal Pseudo-obstruction: Diagnosis and Treatment ~ *Reprint*
Gastroesophageal Reflux in Infants and Children ~ *Brochure*

Concerned with the following diseases or disorders:
Cat Eye Syndrome; Hirschsprung's Disease; Intestinal Pseudoobstruction; Muscular Dystrophy, Oculo-Gastrointestinal

1583 **AMERICAN SELF-HELP CLEARINGHOUSE**

Northwest Covenant Medical Center
25 Pocono Road
Denville, NJ 07834-2995 973-625-3037
Fax: 973-625-8848
TDD: 973-625-9053
E-mail: ashc@cybernex.net
http://www.cmhc.com/selfhelp/

The American Self-Help Clearinghouse is a not-for-profit service organization that increases the awareness, utilization, and development of self-help support groups and networks across the country. Established in 1990, the Clearinghouse provides free consultation assistance to those individuals interested in starting needed new member-run national/international rare disorder support and information-sharing networks that currently do not exist. The Clearinghouse also provides information on existing national/international self-help groups for a wide range of illnesses, disabilities, addictions, and stressful life situations such as bereavement. The Clearinghouse places people in contact with local self-help clearinghouses in many states. In addition, the American Self-Help Clearinghouse provides a variety of educational and support materials including a handout on "Ideas for Starting a Self-Help Group," a brochure on "Developing a Self-Help Support Network for Persons with a Rare Illness," the latest paperback edition of "The Self-Help Sourcebook," and a free listing of phone contacts for self-help clearinghouses across the country.

Executive Director: Edward Madara
Year Established: 1990

Publishes the following materials:
The Self-Help Sourcebook ~ *Book*
Our Clearinghouse Services ~ *Factsheet*
Developing a Self-Help Support Network for Persons with a Rare Illness ~ *Pamphlet*

1584 AMERICAN SOCIAL HEALTH ASSOCIATION (ASHA)

P.O. Box 13827
Resrch Triangle Pk, NC 27709 919-361-8400
Fax: 919-361-8425
http://sunsite.unc.edu/ASHA

The American Social Health Association (ASHA) is a not-for-profit voluntary organization dedicated to stopping sexually transmitted diseases (STDs) and their harmful consequences to individuals, families, and communities. Established in 1914, ASHA provides direct patient support through the Herpes Resource Center/National Herpes Hotline and the HPV Support Group, which coordinate a network of over 100 local support groups and publish quarterly journals. ASHA also operates the National AIDS Hotline and the National STD Hotline, both under contract with the Centers for Disease Control and Prevention (CDC), as well as the FIRST STEP Hotline and Health Check Hotline, components of North Carolina's effort to improve the health and development of children in the state. In addition, ASHA advocates for increased funding for STD programs and public policies on STD control, working through its office in Washington D.C.; provides leadership for the National Coalition to Fight Sexually Transmitted Diseases; and operates the Women's Health Matters program. The organization also administers the ASHA Research Fund, the only privately funded training program for STD research. ASHA's materials include an annual report, quarterly catalog, and pamphlets. ASHA also maintains a web site at [http://sunsite.unc.edu/ASHA/].

President: Linda L. Alexander, Ph.D., FAAN (CEO)
Executive Director: Sharon Broom (Director of Public Relations)
Organization Language: Spanish (written/spoken).
Year Established: 1914
Organization Members: Non-Membership

Publishes the following materials:
Some Questions and Answers about PID ~ *Brochure*
Hepatitis B. The Sexually Transmitted Disease With No Cure ~ *Brochure*
My Health Matters ~ *Brochure*
Sex Talk. Making Love Better, Healthier ~ *Brochure*
Better Sex. Healthy Sex ~ *Brochure*
Stopping Gonorrhea the clap ~ *Brochure*
Condoms, Contraceptives and STDs ~ *Brochure*
Becoming an Askable Parent ~ *Booklet*
For Teens ~ *Leaflet*
Some Questions and Answers about Chlamydia ~ *Brochure*
Questions. HIV/AIDS ~ *Brochure*
Questions. STD(VD) ~ *Brochure*
Questions. Herpes ~ *Brochure*
Some Questions and Answers about HPV and Genital Warts ~ *Brochure*

Concerned with the following diseases or disorders:
AIDS (Acquired Immune Deficiency Syndrome); Chlamydia; Condyloma; Epididymitis; Hepatitis B

1585 AMERICAN SOCIETY FOR DEAF CHILDREN (ASDC)

1820 Tribute Road
Suite A
Sacramento, CA 95815 916-641-6084
800-942-2732
Fax: 916-641-6085
TDD: 916-641-6084
E-mail: ASDC1@aol.com
www.educ.kent.edu/deafed/asdchome.htm

The American Society for Deaf Children, a national not-for-profit self-help organization, consists of parents and families who advocate the full participation of hearing-impaired children in their communities, schools, and families. The organization supports the use of signing and recognizes and respects deaf culture as critical for enhancing and broadening the social, personal, and educational aspects of hearing-impaired children's lives. Educational materials produced by the organization include a variety of patient and professional informational brochures and a regular newsletter.

President: Ms. Benna Timberlake (1993-Present)
Organization Language: Spanish.
Year Established: 1962
Organization Chapters: 100
Organization Members: 20,000

Concerned with the following diseases or disorders:
Alstrom Syndrome; Branchio Oto Renal Syndrome; DOOR Syndrome; Marshall Syndrome; Miller Syndrome; Nager Syndrome; Norrie Syndrome; Smith Magenis Syndrome; Treacher Collins Syndrome; Usher's Syndrome; Wildervanck Syndrome

1586 AMERICAN SOCIETY OF HYPERTENSION (ASH)

515 Madison Avenue
Room 1212
New York, NY 10022 212-644-0650
Fax: 212-644-0658
E-mail: ASHNY@aol.com
http://www.ash-us.org

The American Society of Hypertension (ASH) is a not-for-profit organization dedicated to a clearer understanding, dissemination, and evaluation of the vast accumulation of data on high blood pressure (hypertension) and to provision of a separate forum for those involved in the study of management of hypertension. Established in 1985 by 17 world famous clinicians and scientists, ASH is now the largest U.S. organization devoted exclusively to hypertension and related cardiovascular diseases. Through the years, ASH has become a scientific organization on the cutting edge of education, research, and treatment strategies and has earned the respect of clinicians, scientists, industry, and government agencies. In addition, the organization conducts an annual four-day scientific meeting, presents several awards to young researchers, and holds regional meetings to provide practicing physicians and their staff with the latest and most comprehensive diagnostic and therapeutic options available in the treatment of hypertensive individuals. Consisting of 3,000 members, ASH publishes a monthly journal entitled "American Journal of Hypertension," has a member directory, and provides educational videos on the topic of hypertension. ASH can be reached at its web site on the Internet at [http://www.ash-us.org].

President: Michael Alderman, M.D. (1996 to Present)
Executive Director: Sandra Kuhach
Year Established: 1985
Organization Members: 3,000

Publishes the following materials:
The American Society of Hypertension Presents "Controlling Hypertension: A Team Approach" ~ *Video Tape*
American Journal of Hypertension ~ *Booklet*
American Society of Hypertension ~ *Brochure*

1587 ANOREXIA NERVOSA & RELATED EATING DISORDERS, INC. (ANRED)

665 South Yale Avenue
Tulsa, OK 74136 918-481-4044
www.anred.org and http://www.laureate.com

Anorexia Nervosa & Related Eating Disorders, Inc. is a national not-for-profit organization dedicated to gathering and disseminating information concerning eating and exercise disorders; leading workshops and self-help groups to assist people with these disorders; providing training for human services personnel who work with affected individuals; and providing speakers and programs for schools, agencies, and other groups. Established in 1979, Anorexia Nervosa & Related Eating Disorders serves people with eating and exercise disorders, their families and friends, youth workers, educators, and members of the medical and mental health communities. The organization offers a variety of educational and support materials including fact sheets, brochures, booklets, and a newsletter entitled "Alert," which summarizes research developments and covers special topics concerning eating and exercise disorders. The organization also maintains web sites at [http://www.anred.org] and [http://www.laureate.com].

President: Jean Bradley Rubel (1979-Present)
Year Established: 1979

Publishes the following materials:
Eating and Exercise Disorders ~ *Booklet*

Concerned with the following diseases or disorders:
Anorexia Nervosa; Bulimia

1588 ANXIETY DISORDERS ASSOCIATION OF AMERICA (ADAA)

6000 Executive Boulevard
Suite 513
Rockville, MD 20852 301-231-9350

The mission of the Anxiety Disorders Association of America (ADAA) is to promote the prevention and cure of anxiety disorders and to improve the lives of all affected individuals. ADAA offers several materials concerning anxiety disorders including a quarterly newsletter that contains clinical information and updates, news on the latest events that ADAA is sponsoring, and personal accounts from affected individuals and members who share their experiences. ADAA also sponsors a variety of events each year including "National Anxiety Disorders Screening Day" and an annual national conference.

Concerned with the following diseases or disorders:
Panic Anxiety Syndrome

1589 ARTHRITIS FOUNDATION
1330 West Peachtree Street
Atlanta, GA 30309 404-872-7100
800-283-7800
Fax: 404-872-0457
E-mail: info@arthritis.org
http://ww.arthritis.org

The Arthritis Foundation is a not-for-profit voluntary health organization dedicated to supporting research into the prevention and cure of arthritis and providing services to improve the quality of life for affected individuals. Arthritis, an inflammatory condition of the joints that may result in swelling and pain, is a joint disease that may be due to a number of different underlying causes. Established in 1948, the Arthritis Foundation disseminates information worldwide on how arthritis is diagnosed, how it is inherited, how it affects pregnancy, its potential symptoms, and treatments. The organization works for all people affected by any of the more than 100 forms of arthritis or related diseases. In nationwide chapters, the Foundation helps support research, offers professional and community education programs, provides referral services, engages in government advocacy, and conducts fund-raising activities. Educational materials include a bimonthly magazine entitled "Arthritis Today," regular newsletters, reports, audiovisual aids, and various topical brochures.

President: Don L. Riggin (1965-Present)
Organization Language: Spanish. French.
Year Established: 1948
Organization Chapters: 60
Organization Members: 375500

Publishes the following materials:
Arthritis Information - Services of the Arthritis Foundation ~ *Brochure*

Concerned with the following diseases or disorders:
Ankylosing Spondylitis; Arthritis, Infectious; Arthritis, Psoriatic; Behcet's Syndrome; Chondrocalcinosis, Familial Articular; Dermatomyositis; Farber's Disease; Felty Syndrome; Fibromyalgia; Forestier's Disease; Mixed Connective Tissue Disease (MCTD); Osgood Schlatter's Disease; Osteonecrosis; Polychondritis; Polymyalgia Rheumatica; Polymyositis; Pseudoxanthoma Elasticum (PXE); Reflex Sympathetic Dystrophy Syndrome (RSDS); Sjogren Syndrome

1590 ASSOCIATION FRANCOPHONE DES GLYCOGENOSES (AFG)
La Versaine
16200
Julienne,
France 10330545367238
Fax: 10330545367238
www.infobiogen.fr/agora/associations/AFG/

The Association Francophone Des Glycogenoses (AFG) is a unique organization dedicated to assisting individuals and families affected by a rare group of genetic diseases that impair the body's ability to properly metabolize or break down glycogen (glycogenesis). Termed "glycogen storage diseases," these familial disorders are characterized by the abnormal accumulation of glycogen in various organs of the body. Symptoms vary greatly depending upon the specific organ systems that are affected and may include muscle weakness without loss of muscle mass (atrophy), abnormal enlargement of the heart (cardiomegaly), liver (hepatomegaly), and/or tongue (macroglossia), as well as heart and kidney problems. These diseases include (but are not limited to) Von Gierke Disease (Type 1), Cori Disease (Type III), Andersen Disease (Type IV), and Pompe Disease (Type II). Established in 1992, the Association is dedicated to identifying families affected by these diseases and providing appropriate information about the different forms of the disease. In addition, the Association Francophone Des Glycogenoses is interested in stimulating ongoing research into the treatment and potential cure of these disorders. The organization distributes educational materials on these disorders and publishes a self-titled regular newsletter. Materials are written in French. The Association also maintains a World Wide Web site at [http://www.infobiogen.fr/agora/associations/AFG/].

President: Hugon Anne
Organization Language: French (written/spoken).
Year Established: 1992
Organization Members: 200

Publishes the following materials:
Association Francophone Des Glycogenoses (French) ~ *Mission Statement*
AFG (French) ~ *Newsletter*
Campagne D'information (French) ~ *Pamphlet*
AFG (Groupe d'entraide) (French) ~ *Phamplet*

1591 ASSOCIATION FOR CHILDREN WITH LIFE-THREATENING OR TERMINAL CONDITIONS AND THEIR FAMILIES (ACT)

65 St. Michael's Hill
Bristol, BS2 8DZ
United Kingdom 117-922-1556
Fax: 117-930-4707

The Association for Children with Life-Threatening or Terminal Conditions and their Families (ACT) is an international nonprofit organization dedicated to providing resources for parents and professionals caring for children with life-threatening or terminal conditions. Established in 1993, ACT's mission is to facilitate and encourage provision of the best possible care for affected children and their families by promoting models of good practice, providing information and education, and stimulating research and informed debate. Comprised of 200 members, ACT provides grief and bereavement counseling to family members of children who have life-threatening and terminal illnesses; works to represent the needs of affected children and their families; and facilitates the provision of a flexible network of care and support. ACT also provides a National Information Resource for children, parents, caregivers, and professionals; promotes models of good care and practice; provides conference and study opportunities; and represents the interest of its members. In addition, ACT publishes a newsletter entitled "ACT - NOW," informational brochures, a compendium of children's hospices in the United Kingdom, and a publication entitled "Listen: My Child Has a Lot of Living to Do."

President: Professor David Baum (1995 to Present)
Executive Director: Stella Elston
Year Established: 1993
Organization Members: 200

Publishes the following materials:
What is ACT? ~ *Brochure*
ACT Charter for Children with Life-Threatening Conditions and their Families (ACT) ~ *Booklet*
ACT Charter ~ *Fact Sheet*
ACT Membership ~ *Mission Statement*
Corporate/Group Membership ~ *Membership Form*
ACT (Association for Children with Life-Threatening or Terminal Conditions and their Families) ~ *Brochure*
ACT Publications ~ *Leaflett*
ACT Membership Subscription Form ~ *Order Form*
ACT NOW ~ *Newsletter*

1592 ASSOCIATION FOR GLYCOGEN STORAGE DISEASE (AGSD)

P.O. Box 896
Durant, IA 52747 319-785-6038
Fax: 319-785-6038

The Association for Glycogen Storage Disease is a national not-for-profit organization that acts as a focus for individuals with Glycogen Storage Diseases and their families. Glycogen storage diseases are a group of rare inborn errors of metabolism characterized by deficiencies of certain enzymes involved in the metabolism of glycogen. The Association seeks to foster communication between affected individuals for the purpose of mutual support and information sharing. Other goals include increasing public awareness of these disorders and promoting medical research into the various forms of glycogen storage diseases. Funds have been used to award college grants and scholarships to students with these disorders and award research grants to medical professionals working on glycogen storage diseases. The Association also fosters publicity in local newspapers to make the public more aware of these diseases and to highlight the need for more research and funding for glycogen storage disease. Educational materials include brochures, newsletters, and a parent handbook.

President: Hollie Swain (1979-Present)
Year Established: 1979
Organization Members: 300

Publishes the following materials:
Association for Glycogen Storage Disease - Could Someone You Know be Affected ~ *Brochure*
The Ray ~ *Newsletter*

Concerned with the following diseases or disorders:
Andersen Disease; McArdle Disease; Pompe Disease; Von Gierke Disease

1593 ASSOCIATION FOR MACULAR DISEASES, INC. (AMD)

210 East 64th Street
New York, NY 10021 212-605-3719
Fax: 212-605-3795

The Association for Macular Diseases is a national not-for-profit voluntary organization that seeks to inform, educate, motivate, and give practical advice and coping strategies to people with retinal degeneration due to macular disease. Age-related macular degeneration is the major cause of legal blindness in Americans over the age of 50. Established in 1978, the Association has work space, donated by the Macular Foundation, at the Manhattan Eye, Ear & Throat Hospital. The Association's quarterly newsletter "Eyes Only" informs members of qualified researchers and the most current optical and electronic devices that improve sight. In addition, the group offers referrals for diagnosis and treatment and arranges public seminars with professional specialists. The Association also distributes educational brochures and fact sheets about Macular Degeneration.

President: Nikolai Stevenson
Year Established: 1978
Organization Chapters: 5
Organization Members: 5,000

Concerned with the following diseases or disorders:
Choroiditis, Serpiginous; Cone Dystrophy; Macular Degeneration; Macular Degeneration, Polymorphic; Pars Planitis; Retinoschisis; X-linked Juvenile Retinoschisis

1594 ASSOCIATION FOR NEURO-METABOLIC DISORDERS (ANMD)

5223 Brookfield Lane
Sylvania, OH 43560-1809 419-885-1497

The Association for Neuro-Metabolic Disorders is a national not-for-profit voluntary organization that is composed of families with children who have metabolic disorders that affect the central nervous system and brain. Established in 1981, the Association shares support and information with other members through a variety of activities. These include a yearly parent conference featuring discussions by experts on neuro-metabolic disorders; an annual family picnic; informal meetings; and phone calls with concerned parents. Other activities include formal lobbying and educational efforts; contact with similar organizations throughout the United States and other countries; and expanded efforts in offering support to teens and adults with neuro-metabolic disorders. The Association produces a brochure and regular newsletter.

President: Cheryl Volk
Executive Director: Cheryl Volk
Year Established: 1981
Organization Chapters: 1
Organization Members: 150

Publishes the following materials:
ANMD Support and Education ~ *Brochure*
ANMD ~ *Newsletter*

Concerned with the following diseases or disorders:
Acidemia, Isovaleric; Acidemia, Methylmalonic; Adrenoleukodystrophy; Alexander's Disease; Alpers Disease; Amyloidosis; Arginase Deficiency; Aspartylglycosaminuria; Carbohydrate deficient Glycoprotein Syndrome Type I; Carboxylase Deficiency, Multiple; Carnitine Deficiency Syndromes; Carnitine Palmitoyltransferase Deficiency; Carnosinemia; Cytochrome C Oxidase Deficiency; Fabry Disease; Farber's Disease; Forbes Disease; Fucosidosis; Galactosemia; Glucose-6-Phosphate Dehydrogenase Deficiency; Glycogen Storage Disease VIII; Hers Disease; Histidinemia; Leigh's Disease; Lesch Nyhan Syndrome; Leukodystrophy; Leukodystrophy, Canavan's; Leukodystrophy, Krabbe's; Leukodystrophy, Metachromatic; Long Chain Acyl CoA Dehydrogenase Deficiency (LCAD); Macroglossia; Maple Syrup Urine Disease; Medium Chain Acyl CoA Dehydrogenase Deficiency; N-Acetyl Glutamate Synthetase Deficiency; Niemann Pick Disease; Phosphoglycerate Kinase Deficiency; Polyglucosan Body Disease, Adult; Pompe Disease; Pyruvate Carboxylase Deficiency; Pyruvate Dehydrogenase Deficiency; Refsum Syndrome; Santavuori Disease; Schindler Disease; Shy Drager Syndrome; Tarui Disease; Tay Sachs Disease; Tetrahydrobiopterin Deficiency; Trimethylaminuria; Tyrosinemia, Hereditary; Whipple's Disease

1595 ASSOCIATION FOR PERSONS WITH SEVERE HANDICAPS (TASH)

29 West Susquehanna Avenue
Suite 210
Baltimore, MD 21204 410-828-8274
800-482-8274
Fax: 410-828-6706
TDD: 410-828-1306
E-mail: tash@tash.org
http://www.tash.org

The Association for Persons with Severe Handicaps (TASH) is a civil rights organization for people with disabilities, their families, advocates, and people around the world who work in the disability field. Established in 1975, TASH's primary concerns include advocacy for comprehensive, high quality, inclusive education and rehabilitation; effective use and sharing of experience and expertise; support for educators, parents, and service providers; and full participation in inclusive community settings that support the same quality of life available to people without disabilities. TASH acts as a clearinghouse for reports of unjust treatment towards disabled people, provides information and referral services, and helps chapters to support local and regional concerns. In addition, the organization sponsors an international conference annually and publishes a monthly newsletter along with a quarterly journal entitled "JASH" (Journal of the Association for Persons with a Severe Handicap). The group maintains a site on the World Wide Web at [http://www.tash.org]. Consisting of approximately 5,100 members, TASH has members from the United States, Canada, and 38 countries worldwide.

Executive Director: Nancy R. Weiss
Year Established: 1975
Organization Chapters: 38
Organization Members: 5,100

Publishes the following materials:
TASH's Structure, Purpose, History and Program ~ *Mission Statement*
TASH Newsletter ~ *Newsletter*
JASH: Journal of the Association for Persons with Severe Handicaps ~ *Journal*
TASH Publications ~ *Order Form*

1596 ASSOCIATION FOR SPINA BIFIDA AND HYDROCEPHALUS (ASBAH)

ASBAH House
42 Park Road
Peterborough, PE1 2YQ
United Kingdom

The Association for Spina Bifida and Hydrocephalus (ASBAH) is a voluntary organization dedicated to providing services to people with spina bifida and/or hydrocephalus, and their care providers. Spina Bifida is characterized by malformation of the spinal column in which incomplete closure of certain vertebrae leaves a portion of the spinal cord exposes (spina bifida). Hydrocephalus is a condition characterized by inhibition of the normal flow of cerebrospinal fluid (CSF) and abnormal widening (dilatation) of the cerebral spaces of the brain (ventricles), causing accumulation of CSF in the skull and potentially increased pressure on brain tissue. Established in 1966, ASBAH aims to keep its clients' knowledge up to date, extend their choices, maximize opportunities for independence, and help their integration in society. The organization's unique network of Fieldworkers provides advice and close support at times of special need to individuals and families in England, Wales, and Northern Ireland. The service is backed up by specialist advisers in education, continence, mobility, and medical matters. Through nationwide and regional networks, these professionals develop and maintain expertise in spina bifida and hydrocephalus so that they may inform and assist other professionals in giving the best possible service. Consisting of 70 chapters, the organization produces educational materials including an information sheet entitled "Just What Is ASBAH?" a newsletter, and a journal. Program activities include advocacy and education.

Executive Director: Andrew Russell
Year Established: 1966
Organization Chapters: 70

Publishes the following materials:
Just What is ASBAH? ~ *Mission Statement*
ASBAH Publications Order Form ~ *Order Form*

Concerned with the following diseases or disorders:
Hydrocephalus; Spina Bifida

1597 ASSOCIATION FOR THE CARE OF CHILDREN'S HEALTH (ACCH)

7910 Woodmont Avenue
Suite 300
Bethesda, MD 20814 301-654-6549
Fax: 301-986-4553
E-mail: acch@clark.net
http://www.acch.org

The Association for the Care of Children's Health (ACCH) is a national not-for-profit professional and advocacy organization. Founded in 1965, the Association is a multidisciplinary network dedicated to establishing a significant place for human services in the health care marketplace. The Association promotes policies and practices that address the comprehensive needs of children, youth, and their families. To this end, the organization is concerned with developmental, emotional, and social needs in hospitals, homes, and community programs. The Association publishes journals, books, manuals, and other resource materials. It offers innovative work published by others through its information clearinghouse. In addition, the organization offers a forum for individuals of diverse disciplines including professionals and family members. Activities include sharing knowledge of practice and supporting of established standards and guidelines. Members receive timely research, advocacy services, news publications, and an annual catalogue of resources.

President: Ericka Waidley (1993-Present)
Executive Director: William Sciarillo, RN, MSN, ScD
Year Established: 1965
Organization Chapters: 35
Organization Members: 4,000

Publishes the following materials:
New and Outstanding Resources from The Association for the Care of Children's Health ~ *Resource Listing*
Association for the Care of Children's Health - Your Invitation to Join ~ *Brochure*
1994 ACCH Resource Catalogue ~ *Catalogue*
Healing, Healthcare: Transcending the Psychosocial ~ *Booklet*
Family-Centered Care for Children Needing Specialized Health and Developmental Services ~ *Book*

1598 ASSOCIATION OF BIRTH DEFECT CHILDREN, INC. (ABDC)

827 Irma Avenue
Orlando, FL 32803 407-245-7035
800-313-2232
Fax: 407-245-7087
http://www.birthdefects.org

The Association of Birth Defect Children is a national not-for-profit organization that functions as a clearinghouse, providing parents and professionals with information about birth defects and services for children with disabilities. Founded in 1982, it sponsors the National Birth Defect Registry and a parent matching service. It also studies the links between drugs, radiation, alcohol, chemicals, lead, mercury, dioxin, and birth defects. The Association of Birth Defect Children operates with a staff and community volunteers under the guidance of a board of directors and two professional advisory boards. Newsletters and publications are supplied to parents, professionals, and interested organizations. Free questionnaires and information packets are available through the organization's toll-free Birth Defect Registry Hotline.

President: Betty Mekdeci
Executive Director: Betty Mekdeci
Year Established: 1982

Publishes the following materials:
What is ABCD? ~ *Membership Application*
Neural Tube Defects (NTDs) ~ *Fact Sheet*

Concerned with the following diseases or disorders:
Anencephaly; Congenital Varicella Syndrome; Fahr's Disease; Tethered Spinal Cord Syndrome

1599 ASSOCIATION OF CHILDREN'S PROSTHETIC/ORTHOTIC CLINICS (ACPOC)

6300 North River Road
Suite 727
Rosemont, IL 60018-4226 847-698-1694
Fax: 847-823-0536
E-mail: hohimer@aaos.org
http://www.acpoc.org

The Association of Children's Prosthetic/Orthotic Clinics was established in 1985 for the purpose of supporting clinical teams that treat children with prosthetic or orthotic devices. Goals of the Clinics are achieved through programs of professional education and ongoing clinical research. Annual meetings are also conducted for associated health care professionals to share research advances and new information about children's prosthetics and orthotics.

President: Shiela Hubbard (1995-Present)
Executive Director: Nancy Franzon
Year Established: 1985
Organization Members: 436

Concerned with the following diseases or disorders:
Hanhart Syndrome; Holt Oram Syndrome; Phocomelia Syndrome; Roberts Syndrome; Schinzel Syndrome; Split Hand Deformity

1600 ASSOCIATION OF COMMUNITY CANCER CENTERS (ACCC)

11600 Nebel Street
#201
Rockville, MD 20852 301-984-9496
Fax: 301-770-1949
http://www.assoc-cancer-ctrs.org

The Association of Community Cancer Centers (ACCC) is a not-for-profit organization dedicated to promoting the continuum of quality cancer care (research, prevention, screening, early detection, diagnosis, treatment, psychosocial services, rehabilitation, and hospice) for individuals with cancer and the community. Established in 1978, ACCC consists of 5,000 members and 5 sub-groups. ACCC's educational materials include a brochure entitled "Cancer Treatments Your Insurance Should Cover," reports, and a directory. Program activities include advocacy and lobbying. ACCC maintains a web site at [http://www.assoc-cancer-ctrs.org].

President: James Wade
Executive Director: Lee Mortenson, DPA
Year Established: 1978
Organization Chapters: 5
Organization Members: 5,000

Publishes the following materials:
Cancer Treatments Your Insurance Should Cover. Information For Patients And Their Families ~ *Brochure*

1601 ASTHMA AND ALLERGY FOUNDATION OF AMERICA, INC. (AAFA)

1125 15th Street NW
Suite 502
Washington, DC 20005 202-466-7643
800-727-8462
Fax: 202-466-8950
E-mail: info@aafa.org
http://www.aafa.org

The Asthma and Allergy Foundation of America, Inc. (AAFA) is a voluntary organization dedicated to controlling and finding a cure for asthma and allergic diseases. Asthma is a disease characterized by episodes of difficult or labored breathing due to spasmodic contraction of the lung's airways. Allergies are characterized by hypersensitivity induced by exposure to a certain substance that provokes an immune response (antigen). Established in 1953, AAFA serves an estimated 50 million individuals with asthma and allergic disorders through the support of research, patient and public education programs, public and governmental advocacy, and a nationwide network of chapters and education/support groups. AAFA currently has 10,000 members and 11 chapters. Educational materials include a bi-monthly newsletter "ADVANCE," a support group newsletter, and a resource list brochure. Asthma and Allergy Foundation of America maintains a web site at [http://www.aafa.org].

President: David Schlegel
Executive Director: Mary Wohstell
Organization Language: Spanish (written).
Year Established: 1953
Organization Chapters: 11
Organization Members: 10,000

Publishes the following materials:
How to Reduce Exposure to Allergens. The Bedroom is Your First Line of Defense ~ *Brochure*
Serving Your Special Needs ~ *Brochure*
The Asthma and Allergy Advance ~ *Newsletter*
Asthma and Allergy Foundation of America ~ *Annual Report*
Leaders Link ~ *Leaflet*
AAFA Network. An activities update published exclusively for AAFA Chapters ~ *Fact Sheet*

Concerned with the following diseases or disorders:
Anaphylaxis; Urticaria, Cold

1602 AUDITORY-VERBAL INTERNATIONAL, INC. (AVI)

2121 Eisenhower Avenue
Suite 402
Alexandria, VA 22314 703-739-1049
Fax: 703-739-0395

Auditory-Verbal International, Inc. (AVI), a voluntary not-for-profit organization that was established in 1987, is dedicated to making the auditory verbal approach available to all children who are hearing impaired. Auditory-Verbal International is also committed to promoting the early detection of hearing impairment and the fitting of the most appropriate form of amplification at the earliest age. In addition, AVI is dedicated to teaching affected children to acquire and process language through their remaining hearing; expecting and working toward independent functioning in both learning and living environments; evaluating progress during ongoing therapy; and implementing a certification procedure and standards for Auditory-Verbal clinicians and teachers. AVI sponsors research related to hearing impairment, encourages international communication among parents and professionals, and provides scholarships and awards to support teacher/therapist training. Auditory-Verbal International also provides an office for networking with parents and professionals and offers an annual membership directory. In addition, the group provides a variety of educational materials including a quarterly newsletter called "The Auricle," bulletins, parents' guides, brochures, pamphlets, and audiotapes.

President: James G. Watson, M.Sc, CED, AVT (1993-Present)
Executive Director: Fran Prince
Year Established: 1987
Organization Members: 650

Publishes the following materials:
Children Who Are Hearing Impaired Can Learn To Listen and to Speak ~ *Brochure*
1994 Membership - Won't You Join Us ~ *Application Form*

1603 **BACK PAIN ASSOCIATION OF AMERICA, INC. (BPAA)**

P.O. Box 135
Pasadena, MD 21123-0135 410-255-3633
Fax: 410-255-7338
E-mail: backpainassoc@MSN.COM

The Back Pain Association of America, Inc. (BPAA) is a national nonprofit organization dedicated to providing information and support to people who are affected by back and neck pain, their family members, friends, and health care professionals. Established in 1991 and consisting of nearly 4,000 members, BPAA offers programs and information to help affected individuals learn more about their spinal disorders and ways to cope with them. The organization also has a program to help individuals prevent back injuries. BPAA publishes a self-titled quarterly newsletter that helps readers stay informed of updated information and new forms of treatment. The organization's "Friends Across America" networking program enables affected individuals to exchange information and support via telephone. BPAA also has a physician referral service as well as an information service for physicians who treat back and neck pain. In addition, the Association also promotes research and offers a variety of fact sheets including "The Relationship Between Nerve Damage and Leg Pain," "Urinary Problems and Diseases of the Spine," "Arachnoiditis, Questions and Answers," and "A Guide to Abdominal & Stretching Exercises."

President: Matthew Shimoda, Pharm.D. (1995 to Present)
Executive Director: Margaret A. Hill
Year Established: 1991
Organization Members: 3,805

Publishes the following materials:
Spinal Arachnoiditis: Its Clinical Significance In Regard to Worldwide Spine Care ~ *Video Tape*
Friends Across America Program ~ *Brochure*
Back Pain. Causes-Diagnosis-Treatment ~ *Brochure*
Back Pain Association of America. Services and Support ~ *Brochure*
Fact Sheet #1. Back Pain Association of America Information ~ *Fact Sheet*
Fact Sheet #2. The Relationshlip Between Nerve Damage and Leg Pain ~ *Fact Sheet*
Fact Sheet #3. Urinary Problems and Diseases of the spine ~ *Fact Sheet*
Fact Sheet #4. Diagnostic and Therapeutic Nerve Root Block ~ *Fact Sheet*
Fact Sheet #5. Spinal Nerves, Vertebrae and Nerve Roots ~ *Fact Sheet*
Fact Sheet #6. Myelograms and Contrast Media ~ *Fact Sheet*
Fact Sheet #7. Arachnoiditis—Questions and Answers ~ *Fact Sheet*
Fact Sheet #8. A Guide to Abdominal and Stretching Exercises ~ *Fact Sheet*
Arachnoiditis Report ~ *Reprint*
Back Pain Association of America Newsletter ~ *Newsletter*
Name of Diseases Served By BPAA ~ *Pamphlet*

1604 **BAND-AIDS & BLACKBOARDS: WEB SITE FOR CHILDREN WITH CHRONIC ILLNESS**

c/o Joan Fleitas, Assistant Professor
Fairfield University School of Nursing
Fairfield, CT 06430 203-254-4000
E-mail: fleitas@FAIR1.FAIRFIELD.EDU
www.faculty.fairfield.edu/faculty/fleitas/contents.html

"Band-Aids & Blackboards: When Chronic Illness ... or Some Other Medical Problem ... Goes to School" is a web site on the Internet for children with chronic illnesses or disabilities, other interested children, parents, and educators. Many health care providers such as pediatricians and pediatric nurses; social workers; and many members of the general public may also find this web site helpful. The purpose of this web site is to provide a forum for children with chronic disorders or disabilities to talk about their daily experiences and challenges; to help sensitive other children to what it is like to grow up with a medical problem; to provide information and support for parents of children with such disabilities; and to provide links to age-appropriate teaching progams and to describe classroom activities for teachers to educate children about these essential issues. The web site includes several areas including an invitation to children to tell their stories; a page for parents about the purposes of this web site; special stories for children created for elementary school classroom use that reveal what it is like to grow up with a chronic medical condition; activities for teachers and parents; links to "lots of info about bodies and minds" for children; and a special area entitled "meet some children with medical problems." This site uses a special combination of colorful graphics, music, drawings, children's activities, and more to make this web site visually interesting and fun for child and adult online visitors alike.

1605 **BAZELON CENTER FOR MENTAL HEALTH LAW (BAZELON CENTER)**

1101 15th Street, NW
#1212
Washington, DC 20005-5002 202-467-5730
Fax: 202-223-0409
TDD: 202-467-4232
E-mail: HN1660@handsnet.org
http://www.bazelon.org

The Bazelon Center for Mental Health Law is a national not-for-profit organization that uses litigation and federal policy reform to define and uphold the legal rights of children, adults, and elderly individuals with mental disabilities and to create approaches to meeting their needs that will assure them choice and dignity. Staff attorneys provide training and technical assistance to legal services, protection and advocacy, state ombudsman programs, and other advocates for low income individuals and families. The Center was formed in 1972 as the Mental Health Law Project; however, its name was changed in 1993 to honor the late Chief Justice of the U.S. Court of Appeals of the District of Columbia Circuit, David L. Bazelon, who had pioneered the field of mental health law with groundbreaking decisions that spelled out the constitutional rights of patients with mental illness. The Bazelon Center's goals include full coverage of mental health care in third party payment plans; effective community based alternatives to institutional or nursing home care; access to home support, health care, and SSI benefits for children with disabilities in low income families; expanded housing and employment opportunities for adults with mental disabilities; and protection of individuals' rights in treatment and implementation of the Americans with Disabilities Act, and other civil rights statutes to end discrimination on the basis of perceived mental disability. The Center is governed bya 20 member board of trustees that includes lawyers, consumers, mental health professionals, and members of allied organizations. The Center publishes issue papers, booklets, manuals, and periodic newsletters explaining and interpreting major federal laws and regulations that protect the rights of and make resources available to children and adults with disabilities. The Center maintains a web site on the Internet at [http://www.bazelon.org].

President: Robert Bernstein, Ph.D. (1997 to Present)
Organization Language: Spanish (written/spoken).
Year Established: 1972
Organization Members: Non-Membership

Publishes the following materials:
Facts in Response to Questionnaires ~ *Factsheet*
Publications ~ *Brochure*
Civil Rights and Human Dignity ~ *Booklet*
Lifeline for Children with Disabilities ~ *Booklet*
Links Letter ~ *Newsletter*
For Advocates, Policymakers, Consumers and Families Publications ~ *Leaflet*

1606 **BEACH CENTER ON FAMILIES AND DISABILITY**

3111 Haworth Hall
University of Kansas
Lawrence, KS 66045 785-864-7600
Fax: 785-864-7605
TDD: 785-864-7600
E-mail: Beach@dole.lsi.ukans.edu

The Beach Center on Families and Disability is a research organization that was established in 1988. The Center's central theme is family empowerment through programs of research, training, and information dissemination. These goals are achieved by motivating families to take an active role in finding appropriate services; supporting families to obtain the resources and skills that they and their children need; and building a society that responds to the needs of the family and its children. Current research projects include determining the efficacy of one-to-one parent to parent support programs; understanding statewide parent to parent programs; identifying the role of fathers; evaluating program responsiveness to fathers; and helping parents facilitate friendships. Educational materials are produced and distributed by the organization including booklets and brochures on family support issues, abuse and neglect, emotional skills, and emotional health. The Beach Center of Families and Disability is funded by the University of Kansas, private donations, and the National Institute on Disability and Rehabilitation Research.

President: Ann Turnbull (Co-coordinator)
Executive Director: H. Rutherford Turnbull III (Co-coordinator)
Year Established: 1988
Organization Members: Non-membership.

Publishes the following materials:
Beach Center on Families and Disability Catalog: 1994-1995 ~ *Catalog*
Beach Center on Families and Disabilities ~ *Mission Statement*

1607 **BEREAVEMENT AND HOSPICE SUPPORT NETLINE**

www.ubalt.edu/www/bereavement/#nbo

The Bereavement and Hospice Support Netline is a web site on the Internet. Its goal is to serve as an online directory of bereavement support groups and services and hospice bereavement programs across the United States to help online users find appropriate help and support in coping with issues of loss and grief. Only no-fee bereavement support groups and no-fee or nominal fee bereavement services and newsletters are listed in the Bereavement and Hospice Support Netline. This site also lists other online resources, online bereavement newsletters, and professional associations in the grief and loss field. Direct Internet connections to groups and services are also offered where available. This site provides a listing of specific types of support groups by state, enabling online users to locate specific chapters or local bereavement groups. Bereavement groups within the directory include support groups for pregnancy/infancy loss; groups for parents or children; widow/widower support groups; and support groups for general bereavement, hospices, and more. The site's directory also includes a listing of National Bereavement Organizations and a description of their goals and services; a listing of Professional Organizations and Associations and a description of their goals, membership, publications, and conferences; and an area to alert the site to a bereavement resource or hospice not yet currently listed in the directory.

1608 **BETTER HEARING INSTITUTE (BHI)**

5021-B Backlick Road
Annandale, VA 22003 703-642-0580
800-327-9355
Fax: 703-750-9302
E-mail: mail@betterhearing.org
http://www.betterhearing.org

The Better Hearing Institute (BHI) is a voluntary not-for-profit organization dedicated to providing information and support to people with hearing impairments, their families, and friends. Established in 1973, the Better Hearing Institute provides information concerning surgical therapies for hearing impairments, other medical treatments, amplification techniques and devices, and other rehabilitation. The Better Hearing Institute also uses all forms of media to increase public awareness, provides appropriate referrals, and offers a variety of educational and support materials. Such materials include informational flyers, celebrity-sponsored brochures, public information videos, guides to better hearing, a brochure specifically for children with hearing impairments, and a quarterly newsletter entitled "Better Hearing News."

Executive Director: Michele D. Hartlove
Year Established: 1973

Publishes the following materials:
Facts About the Institute ~ *Fact Sheet*
Better Hearing News ~ *Newsletter*
Public Information Tools ~ *Resource Listing*
Answers to Common Questions About Assistive Technology ~ *Brochure*
Nerve Deafness and You ~ *Brochure*
A Guide to Your Child's Hearing ~ *Brochure*
Tinnitus, or Head Noises ~ *Brochure*
"Descube Un Mundo Donde Se Oye Mejor!" ~ *Brochure*
We Overcame Hearing Loss ~ *Booklet*
Your Guide to Better Hearing ~ *Booklet*
"Discover A World of Better Hearing!" ~ *Brochure*
Overcome Hearing Loss NOW! ~ *Brochure*

Concerned with the following diseases or disorders:
Acoustic Neuroma; Alstrom Syndrome; Bjornstad Syndrome; DOOR Syndrome; Ear, Patella, Short Stature Syndrome; Meniere Disease; Neurofibromatosis Type 2 (NF-2); Patulous Eustachian Tube; Tinnitus

1609 **BIG HEARTS FOR LITTLE HEARTS**

365 Willis Avenue
Mineola, NY 11501 516-741-5522

Big Hearts for Little Hearts, a subgroup of the American Heart Association, is a not-for-profit self-help organization dedicated to providing information and support to families of children with congenital heart disease. Established in 1983, Big Hearts for Little Hearts engages in patient advocacy, provides educational information to affected individuals and family members, and offers support services to the more than 100 member families.

President: Lucy Holtzman Gave (1983-Present)
Executive Director: Edward Webb
Year Established: 1983
Organization Members: 130

Concerned with the following diseases or disorders:
Cat Eye Syndrome; Endocardial Fibroelastosis (EFE); Holt Oram Syndrome; LEOPARD Syndrome

1610 **BLIND CHILDREN'S CENTER (BCC)**

4120 Marathon Street
Los Angeles, CA 90029 213-664-2153
800-222-3566
Fax: 213-665-3828
E-mail: info@blindcntr.org
http://www.blindcntr.org/bcc

The Blind Children's Center, Inc. is a not-for-profit voluntary organization dedicated to serving children with visual impairments from birth to school age. Established in 1938 and consisting of 45 members, the organization has center-based programs and services that facilitate the acquisition of skills and build independence in affected children. The Center utilizes its expertise and experience to serve families and professionals worldwide through support services, education, and research. Program activities include an infant program where parents learn techniques that encourage their children to explore their environment and develop their other senses; individualized preschool educational programs including low vision training, sensory development, orientation and mobility, occupational therapy, and speech/language consultation; and family services including a social services staff, consisting of social workers and a psychologist who provide support for the entire family. All programs are available in Spanish. The organization also provides referrals to early intervention programs, programs for children who are visually impaired, social services agencies, advocacy groups, companies that carry products for visually impaired individuals, self help organizations, and rehabilitation centers. The Blind Children's Center offers several educational materials including brochures, information sheets and booklets, and audiovisual aids. The Blind Children's Center also maintains a web site on the Internet at [http://www.blindcntr.org/bcc].

President: Lynnel P. Munoz (1996 to Present)
Executive Director: Midge Horton
Organization Language: Spanish.
Year Established: 1938
Organization Members: 45

Publishes the following materials:
Blind Children's Center, Inc. ~ *Mission Statement*
Information and Referral Service ~ *Fact Sheet*

Concerned with the following diseases or disorders:
Alstrom Syndrome; Keratomalacia; Leber's Optic Atrophy; Loken Senior Syndrome; Norrie Syndrome; Retinitis Pigmentosa; Septo Optic Dysplasia; Usher's Syndrome

1611 **BLIND CHILDREN'S FUND (BCF)**

4740 Okemos Road
Okemos, MI 48864-1637 517-347-1357
Fax: 517-347-1459
E-mail: blindchfnd@aol.com
http://www.blindchildrensfund.org

The Blind Children's Fund, formerly known as the International Institute for the Visually Impaired, is an international not-for-profit organization that was established in 1978. The Fund was incorporated to respond to the special educational and emotional needs of blind children and their families. The Blind Children's Fund represents a network of parents, professionals, and volunteers throughout the United States and the world who are committed to developing, organizing, and disseminating information and materials for affected families. The Fund develops and distributes educational materials and literature; publishes a quarterly newsletter; and distributes national position papers relative to advocacy and program development for affected children. The Fund organizes International Symposia, conducts workshops and conferences, provides in-service and consultant services, and provides a slide and tape show for UNESCO in four languages that helps train professionals and paraprofessionals who work with infants and young children with blindness.

President: Beulah Gray (1994-Present)
Executive Director: Sherry Raynor
Year Established: 1978
Organization Chapters: 2
Organization Members: 500

Publishes the following materials:
Books From Lilli Nielsen ~ *Order Form*
About the Blind Children's Fund ~ *Fact Sheet*
Materials Order Form ~ *Order Form*
Giving the Infant Blind the Best Chance In Life ~ *Fact Sheet*
Rationale for Incorporation of the Blind Children's Fund ~ *Fact Sheet*

Concerned with the following diseases or disorders:
Aicardi Syndrome; Alstrom Syndrome; Aniridia; Bardet Biedl Syndrome; Cataracts; Choroideremia; Coats' Disease; Hermansky Pudlak Syndrome; Laurence Moon Syndrome; Leber's Congenital Amaurosis; Loken Senior Syndrome; Lowe's Syndrome; Maroteaux Lamy Syndrome; Norrie Syndrome; Refsum Syndrome; Retinoschisis; Rieger Syndrome; Sandhoff Disease; Septo Optic Dysplasia; Usher's Syndrome

1612 BLOOD & MARROW TRANSPLANT NEWSLETTER

1985 Spruce Avenue
Highland Park, IL 60035 847-831-1913
Fax: 847-831-1943
E-mail: help@bmtnews.org
http://www.bmtnews.org

The Blood & Marrow Transplant Newsletter (formerly the BMT Newsletter) is a not-for-profit organization established in 1990 to provide non-technical information to the public on bone marrow/peripheral stem cell transplantation (BMT/PSCT). This is a medical procedure that may be used to treat certain diseases such as cancer, aplastic anemia, immune deficiency diseases, inborn errors of metabolism, and some brain tumors. Published four times annually, the Blood & Marrow Transplant Newsletter describes the BMT/PSCT procedure as well as related psychological, emotional, and financial issues. Readership includes BMT/PSCT patients and survivors, their families and friends, patient support and information groups, medical personnel at BMT cancer centers, and insurance review personnel who handle such cases. In addition to publishing the Newsletter, the organization provides referrals for people having difficulty securing insurance coverage for their BMT/PSCT procedure and offers a patient/survivor link service that enables BMT/PSCT candidates to discuss the procedure with survivors who can describe the experience from a patient's perspective. The organization also produces two books: "Bone Marrow Transplants: A Book of Basics for Patients" and "Mira's Month," a book that chronicles the events and feelings a child experiences from the time her mother is diagnosed with cancer to the day she returns home from the hospital.

President: Susan Stewart (1994-Present)
Executive Director: Susan Stewart
Year Established: 1990
Organization Members: 17,000

Publishes the following materials:
BMT Newsletter ~ *Newsletter*
Mira's Month ~ *Book*
Bone Marrow Transplants: A Book of Basics for Patients ~ *Book*

1613 BRAIN INJURY ASSOCIATION, INC. (BIA)

1776 Massachusetts Avenue NW
Suite 100
Washington, DC 20036-1904 202-296-6443
800-444-6443
Fax: 202-296-8850
http://www.biausa.org

The Brain Injury Association, Inc. (BIA) is a national voluntary health organization dedicated to promoting awareness, understanding, and prevention of brain injuries and ensuring improved outcomes for children and adults with such injuries through education, advocacy, and community support services. Established in 1980, the Brain Injury Association provides information, assistance, and a variety of programs and services to people with brain injuries and their families, health care professionals, and the general public. The BIA networks with and provides guidance to state associations as well as hundreds of chapters and support groups that offer a range of services including care/case management, respite care, recreational opportunities, and, in some cases, housing, transportation, and emergency financial assistance. The BIA also lobbies before Congress and the Administration; encourages state agencies to develop and fund appropriate services for people with brain injuries; offers a toll-free Family Helpline; provides emergency financial assistance through its "Thumbs Up Fund"; and offers the "Brain Injury Resource Center," an interactive multimedia computer system with comprehensive brain injury information that is available at rehabilitation facilities, trauma centers, and hospitals across the country. To increase awareness of brain injuries among professionals, the BIA also participates in and promotes the development of practice guidelines for severe brain injury andrehabilitation; facilitates task forces that address end of life quality, managed care, and pediatric and adolescent issues; sponsors several annual educational conferences; and publishes manuals, directories, magazines, and books including "National Directory of Brain Injury Rehabilitation Services," "Analysis, Understanding, and Presentation of Cases Involving Traumatic Brain Injury," and "An Educator's Manual: What Educators Need to Know About Students with Brain Injury." The BIA also has educational programs to help promote public awareness including a "Wear a Helmet" campaign and a coordinated effort with the National Highway Traffic Safety Administration entitled "Campaign Safe & Sober" focused on reducing impaired driving and increasing safety belt use. The BIA also has a quarterly magazine entitled "TBI Challenge!" that serves as the BIA's main communication vehicle to its over 13,400 members consisting of affected individuals, family members, professionals, and the general public.

President: Dr. George Zitnay
Year Established: 1980
Organization Chapters: 200
Organization Members: 13,400

Publishes the following materials:
Brain Injury Association, Inc. ~ *Mission Statement*
TBI Challelng! ~ *Newsletter*
This "silent epidemic" claims 50,000-60,000 lives each year... ~ *Brochure*
The 1997 National Directory of Brain Injury Rehabilitation Services ~ *Brochure*
Traumatic Brain Injury ~ *Fact Sheet*
Basic Questions about Brain Injury and Disability ~ *Fact Sheet*
Fundamental Principles For Family And Friends ~ *Fact Sheet*
Family News and Views ~ *Reprint*

1614 BRAIN TUMOR FOUNDATION FOR CHILDREN, INC. (BTFC)

2231 Perimeter Park Road
Suite 9
Atlanta, GA 30341 770-458-5554
Fax: 770-458-5467
E-mail: eallman1@Juno.com

The Brain Tumor Foundation for Children, Inc. (BTFC) is a national voluntary organization dedicated to providing emotional and informational support to families of children with brain tumors. Established in 1983 and currently consisting of approximately 1,400 members, BTFC is also committed to promoting public awareness of pediatric brain tumors and raising funds to support research that may discover potential cures and improve the treatment and quality of life of those affected by pediatric brain tumor disease. In addition, the Brain Tumor Foundation for Children has support groups, offers family networking services, and engages in patient education. Educational materials includes brochures, pamphlets, and a regular newsletter.

President: Rick Sauers (1983 to Present)
Executive Director: Elaine Allman
Year Established: 1983
Organization Members: 1,400

Concerned with the following diseases or disorders:
Brain Tumors, General

1615 BRAIN TUMOR FOUNDATION OF CANADA

111 Waterloo Street
Suite 201
London
Ontario, N6B 2M4
Canada 519-642-7755
Fax: 519-642-7192

The Brain Tumor Foundation of Canada is a not-for-profit organization dedicated to funding brain tumor research, providing patient and family support services, and educating the public. Established in 1982, the Brain Tumor Foundation of Canada is committed to raising public awareness about the causes, effects, and treatment of brain tumors; working to support and improve the quality of life of those affected by train tumors; and striving to find a cure for brain tumors. The Foundation's primary educational objective is to meet the information needs of individuals with brain tumors and their families. Educational materials include comprehensive and easy-to-read patient resource handbooks in adult and pediatric versions, which provide information on different types of brain tumors, diagnostic procedures, medications, coping mechanisms, and other helpful material. Other materials include pamphlets designed to alert individuals, parents, educators, and health care professionals to the early warning signs and symptoms of brain tumors; a quarterly newsletter entitled "Brainstorm"; and many books, publications, videos, and audio cassettes. Program activities include support group meetings; a national telephone support system; home and hospital visits; and an annual Adult and Pediatric Brain Tumor Information Day, which provides an opportunity for persons with brain tumors, their families, friends, and health care professionals to meet and discuss issues relating to brain tumors.

President: Mary Anderson (1996 to Present)
Executive Director: Sue Barnes
Organization Language: French (written).
Year Established: 1982

Publishes the following materials:
Information Request - Brain Tumor Foundation of canada ~ *Information Request*
Brain Tumors Strike at Any Age ~ *Brochure*
What is the Goal ~ *Mission Statement*
Brainstorm ~ *Newsletter*
Brain Tumor Patient Resource Handbook - Pediatric Version ~ *Book*
Brain Tumor Patient Resource Handbook - Adult Version ~ *Book*

Brains Tumors strike at any age (French) ~ *Brochure*
We help. We hope. We care. ~ *Brochure*
Brain Tumors strike at any age ~ *Brochure*
Brain Tumor Patient Resource Handbook (Adult Version) ~ *Book*
Brain Tumor Patient Resource Handbook (Adult Version) (French) ~ *Book*
Brain Tumor Patient Resource Handbook (Pediatric Version) ~ *Book*
Brain Tumor Patient Resource Handbook (Pediatric Version) (French) ~ *Book*
Brain Storm ~ *Newsletter*
Sleep Difficulties ~ *Reprint*
Speech and Language ~ *Fact Sheet*
Prevention of Deep Vein Thrombosis. A Post Operative Complication ~ *Newsletter Supplement*
Seizures ~ *Reprint*
Know Your Medication-Decadron ~ *Fact Sheet*
What Makes Brain Tumors Grow? ~ *Reprint*

Concerned with the following diseases or disorders:
Brain Tumors, General

1616 BRAIN TUMOR SOCIETY (TBTS)

84 Seattle Street
Boston, MA 02134-1245 617-783-0340
800-770-8287
Fax: 617-783-9712
E-mail: info@tbts.org
http://www.tbts.org

The Brain Tumor Society is a national voluntary not-for-profit organization dedicated to finding a cure for brain tumors, improving affected individuals' quality of life, disseminating educational information on brain tumors, and providing psychosocial support to affected individuals and their families. The Society raises funds and makes grants to advance carefully selected scientific research projects, improve clinical care, and stimulate and support basic scientific research into various areas of study including gene therapy, immunotherapy, chemotherapy, radiation therapy, and radiosurgery. The Society also encourages participation in support groups and offers a wide range of services to help individuals cope with and manage the problems associated with brain tumors. For example, Patient Inquiry Services, staffed by knowledgeable volunteers, provides up-to-date information, enabling people to make informed decisions about treatment options and recovery. In addition, the Society offers a variety of educational programs to raise public awareness and facilitate early diagnosis and treatment. Educational materials include a newsletter entitled "Heads Up," a booklet on resources, brochures, and special resources for persons with rare brain tumors.

President: G. Bonnie Feldman (1989-Present)
Executive Director: Beth Tishler (Interim)
Year Established: 1989
Organization Members: 15,000

Publishes the following materials:
HEADS UP ~ *Newsletter*
Never Feel Alone ~ *Brochure*
There is Hope ~ *Brochure*
Color Me Hope ~ *Book*
A Guide for People who have a Brain Tumour ~ *Booklet*
What is the Brain Tumour Foundation? ~ *Mission Statement*
Information Resource Library ~ *Information Sheet*
Brain Tumour Foundation Price List ~ *Price List*

Concerned with the following diseases or disorders:
Astrocytoma, Benign; Astrocytoma, Malignant; Brain Tumors, General; Glioblastoma Multiforme; Medulloblastoma; Meningioma

1617 BRAIN AND PITUITARY FOUNDATION OF AMERICA

281 East Moody Avenue
Fresno, CA 93720-1524 209-434-0610

The Brain and Pituitary Foundation of America is a not-for-profit voluntary health organization dedicated to assisting individuals with various brain and pituitary abnormalities such as Acromegaly, Prolactinoma, and Cushing's Syndrome. Established in 1984, this self-help organization also provides patient support and referrals for those seeking medical assistance. Educational materials produced by the organization include various brochures and disease specific literature.

President: Marlene Stephens (1987-Present)
Year Established: 1984
Organization Members: 500

Concerned with the following diseases or disorders:
ACTH Deficiency; Acromegaly; Agenesis of Corpus Callosum; Arachnoid Cysts; Astrocytoma, Malignant; Brain Tumors, General; Cushing Syndrome; Locked In Syndrome; Nelson Syndrome; Precocious Puberty; Pseudotumor Cerebri; Septo Optic Dysplasia; Sheehan Syndrome

1618 BRITISH COALITION OF HERITABLE DISORDERS OF CONNECTIVE TISSUE (BCHDCT)

Rochester House
5 Aldershot Road
Fleet
Hampshire, GU13 9NG
United Kingdom 01252 810472
Fax: 01252 810473
www.Business-Partners.co.uk/marfan

The British Coalition of Heritable Disorders of Connective Tissue (BCHDCT), a not-for-profit coalition, brings together several member organizations that are dedicated to providing information, assistance, and support to individuals and family members affected by various inherited connective tissue disorders. Such disorders include Marfan Syndrome and Ehlers-Danlos Syndrome. Marfan Syndrome is a rare inherited disorder characterized by abnormalities of the heart and blood vessels (cardiovascular system), skeleton, and eyes. Affected individuals may be unusually tall and thin, have abnormally large hands and feet, have malformations of the chest and spine, and experience weakness of the joints, ligaments, and tendons. Ehlers-Danlos Syndrome (EDS) is a group of rare inherited connective tissue disorders characterized by abnormalities of the skin, ligaments, and internal organs. Although symptoms and physical features may vary greatly depending upon the specific form of EDS present, many affected individuals may have thin, fragile, hyperextensible skin that may bruise easily; abnormally loose joints that are prone to recurrent dislocation; widespread tissue fragility with bleeding and poor healing of wounds; and/or other abnormalities. Established in 1990, the BCHDCT enables member organizations to act collectively on important issues, concerns, and goals and to liaison with other coalitions and associations. The Coalition engages in a variety of activities including patient advocacy and lobbying efforts.

President: Diane Rust (Founder/Coordinator) (1990 to Present)
Year Established: 1990
Organization Members: 4 Nat'l Support Grps

Concerned with the following diseases or disorders:
Beals Syndrome; Cutis Laxa; Dermatomyositis; Ehlers Danlos Syndrome; Fibrodysplasia Ossificans Progressiva (FOP); Marden Walker Syndrome; Marfan Syndrome; Mixed Connective Tissue Disease (MCTD); Polymyositis; Pseudoxanthoma Elasticum (PXE); Scleroderma

1619 BURNS UNITED SUPPORT GROUPS, INC. (B.U.S.G., INC.)

P.O. Box 36416
Grosse Pt Farms, MI 48236 313-881-5577
Fax: 313-417-8702
E-mail: 1561@concentric.net

Burns United Support Groups, Inc. (B.U.S.G., Inc.) is a national not-for-profit service organization dedicated to giving emotional support to burn survivors and their families. Established in 1986 by a burn survivor, the Group is open to all burn survivors, family members and friends, physicians, other health care professionals, and all other interested individuals. The Group, which has three chapters and approximately 350 members, offers coping strategies and emotional support to burn survivors and family members, provides referral services, and offers peer counseling and support. Burns United Support Groups also serves as an information center, providing news on fire prevention and the latest techniques in post burn care, a library of videos and books that discuss burn survivors' experiences and positive motivational information, and monthly flyers and quarterly newsletters.

President: Donna Schneck
Year Established: 1986
Organization Chapters: 3
Organization Members: 350

Publishes the following materials:
Children and Adult Burn Survivors ~ *Brochure*
No Matter How "Major" or "Minor" the Burn ~ *Brochure*
History of BUSG, Inc. ~ *Mission Statement*
Burns United Support Groups, Inc. Serving Children and Adult Burn Survivors Since 1986 ~ *Brochure*

1620 C.A.N.D.L.E.

4414 McCampbell Drive
Montgomery, AL 36106 334-271-3947
Fax: 334-271-3947

C.A.N.D.L.E. is an international not-for-profit voluntary support organization composed of parents, families, professionals, and friends of children with neurological disorders. C.A.N.D.L.E. provides educational and medical information and recommendations about all aspects of Childhood Aphasia, Autism, Pervasive Development Disorder, Landau-Kleffner Syndrome, and Epilepsy. The organization's primary focus is to act as a clearinghouse for information on childhood neurological disorders. To this end, the organization accumulates and disseminates information about these neurological disorders. It stimulates increased access to resources, answers questions from parents and professionals concerning identification, evaluation, treatment, and rehabilitation, and encourages scientific research into the causes, control, and cure of such disorders. In addition, C.A.N.D.L.E. seeks to aid parents in understanding treatment options and offer support by listening, sharing experiences, and networking families with similar disorders. Educational materials produced by the organization include brochures, journals, and a regular newsletter.

President: Jane Rudick
Executive Director: Jane Rudick
Year Established: 1989

Concerned with the following diseases or disorders:
Autism; Landau Kleffner Syndrome; MASA Syndrome

1621 **CHERUB—ASSOCIATION OF FAMILIES AND FRIENDS OF CHILDREN WITH LIMB DISORDERS**
936 Delaware Ave.
Buffalo, NY 14209

CHERUB—Association of Family and Friends of Children with Limb Disorders is a voluntary not-for-profit organization dedicated to providing information and support to children with limb disorders (such as congenital absence of limbs), affected families, and friends through organized activities, phone support, correspondence, and visits. CHERUB has over 200 members across the United States and in several other countries. The Association conducts an annual week-long summer camp for affected children from the ages of eight to 18. In addition, CHERUB provides a variety of educational and support materials including a regular newsletter and brochures.

President: Thomas Hauser (1986-Present)
Executive Director: Sandra Richenberg (Secretary)
Year Established: 1986
Organization Members: 200

Concerned with the following diseases or disorders:
Adams Oliver Syndrome; Amniotic Bands; Clubfoot; Congenital Varicella Syndrome; Cornelia de Lange Syndrome; Dysplasia, Epiphysealis Hemimelica; Holt Oram Syndrome; Phocomelia Syndrome; Poland Syndrome; Schinzel Syndrome

1622 **CHERUBS - THE ASSOCIATION OF CONGENITAL DIAPHRAGMATIC HERNIA RESEARCH, ADVOCACY AND SUPPORT (CHERUBS)**
P.O. Box 1150
Creedmore, NC 27522 919-693-8158
E-mail: cherubs@gloryroad.net
www.gloryroad.net/~cherubs

CHERUBS — The Association of Congenital Diaphragmatic Hernia Research, Advocacy and Support is an international support group for the families of children who are born with Congenital Diaphragmatic Hernias (CDH) and their caregivers and physicians. Congenital Diaphragmatic Hernia is a rare condition that is present at birth and characterized by the protrusion of organs from the abdomen into the chest through an abnormal opening (hernia) in the muscle that divides the chest from the abdominal cavity. Established in 1993, CHERUBS is a volunteer organization associated with the March of Dimes, the Association of Birth Defect Children, Inc., and the California Birth Defects Monitoring Program. The Association serves people in the United States, Canada, Great Britain, and Ireland. CHERUBS offers a "Parent Reference Guide," periodic newsletters, and brochures; has a parent-to-parent matchup program; and provides referrals. Memberships are available, although medical professionals are asked to pay a one-time fee. In addition, the organization maintains a research library and compiles data from research surveys (e.g., Congenital Diaphragmatic Hernia Research Survey).

President: Dawn M. Torrence (1995 to Present).
Year Established: 1995
Organization Members: 100

Publishes the following materials:
CHERUBS ~ *Newsletter*

Concerned with the following diseases or disorders:
Pentalogy of Cantrell

1623 **CVS (CHORIONIC VILLUS SAMPLING) PARENT NETWORK SUPPORT GROUP**
15706 Independence Court
Oak Forest, IL 60452 708-535-2864
Fax: 708-535-2864
E-mail: midsun@aol.com

The CVS Parent Network Support Group is a not-for-profit research organization dedicated to giving moral support and medical information to families whose children were born with birth defects caused by the chorionic villus sampling (CVS) prenatal test. During CVS testing, a tissue sample is removed from a portion of the placenta and electron microscopic evaluation and DNA studies are then performed on the sample. Established in 1992, the Network provides information to women considering a CVS test. The organization educates women about its members' experiences with the test and the risks that may be involved. The Network also links affected families and works with the CVS Birth Defects Registry. The organization has support groups, promotes research, offers referrals, and provides information through its registry, database, and brochures.

President: Cynthia Kernats (1992 to Present)
Year Established: 1992
Organization Chapters: 1

Publishes the following materials:
CVS Parent Network Support Group ~ *Brochure*
Morbidity and Mortality Weekly Report. Recommendations and Reports ~ *Pamphlet*
Oromandibular-limb hypogenesis syndrome following chorionic villus sampling ~ *Pamphlet*
Chorionic Villus Sampling and Limb and Other Defects ~ *Pamphlet*
CVS Birth Defects Registry ~ *Fact Sheet*
Is My Baby All Right? ~ *Reprint*
"If Only I'd Known" ~ *Reprint*

1624 CAITLIN RAYMOND INTERNATIONAL REGISTRY OF BONE MARROW DONOR BANKS (CRIR)

University of Massachusetts Medical Center
65 Lake Avenue North
Worcester, MA 01655
508-756-6444
800-726-2824
Fax: 508-752-1496
E-mail: crir@tiac.net
http://www.tiac.net/users/crir

The Caitlin Raymond International Registry (CRIR) of Bone Marrow Donor Banks is a not-for-profit organization founded in 1986 as a coordinating center for conducting national and international searches for unrelated donors for individuals with diseases that are treatable by bone marrow transplantatation or placental blood transfusion. CRIR strives not only to identify potential donors, but to facilitate and coordinate the entire search process. Daily search activities include coordinating existing donor resources and assisting in the development of new bone marrow and cord blood donor sources; developing and maintaining an information service for physicians, transplant coordinators, and affected individuals regarding all available donor sources; and maintaining communications with and problem solving for physicians, transplant coordinators, and affected individuals. The organization also distributes information concerning all available medical, financial, and community support services; monitors search progress and assists in the identification of problems resulting from unnecessary delays, costs, and/or incomplete search results; and works directly with the physician, transplant coordinator, and affected individual to tailor the search process to meet the needs of the individual. The organization produces brochures entitled "The Caitlin Raymond International Registry," "Did You Know That Your Healthy Bone Marrow Could Save This Child's Life?," and "Cord Blood Donors: The Smallest Heroes." The Caitlin Raymond International Registry maintains a web site at [http://www.tiac.net/users/crir].

Executive Director: Joanne Raymond
Year Established: 1986
Organization Members: Non-Membership

Publishes the following materials:
The American Bone Marrow Donor Registry. Search Coordination Center ~ *Brochure*
Cord blood donors: The smallest heroes ~ *Brochure*
Did You Know That Your Healthy Bone Marrow Could Save This Child's Life? ~ *Brochure*

Concerned with the following diseases or disorders:
Graft versus Host Disease

1625 CANADIAN FOUNDATION FOR THE STUDY OF INFANT DEATHS

586 Eglinton Avenue East
Suite 308
Toronto
Ontario, M4P 1P2
Canada
416-488-3260
800-363-7437
Fax: 416-488-3864
E-mail: sidscanada@inforamp.net
http://www.sidscanada.org/sids.html

The Canadian Foundation for the Study of Infant Deaths is a voluntary charitable organization dedicated to responding to the needs of Canadian families affected by Sudden Infant Death Syndrome (SIDS). Sudden Infant Death Syndrome is the sudden death of any infant or young child that is unexpected by history and for which no adequate cause for death can be found. Established in 1973, the Foundation is committed to promoting and supporting research into the causes of Sudden Infant Death Syndrome, facilitating programs of public education, and offering information and emotional support to bereaved families. Informational pamphlets and articles are distributed on request to parents, health professionals, emergency services personnel, and the general public. The Foundation also distributes three videos, "Sam's Story: A Story for Families Surviving Sudden Infant Death Syndrome," "When the Bough Breaks," and "SIDS—Emergency Response." The Foundation maintains a web site at [http://www.sidscanada.org/sids.html].

President: Debra Keays (1996 to Present)
Executive Director: Beverley DeBruyn
Organization Language: French (written/spoken).
Year Established: 1973
Organization Chapters: 15
Organization Members: 250

Publishes the following materials:
Profile of The Canadian Foundation for the Study of Infant Deaths ~ *Fact Sheet*
Goals and Objectives ~ *Mission Statement*
Information about Sudden Infant Death Syndrome (SIDS) ~ *Brochure*
When Your Baby Has Died of Sudden Infant Death Syndrome ~ *Brochure*
Having Another Child after a SIDS Death ~ *Brochure*
The Canadian Foundation For The Study Of Infant Deaths ~ *Brochure*
Sweet Dreams ~ *Brochure*
Some Resources Available From The Canadian Foundation For The Study Of Infant Deaths ~ *Bibliography*

1626 CANADIAN ORGANIZATION FOR RARE DISORDERS (CORD)

P.O. Box 814
Coaldale
Alberta, T1M 1M7
Canada
403-345-4544
Fax: 403-345-3948
E-mail: cord@bulli.com
http://www.bulli.com/~cord

The Canadian Organization for Rare Disorders (CORD) is a not-for-profit organization dedicated to the enhancement of lives of all persons affected by rare disorders through an educational and informational support network. CORD's objectives are the world wide collection and dissemination of information on rare disorders to all interested parties including health care professionals; to identify those specific groups living with a rare disorder and to encourage medical research into the causes and effects of rare disorders; and to work in harmony with the media and medical community to increase public awareness about the existence of rare disorders in Canada. It also provides rare disease information to health care professionals, the media, support groups, and individuals affected by a rare disorder. Upon consent by persons and families with rare disorders, CORD will link other families and individuals with similar rare disorders through a positive and productive networking system. Together they can exchange ideas on how to plan their daily lives, what they can expect to encounter, and offer emotional support so that they can lead productive lives. CORD can be reached at its web site on the Internet at [http://www.bulli.com/~cord].

President: Maureen Gaetz-Faubert
Organization Language: French (spoken).
Year Established: 1996
Organization Members: 40

Publishes the following materials:
Objectives of CORD ~ *Mission Statement*
CORD. Your Link ~ *Brochure*

1627 CANADIAN SOCIETY FOR MUCOPOLYSACCHARIDE AND RELATED DISEASES, INC.

Postal Box #64714
Unionville
Ontario, L3R OM9
Canada
905-479-8701
800-667-1846
Fax: 905-479-8701
neuro-www2mgh.harvard.edu/MPS/mpsmain.html

The Canadian Society for Mucopolysaccharide and Related Diseases, Inc. is an international voluntary health organization based in Ontario, Canada. Founded in 1984, the Society is dedicated to functioning as a parent support group; increasing public awareness of the mucopolysaccharidoses (MPS) and related diseases; and raising funds for further research into MPS. The Mucopolysaccharidoses are a group of rare hereditary diseases of lysosomal storage. These disorders are characterized by the abnormal accumulation of mucopolysaccharides in various tissues of the body such as the central nervous system, respiratory system, cardiovascular system, liver, spleen, and/or other areas. Although symptoms and findings may vary depending upon the form of the disease present, affected children often have distinctive facial abnormalities, skeletal malformations, growth delays, and mental retardation. The Canadian Society for Mucopolysaccharide and Related Diseases works through provincial families to provide local support to families of children who have recently been diagnosed; holds conferences where families and professionals can exchange valuable ideas and information; funds research on MPS disorders; and funds the purchase of equipment for medical research. The Society publishes a regular newsletter and a variety of other educational materials. In addition, the Society maintains a web site at [http://neuro-www2mgh.harvard.edu/MPS/mpsmain.html].

President: Corrina Kaweski (1997 to Present)
Executive Director: Lore Di Ilio
Organization Language: French (written).
Year Established: 1984
Organization Members: 110

Publishes the following materials:
The Genetics and Biochemistry of MPS Diseases ~ *Booklet*
The Canadian Society For Mucopolysaccharide Diseases, Inc. (French) ~ *Brochure*
The Canadian Society For Mucopolysaccharide Diseases, Inc. ~ *Brochure*
Lysosomal Storage Disorders ~ *Brochure*
The Canadian Society For Mucopolysaccharide and Related Diseases, Inc. ~ *Brochure*
Is Your Child Having An Anaesthetic? ~ *Booklet*
Hearing Impairment In MPS Children ~ *Booklet*
The Pattern of Inheritance ~ *Booklet*
Multiple Sulfatase Deficiency ~ *Booklet*
Mucolipidosis Type IV ~ *Booklet*
Mannosidosis ~ *Booklet*
Hunter Syndrome ~ *Booklet*
Morquio Disease ~ *Booklet*
Aspartylglucosaminuria ~ *Booklet*
Mucopolysaccharide Diseases ~ *Booklet*
Maroteaux-Lamy Disease ~ *Booklet*
Sanfilippo Disease ~ *Booklet*
Mucolipidosis II and III. I-Cell Disease ~ *Booklet*
Hurler, Scheie and Hurler/Scheie Diseases ~ *Booklet*
Fucosidosis ~ *Booklet*
Glycosphingolipidoses. GM 2 - Gangliosidosis. Tay-Sachs Disease. Sandhoff Disease ~ *Booklet*

Concerned with the following diseases or disorders:
Hunter Syndrome; Hurler Syndrome; I Cell Disease; Maroteaux Lamy Syndrome; Morquio Syndrome; Mucopolysaccharidosis; Pseudo Hurler Polydystrophy; Sanfilippo Syndrome; Sialidosis; Sly Syndrome

1628 CANCERONLINE

E-mail: cancerinfo@stonecottage.com
www.stonecottage.com/canceronline/

CancerOnline is a nonprofit site on the Internet dedicated to providing individuals with cancer easy access to clinical information and offering extensive practical support and encouragement. CancerOnline collaborates with many different cancer care centers and organizations and provides original material contributed by cancer patients, caregivers, and cancer care specialists in private practice and a variety of cancer centers. CancerOnline's content is overseen by three advisory panels made up of oncologists, radiologists, and clinical care providers who want to help cancer patients become students of their disease; other cancer care specialists and providers of psychosocial support who want to encourage patients to participate actively in their treatment; and patients, survivors, and caregivers who want to help patients live with vitality and hope even in the face of a life-challenging illness. CancerOnline offers several major areas within its site including "About CancerOnline," "Support and Encouragement," "Getting Information," "Participating in This Community," and "Special Features." The site offers several sources of clinical information that can be accessed through a network of subject areas; practical advice before, during, and after treatment; stories from individuals who have triumphed over cancer; opportunities for affected individuals and families to contribute personal stories, creative expressions, commentaries, and questions; hints on how to obtain additional information on and off the Internet; dynamic linkage to additional web sites that provide information and support to those with particular types of cancer; and more. CancerOnline provides information and support to individuals with any type of cancer including Bladder Cancer, Breast Cancer, Colon and Rectal Cancer, Liver Cancer, Lymphoma, Ovarian Cancer, Prostate Cancer, Stomach Cancer, Uterine Cancer, Pediatric Cancers, Brain Tumors, Head and Neck Cancer, Leukemia, Lung Cancer, Melanoma, Pancreatic Cancer, Skin Cancer, Thyroid Cancer, and Rare Adult Cancers.

Concerned with the following diseases or disorders:
Cancer, Breast; Cancer, Colon; Cancer, Lung; Cancer, Prostate; Cancers, Skin, General; Carcinoma, Renal Cell; Carcinoma, Squamous Cell; Nevoid Basal Cell Carcinoma Syndrome; Tongue Carcinoma

1629 CANDLELIGHTERS CHILDHOOD CANCER FOUNDATION (CCCF)

7910 Woodmont Avenue
Suite 460
Bethesda, MD 20814 301-657-8401
800-366-2223
Fax: 301-718-2686
E-mail: info@candlelighters.org
http://www.candlelighters.org

The Candlelighters Childhood Cancer Foundation is a voluntary self-help not-for-profit organization dedicated to providing information, support, and advocacy services to people affected by childhood cancer, their families, and the health care professionals who care for them. Established in 1970 by concerned parents of children with cancer, the Foundation's membership now exceeds 50,000. These members include parents of children who are currently being treated or have been treated for cancer, survivors of childhood cancer, immediate and extended family members, health care professionals, and educators. The Foundation provides a library of 1,000 volumes and 2,800 articles relating to childhood cancer; conducts computerized searches of protocols, treatment options, and literature; matches families with sources of help; and coordinates national and regional conferences. Candlelighters is also a registered lobbyist, advocating on behalf of parents of children with cancer. The Foundation provides a variety of educational and support materials including brochures, pamphlets, books, booklets, videos, guidebooks, and three regular newsletters entitled "The Phoenix," "Candlelighters Youth Newsletter," and a quarterly newsletter.

Executive Director: Laura Lee Lieberman
Year Established: 1970
Organization Chapters: 400
Organization Members: 50,000

Publishes the following materials:
The Candlelighters Childhood Cancer Foundation ~ *Brochure*
Introduction to the Americans with Disabilities Act ~ *Brochure*
Candlelighters Youth Newsletter ~ *Newsletter*
The Phoenix ~ *Newsletter*
Candlelighters List of Publications ~ *Publications List*
Pieces of the Puzzle ~ *Brochure*
Ombudsman Program ~ *Brochure*
Educating the Child with Cancer ~ *Book*
The Candlelighters Guide to Bone Marrow Transplants in Children ~ *Book*
The Candlelighters Bibliography and Resource Guide ~ *Booklet*
Progress Reports ~ *Report*

Concerned with the following diseases or disorders:
Astrocytoma, Benign; Astrocytoma, Malignant; Beckwith Wiedemann Syndrome; Brain Tumors, General; Cancers, Skin, General; Drash Syndrome; Glioblastoma Multiforme; Medulloblastoma; Retinoblastoma; WAGR Syndrome; Wilms' Tumor

1630 CANDLELIGHTERS CHILDHOOD CANCER FOUNDATION CANADA (CCCFC)

55 Eglinton Avenue East
Suite 401
Toronto
Ontario, M4P 1G8
Canada
416-489-6440
800-363-1062
Fax: 416-489-9812
E-mail: staff@candlelighters.ca
http://www.candlelighters.ca

The Candlelighters Childhood Cancer Foundation Canada (CCCFC), a national not-for-profit " volunteer organization, is dedicated to serving families of children and adolescents with cancer by providing educational information, engaging in advocacy, and encouraging and assisting in the development of local parent support groups. Established in 1987, the Foundation has a network of over 50 local support groups across Canada for parents of children with cancer; promotes and supports the development of a long-term survivor network; offers individual and group assistance; and is developing a national financial assistance program. The Foundation's advocacy efforts include communicating the results of patient/family needs surveys to all levels of government; instituting task forces on professional and family issues; and forming coalitions with other organizations to address advocacy issues. The CCCFC also serves as a liaison with professionals and treatment centers, offers a speaker's bureau, and provides a wide variety of educational materials through its national resource library, which currently contains more than 300 books, pamphlets, and videos. In addition, the Foundation offers a school reentry resource kit and manual, provides supportive parent literature, and has several regular newsletters including a quarterly newsletter for families of children with cancer entitled "CONTACT," a quarterly newsletter with information for and by parents and professionals, and a youth newsletter with stories, art, and poetry by children with cancer and their siblings.

President: Christine Wandzura (1995 to Present)
Executive Director: Eleanor G. Pask
Organization Language: (Information available in several languages.)
Year Established: 1987
Organization Chapters: 52

Publishes the following materials:
Candlelighters Childhood Cancer Foundation Canada ~ *Brochure*
The Candlelighters Childhood Cancer Foundation Canada ~ *Fact Sheet*
Facts on Childhood Cancer ~ *Fact Sheet*
Touch the Sky ~ *Brochure*
Help Us to Help Children with Cancer and their families ~ *Brochure*
Helping Your Child Feel Better ~ *Booklet*
Neutropenia. Causes, Consequences, and Care ~ *Booklet*
Chemotherapy and Neutropenia ~ *Booklet*
1995 Annual Report ~ *Booklet*
Resource Catalogue ~ *Booklet*

Concerned with the following diseases or disorders:
Brain Tumors, General; Wilms' Tumor

1631 CARDIAC ARRHYTHMIAS RESEARCH AND EDUCATION FOUNDATION, INC. (CARE FOUNDATION, INC.)
2082 Michelson Drive
#301
Irvine, CA 92612-1212 714-752-2273
800-404-9500
Fax: 714-752-9119
E-mail: care@inconnect.com
http://www.inconnect.com/~care

The Cardiac Arrhythmias Research and Education Foundation, Inc. (CARE Foundation) is a national not-for-profit organization dedicated to promoting physician education and public awareness of the unexpected sudden death of children and young adults due to heart rhythm disorders. Cardiac arrhythmias are disturbances in the heart's natural rhythm. These disturbances are caused by disruptions in the normal conduction of electrical signals within the heart. Due to various reasons, electrical signals may be detoured, slowed, or blocked while traveling through certain parts of the heart. This may cause the heart's natural rhythm to speed up, slow down, or become irregular, affecting the flow of blood to the body's internal organs. The CARE Foundation was founded in 1995 by a group of electrophysiologists and individuals who have been affected by sudden cardiac death. The Foundation's primary goals are to raise funds for clinical research of cardiac arrhythmias and to educate the public and the medical community about the prevention and treatment of arrhythmias. The Foundation promotes screening for at-risk families and participation in ongoing genetic research studies. Foundation activities include providing physician referrals and conducting informational meetings and national seminars for affected families and physicians throughout the country. Publications produced by the CARE Foundation include brochures on various types of cardiac arrhythmias such as right ventriculardysplasia, mitral valve prolapse, hypertrophic cardiomyopathy, neurocardiogenic syncope, atrial fibrillation, and paroxysmal supraventricular tachycardia. The organization also publishes a regular newsletter entitled "CARE" and maintains a web site at [http://www.inconnect.com/~care].

President: David S. Cannom, M.D. (1995 to Present)
Executive Director: Doris Goldman
Organization Language: Spanish.
Year Established: 1995

Publishes the following materials:
The Care Foundation Benefit Video ~ *Video Tape*
Cardiac Arrhtyhmias and the Prevention of Sudden Cardiac Death ~ *Brochure*
AFVD ~ *Fact Sheet*
Atrial Fibrillation ~ *Fact Sheet*
Dilated Cardiomyopathy ~ *Fact Shet*
Hypertrophic Cardiomyopathy ~ *Fact Sheet*
More about Long QT Syndrome ~ *Fact Sheet*
Mitral Valve Prolapse ~ *Fact Sheet*
Neurocardiogenic Syncope ~ *Fact Sheet*
PVST ~ *Fact Sheet*
Wolff-Parkinson-White Syndrome ~ *Fact Sheet*
CARE ~ *Newsletter*

1632 CENTER FOR LOSS IN MULTIPLE BIRTH, INC. (CLIMB)
P.O. Box 1064
Palmer, AK 99645 907-746-6123
E-mail: climb@pobox.alaska.net

The Center for Loss in Multiple Birth, Inc. (CLIMB) is a not-for-profit voluntary organization dedicated to parents who have experienced loss of twins or higher multiples during pregnancy, at birth, in infancy, or in childhood. Established in 1987, CLIMB consists of 750 family members. The organization produces educational materials including numerous brochures and a quarterly newsletter with personal stories and updates, features, and resource information. The organization also provides information on local networks and support efforts, examples of birth and memorial announcements, special issues of its newsletter, and a bibliography of information, articles, and other items in print on various aspects of multiple birth loss. CLIMB also offers support groups, referrals, and networking services. For example, the organization provides a contact list of affected families from the United States, Canada, Australia, and New Zealand.

President: Jean Kollantai (1991 to Present)
Year Established: 1987
Organization Members: 750

Publishes the following materials:
SIDS and Multiples ~ *Brochure*
The Death of Your Twin or Triplet Babies ~ *Leaflet*
CLIMB, Inc. Publications ~ *Bibliography*
Our Newsletter ~ *Newsletter*

1633 **CENTER FOR ASSISTIVE TECHNOLOGY (CAT)**

University at Buffalo
515 Kimball Tower
Buffalo, NY 14214-3079 716-829-3141
800-628-2281
Fax: 716-829-3217
TDD: 800-628-2281
E-mail: jweir@acsu.buffalo.edu
http://wings.buffalo.edu/go?cat

The Center for Assistive Technology (CAT) is a nonprofit organization that conducts research and provides educational and service programs to increase consumer knowledge related to assistive technology for persons with disabilities. Established in 1988, the Center works in five specific areas: research on assistive device use for all aspects of daily living; education for students and clinical professionals; assistive device service provision; development and evaluation of new innovative technology ideas; and public policy analysis, providing information and evaluation data to consumers. CAT is also the Western New York Regional Center for the New York State TRAID Program, for which it coordinates information on technology-related expertise and resources for people with disabilities. In collaboration with private corporations, government agencies, advocacy groups, faculty, and consumers, CAT is involved in a series of ongoing projects for technological assistance and evaluation; works for government and legislation for its causes; strives to educate and inform the general public about devices; and offers referrals to its clientele. It publishes a periodic newsletter, a directory, a journal ("Technology and Disability"), reports, brochures (such as "CAT Brochure," "Project LINK Brochure," and "AZtech Brochure"), and research findings, some of which are available in Spanish.

President: Jennifer Weir, Information Coordinator (1993 to Present)
Executive Director: William C. Mann, Ph.D., OTR
Organization Language: Spanish (written).
Year Established: 1988
Organization Members: Non-Membership

Publishes the following materials:
Media and Publications Catalog on Assistive Technology ~ *Booklet*
Professional Services in Assistive Technology for Persons with Disabilities ~ *Brochure*
Inventors Researchers Companies. Transforming Inventions into Products for Persons with Disabilities ~ *Brochure*
Project LINK. LINK to Assistive Products ~ *Brochure*
Endometriosis Association ~ *Newsletter*

1634 **CENTER FOR CHILDREN WITH CHRONIC ILLNESS AND DISABILITY (C3ID)**

Box 721
420 Delaware Street SE
Minneapolis, MN 55455-0392 612-626-4032
Fax: 612-626-2134
TDD: 612-626-3939
E-mail: C3ID@gold.umn.edu
http://www.peds.umn.edu/Centers

The Center for Children with Chronic Illness and Disability (C3ID) is a pediatric research, training, and rehabilitation center that is committed to fostering the physical, physiological, and social development and well-being of infants, children, and adolescents with chronic illness and disabilities. Founded in 1989, C3ID is supported by the National Institute on Disability and Rehabilitation Research. The Center works to provide opportunities, assistance, improved services and delivery systems, and useful materials and information to children with chronic illnesses and their families through local resources and federal programs. C3ID serves the United States, Canada, Australia, South America, and Western Europe. A periodic newsletter entitled "Children's Health Issues" and various reports and research findings are available in both English and Spanish.

Executive Director: Robert W. Blum, M.D., Ph.D.
Organization Language: Spanish (written/spoken).
Year Established: 1989

Publishes the following materials:
Center for Children with Chronic Illness and Disability ~ *Brochure*
Children's Health Issues ~ *Newsletter*
The First 5 Years ~ *Summary*
Brave New Partnerships: Children with Disabilities. Families and Managed Care ~ *Booklet*

1635 **CENTER FOR MEDICAL CONSUMERS**

237 Thompson Street
New York, NY 10012 212-674-7105
Fax: 212-674-7100
E-mail: artel@compuserve.com

The Center for Medical Consumers is a nonprofit organization dedicated to providing people with the information they need to understand medical conditions and obtain appropriate health care. Established in 1976, the Center for Medical Consumers works in a number of ways to protect people's medical rights. Their ongoing role as a member of the Consumer Consortium put together by the

Food and Drug Administration's Office of Consumer Affairs allows the Center to participate in the selection of consumer representatives to serve on all FDA advisory panels that approve new drugs and devices. In addition to this continuing project, the Center for Medical Consumers was recently chosen to be one of eight national advocacy groups serving on the FDA Steering Committee that designed a new action plan to provide all consumers with useful written information about their prescription drugs. The Center for Medical Consumers has long been an advocate for a universal health insurance system for the United States similar to Canada's, and opposes the growth of profit-making in our health care system. As part of its commitment to upholding the quality and availability of medical insurance, it has led efforts to make managed care organizations more responsible for the quality of health care they provide and to establish meaningful processes for consumers to pursue grievances. It should be noted that while the Center is active in consumer advocacy on the state and national levels, it does not take on individual cases. The organization maintains a free medical library, which is designed especially for lay readers, and which features numerous subject files, books, newsletters, and journals on both conventional and alternative therapies. The organization produces a newsletter entitled "HealthFacts," a monthly publication offering a consumer perspective on medical news. The Center for Medical Consumers can be reached at its e-mail address at [artel@compuserve.com].

Executive Director: Arthur A. Levin
Year Established: 1976
Organization Members: Non-Membership

Publishes the following materials:
Center for Medical Consumers ~ *Brochure*
Center for Medical Consumers Healthfacts ~ *Newsletter*

1636 CENTER FOR REHABILITATION TECHNOLOGY (CRT)

Georgia Institute of Technology
490 Tenth Street
Atlanta, GA 30332-0156 404-894-4960
800-726-9119
Fax: 404-894-9320
TDD: 404-894-9119
www.arch.gatech.edu/crt/crthome.htm/

The Center for Rehabilitation Technology (CRT) is a national not-for-profit research organization dedicated to facilitating the development and application of technology to alleviate problems of human need. Established in 1980 as part of the Georgia Institute of Technology (Georgia Tech), the CRT achieves its mission through expert assessment services, research, design, technological development, information dissemination, and education. The Center works to fulfill six fundamental areas of service: Rehabilitation Engineering and Product Design; Information and Referral Services; Computer-Access Evaluations and Training; Accessibility Evaluations; Technology Demonstrations; and Adult Literacy Training.

Executive Director: Joe Koncelik (Director)
Year Established: 1981
Organization Members: Non-Membership

Publishes the following materials:
Center for Rehabilitation Technology ~ *Mission Statement*
CRT News Update ~ *Newsletter*
Center For Rehabilitation Technology ~ *Booklet*

1637 CENTER FOR RESEARCH IN SLEEP DISORDERS

1275 East Kemper Rd.
Cincinnati, OH 45246 513-671-3101
Fax: 513-671-4159
TDD: 311-111-6111
E-mail: sleepsat1@aol.com

The Center for Research in Sleep Disorders is a not-for-profit organization dedicated to assisting individuals with night tremors, sleep apnea, and other sleep disorders. Established in 1970, the Center seeks to educate affected individuals, physicians, and the public about sleep disorders and their effects and supports ongoing studies into the causes, prevention, and treatment of sleep disorders. In addition, the Center for Research in Sleep Disorders produces educational materials including brochures and fact sheets.

President: Martin Scharf (1970-Present)
Year Established: 1970

Concerned with the following diseases or disorders:
Apnea, Infantile; Apnea, Sleep; Central Hypoventilation Syndrome, Congenital; Narcolepsy

1638 CENTER FOR RESEARCH ON WOMEN WITH DISABILITIES (CROWD)

3440 Richmond Avenue
Suite B
Houston, TX 77046 713-960-0505
800-442-7693
Fax: 713-961-3555
E-mail: mnosek@bcm.tmc.edu

The Center for Research on Women with Disabilities (CROWD) is a research organization dedicated to conducting ongoing research and promoting, developing, and disseminating information to expand the life choices of women with disabilities so that they may fully participate in community life. Established in 1993, the Center conducts research and training activities on issues related to the health, independence, and community integration of women and men with physical disabilities, primarily with funding from federal grants. Sources include the National Institutes of Health and the U.S. Department of Education. The Center has established a database on psychosocial behaviors of women with disabilities compared to able-bodied women based upon 900 responses to a comprehensive national survey. The data has provided the first empirical data on a population of women with physical disabilities ages 18 through 85 years. Findings have been introduced to undergraduate and graduate medical training at Baylor College of Medicine and continuing education courses for a broad range of medical practitioners. The Center fulfills requests for information on its research findings and is expanding its efforts to conduct training and disseminate materials targeting a variety of audiences including medical professionals, allied health professionals, counselors, social workers, educators, policy analysts, and consumers. The Center offers a wide variety of materials including its prospectus, audiovisuals, reports, and a listing of the Center's journal articles concerning women with disabilities, the Americans With Disabilities Act, personal assistance services, and independent living.

Executive Director: Margaret Nosek, Ph.D.
Year Established: 1993
Organization Members: Non-Membership

Publishes the following materials:
Center for Research on Women with Disabilities. A Prospectus ~ *Mission Statement*
CROWD Publications List ~ *Bibliography*

1639 CENTERWATCH, INC.

581 Boylston Street
Suite 407
Boston, MA 02116 617-247-2327
Fax: 617-247-2535
E-mail: cntrwatch@aol.com
http://www.CenterWatch.com

CenterWatch, a publishing company, focuses on the industry of clinical research. It has established a web site to help patients identify ongoing clinical trials. Investigative centers, in turn, can use this web site to recruit patients for their studies. The goal of this site is to serve as an international listing of clinical trials in a broad range of therapeutic areas. The web site provides a searchable clinical trials listing, an e-mail patient notification service, profiles of centers conducting clinical research, resource information about drug therapies newly approved by the Food and Drug Administration (FDA), background information on clinical research, and additional resources.

President: Ken Getz
Executive Director: Ann Kennon (Contact Person) (Web Manager)
Year Established: 1994
Organization Members: Non-Membership

Publishes the following materials:
CenterWatch Clinical Trials Listing Service ~ *Leaflet*

1640 CENTRE FOR RARE DISORDERS (NORWAY)

E-mail: ssss@rh.uio.no
rhpc205.uio.no/ssss/English/engindex.htm

The Centre for Rare Disorders (Norway) at The National Hospital in Oslo is a project under the Government Action Plan for the Handicapped. The objective of the project is to develop a model for improving the organization and implementation of the services available for persons with rare disorders in Norway. The Centre has been a trial project from 1994-1995. The Ministry of Health and Social Affairs prolonged the project by two years so that the present activities will continue through 1997. Within this period, the Government will have approved the subsequent mode of operation. The Centre currently has responsibilities related to 15 rare disorders and syndromes. The Centre is located in The National Hospital since many patients with these disorders visit this hospital concerning diagnosis, treatment, and/or follow-up. Use is made of the medical expertise at the hospital when the Centre works on the disorders. The Centre also establishes close cooperation with other regional hospitals, central hospitals, and rehabilitation services. The Centre's main goals are to disseminate information and coordinate assistance given to affected individual and their families. The Centre is a source of information and knowledge that affected individuals, relatives, and professionals at all levels can contact about facts related to a disorder. The information is collected, systematized, edited, and disseminated by the Centre, thus increasing local qualifications in relation to a raredisorder. The Centre is not meant to replace existing offers of treatment, but supplements the municipal and regional services. The Centre's web site includes detailed information on the 15 rare disorders and syndromes it is dedicated to supporting; includes links to information on several resources including habilitation services, family counseling, mental health services, special education, etc.; and includes dynamic links to several additional web sites that may provide additional helpful information.

Organization Language: Norwegian.

1641 **CHALLENGE AIR FOR KIDS AND FRIENDS (CHALLENGE AIR)**

Love Field North Concourse
8008 Cedar Springs Road
Suite N106 LB24
Dallas, TX 75235 214-351-3353
Fax: 214-351-4565
E-mail: lharris@cyberramp.net
http://www.challengeair.com

Challenge Air for Kids and Friends is a national nonprofit organization dedicated to providing motivational, occupational, recreational, and educational therapy to disabled, disadvantaged, and seriously ill children through the experience of flight with a disabled pilot free of charge. Challenge Air was established in 1993 by a pilot who lost the use of his legs when his plane crashed while returning from a combat mission over Vietnam. The purpose of the flights is to provide enjoyable experiences and to demonstrate that the human spirit can prevail over any physical or mental obstacle. Challenge Air organizes day long events that allow groups of children to enjoy motivational flights, food, and other fun. Events have include handicapped athletic groups, therapy programs, social service organizations, and more. A typical Challenge Air fly day serves more than 150 children and their families. Each program is underwritten by individual, corporate, and philanthropic donations. Challenge Air has flown over 4,000 children in 15 states as well as Canada. Challenge Air has several materials available including brochures, pamphlets, videos, and a newsletter. Challenge Air also has a web site at [http://www.challengeair.com].

President: Lonna Harris (Marketing Director)
Executive Director: Johnnie Hitt (1997 to Present)
Year Established: 1993
Organization Members: 4

Publishes the following materials:
Challenge Air. Rick Amber ~ *Video Tape*
Challenge Air. Hopes of Special Children Soar High.
Disabled Pilots Arrange Thousands of Free Flights For Kids ~ *Mission Statement*
Challenge Air For Kids & Friends "The Sky is the Limit" ~ *Brochure*
Rick Amber. Founder of Challenge Air For Kids & Friends ~ *Biography*
Challenge Air Programs ~ *Fact Sheet*
More Fun ~ *Newsletter*
Plane ride gives kids a real lift ~ *Reprint*

1642 **CHEMOCARE**

2 North Road
Suite A
Chester, NJ 07930 908-879-4039
800-552-4366
Fax: 908-879-6518
E-mail: chemocare@aol.com

Chemocare is a not-for-profit volunteer organization dedicated to providing one-on-one support to people undergoing treatment for cancer and their families. The organization provides this support by training individuals who have recovered from cancer and matching them with individuals with cancer who are currently undergoing a similar experience. Such pairings are treatment specific. Through this matching process, Chemocare strives to instill hope and to make a difference in an affected individual's fight against cancer. Established in 1981, Chemocare is a free and confidential service providing one-to-one emotional support for individuals with cancer and their families. Chemocare's educational materials include a newsletter entitled "Chemocare"; brochures for patients, medical professionals, and corporations; and videotapes.

President: Ken Bertaccini
Executive Director: Randi F. Schayowitz, A.C.S.W.
Organization Language: Spanish (written).
Year Established: 1981
Organization Members: 325

Publishes the following materials:
Stand Behind a Cancer Patient During Treatment ~ *Brochure*
No One Knows More About Cancer ~ *Brochure*
Support a Cancer Patient During Treatment ~ *Brochure*
Chemocare ~ *Newsletter*
Chemocare...because no one knows more about cancer than someone who has been through it. ~ *Mission Statement*
Chemocare...Making a Difference ~ *Fact Sheet*
Frequently Asked Questions About Chemocare ~ *Leaflet*

1643 CHILD CARE ACTION CAMPAIGN (CCAC)

330 Seventh Avenue
17th Floor
New York, NY 10010 212-239-0138
Fax: 212-268-6515
E-mail: hn5746@handsnet.org
http://www.usakids.org/sites/ccac.html

The Child Care Action Campaign (CCAC) is a not-for-profit organization dedicated to stimulating and supporting the development of policies and programs that will increase the availability of quality, affordable child care for the benefit of children, their families, and the economic well-being of the nation. Established in 1984, CCAC provides information and original research to parents, the general public, and government and corporate policy makers about the needs of families and children. CCAC emphasizes the connection between these needs and the nation's prosperity and advocates for additional investment in child care by employers, labor, and federal, state, and local governments. Consisting of 1,500 members, the organization produces educational materials including a newsletter and brochures. CCAC maintains as web site on the Internet at [http://www.usakids.org/sites/ccac.html].

President: Richard B. Stolley
Executive Director: Gail Richardson
Year Established: 1984
Organization Members: 1,500

Publishes the following materials:
Child Care Action Campaign ~ *Mission Statement*
CCAC Publications ~ *Bibliography*

1644 CHILDHELP USA

15757 North 78th Street
Scottsdale, AZ 85260 602-922-8212
800-422-4453
Fax: 602-922-7061
TDD: 800-222-4453
http://www.childhelp.org

Childhelp USA is a national not-for-profit organization dedicated to meeting the physical, emotional, educational, and spiritual needs of abused and neglected children. Established in 1959, Childhelp USA focuses its efforts and resources in the areas of treatment, prevention, and research. There are 10 chapters across the United States with approximately 1,000 voluntary members. In 1978, Childhelp USA began a residential treatment program designed to help abused children and their families. The program is known as the Village of Childhelp USA and is located in Beaumont, California. In 1993, Childhelp USA opened a second "village" in Culpeper, Virginia. In addition, in 1987, the organization established group homes that are located in residential neighborhoods. These homes provide a place of transition and a safe and nurturing refuge until foster or adoptive parents can be found for affected children. To ensure that the children of Childhelp USA continue to receive special care when placed in a private home environment, Childhelp USA follows up residential treatment at the "villages" or group homes with its own extensive therapeutic foster home program. The foster family is monitored and supported (e.g., with counseling services and financial assistance) while fulfilling the child care role. In addition, Childhelp USA maintains a 24-hour, toll-free hotline that provides crisis intervention, information, and referrals. The hotline offers referrals to over 65,000 agencies nationwide and has the ability to communicate with callers in approximately 140 different languages. The organization also sponsors two advocacy centers that serve as one-stop centers for examining and interviewing young victims of sexual abuse. Childhelp USA produces educational materials including a newsletter, brochures, and Spanish language materials. Childhelp USA also maintains a web site at [http://www.childhelp.org].

President: Sara O'Meara / Yvonne Fedderson (Founders)
Executive Director: Chris Monaco, Ph.D. (Hotline Director)
Organization Language: Spanish (written/spoken).
Year Established: 1959
Organization Chapters: 10
Organization Members: 1,000

Publishes the following materials:
Childhelp USA ~ *Mission Statement*
Childhelp USA. Child Abuse In America ~ *Fact Sheet*
Child Abuse ~ *Fact Sheet*
Survivor: One who continues to live or exist despite traumatic life events. ~ *Fact Sheet*
Tips For Positive Parenting ~ *Fact Sheet*

1645 CHILDREN ANGUISHED WITH LYMPHATIC MALFORMATIONS (CALM)

16 River Bend Road
Montgomery, IL 60538 630-906-9028

Children Anguished with Lymphatic Malformations (CALM) is a national not-for-profit voluntary organization established in 1993 to offer support and information to families affected by lymphatic malformations such as Cystic Hygroma and Lymphangioma. The goals of CALM include the education of affected families, their physicians, and the public. The group sponsors a conference, engages in fund-raising activities to promote research into the treatment of lymphatic malformations, and produces a regular newsletter.

President: Tina Baalman (1993-Present)
Executive Director: Tina Baalman
Year Established: 1993
Organization Members: 36

Publishes the following materials:
My Name is Tina Baalman ~ *Letter*
Children Anguished with Lymphatic Malformations ~ *Newsletter*

Concerned with the following diseases or disorders:
Cystic Hygroma

1646 CHILDREN'S BLOOD FOUNDATION (CBF)

333 East 38th Street
Room 830
New York, NY 10016-2745 212-297-4336
Fax: 212-297-4340
E-mail: cbf@nyh.med.cornell.edu

The Children's Blood Foundation (CBF) is a nonprofit organization dedicated to promoting and/or supporting research, medical training of physicians, and care of children with leukemia, thalassemia, hemophilia, anemia, cancer, immune disorders, and AIDS. Established in 1952, the CBF has the largest hemophilia center in the New York area and the largest thalassemia center in North America, receiving more than 5,000 patient visits every year. All affected children are served, regardless of the family's ability to pay. Educational materials include a self-titled brochure, a regular newsletter entitled "The Key to Life for a Child," and a booklet entitled "What's It Called Again? — Answers to the Most Commonly Asked Questions About Idiopathic Thrombocytopenic Purpura (ITP) In Children." CBF has support groups, offers networking services, and engages in educational activities.

President: Margaret W. Hilgartner, M.D. (1996 to Present)
Executive Director: Susan R. Byrne
Year Established: 1952
Organization Chapters: 3
Organization Members: 75

Publishes the following materials:
Children's Blood Foundation Benefit Tape ~ *Video Tape*
Diseases Treated At The Division ~ *Fact Sheet*
What Does It Stand For? ~ *Booklet*
What's It Called Again? ~ *Booklet*
Children's Blood Foundation. The Key to Life for a Child ~ *Brochure*
Explaining Immune Thrombocytopenia Purpura ~ *Brochure*
The Key ~ *Newsletter*

Concerned with the following diseases or disorders:
Thalassemia Major

1647 CHILDREN'S BRAIN TUMOR FOUNDATION (CBTF)

274 Madison Avenue
Suite 1301
New York, NY 10016 212-448-9494
Fax: 212-448-1022
http://childrensneuronet.org

The Children's Brain Tumor Foundation, a nonprofit organization, was founded by parents, physicians, and interested individuals to take action concerning the impact of brain and spinal cord tumors in children, to provide funding for research, and to offer avenues to support. Established in 1988, the Foundation funds free monthly support groups; offers a parent-to-parent network; funds the initial costs of individual counseling for parents by certified specialists who are experienced in this area; raises private funds for ongoing research; and awards grants for basic, clinical, and psychosocial research. The organization also publishes a free "Resource Guide" for parents and cosponsors conferences for people affected by brain tumors and their families. The conferences address issues related to the latest research, treatment for brain tumors, and improvement of quality of life.

President: Joel Shiff (1996 to Present)
Executive Director: Susan L. Weiner, Ph.D.
Year Established: 1988

Publishes the following materials:
The Children's Brain Tumor Foundation ~ *Fact Sheet*
A Resource Guide For Parents of Children With Brain or Spinal Cord Tumors ~ *Booklet*

Concerned with the following diseases or disorders:
Brain Tumors, General

1648 CHILDREN'S CRANIOFACIAL ASSOCIATION (CCA)

P.O. Box 280297
Dallas, TX 75228 972-240-7730
800-535-3643
Fax: 972-240-7607
http://www.masterlink.com/children

The Children's Craniofacial Association (CCA) is a not-for-profit organization dedicated to improving the quality of life for individuals with craniofacial disorders and their families. Established in 1989, CCA is devoted to addressing the medical, financial, psychosocial, emotional, and educational concerns relating to craniofacial conditions. In addition, the Association advocates on behalf of affected individuals and promotes public awareness of craniofacial disorders. Through the combined efforts of its medical and parental advisory boards, CCA provides referral services and a support network for affected children and their families. The organization also provides financial assistance; sponsors workshops to help educate parents about psychosocial, medical, and insurance issues related to their children's care; and refers patients to appropriate support groups and outreach programs. The group engages in patient advocacy to ensure quality care and appropriate health care standards and offers an annual weekend retreat for affected individuals and their families. The Children's Craniofacial Association also provides a variety of educational materials including a regular newsletter, brochures, and a booklet series on a variety of craniofacial conditions.

President: Mike Clay (1992-Present)
Executive Director: Charlene Smith
Year Established: 1989
Organization Chapters: 1

Publishes the following materials:
A Guide to Understanding Craniosynostosis ~ *Booklet*
A Guide to Understanding Apert Syndrome ~ *Booklet*
Children's Craniofacial Association ~ *Brochure*
A Guide to Understanding Hemifacial Microsomia ~ *Booklet*
A Guide to Understanding Treacher Collins Syndrome ~ *Booklet*
A Guide to Understanding Microtia ~ *Booklet*

Concerned with the following diseases or disorders:
Ablepharon Macrostomia Syndrome; Antley Bixler Syndrome; Apert Syndrome; Baller Gerold Syndrome; Blepharophimosis, Ptosis, Epicanthus Inversus Syndrome; Cerebro Oculo Facio Skeletal Syndrome; Chromosome 10, Distal Trisomy 10q; Chromosome 11, Partial Monosomy 11q; Chromosome 13, Partial Monosomy 13q; Chromosome 15, Distal Trisomy 15q; Chromosome 4, Partial Trisomy Distal 4q; Chromosome 7, Monosomy 7p2; Chromosome 9, Partial Monosomy 9p; Cleft Palate and Cleft Lip; Cleidocranial Dysplasia; Cornelia de Lange Syndrome; Craniofrontonasal Dysplasia; Craniometaphyseal Dysplasia; Craniosynostosis, Primary; Crouzon Disease; Encephalocele; Fraser Syndrome; Frontofacionasal Dysplasia; Frontonasal Dysplasia; Goldenhar Syndrome (Oculo Auriculo Vertebral Spectrum); Goodman Syndrome; Gorlin Chaudhry Moss Syndrome; Greig Cephalopolysyndactyly Syndrome; Hallermann Streiff Syndrome; Hyperostosis Frontalis Interna; Jackson-Weiss Syndrome; Marshall Syndrome; Maxillofacial Dysostosis; Maxillonasal Dysplasia, Binder Type; Megalocornea Mental Retardation Syndrome; Miller Syndrome; Moebius Syndrome; Nager Syndrome; Oral Facial Digital Syndrome; Orocraniodigital Syndrome; Oto Palato Digital Syndrome Type I and II; Pallister W Syndrome; Pfeiffer Syndrome; Popliteal Pterygium Syndrome; Pyknodysostosis; Rapp Hodgkins Syndrome; Roberts Syndrome; Robinow Syndrome; Rubinstein Taybi Syndrome; Saethre Chotzen Syndrome; Sakati Syndrome; Scott Craniodigital Syndrome With Mental Retardation; Seckel Syndrome; Se tleis Syndrome; Simpson Dysmorphia Syndrome; Summitt Syndrome; Telecanthus with Associated Abnormalities; Three M Syndrome; Treacher Collins Syndrome; Tricho Dento Osseous Syndrome

1649 CHILDREN'S HOPES & DREAMS FOUNDATION

280 Route 46
Dover, NJ 07801 973-361-7366
800-437-3262
Fax: 973-361-6627

The Children's Hopes & Dreams Foundation, an international nonprofit voluntary organization, is dedicated to fulfilling the dreams of children who are affected by life-threatening or chronic illnesses or disabilities. Established in 1983, the Foundation also provides continual support for these children and their families through the International Pen-Pal Program and the "Kid's Kare Packages" program. The Foundation's Dream Fulfillment Program is designed to fulfill the special dreams of children between the ages of four and seventeen whose parents are unable to fulfill such a dream request due to finances or lack of necessary connections. The entire family is involved in the fulfillment of a dream, since the illness or disability affects the entire family. Dreams may range in expense from the gift of a puppy to a family trip to the Olympics. The Pen-Pal Program, begun in 1990, now includes over 6,000 children between the ages of four and seventeen and provides children with the opportunity to communicate with others who share similar experiences. Children are matched by age, gender, and category of illness or disability with a child from a different state or one of 39 countries. Thousands of children's hospitals, national health organizations, serious illness camps, hospices, and Ronald McDonald Houses participate in the Pen-Pal Program by making free enrollment cards available to children who are affected by life-threatening or chronic illnesses or disabilities. The Foundation also provides "Kid's Kare Packages," sending donated gifts from a variety of companies, organizations, and individuals year round to the children to reassure them of the Foundation's continued support and concern. The Children's Hopes & Dreams Foundation publishes brochures, pamphlets, information packets, and a regular newsletter.

President: Victor Franklin, Jr. (1983 to Present) (Founder)
Year Established: 1983
Organization Members: Non-Membership

Publishes the following materials:
Fulfilling The "Dreams" Of Children With Life Threatening Illnesses ~ *Brochure*
Children's Hopes & Dreams Foundation. Dream Fulfillment. Pen-Pal Program. Kid's Kare Packages ~ *Pamphlet*

1650 CHILDREN'S HOSPICE INTERNATIONAL (CHI)

2202 Mt. Vernon Avenue
Suite 3C
Alexandria, VA 22301 703-684-0330
800-242-4453
Fax: 703-684-0226
E-mail: chiorg@aol.com
http://www.chionline.org

The Children's Hospice International (CHI) is a not-for-profit organization dedicated to providing a network of support and care for children with life-threatening conditions and their families. The hospice approach for children is a team effort that provides medical, psychological, social, and spiritual expertise and information in the United States and abroad. Established in 1983, the goals of Children's Hospice is to enhance the quality of life each day. The child and the family are included to the fullest degree possible in the decision making process concerning treatment and choices. CHI works to ensure continuity and consistency of care through the coordination of a team of professional support including medical, nursing, psychological, spiritual, and trained volunteers, and other appropriate services. CHI provides support that enables the family to cope more effectively, dramatically reducing job loss and potential substance abuse. Consisting of 400 members, the organization supports several program activities including a national telephone hotline serving the needs of terminally ill children and teens; educational programs; seminars; and workshops. CHI maintains a web site at [http://www.chionline.org].

President: Ann Armstrong-Dailey
Year Established: 1983
Organization Members: 400

Publishes the following materials:
My Life. Melinda's Story ~ *Booklet*
Background Information ~ *Mission Statement*
Children's Hospice International ~ *Fact Sheet*
Standards of Hospice Care for Children ~ *Fact Sheet*
Children's Hospice International. Vision Statement, Mission and Goals ~ *Fact Sheet*
Definition of Children's Hospice Care ~ *Reprint*

1651 CHILDREN'S LIVER ALLIANCE (CLA)

3835 Richmond Avenue
Box 190
Staten Island, NY 10312-0190 718-987-6200
Fax: 718-987-6200
E-mail: livers4kids@earthlink.net
http://www.livertx.org

The Children's Liver Alliance (formerly the Biliary Atresia & Liver Transplant Network) is an international not-for-profit voluntary health organization that was established in 1995. The mission of the Children's Liver Alliance (CLA) is to empower the hearts and minds of children with liver disease, their families, and the medical professionals who care for them. CLA disseminates educational information about pediatric liver diseases and transplantation via written publications, seminars, and the Internet. CLA provides a support network for families of children with liver disease (both pre- and post-liver transplantation), acts as liaison between families and health care professionals, offers networking services, and promotes the importance of organ donation and tranplantation. CLA's publications include the bimonthly newsletter "The Biliary Tree."

President: Patricia Zervanos
Executive Director: Lisa L. Carroccio
Organization Language: Spanish.
Year Established: 1995
Organization Chapters: Several
Organization Members: 4,000

Publishes the following materials:
The Biliary Tree ~ *Newsletter*
The Biliary Tree Parent Questionnaire ~ *Questionnaire/Flyer*

Concerned with the following diseases or disorders:
Alagille Syndrome; Alpha-1-Antitrypsin Deficiency; Biliary Atresia, Extrahepatic; Cat Eye Syndrome; Galactosemia; Glycogen Storage Disease VIII; Hepatitis, Neonatal; Hyperoxaluria, Primary (Type I); Tyrosinemia, Hereditary; Wilson's Disease

1652 CHILDREN'S LIVER ASSOCIATION FOR SUPPORT SERVICES (CLASS)

26444 Emerald Dove Drive
Valencia, CA 91355-3514 805-255-0353
E-mail: SupportSrv@aol.com
http://www.transweb.org/class

The Children's Liver Association for Support Services (CLASS) is an all volunteer organization dedicated to addressing the emotional, educational, and financial needs of families with children affected with liver disease and liver transplantation. Established in 1995, CLASS distributes educational materials about pediatric liver disease; offers a support network for families of children with liver disease via a telephone hotline, newsletters, and educational seminars; provides direct financial assistance to families in need due to their child's liver disease; and funds seed grants for research into causes, diagnosis, detection, treatment, and prevention of pediatric liver diseases. In addition, the Association is dedicated to sponsoring educational seminars on the medical and social issues related to liver disease in children; maintaining a database of literature related to liver disease and associated topics; increasing public awareness of the importance of organ donation; soliciting funds from private and public sources; and administering and dispersing such funds to further their mission.

President: Diane Sumner (1995 to Present)
Organization Language: Spanish (spoken).
Year Established: 1995

Publishes the following materials:
Class Notes (Spring 1997) ~ *Newsletter*
Children's Liver Association for Support Services. Alagille Syndrome ~ *Brochure*
Children's Liver Association for Support Services ~ *Brochure*
CLASS. Your Child and Prednisone. Answers to parents' questions about prednisone ~ *Booklet*

Concerned with the following diseases or disorders:
Cholestasis

1653 CHILDREN'S LIVER DISEASE FOUNDATION (CLDF)

1st Floor, 138 Digbeth
Birmingham, B5 6DR
United Kingdom 0121 643 7282
Fax: 0121 643 8262

The Children's Liver Disease Foundation (CLDF) is a voluntary organization dedicated to caring for children and families around the world who are affected by liver disease. Established in 1980 and consisting of 30 chapters, CLDF is dedicated to educating the medical profession and the general public about childhood liver disease; promoting research into early diagnosis, treatments, and cure; providing new facilities and trained staffs; and giving emotional support to children and families affected by pediatric liver disease. CLDF also publishes a newsletter, reports, and brochures; offers a referral service, a database, and a directory; and offers translations of various educational materials.

President: David Bullough
Executive Director: Catherine Arkley
Year Established: 1980
Organization Chapters: 30
Organization Members: 3,000

Publishes the following materials:
Children's Liver Disease Foundation Publications List ~ *Publications List*
One of These Children Has Liver Disease ~ *Brochure*
A Guide to the Liver ~ *Brochure*
Children's Liver Disease Foundation Annual Review ~ *Booklet*
DELIVERY ~ *Newsletter*

Concerned with the following diseases or disorders:
Alpha-1-Antitrypsin Deficiency; Biliary Atresia, Extrahepatic; Cat Eye Syndrome; Gilbert Syndrome

1654 CHILDREN'S MOTILITY DISORDER FOUNDATION, INC. (CMDF)

1534 Dunwoody Village Parkway
Suite 104
Atlanta, GA 30303-1729 770-395-1050
800-809-9492
Fax: 770-395-1025
E-mail: info@motility.org
http://www.motility.org

The Children's Motility Disorder Foundation, Inc. (CMDF) is a national not-for-profit organization dedicated to increasing awareness of pediatric motility disorders among the general public and among the physicians most likely to encounter children affected by these conditions, such as pediatricians and family practice physicians. Gastrointestinal motility refers to a series of wave-like contractions (peristalsis) that move the digested food along an individual's gastrointestinal tract. Pediatric gastrointestinal disorders include a range of neuromuscular disorders that affect a child's ability to eat and appropriately digest and eliminate food materials. Children affected by motility disorders often cannot eat food and must be nourished by other means, such as feeding tubes implanted in the stomach or intestines or central intravenous lines. Founded in 1994, CMDF maintains an updated list of reprints of medical journal articles, offers brochures, and supports medical research into the causes, treatment, and possible cure of these rare disorders.

President: Daniel Grossman (1994 to Present).
Executive Director: Laura E. Bliss (Associate Director)
Year Established: 1994

Publishes the following materials:
Gastroduodenal Motility and Dysmotility: An Update on Techniques Available for Evaluation ~ *Reprint*
Journal Articles Available To Health Care Professionals ~ *Request Form*
Promoting Greateer Awareness, and Someday...a Cure ~ *Brochure*

1655 CHILDREN'S ORGAN TRANSPLANT ASSOCIATION, INC. (COTA)

2501 COTA Drive
Bloomington, IN 47403 812-336-8872
800-366-2682
Fax: 812-336-8885
E-mail: cota@cota.org
http://www.cota.org

Children's Organ Transplant Association, Inc. (COTA) is a voluntary health organization dedicated to ensuring that no individual is excluded from a life-saving organ transplant due to a lack of funding. COTA works with individuals of all ages, not just children. COTA's goals are to assist the families and communities of affected individuals in raising the necessary funds for transplant expenses and to educate the general public on the need for organ donors and organ transplants. COTA provides local campaigns with on-site staff assistance for start up; free donation containers and COTA flyers; fund-raising advice and support; and campaign start-up kits. Founded in 1986, the Association assists in the coordination of hospital selection, patient transportation, and other transplant needs as requested. In order to qualify for COTA assistance, an individual must be a U.S. citizen and in need of a life-saving transplant. Educational materials include brochures and fact sheets.

President: David Cain (1985 to Present)
Executive Director: David Speicher
Year Established: 1986

Publishes the following materials:
COTA History And Program Objectives ~ *Pamphlet*
COTA Touch...And Let Live ~ *Brochure*
COTA Transplant News Coverage ~ *Phamphlet*
Touch and Let Live ~ *Video Tape*
COTA Letters and Commendations ~ *Pamphlet*
Children's Organ Transplant Association, Inc. ~ *Fact Sheet*
COTA Quick Facts ~ *Fact Sheet*
History. Children's Organ Transplant Association ~ *Mission Statement*
COTA Headquarters ~ *Fact Sheet*
David Cain. COTA Chairman and Founder ~ *Biography*

1656 CHILDREN'S WISH FOUNDATION INTERNATIONAL, INC. (CWFI)

P.O. Box 28785
Atlanta, GA 30358 770-393-9474
800-323-9474
Fax: 770-393-0683
E-mail: childrenswish@mindspring.com

The Children's Wish Foundation International (CWFI) is a nonprofit voluntary organization dedicated to fulfilling wishes for children with life-threatening and terminal illnesses. The Foundation was formed in 1985 in memory of 14-year-old Susan Dozoretz, a young girl with Ewing's Sarcoma who dreamed of having her driver's license. Because Susan was unable to fulfill her wish, those who loved her vowed that they would help ensure that other children with life-threatening illnesses could have a favorite wish or dream fulfilled. Since then, the Foundation has grown and thousands of wishes have been fulfilled. The Foundation will grant any wish for any terminally ill child under the age of 18, regardless of where the child lives or where he or she is undergoing treatment. When wishes are fulfilled, the immediate family is included so that the child and the family can create happy memories together. In addition, all expenses are covered for the family including airline tickets, rental cars, meals, spending money, and any salary potentially lost as a result of parents' taking time off from their jobs to share their child's wish. CWFI's materials include brochures, pamphlets, an informational video, a press kit, and a quarterly newsletter entitled "Wishing Well."

President: Arthur J. Stein (1985 to Present)
Executive Director: Linda Dozoretz
Year Established: 1985
Organization Members: Non-Membership

Publishes the following materials:
Children's Wish Foundation International. Presentation Video ~ *Video Tape*
Children's Wish Foundation International ~ *Mission Statement*
Lee Katherine ~ *Fact Sheet*
Katie ~ *Fact Sheet*
Julie ~ *Fact Sheet*
Brady ~ *Fact Sheet*
Children's Wish Foundation ~ *Brochure*
Wishing Well ~ *Newsletter*

1657 CHOICE IN DYING (CID)

200 Varick Street
10th Floor
New York, NY 10014-4810 212-366-5540
800-989-9455
Fax: 212-366-5337
E-mail: cid@choices.org
http://www.choices.org

Choice In Dying is a national not-for-profit organization dedicated to serving the needs of people with a terminal illness and their families. The organization developed the first living will 25 years ago and has distributed approximately 10 million living wills to date. Established in 1940 and consisting of 45,000 members, Choice In Dying advocates the right of individuals to participate fully in decisions about their medical treatment at the end of life. The organization deals broadly with end of life issues and provides public and professional education and counseling about the preparation and use of advance directives. Advance directives is the general term for two types of legal documents, a living will and a medical power of attorney. A living will allows individuals to state their wish about medical treatment at the end of life. A medical power of attorney is a legal document that allows individuals to appoint someone they trust, such as a spouse, adult child, or close friend, to make medical treatment decisions in the event they cannot speak for themselves. Choice in Dying's program activities include staffing a counseling service to answer questions about end of life issues; making available state-specific advance directives to individuals; working with state and federal legislators concerning laws related to patient rights; helping health care facilities comply with patient wishes and with state and federal laws; preparing and distributing educational publications; and offering public education through a network of volunteer speakers. Choice In Dying maintains a web site at [http://www.choices.org].

President: Karen Orloff Kaplan, MPH SCD (Executive Director) (1993 to Present)
Organization Language: Spanish (written).
Year Established: 1940
Organization Members: 45,000

Publishes the following materials:
Choice In Dying - Descriptive Content ~ *Mission Statement*
Dying At Home ~ *Brochure*
CHOICES ~ *Newsletter*
Q and A. You and Your Choices ~ *Brochure*
Choice in Dying. Products and Services ~ *Brochure*
Whose Death Is It, Anyway? ~ *Brochure*
You know where your advance directive documents are. But will you have them when you need them? ~ *Brochure*
Choice in Dying ~ *Mission Statement*
Descriptive Content ~ *Fact Sheet*

1658 CHROMOSOME 18 REGISTRY AND RESEARCH SOCIETY

6302 Fox Head
San Antonio, TX 78247 210-657-4968
Fax: 210-657-4968
E-mail: cody@uthscsa.edu
http://chr18.uthscsa.edu

The Chromosome 18 Registry and Research Society is a not-for-profit self-help organization dedicated to maintaining a registry of individuals affected by Chromosome 18 abnormalities; educating affected families and the public; and encouraging, conducting, and publishing research in areas impacting affected families. The Society seeks to link affected families and their physicians to the research community. Established in 1990, the Chromosome 18 Registry and Research Society promotes patient advocacy, provides phone support to affected families, offers appropriate referrals, provides a pen pal program, and offers educational and support materials. These include a regular newsletter, reports, and brochures.

President: Jannine Cody (1989-Present)
Executive Director: Gloria Ellwanger (Administrative Director)
Year Established: 1990

Concerned with the following diseases or disorders:
Chromosome 18, Monosomy 18p; Chromosome 18, Ring; Chromosome 18, Tetrasomy 18p; Chromosome 18q- Syndrome

1659 CHROMOSOME DELETION OUTREACH (CDO)

P.O. Box 724
Boca Raton, FL 33429 561-391-5098
Fax: 561-395-4252
E-mail: cdo@worldnet.att.net
http://members.aol.com/cdousa/cdo.htm

The Chromosome Deletion Outreach is a national not-for-profit organization dedicated to providing support to people affected by chromosomal deletions and their families and promoting education of the medical community and the general public about chromosomal deletions (monosomies). Established in 1992, the Chromosome Deletion Outreach provides a phone network for parents, referrals to medical professionals, a lending library, and a quarterly newsletter for members. The newsletter includes letters from families affected by chromosomal deletions, birthday listings of members, and news about chromosomal deletions. Although the organization's main focus is on chromosomal deletions, the organization also has some members who are affected by or interested in chromosomal duplications (trisomies).

President: Linda Sorg
Year Established: 1992
Organization Members: 250

Publishes the following materials:
Chromosome Deletion Outreach Membership Form ~ *Membership Form*
Chromosome Deletion Outreach Newsletter ~ *Newsletter*

Concerned with the following diseases or disorders:
Chromosome 10, Monosomy 10p; Chromosome 11, Partial Monosomy 11q; Chromosome 13, Partial Monosomy 13q; Chromosome 14 Ring; Chromosome 15 Ring; Chromosome 18, Monosomy 18p; Chromosome 18, Ring; Chromosome 18q- Syndrome; Chromosome 21 Ring; Chromosome 22 Ring; Chromosome 3, Monosomy 3p2; Chromosome 4 Ring; Chromosome 4, Monosomy 4q; Chromosome 4, Monosomy Distal 4Q; Chromosome 6 Ring; Chromosome 7, Monosomy 7p2; Chromosome 8, Monosomy 8p2; Chromosome 9 Ring; Chromosome 9, Partial Monosomy 9p; Cri du Chat Syndrome; Smith Magenis Syndrome; Wolf Hirschhorn Syndrome

1660 CITIZENS FOR INDEPENDENCE IN LIVING AND BREATHING (CILB)

78 Golfwood Heights
Toronto
Ontario, M9P 3M2
Canada 416-244-2248
Fax: 416-244-2248

The Citizens For Independence In Living and Breathing (CILB) is a not-for-profit organization dedicated to promoting choice, control, and independence through education and information for both current and prospective ventilator users with neuromuscular disorders. CILB was established in 1988, when community action funding enabled the Canadian Paraplegic Association to investigate the needs of severely disabled individuals including ventilator users. CILB assists the community by providing information concerning the choice of independent living options available to individuals who are capable of directing their own services; publishing and disseminating information about living with a ventilator and alternative ventilation techniques; providing information about available community services, attendant services, health care, education, employment, and recreation; providing information regarding funding for the hiring and training of attendants; and assisting in the development of support networks for users, families, and others who require assistance. CILB consists of 65 active members who participate in various advisory committees and groups such as Ontario Ministries including Health, Community and Social Services, Housing, and Education and Citizenship; the Canadian Standards Association; and District Health Councils. Educational materials include pamphlets, CILB conference session tapes, and videotapes.

President: Laura Forma (1997 - 1999)
Executive Director: Margaret Wagner (Contact Person)
Year Established: 1988
Organization Members: 65

Publishes the following materials:
Citizens for Independence in Living and Breathing ~ *Pamphlet*
Citizens for Independence in Living and Breathing. Choice. Control Independence. ~ *Brochure*
Citizens for Independence in Living and Breathing Values and Beliefs ~ *Fact Sheet*
CILB Library Holdings ~ *Pamphlet*

1661 **CLEFT PALATE FOUNDATION (CPF)**
1829 East Franklin Street
Suite 1022
Chapel Hill, NC 27514 919-933-9044
800-242-5338
Fax: 919-933-9604
E-mail: cleftline@aol.com
http://www.cleft.com

The Cleft Palate Foundation was founded by its parent organization, the American Cleft Palate Craniofacial Association, as the public service arm of this professional organization. The purpose of the Foundation is to educate and assist the public concerning cleft lip, cleft palate, and other related craniofacial anomalies. The Foundation also seeks to encourage medical research in the field of craniofacial anomalies. The Foundation operates the CLEFTLINE, a toll-free service that provides information and referrals for parents with newborns who have cleft lip and/or cleft palate and for adults affected by these abnormalities. The Foundation also offers free brochures and fact sheets on various aspects of these birth defects.

Executive Director: Nancy Smythe
Year Established: 1973

Concerned with the following diseases or disorders:
Catel Manzke Syndrome; Cerebrocostomandibular Syndrome; Chromosome 4, Monosomy Distal 4Q; Cleft Palate and Cleft Lip; Fetal Hydantoin Syndrome; Orocraniodigital Syndrome; Popliteal Pterygium Syndrome

1662 **CLOACA CONNECTION**
6530 Highway 78
Mazomanie, WI 53560 608-795-2665

The Cloaca Connection is a voluntary self-help organization dedicated to providing information and assistance to parents of children with malformations of the cloaca, the structure that normally gives rise to the bladder, the rectum, and the genitals during fetal development. Such abnormalities may include failure of cloacal development (cloacal atresia) or a condition in which the two segments of the bladder are divided by abnormal protrusion of a segment of the intestine, appearing as a large red tumor-like structure in the middle of the lower abdomen (cloacal exstrophy). Such cloacal malformations may occur as isolated conditions or may be due to or occur in association with a number of different underlying disorders. The Cloaca Connection is committed to providing parents of affected children with information concerning available medical options to help them make the best choices for their child's specific situation. The organization provides support, offers patient networking opportunities, and provides a variety of educational materials.

President: Laurie Schall (1990 to Present)
Year Established: 1990

Concerned with the following diseases or disorders:
VACTERL Association

1663 **COBALAMIN NETWORK**
P.O. Box 174
Thetford Cntr, VT 05075-0174 802-785-4029
E-mail: SueBee18@valley.net

The Cobalamin Network in an informal network of parents with children who have been diagnosed with errors in the metabolism of cobalamin (Vitamin B12). The Cobalamin Network enables affected families to exchange information, support and resources through phone calls, letters, and videotapes. Some informal gatherings have also been scheduled among affected families.

President: Susan L. Rump (Contact Person)
Year Established: 1988

Concerned with the following diseases or disorders:
Vitamin B12 Deficiency

1664 **COCHLEAR IMPLANT CLUB INTERNATIONAL (CICI)**
P.O. Box 464
Buffalo, NY 14223-0464 716-838-4662
Fax: 716-838-4662
TDD: 716-838-4662
E-mail: 76207.3114@compuserve.com

The Cochlear Implant Club International (CICI) is a not-for-profit voluntary organization dedicated to serving implant users, candidates, their families, and professional supporters. A cochlear implant is a small artificial device (prosthesis) placed in the inner ear that provides a sensation of hearing for profoundly deaf individuals. CICI was established in 1981 by a small group of implant users in Nashville, Tennessee. Their original purpose was to help one another cope with the daily challenges of hearing impairment. Today, CICI has 1,500 members including adults, children, families, medical and therapeutic professionals, educators, and other interested individuals. The purposes of CICI are to promote the opportunities afforded by the use of cochlear implants through mutual sharing of ideas and personal experiences; to function as a support group for cochlear implant candidates at both the pre- and postoperative stages; to enhance community awareness of hearing impairment and to promote a better understanding of cochlear implants; to promote improved financial support for cochlear implants; and to support and encourage the development of local CICI chapters. CICI's educational materials include a newsletter entitled "Contact," brochures, audiovisual aids, and a library of relevant publications.

President: Bev Fish
Executive Director: Craig G. Carpenter
Year Established: 1981
Organization Chapters: 25
Organization Members: 1,500

Publishes the following materials:
Cochlear Implant Club International. An Overview ~ *Brochure*
Cochlear Implant Club International on the move! ~ *Brochure*
When Insurance Companies Deny Benefits for a Cochlear Implant ~ *Brochure*

1665 COMA RECOVERY ASSOCIATION, INC. (CRA)

100 East Old Country Road
Suite 9
Mineola, NY 11501 516-746-7714
Fax: 516-746-7706

The Coma Recovery Association (CRA) is a not-for-profit organization dedicated to acting as a support group for friends and families of individuals who have survived coma and head injury. Established in 1980, CRA works to provide information and referrals to affected families to offer support and enable them to make informed choices regarding treatment, rehabilitation, and socialization alternatives. CRA is also an advocate for higher quality care, education, and research for individuals and families affected by coma and/or head injury. The Association also hosts conferences and offers educational materials including a regular newsletter entitled "Coma Recovery Association" and brochures entitled "Traumatic Brain Injury" and "Neurological Dysfunctions."

President: Florence Manginaro
Executive Director: Philip Mickulas
Year Established: 1980

Publishes the following materials:
Coma Recovery Association Membership Application ~ *Membership Application*
Coma Recovery Association Newsletter ~ *Newsletter*
Coma Recovery Association, Inc. ~ *Brochure*

1666 COMPASSION IN DYING (CID)

410 East Denny Way
Suite 111
Seattle, WA 98122 206-624-2775
Fax: 206-624-2673
E-mail: info@compassionindying.org
http://www.compassionindying.org

Compassion in Dying is a national not-for-profit service organization dedicated to providing information, counseling, and emotional support to terminally ill individuals. Established in 1993, the organization is committed to counseling affected individuals and family members about intensive pain management, comfort or hospice care, and other options. Compassion in Dying offers patient advocacy services; promotes research; engages in patient, professional, and general education; and offers a variety of materials including brochures, pamphlets, and a regular newsletter.

President: Susan J. Dunshee
Executive Director: Barbara Coombs Lee
Year Established: 1993

Publishes the following materials:
Compassion in Dying ~ *Brochure*

1667 COMPASSIONATE FRIENDS, INC. (TCF)

P.O. Box 3696
Oak Brook, IL 60522-3696 630-990-0010
Fax: 630-990-0246
E-mail: TCF_National@prodigy.com
http://www.jjt.com/~tcf_national

The Compassionate Friends, Inc. (TCF) is a national mutual assistance, self-help organization dedicated to assisting in the positive resolution of grief following the death of a child or sibling, supporting the efforts of families or individuals to achieve physical and emotional health, and providing information about parental and sibling grief to families, professionals, and the community. Established in 1969 and consisting of 600 chapters, TCF offers support to family members who have experienced the death of a child including parents, grandparents, and siblings. The organization has support groups, a pen pal program for children who have lost siblings, and a large resource department that offers books, brochures, audiotapes, videotapes, and fact sheets.

President: Karen Snepp
Executive Director: Diana K. Cunningham
Organization Language: Spanish (written).
Year Established: 1969
Organization Chapters: 600

Publishes the following materials:
We Need Not Walk Alone ~ *Newsletter Spring 1997*
The Compassionate Friends ~ *1997 Fact Sheet*
Understanding Grief ~ *Fact Sheet*
Suggestions for the Friends and Relatives of the Grieving Survivor ~ *Fact Sheet*
Understanding Grief. When a Child Dies ~ *Brochure*
Principles of The Compassionate Friends ~ *Brochure*
When a Brother or Sister Dies ~ *Brochure*
The Grief Of Stepparents. When a Child Dies ~ *Brochure*
When a Child Dies ~ *Brochure*
Understanding Grief. When a Grandchild Dies ~ *Brochure*
Caring For Surviving Children. When a Child Dies ~ *Brochure*
Parents Who Are Now Childless ~ *Brochure*
Stillbirth, Miscarriage and Infant Death. Understanding Grief ~ *Brochure*
Surviving Your Child's Suicide ~ *Brochure*
When an Employee Is Grieving. The Death of a Child ~ *Brochure*
When a Co-Worker Is Grieving. The Death Of a Child ~ *Brochure*
For First Responders: Dealing With The Sudden Death of a Child ~ *Brochure*
Suggestions For Medical Personnel. When a Child Dies ~ *Brochure*
Suggestions For Clergy. When a Child Dies ~ *Brochure*
Suggestions for Funeral Directors. When a Child Dies ~ *Brochure*
Suggestions for Teachers and School Counselors. When a Child Dies ~ *Brochure*
How Can I Help? When a Child Dies ~ *Brochure*

1668 CONGENITAL HEART ANOMALIES, SUPPORT, EDUCATION, & RESOURCES (CHASER)

2112 North Wilkins Road
Swanton, OH 43558 419-825-5575
Fax: 419-825-2880
E-mail: myer106w@wonder.em.cdc.gov or chaser@compuserve.co
http://www.csun.edu/~hfmth006/chaser/

Congenital Heart Anomalies, Support, Education, and Resources (CHASER) is a not-for-profit voluntary health organization whose primary purpose is patient and family support for children with congenital heart disease and acquired heart disorders. Established in 1993, the organization seeks to increase public awareness about these disorders and provide educational materials to affected individuals, their families, and physicians. In addition, this self-help organization provides a networking program for both parents and young adults. Educational materials include a quarterly publication, newsletters, a variety of informational brochures, updates on medical research, and a directory of pediatric heart surgeons and treatment facilities. CHASER also maintains an international directory of individuals diagnosed with congenital and/or acquired heart defects.

President: James H. Myers (1993-Present)
Executive Director: Anita K. Myers
Year Established: 1993

Publishes the following materials:
CHASER News ~ *Newsletter*

Concerned with the following diseases or disorders:
Apert Syndrome; Atrial Septal Defects; Atrioventricular Septal Defect; CHARGE Syndrome; Cat Eye Syndrome; Catel Manzke Syndrome; Cayler Syndrome; Chromosome 10, Distal Trisomy 10q; Chromosome 11, Partial Monosomy 11q; Chromosome 13, Partial Monosomy 13q; Chromosome 15, Distal Trisomy 15q; Chromosome 4, Partial Trisomy Distal 4q; Chromosome 7, Monosomy 7p2; Chromosome 8, Monosomy 8p2; Cor Triatriatum; Cornelia de Lange Syndrome; Dextrocardia with Situs Inversus; Eisenmenger Syndrome; Endocardial Fibroelastosis (EFE); Endomyocardial Fibrosis; Goldenhar Syndrome (Oculo Auriculo Vertebral Spectrum); Goodman Syndrome; Heart Block, Congenital; Holt Oram Syndrome; Hypoplastic Left Heart Syndrome; Johanson Blizzard Syndrome; LEOPARD Syndrome; Pierre Robin Syndrome; Robinow Syndrome; Rubinstein Taybi Syndrome; Sakati Syndrome; Singleton Merten Syndrome; Tetralogy of Fallot; Ventricular Septal Defects

1669 CONGENITAL HEART DISEASE RESOURCE PAGE

E-mail: sheri.berger@csun.edu
http://www.csun.edu/~hcmth011/heart/

The Congenital Heart Disease Resource Page is a home page on the World Wide Web on the Internet. The site's purpose is to give parents of children with congenital heart disease a place to find information about specific diseases and other support resources. The site's home page includes the following headings: Books (on congenital heart disease); links (dynamic links to other sources of information); ListServs (e-mail discussion groups); Newsgroups (on associated topics); Personal (links to personal home pages regarding congenital heart disease); Support (links to organizations that may provide further information and support); Transplant (links to resources regarding heart transplantation); and "What Is ...?" (information on specific types of heart disease).

Concerned with the following diseases or disorders:
Cornelia de Lange Syndrome; Heart Block, Congenital; Holt Oram Syndrome; Singleton Merten Syndrome

1670 CONTACT A FAMILY (CAF)

170 Tottenham Court Road
London, W1P 0HA
United Kingdom 171-383-3555
Fax: 171-383-0259

Contact a Family (CaF) is a registered charity in the United Kingdom that provides support, advice, and aid to families caring for children with any disability, illness, or special need. The organization's networking program establishes links and enables communication between families affected by the same conditions. CaF has also developed support groups for various conditions, is a non-political lobbyist for patient rights, and is affiliated with hundreds of similar government, genetic, and charitable organizations throughout the United Kingdom. Contact a Family publishes a newsletter, a directory, reports, and brochures for all interested individuals; however, the organization's direct patient/family services are only available to people living in the UK.

President: Carol Youngs
Year Established: 1979
Organization Chapters: 1000

Publishes the following materials:
Have You a Child with Special Needs on Your Caseload: ~ *Brochure*
Are You Caring for a Child with Special Needs: ~ *Brochure*
Contact A Family Annual Report 1995/6 ~ *Annual Report*
The CaF Directory ~ *Pamphlet*
Share an Idea ~ *Newsletter*

1671 COUNCIL FOR EXCEPTIONAL CHILDREN (CEC)

1920 Association Drive
Reston, VA 20191-1589 703-620-3660
Fax: 703-264-9444
TDD: 703-264-9446
E-mail: cec@cec.sped.org
http://www.cec.sped.org

The Council for Exceptional Children (CEC) is a national, not-for-profit, professional organization dedicated to improving educational outcomes for individuals with exceptionalities — individuals with disabilities, gifts, and/or talents. Established in 1922, the Council accomplishes its mission, which is carried out in support of special education professionals and others working on behalf of individuals with exceptionalities, by advocating for appropriate government policies; setting professional standards; providing continuing professional development; advocating for newly and historically under-served individuals with exceptionalities; and assisting professionals achieve the conditions and resources necessary for effective professional practice. The CEC consists of 17 specialized divisions that provide additional focus and depth of information on a particular exceptionality or interest area in special education, such as The Council for Educational Diagnostic Services or the Division for Physical and Health Disabilities. Each of the 17 divisions publishes educational materials including journals, newsletters, books, and monographs; sponsors conferences and other professional developmental programs; and provides unique networking opportunities. The Council for Exceptional Children also produces educational materials including pamphlets; a research journal entitled "Exceptional Children"; a quarterly, classroom oriented magazine entitled "TEACHING Exceptional Children";and a newsletter entitled "CEC Today," which provides news on special education at the local, state/provincial, national, and international levels. In addition, CEC maintains a database of more than 70,000 print and non-print resources.

President: Linda Marsal
Executive Director: Nancy Safer
Year Established: 1922
Organization Chapters: 17
Organization Members: 52,000

Publishes the following materials:
The Council for Exceptional Children ~ *Brochure*
Today ~ *Newsletter*
Teaching ~ *Magazine*

1672 COUNCIL OF FAMILIES WITH VISUAL IMPAIRMENT (CFVI)

6212 West Franklin Street
Richmond, VA 23226 804-288-0395

The Council of Families with Visual Impairment is a national not-for-profit health organization dedicated to providing advocacy services on behalf of children with visual impairments or blindness to ensure that they receive appropriate public education. Established in the late 1970s, the Council of Families with Visual Impairment provides information and appropriate referrals to affected families. Educational materials include a regular newsletter, audiovisual aids, and comprehensive brochures on a variety of visual impairments.

President: Roy Ward (Treasurer)
Year Established: 1979
Organization Members: 125

Concerned with the following diseases or disorders:
Cat Eye Syndrome; Cataract Dental Syndrome; Choroideremia; Coats' Disease; Laurence Moon Syndrome; Leber's Optic Atrophy; Lenz Microphthalmia Syndrome; Macular Degeneration; Macular Degeneration, Polymorphic; Megalocornea Mental Retardation Syndrome; Norrie Syndrome; Retinitis Pigmentosa; Retinopathy, Arteriosclerotic; Retinopathy, Hypertensive; Retinoschisis; Septo Optic Dysplasia; Treacher Collins Syndrome; Usher's Syndrome; Waardenburg Syndrome

1673 CRANIOFACIAL FOUNDATION OF AMERICA (CFA)

Tennessee Craniofacial Center
975 East Third Street
Chattanooga, TN 37403 423-778-9192
800-418-3223
Fax: 423-778-8172
E-mail: farmertm@erlanger.org
http://www.erlanger.org/cranio

The Craniofacial Foundation of America (CFA) is a not-for-profit organization dedicated to improving the quality of life for individuals and families affected by head and/or facial difference(s) as a result of birth defect, tumor, or trauma-related injury. Established in 1989, the Foundation provides financial assistance for food, travel, and lodging expenses to qualified families traveling to the Tennessee Craniofacial Center for evaluation and treatment. The Foundation provides support services for both affected individuals and their families including regularly scheduled support group meetings and a parent to parent network. CFA also maintains a toll-free hotline and offers educational materials including brochures on "The History of Craniofacial Surgery" and "Post Traumatic Deformities and Facial Reconstruction in Treacher Collins Syndrome."

President: Judy Bellenfant (1990 to Present)
Executive Director: Terri Farmer
Organization Language: Spanish (written).
Year Established: 1989
Organization Members: Non-Membership

Publishes the following materials:
Craniofacial Surgery Treatment of Deformities of the Face and Skull ~ *Book*
Craniosynostosis Diagnosis and Current Surgical Treatment ~ *Booklet*
New Hope. New Promise. New Tomorrows. ~ *Brochure*
New Hope for Facial Deformities Craniofacial Surgery ~ *Leaflet*
The Craniofacial Center: Advances in The Treatment of Facial Deformities ~ *Leaflet*
Choosing A Craniofacial Team For Your Child ~ *Reprint*
Hemifacial Microsomia ~ *Reprint*
Post-Traumatic Facial Deformities ~ *Reprint*
Ear Reconstruction ~ *Reprint*
Mobius Syndrome: Congenital Facial Paralysis ~ *Reprint*
Facial Reconstruction in Treacher Collins Syndrome ~ *Reprint*
Apert Syndrome ~ *Reprint*
Traumatic Facial Deformities ~ *Reprint*
The History Of Craniofacial Surgery ~ *Reprint*
Clefts of the Lip and Palate ~ *Reprint*
Nasal Encephaloceles ~ *Reprint*
Orthognathic Surgery ~ *Reprint*
Craniofacial Surgery ~ *Book*

Concerned with the following diseases or disorders:
Chromosome 10, Distal Trisomy 10q; Chromosome 11, Partial Monosomy 11q; Chromosome 13, Partial Monosomy 13q; Jansen Type Metaphyseal Chondrodysplasia; Megalocornea Mental Retardation Syndrome; Robinow Syndrome; Scott Craniodigital Syndrome With Mental Retardation; Seckel Syndrome; Setleis Syndrome; Three M Syndrome; Treacher Collins Syndrome; Tricho Dento Osseous Syndrome

1674 CRANIOFACIAL SUPPORT GROUP (CFSG)

44 Helmsdale Road
Leamington Spa, CV32 7DW
United Kingdom 44 1926 334629
E-mail: SJMoody@compuserve.com
http://www.hopwood.ac.uk/~cranio

The Craniofacial Support Group (CFSG) is an international self-help organization dedicated to providing support and information to individuals who have craniofacial differences and their families. Consisting of 2,200 members, the organization was established in 1993 by a group of parents whose children were affected by a variety of conditions involving craniosynostosis, premature closure of the fibrous joints between certain bones in the skull. In addition to providing support for families, the Group aims to raise awareness and understanding of craniofacial conditions among the general public and in the medical community. CFSG publishes a quarterly newsletter entitled "Headlines" and a variety of brochures including "The Genetic Background of Craniosynostosis," "Your Child In Hospital," "Crouzon Syndrome," "Pfeiffer Syndrome," "Saethre-Chotzen Syndrome," and "The Surgical Treatment of Hand Anomalies Associated with Craniofacial Conditions." Additionally, the Group facilitates a networking program for affected individuals and their families and has developed an outreach program for use in the school system that explores physical appearance and the effects of facial differences.

President: Steve Moody (1993 to Present)
Organization Language: Greek (written/spoken). Spanish (written/spoken). French (written/spoken). Portuguese (written/spoken). Italian (written/spoken).
Year Established: 1993
Organization Members: 2,200

Publishes the following materials:
The Craniofacial support Group. The Surgical Treatment of Hand Anomalies Associated with Craniofacial Conditions ~ *Leaflet*
Craniofacial Support Group. The Genetic Background to Craniosynostosis ~ *Leaflet*
Craniofacial Support Group. Your Child in Hospital ~ *Leaflet*
Craniofacial Support Group. Crouzon Syndrome ~ *Leaflet*
Craniofacial Support Group. Pfeiffer Syndrome ~ *Leaflet*
Craniofacial Support Group. Saethre-Chotzen Syndrome ~ *Leaflet*
The Craniofacial Support Group. Resources List ~ *Pamphlet*

Concerned with the following diseases or disorders:
Apert Syndrome; Craniosynostosis, Primary; Crouzon Disease; Pfeiffer Syndrome; Saethre Chotzen Syndrome

1675 CROHN'S AND COLITIS FOUNDATION OF AMERICA (CCFA)

386 Park Avenue South
17th Floor
New York, NY 10016-7374 212-685-3440
800-932-2423
Fax: 212-779-4098
E-mail: mhda37b@prodigy.com
http://www.ccfa.org

The Crohn's and Colitis Foundation of America is a not-for-profit voluntary health organization dedicated to raising funds for research to determine the cause of and the cure for Crohn's Disease and colitis. Crohn's Disease and ulcerative colitis, collectively known as inflammatory bowel disease, are chronic digestive diseases of unknown cause. While Crohn's Disease may affect any part of the gastrointestinal tract and often results in swelling, soreness, and inflammation of layers of the large and/or small intestinal wall, Ul uerative colitis affects only the colon (large intestine), causing inflammation of the inner lining and resulting in diarrhea, often mixed with blood, cramping abdominal pain, and other symptoms. Established in 1967, the Crohn's and Colitis Foundation of America seeks to educate affected individuals, physicians, and the public about these disorders in order to increase awareness about the nature of these chronic disorders and help affected individuals confront their unique problems. In addition, the Foundation establishes support groups, engages in patient advocacy, plays an active role in government legislation, and provides medical referrals. Educational materials produced by the organization include a regular newsletter, reports, and informative brochures.

President: Robert Brine
Year Established: 1967
Organization Chapters: 72
Organization Members: 30,000

Publishes the following materials:
A Teacher's Guide to Crohn's Disease & Ulcerative Colitis ~ *Brochure*
Questions & Answers about Diet & Nutrition ~ *Brochure*
Questions and Answers about Complications ~ *Brochure*
Questions and Answers about Emotional Factors ~ *Brochure*
A Guide for Children & Teenagers to Crohn's Disease & Ulcerative Colitis ~ *Brochure*
Questions and Answers About Pregnancy ~ *Brochure*
Questions & Answers about Crohn's Disease & Ulcerative Colitis, Including a Glossary of IBD Terms ~ *Brochure*
Question & Answers about Surgery ~ *Brochure*
Crohn's Disease, Ulcerative Colitis & Your Child ~ *Brochure*
Attention PC Users ~ *Brochure*
Coping with Crohn's and Colitis is Tough ~ *Brochure*

Concerned with the following diseases or disorders:
Colitis, Collagenous; Colitis, Ulcerative; Crohn's Disease; Gastritis, Chronic, Erosive; Irritable Bowel Syndrome; Pyoderma Gangrenosum

1676 CROUZON'S/MENIERE'S SUPPORT NETWORK (CMSN)

3757 North Catherine Drive
Prescott Valley, AZ 86314-8320 520-772-1784
TDD: 800-842-4681
E-mail: katy@northlink.com

The Crouzon's/Meniere's Support Network (CMSN) is a not-for-profit self-help organization that reaches out to individuals and families affected by Crouzon Disease and Meniere Disease. Crouzon Disease is a rare genetic disorder characterized by premature closure of fibrous joints between certain bones in the skull (craniosynostosis), causing the head to appear abnormally long (acrocephaly); widely spaced eyes; crossing of the eyes; underdevelopment of the upper jaw; and/or other abnormalities. Meniere's Disease is a disorder characterized by recurrent dizziness, possible hearing loss, and ringing in the ears associated with abnormal widening (dilation) of the membranous labyrinth of the ear. Founded in 1991, CMSN's goal is to provide information, networking services and support to individuals affected by Crouzon Disease or Meniere's Disease. A secondary goal is to identify any link between these two hereditary syndromes and to encourage genetic research in these areas.

President: Kathleen Handsaker (1992 to present)
Organization Language: French (spoken).
Year Established: 1991

Publishes the following materials:
Crouzon's/Meniere's Support Network ~ *Brochure*

Concerned with the following diseases or disorders:
Crouzon Disease; Meniere Disease

1677 CRUSE—BEREAVEMENT CARE (CRUSE)

126 Sheen Road
Richmond
Surrey, TW9 1UR
United Kingdom 01819404818
Fax: 01819407638

Cruse—Bereavement Care is a voluntary organization based in England that offers personal and confidential help to bereaved people and those who care for them. Established in 1959, Cruse has grown to include 194 branches throughout the United Kingdom. As a non-denominational organization, Cruse provides free counseling, social support groups, and information to people of all religions and beliefs (although there is a small membership fee). All counselors are trained by the organization. In addition to speaking English, some staff members are fluent in French, Farsi, Assyrian, Urdu, Hindu, and Punjabi. Cruse also offers training courses for firms and organizations; journals, books, videos, training manuals, and brochures for those interested in participating in Cruse's work; and a newsletter for its members. Cruse also advocates on behalf of bereaved people.

Executive Director: Rosemary Pearce
Organization Language: French. Farsi. Assyrian. Urdu. Hindu. Punjabi.
Year Established: 1959
Organization Chapters: 194
Organization Members: 6,000

Publishes the following materials:
Cruse Publication List ~ *Publication List*
Helping the Bereaved ~ *Brochure*

1678 CYSTIC FIBROSIS TRUST (CF TRUST)

Alexandria House
5 Blyth Road
Bromley
Kent, BR1 3RS
United Kingdom 0181 464 7211
Fax: 0181 313 0472

The Cystic Fibrosis Trust is a voluntary organization in the United Kingdom dedicated to raising funds for hospital and medical research into improved treatment and prevention of cystic fibrosis (CF), a rare inherited disorder that affects many exocrine ("outwardly-secreting") glands of the body including the sweat glands, salivary glands, and those within the pancreas and respiratory system. Established in 1964, the Cystic Fibrosis Trust has approximately 16,000 members in 300 chapters throughout the United Kingdom. The CF Trust provides a network of support groups for affected individuals and family members and offers several materials including brochures, pamphlets, fact sheets, and videos.

President: Rosie Barnes (Chief Executive) (1996 to Present)
Year Established: 1964
Organization Chapters: 300
Organization Members: 16,000

Publishes the following materials:
Understanding Cystic Fibrosis. Publications List ~ *Pamphlet*
What do you know about Cystic Fibrosis? ~ *Brochure*
We're making great progress but.... ~ *Brochure*
Help for People with cystic fibrosis and their families ~ *Brochure*
Growing up with cystic fibrosis. A guide for young people ~ *Booklet*
Cystaic fibrosis and you ~ *Booklet*
Finding out about cystic fibrosis ~ *Booklet*
Eating will with cystic fibrosis. A guide for children and parents ~ *Booket*
The physical treatment of cystic fibrosis ~ *Booklet*
Genetics, carrier tests and tests during pregnancy ~ *Booklet*
Diabetes mellitus in cystic fibrosis ~ *Booklet*
The Cystic Fibrosis Trust ~ *Mission Statement*
CF News ~ *Magazine*

Concerned with the following diseases or disorders:
Cystic Fibrosis

1679 DB-LINK

Teaching Research
345 North Monmouth Avenue
Monmouth, OR 97361 503-838-8403
800-438-9376
Fax: 503-838-8150
TDD: 800-854-7013
E-mail: dblink@tr.wou.edu
http://www.tr.wou.edu/dblink

DB-LINK is a national not-for-profit service organization that functions as a clearinghouse for information concerning children and youth who are deaf and blind. Educational materials are available to affected individuals, their families, their physicians, their communities, and the public. DB-LINK strives to provide access to information through a balanced presentation of resources to meet the unique informational needs of affected individuals. The organization believes that information access and ongoing education are essential to the realization of each affected individual's basic right to lead a fulfilling life. In addition to providing a wide variety of educational materials, DB-LINK also offers referrals to appropriate regional services.

Executive Director: John Reiman
Year Established: 1992

1680 DANISH CENTRE FOR RARE DISEASES AND DISABILITIES (CSH)

Bredgade 25
Sct. Annae Passage, Opg. F.
Copenhagen K, DK-1260
Denmark 00 453 3914020
Fax: 00 453 3914019
E-mail: csh-kbh@inet.uni-c.dk

The Danish Centre for Rare Diseases and Disabilities is a nonprofit government organization that is concerned primarily with severe physical or mental disabilities that affect a population of less than one person in every 10,000. Most of these disorders are congenital or hereditary in nature. Founded in 1990, the Centre's objectives are to offer nationwide support to adults and families who have children with rare disabilities or special needs and to ensure their access to highly qualified information and counseling services; to network affected individuals and family members with other affected families thus promoting mutual support and self-help groups; to network health care professionals; and to promote dialogue and research and thus improve public knowledge and awareness of issues concerning rare diseases and disabilities. A wide range of information and counseling services is offered to all who, either as health professionals or as private persons, need information on rare diseases. Target groups are local professionals and authorities involved in the provision and coordination of counseling, treatment, education and support for persons affected by a rare disease and their families. Educational materials include pamphlets, brochures, and books in Danish.

Executive Director: Terkel Andersen
Organization Language: Danish (written/spoken).
Year Established: 1990

Publishes the following materials:
The Danish Centre for Rare Diseases and Disabilities ~ *Brochure*

1681 DEAFNESS RESEARCH FOUNDATION (DRF)

9 East 38th Street
7th Floor
New York, NY 10016-0003 212-684-6556
800-535-3323
Fax: 212-779-2125
TDD: 800-535-3323

The Deafness Research Foundation is a national voluntary health organization that offers seed research grants to help solve the problems of deafness and other serious ear disorders. Founded in 1958, the Deafness Research Foundation is committed to increasing public awareness about hearing health. The four primary objectives of the Deafness Research Foundation include fostering innovative research and education into the causes, treatments, and prevention of hearing loss and other dysfunctions of the auditory and balance systems; increasing awareness of measures to prevent hearing loss and the need to support research; creating greater understanding about the effect of hearing loss on people's lives; and increasing the number of scientists who are committed to hearing health. The Deafness Research Foundation also publishes materials including brochures on deafness and a grants policy fact sheet.

President: James H. Rand (1993-Present)
Year Established: 1958
Organization Members: 2,300

Publishes the following materials:
Don't Let Noise Damage Your Hearing ~ *Brochure*
Hearing Health: Have You Heard the Latest Facts? ~ *Brochure*
Otitis Media ~ *Brochure*
A Few Short Years That Can Last A Lifetime ~ *Brochure*
DRF Receiver ~ *Annual Report*

Concerned with the following diseases or disorders:
Acoustic Neuroma; Cardio Auditory Syndrome; Norrie Syndrome; Usher's Syndrome; Wildervanck Syndrome

1682 **DELTA SOCIETY**
289 Perimeter Road East
Renton, WA 98055-1329 425-226-7357
800-869-6898
Fax: 425-235-1076
TDD: 800-809-2714
E-mail: deltasociety@cis.compuserve.com
http://www.deltasociety.org

The Delta Society is a not-for-profit, voluntary organization dedicated to bringing pets into the lives of people who are ill in an effort to improve healing and to helping individuals with disabilities overcome barriers and lead healthier lifestyles. The Society's Pet Partners Program was established in 1977 to train volunteers and screen their pets for visiting animal programs in hospitals, nursing homes, rehabilitation centers, and schools. The organization currently consists of 5,000 members with 2,000 pet partners teams operating in 45 states. Animal assisted therapy is incorporated as part of the treatment program for depression, attention deficit hyperactivity disorder, head injuries, and speech disorders as well as many other conditions. Training is provided through Delta certified instructors, a home study course and videotape, and a continuing education newsletter. In addition, the Society offers an 800 Action Line, which provides immediate and comprehensive assistance to people with service dogs who are denied access to places of public accommodation, housing, and employment.

President: Sophie Engelhard Craighead (Chairperson)
Executive Director: Linda M. Hines
Year Established: 1977
Organization Members: 5,000

Publishes the following materials:
Delta Society. Animals Helping People. People Helping Animals ~ *Mission Statement*
Anthrozoos ~ *Book*
Pet Partners ~ *Newsletter*
Delta Society ~ *Brochure*
Welcome to the National Service Dog Center ~ *Brochure*
Facts you should know about Service Dogs ~ *Brochure*
Healthcare Options: Service Dogs for people who have disabilities ~ *Brochure*
Delta Society Pet Loss Bibliography ~ *Brochure*

1683 **DEPRESSION AFTER DELIVERY, INC. (DAD)**
P.O. Box 278
Bellemead, NJ 08502 215-295-3994
800-944-4773
http://www.behavenet.com/DADINC

Depression After Delivery, Inc. is a self-help organization dedicated to providing support, information, and referrals to women and families coping with anxiety or depression associated with the arrival of a newborn. Established in 1985, the organization provides support groups, engages in patient advocacy, offers networking services, and provides referrals. Consisting of 700 members and 100 chapters, the organization provides a variety of educational materials including the "Heart Strings" newsletter, brochures, and audiovisual aids.

President: Susan B. Feingold, M.D. (1996 to Present)
Executive Director: Trish Bukowski (Operations Director)
Organization Language: Spanish (written).
Year Established: 1985
Organization Chapters: 100
Organization Members: 700

Publishes the following materials:
D.A.D. ~ *Information Packet*
Feelings After Birth ~ *Broshure*
Heart Strings ~ *Newsletter*

1684 **DEPRESSION AND RELATED AFFECTIVE DISORDERS ASSOCIATION (DRADA)**
Meyer 3-181
600 North Wolfe Street
Baltimore, MD 21287-7381 410-955-4647
Fax: 410-614-3241
infonet.welch.jhu.edu/departments/drada/def

The Depression and Related Affective Disorders Association (DRADA) is a nonprofit organization uniting the efforts of persons with affective disorders, family members, and mental health professionals. The mission of the organization is to provide information, assistance, and support to those with depression and manic depression by assisting self-help groups. In addition, the Association lends support to research programs. Educational materials produced by the Depression and Related Affective Disorders Association include a variety of pamphlets, books, and videos.

President: J. Raymond DePaulo Jr., M.D. (1995-Present)
Executive Director: Paul Hoagberg
Year Established: 1986
Organization Members: 800

Publishes the following materials:
Depression & Related Affective Disorders Association ~ *Brochure*

Support Services Programs ~ *Brochure*
Books and Videos about Affective Disorders ~ *Brochure*
I Am The Greatest I Am Depressed ~ *Brochure*
Smooth Sailing ~ *Newsletter*
Adolescent Depression. A Counselor's Guide. ~ *Factsheet*
Impact of Maryland Health Insurance Reform Laws on Mental Health Coverage ~ *Brochure*
How to Evaluate Your Psychiatrist or Other Therapist If You Have (Or Possibly Have) a Depressive Disorder ~ *Factsheet*
What You Need to Know About Psychiatric Medications ~ *Brochure*
Book, Pamphlets, and Audiovisual Materials about Depressive Illness (Unipolar Affective Disorder) and Manic-Depress ~ *Brochure*
Books and Videos ~ *Brochure*
I Wish I Was Never Born. I Really Hate Myself. ~ *Pamphlet*

Concerned with the following diseases or disorders:
Anorexia Nervosa; Manic Depression, Bipolar; Panic Anxiety Syndrome

1685 DIABETES INSIPIDUS AND RELATED DISORDERS (DIARD)

535 Echo Court
Saline, MI 48176 734-944-0078
Fax: 734-944-0078
E-mail: GSMAYES@aol.com
http://members.aol.com/ruudh/dipage1.htm

Diabetes Insipidus and Related Disorders Network (DIARD) is a voluntary organization dedicated to providing informational support to families affected by central diabetes insipidus and nephrogenic diabetes insipidus. Diabetes insipidus is a rare metabolic disease that is characterized by a deficiency of the anti-diuretic hormone (ADH), a hormone stored in the posterior lobe of the pituitary gland. Excessive thirst and excessive urination are the major symptoms of this disorder. Founded in 1988, DIARD publishes a quarterly self-titled newsletter and maintains a home page on the World Wide Web. DIARD can be reached toll-free at (800) 484-3508, then dial 9070*2.

Executive Director: Gwen Mayes (Contact Person)
Organization Language: Spanish (written).
Year Established: 1988
Organization Chapters: 1
Organization Members: 300

Concerned with the following diseases or disorders:
Diabetes Insipidus

1686 DIABETES INSIPIDUS FOUNDATION, INC. (DI FOUNDATION)

4533 Ridge Drive
Baltimore, MD 21229 410-247-3953

The Diabetes Insipidus Foundation is concerned with all forms of diabetes insipidus (DI), namely neurogenic, nephrogenic, gestagenic (gestational DI), and dipsogenic. The three major goals of the Foundation include promoting research, providing information, and offering support to affected individuals and their families. In the area of research, the Foundation strives to increase research dollars by educating the biomedical community about the prevalence of diabetes insipidus and its numerous extra-urinary manifestations. The Foundation also strives for more accurate diagnosis, more specific therapy, and, ultimately, the prevention and cure diabetes insipidus. In addition, the Foundation strives for greater public awareness and understanding of the disease by promoting public education and offering informational material such as a quarterly newsletter.

President: Mrs. Marian C. Arminger
Executive Director: Marian C. Arminger
Organization Language: Spanish. Portuguese. Russian.
Year Established: 1988

Concerned with the following diseases or disorders:
Diabetes Insipidus; Septo Optic Dysplasia; Wolfram Syndrome

1687 DIGESTIVE DISEASE NATIONAL COALITION (DDNC)

507 Capitol Court
Suite 200
Washington, DC 20002 202-544-7497
Fax: 202-546-7105

The Digestive Disease National Coalition (DDNC) is a not-for-profit voluntary organization dedicated to promoting federal investment in biomedical research, representing the digestive disease community in the public arena; and serving as a resource for consumer-directed educational information. Established in 1978, DDNC is comprised of 22 patient and professional organizations concerned with diseases of the digestive tract. DDNC has local support groups, offers a toll-free hotline to serve the community, provides patient networking services, and has several educational materials such as brochures and pamphlets on digestive disorders.

President: William Mahood, M.D. (1996 to Present)
Executive Director: Dale P. Dieks
Year Established: 1978
Organization Members: 22

Concerned with the following diseases or disorders:
Alagille Syndrome; Barrett Esophagus; Cholecystitis; Colitis, Collagenous; Degos Disease; Diverticulitis;

Diverticulosis; Duodenal Atresia or Stenosis; Gastritis, Chronic, Erosive; Gastroenteritis, Eosinophilic; Gastroesophageal Reflux; Gastroschisis; Hyperkalemia; Hypokalemia; Irritable Bowel Syndrome; Mallory Weiss Syndrome; Mesenteritis, Retractile; Prune Belly Syndrome

1688 DISABILITY INFORMATION & RESOURCE CENTRE, INC., SOUTH AUSTRALIA (DIRC)

195 Gilles Street
Adelaide, SA 5000
Australia
088-223-7522
Fax: 088-223-5082
TDD: 088-223-7579
E-mail: dirc@dircsa.org.au
http://www.dircsa.org.au/

The Disability Information & Resource Centre (DIRC), Inc., South Australia, was founded in 1982 to provide a centralized, independent organization capable of providing information relating to any aspect of disability. DIRC is an Incorporated body funded by the State Government. The Management Committee includes people with disabilities and representatives of organizations that provide services to people with disabilities. DIRC's role is to "point people in the right direction" to end the confusion concerning where to go for information about disability and to refer people to the most appropriate places to meet their special needs. DIRC's resources are available to all people with disabilities and to organizations and persons involved in providing services to people with disabilities. The organization offers information services to affected individuals, disability organizations, professionals, government departments, and any member of the public. DIRC provides a computerized information retrieval system as well as a library of books, videos, newsletters, and journals that offer information on disabilities in easy to understand language. Copies of journals and newsletters dealing with the majority of disabilities are received by DIRC from hundreds of organizations in Australia and overseas. The organization also provides details of services provided by over 600 Australian disability organizations concerning accommodation, access, mobility, employment, transport, holidays, recreation, sport, community services, building design, discrimination, education, disability publications, benefits, etc.. DIRC offers an annual directory containing such organizational information that may be purchased at the Centre or by mail order. The organization also has a web site on the Internet that outlines its many services, provides access to information on disabilities, and includes links to many disability newsletters and other web sites. DIRC also offers a computer bulletin board service, called "Common Ground," that gives access to a wide range of information on all aspects of disability. A host computer at DIRC acts as a storage facility for the bulletin board's messages, files, and information databases. Other computers can access this information through the telephone system. When users log on to Common Ground, they may read messages that other users have "pinned" to the board, leave public or private messages for other users of the service, and chat online directly with others. Users may also use the bulletin board to access information about a particular disability topic or to ask for help, support, or ideas on a particular topic. DIRC's web site provides additional information on how online users may be able to participate in the Common Ground Bulletin Board Service.

Year Established: 1982

1689 DISABILITY RIGHTS EDUCATION AND DEFENSE FUND, INC. (DREDF)

2212 Sixth Street
Berkeley, CA 94710
510-644-2555
800-466-4232
Fax: 510-841-8645
TDD: 800-466-4232

The Disability Rights Education and Defense Fund (DREDF) is a nonprofit national law and policy center dedicated to furthering the civil rights of people with disabilities. Managed and directed by people with disabilities and parents of children with disabilities, DREDF is an advocate for the rights of all people with disabilities. Established in 1979, the organization promotes the full integration of people with disabilities into the mainstream of society. Programs and services provided by DREDF include technical assistance, information, and referrals on disability rights, laws, and policies; training of and legal advocacy for parents of children with disabilities to help them secure the education and services guaranteed to their children by law; and legal representation to adults and children with disabilities in cases involving their rights to employment, education, transportation, housing, and access to public accommodations. Additional services include training and speakers for the disability community, public entities, and private businesses on the provisions of the Americans with Disabilities Act (ADA) and its relationship to other state and federal laws; education for legislators and policy makers on issues affecting the rights of people with disabilities; and a toll-free hot line that provides information concerning the ADA. DREDF also provides a blue book that offers a detailed analysis of the ADA and offers a video entitled "Open For Business," which depictsthe disability and business communities of one small town working together.

Executive Director: Susan Henderson
Year Established: 1979
Organization Members: Non-Membership

Publishes the following materials:
"Myths and fears about disability are as handicapping as are the physical limitations that flow from the actual imp ~ *Brochure*
What DREDF is and does ~ *Mission Statement*

1690 DISABLED AMERICAN VETERANS (DAV)

National Service and Legislative Headquarters
807 Main Avenue SW
Washington, DC 20024 202-554-3501
Fax: 202-554-3581
http://www.dav.org

The Disabled American Veterans (DAV) is a service organization dedicated to building better lives for all our nation's disabled veterans and their families. Established in 1920, its mission is carried forward by providing free, professional assistance to veterans and their families in obtaining benefits and services earned through military service and provided by the Department of Veterans Affairs (VA) and other agencies of government; representing the interests of disabled veterans, their families, their widowed spouses, and their orphans before Congress, the White House, and the Judicial Branch, as well as state and local government; extending the DAV's mission of hope into the communities where these veterans and their families live through a network of state-level departments; and providing a structure through which disabled veterans can express their compassion for their fellow veterans through a variety of volunteer programs. These programs include the DAV's National Legislation Program; the DAV's National Employment Program; and the DAV's National Voluntary Service Program. Consisting of one million members and over 2,000 chapters, DAV produces educational materials including a brochure entitled "DAV Legislative Goals for 1996," a fact sheet, and a magazine entitled "DAV." Program activities include government legislation, lobbying, and research. DAV can be reached at its web site on the Internet at [http://www.dav.org].

President: Harry McDonald
Executive Director: David W. Gorman
Year Established: 1920
Organization Chapters: 2,000
Organization Members: 1,000,000

Publishes the following materials:
DAV Gives You Straight Answers About Your Rights And Benefits ~ *Brochure*
Background Information on the Disabled American Veterans ~ *Mission Statement*

1691 DISABLED CHILDREN'S RELIEF FUND (DCRF)

402 Pennsylvania Avenue
Freeport, NY 11520 516-377-1605
Fax: 516-377-3978

The Disabled Children's Relief Fund (DCRF) is a national not-for-profit organization dedicated to acting as an advocate for the rights and needs of children with disabilities. Founded in 1990, DCRF provides cash grants for disabled children, with preference given to families who do not have health insurance. Grants are provided for assistive devices, equipment, and rehabilitative services, as well as for innovative arts and humanitarian services for children with disabilities. DCRF publishes a regular newsletter entitled "The Challenger."

President: Jerome H. Blue, Ph.D. (1994 to present)
Year Established: 1990
Organization Members: Non-Membership

Publishes the following materials:
A Safety Net for Children with Disabilities ~ *Brochure*
1995 Grant Applications - Disabled Children's Relief Fund ~ *Application Form*
Disabled Children's Relief Fund - Annual Report ~ *Report*
The Challenger ~ *Newsletter*
A Major Advocate for Children with Disabilities ~ *Reprint*

1692 **DISABLED PEOPLES' INTERNATIONAL (DPI)**
101-7 Evergreen Place
Winnipeg
Manitoba, 43L 2T3
Canada
204-287-8010
800-749-7773
Fax: 204-453-1367
TDD: 204-453-1367
E-mail: DPI@DPI.ORG
http://www.dpi.org.html

Disabled Peoples' International (DPI) is an international not-for-profit self-help group that is dedicated to the enhancement of the rights and opportunities of all disabled people. Established in 1981, DPI is dedicated to the philosophy that disabled persons are citizens with equal rights and hence should achieve full participation and equalization of opportunity with their fellow citizens in all societies. Consisting of 114 members, the organization provides several materials including a newsletter entitled "Disability International," numerous reports, and a publications listing. DPI offers several services including networking and lobbying. Disabled Peoples' International maintains a web site at [http://www.dpi.org.html].

President: Kalle Konkkola (Chairperson)
Executive Director: Lucy Wong-Hernandez
Organization Language: French. (written/spoken). Spanish (written/spoken).
Year Established: 1981
Organization Members: 114

Publishes the following materials:
Free Information...about disability ~ *Brochure*
Publications - Disabled Peoples' International ~ *Publications List*
DPI Overview ~ *Reprint*
Disability International ~ *Newsletter*
Disabled Peoples' International ~ *Mission Statement*

1693 **DISABLED SPORTS USA (DS/USA)**
451 Hungerford Drive
Suite 100
Rockville, MD 20850
301-217-0960
Fax: 301-217-0968
TDD: 301-217-0963
E-mail: dsusa@dsusa.org
http://www.dsusa.org/~dsusa/dsusa.html

Disabled Sports USA (DS/USA) is a not-for-profit organization dedicated to ensuring that disabled people have access to sports, recreation, and physical education programs from preschool through college to elite sports levels. Established in 1967 by disabled Vietnam veterans, DS/USA serves people with physical disabilities that restrict mobility, including amputations, weakness or paralysis of both legs (paraplegia), paralysis of all four limbs (quadriplegia), cerebral palsy, head injury, multiple sclerosis, muscular dystrophy, spina bifida, stroke, and visual impairment. DS/USA consists of more than 60,000 members and 80 chapters around the United States. Educational materials include a general information packet, a newsletter entitled "Disabled Sports USA Update," and a sports magazine entitled "Challenge." Program activities include sporting activities and events, patient education (e.g., workshops), and patient networking. DS/USA maintains a web site at [http://www.dsusa.org/~dsusa/dsusa.html].

Executive Director: Kirk M. Bauer
Year Established: 1967
Organization Chapters: 80
Organization Members: 60,000

Publishes the following materials:
Disabled Sports USA Update (Summer/Fall 1996) ~ *Newsletter*
Premiere Issue. Challenge ~ *News Magazine*
DS/USA Chapter Roster ~ *List*
Summer Competition Schedule ~ *Schedule*
Skitour Schedule of Events ~ *Schedule*

1694 **DISABLED AND ALONE/LIFE SERVICES FOR THE HANDICAPPED, INC. (LIFE SERVICES)**
352 Park Avenue South
Suite 703
New York, NY 10010
212-532-6740
800-995-0066
Fax: 212-532-6740

Disabled and Alone/Life Services for the Handicapped, Inc. is a not-for-profit voluntary organization dedicated to providing direct services to persons with disabilities and their families and the organizations that serve them. Established in 1988, Life Services provides a program that assists parents in planning for their children's future when the parents will no longer be available as caregivers; serves as an alternative service program if private or family arrangements cannot be made; advises parents, relatives, attorneys, and financial planners concerning long-term care disability; and provides direct services to affected individuals whose families have left funds for their care. The organization also provides referrals and seminars, has meetings in local communities, and offers a variety of materials including brochures and a quarterly newsletter entitled "Lifelines."

President: Leslie D. Park (1988 to Present)
Executive Director: Roslyn Brilliant
Year Established: 1988
Organization Members: 12

Publishes the following materials:
Alone! Without Family Without Friends Without Hope ~ *Brochure*
LifeLines ~ *Newsletter*
"Disabled and Alone" Life Services for the Handicapped, Inc.
1996 Annual Report-Eighth Anniversary ~ *Annual Report*
"After We're Gone" ~ *Booklet*
Partnership Plan ~ *Booklet*

1695 DOGS FOR THE DEAF, INC. (DFD)

10175 Wheeler Road
Central Point, OR 97502 541-826-9220
Fax: 541-826-6696
TDD: 541-826-9220

Dogs for the Deaf, Inc. is a not-for-profit organization dedicated to providing professionally trained "hearing dogs" free of charge to qualified applicants nationwide. Established in 1977, Dogs for the Deaf is the oldest and largest hearing dog training center in the United States. Dogs for the Deaf selects dogs from adoption shelters. The dogs are usually mixed breeds, small to medium sized, and eight to 24 months of age. All dogs are spayed or neutered; thereafter, they begin four to six months of intensive specialized training. The dogs are taught to respond to verbal commands and hand signals and are trained to alert their partners to household sounds such as smoke alarms, doorbells, crying babies, telephones, alarm clocks, etc. Dogs for the Deaf provides educational materials including a general brochure and a regular newsletter entitled "Canine Listener." All applicants must meet certain requirements before receiving a dog. Dogs for the Deaf has more than 600 recipients of hearing dogs. All applicants must agree to certain requirements including regular training sessions to keep appropriate obedience and alert responses to sound, a fenced yard or area, and no other dogs in the household.

President: Robin Dickson
Organization Language: American Sign Language.
Year Established: 1977
Organization Members: 250

Publishes the following materials:
Dogs for the Deaf, Inc. ~ *Newsletter*
Canine Listener ~ *Newsletter*
Dogs For The Deaf, Inc. ~ *Brochure*
Dogs For The Deaf, Inc. Descriptions and Requirements ~ *Pamphlet*

1696 DYSTONIA MEDICAL RESEARCH FOUNDATION

1 East Wacker Drive
Suite 2430
Chicago, IL 60601-1905 312-755-0198
800-377-3978
Fax: 312-803-0138
E-mail: dystfndt@aol.com
www.dystonia-foundation.org/~dystonia/

The Dystonia Medical Research Foundation is an international not-for-profit voluntary organization dedicated to serving people with all forms of dystonia. Dystonia is a neurological condition characterized by involuntary sustained muscle spasms. Dystonia may affect various parts of the body and can cause abnormal movements and postures. Foundation goals include the advancement of medical research to determine the cause, treatment, and cure of dystonia. Founded in 1976, the Dystonia Medical Research Foundation seeks to increase physician and public awareness of the dystonias by distributing educational materials and informational videotapes on these disorders. The Foundation also conducts symposia on this group of movement disorders and sponsors support groups for affected individuals and their families. The Dystonia Medical Research Foundation has more than 100 local groups and 100 area contacts.

President: Dennis Kessler (1989-Present)
Executive Director: Valerie F. Levitan, Ph.D.
Organization Language: French. Spanish.
Year Established: 1976
Organization Chapters: 90
Organization Members: 25,000

Publishes the following materials:
Highlights Excerpted from the Dystonia Medical Awareness Video ~ *Factsheet*
Support Group Manual ~ *Brochure*
Strategies: Obtaining Social Security Disability Benefits ~ *Brochure*
Guidebook for Families: Special Education Rights ~ *Brochure*
Social Security Ruling 1983 SSR 83-20 ~ *Pamphlet*
Dystonia Directions ~ *Pamphlet*
Botulinum Toxin Injections ~ *Pamphlet*
Writer's Cramp ~ *Pamphlet*
Childhood Dystonia ~ *Pamphlet*
Oromandibular Dystonia ~ *Pamphlet*
1995 General Dystonia Grant Policies ~ *Pamphlet*
1995 Special Focal Dystonia Grant Policies ~ *Pamphlet*
Dystonia What Now? ~ *Brochure*
ANDA Dystonia Awareness Video ~ *Videotape*
What is Dystonia? ~ *Brochure*
Is Dystonia a Genetic Disorder? ~ *Brochure*
Spasmodic Dysphonia ~ *Brochure*
Spasmodic Torticollis (Cervical Dystonia) ~ *Brochure*

Blepharospasm ~ *Brochure*
Dystonia Dialogue ~ *Brochure*
Dystonia Dialogue Canadian Supplement ~ *Brochure*
Moving Together ~ *Brochure*

Concerned with the following diseases or disorders:
Blepharospasm, Benign Essential; Dysphonia, Chronic Spasmodic; Dystonia, Torsion; Hallervorden Spatz Disease; Meige Syndrome; Spasmodic Torticollis; Tardive Dyskinesia

1697 DYSTONIA SOCIETY

Weddel House
13-14 West Smithfield
London, EC1A 9HY
United Kingdom 01713290797
Fax: 01713290689

The Dystonia Society is a voluntary, self-help support organization dedicated to promoting greater awareness of dystonia within the medical community and the general public. Dystonia is a neurological condition characterized by involuntary sustained muscle spasms. These can affect various parts of the body and cause abnormal movements and postures. Established in 1983, the Society disseminates information on available treatments to individuals affected by dystonia; provides emotional and informational support through a network of approximately 27 support groups; and helps to fund research into the causes, treatments, and eventual cure of dystonia. The Society publishes a self-titled newsletter and several informational brochures including "Dystonia: Your Questions Answered," "Hemifacial Spasm: Your Questions Answered," and "Blepharospasm: Your Questions Answered." The Dystonia Society also produces audiovisual aids, offers a referral service, and maintains a database of patients, physicians, and treatment centers. The Dystonia Society is affiliated with the Dystonia Medical Research Foundation USA and the European Dystonia Federation.

President: Stan Dutton (Chairman) (1991 to present).
Executive Director: Alan Leng
Organization Language: French (written/spoken). German (written/spoken). Spanish (written/spoken).
Year Established: 1983
Organization Chapters: 19
Organization Members: 2,250

Publishes the following materials:
What is Dystonia? ~ *Pamphlet*
Dystonia - Your Questions Answered ~ *Information Packet*
European Dystonia Federation ~ *Membership Directory*
TDS Publications List ~ *Publications List*
The Dystonia Society Newsletter ~ *Newsletter*

Concerned with the following diseases or disorders:
Blepharospasm, Benign Essential; Dysphonia, Chronic Spasmodic; Dystonia, Torsion

1698 DYSTROPHIC EPIDERMOLYSIS BULLOSA RESEARCH ASSOCIATION OF AMERICA, INC. (DEBRA OF AMERICA)

40 Rector Street
14th Floor
New York, NY 10006 212-513-4090
Fax: 212-513-4099
E-mail: debraorg@ix.netcom.com
http://www.debra.org

The Dystrophic Epidermolysis Bullosa Research Association of America (DEBRA) is a national voluntary health organization dedicated to achieving a cure for Epidermolysis Bullosa (EB) and improving the care and quality of life for people with this disorder and their families. EB is a group of genetic disorders in which there is a defect causing the skin layers to separate and blister either spontaneously or at the slightest friction. Symptoms usually are apparent at or shortly after birth. The Association promotes and supports scientific research on the cause, diagnosis, treatment, and cure of this disorder. DEBRA seeks to meet the unique needs of affected individuals and their families through programs that supply information, assistance, support, and guidance. DEBRA is also committed to raising public awareness about the nature of Epidermolysis Bullosa and to representing the special concerns of affected individuals and their families to government officials. The organization offers a variety of educational materials including brochures entitled "Time Does Not Heal All Wounds" and "Hope Through Research."

President: Faith Daniels (1994-Present)
Executive Director: Miriam Feder
Organization Language: Spanish.
Year Established: 1980
Organization Chapters: 8
Organization Members: 3,500

Publishes the following materials:
Vision and Mission of the D.E.B.R.A. Association of America, Inc. ~ *Factsheet*
Living with Epidermolysis Bullosa ~ *Brochure*
Hope Through Research ~ *Brochure*
Time Does Not Heal All Wounds ~ *Brochure*
List of DEBRA Publications ~ *Publication List*

Concerned with the following diseases or disorders:
Epidermolysis Bullosa; Lyelles Syndrome

1699 EA/TEF CHILD AND FAMILY SUPPORT CONNECTION, INC. (EA/TEF)

921 Acorn Drive
Suite 100
Sleepy Hollow, IL 60118-2678 847-426-0414
Fax: 847-426-9486
E-mail: eatef2@aol.com

The EA/TEF (Esophageal Atresia and Tracheoesophageal Fistula) Child and Family Support Connection is a nonprofit organization dedicated to providing educational resources as well as emotional and practical support to aid in the daily care of children affected by esophageal atresia or tracheoesophageal fistula. Esophageal Atresia (EA) is a congenital birth defect characterized by lack of continuity of the esophagus (which is normally a single passage extending from the throat to the stomach). Tracheoesophageal Fistula (TEF) is a birth defect characterized by the presence of an abnormal passage between the esophagus and the windpipe. Established in 1992, eight families in the Chicago area joined forces to create a support network of parents of children born with EA/TEF. Their shared experiences were made easier with the support of others who faced similar situations and had similar questions. The network of information and support that they created was the seed for the EA/TEF Child and Family Support Connection. The organization, which currently consists of 1,200 members and 10 chapters, has become a national clearinghouse for information on these birth defects. EA/TEF provides a variety of materials through its Family Orientation Packet, a Lending Library of books and videos, educational brochures and flyers, and a regular newsletter. The organization has a national database that provides important information to parents as well as health care professionals; has a family directory containing a listing of families for the purpose of telephone networking; and offers the "Sunshine Program" which sends special gifts to affected children who are hospitalized or ill, sends birthday greetings, and acknowledges achievement of developmental milestones.

President: Bruce Davis (1997 - 2000)
Executive Director: Sandi Masi
Year Established: 1993
Organization Chapters: 10
Organization Members: 1,200

Publishes the following materials:
EA/TEF Child And Famlily Support Connection ~ *Newsletter*
EA/TEF. Esophageal Atresia/Tracheoesophageal Fistula. A Guide for Teachers. ~ *Brochure*
A Parent's Guide to the EA/TEF Child and Family Support Connection, Inc. ~ *Brochure*
EA/TEF A Guide for Caregivers. ~ *Brochure*
Proper Care of Your Child's Gastrostomy Tube/Button ~ *Brochure*
Helping Your Child Cope with Painful Medical Procedures ~ *Brochure*
Helping Helathy Siblings Adjust to a Child's Illness ~ *Brochure*
Switching from Tube Feeding to Oral Feeding ~ *Brochure*
Guidelines for the Progression of Food Textures ~ *Brochure*
EA/TEF Family Directory ~ *Booklet*
Survival Tips for Parents of Babies Born with Esophageal Atresia and TEF ~ *Fact Sheet*
Henschel Lending Library ~ *Book/Video List*
Supply Sharing ~ *Medical Supply List*
Food for Thought ~ *Fact Sheet*

Concerned with the following diseases or disorders:
Esophageal Atresia and/or Tracheoesophageal Fistula; Goldenhar Syndrome (Oculo Auriculo Vertebral Spectrum); VACTERL Association

1700 EAR (EDUCATION AND AUDITORY RESEARCH) FOUNDATION (TEF)

1817 Patterson Street
Nashville, TN 37203 615-329-7807
800-545-4327
Fax: 615-329-7935
TDD: 615-329-7849
E-mail: theearfd@aol.com
http://www.theearfound.com or
http://www.theea

The EAR (Education and Auditory Research) Foundation is a not-for-profit organization dedicated to integrating persons who have hearing impairments into the mainstream of society through public awareness and medical education. The Foundation administers the Meniere's Network, a national network of patient support groups that provides people with the opportunity to share experiences and coping strategies. Meniere's Disease is characterized by episodic vertigo, hearing loss, and ringing or roaring in the ear. Established in 1971, the EAR Foundation sponsors a variety of programs in addition to the Meniere's Network including a medical education program that offers continuing medical education (CME) courses to physicians; the "young ears" program, which focuses on raising the level of awareness among children, parents, and physicians regarding hearing preservation; and the "Minnie Pearl Scholarship Fund," which helps many hearing-impaired high school and college students further their education. The Foundation publishes "STEADY," the Meniere's Network newsletter and several brochures and booklets for both consumers and medical professionals. The EAR Foundation also maintains a web site.

Executive Director: Eddie Thompson, Ed.D.
Year Established: 1971
Organization Members: Non-Membership

Publishes the following materials:
The GIFT of Hearing ~ *Brochure*
MINNIE PEARL SCHOLARSHIP PROGRAM ~ *Brochure*
Four Questions to Ask About Your Child's Hearing ~ *Brochure*
OTOSCOPE ~ *Newsletter*
INSTRUCTIONAL PROGRAM AND AUDIOVISUAL CATALOG ~ *Brochure*
Communicating with the Hearing Impaired ~ *Factsheet*
STEADY ~ *Brochure*

Concerned with the following diseases or disorders:
Cardio Auditory Syndrome; Meniere Disease; Nystagmus, Benign Paroxysmal Positional

1701 EURORDIS EUROPEAN ORGANIZATION FOR RARE DISEASES (EURORDIS)

Institut de Myologie - Batiment Babinski
Groupe hospitalier Pitie'-Salpetriere
75651 Paris Cedex 13,
France 01133142165862
Fax: 01133142165887
E-mail: yjeronym@myologie.infobiogen.fr

EURORDIS, the European Organization for Rare Diseases, is a voluntary organization that is dedicated to improving the quality of life of all those affected by rare disorders. The purpose of the organization is to propose and lobby for new European regulations designed to increase research and development of promising therapeutic options for the treatment of rare diseases; to insure the best possible health care throughout the European Union for those affected by rare disorders; and to improve the overall quality of life of those affected by rare diseases. Additional goals include the stimulation of coordinated research efforts at the European level to increase the knowledge of rare disorders, their causes, and new and effective treatments; the provision of a European platform to a wide variety of national patient organizations to coordinate their actions at the European level; and the provision of a patient interest-driven mediator between all the various European structures and institutions that are involved in public health responses to the needs of persons with rare disorders. Information is available English, Italian, Spanish, and French.

President: Marie-Claude Lagrange (1997)
Executive Director: Stephane Korsia
Organization Language: French (written/spoken). Spanish (written). Italian (written).
Year Established: 1997
Organization Members: 50

1702 EAR ANOMALIES RECONSTRUCTED: ATRESIA/MICROTIA SUPPORT GROUP

72 Durand Road
Maplewood, NJ 07040 201-761-5438
Fax: 201-378-8930

Ear Anomalies Reconstructed: Atresia/Microtia Support Group is an international not-for-profit self-help organization dedicated to providing information and support to individuals affected by congenital ear anomalies such as aural atresia, microtia, and craniofacial microsomia. In affected infants and children, abnormally small, underdeveloped (hypoplastic), and/or malformed (dysplastic) ears (pinnae) with blind ending or absent external ear canals (microtia) may result in hearing impairment (conductive hearing loss). The organization offers networking services, conducts conferences that feature leading plastic surgeons and otolaryngologists, and offers regular support group meetings in the New York City area.

President: Jack Gross (contact)
Executive Director: Betsy Old
Year Established: 1986

Concerned with the following diseases or disorders:
Ear, Patella, Short Stature Syndrome; Goldenhar Syndrome (Oculo Auriculo Vertebral Spectrum); Treacher Collins Syndrome

1703 EATING DISORDERS AWARENESS AND PREVENTION, INC. (EDAP)

603 Stewart Street
Suite 803
Seattle, WA 98101 206-382-3587
Fax: 206-292-9890
http://members.aol.com/edapinc

Eating Disorders Awareness and Prevention, Inc. (EDAP) is a not-for-profit organization that serves the United States and Canada and is dedicated to increasing awareness of and preventing eating disorders. Eating disorders include self-starvation and excessive weight loss (anorexia nervosa), a secretive cycle of binge eating followed by purging (bulimia nervosa), and compulsive overeating. Established in 1987, EDAP is dedicated to challenging cultural attitudes that may promote the development of eating disorders; advocating the importance of self-esteem based on inner beauty and personal strengths, rather than on appearance or weight; enhancing public and professional awareness of the signs and symptoms of eating disorders and treatment options; emphasizing that early detection and prompt treatment may help to speed the recovery process; and encouraging public understanding of eating disorders to facilitate compassionate, supportive attitudes. Comprised of 750 members, EDAP disseminates information about prevention, early detection, and awareness of eating disorders; maintains a centralized database of information on prevention and health promotion; offers curricula and information to schools and universities across the country; provides information to parents, families, and the organizations that reach them; and provides information to professionals such as nurses, dentists, dietitians, physicians, attorneys, teachers, health educators, coaches, health and fitness instructors, pharmacists, psychotherapists, social workers, and counselors. The organization's materials include brochures, videos, fact sheets, and a regular newsletter entitled "EDAP Matters." Other programs and activities include the sponsorship of Eating Disorders Awareness Week, the EDAP puppet project for schools, and national conferences. EDAP also maintains a web site at [http://members.aol.com/edapinc].

President: Michael Levine, Ph.D. (1997 to 1999)
Executive Director: Jennifer Biely, J.D.
Year Established: 1987
Organization Chapters: 250
Organization Members: 750

Publishes the following materials:
Eating Disorders Awareness and Prevention ~ *Brochure*
A Guide to the Primary Prevention of Eating Disorders ~ *Brochure*
EDAP Matters ~ *Newsletter*

Concerned with the following diseases or disorders:
Anorexia Nervosa; Bulimia

1704 EDUCATIONAL EQUITY CONCEPTS (EEC)

114 East 32nd Street
Suite 701
New York, NY 10016 212-725-1803
Fax: 212-725-0947
TDD: 212-725-1803
E-mail: 75507.1306@compuserve.com

Educational Equity Concepts is a national nonprofit advocacy organization dedicated to decreasing and eventually eliminating discrimination from all school systems. The EEC believes in the inclusive education approach and has implemented this technique in many school systems. Established in 1982, EEC embraces and instills the concept that understanding the connections between gender, racial, and disability biases can enhance the quality and success of an educational program as well as create emotional security, stability, and open-mindedness in both disabled and non-disabled students. The organization's main objectives focus on equity and integration and include developing early childhood education programs; creating equity-based hands-on science programs for teachers, parents, and children from pre-kindergarten through third grade; and promoting integration of people with disabilities into all educational levels, specifically addressing the needs and rights of females with disabilities. EEC publishes brochures and reports on various issues as well as a curriculum guide for teachers. They also offer networking services, referrals, educational services, and a directory.

President: Ellen Rubin (Coordinator)
Executive Director: Barbara Sprung and Merle Froschl (Co-Directors)
Organization Language: Hebrew (written/spoken). Spanish (written/spoken).
Year Established: 1982
Organization Members: Non-Membership

Publishes the following materials:
Alliance for Mainstreaming Youth with Disabilities ~ *Brochure*
Issue Paper Number 2 ~ *Factsheet*
Educational Equity Concepts ~ *Mission Statement*
Educational Equity Concepts, Inc. ~ *Brochure*

1705 EHLERS-DANLOS NATIONAL FOUNDATION (EDNF)

6399 Willshire Boulevard
Suite 510
Los Angeles, CA 90048 213-651-3038
Fax: 213-651-1366
E-mail: loosejoint@aol.com
http://www.ednf.org

Ehlers-Danlos National Foundation is a voluntary self-help not-for-profit organization that is dedicated to providing emotional support and updated information to individuals affected by Ehlers-Danlos Syndrome (EDS) and their families. Ehlers-Danlos Syndrome is a group of inherited connective tissue disorders characterized by abnormalities of the skin, ligaments, and internal organs. Although symptoms and physical features may vary greatly depending upon the specific form of EDS present, many affected individuals may have thin, fragile, hyperextensible skin that may bruise easily; abnormally loose joints that are prone to dislocation; and widespread tissue fragility with bleeding and poor healing of wounds. Established in 1985, the Foundation serves as an informational link to the medical and research community on behalf of affected individuals. The Ehlers-Danlos National Foundation has worked to raise funds to support ongoing medical research and fund the Ehlers-Danlos Syndrome Database Manager, which was established to accumulate data on EDS. The Foundation produces educational and support materials including pamphlets, brochures, audiovisual aids, journal article reprints, and a newsletter entitled "Loose Connections." The Foundation also offers a physician referral service and holds learning conferences.

President: Nancy Regas
Executive Director: Linda Neumann-Potash
Year Established: 1985
Organization Chapters: 20
Organization Members: 1,500

Publishes the following materials:
A Survey of Patients with Ehlers-Danlos Syndrome ~ *Reprint*
The Skin In Ehlers-Danlos Syndrome ~ *Brochure*
Ehlers-Danlos Syndrome Type IV ~ *Brochure*
The Facts About Ehlers-Danlos Syndrome ~ *Brochure*
Podiatric Management of Ehlers-Danlos Syndrome ~ *Brochure*
Loose Connections ~ *Newsletter*
Ehlers-Danlos National Foundation Membership Form ~ *Membership Form*
Ehlers-Danlos National Foundation Family History Form ~ *Family History Form*
Ehlers-Danlos Syndrome ~ *Newletter Reprints*
What's Wrong with Me? ~ *Article Reprint*
Understanding Ehlers-Danlos Syndrome ~ *Reprint*
Arthritis Information Ehlers-Danlos Syndrome (EDS) ~ *Brochure*

Concerned with the following diseases or disorders:
Ehlers Danlos Syndrome

1706 ELDERCARE AMERICA, INC.

1141 Loxford Terrace
Silver Spring, MD 20901 301-593-1621
Fax: 301-593-1621

Eldercare America, Inc. is a nonprofit organization dedicated to advocating on behalf of the millions of family caregivers of the elderly and to promoting more responsive legislative changes for their benefit. Established in 1983, Eldercare America is a national organization that focuses exclusively on family eldercare; stimulates, supports, and strengthens local self-help and community based service initiatives; promotes the well-being, dignity, and independence of older persons and the families who care for them; and acts as a focal point for empowerment, advocacy, and networking. The organization produces videotapes including "Eldercare in the Workplace" and "Caregivers! What They Do and Why They Do It." The organization also supplies a summary of recommendations from the mini-conference on Family Caregiving and Corporate Eldercare. This event was officially recognized as a "White House Conference on Aging" activity.

President: Andrew Hofer
Year Established: 1983
Organization Members: Non-Membership

Publishes the following materials:
Eldercare America, Inc. ~ *Mission Statement*

1707 ENDOMETRIOSIS ASSOCIATION (EA)

International Headquarters
8585 North 76th Place
Milwaukee, WI 53223 414-355-2200
800-992-3636
Fax: 414-355-6065

The Endometriosis Association is a not-for-profit self-help organization dedicated to providing support and education to women affected by endometriosis and their families. Endometriosis is a prevalent gynecological condition characterized by an inability to shed the build-up of bloody tissue that normally forms on the lining of the uterus (endometrium) before menstruation. Established in 1980, the organization provides support for women with endometriosis and their families; educational materials for the public and medical professionals about the disease; and promotes and carries out research on the disease. As part of its Research Program, the Association conducts research on endometriosis, including a special program at Dartmouth Medical School and continuing work on the relationship between dioxin and endometriosis. Consisting of 10,000 members and 250 chapters, the organization produces educational materials including "What is Endometriosis?" written in several languages; the "Endometriosis Association Newsletter" published six times a year; and a book entitled "The Endometriosis Sourcebook." Program activities include "The Support Program" with a wide range of services including support groups, formal and informal counseling, crisis call assistance, networking, and other forms of support.

President: Mary Lou Ballweg (1980 to Present).
Organization Language: French (written). Spanish (written/spoken). Chinese (written). Japanese (written). Italian (written). German (written). Dutch (written). Portuguese (written/spoken). Arabic (written). Russian
Year Established: 1980
Organization Chapters: 250
Organization Members: 10,000

Publishes the following materials:
Endometriosis Association - Materials To Help You ~ *Booklet*
Endometriosis Association ~ *Pamphlet*
The 1994-95 Endometriosis Association Journalism Awards ~ *Brochure*
Endometriosis and the Black Female ~ *Factsheet*
Facts and Figures on Endometriosis ~ *Factsheet*
The Endometriosis Association's Accomplishments——-1980-1994 ~ *Factsheet*
Endometriosis Association Advisors ~ *Directory*
Mary Lou Ballwig ~ *Profile*
Characteristics of Women with Endometriosis ~ *Fact Sheet*
Case History ~ *Pamphlet*
Endometriosis Association. Education Support Research ~ *Brochure*
Endometriosis Association. Materials to Help You ~ *Brochure*
Endometriosis Association. Facts and Figures on Endometriosis ~ *Fact Sheet*
Case History: Puzzling illness almost ruins student's college experience ~ *Fact Sheet*
Characteristics of Women with Endometriosis ~ *Fact Sheet*
Facts about Endometriosis and the Black Female ~ *Fact Sheet*
Case History: Mother who suffered endometriosis recognizes daughter's symtoms ~ *Fact Sheet*
Case History: Career impacted by endometriosis ~ *Fact Sheet*
The Anguish of Endometriosis. Excerpts from our Mailbox ~ *Fact Sheet*
Case History: Endometriosis in African-American women often misdiagnosed ~ *Fact Sheet*
Endometriosis Association. Education Support Research (Japanese) ~ *Brochure*
Endometriosis Association. Education Support Research (Arabic) ~ *Brochure*

Concerned with the following diseases or disorders:
Endometriosis

1708 EPILEPSY FOUNDATION OF AMERICA (EFA)
4351 Garden City Drive
Landover, MD 20785
301-459-3700
800-332-1000
Fax: 301-577-2684
TDD: 800-332-2070
E-mail: postmaster@efa.org
http://www.efa.org/

The Epilepsy Foundation of America is a national not-for-profit voluntary organization that works for people affected by seizures through programs of research, education, advocacy, and service. Established in 1968, the Foundation has a national office outside of Washington, D.C. and a network of over 60 affiliated organizations offering services in 125 communities nationwide. The Foundation seeks to improve the quality of life for people affected by seizures; facilitate access to reliable information about epilepsy; and act as a voice for people affected by seizures. National programs include a toll-free information service, research studies, professional education programs, public and family education programs, legal and legislative advocacy programs, and career choice and employment assistance. Local programs include outreach programs to schools and community centers, support groups, camping trips, employment services, respite care for families, and help with living arrangements. The Foundation supplies informational materials to the public and health care professionals. In addition, the National Epilepsy Library and Resource Center provides authoritative information to professionals and the public by means of computer access to major collections of medical information.

President: Jeanne Carpenter, Esq.
Executive Director: Paulette V. Maehara
Organization Language: Spanish.
Year Established: 1968
Organization Chapters: 64
Organization Members: 16,000

Publishes the following materials:
Epilepsy Foundation of America - Annual Report 1993 ~ *Report*

Concerned with the following diseases or disorders:
Acrocallosal Syndrome, Schinzel Type; Alpers Disease; Chromosome 14 Ring; DOOR Syndrome; Epilepsy; Epilepsy, Myoclonic Progressive Familial; Fountain Syndrome; Galloway Mowat Syndrome; Hypomelanosis of ITO; Lennox Gastaut Syndrome; MELAS Syndrome; MERRF Syndrome; Myoclonus, General; Oculocerebrocutaneous Syndrome; Perisylvian

Syndrome, Congenital Bilateral; Santavuori Disease; Tuberous Sclerosis; West Syndrome

1709 ERYTHROMELALGIA AND RELATED DISORDERS ASSOCIATION OF AMERICA

P.O. Box 4046
Portland, OR 97208

The Erythromelalgia and Related Disorders Association of America is a voluntary not-for-profit organization dedicated to providing information and support to individuals with Erythromelalgia and related disorders. Erythromelalgia is a rare vascular disorder that affects the skin of the feet and/or hands and is characterized by episodes of sudden widening of the blood vessels in these areas. Symptoms may include severe burning pain, redness, and/or increased temperature. Established in 1988, the Association responds to inquiries through the mail with a letter discussing the organization, its history, its mission, and information concerning Erythromelalgia. The Association also sends research article reprints as well as a bibliography of additional published materials. The Association's goals include creating a registry of individuals with Erythromelalgia.

Executive Director: Elizabeth Duncan, RN, MN, (Contact Person)
Year Established: 1988

Concerned with the following diseases or disorders:
Erythromelalgia

1710 EXTRACORPOREAL MEMBRANE OXYGENATION SUPPORT GROUP (ECMO)

Department of Pediatrics
4th and Indiana
Texas Tech HSC
Lubbock, TX 79430 806-743-2284
Fax: 806-743-2314

The Extracorporeal Membrane Oxygenation (ECMO) Support Group is a not-for-profit self-help organization dedicated to providing information and support to parents of children facing surgery for ECMO. This is a technique that provides respiratory support by oxygenating the blood outside the body and then returning it to the circulatory system. Established in 1987, the ECMO Support Group provides educational and supportive information through a regular newsletter and materials discussing surgery for ECMO.

President: Gayle Willson
Executive Director: Mary Ann Rogers
Organization Language: Spanish.
Year Established: 1987

1711 EYE BANK ASSOCIATION OF AMERICA (EBAA)

1001 Connecticut Avenue, NW
Suite 601
Washington, DC 20036 202-775-4999
Fax: 202-429-6036
E-mail: sightebaa@aol.com
http://www.restoresight.org/

The Eye Bank Association of America (EBAA) is a not-for-profit organization dedicated to the restoration of sight through the promotion and advancement of eye banking. An eye bank retrieves, evaluates, and distributes eyes donated for corneal transplantation, research, and education. Member eye banks around the world make possible thousands of corneal transplants annually. The cornea is the front, clear portion of the eye through which light passes. Corneal blindness is a form of visual impairment caused when the cornea becomes clouded, scarred, or misshapen. This condition may be the result of disease, infection, or injury. Established in 1961 and consisting of 108 members, EBAA promotes research and professional education and provides a newsletter, brochures, and pamphlets. EBAA also maintains a web site at [http://www.restoresight.org].

President: Particia Acken-O'Neil
Year Established: 1961
Organization Members: 108

Publishes the following materials:
Questions and Answers About Eye Donation and Corneal Transplantation ~ *Brochure*

Concerned with the following diseases or disorders:
Corneal Dystrophy; Keratoconus

1712 FACES: THE NATIONAL CRANIOFACIAL ASSOCIATION (FACES)

P.O. Box 11082
Chattanooga, TN 37401 423-266-1632
800-332-2373
Fax: 423-267-3124
E-mail: faces@mindspring.com

FACES: The National Craniofacial Association is a not-for-profit organization whose purpose is to provides families with financial assistance for travel to major medical centers for reconstructive surgery; offer information and support to affected families; and increase public awareness and understanding of facial abnormalities. Educational materials produced by FACES include brochures, a quarterly newsletter, and a statement of services and other resources.

President: Susan T. Johnson (1994-Present)
Executive Director: Lynne G. Mayfield
Year Established: 1969

Publishes the following materials:
Questions and Answers about FACES ~ *Brochure*
FACES ~ *Newsletter*
Traumatic Facial Deformities ~ *Reprint*
Craniosynostosis Part I ~ *Reprint*
Craniosynostosis Part II ~ *Reprint*

Concerned with the following diseases or disorders:
Ablepharon Macrostomia Syndrome; Antley Bixler Syndrome; Apert Syndrome; Baller Gerold Syndrome; Blepharophimosis, Ptosis, Epicanthus Inversus Syndrome; Branchio Oculo Facial Syndrome; C Syndrome; Carpenter Syndrome; Cerebro Oculo Facio Skeletal Syndrome; Chromosome 10, Distal Trisomy 10q; Chromosome 11, Partial Monosomy 11q; Chromosome 13, Partial Monosomy 13q; Chromosome 4, Monosomy Distal 4Q; Chromosome 4, Partial Trisomy Distal 4q; Chromosome 7, Monosomy 7p2; Cleidocranial Dysplasia; Cornelia de Lange Syndrome; Craniofrontonasal Dysplasia; Craniometaphyseal Dysplasia; Craniosynostosis, Primary; Crouzon Disease; Encephalocele; Fraser Syndrome; Frontofacionasal Dysplasia; Frontonasal Dysplasia; Goodman Syndrome; Gorlin Chaudhry Moss Syndrome; Greig Cephalopolysyndactyly Syndrome; Hallermann Streiff Syndrome; Hanhart Syndrome; Hyperostosis Frontalis Interna; Jackson-Weiss Syndrome; Johanson Blizzard Syndrome; Maxillofacial Dysostosis; Maxillonasal Dysplasia, Binder Type; Miller Syndrome; Moebius Syndrome; Nager Syndrome; Oral Facial Digital Syndrome; Orocraniodigital Syndrome; Oto Palato Digital Syndrome Type I and II; Pallister W Syndrome; Parry Romberg Syndrome; Pfeiffer Syndrome; Pierre Robin Syndrome; Roberts Syndrome; Rubinstein Taybi Syndrome; Saethre Chotzen Syndrome; Sakati Syndrome; Scott Craniodigital Syndrome With Mental Retardation; Simpson Dysmorphia Syndrome; Summitt Syndrome; Telecanthus with Associated Abnormalities; Treacher Collins Syndrome; Tricho Dento Osseous Syndrome; Velocardiofacial Syndrome; Waardenburg Syndrome

1713 FOCUS—FOR OUR CHILDREN'S UNIQUE SIGHT (FOCUS)

2571 Pico Place
San Diego, CA 92109 619-273-1473
Fax: 619-273-1473
E-mail: daphari@adnc.com

F.O.C.U.S.—For Our Children's Unique Sight is a national not-for-profit voluntary self-help organization dedicated to providing information, assistance, and support to families whose children are affected by rare visual syndromes. Headquartered in San Diego, California, the organization distributes current medical literature regarding specific visual disorders; provides information on community resources; conducts parent meetings and social events; and publishes a bimonthly newsletter entitled "Focal Points." For those families who choose to participate, there is a registry of members for the purpose of diagnosis matching.

Executive Director: Pilar Hari
Year Established: 1993
Organization Members: 100

Publishes the following materials:
F.O.C.U.S For Our Children's Unique Sight ~ *Brochure*

1714 FOD (FATTY OXIDATION DISORDER) FAMILY SUPPORT GROUP (FOD FAMILY SUPPORT GROUP)

805 Montrose Drive
Greensboro, NC 27410 910-547-8682
E-mail: GouldDan@aol.com
http://www.cinternet.net/FOD

The Fatty Oxidation Disorders (FOD) Family Support Group is a self-help organization dedicated to providing emotional and informational support to families who have been affected by this rare group of inherited metabolic disorders. Established in 1991 and currently consisting of 150 members and 150 professionals, the group is dedicated to providing phone support and referrals to families across the country. The Network's educational materials include "FOD Communication Network," a biannual newsletter that provides practical information about coping with FOD as well as updates on medical research and pharmaceutical news. A "family list" is also provided so that members may call or write other families affected by FOD.

Executive Director: Deb Lee Gould (1991 to Present)
Year Established: 1991
Organization Members: 150

Publishes the following materials:
Professional List ~ *Fact Sheet*
FOD (Fatty Oxidation Disorder) Communication Network. "All In This Together" ~ *Newsletter*

Concerned with the following diseases or disorders:
Carnitine Deficiency Syndromes; Carnitine Palmitoyltransferase Deficiency; Glutaricaciduria II; Long Chain Acyl CoA Dehydrogenase Deficiency (LCAD); Medium Chain Acyl CoA Dehydrogenase

Deficiency; Short Chain Acyl CoA Dehydrogenase Deficiency (SCAD)

1715 FAMILIES OF SPINAL MUSCULAR ATROPHY

P.O. Box 196
Libertyville, IL 60048 847-367-7620
800-886-1762
Fax: 847-367-7623
E-mail: sma@interaccess.com
http://www.fsmc.org

Families of Spinal Muscular Atrophy (SMA) is a voluntary not-for-profit organization dedicated to promoting and supporting research, offering support to families affected by spinal muscular atrophy, and educating the public. Spinal muscular atrophy is the name given to a group of inherited disorders that result in the progressive deterioration of the spinal nerves controlling voluntary movement. Established in 1984 by a group of concerned parents, Families of Spinal Muscular Atrophy enables affected families to share information, support, and resources through its networking program. The organization also provides families with financial assistance to enable them to purchase necessary equipment; funds several full-time researchers including a roster at Indiana University that provides researchers with a central location to access necessary family information; and offers referrals to genetic counseling, support groups, and other services. SMA provides a variety of educational and support materials including a quarterly newsletter entitled "Direction," brochures, pamphlets, and videotapes. The organization supports several languages including Spanish, Italian, German, Polish, Greek, and Yiddish.

President: Audrey Lewis
Executive Director: Audrey Lewis
Organization Language: Spanish. Italian. German. Polish.
Year Established: 1984
Organization Chapters: 9
Organization Members: 800

Publishes the following materials:
Spinal Muscular Atrophy ~ *Brochure*
Direction ~ *Newsletter*

Concerned with the following diseases or disorders:
Amyotrophic Lateral Sclerosis; Brown Sequard Syndrome; Hypotonia, Benign Congenital; Kennedy Disease; Kugelberg Welander Syndrome; Motor Neuron Disease; Werdnig Hoffman Disease

1716 FAMILY RESOURCE CENTER ON DISABILITIES (FRCD)

20 East Jackson
Room 900
Chicago, IL 60604 312-939-3513
800-952-4199
Fax: 312-939-7297
TDD: 312-939-3519

The Family Resource Center on Disabilities (FRCD), formerly the Coordinating Council for Handicapped Children, is a not-for-profit advocacy organization. Established in 1969, the Center is dedicated to improving services for all children with disabilities by providing support and services to affected families, informing parents of their rights under the law, and helping parents become advocates for their children. The Center also seeks to educate and train health care professionals and volunteers. In 1976, the Family Resource Center on Disabilities was one of five pilot programs to operate a parent center funded by the U.S. Department of Education's Office of Special Education Programs. There are now more than 65 federally funded Parent Centers in the United States. The Center offers family support services, information and referral services, and transition services that prepare disabled high school students for adulthood. Special education rights training and the Parent-to-Parent Training Project help parents become effective advocates in their communities. The Center also offers a variety of educational and support materials. These include a regular newsletter, a pamphlet series, and manuals concerning the basics of organizing parent advocacy groups. Other publications distributed by the Center include the provisions of the Federal Rehabilitation Act and its amendments and current federal and state special education rules.

President: Bobbye Watts (1997-Present)
Executive Director: Charlotte Des Jardins
Organization Language: Spanish. French. Polish.
Year Established: 1969
Organization Chapters: 80
Organization Members: 600

Publishes the following materials:
Third Decade of Service ~ *Brochure*
How to Participate Effectively in Your Child's IEP Meeting ~ *Brochure*
How to Prepare for a Successful Due Process Hearing ~ *Brochure*
Rehabilitation Win-Mill ~ *Brochure*
They're Here! ~ *Brochure*
Tax Guide for Parents ~ *Brochure*
FRCD Newsletter ~ *Newsletter*

Introducing FRCD's Special Education Manual ~ *Order Form*
Introduciong FRCD's Rehabilitation Act Manual ~ *Order Form*

1717 FAMILY RESOURCE LIBRARY/CENTER FOR PERSONS WITH DISABILITIES (FRL)

1780 North Research Parkway
Suite 112
North Logan, UT 84341 801-752-0238
Fax: 801-753-9750
TDD: 801-753-9750
E-mail: cope@cc.usu.edu

The Family Resource Library (FRL) is a not-for-profit service organization dedicated to collecting materials containing practical and useful information for families of persons with disabilities. Established in 1948, the Family Resource Library primarily serves persons with disabilities and their families in the four-state area of Utah, Idaho, Wyoming, and Nevada and is located at the Mountain Plains Regional Resource Center, Utah State University in Logan. However, information will be provided to all individuals regardless of disability or location. Educational materials include more than 600 books, booklets, videotapes, and audiotapes on a wide variety of topics.

President: Marilyn Thomas (Librarian) (1975 to Present)
Executive Director: Julia Burnham (Library Coordinator)
Year Established: 1948
Organization Members: Non-Membership

Publishes the following materials:
Family Resource Library ~ *Brochure*
Family Resource Library/Center for Persons with Disabilities ~ *Brochure*
Family Resource Library. Material Catalog ~ *Catalog*

1718 FAMILY VOICES, INC. (FV)

P.O. Box 769
Algodones, NM 87001 505-867-2368
Fax: 505-867-6517
E-mail: famvoi@usa.net
www.ichp.ufl.edu/MCHNetLink/FamilyVoices/

Family Voices (FV) is a not-for-profit voluntary organization dedicated to ensuring that children's health issues are addressed as public and private health care systems undergo change in communities, states, and the nation. Established in 1995, Family Voices, which currently consists of 12,200 members and 50 chapters, is a national grassroots clearinghouse for information and education about ways to assure and improve health care for children with disabilities and chronic conditions. Family Voices is dedicated to the principle that every child deserves quality primary and specialty health care that is affordable and within geographic reach as well as the principle that families are the core of this nation's health system, functioning as their children's most important health providers and caregivers. Family Voices encourages and provides support to families who want to play a role in their child's health care whether in a clinic, hospital, board room, agency, office, or legislative hearing. The organization also encourages partnerships between families and their child's health practitioner, policy makers, the media, and other advocates who also care about children. Family Voices provides a variety of materials including pamphlets, a newsletter entitled "Voices," and frequent one page papers on important topics. FV maintains a web site at [http://www.ichp.ufl.edu/MCHNetLink/FamilyVoices/].

Executive Director: Polly Arango
Organization Language: Spanish (written/spoken).
Year Established: 1995
Organization Chapters: 50
Organization Members: 12,200

Publishes the following materials:
Family Voices ~ *Mission Statement*
Family Voices (Spanish) ~ *Mission Statement*
Family Voices. Questions To Ask and Answer ~ *Fact Sheet*
Family Voices. Questions To Ask and Answer (Spanish) ~ *Fact Sheet*
Alphabet Soup: Health Care Definitions ~ *Fact Sheet*
Important Information About The SSI Children's Program ~ *Fact Sheet*
Family Voices Discusses: Managed Care ~ *Fact Sheet*
Ten Promises To Our Children In 1997 ~ *Fact Sheet*
Children With Spoecial Health Care Needs: Is There A Federal Responsibility? ~ *Fact Sheet*
Guidelines For Organizing ~ *Fact Sheet*
Tips for Testifying ~ *Reprint*
Waivers: The Katie Beckett Waivers and The 1115 Waivers ~ *Fact Sheet*
Children with Special Health Care Needs and Title V Programs ~ *Fact Sheet*
How To Help Kids and Families Undergoing SSI Review ~ *Fact Sheet*
Family Voices: A national grassroots network of families and friends speaking on behalf of children with special h ~ *Fact Sheet*
Voices ~ *Fact Sheet*
Famlily Voices ~ *Brochure*

1719 **FEDERATION FOR CHILDREN WITH SPECIAL NEEDS (FCSN)**

95 Berkeley Street
Suite 104
Boston, MA 02116 617-482-2915
800-331-0688
Fax: 617-695-2939
TDD: 617-482-2915
E-mail: fcsninfo@bitwise.net
http://www.fcsn.org

The Federation for Children with Special Needs is a voluntary organization dedicated to providing information, support, and assistance to parents of children with disabilities, their professional partners, and their local communities. The Federation is committed to listening to and learning from families about their special needs and to encouraging full participation in community life by all people including those with disabilities. The organization has support groups; engages in patient, professional, and general education; offers referrals; and engages in lobbying. Educational materials include a newsletter entitled "News Line"; a journal from the Technical Assistance for Parent Programs (TAPP) Project entitled "Coalition Quarterly"; and a report entitled "Families in Program and Policy: Report of a 1992 Survey of Family Participation in State Title V Programs for Children with Special Health Care Needs." The Federation also conducts a variety of workshops including "Transition from School to Work," "Father's Workshop," and "Family Issues." Please note that the toll free number listed above is for Massachusetts residents only.

Executive Director: Martha Ziegler (Director of Public Policy) (Founde
Organization Language: Spanish (written).

Publishes the following materials:
Federation For Children With Special Needs ~ *Brochure*
We Believe... ~ *Mission Statement*

1720 **FEDERATION OF FAMILIES FOR CHILDREN'S MENTAL HEALTH (FFCMH)**

1021 Prince Street
Alexandria, VA 22314 703-684-7710
Fax: 703-836-1040
E-mail: ffcmh@crosslink.net
http://www.ffcmh.org

The Federation of Families for Children's Mental Health is a not-for-profit, parent-run, advocacy organization focused on the needs of children and youth with emotional, behavioral, or mental disorders. The Federation's mission is to provide leadership in the field of children's mental health and develop necessary human and financial resources to meet its goals. The Federation addresses the unique needs of children and youth with emotional, behavioral, or mental disorders from birth through the transition to adulthood. It works to ensure the rights to full citizenship, support, and access to community-based services for all affected children and their families. The Federation also seeks to provide information and engage in advocacy regarding research, prevention, early intervention, family support, education, transition services, and other services. Established in 1988, the Federation distributes a variety of educational materials including brochures, a philosophy statement, and a "Principles on Family Support" statement.

President: Gail Daniels
Executive Director: Barbara Huff
Organization Language: Spanish.
Year Established: 1988
Organization Chapters: 125
Organization Members: 5,000

Publishes the following materials:
The Federation of Families for Children's Mental Health ~ *Brochure*
Principles on Family Support ~ *Fact Sheet*
Philosophy Statement ~ *Mission Statement*

Concerned with the following diseases or disorders:
Autism; Pica; Trichotillomania

1721 **FIGHT FOR SIGHT, INC.**

160 East 56th Street
8th Floor
New York, NY 10022 212-751-1118
Fax: 212-688-9641

Fight For Sight, Inc., once known as the National Council to Combat Blindness, is a voluntary not-for-profit organization dedicated to the restoration and preservation of sight through eye research and treatment. Established in 1946, and consisting of approximately 500 members, Fight For Sight provides awards, grants, and fellowships to accredited medical colleges, hospitals, and eye centers throughout the nation and in foreign countries; supports eye clinics at leading institutions, enabling thousands of disadvantaged youngsters to receive quality eye care; and has support groups. The organization also offers a variety of educational materials.

President: Kenneth Barasch, M.D.
Executive Director: Mildred Weisenfeld
Year Established: 1946
Organization Members: 500

Publishes the following materials:
"I can't wake up, mommy. I just can't wake up." ~ *Brochure*
Perceiver. The Sights and souinds of the American Academy of Ophthalmology and Otolaryngology ~ *Reprint*

1722 FIGHTERS FOR ENCEPHALY SUPPORT GROUP

332 Brereton Street
Pittsburgh, PA 15219 412-687-6437

The Fighters for Encephaly Support Group is a not-for-profit national health organization dedicated to providing information and support to families affected by disorders involving the brain. Established in 1988, this parent-to-parent support group disseminates information to physicians, other health care professionals, clinics, affected families, and others who are interested in or affected by encephaly-related disorders. In addition, the group promotes patient and family advocacy, provides referrals, and publishes a regular newsletter as well as various disorder-related brochures.

President: Nancy Gomski (1988-Present)
Year Established: 1988
Organization Members: 275

Concerned with the following diseases or disorders:
Anencephaly; Encephalocele; Holoprosencephaly; Perisylvian Syndrome, Congenital Bilateral

1723 FOOD ALLERGY NETWORK (FAN)

10400 Eaton Place
Suite 107
Fairfax, VA 22030-2208 703-691-3179
800-929-4040
Fax: 703-691-2713
E-mail: fan@worldweb.net
http://www.foodallergy.org/

The Food Allergy Network (FAN) is a not-for-profit service organization dedicated to bringing about a clearer understanding of the issues surrounding food allergies and to helping affected individuals lead a normal life while following restricted diets. Established in 1991 and consisting of 11,000 members, FAN is committed to increasing public awareness about food allergies and anaphylaxis, a severe, life-threatening reaction, and providing emotional support and coping strategies to affected individuals. While FAN's membership includes people of all ages, the organization's main focus is on children since they are the largest population group affected by food allergies. FAN has a regular newsletter containing recipes, practical tips, consumer alerts, and medical and dietary information. FAN also offers a brochure entitled "The Food Allergy Network," which details the full range of the Network's services and provides information on food allergies.

President: Anne Munoz-Furlong (1991 to Present).
Year Established: 1991
Organization Members: 11,000

Publishes the following materials:
The Food Allergy Network ~ *Mission Statement*
Food Allergy News ~ *Newsletter*

1724 FORWARD FACE, INC.

317 East 34th Street
Room 901
New York, NY 10016 212-684-5860
800-393-3223
Fax: 212-684-5864

Forward Face, Inc. is a self-help group affiliated with the Institute of Reconstructive Plastic Surgery at the New York University Medical Center and the National Foundation for Facial Reconstruction. Established in 1978, Forward Face is dedicated to helping affected individuals and family members successfully cope with craniofacial disorders. Forward Face networks affected individuals and families with similar conditions and offers a comprehensive support system including medical, psychological, and financial services. The organization works to facilitate communication between affected families and their physicians, conducts workshops, and distributes a variety of resource materials. Forward Face also funds pediatric projects at New York University, conducts community outreach programs, publishes periodic newsletters, and holds quarterly membership meetings to promote education and networking opportunities.

President: Barbara Robertson
Executive Director: Kristin Ronelli
Year Established: 1978
Organization Members: 500

Publishes the following materials:
Forward Face ~ *Newsletter*
Forward Face A Support Group For Patients With Crainofacial Disorders ~ *Brochure*

Concerned with the following diseases or disorders:
Ablepharon Macrostomia Syndrome; Apert Syndrome; Baller Gerold Syndrome; Blepharophimosis, Ptosis, Epicanthus Inversus Syndrome; Cardio Facio Cutaneous Syndrome; Carpenter Syndrome; Cerebro Oculo Facio Skeletal Syndrome; Chromosome 10, Distal Trisomy

10q; Chromosome 4, Partial Trisomy Distal 4q; Cleft Palate and Cleft Lip; Cornelia de Lange Syndrome; Craniofrontonasal Dysplasia; Craniometaphyseal Dysplasia; Craniosynostosis, Primary; Crouzon Disease; Encephalocele; Fraser Syndrome; Frontofacionasal Dysplasia; Frontonasal Dysplasia; Goodman Syndrome; Gorlin Chaudhry Moss Syndrome; Greig Cephalopolysyndactyly Syndrome; Hallermann Streiff Syndrome; Hanhart Syndrome; Jackson-Weiss Syndrome; Maxillofacial Dysostosis; Moebius Syndrome; Nager Syndrome; Oral Facial Digital Syndrome; Orocraniodigital Syndrome; Pallister W Syndrome; Pfeiffer Syndrome; Popliteal Pterygium Syndrome; Rapp Hodgkins Syndrome; Roberts Syndrome; Saethre Chotzen Syndrome; Sakati Syndrome; Scott Craniodigital Syndrome With Mental Retardation; Seckel Syndrome; Setleis Syndrome; Summitt Syndrome; Telecanthus with Associated Abnormalities; Treacher Collins Syndrome

1725 FOUNDATION FIGHTING BLINDNESS (FFB)

Executive Plaza 1
11350 McCormick Road, Suite 800
Hunt Valley, MD 21031-1014 410-785-1414
888-394-3937
Fax: 410-771-9470
TDD: 800-683-5551
http://www.blindness.org

The Foundation Fighting Blindness is dedicated to funding research that investigates the cause, cure, and prevention of Retinitis Pigmentosa (RP) and other related forms of retinal degeneration. Established in 1971, the Foundation also engages in patient and professional education; provides appropriate referrals; and promotes public awareness. In addition, the Foundation has several Self-Help Networks (Usher Syndrome, Bardet-Biedl Syndrome, and Young Adult Self-Help Networks) to enable members to exchange information, mutual support, and resources. The Foundation also produces a variety of educational materials including booklets, large print information sheets, cassette tapes, and braille booklets.

President: Gordon Gund
Executive Director: Robert M. Gray
Year Established: 1971
Organization Chapters: 40
Organization Members: 60,000

Publishes the following materials:
RP Foundation Fighting Blindness Publication List ~ *Publication List*
Information about RP and Allied Degenerative Diseases ~ *Pamphlet*
Information about Retinitis Pigmentosa ~ *Factsheet*
Information about Usher Syndrome. ~ *Booklet*
Information about Usher Syndrome ~ *Factsheet*
The Inheritance of RP and Allied Retinal Degenerative Diseases ~ *Brochure*
Information about Bardet-Biedl Syndrome ~ *Factsheet*
Information about Choroideremia ~ *Factsheet*
Information about Stargardt Disease ~ *Factsheet*
1994 Annual Report ~ *Brochure*
Fighting Blindness News ~ *Newsletter*
Keeping the Future in Sight ~ *Factsheet*
Tips For Teachers ~ *Factsheet*
Tips For Travelers ~ *Factsheet*

Concerned with the following diseases or disorders:
Acanthocytosis; Alstrom Syndrome; Bardet Biedl Syndrome; Coats' Disease; Cone Dystrophy; Kearns Sayre Syndrome (KSS); Leber's Congenital Amaurosis; Loken Senior Syndrome; Norrie Syndrome; Refsum Syndrome; Retinitis Pigmentosa; Retinoschisis; Septo Optic Dysplasia; Usher's Syndrome

1726 FOUNDATION FOR ICHTHYOSIS & RELATED SKIN TYPES (FIRST)

P.O. Box 669
Ardmore, PA 19003 610-789-3995
800-545-3286
Fax: 610-789-4366
E-mail: ichthyosis@aol.com
http://www.libertynet.org/~ichthyos/

The Foundation for Ichthyosis & Related Skin Types (FIRST) is a voluntary organization dedicated to helping individuals and families affected by the inherited skin diseases collectively called the "Ichthyoses." The Ichthyoses are a group of rare, inherited disorders characterized by abnormally dry, scaly, thickened skin due to abnormalities in the production of the protein keratin. FIRST provides support, information, education, and advocacy for individuals and families affected by ichthyosis. FIRST supports research into the causes, treatment, and ultimate cure for ichthyosis.

President: Donna Rice
Executive Director: Mark Levitan
Year Established: 1981
Organization Members: 8,000

Publishes the following materials:
F.I.R.S.T. Foundation for Icthyosis and Related Skin Types ~ *Brochure*
Foundation for Ichthyosis & Related Skin Types (F.I.R.S.T.) ~ *Newsletter*

Concerned with the following diseases or disorders:
Cardio Facio Cutaneous Syndrome; Darier Disease; Epidermal Nevus Syndrome; Epidermolytic Hyperkeratosis; Erythrokeratodermia with Ataxia; Ichthyosis; Ichthyosis Congenita; Ichthyosis Hystrix, Curth Macklin Type; Ichthyosis Vulgaris; Ichthyosis, CHILD Syndrome; Ichthyosis, Chanarin Dorfman Syndrome; Ichthyosis, Erythrokeratodermia Progressiva Symmetrica; Ichthyosis, Erythrokeratodermia Variabilis; Ichthyosis, Erythrokeratolysis Hiemalis; Ichthyosis, Harlequin Type; Ichthyosis, Keratosis

Follicularis Spinulosa Decalvans; Ichthyosis, Lamellar Recessive; Ichthyosis, Netherton Syndrome; Ichthyosis, Sjogren Larsson Syndrome; Ichthyosis, Tay Syndrome; Ichthyosis, X-Linked; Keratitis Ichthyosis Deafness Syndrome; Peeling Skin Syndrome; Pityriasis Rubra Pilaris

1727 FOUNDATION FOR NAGER AND MILLER SYNDROMES (FNMS)

1827 Grove Street
#2
Glenview, IL 60025-2913 708-724-6449
800-507-3667
Fax: 708-724-6449
http://www.nagerormillersynd.com

The Foundation for Nager and Miller Syndromes is an international not-for-profit organization that functions as a support group for people affected by two similar genetic conditions (Nager and Miller Syndromes) involving severe facial and limb abnormalities. The Foundation serves as an information clearinghouse that links other similarly challenged families. An extensive library of resources and medical reports is available to those with Nager and Miller Syndromes and their physicians. The organization has initiated and is involved in a genetic research project that is working to locate the genes responsible for these disorders. This study is being conducted at the University of Maryland in Baltimore. The Foundation also provides scholarships to children between the ages of 8 and 18 years who wish to attend a summer camp program in Indiana called About Face. This camp allows children to experience independence and to meet others with similar problems. The Foundation publishes a biannual newsletter entitled "All About Me." Articles from this newsletter are regularly reprinted in various other publications. Interpreters are available for written correspondence in German, Portuguese, French, Italian, Spanish, and Polish.

President: Margaret Ieronimo (1992-Present)
Executive Director: Margaret Ieronimo
Organization Language: German (written). Portuguese (written). French (written). Italian (written). Spanish (written). Polish (written).
Year Established: 1992
Organization Members: 40

Publishes the following materials:
FNMS ~ *Brochure*
All About Me ~ *Newsletter*

Concerned with the following diseases or disorders:
Miller Syndrome; Nager Syndrome

1728 FOUNDATION FOR SPINAL CORD INJURY PREVENTION (FSCIP)

1310 Ford Building
Detroit, MI 48226 313-963-1600
800-342-0330
Fax: 313-963-1330

The Foundation for Spinal Cord Injury Prevention (FSCIP) is a voluntary organization that promotes public awareness and prevention of spinal cord injuries from various causes. Founded in 1988, FSCIP disseminates information; shares information with other organizations; and creates public service and safety announcements on the prevention, treatment, rehabilitation, research, and overall physical, mental, and emotional effects of spinal cord injury. In addition, FSCIP facilitates a networking service for affected individuals. FSCIP is a member of the National Safety Council, the MRPA, and a number of other organizations that are interested in safety and the prevention of spinal cord injury. The organization produces several educational materials including "Myths of Diving and Drowning," "No Diving Signs," and "Diving is Deadly."

President: Ronald R. Gilbert (1988 to present)
Year Established: 1988
Organization Members: 6

Publishes the following materials:
Ronald R. Gilbert. Foundation for Spinal Cord Injury Prevention ~ *Booklet*
Spinal Arachnoiditis ~ *Video Tape*
Some Myths and Facts About Children's Drowning ~ *Reprint*
Ronald R. Gilbert! A Uniform Minimum Safe Diving Depth for Swimming Facilities ~ *Pamphlet*
Myths of Diving ~ *Reprint*

1729 FRIENDS NETWORK "FUNLETTERS" (FN)

P.O. Box 4545
Santa Barbara, CA 93140 805-565-7031

The Friends Network "Funletters" is a nonprofit organization established in 1992 that is dedicated to encouraging children to fight cancer with hope. "Funletters," an upbeat, creative outlet for children fighting cancer, is available to all whom request it. The Friends Network, which currently consists of 3,700 members, provides support and resources to individual families, hospitals, and clinics. In addition to providing "Funletters," the Friends Network offers a newsletter called "Updates" and provides networking services.

President: Kenon Neal (1991 to Present)
Year Established: 1992
Organization Chapters: 650
Organization Members: 3,700

Publishes the following materials:
Funletter Update (Spring 1997) ~ *Newsletter*
Funletter (July/August) ~ *Newsletter*

1730 FRIENDS OF DISABLED ADULTS AND CHILDREN, INC. (FODA)

4900 Lewis Road
Stone Mountain, GA 30083 770-491-9014
Fax: 770-491-0026
http://www.foda.org

Friends of Disabled Adults and Children, Inc. (FODA) is a not-for-profit organization dedicated to providing necessary services and support to physically and mobility impaired people of all ages. Established in 1986, the organization provides free mobility impairment, rehabilitative, and home health care equipment, clothing, and household essentials. FODA also provides individual and group counseling; offers employment opportunities by working closely with potential employers and conducting vocational assessments; and provides entry-level job skills training, aid in learning interview techniques, and on-the-job mentoring. Friends of Disabled Adults provides a variety of brochures and pamphlets.

President: Ed Butchart (1986-Present)
Executive Director: Ed Butchart
Organization Language: Spanish. German.
Year Established: 1986

Publishes the following materials:
What is Friends of Disabled Adults? ~ *Brochure*
Tom Brokaw Called Him "The Real Thing" ~ *Brochure*
Picture Yourself as a FODA Volunteer ~ *Brochure*
The Enabler ~ *Brochure*
Industrial Development Program ~ *Brochure*
FODA 1993 Annual Report ~ *Report*
Are Assisted By Miracles ~ *Article*
Wheelchairs, vans all it takes to keep disabled on the go ~ *Article*
Santa Needs A Few More Eyes ~ *Article*
DeKalb Extra ~ *Article*
For this "Santa," helping others isn't bottom line, it's the only line ~ *Article*
Friends of Disabled Adults Fall Update ~ *Article*
Spineline ~ *Fact Sheet*

1731 GASTRO-INTESTINAL RESEARCH FOUNDATION (GIRF)

70 East Lake Street
Suite 1015
Chicago, IL 60601 312-332-1350
Fax: 312-332-4757

The Gastro-Intestinal Research Foundation (GIRF) is a not-for-profit voluntary organization dedicated to raising funds to help promote ongoing gastroenterologic research. Gastroenterology is the study of the digestive system and the disorders that affect the digestive tract. Established in 1962 and consisting of 600 members, the Foundation has a registry and provides information to interested individuals. The Foundation also conducts two seminars on gastro-intestinal health issues each year. These seminars are free and open to the public. The Foundation has a variety of educational materials including a regular newsletter and produces brochures on inflammatory bowel disease and women's health issues relating to gastro-intestinal conditions.

President: Joel Cohen
Executive Director: Judith C. McArdle
Year Established: 1962
Organization Chapters: 2
Organization Members: 600

Publishes the following materials:
Nutrition and Your Health: Dietary Guidelines for Americans ~ *Booklet*
Isues in Women's Gastro-Intestinal Health ~ *Booklet*
Inflammatory Bowel Diseases ~ *Booklet*

Concerned with the following diseases or disorders:
Colitis, Collagenous; Colitis, Ulcerative; Crohn's Disease

1732 GAZETTE INTERNATIONAL NETWORKING INSTITUTE (GINI)

4207 Lindell Boulevard
#110
St. Louis, MO 63108-2915 314-534-0475
Fax: 314-534-5070
E-mail: gini_intl@msn.com

The Gazette International Networking Institute (GINI) is a voluntary not-for-profit organization dedicated to supporting the independent living, self-direction, dignity, and personal achievement of people with disabilities. Established in 1960, the Institute is a primary source of information about independent living, polio and its late effects, home mechanical ventilation, and ventilation equipment. In addition to compiling and disseminating information, the Institute enables people to network with one another to exchange information, resources, and support. The organization also conducts advocacy efforts related to poliomyelitis and late effects of poliomyelitis through its coordination of the International Polio Network. The Institute has expanded its role to assist additional ventilation users through the International Ventilator Users Network. The Gazette International Networking Institute also conducts conferences and workshops; provides directories listing appropriate clinics, health care professionals, and support groups; and publishes a listing of sources for oral and nasal face masks. GINI offers a variety of additional educational and support materials including handbooks, regular newsletters, pamphlets, brochures, and proceedings from the Institute's conferences.

President: Martin B. Wice, M.D.
Executive Director: Joan L. Hedley
Year Established: 1960

Publishes the following materials:
I.V.U.N. News ~ *Newsletter*
Polio Network News ~ *Newsletter*
Post-Polio Directory 1994 ~ *Directory*
Rehabilitation Gazette Resources ~ *Journal*
The Late Effects of Polio An Overview ~ *Brochure*
Gazette International Networking Institute (G.I.N.I.) ~ *Brochure*

1733 GUIDING EYES FOR THE BLIND, INC.

611 Granite Springs Road
Yorktown Heights, NY 10598 914-245-4024
800-942-0149
Fax: 914-245-1609
E-mail: geb@westnet.com
http://www.guiding-eyes.org

Guiding Eyes For The Blind is an international nonprofit service organization and residential training facility dedicated to providing visually impaired individuals with a sense of independence and security through the assistance of professionally-trained guide dogs. Guiding Eyes applicants must be legally blind and at least 16 years of age. There is no maximum age limit, though applicants must be physically and psychologically able to handle and care for a dog. Each month, students from all over the world who are blind or visually impaired come to Guiding Eyes for the Blind's Training Center in Yorktown Heights, New York for an intensive 26-day course to learn to work with and care for a guide dog. Guiding Eyes also provides follow-up services to ensure that graduates and dogs are doing well. The approximately $25,000 cost of the residential training program and follow-up services is paid for through private donations from individuals, corporations, philanthropies, and bequests. The dogs that most consistently exhibit the characteristics of a superior guide dog are labrador retrievers, German shepherds, and golden retrievers. More than 90 percent of the guide dogs that go through training come from Guiding Eyes' own Breeding Center. Guide dogs spend the first year of their lives with volunteer "raisers" who nurture the puppies and familiarize them with everyday life situations, ensuring that they grow into mannerly, well-adjusted adult dogs. After a year with the families, the dogs are returned to Guiding Eyes for evaluation and medical check-ups. Those that pass their tests begin formal training with professional instructors and are taught over several months to assume responsibility for their owner's safe travel. Those dogs not deemed suitable for guide training are often adopted by their puppy-raising families or by others on a long waiting list of people who are eager to adopt the dogs as pets.

President: William Badser
Organization Language: Spanish (written).
Year Established: 1954
Organization Members: Non-Membership

Publishes the following materials:
When You Meet a Person with a Guide Dog ~ *Book Mark*
Guiding Eyes For The Blind ~ *Brochure*
Insight ~ *Newsletter*

Concerned with the following diseases or disorders:
Leber's Optic Atrophy

1734 H.O.R.S.E.S. FOR THE PHYSICALLY CHALLENGED (HORSES, LTD.)

23807 Moss Lane North East
P.O. Box 280
Scotts Mills, OR 97375 503-873-3890
E-mail: horses@open.org
http://www.open.org/horses88/

H.O.R.S.E.S. for the Physically Challenged is a voluntary not-for-profit organization that provides wilderness and recreational horseback riding activities and services for people with disabilities. The organization's belief is that these life-enriching experiences should be available to all people regardless of physical ability and that any person who has the desire to pursue such activities also has the right to pursue that desire. H.O.R.S.E.S., which was established in 1988, provides private and group lessons, adaptive riding equipment, and specialized horse training tailored to the needs of the challenged rider. The organization also produces educational materials including "Mount Up to a World of Adventure," a program brochure, and "Kerry," a program video. H.O.R.S.E.S. maintains a web site at [http://www.open.org/horses88].

President: Kerrill L. Knaus-Hardy (1990 to Present)
Year Established: 1988
Organization Members: Non-Membership

Publishes the following materials:
Mount Up To A World Of Adventure ~ *Brochure*
The Latham Foundation presents: "KERRY" ~ *Video Tape*

1735 HEAR NOW

9745 East Hampden Avenue
Suite 300
Denver, CO 80231 303-695-7797
800-648-4327
Fax: 303-695-7789
TDD: 800-648-4327
E-mail: HEARNOW@charitiesusa.com

HEAR NOW is a voluntary not-for-profit health organization dedicated to helping those who cannot otherwise afford assistance for hearing and cochlear disorders. Established in 1988, this national service organization provides applications for medical assistance to those affected by hearing disorders. In addition, the organization refers individuals to local audiologists. HEAR NOW publishes a newsletter entitled "Hear Now."

President: Dr. Bernice Dinner
Executive Director: MaryAnn Fleet
Year Established: 1988

Concerned with the following diseases or disorders:
Patulous Eustachian Tube

1736 HEATH RESOURCE CENTER

One Dupont Circle NW, Suite 800
Washington, DC 20036-1193 202-939-9320
800-544-3284
Fax: 202-833-4760
TDD: 202-939-9320
E-mail: heath@ace.nche.edu
http://www.acenet.edu

The HEATH Resource Center of the American Council on Education is a national not-for-profit clearinghouse for information on postsecondary education for individuals with disabilities. Established in 1984, HEATH responds to approximately 30,000 electronic, mail, and telephone inquiries per year. The Center serves as an information exchange regarding educational support services, policies, procedures, adaptations, and opportunities at American campuses, vocational-technical schools, and other postsecondary training entities. Educational materials produced by the HEATH Resource Center include a newsletter, guides, directories, and reports that often deal with vision, hearing, mobility, and learning disabilities; independent living; severe or multiple disabilities; and other pertinent topics. The HEATH Resource Center is supported in part by the United States Department on Education.

President: Rhona Hartman
Executive Director: Vicki Barr
Year Established: 1984

Concerned with the following diseases or disorders:
Dyslexia

1737 HASTINGS CENTER

255 Elm Road
Briarcliff Manor, NY 10510 914-762-8500
Fax: 914-762-2124

The Hastings Center is a not-for-profit, nonaffiliated bioethics research center dedicated to studying the ethical issues that arise in health care, medical, scientific, and environmental fields. Established in 1969, the Center carries out an active research program on such subjects as priorities in mental health and justice in health care delivery. Drawing upon a variety of disciplines, the Center's research work strives to provide nonpartisan information, analysis, and recommendations. The Center also engages in educational efforts such as sponsoring programs for individuals and professional groups. In addition, staff members have served as consultants to educators, professional and community groups, policy makers, and the media. The Center publishes two bimonthly journals entitled "Hastings Center Report" and "IRB: A Review of Human Subjects Research." In addition, the Center's research groups produce various other publications including supplements, books, and instructional packets.

President: Daniel Callahan (1969 to Present)
Executive Director: Bruce Jennings
Year Established: 1969
Organization Members: Non-Membership

Publishes the following materials:
Independent Study at The Hastings Center ~ *Brochure*
The Hastings Center ~ *Brochure*
Bioethics and Our Lives ~ *Booklet*
Publications ~ *Order Form*
The Hastings Center Annual Report ~ *Booklet*
The Hastings Center Report. Is There A Duty to Die? ~ *Booklet*
IRB A Review of Human Subjects Research ~ *Newsletter*

1738 **HEAD INJURY HOTLINE**

P.O. Box 84151
Seattle, WA 98124 206-329-1371
Fax: 206-623-4251
E-mail: brain@headinjury.com
http://www.headinjury.com/brain

Head Injury Hotline is a not-for-profit clearinghouse for information and referrals regarding brain injury that results from head injury. Founded and operated by head injury survivors since 1985, the Head Injury Hotline answers questions and makes referrals to health care and legal professionals as well as to support groups. Head Injury Hotline offers advice and seminars to help consumers maximize available professional services. Informational brochures include "From The Ashes, A Head Injury Self-Advocacy Guide" and "What You Should Know About Head Injury."

President: Constance Miller (1985 to Present)
Year Established: 1985

Publishes the following materials:
From The Ashes. A Head Injury Self-Advocacy Guide ~ *Brochure*
What You Should Know About Head Injury ~ *Brochure*
Head Injury Hotline ~ *Fact Sheet*

1739 **HEALING THE CHILDREN NORTHEAST, INC. (HTCNE)**

21 Main Street
Suite 4
P.O. Box 129
New Milford, CT 06776 860-355-1828
Fax: 860-350-6634
E-mail: htcne.inc@worldnet.att.net

Healing The Children Northeast, Inc. (HTCNE) is an international voluntary organization dedicated to providing medical and surgical treatment to children from impoverished backgrounds. Established in 1985 and currently consisting of approximately 2,000 members and 14 chapters, HTCNE assembles volunteer teams of medical and surgical health professionals to travel to host countries where children and young adults are treated free of charge. HTCNE's "Medical Missions Abroad" program serves over 3,000 children annually and provides over three million dollars in donated services. Healing The Children Northeast is committed to expanding the Medical Missions Abroad program to meet the increasing needs of children worldwide. HTCNE provides referrals to appropriate health care agencies, has a database, and offers a variety of materials including brochures, pamphlets, booklets, reports, Spanish language materials, videos, and a quarterly newsletter entitled "Healing."

President: Steve Nargiso (January 1997 to Present)
Executive Director: Angeles Glick
Organization Language: Spanish (written/spoken). Russian (written).
Year Established: 1985
Organization Chapters: 14
Organization Members: 2,000

Publishes the following materials:
Healing ~ *Newsletter Spring 1997*
Missions Abroad Program ~ *Booklet*

1740 **HEALTH RESOURCE CENTER FOR WOMEN WITH DISABILITIES (HRCWD)**

Rehabilitation Institute of Chicago
345 E. Superior Street
Chicago, IL 60611 312-908-7997
Fax: 312-908-1087
TDD: 312-908-8523

The Health Resource Center for Women with Disabilities (HRCWD) is a national, not-for-profit, general health and service center that provides accessible medical services for women with disabilities, conducts research into health issues concerning disabled women, and offers educational resources for health care professionals and women with disabilities. Established in 1991 by the Rehabilitation Institute of Chicago, the HRCWD uses an interdisciplinary team approach that addresses the wide range of physical, psychosocial, and emotional issues that may affect women with disabilities. The Center is governed by a Peer Advisory Board, consisting of a council of women with disabilities, that guides the Center's structure for health service delivery and determines priorities for research, education, and resource development. The HRCWD's medical services for women with disabilities include consultative pregnancy services, family planning, mammography referrals, preventive health care counseling, parenting support, peer counseling, psychological and psychosocial services, and support groups. The Center's research initiatives have included exploration of factors that may affect disabled women's levels of satisfaction with medical services, birth control options for women with disabilities, and the effects of osteoporosis on disabled women. In addition, the HRCWD also provides a variety of materials and educational opportunities through its library and resource center, its quarterly newsletter entitled "Resourcesful Women," information sheets, brochures, videos, and free quarterly seminars for women and their health care providers on such topics as parenting, sexuality, employment, and aging.

President: Judy Panko Reis
Year Established: 1991
Organization Members: 90

Publishes the following materials:
The Health Resource Center for Women with Disabilities ~ *Brochure*
Rehabilitation Institute of Chicago ~ *Mission Statement*
Resourceful Woman ~ *Newsletter*

1741 HELPING HANDS: MONKEY HELPERS FOR THE DISABLED

1505 Commonwealth Avenue
Boston, MA 02135 617-787-4419
Fax: 617-787-5665

Helping Hands: Monkey Helpers for the Disabled is a national not-for-profit organization dedicated to training capuchin monkeys to assist severely disabled individuals. The monkeys are raised in a nationwide network of volunteer foster families as though they were human. At five years of age, young monkeys are mature enough to begin their training. Monkeys are then trained to accomplish the chores of everyday living including feeding, retrieving fallen objects, turning the lights on and off, and loading a floppy disk or videotape. At the end of the training phase, each monkey is placed with an individual who has lost the ability to use his or her limbs (paraplegia). Educational materials produced by Helping Hands include brochures and fact sheets detailing the program and its requirements.

President: Judi Zazula
Year Established: 1983
Organization Members: Non-Membership

Publishes the following materials:
Helping Hands Monkey Helpers for the Disabled ~ *Mission Statement*
Helping Hands Selection Criteria for Potential Monkey Helper Recipients ~ *Fact Sheet*

1742 HEREDITARY DISEASE FOUNDATION, INC. (HDF)

1427 Seventh Street
Suite 2
Santa Monica, CA 90401-9798 310-458-4183
Fax: 310-458-3937
E-mail: cures@hdfoundation.org
http://www.hdfoundation.org

The Hereditary Disease Foundation is a national not-for-profit voluntary organization that was established in 1971. Focusing on Huntington's Disease as a model for genetic diseases, the Foundation conducts an interdisciplinary workshop program that recruits scientists to develop and apply new technologies; supports basic research on genetic illness through grant and postdoctoral fellowship programs at major universities; and provides research tissue to medical investigators. The Hereditary Disease Foundation is supported and guided by a Scientific Advisory Board and a Board of Trustees. Educational materials produced by the Foundation include booklets entitled "Care of the Patient and Family with Huntington's Disease: A Guide for Clinicians," "A Family Member Speaks About Huntington's Disease," and "A Neurologist Speaks About Huntington's Disease." Other materials include reprints of medical journal articles about Huntington's Disease.

President: Nancy S. Wexler, PhD (1983-Present)
Executive Director: Ellen Robinson
Year Established: 1971
Organization Members: 2,500

Publishes the following materials:
Hereditary Disease Foundation - Board of Trustees - Scientific Advisory Board ~ *Trustee List*
Testing for the Huntington's Disease Gene ~ *Medical Center Listing*
Hereditary Disease Foundation-The Story ~ *Fact Sheet*
To Catch a Killer Gene ~ *Article Reprint*
Rejoice The Huntingon's Disease Gene Has Been Found ~ *Fact Sheets*
Discover: Hunting Down Huntington's ~ *Reprint*

Concerned with the following diseases or disorders:
Huntington's Disease

1743 HEREDITARY NEPHRITIS FOUNDATION (HNF)

P.O. Box 57294
Murray, UT 84157-0294 801-262-5901

The Hereditary Nephritis Foundation is a not-for-profit voluntary health organization that was founded in 1978. The Foundation seeks to inform the public about Hereditary Nephritis (HN), a group of rare kidney diseases; raise money for continued research into potential treatments; and provide support to affected families. The Hereditary Nephritis Foundation produces a semi-annual newsletter that provides up-to-date information and offers avenues to networking and mutual support for affected individuals and family members.

President: Kay R. Johnson (1978-Present)
Year Established: 1978
Organization Members: 100

Publishes the following materials:
Newsletter Hereditary Nephritis Foundation ~ *Newsletter*

Concerned with the following diseases or disorders:
Alport Syndrome

1744 HISTIOCYTOSIS ASSOCIATION OF AMERICA

302 North Broadway
Pitman, NJ 08071 609-589-6606
800-548-2758
Fax: 609-589-6614
E-mail: histiocyte@aol.com
http://www.histio.org

The Histiocytosis Association of America is a national not-for-profit organization committed to the promotion of scientific research into the Histiocytoses and the development of improved control and management of these diseases. The ultimate goal is medical research leading to the prevention and cure of Histiocytosis. Established in 1986, the Association seeks to provide solutions to problems that are specific to people who have Histiocytosis and offers support to affected individuals and their families. The Histiocytosis Association of America promotes public education and produces educational materials. These include brochures, a networking directory, and "white papers" that are used in the evaluation of children with Langerhans Cell Histiocytosis (LCH) and other Histiocytoses. Diseases that are represented by the Association include Histiocytosis X, Langerhans Cell Histiocytosis, Letterer-Siwe Disease, Hand-Schuller-Christian Syndrome, Eosinophilic Granuloma, Pulmonary Granuloma, Hashimoto-Pritzker Syndrome, Langerhans Cell Granulomatosis, Familial Hemophagocytic Lymphohistiocytosis, Virus-Associated Hemophagocytic Lymphohistiocytosis, Xanthogranuloma, and Diabetes Insipidus with Langerhans Cell Histiocytosis.

President: Jeffrey M. Toughill (1993-Present)
Executive Director: Jeffrey M. Toughill
Year Established: 1986
Organization Members: 3,500

Publishes the following materials:
Histiocytosis Syndromes in Children ~ *Booklet*
Histiocytosis Association of America Research Progress Report ~ *Report*
Histiocitosis de Celulas Langerhans ~ *Brochure*
Histiocytosis Association Parent/Patient Networking Directory ~ *Directory*
Family Circle ~ *Reprint*
Histiocytosis Syndromes in Children ~ *Booklet*
The Facts About Langerhans Cell Histiocytosis ~ *Brochure*
The Facts About Diabetes Insipidus and Langerhans Cell Histiocytosis ~ *Brochure*
Advancing into 1994 Research and Membership Services ~ *Newsletter*

Concerned with the following diseases or disorders:
Histiocytosis X

1745 HOSPICE FOUNDATION OF AMERICA

2001 South Street NW
#300
Washington, DC 20009 202-638-5419
Fax: 202-638-5312
E-mail: hospicefnd@charitiesusa.com
http://www.hospicefoundation.org/

The Hospice Foundation of America is a not-for-profit public charity whose sole mission is to promote the hospice concept of care. The Foundation acts as an advocate for the hospice concept of care by conducting programs of public education and information related to hospice; offering professional development and educational opportunities to hospice and other health care workers; sponsoring research on ethical issues; participating in public policy initiatives; providing technical assistance to organizations; and serving as a philanthropic presence within the national hospice community. The Hospice Foundation of America provides a web site on the Internet that explains the purpose of and services provided by hospice care; offers links to other hospice sites that enable online users to locate hospices in their area; discusses upcoming Foundation programs; includes an area entitled "Hospice Stories"; and provides dynamic links to additional sources of hospice information, bereavement support, nonprofit sites, and other helpful sources of information, services, and support on the Internet.

1746 **HOSPICE HANDS**

Hospice Hands
c/o Hospice of North Central Florida (HNCF)
P.O. Box 15235
Gainesville, FL 32604 352-378-2121
Fax: 352-378-4111
E-mail: healing@hospice-cares.com
http://hospice-cares.com/

Hospice Hands, an international online resource, was created and is maintained by Hospice of North Central Florida (HNCF). The HNCF is dedicated to serving people and their communities affected by life limiting illness and loss by providing comprehensive, compassionate care, while respecting each person's needs, beliefs, and wishes. The purpose of the Hospice Hands' web site is twofold. Locally, they intend to provide information on their organizational history and current services. Their larger purpose is to promote the hospice philosophy by providing an interactive gathering place for the online hospice community, offering a comprehensive index of the hospice related information available over the Internet, and adding to such knowledge by providing original articles. The Hospice Hands' web site also contains dynamic linkage to basic information on hospice and the disorders most common to hospice patients; sites pertaining to children as patients or grievers; children's hospices; national organizations, hospice mailing lists, and articles on issues of interest to the hospice community; additional sources of support for those giving care to hospice patients as well as for those mourning the loss of loved ones; and home pages for individual hospices. The Hospice Hands' web site also provides a hospice chat room, a hospice Q & A forum, a hospice education bulletin board, a Hospice Hands mailing list, and other sources of information and support.

1747 **HOSPICE WEB**

E-mail: hospice@teleport.com
www.teleport.com/~hospice/index.htm

Hospice Web, a web site on the Internet, explains the purpose of and unique services provided by hospice care. Hospice Web also provides a searchable online directory of the over 2,500 hospices in the United States, helping online users quickly locate hospices in their local areas; a "Frequently Asked Questions" (FAQ) area; dynamic links to other hospice sites on the Internet; a bulletin board area called "Hospice Talk" where online users can post, respond to, or simply read other online users' hospice-related questions; and more.

1748 **HUMAN GROWTH FOUNDATION (HGF)**

7777 Leesburg Pike
Suite 202 South
Falls Church, VA 22043 703-883-1773
800-451-6434
Fax: 703-883-1776
E-mail: hgfound@erols.com
http://www.genetic.org/hgf/

The Human Growth Foundation is a national voluntary not-for-profit organization that was established in 1965. The Foundation is dedicated to expanding and accelerating medical research into growth and growth disorders. Composed of concerned parents, friends of children with growth problems, and interested health professionals, the Human Growth Foundation supports family education and service, public education, support for training of growth specialists, and education of medical professionals. The Foundation conducts national education conferences, makes starter research grants to investigators, and coordinates Human Growth Month. The Foundation also publishes informational pamphlets, booklets, and a monthly newsletter and serves as an information clearinghouse for families of children who have growth disorders.

President: Campbell P. Howard, M.D. (1990-Present)
Executive Director: Kimberly Frye
Organization Language: Spanish.
Year Established: 1965
Organization Chapters: 42
Organization Members: 1,000

Publishes the following materials:
Help The Children Grow ~ *Brochure*
Short Stuff ~ *Brochure*
Patterns of Growth ~ *Brochure*
Intrauterine Growth Retardation ~ *Brochure*
Growth Hormone Deficiency ~ *Brochure*
Turner Syndrome ~ *Brochure*
A Guidebook for Patients ~ *Brochure*
Short & OK. A Guide for Parents of Short Children ~ *Brochure*
My Child's Growth ~ *Factsheet*
Deficiencia de la Hormona del Crecimiento (Growth Hormone

Deficiency) ~ *Brochure*
Patrones del Crecimiento (Patterns of Growth) ~ *Brochure*

Concerned with the following diseases or disorders: Achondrogenesis; Achondroplasia; Acromicric Dysplasia; Arthrogryposis Multiplex Congenita; Bloom Syndrome; Camptomelic Syndrome; Cardio Facio Cutaneous Syndrome; Cockayne Syndrome; Conradi Hunermann Syndrome; Costello Syndrome; Diastrophic Dysplasia; Dyggve Melchior Clausen Syndrome; Dyschondrosteosis; Dystrophy, Asphyxiating Thoracic; Ear, Patella, Short Stature Syndrome; Ellis Van Creveld Syndrome; Fairbank Disease; Floating-Harbor Syndrome; Froelich's Syndrome; Growth Delay, Constitutional; Growth Hormone Deficiency; Hypochondroplasia; Jansen Type Metaphyseal Chondrodysplasia; Kenny Caffe Syndrome; Kniest Syndrome; LEOPARD Syndrome; Laron Dwarfism; Leri Pleonosteosis; Marshall Smith Syndrome; McKusick Type Metaphyseal Chondrodysplasia; Megalocornea Mental Retardation Syndrome; Metatropic Dysplasia I; Mulibrey Nanism Syndrome (Perheentupa Syndrome); Myhre Syndrome; Noonan Syndrome; Robinow Syndrome; Rothmund Thomson Syndrome; Russell Silver Syndrome (RSS); SHORT Syndrome; Seckel Syndrome; Septo Optic Dysplasia; Spondyloepiphyseal Dysplasia Tarda; Spondyloepiphyseal Dysplasia, Congenital; Trichorhinophalangeal Syndrome Type I; Trichorhinophalangeal Syndrome Type III; Turner Syndrome; Weaver Syndrome; Weill Marchesani Syndrome; Weismann Netter Stuhl Syndrome

1749 HYGEIA: AN ONLINE JOURNAL FOR PREGNANCY AND NEONATAL LOSS

P.O. Box 3943
Amity Station
New Haven, CT 06525
E-mail: hygeia@connix.com
http://www.connix.com/~hygeia

Hygeia, An Online Journal for Pregnancy and Neonatal Loss, is a Home Page on the World Wide Web. Established in 1995, Hygeia is an interactive online journal that offers online users educational materials, medical news, poetry to help with grieving, and networking opportunities with others who have experienced grieving and loss as it pertains to pregnancy loss, miscarriage, neonatal loss, poor neonatal outcome, and voluntary terminations of abnormal pregnancies. The Hygeia Web Site provides a monthly Journal offering updates of current medical news, periodic subject reviews, and comprehensive, multidisciplined insights into the nature of pregnancy and perinatal and neonatal loss. (Past topics have included genetic disorders, Anti-Phospholipid Syndrome, Congenital Heart Disease, and Molar Pregnancy.) Each journal article is accompanied by an original poem or citation from the world literature. Other features include a volume of original poems with annotations entitled "Cherished Purposes: Poems of Grieving and Hope"; a Visitors Contribution area where letters and stories are submitted and posted; a "Grieving and Sharing Registry" that serves as a networking e-mail service through which online users can exchange information, experiences, support, and resources; and a "Grieving and Sharing Registry for Caregivers," a similar networking e-mail service for health care professionals and family members. Hygeia also provides linkage to many additional Internet sites for pregnancy and neonatal loss; linkage to other helpful Internet sites; listings of major university obstetrical, genetic, and newborn centers; a listing of books and periodicals; and an extensive listing of organizations and support groups that may provide additional information, support, resources, and services. Hygeia, An Online Journal for Pregnancy and Neonatal Loss, can be located at [http://www.connix.com/~hygeia].

Year Established: 1995
Organization Members: Non-Membership

1750 HYSTERECTOMY EDUCATIONAL RESOURCES AND SERVICES FOUNDATION (HERS FOUNDATION)

422 Bryn Mawr Avenue
Bala Cynwyd, PA 19004 610-667-7757
Fax: 610-667-8096
E-mail: HERSFdn@aol.com
http://www.dca.net/~hers/

The Hysterectomy Educational Resources and Services Foundation (HERS) is a not-for-profit voluntary organization dedicated to the ideal that every woman should have available to her full, accurate information about the alternatives to and possible consequences of a hysterectomy. Established in 1982, HERS provides an initial free packet of information, counseling by telephone, assistance in determining whether proper, complete evaluation of symptoms has been obtained, referral to physicians nationwide, and liaison with physicians as needed. Educational materials include a newsletter, a resource list, and a HERS publications list. The organization also offers a support group, engages in patient advocacy, and offers networking services. HERS maintains a web site at [http://www.dca.net/~hers/].

President: Nora Weisberg-Coffey (1985 to Present)
Organization Language: Spanish (written).
Year Established: 1982
Organization Members: Non-Membership

Publishes the following materials:
HERS Foundation ~ *Pamphlet*

1751 IMMUNE DEFICIENCY FOUNDATION (IDF)

25 West Chesapeake Avenue
Suite 206
Towson, MD 21204 410-321-6647
800-296-4433
Fax: 410-321-9165
E-mail: idf@clark.net
http://www.clark.net/pub/idf

The Immune Deficiency Foundation is a national not-for-profit voluntary health organization that was founded in 1980 by a group of parents with children affected by primary immune deficiency diseases. The Foundation has concentrated on creating a national focus for these disorders by supporting research, physician training, and patient and family education. The objectives of the Foundation are to promote and support scientific research into the causes, prevention, treatment, and cure of primary immune deficiency diseases; to promote training in medical research and clinical treatment; to gather, coordinate, and disseminate information concerning research and treatment of these disorders; to conduct education campaigns to increase public awareness; and to establish support systems for affected individuals and families throughout the United States. The Foundation produces a variety of educational materials including general information booklets, illustrated booklets for children, and a slide set entitled "Our Immune System."

President: Marcia Boyle (1993-Present)
Executive Director: Thomas E. Moran
Year Established: 1980
Organization Chapters: 22
Organization Members: 10,000

Publishes the following materials:
A Guide for Nurses ~ *Booklet*
Immune Deficiency Foundation ~ *Brochure*
Primary Immune Deficiency Diseases: An Overview ~ *Pamphlet*
The Clinical Presentation of the Primary Immunodeficiency Diseases ~ *Booklet*
Our Immune System ~ *Booklet*
Nuestro Sistema Inmunitario ~ *Booklet*
The Immune Deficiency Foundation National Newsletter ~ *Newsletter*
Patient and Family Handbook ~ *Book*
Immune Deficiency and Alllied Disorders Clinical Updates ~ *Pamphlet*

Concerned with the following diseases or disorders:
Agammaglobulinemias, Primary; DiGeorge Syndrome; Goodpasture Syndrome; Granulomatous Disease, Chronic; Hyper IgM Syndrome; Job Syndrome; Lymphadenopathy, Angioimmunoblastic with Dysproteinemia; McKusick Type Metaphyseal Chondrodysplasia; Nezelof's Syndrome; Severe Combined Immunodeficiency; Wiskott Aldrich Syndrome; X-Linked Lymphoproliferative Syndrome

1752 IMMUNIZATION ACTION COALITION/HEPATITIS B COALITION (IAC)

1573 Selby Avenue
St. Paul, MN 55104 612-647-9009
Fax: 612-647-9131
E-mail: editor@immunize.org
http://www.immunize.org

The Immunization Action Coalition/Hepatitis B Coalition (IAC) is a nonprofit organization dedicated to boosting immunization rates and promoting Hepatitis B vaccinations. Established in 1990, the Immunization Action Coalition promotes physician, community, and family awareness of and responsibility for appropriate immunization of all people of all ages against all vaccine-preventable diseases. The Hepatitis B Coalition, a program of the Immunization Action Coalition, promotes Hepatitis B vaccination for all infants, children, and adolescents. Hepatitis B is one of several viral agents that cause inflammation of the liver known as "hepatitis" or "diffuse hepatocellular inflammatory disease." Hepatitis B is characterized by fever, nausea, vomiting, and persistent yellowing of the skin, mucous membranes, and whites of the eyes (jaundice). The IAC's educational materials include a newsletter, brochures, and audiovisual aids. IAC also maintains a web site on the Internet at [http://www.immunize.org].

President: Deborah L. Wexler, M.D.
Executive Director: Lynn Bahta (Health Educator)
Organization Language: Spanish (written). Cambodian (written). Vietnamese (written). Laotian (written). Korean (written). Chinese (written). Russian (written). Mien (written).
Year Established: 1990
Organization Members: 1,000

Publishes the following materials:
Letters to the Editor ~ *Mission Statement*

Concerned with the following diseases or disorders:
Hepatitis B

1753 IN TOUCH TRUST (IN TOUCH)

10 Norman Road
Sale
Cheshire, M33 3DF
United Kingdom 0161 905 2440
Fax: 0161 718 5787

The In Touch Trust is a not-for-profit organization dedicated to bringing together parents of children with similar special needs such as learning and/or physical disabilities. The Trust has a particular interest in assisting those caring for children affected by rare and complex conditions. Established in 1968 and consisting of approximately 1,400 members, In Touch enables parents to network with others whose children may have the same or similar conditions. The Trust also provides information concerning a wide range of support groups for specific disorders, many of which help families to come together for the purpose of mutual support. Many of these groups have grown out of the contacts provided by In Touch and are able to offer advice to anyone wishing to set up a new group. In Touch is primarily a service for parents. All inquiries are answered personally by the organizer or her assistant and aim to provide encouragement, support, and information. Educational materials include a newsletter entitled "In Touch" and a general information sheet.

President: Ann Worthington (1968 to Present)
Year Established: 1968
Organization Members: 1,400

Publishes the following materials:
In Touch - Information and Contacts for Parents of Children with Special Needs ~ *Brochure*
In Touch ~ *Newsletter Spring 1997*
Information and Contacts for Parents of Children with Special Needs ~ *Mission Statement*

1754 INSTITUTE FOR FAMILIES OF BLIND CHILDREN

P.O. Box 54700
Mailstop #111
Los Angeles, CA 90054-0700 213-669-4649

The Institute for Families of Blind Children is a not-for-profit voluntary organization dedicated to providing support, information, and understanding to families affected by blindness. All services are provided at no cost to families and professionals. Funding is provided by private donations. Established in 1987, the Institute provides consultation and therapy for parents, siblings, and extended family members and refers parents and physicians to organizations specializing in meeting the needs of children with visual impairment. Educational materials include regularly published journal articles, booklets, a regular newsletter, and videotapes that offer practical suggestions and coping strategies for individuals who are blind. The Institute also provides nationwide "in service training" for physicians, residents, medical students, nurses, and other health care workers to enhance their understanding of issues facing affected families.

Executive Director: Nancy Mansfield, M.A.
Year Established: 1987

Publishes the following materials:
When a Family First Learns that Their Child Has a Serious Visual Problem ~ *Brochure*
The Institute for Families of Blind Children ~ *Brochure*
The Institute for Families of Blind Children ~ *Brochure*

Concerned with the following diseases or disorders:
Cataract Dental Syndrome; Chromosome 13, Partial Monosomy 13q; Retinoblastoma

1755 INSTITUTE FOR HEALTH AND DISABILITY

University of Minnesota
Box 721
420 Delaware Street SE
Minneapolis, MN 55455-0392 612-624-3939
Fax: 612-626-2134
TDD: 612-624-3939
E-mail: instihd@c.umn.edu
http://www.peds.umn.edu/Centers/ihd

The Institute for Health and Disability is a national organization that is housed in the University of Minnesota's Division of Pediatrics and Adolescent Health. The Institute brings together research, training, and information dissemination projects and centers dedicated to the study and promotion of the psychological and social well-being of children with disabilities and their families. There are several branches of the Institute for Health and Disability. The Center for Children with Chronic Illness and Disability (C3ID) functions as a rehabilitation, research, and training center committed to increasing and applying knowledge that fosters the physical, psychological, and social development and confidence of children and adolescents with chronic illness and disability. The National Center for Youth with Disabilities (NCYD) is an information dissemination and resource center focusing on adolescents with chronic illnesses and disabilities and the issues involved in their transition to adulthood. Project Connect is a health care reform personnel preparation project focusing on meeting the needs of children and youth with disabilities in managed care settings. Project Resilience is a longitudinal study of factors predicting competence in children with chronic conditions, and Special Ukids is a clinic-based demonstration project that provides coordination for children with complex medical conditions. Additional projects include Project Launch; Children, Youth, and Families: Building on Cultural Strengths; Family Stories, An American Indian Family Project; and Parents-as-Teachers. The Institute for Health and Disability provides a variety of resources for families, professionals, and agencies including The National Resource Library, a newsletter called "Health Issues," special reports, monographs, and a series of annotated bibliographies detailing research and resource information known as "CYDLINE Reviews."

President: Robert Blum, M.D., M.P.H., Ph.D. (Director)
Executive Director: Marty Smith, M.A. (Executive Director)
Organization Language: Spanish (written/spoken).
Year Established: 1996
Organization Members: Non-Membership

Publishes the following materials:
Health Issues (February 1997) ~ *Newsletter*
Promoting Resilience in Your with Chronic Conditions and Their Families ~ *Booklet*
Transition Planning for the 21st Century: A Call to Action ~ *Booklet*
Institute for Health and Disability. A Network of programs for children and youth and their families ~ *Fact Sheet*
National Center for Youth with Disabilities. Publications List ~ *Pamphlet*

1756 INTERNATIONAL ALLIANCE OF ALS/MND ASSOCIATIONS

Secretariat
P.O. Box 246
Northampton, NN1 2PR
United Kingdom 44 1604 250505
Fax: 44 1604 24726
http://www.alsmndalliance.org/

The International Alliance of ALS/MND Associations is a self-help organization dedicated to representing the views of people affected by Amyotrophic Lateral Sclerosis (ALS) and Motor Neuron Disease (MND) and to providing an international forum for the support and exchange of information. ALS/MND is a rare disorder characterized by progressive degeneration and eventual loss of function of both upper and lower motor neurons resulting in progressive muscular wasting and weakness. Established in 1992, the organization is committed to increasing awareness of ALS/MND worldwide, exchanging and disseminating information, improving quality of care for affected individuals, stimulating and supporting research, and providing an international identity for affected individuals. The Alliance, which consists of 23 sister associations, has regular support group meetings, offers family networking services, and produces educational materials including bulletins, a yearly directory, and fact sheets. In addition, Alliance members host the annual "International Symposium on ALS/MND," which brings together leading researchers and health care providers from around the world. The Alliance also maintains a web site at [http://www.alsmndalliance.org].

President: Mavis Gallienne (General Secretary) (1996 to Present)
Executive Director: George Levvy
Organization Language: French (spoken). Spanish (spoken).
Year Established: 1992
Organization Chapters: 23
Organization Members: Non-Membership

Publishes the following materials:
Information Exchange Bulletin ~ *Newsletter*
1995 Directory of Associations for People with ALS/MND ~ *Directory*
1997 Directory of Associations for People with Amyotrophic Lateral Sclerosis/Motor Neurone Disease ~ *Booklet*
International Alliance of ALS/MND Associations Information Sheet ~ *Mission Statement*

1997 Directory ~ *Booklet*
Information Exchange Bulletin (January 1997) ~ *Booklet*

Concerned with the following diseases or disorders:
Amyotrophic Lateral Sclerosis; Motor Neuron Disease

1757 INTERNATIONAL ALSTROM'S SYNDROME NEWSLETTER

1006 Howard Road
Warminster, PA 18974-2749 215-674-1936
E-mail: sasf@voicenet.com
http://www.jax.org/alstrom

The International Alstrom's Syndrome Newsletter is a voluntary organization dedicated to providing support to and avenues of communication for families who have a child with Alstrom's Syndrome. Alstrom's Syndrome is a rare inherited disorder characterized by progressive loss of vision and hearing beginning in early childhood, diabetes mellitus, and obesity. Founded in 1991, the organization publishes a newsletter that contains personal accounts from families affected by this disorder. The organization also provides reprints of medical articles on Alstrom's Syndrome.

President: Janet Seeger
Executive Director: Janet Seeger
Year Established: 1991
Organization Members: 20

Concerned with the following diseases or disorders:
Alstrom Syndrome

1758 INTERNATIONAL BONE MARROW TRANSPLANT REGISTRY (IBMTR/ABMTR)

Autologous Blood & Marrow Transplant Registry (ABMTR)
Statistical Center
Medical College of Wisconsin
8701 Watertown Plank Road
Milwaukee, WI 53226 414-456-8325
Fax: 414-456-6530
E-mail: nuge@post.its.mcw.edu
www.biostat.mcw.edu/ibmtr or
http://www.bio

The International Bone Marrow Transplant Registry (IBMTR) and Autologous Blood and Marrow Transplant Registry (ABMTR) are voluntary research organizations that collect, organize, and collaborate information on blood and bone marrow transplants. Comprised of over 300 worldwide transplant institutions, IBMTR/ABMTR have worked since 1972 to study transplantation, cancer treatments, and other related issues and medical possibilities. IBMTR/ABMTR also offer educational programs for both the professional and public communities, publish reports and a regular newsletter entitled "IBMTR Newsletter," and offer a selection of audiovisual aids.

President: Mary M. Horowitz, M.D., M.S. (Scientific Director) (1985 to Present).
Executive Director: Melodee L. Nugent (Contact Person)
Year Established: 1972
Organization Members: 300

Publishes the following materials:
List of Centers Reporting Patient Data to IBMTR ~ *Directory*
IBMTR Newsletter ~ *Newsletter*
1995 IBMTR/ABMTR Summary Slides ~ *Slides*
Sharing Knowledge. Sharing Hope ~ *Booklet*
ABMTR Newsletter ~ *Newsletter*
1996 IBMTR/ABMTR Summary Slides ~ *Slides*

Concerned with the following diseases or disorders:
Hyper IgM Syndrome; Wiskott Aldrich Syndrome

1759 INTERNATIONAL CHILDREN'S ANOPHTHALMIA NETWORK (ICAN)

Center for Developmental Medicine & Genetics
Albert Einstein Medical Center
5501 Old York Road
Philadelphia, PA 19141 215-456-8722
800-580-4226
Fax: 215-456-2356
E-mail: aemcgenetics@icdc.com
http://www.ioi.com/ican

The International Children's Anophthalmia Network (ican), a voluntary not-for-profit organization, is a group of families and professionals dedicated to lending support to individuals who want to learn more about microphthalmia and anophthalmia (eyes that are abnormally small, completely absent, or consist only of vestigial portions). Members of ican are offered the opportunity to enroll in the Anophthalmia/Microphthalmia Registry, which was established to identify all syndromes associated with anophthalmia/ microphthalmia, describe the spectrum of associated anomalies, and investigate whether any teratogens are involved in the etiology of anophthalmia/microphthalmia. Established in 1993, ican also enables parents with affected children to share personal experiences, information, and support; take advantage of the Network's database of physicians and educational resources; and learn about ongoing research and medical issues. ican provides referrals to genetic counseling, support groups, and other services and promotes professional and patient education. It provides a variety of educational and support materials through its computer database, directory, and regular newsletter.

President: Sandy Gomberg (1993-Present)
Year Established: 1993
Organization Members: 100

Concerned with the following diseases or disorders:
Goldenhar Syndrome (Oculo Auriculo Vertebral Spectrum); Lenz Microphthalmia Syndrome; Schwartz Jampel Syndrome

1760 INTERNATIONAL FOUNDATION FOR FUNCTIONAL GASTROINTESTINAL DISORDERS (IFFGD)

P.O. Box 17864
Milwaukee, WI 53217 414-964-1799
888-964-2001
Fax: 414-964-7176
E-mail: iffgd@execpc.com
http://www.execpc.com/iffgd

The International Foundation for Functional Gastrointestinal Disorders (IFFGD) is a non-profit educational and research organization dedicated to addressing the issues affecting individuals with functional gastrointestinal (GI) disorders. These disorders include irritable bowel syndrome (IBS), incontinence, diarrhea, constipation, pelvic floor pain, anorectal pain, abdominal bloating or pain, esophageal disorders, gastroduodenal disorders, and biliary disorders. Founded in 1990 and consisting of approximately 20,000 members, IFFGD offers support to affected individuals and their families. The Foundation also works with the medical, health care, and research communities to increase awareness of these disorders and to promote research efforts to improve diagnosis and treatment. Educational materials include a quarterly newsletter entitled "Participate" and several fact sheets on various gastrointestinal disorders and their treatment alternatives. IFFGD also distributes a "Personal Daily Diary" that is designed to help individuals with gastrointestinal disorders gain a more complete understanding of their condition through the regular recording of important details.

President: Nancy J. Norton (1989 to Present)
Organization Language: French (written).
Year Established: 1990
Organization Chapters: 4
Organization Members: 20,000

Publishes the following materials:
Participate ~ *Newsletter*
Who We Are ~ *Brochure*
Irritable Bowel Syndrome ~ *Brochure*
Personal Daily Diary ~ *Booklet*
A Biopsychosocial Approach to Irritable Bowel Syndrome ~ *Leaflet*
Report from the 1st International Symposium on Functional Gastrointestinal Disorders ~ *Booklet*
The IBS Anxiety Profile ~ *Reprint*
Quality of Life Assessment ~ *Reprint*
Incontinence-Radiation Proctitis ~ *Reprint*
Abdominal Bloating ~ *Reprint*
Visceral Sensations and Brain-Gut Mechanisms ~ *Reprint*
Inflammatory Bowel Disease ~ *Reprint*
Irritable Bowel Syndrome Research-What is Being Done ~ *Reprint*
IBS Research ~ *Reprint*
Gynecological Aspects of IBS ~ *Reprint*
Motility ~ *Reprint*
Dyspepsia ~ *Reprint*
Malabsorption ~ *Reprint*
Evaluation and Treatment of Constipation ~ *Reprint*
The Etiology of Fecal Incontinence: Causes and Diagnosis ~ *Reprint*
Doctor-Patient Communication ~ *Reprint*
Common Questions about Gas ~ *Reprint*

Concerned with the following diseases or disorders:
Colitis, Collagenous; Colitis, Ulcerative; Crohn's Disease; Irritable Bowel Syndrome

1761 INTERNATIONAL HEARING DOG, INC. (IHDI)

5901 East 89th Avenue
Henderson, CO 80640 303-287-3277
Fax: 303-287-3425
TDD: 303-287-3277

International Hearing Dog, Inc. (IHDI) is a nonprofit organization dedicated to training dogs to assist people who are deaf or have hearing impairment. The dogs are trained to recognize and to alert their masters to certain sounds. Once the 90-day probation period is completed, the dog has legal access to all public places when it is accompanied by its master. A professionally trained hearing dog can restore an individual's independence and awareness by alerting its master to such sounds as ringing telephones, doorbells, knocks, smoke alarms, alarm clocks, baby cries, security buzzers, and any unusual sounds that may indicate danger. Established in 1979, the organization also trains dogs to assist individuals who are blind and deaf or who use wheelchairs. All dogs are trained to meet the special needs and lifestyle of each applicant and are placed in an applicant's home at no charge. The organization's materials include brochures and a regular newsletter entitled "Paws for Silence."

President: Martha A. Foss (1986 to Present)
Organization Language: American Sign Language.
Year Established: 1979
Organization Members: Non-Membership

Publishes the following materials:
Paws for Silence ~ *Newsletter*
Training Other Ears to Hear... ~ *Brochure*

1762 INTERNATIONAL INSTITUTE OF RECONSTRUCTIVE MICROSURGERY (IIRM)

330 West Brambleton Avenue
Norfolk, VA 23510 757-625-6347
Fax: 757-625-2131

The International Institute of Reconstructive Microsurgery (IIRM) is a voluntary organization dedicated to research and education in the area of reconstructive microsurgery. Established in 1992, IIRM has a fellowship program that trains three to five fellows each year in microsurgery; supports clinical research on procedures to correct facial paralysis, infant injuries at birth, nerve damage, etc.; and offers patient care programs that provide necessary surgery for children who are medically needy. The organization produces a regular newsletter entitled "International Institute of Reconstructive Microsurgery."

President: Julia K. Terzis, M.D., Ph.D. (1992 to Present)
Executive Director: Mary Vander Veen, C.P.A. (Treasurer)
Organization Language: Greek (written/spoken).
Year Established: 1992
Organization Members: Non-Membership

Publishes the following materials:
IIRM ~ *Newsletter*

1763 INTERNATIONAL ORGANIZATION OF GLUTARIC ACIDURIA (IOGA)

167A RR3
Jersey Shore, PA 17740 717-321-6487
Fax: 717-322-7375

The International Organization of Glutaric Aciduria (IOGA) is an international voluntary nonprofit organization dedicated to promoting early detection, preventing neurological damage, and assisting in the treatment and rehabilitation of those affected by Glutaric Aciduria Type I (GA1) and other neurologic diseases. GA1, an autosomal recessive genetic disorder, is an inborn error of metabolism in which deficiency of the enzyme glutaryl-CoA dehydrogenase results in abnormal accumulation and excretion of glutaric acid. Symptoms and physical findings may include motor delays; mental retardation; abnormally diminished muscle tone (hypotonia); progressive involuntary irregular muscle movements (e.g., dystonia, choreoathetosis); impairment or distortion of voluntary movements (dyskinesia); unusually low levels of glucose in the blood (hypoglycemia); and/or other symptoms and findings. Established in 1995 and consisting of approximately 100 members, IOGA engages in patient advocacy, offers family networking services, promotes research, offers referrals, and engages in patient education. Educational materials include medical journal article reprints, brochures, and a regular newsletter.

President: Michael Metil (1996 to Present)
Executive Director: Cay Welch (Co-Founder and Contact Person)
Organization Language: German (spoken).
Year Established: 1995
Organization Members: 100

Publishes the following materials:
IOGA Newsletter ~ *Newsletter*
Glutaric Aciduria Type I ~ *Reprint*

Concerned with the following diseases or disorders:
Glutaricaciduria I; Glutaricaciduria II

1764 INTERNATIONAL PATIENT ADVOCACY ASSOCIATION

800 Bellevue Way
MGM Building, Suite 400
Bellevue, WA 98004 206-462-4037
Fax: 206-462-9532
E-mail: 75713.2275@compuserve.com

The International Patient Advocacy Association is a not-for-profit organization dedicated to providing resources and support for individuals facing a chronic, genetic illness and their families and medical support teams. Established in 1986, the International Patient Advocacy Association also provides assistance to individuals confronting legal issues concerning their disorders. On a pro bono basis, the Association assists affected individuals with concerns regarding employment issues, medical records, patient confidentiality, and other legal matters. In addition, the Association enables affected individuals to network via mail or telephone or in person. The Association has volunteers in every state in the United States and in 33 countries. Educational materials include brochures and Spanish language materials.

President: Lenny Van Pelt, Attorney (Founder)
Organization Language: Spanish (written).
Year Established: 1986
Organization Members: Non-Membership

Publishes the following materials:
Dear Senator: ~ *Letter*
If Not Us, Who? If Not Now, When? ~ *White Papers*
Lenny Van Pelt. Your Advocate in Washington ~ *Reprint*
Legal Rights for the Human Clone ~ *White Papers*
Lenny Van Pelt, M.A., J.D. ~ *Biography*
International Patient Advocacy Association. List of member organizations ~ *List Sheet*
Curriculum Vitae ~ *Fact Sheet*

Concerned with the following diseases or disorders:
Hepatic Fibrosis, Congenital; Polycystic Kidney Diseases

1765 INTERNATIONAL PATIENT ORGANIZATION FOR PRIMARY IMMUNODEFICIENCIES (IPOPI)

http://ipopi.org/

The International Patient Organization for Primary Immunodeficiencies (IPOPI) is an international organization whose members are national patient organizations for the Primary Immunodeficiencies (PIDs). The organization was formed to benefit and serve its members and individuals with Primary Immunodeficiencies. Its purpose is to unite the experience, expertise, resources, and influence of its members in order to achieve worldwide improvement in the care and treatment of individuals with Primary Immunodeficiency Disorders. IPOPI strives to be responsive on an international level to the issues of greatest concern to its members. These issues include blood product safety, improving patient diagnosis, gene therapy, immunoglobulin therapy, patient organization development, patient and professional education, and prospects from mapping the human genome. The IPOPI's web site includes a listing of all IPOPI Member Organizations and International Support Groups, patient and family information on various Primary Immunodeficiency Disorders, the IPOPI current newsletter and archives, and an international listing of clinical services. The site also provides access to the IPOPI's ListServ and Fax Service, an interactive area consisting of a chat line and discussion forums, clinical updates, a patient family handbook for the Primary Immunodeficiency Disorders, other educational materials, the ability to search the entire web site by specific keywords, and an area containing dynamic linkage to related immunological web sites.

Organization Language: Swedish. German. French. Italian.

Concerned with the following diseases or disorders:
Agammaglobulinemias, Primary; Chediak Higashi Syndrome; DiGeorge Syndrome; Granulomatous Disease, Chronic; Hyper IgM Syndrome; Job Syndrome; Lymphadenopathy, Angioimmunoblastic with Dysproteinemia; Nezelof's Syndrome; Severe Combined Immunodeficiency; Wiskott Aldrich Syndrome; X-Linked Lymphoproliferative Syndrome

1766 INTERNATIONAL PROGERIA REGISTRY

Human Genetics
Institute for Research
1050 Forest Hill Road
Staten Island, NY 10314 718-494-5333
Fax: 718-494-1026

The International Progeria Registry, associated with the Institute for Basic Research's Department of Human Genetics, is a research organization whose primary purpose is to learn more about the natural history of progeria. Progeria is a rare condition characterized by premature aging, small stature, and coronary artery disease. There are different forms of the condition including Hutchinson-Gilford Progeria Syndrome, which becomes apparent during early childhood, and Werner Syndrome, which starts in adolescence or early adulthood. There are several additional disorders that may also be characterized by a progeroid appearance in association with other distinct abnormalities. Established in 1983, the International Progeria Registry also serves as a consultation service to physicians and provides information to affected families.

President: W. Ted Brown, M.D. Ph.D.
Year Established: 1983

Concerned with the following diseases or disorders:
Cockayne Syndrome; Gottron's Syndrome; Hutchinson Gilford Progeria Syndrome; Werner Syndrome; Wiedemann Rautenstrauch Syndrome

1767 INTERNATIONAL TREMOR FOUNDATION (ITF)

833 West Washington Boulevard
Chicago, IL 60607 312-733-1893
Fax: 312-733-1896

The International Tremor Foundation is an international not-for-profit organization that derives its support entirely from its membership and the general public. Members can call or write for a personal response to specific questions about tremor. A Medical Advisory

Board is accessible for consultation to the staff; the Board also supervises the preparation and content of the Foundation's publications. In addition, an extensive referral service is maintained to guide affected individuals and families to appropriate clinical care. The International Tremor Foundation has a program of educational symposia during which experts in the field of tremor research and care address affected individuals and family members. Educational materials produced by the Foundation include quarterly newsletters and a booklet that informs newly diagnosed patients and their families about tremor.

President: William C. Koller, M.D., Ph.D.
Executive Director: Ms. Judy Rosner
Year Established: 1988
Organization Chapters: 3
Organization Members: 25,000

Concerned with the following diseases or disorders:
Benign Essential Tremor; Pancreatic Islet Cell Tumor; Parkinson's Disease

1768 INTERNATIONAL VENTILATOR USERS NETWORK (IVUN)

4207 Lindell Boulevard
Suite #110
St. Louis, MO 63108-2915 314-534-0475
Fax: 314-534-5070
TDD: 800-735-2966
E-mail: gini_intl@msn.com

The International Ventilator Users Network (IVUN) is an international nonprofit organization dedicated to supporting the independent living, self direction, dignity, and personal achievement of ventilator users. Established in 1987, IVUN endeavors to network ventilator users and their families with other affected families and with health care professionals committed to home mechanical ventilation. The organization also compiles and disseminates information including a biannual newsletter entitled "IVUN News." IVUN is coordinated by Gazette International Networking Institute, which was founded in 1960 as a source of information about polio and its late effects.

President: Martin B. Wice, M.D. (1993 to Present)
Executive Director: Joan L. Headley
Year Established: 1987
Organization Members: Non-Membership

Publishes the following materials:
International Ventilator Users Network (IVUN) ~ *Brochure*
IVUN News ~ *Newsletter*

1769 INTESTINAL DISEASE FOUNDATION (IDF)

1323 Forbes Avenue
Suite 200
Pittsburgh, PA 15219 412-261-5888
Fax: 412-471-2722

The Intestinal Disease Foundation (IDF) is an international not-for-profit organization dedicated to providing information, assistance, and mutual support to individuals with chronic intestinal illnesses including irritable bowel syndrome, diverticular disease, ulcerative colitis, Crohn's disease, short-bowel syndrome, lactose intolerance, chronic constipation, chronic gas, fecal incontinence, and diarrhea. Established in 1986 and consisting of 1,400 members in the United States, IDF promotes healing by encouraging individuals to assume an active role in their own treatment through a positive mental attitude founded on shared experiences. This is facilitated by a telephone network of individuals with intestinal illnesses who provide support, encouragement, and information to others in similar situations. The Foundation publishes a quarterly newsletter entitled "Intestinal Fortitude" as well as a variety of informational brochures and educational materials on chronic intestinal diseases and conditions. Titles include "Tips for Controlling Diarrhea," "Intestinally Friendly Foods," "Dietary Strategies for Coping with the Gastrointestinal Discomforts of Therapy," "Relieving the Psychological Symptoms of IBD and IBS," "Antidepressant Medications: Do They Have a Role in Treating Irritable Bowel," "Bloating—What To Do," and "Laxatives—The Inside Scoop." IDF also provides assistance to individuals interested in establishing local support groups and provides physician referrals.

President: Mary McCrory (1996 to Present)
Executive Director: Linda E. Schorr, M.S.Ed., NCC
Year Established: 1986
Organization Members: 1,400

Publishes the following materials:
Tips For Controlling Diarrhea ~ *Brochure*
Intestinally Friendly Foods ~ *Fact Sheet*
Dietary Strategies For coping With The Gastrointestinal Discomforts Of Therapy ~ *Fact Sheet*
Miracle Food Hits the Market ~ *Pamphlet*
Relieving the Psychological Symptoms of IBD and IBS ~ *Reprint*
Inflammatory Bowel Disease: Drug Therapy ~ *Pamphlet*
Treating Irritable Bowel Symptoms of Crohn's and Colitis ~ *Pamphlet*
Constipation. Causes, Treatment and Prevention ~ *Pamphlet*
Intestinal Fortitude ~ *Newsletter*
Controlling Incontinence by Controlling Diarrhea: The Role of

Diet ~ *Reprint*
When Incontinence Hits ~ *Pamphlet*
Intestinal Gas: It's No Joke ~ *Pamphlet*
Bloating. What To Do? ~ *Reprint*
Laxatives. The Inside Scoop ~ *Reprint*
Intestinal Disease Foundation, Inc. ~ *Pamphlet*
Inflammatory Bowel Disease (IBD) Crohn's Disease. Ulcerative Colitis. Proctitis ~ *Pamphlet*
Diverticular Disease (Diverticulosis and Diverticulitis) ~ *Pamphlet*
The Intestinal Tract: When It Functions Right and When It Functions Wrong ~ *Pamphlet*
Intestinal Fortitude ~ *Newsletter*

Concerned with the following diseases or disorders:
Colitis, Collagenous; Colitis, Ulcerative; Crohn's Disease; Diverticulitis; Diverticulosis; Irritable Bowel Syndrome

1770 INTESTINAL MULTIPLE POLYPOSIS AND COLORECTAL CANCER REGISTRY (IMPACC)

P.O. Box 11
Conyngham, PA 18219 717-788-3712
Fax: 717-788-4046
E-mail: user291524@aol.com

The Intestinal Multiple Polyposis and Colorectal Cancer Registry, also known as IMPACC, is a not-for-profit self-help service organization that was established in 1986. The purpose of the group is to provide information and support to people affected by Multiple Polyposis or Hereditary Colorectal Cancer, their families, and their physicians. Multiple Familial Polyposis is a group of rare inherited conditions of the gastrointestinal system characterized by benign growths (adenomatous polyps) lining the mucous membrane of the intestine. Because such growths have high malignant potential, affected individuals may potentially develop cancer of the colon and/or rectum. The Registry promotes ongoing medical research into the causes, treatment, and prevention of these disorders. IMPACC also offers a variety of services including genetic counseling, referrals to appropriate avenues of treatment, and a quarterly newsletter.

President: Ann Fagan
Year Established: 1986

Concerned with the following diseases or disorders:
Cronkhite Canada Disease; Gardner Syndrome; Polyposis, Familial

1771 INVERTED DUPLICATION EXCHANGE, ADVOCACY AND SUPPORT (IDEA)

RD #1
Box 260B
Thomasville, PA 17364-9768 717-225-5229

Inverted Duplication Exchange and Advocacy (IDEA) is a national not-for-profit self-help organization that was founded in 1994. The group was established to support families of children with an inverted duplication of chromosome 15 and the health care professionals who work with them. An inverted duplication of Chromosome 15 is a rare chromosomal disorder that may result in mental retardation, learning disabilities, neurological problems, and autistic-like behaviors. The organization provides current information on this disorder and offers support to affected families and other interested individuals. The group also functions as an advocate for children and adults affected by this chromosomal disorder. Inverted Duplication Exchange and Advocacy publishes a newsletter entitled "The Mirror" that offers information on current research along with family profiles and the "IDEA Corner."

Executive Director: Donna Bennett
Year Established: 1994
Organization Members: 105

Publishes the following materials:
The Mirror ~ *Newsletter*

Concerned with the following diseases or disorders:
Cat Eye Syndrome

1772 IRON OVERLOAD DISEASES ASSOCIATION, INC.

433 Westwind Drive
North Palm Beach, Fl 33408 407-840-8512
Fax: 407-842-9881

Iron Overload Diseases Association, Inc. is a voluntary not-for-profit organization dedicated to leading the search for individuals who have undiagnosed Hemochromatosis and preventing the health problems that may result. Hereditary Hemochromatosis is a metabolic disorder characterized by increased absorption of dietary iron. Without appropriate treatment, excessive iron may accumulate in the liver, heart, pancreas, and other organs, causing organ dysfunction and tissue damage. Established in 1981, the Association is also committed to providing information and support to affected individuals and their families; educating the general public; promoting and supporting research; and pressing for earlier diagnosis and more effective treatment for Hemochromatosis. The Association acts as a clearinghouse for affected individuals, family members, and physicians; provides telephone consultations; offers referrals to genetic counseling and support groups; promotes patient advocacy; and conducts an annual medical symposium as well as conference meetings between patients and health care professionals. The Iron Overload Diseases Association also provides a variety of educational and support materials including books, brochures, fact sheets, and a bimonthly newsletter entitled "Ironic Blood."

President: Roberta Crawford
Executive Director: Roberta Crawford
Year Established: 1981
Organization Chapters: 4
Organization Members: 2,000

Publishes the following materials:
Overload - An Iron Disease ~ *Brochure*
Iron Overload Alert ~ *Brochure*
Hemochromatosis Fact Sheet ~ *Fact Sheet*
Ironic Blood ~ *Newsletter*

Concerned with the following diseases or disorders:
Hemochromatosis, Hereditary

1773 JEFFREY MODELL FOUNDATION (JMF)

43 West 47th Street
2nd Floor
New York, NY 10036 212-575-1122
800-533-3544
Fax: 212-764-4180
E-mail: jmfworld@aol.com
http://www.mssm.edu/peds/modell/

The Jeffrey Modell Foundation (JMF) is a national not-for-profit research foundation dedicated to helping individuals and family members affected by primary immune deficiency disorders. The Foundation is active in four main areas: research, physician and patient education, patient support, and public awareness of primary immune deficiency. The Foundation provides funding of research fellowships and laboratory facilities; sponsors physician symposia in the United States, Canada, and Europe as well as grand rounds, seminars, and other educational activities for physicians; offers publications for both the lay and medical communities; and provides affected individuals with access to leading medical centers with departments of clinical immunology. The JMF also sponsors K.I.D.'s (Kids with Immunodeficiency) Days for affected children and their families; has insurance reimbursement workshops for affected individuals and family members; is engaged in ongoing education campaigns to promote awareness of primary immune deficiency (PID) in the general public; conducts advocacy on behalf of affected individuals by lobbying the U.S. Congress; and is committed to ongoing biomedical research into primary immune deficiency at the National Institutes of Health. The JMF also publishes a regular newsletter for affected individuals and family members, physicians, and researchers; offers general materials on the primary immune deficiency disorders as well as materials on specific PID disorders for lay and medical audiences; and has a 24-hour JMF Hotline at (800) Jeff-844, which has assisted thousands of families throughout the United States. The JMF also has a web site on the Internet at [http://www.mssm.edu/peds/modell/].

President: Frederick Modell (1987 to Present)
Executive Director: Christine O'Leary
Year Established: 1987

Publishes the following materials:
Understanding Primary Immune Deficiency ~ *Brochure*
The Jeffrey Modell Center. For Research and Comprehensive Care In Primary Immune Deficiency ~ *Brochure*
The Jeffrey Modell Foundation. The First Ten Years ~ *Booklet*
Primary Immune Deficiency ~ *Booklet*
Discovering Causes, Improving Lives, Working Toward A Cure ~ *Booklet*

Concerned with the following diseases or disorders:
Agammaglobulinemias, Primary; Chediak Higashi Syndrome; Granulomatous Disease, Chronic; Hyper IgM Syndrome; Nezelof's Syndrome; Severe Combined Immunodeficiency; Wiskott Aldrich Syndrome; X-Linked Lymphoproliferative Syndrome

1774 JOB ACCOMMODATION NETWORK (JAN)

918 Chestnut Ridge Road
Suite 1
P.O. Box 6080
Morgantown, WV 26506-6080 304-293-7186
800-526-7234
Fax: 304-293-5407
E-mail: jan@jan.icdi.wvu.edu
http://janweb.icdi.wvu.edu

The Job Accommodation Network (JAN) is an international information network and consulting resource that promotes the hiring of qualified workers with disabilities by bringing together information from several sources concerning practical ways of making accommodations for employees and applicants with disabilities. Established in 1982, JAN offers comprehensive information on methods and available equipment that have proven effective for a wide range of accommodations. JAN also publishes a regular newsletter, reports, and brochures. JAN maintains a web site at [http://janweb.icdi.wvu.edu].

Executive Director: Barbara Judy
Organization Language: Spanish (written/spoken). French (written/spoken).
Year Established: 1982
Organization Chapters: 1

Publishes the following materials:
JAN. Job Accommodation Network ~ *Booklet*
Job Accommodation Network ~ *Brochure*

1775 JOHNS HOPKINS HEREDITARY COLORECTAL CANCER REGISTRY

Johns Hopkins Hospital
550 North Broadway
#108
Baltimore, MD 21205-2011 410-955-3875
888-772-6566
Fax: 410-614-9544
E-mail: hccregistry@wpmail.onc.jhu.edu

The Johns Hopkins Hereditary Colorectal Cancer Registry is a research organization that maintains a registry of families affected by different forms of Hereditary Colorectal Cancer including Hereditary Colon Cancer, Familial Adenomatous Polyposis, Hereditary Nonpolyposis Colorectal Cancer, Juvenile Polyposis, and Peutz-Jeghers Syndrome. Established in 1973, the Registry currently includes hundreds of families affected by these disorders. Interested individuals are offered the opportunity to participate in ongoing research studies. The Registry also offers educational materials to people affected by hereditary forms of colon cancer, their families, and physicians.

President: Judy Bacon (Coordinator)
Executive Director: Francis M. Giardiello, M.D.
Year Established: 1973

Publishes the following materials:
Familial Adenomatous Polyposis ~ *Booklet*

Concerned with the following diseases or disorders:
Cancer, Colon

1776 KENT WALDREP NATIONAL PARALYSIS FOUNDATION (NPF)

16415 Addison Road
Suite 550
Dallas, TX 75248 972-248-7100
800-925-2873
Fax: 972-248-7313
E-mail: npf@compugen.net
http://www.kwnpf.org

The Kent Waldrep National Paralysis Foundation (NPF) is a not-for-profit organization dedicated to raising funds for research to find a cure for paralysis caused by brain injury, spinal cord injury, or stroke. Established in 1985, NPF provides funding to support a comprehensive paralysis research center at UT-Southwestern in Dallas; the Research Scholars Program to attract and train new scientists; Research Grant Programs to support leading edge research; the Medical Symposium Fund to support national and international medical education and information sharing programs; and community service activities for affected individuals to promote a better quality of life through education, employment, and recreational sports opportunities. The Foundation's educational materials include brochures and a regular newsletter. NPF also maintains a web site at [http://www.kwnpf.org].

President: Kent Waldrep (1985 to Present)
Executive Director: Kathy Smith (Director of Finance)
Year Established: 1985
Organization Chapters: 1
Organization Members: 40

Publishes the following materials:
Paralysis: An Epidemic ~ *Brochure*
One Step ~ *Newsletter Spring 1997*
Paralysis: An Epidemic. Spinal Victory: Our Mission ~ *Brochure*

1777 KIDSCOPE

3400 Peachtree Road NE
Suite 703
Atlanta, GA 30326 404-233-0001
Fax: 404-233-3756
http://www.kidscope.org

KidsCope is a voluntary nonprofit organization dedicated to creating and providing educational materials to help children cope with changes in the family when a parent has cancer. Established in 1995, the organization was formed by individuals who discovered the need for educational materials for children during their family's experience with breast cancer. The goal of KidsCope is to fulfill the need for materials from a child's perspective that help kids cope with the effects of cancer in the family and changes in everyday life during chemotherapy and beyond. The organization's belief is that the key to adapting to these lifestyle and personal changes is education. The organization's materials include brochures; pamphlets; a videotape entitled "My Mom Has Breast Cancer—A Guide For Families," which includes interviews with four mothers who have survived breast cancer as well as interviews with their seven children; and a special comic book for children entitled "Kemo Shark." KidsCope also has a web site on the Internet at [http://www.kidscope.org].

President: Charles N. Center (1995 to Present)
Organization Language: Spanish (written).
Year Established: 1995
Organization Members: Non-Membership

Publishes the following materials:
"My Mom Has Breast Cancer" ~ *Brochure*
Kemo Shark ~ *Booklet*

1778 LACTIC ACIDOSIS SUPPORT TRUST (LAST)

1A Whitley Close
Middlewich
Cheshire, CW10 0NQ
United Kingdom 01606837198
Fax: 01606837198

The Lactic Acidosis Support Trust is a not-for-profit voluntary health organization located in the United Kingdom. Established in 1993, the Trust works toward its goal of promoting research into the cause, treatment, and prenatal diagnosis of lactic acidosis and mitochondrial cytopathies. The Support Trust provides counseling, advice, and support to parents and caregivers of children with these rare conditions; and encourages health care professionals to become specialists in this field of medicine. The Trust seeks to provide information to parents or other relatives on a 24 hour basis and to provide physicians with financial support and grants to further their research. Fund-raising events include dances, coffee mornings, and other sponsored activities. The Lactic Acidosis Support Trust produces several educational materials including pamphlets, brochures, and a newsletter.

President: Paul Preston
Year Established: 1993
Organization Members: 50

Publishes the following materials:
MELAS ~ *Fact Sheet*
Lactic Acidosis Support Trust Factsheet ~ *Disease Listing/Fact Sheet*
Lactic Acidosis Support Trust ~ *Brochure*
Specific Condition Group News - 11 ~ *Fact Sheet*
Playing a Waiting Game ~ *Article Reprint*
Baby Death Couple Face Test Agony Over Child ~ *Article Reprint*
Mitochondrial Myopathy, Mitochondrial Cytopathy, Mitochodrial Encephalomyopathy and Congenital Lactic Acidosis ~ *Fact Sheet*
Lactic Acidaemia in Infancy ~ *Fact Sheets*

Concerned with the following diseases or disorders:
Cytochrome C Oxidase Deficiency; Glutaricaciduria I; Glutaricaciduria II; Leigh's Disease; MELAS Syndrome; MERRF Syndrome; Medium Chain Acyl CoA Dehydrogenase Deficiency; PEPCK Deficiency, Mitochondrial; Pyruvate Carboxylase Deficiency; Pyruvate Dehydrogenase Deficiency; Pyruvate Kinase Deficiency

1779 LASTING CONNECTIONS, INC. (LC)

277 Fairfield Road
Suite 132
Fairfield, NJ 07004 201-575-2903
Fax: 201-575-1485
E-mail: camelotgrp@aol.com
http://www.camelotgrp.com/

Lasting Connections, Inc. is a nonprofit foundation dedicated to helping families maintain communication in times of medical crisis. Established in 1992, Lasting Connections provides financial assistance for telephone or telecommunications services, direct service such as debit calling cards, and guidance on how best to stretch telecommunications capabilities. The foundation's grant process is based on specific criteria including financial circumstances of the family; severity and duration of the medical crisis; geographical distance between family members; and analysis of the family's communication needs. Lasting Connections will grant up to $500 per family with payments made directly to the serving telephone company. Lasting Connections assists families in the United States, Puerto Rico, Canada, and the US Virgin Islands through dispensation of grants in times of medical crisis. Lasting Connections also distributes prepaid calling cards, often used by families in hospital or clinical treatment settings. The organization places no restriction on the type or scope of medical crisis considered, nor are there geographic limits on calling areas. Lasting Connections receives its revenue from corporate contributions, foundation grants, and individual support. The organization also has a web site on the Internet.

President: Susan Marc Lawley (1992 to Present)
Year Established: 1992
Organization Members: 15

Publishes the following materials:
History and Mission of the Foundation ~ *Mission Statement*
Criteria for Grants to Families ~ *Criteria*
Keeping the Lines Open ~ *Reprint*
Helping Families Talk When Someone Is Ill ~ *Reprint*

10 Tips for Smart Phoning During the Cancer Crisis ~ *Reprint*
Lasting Connections, Inc., Application Form ~ *Application Form*
Help Us Help Them Keep in Touch! ~ *Brochure*
Charity helps connect sick with outside world ~ *Reprint*
Communication ~ *Reprint*
Making a Difference. Helping Families Talk When Someone Is Ill ~ *Reprint*
Keeping the lines open. Help for families in distress ~ *Reprint*

1780 LEARNING DISABILITIES ASSOCIATION OF AMERICA (LDA)

4156 Library Road
Pittsburgh, PA 15234-1349 412-341-1515
Fax: 412-344-0224
E-mail: ldanatl@usaor.net
http://www.ldanatl.org/

The Learning Disabilities Association of America (LDA) is a national not-for-profit voluntary and advocacy organization that was established in 1964 by a group of concerned parents. The only organization of its kind, the Association is dedicated to defining and finding solutions for the broad spectrum of learning disabilities (e.g., visual, auditory, motor, communication, and logical thinking problems). The Association has 50 state affiliates and more than 775 local chapters. Members include parents, professionals from many different disciplines, and other concerned citizens. The Association works directly with school systems in planning and implementing programs for the early identification and diagnosis of children with learning disabilities. The Learning Disabilities Association's Governmental Affairs Committee provides information and recommends action on pending legislation that may affect children with learning disabilities and/or their families. Educational materials produced by the Association include a newsletter published six times a year and numerous brochures, pamphlets, and books related to a variety of topics including adolescents with learning disabilities, LD assessment, and Attention Deficit Hyperactivity Disorder.

President: Sandra Britt
Executive Director: Jean Peterson
Year Established: 1964
Organization Chapters: 775
Organization Members: 55,000

Concerned with the following diseases or disorders:
Attention Deficit Hyperactivity Disorder; Dubowitz Syndrome; Dyslexia; Gerstmann Syndrome; Triplo X Syndrome

1781 LEARNING DISABILITIES ASSOCIATION OF CANADA (LDAC)

323 Chapel Street
Suite 200
Ottawa
Ontario, K1N 7Z2
Canada 613-238-5721
Fax: 613-235-5391
E-mail: ldactaac@fox.nstn.ca
http://educ.queensu.ca/~lda

The Learning Disabilities Association of Canada (LDAC) is a not-for-profit organization dedicated to advancing the education, employment, social development, legal rights, and general well-being of people with learning disabilities. Established in 1963, LDAC consists of 10,000 members and 140 chapters. Educational materials include a quarterly newsletter entitled "LDAC," which features articles for parents, teachers, other professionals, and individuals with learning disabilities; a chapter development manual, which is a useful guide for groups interested in setting up local LDAC chapters in their area; and a video entitled "About Us: Adults With Learning Disabilities" that consists of four adults with learning disabilities who speak about the difficulties, challenges, and achievements they have experienced. Program activities include patient advocacy, government legislation, and a database. LDAC can be reached at its e-mail address at [ldactaac@fox.ntn.ca] or its web site at [http://educ.queensu.ca/~lda].

President: James Horran (1996 to Present)
Executive Director: Pauline Mantha
Organization Language: French (written/spoken).
Year Established: 1963
Organization Chapters: 140
Organization Members: 10,000

Publishes the following materials:
National ~ *Newsletter Spring 1997*
Social Skills Development (French) ~ *Fact Sheet*
Social Skills Development ~ *Fact Sheet*
Employing People with Learning Disabilities is Good Business. An Employer's Perspective (French/English) ~ *Brochure*
Please Listen. We Have Something to Tell You (French/English) ~ *Booklet*

1782 LET'S FACE IT, INC.

P.O. Box 711
Concord, MA 01742 508-371-3186

Let's Face It, Inc. is the United States branch of an international voluntary not-for-profit organization dedicated to helping people with facial differences, their families, health care professionals, and their communities understand and solve the problems of living with facial differences. Established in the United Kingdom in 1984 and in the United States in 1987, Let's Face It is committed to networking affected individuals, family members, friends, and health care professionals and educating the public about facial differences. It also seeks to enable people who are facially different to share their experiences through a mutual help network and provide continuing education to medical, nursing, and allied health professionals. Let's Face It provides a variety of educational and support materials to affected individuals, family members, health care professionals, educators, and the general public. These include a yearly Resource Directory, pamphlets, medical articles, and videos. A computer database is also maintained by the organization.

President: Betsy Wilson (1987-Present)
Executive Director: Betsy Wilson
Year Established: 1987

Concerned with the following diseases or disorders:
Apert Syndrome; Baller Gerold Syndrome; Branchio Oculo Facial Syndrome; Carpenter Syndrome; Cleft Palate and Cleft Lip; Crouzon Disease; Goodman Syndrome; Marshall Syndrome; Maxillofacial Dysostosis; Nager Syndrome; Oral Facial Digital Syndrome; Oto Palato Digital Syndrome Type I and II; Pallister W Syndrome; Pfeiffer Syndrome; Saethre Chotzen Syndrome; Sakati Syndrome; Summitt Syndrome; Treacher Collins Syndrome

1783 LIGHTNING STRIKE & ELECTRIC SHOCK SURVIVORS INC. (LS&ESSI, INC.)

P.O. Box 1156
Jacksonville, NC 28541-1156 910-346-4708
Fax: 910-346-4708
E-mail: lightning@nternet.net
www.mindspring.com/~lightningstrike

Lightning Strike & Electric Shock Survivors Inc. is an international group for those who have been stuck by lightning or have received a damaging electrical shock. Established in 1989, the group's mission is to communicate with other members by acting as a resource for information and encouraging family members to better understand the physical, emotional, and psychological symptoms associated with lightning strikes and damaging electrical shocks. The organization supports survivors by listening to their health issues and concerns and providing an avenue for members to express their feelings, fears, and emotions. The group also supports the study of long-term physical and emotional consequences of exposure to lightning strikes and damaging electrical shock. In addition, Lightning Strike and Electric Shock Survivors, Inc. publishes a newsletter entitled "Hit & Miss Newsletter" and informational brochures, which are available at no cost.

President: Steve Marshburn, Sr. (1989 to present)
Executive Director: Gerolf H. Enqelstatter, Ph.D., ABMP, IABCP
Year Established: 1989
Organization Chapters: 2
Organization Members: 543

Publishes the following materials:
Hit & Miss Newsletter ~ *Newsletter*
Life After Shock ~ *Book*
Can Long Term Cognitive and Emotional Problems Be Caused By Electric Shock and Lightning Strike Accidents or is Any ~ *Booklet*
Psychological & Neuropsychological Sequelae to Lightning Strike and Electric Shock Injuries Behavioral Consequence ~ *Booklet*
Emergent Care of Lightning and Electrical Injuries ~ *Booklet*
Lightning Strike and Electric Shock Victims International ~ *Mission Statement*
Basic Facts About Lightening ~ *Fact Sheet*
Clinical Effects - Symptoms ~ *Fact Sheet*
Areas of the Brain ~ *Fact Sheet*
What Happens in Electrical Burns ~ *Fact Sheet*

1784 LITTLE PEOPLE OF AMERICA (LPA)

P.O. Box 9897
Washington, D.C. 20016 301-589-0730
888-572-2001
www.bfs.ucsd.edu/dwarfism/contracts.htm

Little People of America (LPA) is a voluntary not-for-profit self-help organization dedicated to providing support and information to people of short stature, their families, and health care professionals. Short stature is generally caused by one of the more than 200 medical conditions known as dwarfism. Established in 1957, the organization provides support and guidance to affected individuals of all ages; offers medical, environmental, educational, vocational, and parental guidance; and networks with national and international growth-related and genetic support groups. The organization's Parents Group gives parents of short-statured individuals the opportunity to exchange ideas about health care, adapting the home and school, laws that address their children's needs, and everyday community experiences. Little People of America also offers information on employment, education, disability rights, adoption of short-statured children, medical issues, clothing, adaptive devices, and parenting tips. In addition, the organization conducts seminars and workshops and provides educational scholarships and medical assistance grants. Little People of America provides appropriate referrals; offers information to local physicians who are working with short-statured individuals for the first time; and provides a variety of educational and support materials such as brochures and regular newsletters.

President: Ruth Ricker (1994-Present)
Organization Language: Spanish.
Year Established: 1957
Organization Chapters: 13
Organization Members: 5,000

Publishes the following materials:
An Organization for People of Short Stature ~ *Pamphlet*

Concerned with the following diseases or disorders:
Achondrogenesis; Achondroplasia; Acrodysostosis; Acromesomelic Dysplasia; Acromicric Dysplasia; Alstrom Syndrome; Camptomelic Syndrome; Conradi Hunermann Syndrome; Costello Syndrome; Diastrophic Dysplasia; Dyschondrosteosis; Ear, Patella, Short Stature Syndrome; Growth Delay, Constitutional; Growth Hormone Deficiency; Hypochondroplasia; Jansen Type Metaphyseal Chondrodysplasia; Kenny Caffe Syndrome; Kniest Syndrome; Laron Dwarfism; Leri Pleonosteosis; Marshall Smith Syndrome; McKusick Type Metaphyseal Chondrodysplasia; Metatropic Dysplasia I; Mulibrey Nanism Syndrome (Perheentupa Syndrome); Myhre Syndrome; Robinow Syndrome; Rothmund Thomson Syndrome; Russell Silver Syndrome (RSS); SHORT Syndrome; Seckel Syndrome; Spondyloepiphyseal Dysplasia Tarda; Spondyloepiphyseal Dysplasia, Congenital; Three M Syndrome; Trichorhinophalangeal Syndrome Type I; Trichorhinophalangeal Syndrome Type II; Trichorhinophalangeal Syndrome Type III; Weaver Syndrome; Weill Marchesani Syndrome; Weismann Netter Stuhl Syndrome

1785 LITTLE PEOPLE'S RESEARCH FUND, INC. (LPRF)

80 Sister Pierre Drive
Towson, MD 21204 410-494-0055
800-232-5773
Fax: 410-494-0062

The Little People's Research Fund was established in 1980 as a not-for-profit health organization dedicated to raising funds for patient care, medical research into dwarfism, and education of the medical community and the general public. The organization's goals include funding research on orthopedic disabilities associated with dwarfism; providing funds for direct patient care/services; working to establish a training program for medical professionals; and supporting the Pierre House for families affected by dwarfism. Besides raising funds, the organization sponsors clinics througout the country, works to educate the community about dwarfism, and assists indigent families with medical expenses, transportation, and housing while in Baltimore for treatment. The Little People's Research Fund produces educational materials including brochures, pamphlets, audio-visual aids, and a newsletter.

President: Charles E. McElwee (1980-Present)
Executive Director: Charles E. McElwee
Year Established: 1980
Organization Members: 1,960

Publishes the following materials:
Make a Big Difference To a Little Person ~ *Brochure*
The Little People's Research Fund ~ *Brochure*
Little People's Research Fund, Inc. ~ *Videotape*

Concerned with the following diseases or disorders:
Achondrogenesis; Achondroplasia; Conradi Hunermann Syndrome; Diastrophic Dysplasia; Dyschondrosteosis; Growth Delay, Constitutional; Growth Hormone Deficiency; Hypochondroplasia; Kenny Caffe Syndrome; Kniest Syndrome; Laron Dwarfism; Leri Pleonosteosis; Marshall Smith Syndrome; Metatropic Dysplasia I; Mulibrey Nanism Syndrome (Perheentupa Syndrome); SHORT Syndrome; Spondyloepiphyseal Dysplasia Tarda; Spondyloepiphyseal Dysplasia, Congenital; Weaver Syndrome; Weill Marchesani Syndrome; Weismann Netter Stuhl Syndrome

1786 LIVING BANK INTERNATIONAL

P.O. Box 6725
Houston, TX 77265-6725 713-961-9431
800-528-2971
Fax: 713-961-0979
E-mail: info@livingbank.org
http://www.livingbank.org

The Living Bank International is a nonprofit organization dedicated to the enhancement of organ and tissue donorship and transplantation. Established in 1968, Living Bank International works toward its goal of motivating and facilitating the commitment of enough organ and tissue donors so that no one must die or suffer for lack of a donation. The functions of the Living Bank are educating the public regarding the donation and utilization of organs and tissues; providing international donor commitment and automated registration services; and providing an information center to support appropriate agencies in maximum utilization of donated organs and tissues. Consisting of 350,000 members, the organization produces educational materials including a newsletter entitled "The Bank Account" and an annual report entitled "The Living Bank." Programs include the Donor Education Program, which develops public service messages and supplies information for articles, newspapers, magazines, radio and television shows; the Local Living Banker Program, which recruits volunteers from all across America to work in the communities; and the Corporate and Association Program in which the leadership of large national corporations are approached to encourage their employees or members and their families to register. The Living Bank International can be reached at its e-mail address at [info@livingbank.org] or its web site address at [http://www.livingbank.org].

President: Bruce B. Conway (President & CEO) (1988 to Present)
Organization Language: Spanish (written/spoken).
Year Established: 1968
Organization Members: 350,000

Publishes the following materials:
Over 47,000 Americans Need A Lifesaving Donor Organ (1995-1996 Annual Report) ~ *Brochure*
Facts About Organ & Tissue Donation & Transplantation ~ *Fact Sheet*
To Remember Me ~ *Fact Sheet*
The Bank Account ~ *Newsletter*
Religious Views on IOrgan Donation & Transplantation ~ *Fact Sheet*
Questions Most Frequently asked about Eye Donation and Corneal Transplantation ~ *Fact Sheet*
Questions and Answers About "Brain Death" ~ *Fact Sheet*
The Living Bank ~ *Fact Sheet*
Bone Donation ~ *Fact Sheet*
National Marrow Donor Program ~ *Fact Sheet*
Tissue Donation ~ *Fact Sheet*
Cancer ~ *Fact Sheet*
Dear Friend ~ *Fact Sheet*
Bereaved kin balk at organ donations ~ *Reprint*

1787 LOIS JOY GALLER FOUNDATION FOR HEMOLYTIC UREMIC SYNDROME, INC.

734 Walt Whitman Road
Melville, NY 11747 516-673-3017
Fax: 516-673-3025
E-mail: FJEC01A@prodigy.com
http://www.comed.com/galler/

The Lois Joy Galler Foundation for Hemolytic Uremic Syndrome, Inc. is a national research foundation dedicated to raising public awareness, providing a supportive community for the families of children with Hemolytic Uremic Syndrome, and acquiring funds needed to enable physicians and scientists to conduct research and develop methods of preventing or curing Hemolytic Uremic Syndrome. Hemolytic-Uremic Syndrome (HUS), a rare disorder that primarily affects young children, is often preceded by a flu-like illness (gastroenteritis) characterized by vomiting, abdominal pain, fever, and diarrhea, which, in some cases, may be bloody. Symptoms of Hemolytic-Uremic Syndrome usually become apparent three to 10 days after the development of gastroenteritis and may include sudden paleness, irritability, weakness, lack of energy, and/or excretion of abnormally diminished amounts of urine. The disease typically progresses to include inability of the kidneys to process waste products from the blood and excrete them into the urine (acute renal failure); a decrease in circulating red blood cells (microangiopathic hemolytic anemia); a decrease in circulating blood platelets (thrombocytopenia); and the abnormal accumulation of platelets within certain blood vessels (microthrombi), reducing the blood flow to several organs (e.g., kidneys, pancreas, brain) potentially leading to multiple organ dysfunction or failure. The onset of Hemolytic-Uremic Syndrome is most frequently associated with infection by a particular strain (O157:H7) of Escherichia coli (E. coli) bacterium. The Lois Joy Galler Foundation for Hemolytic Uremic Syndrome, Inc. was founded by Mr. and Mrs. Robert C. Galler in memory of their daughter, Lois Joy. In addition to offering support to affected families and promoting research, the Foundation provides information concerning HUS in easy-to-understand lay terminology. The Foundation also has a web site on the Internet at [http://www.comed.com/galler/] that discusses the organization's goals, has a listing of its Board of Directors and Medical Research Council (MRC), and provides understandable information on HUS.

President: Robert C. Galler (and Chairman of the Board)
Executive Director: Bernard S. Kaplan, M.B., B.Ch. (V.P., Ch., MRC)

Concerned with the following diseases or disorders:
Hemolytic Uremic Syndrome

1788 MAGIC FOUNDATION FOR CHILDREN'S GROWTH

1327 North Harlem Avenue
Oak Park, IL 60302 708-383-0808
800-362-4423
Fax: 708-383-0899
E-mail: mary@magicfoundation.org
http://www.magicfoundation.org

The MAGIC Foundation for Children's Growth is a national non-profit organization dedicated to helping children whose physical growth is affected by a medical problem. Established in 1989, the MAGIC Foundation for Children's Growth assists families of affected children through local support groups, public education and awareness, newsletters, specialty divisions, and programs for children, such as pen pals and birthday clubs. The Main Division of the MAGIC Foundation serves people with all growth disorders not covered in the specialty divisions. The speciality divisions include Congenital Adrenal Hyperplasia, Precocious Puberty, McCune Albright Syndrome, Congenital Hypothyroidism, Russell-Silver Syndrome, and Down's Syndrome with Growth Deficiency, Adults with Growth Hormone Deficiency, and Turner Syndrome. Educational materials produced by the Foundation include brochures, networking form, disease specific brochures, and a video entitled Just Say Yes to Growth Hormone.

President: Teresa Tucker (1991-Present)
Executive Director: Mary Andrews
Year Established: 1989
Organization Chapters: 16
Organization Members: 5,000

Concerned with the following diseases or disorders:
Achondrogenesis; Achondroplasia; Acrodysostosis; Acromesomelic Dysplasia; Acromicric Dysplasia; Adrenal Hyperplasia, Congenital (General); Arthrogryposis Multiplex Congenita; Bloom Syndrome; Cardio Facio Cutaneous Syndrome; Cat Eye Syndrome; Cockayne Syndrome; Conradi Hunermann Syndrome; Costello Syndrome; Diastrophic Dysplasia; Dyggve Melchior Clausen Syndrome; Dyschondrosteosis; Dystrophy, Asphyxiating Thoracic; Ellis Van Creveld Syndrome; Fairbank Disease; Froelich's Syndrome; Growth Delay, Constitutional; Growth Hormone Deficiency; Hypochondroplasia; Hypophosphatasia; Jansen Type Metaphyseal Chondrodysplasia; Johanson Blizzard Syndrome; Kniest Syndrome; LEOPARD Syndrome; Laron Dwarfism; Marshall Smith Syndrome; McCune Albright Syndrome; McKusick Type Metaphyseal Chondrodysplasia; Metatropic Dysplasia I; Noonan Syndrome; Robinow Syndrome; Rothmund Thomson Syndrome; Russell Silver Syndrome (RSS); SHORT Syndrome; Septo Optic Dysplasia; Spondyloepiphyseal Dysplasia Tarda; Spondyloepiphyseal Dysplasia, Congenital; Three M Syndrome; Weaver Syndrome; Weill Marchesani Syndrome

1789 MPD (MYELOPROLIFERATIVE DISEASE) RESEARCH CENTER, INC.

115 East 72nd Street
New York, NY 10021 212-535-8181
800-435-7673
Fax: 212-535-7744
E-mail: Editormpd@aol.com
http://www.acor.org/diseases/hematology/MPD

The Myeloproliferative Disease Research Center, Inc. is a not-for-profit voluntary organization established in 1989. One of the major goals of the organization is to establish a support network for people with myeloproliferative diseases for the purpose of sharing problems and experiences that are unique to these diseases. The Research Center seeks to produce and distribute educational understandable materials that pertain to myeloproliferative diseases and to sponsor educational activities for the general public. Other goals include the establishment of a Myeloproliferative Diseases Physician's Network; enhancement of professional awareness of these diseases; and maintenance of a database that provides updated medical information to both affected individuals and physicians. The Center supports research that promotes understanding of these diseases and improvement of the care of affected individuals including advanced diagnostic techniques and therapeutic services.

President: Harriet S. Gilbert M.D.
Executive Director: Harriet S. Gilbert M.D.
Year Established: 1989
Organization Members: 1,000

Concerned with the following diseases or disorders:
Anemia, Aplastic; Leukemia, Chronic Myelogenous; Myelofibrosis, Idiopathic; Polycythemia Vera; Thrombocythemia, Essential

1790 MACULAR DEGENERATION FOUNDATION, INC. (MDF)

P.O. Box 9752
San Jose, CA 95157 408-260-1335
888-633-3937
Fax: 408-260-1336
E-mail: eyesight@eyesight.org
http://www.eyesight.org

The Macular Degeneration Foundation, Inc. (MDF) is a nonprofit voluntary organization dedicated to gathering and disseminating information about macular degeneration, and to increase the scope, scale, and pace of research addressing this public health problem. Macular degeneration is a common hereditary eye disorder characterized by a gradual bilateral decrease of vision. Central vision is impaired or absent in macular degeneration while peripheral vision remains normal. A vision disturbance in which shapes seem distorted or changing (metamorphopsia) can occur. An area of depressed vision within the visual field surrounded by an area of normal vision (central scotoma) is also symptomatic of this disorder. Established in 1993, the Foundation supports research that attempts to find new tools for the management of macular degeneration. Educational materials include a periodic newsletter and reports. Program activities include support of ongoing research and educational activities. MDF can be reached at its e-mail address at [eyesight@eyesight.org] or its web site on the Internet at [http://www.eyesight.org].

President: Edmund J. Aleksandrovich (1993 to Present)
Year Established: 1993
Organization Members: Non-Membership

Publishes the following materials:
Macular Degeneration Foundation, Inc. ~ *Mission Statement*
The Magnifier (Volumes 1-4) ~ *Newsletter*
The Magnifier (Volume 5) ~ *Newsletter*
The Magnifier (Volume 6) ~ *Newsletter*

Concerned with the following diseases or disorders:
Macular Degeneration

1791 MACULAR DEGENERATION INTERNATIONAL (MDI)

2968 West Ina Road
#106
Tucson, AZ 85741 520-797-2525
800-393-7634
Fax: 520-797-8018
E-mail: TPerski@aol.com

Macular Degeneration International is a national not-for-profit self-help service organization that was established in 1993. The mission of the organization is to foster scientific research into the nature of the Juvenile Macular Dystrophies and age-related macular degeneration. The organization also provides educational and support programs to help affected individuals cope with their vision related problems. Macular Degeneration International maintains a database, publishes a quarterly newsletter, hosts conferences, and makes referrals to physicians who are familiar with macular dystrophies. Brochures and reports are also available from the organization.

Executive Director: Thomas B. Perski, M.A.
Year Established: 1993
Organization Members: 4,500

Concerned with the following diseases or disorders:
Macular Degeneration; Macular Degeneration, Polymorphic

1792 MAINSTREAM, INC.

3 Bethesda Metro Center
Suite 830
Bethesda, MD 20814 301-654-2400
Fax: 301-654-2403
E-mail: mainstrm@aol.com

Mainstream, Inc. is a nonprofit organization dedicated to improving competitive employment opportunities for persons with disabilities. Established in 1975, Mainstream was founded by Harold E. Krents, a graduate of Harvard Law School. His credentials and talents were seemingly useless in a business environment that judged him by his disability (blindness). He decided to change this for himself and all persons with disabilities by establishing Mainstream. Mainstream provides specialized services and acts as a bridge that links service providers, employers, and persons with disabilities. To achieve its goals, the organization provides its constituents with training, educational publications, and videos on disability employment issues. Educational materials include a magazine entitled "Employment In the Mainstream" that reports on the latest trends and developments affecting the employment of Americans with disabilities. A brochure and audio-visual aids are also available. Programs include Project LINK, a model employment service program for persons with disabilities in Dallas, TX and Washington D.C., as well as the Disability Employment Network, a pilot program that provides counseling and referral services to job hunters in the New York City area.

Executive Director: Patricia M. Jackson
Year Established: 1975

Publishes the following materials:
Project Link. Moving People with Disabilities into the Workplace ~ *Fact Sheet*
About Mainstream, Inc. ~ *Mission Statement*
Employment in the Mainstream (Spring 1997) ~ *News Magazine*

1793 MARCH OF DIMES BIRTH DEFECTS FOUNDATION

1275 Mamaroneck Avenue
White Plains, NY 10605 914-428-7100
888-663-4637
Fax: 914-997-4763
TDD: 914-997-4764
E-mail: resourcecenter@modimes.org
http://www.modimes.org

The March of Dimes Birth Defects Foundation is a national not-for-profit organization that was established in 1938. The mission of the Foundation is to improve the health of babies by preventing birth defects and infant mortality. Through the Campaign for Healthier Babies, the March of Dimes funds programs of research, community services, education, and advocacy. Educational programs that seek to prevent birth defects are important to the Foundation and to that end it produces a wide variety of printed informational materials and videos. The March of Dimes public health educational materials provide information encouraging health-enhancing behaviors that lead to a healthy pregnancy and a healthy baby.

President: Jennifer L. Howse, PhD
Organization Language: Spanish.
Year Established: 1938
Organization Chapters: 104

Publishes the following materials:
Teresa come por dos ~ *Brochure*
Eating for Two ~ *Brochure*
Jorge, tu tambien vas a tener un bebe! ~ *Brochure*
"Dad, it's your baby, too," ~ *Brochure*
Trate bien a su bebe antes de que nazca ~ *Brochure*
Be Good to Your Baby Before It Is Born ~ *Brochure*
Deje De Fumar ~ *Brochure*
Stop Smoking ~ *Brochure*
Teresa presencia el milagro de la vida ~ *Brochure*
How Your Baby Grows ~ *Brochure*
Catalog of Public Health Education Materials ~ *Brochure*
Public Health Education Information Sheet Tay-Sachs Disease ~ *Information Sheet*
Public Health Education Information Sheet Genetic Series Thalassemia ~ *Fact Sheet*
Public Health Education Information Sheet Genetic Series Sickle Cell Disease ~ *Fact Sheet*
Public Health Education Information Sheet Genetic Series PKU ~ *Fact Sheet*
Public Education Information Sheet Marfan Syndrome ~ *Fact Sheet*
Public Health Education Information Sheet - Congenital Heart Defects ~ *Fact Sheet*
Public Health Education Information Sheet - Down Syndrome ~ *Fact Sheet*
Public Health Education Information Sheet - The Neurofibromatoses ~ *Fact Sheet*
Public Health Education Information Sheet - Perinatal AIDS ~ *Fact Sheet*
Public Health Education Information Sheet - Spina Bifida ~ *Fact Sheet*

Concerned with the following diseases or disorders:
Aase Syndrome; Acanthosis Nigricans; Achalasia; Achondroplasia; Adrenal Hyperplasia, Congenital (General); Adrenoleukodystrophy; Agammaglobulinemias, Primary; Aicardi Syndrome; Albinism; Alexander's Disease; Alkaptonuria; Alpha-1-Antitrypsin Deficiency; Alzheimer's Disease; Amyloidosis; Anemia, Fanconi's; Anemia, Hereditary Nonspherocytic Hemolytic; Anemia, Hereditary Spherocytic Hemolytic; Anemia, Pernicious; Angioedema, Hereditary; Ankylosing Spondylitis; Antithrombin III Deficiency; Arnold Chiari Syndrome; Ataxia, Friedreich's; Atrial Septal Defects; Autism; Beckwith Wiedemann Syndrome; Benign Essential Tremor; Bloom Syndrome; Blue Diaper Syndrome; Broad Beta Disease; Carnitine Deficiency Syndromes; Carnosinemia; Central Core Disease; Cerebral Palsy; Chediak Higashi Syndrome; Cleft Palate and Cleft Lip; Cornelia de Lange Syndrome; Cri du Chat Syndrome; Crohn's Disease; Cystic Fibrosis; Cystinosis; Cystinuria; DiGeorge Syndrome; Down Syndrome; Dystonia, Torsion; Ectodermal Dysplasias; Epidermolysis Bullosa; Epilepsy; Factor XIII Deficiency; Fucosidosis; Gardner Syndrome; Gaucher Disease; Gottron's Syndrome; Hemochromatosis, Hereditary; Hemophilia; Huntington's Disease; Hydrocephalus; Joseph's Disease; Joubert Syndrome; Klinefelter Syndrome; Lactose Intolerance; Laurence Moon Syndrome; Leukodystrophy, Canavan's; Lowe's Syndrome; Malignant Hyperthermia; Maple Syrup Urine Disease; Marfan Syndrome; May Hegglin Anomaly; Mediterranean Fever, Familial; Muscular Dystrophy, Duchenne; Myoclonus, General; Myopathy, Congenital, Batten Turner Type; Nemaline Myopathy; Neurofibromatosis Type 1 (NF-1); Nezelof's Syndrome; Niemann Pick Disease; Osteogenesis Imperfecta; Pelizaeus Merzbacher Brain Sclerosis; Pemphigus; Peutz Jeghers Syndrome; Phenylketonuria; Polyposis, Familial; Prader Willi Syndrome; Retinitis Pigmentosa; Sandhoff Disease; Severe Combined Immunodeficiency; Sickle Cell Disease; Spina Bifida; Tay Sachs Disease; Thalassemia Major; Thalassemia Minor; Thrombasthenia of Glanzmann and Naegeli; Tourette Syndrome; Tuberous Sclerosis; Turner Syndrome; Waldmann Disease; Werdnig Hoffman Disease; Werner Syndrome; Wilson's Disease; Wiskott Aldrich Syndrome

1794 MEDICARE RIGHTS CENTER (MRC)

1460 Broadway, 8th Floor
New York, NY 10036-7393 212-869-3850
Fax: 212-869-3532

Medicare Rights Center (MRC) is a national, not-for-profit organization exclusively dedicated to ensuring that seniors and people with disabilities on Medicare have access to quality, affordable health care. Through direct services, publications and public policy programs, Medicare Rights Center empowers people on Medicare to make informed choices regarding their health care benefits—e.g., choosing a Medicare Supplemental Insurance policy, learning about HMOs, or understanding how Medicare works in conjunction with an employer's health plan.

Year Established: 1989

Publishes the following materials:
Medicare Rights Center ~ *Brochure*
Medicare Appeals and Grievances: Strategies for System Simplification and Informed Consumer Decisionmaking ~ *Booklet*
MRC News ~ *Newsletter*
Money and Investing ~ *Reprint*
HMOs May Not Always Be Best for Long-Term Ils ~ *Reprint*
Senior Membership Horizons ~ *Reprint*
Statement of Diane Archer, Exq., Medicare Rights Center Before the U.S. House of Representatives Subcommittee on He ~ *Pamphlet*
Medicare Basics: 1996 ~ *Leaflet*
Medicare Beneficiaries Defense Fund ~ *Leaflet*
Questions to Ask Before Choosing an HMO ~ *Fact Sheet*
Your Doctor's Bills: A Medicare Road Map ~ *Brochure*
Medicare and Employer Health Insurance: How They Work Together ~ *Brochure*
How To Receive The Medicare Home Health Benefit ~ *Brochure*
Your Appeal Rights Under Medicare Part B ~ *Brochure*
How To Avoid Overpaying Your Doctor Under Medicare Part B ~ *Brochure*

1795 MENTAL HEALTH NET

http://www.cmhc.com/

Mental Health Net, Inc., a not-for-profit mental health organization, provides online information and educational resources to the global community. Its web site, Mental Health Net, serves as a comprehensive guide to mental health information on the Internet. The site, which features over 6,000 individual resources, provides information for affected individuals, family members, and health care professionals. Such information includes material on specific mental health disorders and other health conditions; information on organizations that may provide additional support and information; professional resources; the organization's mental health magazine entitled "Perspectives," which is directed toward patients, family members, consumers, mental health professionals, administrators, and others associated with the mental health field; journals; and more. Mental Health Net also provides dynamic links to other helpful mental health and general health-related sites on the Web. It uses its own four-star rating system for such sites to rate the quality of their content, their presentation, their ease of use, and online users' overall experience when visiting the site. Mental Health Net also includes discussion forums, opinion polls, and other interactive opportunities for online visitors.

1796 METABOLIC INFORMATION NETWORK (MIN)

P.O. Box 670847
Dallas, TX 75367-0847 214-696-2188
800-945-2188
Fax: 214-696-3258
E-mail: mizesg@ix.netcom.com

The Metabolic Information Network (MIN) is a not-for-profit organization dedicated to facilitating research and enhancing care of families affected by inborn errors of metabolism. Established in 1989, the organization publishes a newsletter, a directory, and reports. The Network maintains a Case Register for 10 groups of disorders (representing 86 diagnoses); a physician directory for 200 inborn efforts of metabolism; and a listing of worldwide genetic metabolic patient registries and patient databases. Information for any genetic metabolic disorder includes contact information, relevant diagnoses based on McKusick Codes, 1CD9 codes, and whether tracking/outcome assessment is performed. The MIN case and master databases contain no patient names. Research investigators and other professionals may obtain individual case details by contacting physicians associated with a particular case. Program activities include research and information resource and retrieval systems for physicians and scientists. These systems contain selected case data for patients with specified disorders, including case physicians, and identifies researchers studying these disorders. The progress of these cases is tracked on an annual basis.

President: Susan G. Mize (1989 to Present)
Year Established: 1989
Organization Members: Non-Membership

Publishes the following materials:
MIN ~ *Brochure*
Metabolic Information Network ~ *Mission Statement*

Concerned with the following diseases or disorders:
5 Oxoprolinuria; Acanthocytosis; Acidemia, Isovaleric; Acidemia, Methylmalonic; Acidemia, Propionic; Acrodermatitis Enteropathica; Adrenal Hyperplasia, Congenital (General); Adrenoleukodystrophy;

Alexander's Disease; Alkaptonuria; Alpha-1-Antitrypsin Deficiency; Amyloidosis; Andersen Disease; Arginase Deficiency; Arginino Succinic Aciduria; Aspartylglycosaminuria; Bartter's Syndrome; Batten Disease; Blue Diaper Syndrome; Carbamyl Phosphate Synthetase Deficiency; Carboxylase Deficiency, Multiple; Carnitine Deficiency Syndromes; Carnitine Palmitoyltransferase Deficiency; Carnosinemia; Chondrocalcinosis, Familial Articular; Citrullinemia; Cockayne Syndrome; Cystinosis; Cystinuria; Diabetes Insipidus; Erythropoietic Protoporphyria (EPP); Fabry Disease; Farber's Disease; Forbes Disease; Fructosuria; Galactosemia; Gilbert Syndrome; Glucose-6-Phosphate Dehydrogenase Deficiency; Glutaricaciduria I; Glutaricaciduria II; Glycogen Storage Disease VIII; Hallervorden Spatz Disease; Hartnup Disease; Hemochromatosis, Hereditary; Hers Disease; Histidinemia; Hunter Syndrome; Hurler Syndrome; Hutchinson Gilford Progeria Syndrome; Hyperchylomicronemia; Hyperlipoproteinemia Type IV; Hyperoxaluria, Primary (Type I); Hyperprolinemia Type I; Hyperprolinemia Type II; Hypokalemia; Hypophosphatasia; I Cell Disease; Leigh's Disease; Leprechaunism; Lesch Nyhan Syndrome; Leukodystrophy; Leukodystrophy, Krabbe's; Leukodystrophy, Metachromatic; Lipodystrophy; Long Chain Acyl CoA Dehydrogenase Deficiency (L CAD); Lowe's Syndrome; MELAS Syndrome; MERRF Syndrome; Mannosidosis; Maple Syrup Urine Disease; Maroteaux Lamy Syndrome; McArdle Disease; Medium Chain Acyl CoA Dehydrogenase Deficiency; Morquio Syndrome; Multiple Sulfatase Deficiency; N-Acetyl Glutamate Synthetase Deficiency; Niemann Pick Disease; Non-Ketotic Hyperglycinemia; Ornithine Transcarbamylase Deficiency; Osteopetrosis; PEPCK Deficiency, Mitochondrial; Pelizaeus Merzbacher Brain Sclerosis; Phenylketonuria; Phosphoglycerate Kinase Deficiency; Pompe Disease; Pyruvate Carboxylase Deficiency; Pyruvate Dehydrogenase Deficiency; Refsum Syndrome; Renal Glycosuria; Schindler Disease; Sialidosis; Sly Syndrome; Sucrose Isomaltose Malabsorption, Congenital; Tarui Disease; Tay Sachs Disease; Tetrahydrobiopterin Deficiency; Trimethylaminuria; Tyrosinemia, Hereditary; Valinemia; Von Gierke Disease

1797 MICRO & ANOPHTHALMIC CHILDREN'S SOCIETY (MACS)

1 Skyrmans Fee
Kirby Cross
Frinton-on-Sea
Essex, C013 ORN
United Kingdom 44 1255677511
Fax: 44 1255677511
E-mail: macs.uk@btinternet.com
http://www.btinternet.com/~macsnet

The Micro and Anophthalmic Children's Society (MACS) is a not-for-profit organization in the United Kingdom dedicated to providing information, assistance, and support to families of children with Microphthalmia or Anophthalmia. Microphthalmia is a developmental abnormality characterized by abnormal smallness of one or both eyes. Individuals with Anophthalmia exhibit absence of rudimentary (vestigial) portions of the eyes. Established in 1993, MACS, which includes approximately 200 families, is dedicated to providing networking services; arranging yearly gatherings for affected families; raising awareness concerning the needs of visually impaired and blind children; providing a resource library containing videos, books, toys, and information materials; and acquiring computer technology for the production of large print and Braille books for the benefit of affected children. MACS offers a variety of educational materials including brochures, pamphlets, and a regular newsletter. The Society also has a web site on the Internet at [http://www.btinternet.com/~macsnet].

President: Juveria Memon (1993 to Present)
Executive Director: Maggie Bourne
Year Established: 1993
Organization Members: 200

1798 MIRACLE-EAR CHILDREN'S FOUNDATION

P.O. Box 59261
Minneapolis, MN 55459-5422 612-520-9550
800-234-5422
Fax: 612-520-9793
TDD: 612-520-9791
http://www.miracle-ear.com

The Miracle-Ear Children's Foundation is a nonprofit organization that provides hearing aids to children whose families do not qualify for public assistance. Established in 1990, the Foundation also provides hearing aid fittings and follow-up care and service free of charge through Miracle-Ear Hearing Centers across the country. The Foundation also provides information on alternative communication and offers a variety of educational materials and brochures including "You Have a Hearing Loss," "Your Child's Hearing Loss," and "First Steps for You and Your Family." Such materials are also available in Spanish.

President: Jerry Krbec (1994 to Present)
Executive Director: Richard C. Brandt
Organization Language: Spanish (written).
Year Established: 1990

Publishes the following materials:
Your Child's Hearing Loss ~ *Booklet*
What You Need To Know. You have a hearing loss. ~ *Booklet*

Helping Children Listen to Life ~ *Brochure*
Your Child/s Hearing Loss (Spanish) ~ *Booklet*
Miracle-Ear Children's Foundation Gives The Gift Of Sound ~ *Mission Statement*
Reading Material For Hearing Impaired Children ~ *List*
Miracle-Ear Children's Foundation. Program Description ~ *Fact Sheet*

1799 MOBILITY INTERNATIONAL USA (MIUSA)

P.O. Box 10767
Eugene, OR 97440 541-343-1284
Fax: 541-343-6812
TDD: 541-343-1284
E-mail: info@miusa.org
http://www.miusa.org

Mobility International USA (MIUSA) is a not-for-profit organization dedicated to ensuring equal opportunities for people with disabilities in international educational exchange, leadership development, disability rights training, travel, and community service. Established in 1981, Mobility International USA coordinates international educational exchanges that specialize in leadership training, community service, cross-cultural experiential learning, and advocacy for the rights of disabled individuals. The organization works toward the full participation of people with disabilities in all educational exchange and leadership programs. It offers a referral service to disabled and non-disabled individuals and organizations. Mobility International USA provides a wealth of information through resource files, contacts with other organizations throughout the world, training workshops, and educational and resource materials. These materials include travel information sheets, a quarterly newsletter called "Over the Rainbow," manuals, curriculum guides, reports, directories, brochures, and videos.

Executive Director: Susan Sygall
Organization Language: Spanish.
Year Established: 1981
Organization Members: 500

Publishes the following materials:
Mobility International USA ~ *Fact Sheet*
Mobility International USA Recruits Participants for Summer 1995 International Exchange Programs ~ *Flier*

1800 MOTOR NEURONE DISEASE ASSOCIATION (MND ASSOCIATION)

P.O. Box 246
Northampton, NN1 2PR
United Kingdom 44 1604 250505
Fax: 44 1604 24726
http://www.businessconnections.com/mnd

The Motor Neurone Disease Association (MND Association) is a voluntary organization dedicated to bringing together all people concerned with Motor Neurone Disease (MND) including people living with the disease, their care givers, and health and social care professionals. Motor Neurone Disease is the name given to a group of related diseases affecting the motor neurons in the brain and spinal cord. Motor neurons are nerve cells that control muscles. The degeneration of motor neurons leads to weakness and wasting of muscles. Established in 1979, the MND Association aims to ensure that every person affected by MND secures the care and support they need; promotes research that will lead to an effective treatment for MND; and improves public and professional awareness of MND. Consisting of 6,000 members and 100 chapters, the organization provides educational materials including a booklet entitled "Motor Neurone Disease: An Introduction," a magazine entitled "Thumb Print," leaflets describing all aspects of the condition both for people affected by the disease and professionals involved in their care or in research of the disorder, and a publications list. Program activities include regional care advisers who are in regular contact with families and individuals coping with MND. These advisers work very closely with local statutory health and community care providers to ensure the needs of these individuals and families are met. The MND Association also maintains a National-Helpline, which is considered a lifeline by those who need information or someone to talk to. MND Association can be reached at its web site at [http://www.businessconnections.com/mnd].

President: Lady Halifax
Executive Director: George Levvy
Year Established: 1979
Organization Chapters: 100
Organization Members: 6,000

Publishes the following materials:
"Motor Neurone Disease took my legs, my arms, my voice" ~ *Brochure*
What is the MND Association ~ *Brochure*

Motor Neurone Disease: An Introduction ~ *Brochure*
Thumb Print ~ *Magazine*
Annual Review (1995/1996) ~ *Booklet*

Concerned with the following diseases or disorders:
Motor Neuron Disease

1801 MOVING FORWARD

2934 Glenmore Avenue
Kettering, OH 45409 937-293-0409

Moving Forward is a voluntary not-for-profit self-help organization dedicated to disseminating information and resources concerning Myoclonus to affected individuals and their families. Myoclonus, a syndrome with more than 75 classifications, is a neurological movement disorder characterized by sudden, shock-like, involuntary contractions of muscles. The disorder may interfere with walking, speech, and/or manual activities. Myoclonus may be caused by a chemical imbalance, a brain or spinal cord injury, a stroke, epilepsy, or another underlying disorder. Established in 1995, Moving Forward is a networking group that promotes awareness of Myoclonus and its many different forms; engages in patient and professional education; and promotes and supports research. The organization offers brochures as well as a resource list of books, articles, and videos. Moving Forward also provides a listing of movement disorder clinics throughout the country as well as several organizations that can offer further information, assistance, networking services, and additional support.

Executive Director: Pauline F. Dill, Ed.S
Year Established: 1995

Publishes the following materials:
What is Myoclonus? ~ *Brochure*

Concerned with the following diseases or disorders:
Myoclonus, General

1802 MUSCULAR DYSTROPHY ASSOCIATION (MDA)

3300 East Sunrise Drive
Tucson, AZ 85718-3208 520-529-2000
800-572-1717
Fax: 520-529-5300
E-mail: mda@mdausa.org
http://www.mdausa.org

Established in 1950, the Muscular Dystrophy Association (MDA) is a non-profit, voluntary health agency dedicated to providing comprehensive medical services to individuals affected by neuromuscular diseases. MDA provides these services at 240 hospital-affiliated clinics across the United States. The Association's worldwide research program, which funds approximately 500 individual scientific investigations each year, represents the largest single initiative to advance current knowledge of neuromuscular diseases and to find cures and treatments for this group of diseases. At facilities in MDA's hospital-affiliated clinics, affected individuals receive diagnosis and follow-up care from specialists in neuromuscular diseases. In addition to its medical services and research programs, MDA conducts educational programs for the public and for medical professionals. The Association publishes and distributes a wide variety of print and audio-visual materials. MDA also sponsors scientific symposia as well as other meetings of specialists in the field of neuromuscular disorders.

President: Lois R. West
Executive Director: Robert Ross
Year Established: 1950
Organization Members: Non-Membership

Publishes the following materials:
MDA Services for the Individual, Family and Community ~ *Booklet*
Facts About Muscular Dystrophy ~ *Booklet*
A Teacher's Guide to Duchenne Muscular Dystrophy ~ *Booklet*
A Do-It-Yourself Owner's Guide ~ *Booklet*
Learning to Live with Neuromuscular Disease ~ *Booklet*
Bibliography of MDS Publications ~ *List*
Facts About Charcot-Marie-Tooth ~ *Booklet*
Facts About Myopathies ~ *Booklet*
Facts About Myasthenia Gravis ~ *Booklet*
Facts About Polymyositis/Dermatomyositis ~ *Booklet*
Facts About spinal Muscular Atrophy ~ *Booklet*
Facts About Friedreich's Ataxia ~ *Booklet*
Facts About Metabolic Diseases of Muscle ~ *Booklet*
Facts About Amyotrophic Lateral Sclerosis ~ *Booklet*
Hey! I'm Here, Too! ~ *Booklet*

Concerned with the following diseases or disorders:
Amyotrophic Lateral Sclerosis; Ataxia, Friedreich's; Ataxia, Marie's; Carnitine Deficiency Syndromes; Carnitine Palmitoyltransferase Deficiency; Central Core Disease; Charcot Marie Tooth Disease; Dejerine Sottas Disease; Dermatomyositis; Dystrophy, Myotonic; Eaton Lambert Syndrome; Fiber Type Disproportion, Congenital; Forbes Disease; Hypotonia, Benign Congenital; Kugelberg Welander Syndrome; McArdle Disease; Motor Neuron Disease; Muscular Dystrophy, Becker; Muscular Dystrophy, Duchenne; Muscular Dystrophy, Emery Dreifuss; Muscular Dystrophy, Fukuyama Type; Muscular Dystrophy, Landouzy Dejerine; Muscular Dystrophy, Limb Girdle; Muscular Dystrophy, Oculo-Gastrointestinal; Myasthenia Gravis; Myopathy, Myotubular; Myopathy, Scapuloperoneal; Myositis, Inclusion Body; Myotonia Congenita; Nemaline Myopathy; Paramyotonia Congenita; Phosphoglycerate Kinase Deficiency; Polymyositis;

Pompe Disease; Tarui Disease; Walker Warburg Syndrome; Werdnig Hoffman Disease

1803 **MUSCULAR DYSTROPHY ASSOCIATION OF CANADA (MDAC)**

2345 Yonge Street
Suite 901
Toronto
Ontario, M4P 2E5
Canada 416-488-2699
800-567-2873
Fax: 416-488-0107

The Muscular Dystrophy Association of Canada (MDAC) is not-for-profit voluntary organization dedicated to eliminating neuromuscular disorders and alleviating the associated symptoms. "Neuromuscular disorders" are a group of diseases affecting the body's ability to move due to an underlying neurological disease. Whether the problem originates within the motor nerve cell, the nerve, or the muscle, the most commonly experienced symptoms are varying degrees of progressive muscle weakness and wasting. There are over 40 nerve and muscle disorders covered under the umbrella of the Muscular Dystrophy Association of Canada. Founded in 1954, the Association's three main goals are funding research that will ultimately result in discovering the causes, treatments, and cures for muscular dystrophy and other neuromuscular disorders; providing support services that assist individuals and families affected by neuromuscular disorders; and providing information to affected individuals, their families, health care professionals, educators, and the general public as to the nature and management of neuromuscular disorders. Services provided by MDAC include the dissemination of information, advocacy, referrals, medical equipment, and travel assistance. Informational brochures include "What Is Spinal Muscular Atrophy?," "What Is Myotonic Dystrophy?," and "What Is Muscular Dystrophy?". MDAC also publishes a news magazine entitled "CONNECTIONS" that features information and articles on various neuromuscular disorders and on related topics such as research, genetics, parenting, and coping with a disability. Additionally, the organization provides advocacy services in resolving individual or community problems. Such issues might involve education, employment, or transportation.

President: Chad Hanna
Organization Language: French (written/spoken).
Year Established: 1954
Organization Members: Non-Membership

Publishes the following materials:
Charcot-Marie-Tooth Disease also known as Peroneal Muscular Atrophy and Hereditary Motor and Sensory Neuropathy ~ *Brochure*
Guillain-Barre Syndrome ~ *Brochure*
FAME. Friedreich's Ataxia Made Easier ~ *Brochure*
Citizens for Independence in Living and Breathing ~ *Brochure*
What is Muscular Dystrophy? ~ *Brochure*
MDAC Services (English/French) ~ *Booklet*
What is Spinal Muscular Atrophy? ~ *Booklet*
What is Myotonic Dystrophy? ~ *Booklet*

Concerned with the following diseases or disorders:
Muscular Dystrophy, Duchenne

1804 **MUSCULAR DYSTROPHY GROUP OF GREAT BRITAIN AND NORTHERN IRELAND (MDG)**

7-11 Prescott Place
London, SW4 6BS
United Kingdom 0171 720 8055
Fax: 0171 498 0670
http://www.sonnet.co.uk/rupert/index.htm

The Muscular Dystrophy Group of Great Britain and Northern Ireland (MDG) is a voluntary research organization dedicated to identifying the causes of muscular dystrophy and allied conditions in order to develop treatments that will alleviate symptoms while working to discover a cure. Muscular Dystrophy (MD) is a group of rare inherited muscle wasting diseases. In some forms of MD, muscles of the hips and shoulders are weakened, walking abnormalities (ataxia) develop, and mild mental retardation may be present. MDG was established in 1959 and is affiliated with two other organizations, the European Alliance of MDA and the World Alliance of MDA. The MDG currently provides funding for eight Muscle Centers that are designed to provide comprehensive medical care to individuals with neuromuscular conditions, and to provide researchers within and between the Centers with medical data and samples that will assist research. There are two types of MDG grants to centers, a Research Servicing Grant which supports costs such as equipment servicing, specialist technicians, secretarial staff, etc. and a Medical Services Grant which provides computing facilities and secretarial staff. Educational materials include an annual review covering different areas of concern for people affected by Muscular Dystrophy. MDG can be reached on the world wide web at [http://WWW.sonnet.co.uk/rupert/index.htm].

President: Lort Attenborough of Richmond Upon Thames
Executive Director: Fergus Logan
Year Established: 1959

Publishes the following materials:
Medical Conditions Covered by the Muscular Dystrophy Group ~ *Fact Sheet*
Research and Medical Service Grants ~ *Leaflet*
Annual Review ~ *Booklet*
The Search ~ *Magazine*

Concerned with the following diseases or disorders:
Muscular Dystrophy, Becker; Muscular Dystrophy, Duchenne; Muscular Dystrophy, Emery Dreifuss; Muscular Dystrophy, Fukuyama Type; Muscular Dystrophy, Landouzy Dejerine; Muscular Dystrophy, Limb Girdle; Muscular Dystrophy, Oculo-Gastrointestinal; Werdnig Hoffman Disease

1805 MYOCLONUS RESEARCH FOUNDATION

200 Old Palisade Road
Suite 17D
Fort Lee, NJ 07024 201-585-0770
Fax: 201-585-0770

The Myoclonus Research Foundation is a national non-profit foundation dedicated to supporting clinical and basic research into the cause and treatment of myoclonus. Myoclonus is a neurological movement disorder characterized by sudden, involuntary jerking movements that can interfere with walking, speech and manual activities. Established in 1980, the Foundation hopes that ongoing research may also help provide clues to other types of movement and neurological disorders such as epilepsy, Parkinson's disease and Alzheimer's disease. The Myoclonus Research Foundation supported four international workshops that brought together and facilitated the sharing of information by physicians, scientists, and investigators active in the field. The proceedings of these meetings have resulted in three publications entitled "Cerebral Hypoxia and Its Consequences," "Myoclonus," and "Negative Motor Phenomena." The Myoclonus Research Foundation currently supports promising research projects, clinical neurological fellows, and student summer fellows in the field of myoclonus, with special emphasis on posthypoxic myloclonus. In addition, the Foundation encourages the participation and support of all who are interested in furthering the understanding, treatment, and cure of myoclonus.

President: Pearl Seiden
Executive Director: Theodora Mason
Year Established: 1978

Publishes the following materials:
Myoclonus Research Foundation ~ *Brochure*
Myoclonus. Patient Information ~ *Fact Sheet*

Concerned with the following diseases or disorders:
Epilepsy, Myoclonic Progressive Familial; Kinsbourne Syndrome; Myoclonus, General; Santavuori Disease

1806 MYOSITIS ASSOCIATION OF AMERICA, INC. (MAA)

1420 Huron Court
Harrisonburg, VA 22801 540-433-7686
Fax: 540-432-0206
E-mail: maa@myositis.org
http://www.myositis.org

The Myositis Association of America is a national not-for-profit organization dedicated to helping people with inflammatory myopathies through a variety of programs. Inflammatory myopathies are a group of muscle disorders characterized by inflammation and degeneration of the skeletal muscles. These disorders include dermatomyositis, polymyositis and inclusion body myositis. Established in 1993, the Association sponsors numerous programs including Research Updates, in which it publishes abstracts of medical journal articles concerning inflammatory myopathies. The Association also provides continuing education on inflammatory myopathies to physicians through symposia, maintains an extensive database for collaboration with medical scientists, coordinates national conferences featuring world renown speakers, and produces a newsletter entitled "The Outlook for Inflammatory Myopathies," which provides education, support, and articles that enhance the lives of individuals with inflammatory myopathies. The Association produces educational materials including brochures and audio visual aids.

President: Betty N. Curry (1993-Present)
Year Established: 1993
Organization Members: 400

Concerned with the following diseases or disorders:
Dermatomyositis; Fibromyalgia; Myositis, Inclusion Body; Polymyositis

1807 NIDCD NATIONAL TEMPORAL BONE, HEARING AND BALANCE PATHOLOGY RESOURCE REGISTRY (THE REGISTRY)

Massachusetts Eye & Ear Infirmary
243 Charles Street
Boston, MA 02114-3096 617-573-3711
800-822-1327
Fax: 617-573-3838
TDD: 617-573-3888
E-mail: tbregistry@meei.harvard.edu
http://www.tbregistry.org

The NIDCD National Temporal Bone, Hearing and Balance Pathology Resource Registry is a not-for-profit research organization that serves as a national resource for researchers and the public to promote research into human temporal bone and balance disorders. The Registry continues and expands upon the activities of the former National Temporal Bone Banks Program established by the Deafness Research Foundation in 1960. The Registry seeks individuals with ear disorders such as hearing loss or balance problems to make an anatomical gift of their temporal bones and associated brain structures. These donations are vital for the advancement of knowledge and understanding of hearing and balance disorders. Established in 1992, the NIDCD National Temporal Bone Hearing and Balance Pathology Resource Registry produces a quarterly newsletter and brochures. In addition, the Registry maintains a computerized database of human temporal bone and associated brain stem collections in the United States.

President: Sumiko M. Goldbaum (Registry Coordinator)
Executive Director: Saumil N. Merchant, M.D. (Co-Director)
Year Established: 1992

Publishes the following materials:
That Others May Hear ~ *Brochures*
The Gift of Hearing ~ *Booklet*
The Registry ~ *Newsletter*

1808 NARCOLEPSY AND CATAPLEXY FOUNDATION OF AMERICA (NCFA)

445 E. 68th Street
L12
New York, NY 10021 212-570-5506

The Narcolepsy and Cataplexy Foundation of America (NCFA) is a voluntary not-for-profit self-help organization dedicated to providing information on Nacrolepsy and Cataplexy to affected individuals, the medical community, and the general public. Current information on treatment options and current research is available from the Foundation. Narcolepsy is a rare disorder characterized by abnormal drowsiness during the day, sudden extreme muscle weakness (cataplexy), hallucinations, paralysis while sleeping, and disrupted sleep during the night. Established in 1976, the Narcolepsy and Cataplexy Foundation of America provides referrals to physicians and treatment centers; promotes research into narcolepsy; provides referrals to support groups; and offers educational information through brochures.

President: Dr. Helen Demitroff (1976-Present)
Year Established: 1976
Organization Members: 200

Concerned with the following diseases or disorders:
Apnea, Sleep; Narcolepsy

1809 NATIONAL ADRENAL DISEASES FOUNDATION (NADF)

505 Northern Bloulevard
Great Neck, NY 11021 516-487-4992
E-mail: nadf@aol.com
http://medhelp.org/www/nadf.htm

The National Adrenal Diseases Foundation (NADF) is a not-for-profit organization dedicated to serving the needs of those with adrenal diseases such as Addison's Disease, Cushing's Syndrome, and Congenital Adrenal Hyperplasia. The Foundation also services the needs of affected families and related health care professionals. To this end, the Foundation provides educational materials, makes referrals to support groups, and, when possible, networks consenting members with one another within their local areas. Established in 1985, NADF provides appropriate referrals to affected individuals, including support groups, and offers a variety of educational and support materials to affected individuals, family members, health care professionals, and the general public. These materials include quarterly newsletters, a pamphlet and fact sheet series, and an audio tape series of talks given by physicians to various support groups.

President: Patti Gelman (1994-Present)
Executive Director: Joyce Mullen
Year Established: 1985
Organization Chapters: 12
Organization Members: 700

Publishes the following materials:
NADF News ~ *Newsletter*
Addison's Disease ~ *Brochure*
Congenital Adrenal Hyperplasia ~ *Brochure*

Cushing's Syndrome, The Facts You Need to Know ~ *Brochure*
Cushing's Syndrome: The Facts You Need to Know ~ *Brochure*
NADF News ~ *Newsletter*
Addison's Disease: The Facts You Need to Know ~ *Brochure*
Congenital Adrenal Hyperplasia ~ *Brochure*
Addison's Disease, An Overview ~ *Fact Sheet*

Concerned with the following diseases or disorders:
ACTH Deficiency; APECED Syndrome; Achard Thiers Syndrome; Addison's Disease; Adrenal Hyperplasia, Congenital (General); Amenorrhea, Primary; Conn Syndrome; Cushing Syndrome; Pheochromocytoma; Precocious Puberty; Schmidt Syndrome; Triploid Syndrome

1810 NATIONAL ADVISORY CENTER FOR PARENTS OF CHILDREN WITH A STOMA (NASPCS)

51 Anderson Drive
Valley View Park
Darvel
Ayrshire, KA17 ODE
Scotland 156-032-2024

The National Advisory Service For Parents Of Children With A Stoma (NASPCS) is a not-for-profit self help organization dedicated to helping parents of children born with a wide variety of bowel and bladder problems. Established in 1984, NASPCS aims to provide a contact and information service for parents on the practical day-to-day management of all aspects of coping with a child who has had an operation involving removal of the part of the gastrointestinal tract (i.e., a colostomy, ileostomy or urostomy); give advice on the incontinence often encountered with bowel and bladder problems; and distribute information on the support available from the social services and other agencies and to advise on educational problems. Support is offered to parents through the organization's parent-contact service, enabling families to contact others in a similar situation for mutual support and advice. Consisting of 630 members, the organization produces educational materials including a quarterly newsletter containing information on a wide variety of topics including contributions from parents within the group, and an update on its contact list. NASPCS also has a booklet called "Our Special Children" which is a practical guide to stoma care in infants and young children. Program activities include a support group, patient networking, and educational programs.

President: John B. Malcolm (1990 to Present)
Year Established: 1987
Organization Members: 630

Publishes the following materials:
Our Special Children ~ *Booklet*
NASPCS ~ *Leaflet*
Me and My Mitrofanoff ~ *Brochure*
NASPCS Information Sheet 1 - Intestinal Neuronal Dysplasia ~ *Information Sheet*
NASPCS Information Sheet 2 - Hirschspring's Disease ~ *Information Sheet*
NASPCS Information Sheet 3 - Gastroschisis ~ *Information Sheet*
My Child Has Hirschsprung's Disease ~ *Booklet*
My Child has an Imperforate Anus ~ *Pamphlet*
Beating Sneaky Poo. Ideas for Faecal Soiling ~ *Booklet*
My Child Has An Imperforate Anus ~ *Booklet*
Ace Procedure. A guide for Nurses ~ *Leaflet*
NASPCS Information Sheet 1 ~ *Brochure*
NASPCS Information Sheet 2 ~ *Brochure*
NASPCS Information Sheet 3 ~ *Brochure*
NASPCS Information Sheet 4 ~ *Brochure*
NASPCS Information Sheet 5 ~ *Brochure*
NASPCS Information Sheet 6 ~ *Brochure*
NASPCS Information Sheet 7 ~ *Brochure*
Our Special Children. A practical guide to stoma care in babies and young children ~ *Booklet*

1811 NATIONAL ALLIANCE FOR RESEARCH ON SCHIZOPHRENIA & DEPRESSION (NARSAD)

60 Cutter Mill Road, Suite 404
Great Neck, NY 11021 516-829-0091
800-829-8289
Fax: 516-487-6930
http://www.mhsource.com/narsad

The National Alliance for Research on Schizophrenia & Depression (NARSAD) is a national not-for-profit organization dedicated to research into causes, treatments, prevention, and the eventual cure of schizophrenia and the various forms of depression. Schizophrenia is a brain disorder that makes it difficult for a person to distinguish between reality and fantasy; to think logically; to have appropriate emotional responses to others, and to adapt to social situations. People with schizophrenia may also have difficulty in remembering, talking, and behaving appropriately. Bipolar Manic Depression is a mental illness in which intense mood swings occur, usually with remissions and recurrences. Depressive symptoms may be most common and can last at least a full day and perhaps several weeks or longer. Manic symptoms may involve hyperactivity and feelings of invincibility, happiness, and restlessness. Established in 1986, NARSAD was founded by family members and professionals with the primary objective of raising funds to find the causes, cures, improved treatments, and prevention of these mental illnesses. Consisting of 40,000 members, NARSAD publishes a newsletter entitled "Research Newsletter," which focuses on the newest developments in treatments. It also provides several educational brochures including "Conquering Depression," "Understanding Schizophrenia," "The Search for Cures," and "Finally, 18 Million Americans Suffering from Depression Have Something to Look Forward to." In 1995, NARSAD launched its "Depression...A flaw in chemistry, not character" educational campaign to enhance public understanding of this disorder. NARSAD also awards two grants each year for outstanding progress in research into schizophrenia and depression.

President: Constance E. Lieber (1989 to present)
Executive Director: Anne Brown (Director of Communication & Education)
Organization Language: Spanish (written).
Year Established: 1986
Organization Members: 40,000

Publishes the following materials:
Conquering Depression ~ *Brochure*
Understanding Schizophrenia ~ *Brochure*
Finally, 18 million Americans Suffering From Depression Have something to Look Forward To ~ *Leaflet*
NARSAD Research Newsletter (1997) ~ *Newsletter*

1812 NATIONAL ALLIANCE FOR THE MENTALLY ILL (NAMI)

200 North Glebe Road
#1015
Arlington, VA 22203-3754 703-524-7600
800-950-6264
Fax: 703-524-9094
TDD: 703-516-7991
E-mail: membership@nami.org
http://www.nami.org

The National Alliance for the Mentally Ill (NAMI) is a not-for-profit voluntary health organization dedicated to providing mutual support, education, advocacy, and research funding for people affected by mental illness, their families, and friends. The organization also serves those who have been diagnosed with schizophrenic depression and other related disorders. Established in 1979, this self-help organization refers individuals to nationwide support groups, services, and outreach programs. Educational materials produced by the organization include a database, directories, annual reports, informational brochures, pamphlets, a bimonthly newsletter entitled "The Advocate," and "The Decade of the Brain," NAMI's quarterly publication for presenting research, clinical practices and advances, and policy updates relevant to serious brain disorders.

President: Annie Saylor
Executive Director: Laurie Flynn
Year Established: 1979
Organization Chapters: 1,160
Organization Members: 186,000

Concerned with the following diseases or disorders:
Anorexia Nervosa; Antisocial Personality Disorder; Attention Deficit Hyperactivity Disorder; Autism; Bulimia; Conversion Disorder; Depersonalization Disorder; Dysthymia; Fetal Alcohol Syndrome; Manic Depression, Bipolar; Mutism, Selective; Neurasthenia; Neuroleptic Malignant Syndrome; Organic Mood Syndrome; Organic Personality Syndrome; Panic Anxiety Syndrome; Pica; Trichotillomania; XYY Syndrome

1813 NATIONAL AMPUTATION FOUNDATION, INC. (NAF)

38-40 Church Street
Malverne, NY 11565 516-887-3600
Fax: 516-887-3667

The National Amputation Foundation, Inc. (NAF) is a not-for-profit organization comprised of amputee volunteers who offer their support to people who have had an amputation and their families. People with amputations that were present at birth (congenital) are also served by the Foundation. NAF's objective is to aid a new amputee in returning to as normal a life as possible within the sphere of his or her potential. Established in 1919, the Foundation provides affected individuals with appropriate referrals to support groups, and promotes education of amputees, family members, health care professionals, and the general public. The Foundation produces a regular newsletter as well as brochures, reprints of medical articles, and pamphlets on a variety of issues. These issues include health, psychological, and daily care concerns; questions concerning devices and prosthetics, sports and exercise, and driving; legal issues; and specific concerns regarding children or adolescents with limb loss.

President: Henry Potten
Executive Director: Sol Kaminsky
Year Established: 1919
Organization Members: 2,000

Publishes the following materials:
Order Form for Topical and Special Interest Pamphlets ~ *Order Form*

National Amputation Foundation ~ *Brochure*
The AMP ~ *Newsletter*

1814 NATIONAL ARTS & DISABILITY CENTER (NADC)

UCLA University Affiliated Program
300 UCLA Medical Plaza
Suite 3330
Los Angeles, CA 90024-6967 310-794-1141
Fax: 310-794-1143
E-mail: oraynor@npia.mednet.
http://www.dcp.ucla.edu/nadc/

The National Arts and Disability Center (NADC) is a federally funded project of the University of California, Los Angeles. Established in 1984, the NADC is an information and resource center focusing on promoting the full inclusion of children and adults with disabilities into the art community. NADC disseminates information and training to artists, families with a child with a disability, the art community, and community support personnel. Major activities of NADC are developing a database that contains listings of art centers, organizations, associations, art schools, programs, museums, libraries, foundations, and city, state, and federal departments concerned with the arts and disability; writing a curriculum for the provision of outreach training; and developing a reference library and database of books, videos, products, and other relevant literature. NADC maintains a web site at [http://www.dcp.ucla.edu/nadc/]. The organization may be reached at its e-mail address at [oraynor@npia.mednet.ucla.edu].

Executive Director: Olivia Raynor, Ph.D.
Year Established: 1984
Organization Members: Non-Membership

Publishes the following materials:
National Arts and Disability Center ~ *Mission Statement*
National Arts and Disability Center. Goals and Objectives ~ *Fact Sheet*
NADC ~ *Brochure*

1815 NATIONAL ASSOCIATION FOR ADULTS WITH SPECIAL LEARNING NEEDS (NAASLN)

P.O. Box 716
Bryn Mawr, PA 19010 610-446-6126
Fax: 610-446-6129
E-mail: 75250.1273@compuserve.com

The National Association For Adults With Special Learning Needs (NAASLN) is a professional organization dedicated to organizing, establishing, and promoting an effective national and international coalition of professionals, advocates, and consumers of lifelong learning for the purpose of educating adults with special learning needs. Established in 1987, NAASLN is governed by a volunteer board of directors comprised of adult education, human service, and rehabilitation professionals; advocates; and consumers representing public and private schools, colleges and universities, correction facilities, government agencies, community organizations, businesses and industry, and a host of adult education and literacy programs. The NAASLN hopes to achieve its mission through its commitment to provide leadership in the advancement of education and lifelong learning opportunities; to unify the adult education profession; to foster development and implementation of exemplary programs and practices; to encourage research and communicate the results of research to the professional and public communities; and to facilitate and promote a global exchange of information and knowledge between consumers, advocates, and professionals. The organization also strives to assist consumers to full participation in lifelong learning opportunities that result in self-sufficiency, productivity, and an improved quality of life; to provide opportunities for professional development; to promote all adulteducation programs that enable consumers to benefit from lifelong learning opportunities; to represent and communicate interests and needs of members and consumers to professional groups, legislative bodies, and community and business organizations; and to serve as the unified voice for all adults with special learning needs. Consisting of 300 members, the organization produces educational materials including a brochure entitled “National Association For Adults With Special Learning Needs,” a newsletter entitled “Learning disAbilities Newsletter,” and a pamphlet entitled “Services for Families.”

President: William R. Langner (1996 to Present)
Executive Director: Richard Cogen, Ph.D.
Organization Language: Spanish (spoken).
Year Established: 1987
Organization Members: 300

Publishes the following materials:
Learning Disabilities. What is it? ~ *Leaflet*
NAASLN ~ *Brochure*
On The Cutting Edge ~ *Newsletter*

1816 **NATIONAL ASSOCIATION FOR CONTINENCE (NAFC)**

P.O. Box 8306
Spartanburg, SC 29305 864-579-7900
800-252-3337
Fax: 864-579-7902

National Association for Continence (NAFC), originally known as Help for Incontinent People, is a not-for-profit self-help organization dedicated to improving the quality of life for people with urinary incontinence. Incontinence is a condition in which one loses bladder control. Established in 1982, the organization is a leading source of education, advocacy, and support to the public and to health care professionals regarding the causes, prevention, diagnosis, treatment, and management alternatives for incontinence. NAFC's purpose is to be the leading source of education, advocacy and support to the public and to the health professional about the causes, prevention, diagnosis, treatments, and management alternatives for incontinence. The NAFC's objectives are to destigmatize incontinence; to provide consumer information; and to provide advocacy and service for those who are affected by this problem. To achieve its objectives, NAFC offers a wide variety of publications and services, such as "Quality Care," a quarterly newsletter that provides moral support and practical information to over 100,000 subscribers; "The Resource Guide - Products and Services for Incontinence," which assists people in finding the most helpful product for their type of incontinence; pamphlets; audio visuals aids; and books designed to educate the general public and health care professionals.

Executive Director: Linda G. Christison, MPA
Organization Language: Spanish.
Year Established: 1982
Organization Members: 90,000

Concerned with the following diseases or disorders:
Binswanger's Disease; Exstrophy of the Bladder

1817 **NATIONAL ASSOCIATION FOR PARENTS OF THE VISUALLY IMPAIRED (NAPVI)**

P.O. Box 317
Watertown, MA 02272-0317 617-972-7441
800-562-6265
Fax: 617-972-7444

Established in 1979, the National Association for Parents of the Visually Impaired, Inc. (NAPVI) is a voluntary not-for-profit organization dedicated to providing support to the parents of children with visual impairment. The Association enables parents to find information and resources for their blind or visually impaired child; helps parents to address the unique needs of visually impaired children who have additional disabilities; and provides parents with leadership, support, and training that enables them to help their child reildren reach their fullest potential. The Association also promotes outreach and networking programs; advocates the educational needs and welfare of affected children; and provides referrals to needed services. In addition, the Association promotes the development of state and local organizations by and for parents of visually impaired children and fosters communication and coordination of services among federal, state, and local agencies. The Association offers a variety of educational and support materials including its database; quarterly newsletter "Awareness"; books; handbooks and guides for parents and teachers; a listing of resources for teachers; brochures; and other publications.

President: Donna Stryker
Executive Director: Susan LaVenture
Year Established: 1979
Organization Members: 2,000

Concerned with the following diseases or disorders:
Alstrom Syndrome; Aniridia; Aniridia Cerebellar Ataxia Mental Deficiency; Bardet Biedl Syndrome; CHARGE Syndrome; Carbohydrate deficient Glycoprotein Syndrome Type I; Cat Eye Syndrome; Cataract Dental Syndrome; Cataracts; Chandler's Syndrome; Choroideremia; Coats' Disease; Essential Iris Atrophy; Goldenhar Syndrome (Oculo Auriculo Vertebral Spectrum); Hermansky Pudlak Syndrome; Laurence Moon Syndrome; Leber's Congenital Amaurosis; Leber's Optic Atrophy; Lenz Microphthalmia Syndrome; Loken Senior Syndrome; Macular Degeneration, Polymorphic; Megalocornea Mental Retardation Syndrome; Norrie Syndrome; Oculocerebral Syndrome with Hypopigmentation; Retinitis Pigmentosa; Retinoschisis; Retrolental Fibroplasia; Rieger Syndrome; Rothmund Thomson Syndrome; Schwartz Jampel Syndrome; Septo Optic Dysplasia; Usher's Syndrome; Wolfram Syndrome

1818 **NATIONAL ASSOCIATION FOR VENTILATOR DEPENDENT INDIVIDUALS (NAVDI)**

P.O. Box 341
Medina, OH 44258 216-778-3612
Fax: 216-778-4321
E-mail: jpetro@ohio.net

The National Association for Ventilator Dependent Individuals, Inc. (NAVDI) is a not-for-profit social service organization committed to the belief that individuals requiring long term or permanent assistance of mechanical ventilation should be afforded every opportunity to improve their quality of life and be provided with a mechanism of support for themselves and their families. Founded in 1990 and consisting of 80 ventilator users, the NAVDI works toward its goals: to educate ventilator dependent individuals and their families through information sharing, networking, programming, and supplying educational materials; to provide educational services focused on developing professional expertise related to improving health care delivery to ventilator dependent individuals and their families; to heighten public awareness related to the unique needs of ventilator dependent individuals and their families; to gather, organize, and disseminate current information related to ventilator dependency services, resources, and education; and to support research and investigation directed toward meeting the needs of ventilator dependent individuals and their families. NAVDI publishes a periodic self-titled newsletter and sponsors a yearly day-long conference for ventilator dependent individuals, their families, and medical and health delivery professionals. NAVDI can be reached via e-mail at [jpetro@ohio.net].

President: Daniel Durowski (1990 to Present)
Executive Director: Janet Petro (Contact Person)
Year Established: 1990
Organization Members: 80

Publishes the following materials:
NAVDI (1997) ~ *Newsletter*
National Association for Ventilator Dependent Individuals, Inc. ~ *Brochure*

1819 NATIONAL ASSOCIATION FOR VISUALLY HANDICAPPED (NAVH)

22 West 21st Street
New York, NY 10010 212-889-3141
Fax: 212-727-2931
E-mail: staff@navh.org
http://www.navh.org

The National Association for Visually Handicapped is a national voluntary health agency dedicated to advancing the welfare of the partially seeing, stimulating medical research, and providing standards for editing reading materials and texts for people who are partially sighted. Founded in 1954, the organization also promotes the publication of educational materials and their distribution to schools, libraries, social institutions, and individuals. The Association seeks to plan and assist in programs of parent and adult education relating to persons with partial seeing and to assist and encourage the partially seeing to integrate into the mainstream of society. The National Association for Visually Handicapped strives to educate the public on the unique needs of the partially seeing. To this end, the Association publishes brochures, a publications listing, and other notices.

President: James Slabe
Executive Director: Lorraine H. Marchi
Organization Language: Yiddish.
Year Established: 1954

Publishes the following materials:
MEMBERSHIP INFORMATION ~ *Factsheet*
National Association for Visually Handicapped Publications List ~ *Publications List*
Eye-Q-Test ~ *Factsheet*
Why NAVH Stands Alone ~ *Pamphlet*
Become a Friend of NAVH ~ *Factsheet*
Providing Services for the Hard of Hearing for over 40 Years ~ *Factsheet*
About Children's Vision - A Guide for Parents ~ *Booklet*
About Children's Eyes ~ *Factsheet*
How to Use Your Low Vision Glasses ~ *Factsheet*
Sensitivity to People with Partial Eyesight ~ *Factsheet*
Classification of Impaired Vision ~ *Factsheet*
Bulletin - Annual Program Report 1993-94 ~ *Newsletter*
The Adult Partially Seeing - A Professional Guide ~ *Booklet*
About Children's Vision - A Guide for Parents ~ *Booklet*
Family Guide - Growth and Development of the Partially Seeing Child ~ *Booklet*
The Heartbreak of Being "A Little Bit Blind" ~ *Brochure*
Problems of the Partially Seeing ~ *Booklet*
A Patient's Guide to Visual Aids and Illumination ~ *Pamphlet*
Visual Aids and Informational Material ~ *Catalog*
Visual Aids Catalog - Price List 1994-1995 ~ *Price List*
Large Print Loan Library 1993 ~ *Catalog*
Visual Aids Catalog ~ *Price List*

Concerned with the following diseases or disorders:
Aicardi Syndrome; Alpers Disease; Alstrom Syndrome; Aniridia; Aniridia Cerebellar Ataxia Mental Deficiency; Bardet Biedl Syndrome; Behcet's Syndrome; Carbohydrate deficient Glycoprotein Syndrome Type I; Cataract Dental Syndrome; Cataracts; Chandler's Syndrome; Choroideremia; Choroiditis, Serpiginous; Coats' Disease; Cogan Reese Syndrome; Corneal Dystrophy; Dandy Walker Malformation; Epitheliopathy, Acute Posterior Multifocal Placoid Pigment; Essential Iris Atrophy; Hermansky Pudlak Syndrome; Kearns Sayre Syndrome (KSS); Keratoconus; Keratomalacia; Laurence Moon Syndrome; Leber's Congenital Amaurosis; Leber's Optic Atrophy; Lenz Microphthalmia Syndrome; Loken Senior Syndrome; Lowe's Syndrome; Macular Degeneration; Macular Degeneration, Polymorphic; Maroteaux Lamy Syndrome; Megalocornea Mental

Retardation Syndrome; Norrie Syndrome; Oculo Dento Digital Dysplasia; Oculocerebral Syndrome with Hypopigmentation; Papillitis; Refsum Syndrome; Retinitis Pigmentosa; Retinopathy, Arteriosclerotic; Retinopathy, Diabetic; Retinopathy, Hypertensive; Retinoschisis; Retrolental Fibroplasia; Rieger Syndrome; Rosenberg Chutorian Syndrome; Rothmund Thomson Syndrome; Sandhoff Disease; Schwartz Jampel Syndrome; Tolosa Hunt Syndrome; Usher's Syndrome; Vogt Koyanagi Harada Syndrome; Waardenburg Syndrome; Weill Marchesani Syndrome; Wolfram Syndrome; X-linked Juvenile Retinoschisis

1820 NATIONAL ASSOCIATION FOR THE DUALLY DIAGNOSED (NADD)

132 Fair Street
Kingston, NY 12401-4082 914-331-4336
800-331-5362
Fax: 914-331-4569

The National Association for the Dually Diagnosed seeks to stimulate the public and professional awareness regarding the dually diagnosed (mental retardation/mental illness) population. Through encouraging the dissemination and exchange of pertinent information, promoting educational and training programs, advocating for appropriate governmental policies, supporting research focused on identification, diagnosis, and treatment, and fostering the development of resources and services, NADD hopes to encourage a greater awareness and education among the general public and those affected by a dual diagnosis.

President: Terrence McNelis, MPA
Executive Director: Robert J. Fletcher, DSW
Year Established: 1983
Organization Chapters: 4
Organization Members: 1200

Publishes the following materials:
Meetiang the Mental Needs of Persons who have Mental Illness and Mental Retardation ~ *Mission Statement*
NADD Product Publications Catalog ~ *Catalog*

1821 NATIONAL ASSOCIATION OF ANOREXIA NERVOSA AND ASSOCIATED DISORDERS, INC. (ANAD)

Box 7
Highland Park, IL 60035 847-831-3438
Fax: 847-433-4632
E-mail: anad20@aol.com
http://members.aol.com/ANAD20/index.html

The National Association of Anorexia Nervosa and Associated Disorders, Inc. (ANAD) is a national not-for-profit self-help organization dedicated to increasing understanding of eating disorders and to alleviating the problems of eating disorders, especially anorexia nervosa and bulimia. The Association seeks to educate the general public and professionals in the health field to become more aware of eating disorders and appropriate methods of treatment. In addition, the organization encourages and promotes research to discover the causes of eating disorders, methods of prevention, types of treatments and their effectiveness, and to formulate relevant statistics. The National Association of Anorexia Nervosa and Associated Disorders acts as a resource center by gathering and providing educational materials about eating disorders. Other activities sponsored by the organization include networking for mutual support, providing funds to aid those with eating disorders, and encouraging interested individuals and groups to join in seeking cures for these disorders.

President: Vivian Hanson Meehan (1976-Present)
Executive Director: Vivian Hanson Meehan
Year Established: 1976
Organization Members: 4,500

Publishes the following materials:
Working Together ~ *Newsletter*
Brief Description of Some Therapies Used in Anorexia Nervosa and Bulimia ~ *Fact Sheet*
Anorexia Nervosa - Bulimia ~ *Fact Sheet*
ANAD - Dear Friend ~ *Information Packet*
Eating Disorders - Danger Signals and Treatment ~ *Brochure*
Confronting a Person with Anorexia or Bulimia ~ *Information Sheet*

Concerned with the following diseases or disorders:
Anorexia Nervosa; Bulimia

1822 NATIONAL ASSOCIATION OF CHILD ADVOCATES (NACA)

1522 K Street NW
Suite 600
Washington, DC 20005 202-289-0777
Fax: 202-289-0776
E-mail: HN1315@handsnet.org
http://www.childadvocacy.org

The National Association of Child Advocates (NACA) is a national not-for-profit advocacy organization dedicated to improving the lives and living conditions of children by strengthening child advocacy organizations in states and communities. Established in 1984, NACA is committed to the creation and sustenance of state and community based child advocacy organizations and serves as the collective voice of these organizations working on the front lines to ensure the safety, security, health, and education of America's children. Consisting of approximately 51 member organizations in 39 states, NACA connects state and local advocates with national experts, acts as a clearinghouse for child advocacy information, and provides organizational development assistance in such areas as board development, program building, and fund-raising. NACA's materials include a manual entitled "Medicaid Managed Care: An Advocate's Guide for Protecting Children" and reports. NACA also has a web site on the Internet at [http://www.childadvocacy.org].

President: Tamara Copeland
Year Established: 1984
Organization Members: 51

Publishes the following materials:
Medicaid Managed Care. An Advocate's Guide for Protecting Chldren ~ *Book*

1823 NATIONAL ASSOCIATION OF HOSPITAL HOSPITALITY HOUSES, INC. (NAHHH)

4915 Auburn Avenue
#303
Bethesda, MD 20814 301-961-5264
800-542-9730
Fax: 301-961-3094
E-mail: nahhhcom@aol.com
http://visit-usa.org/hhh

The National Association of Hospital Hospitality Houses (HHH), Inc. is a not-for-profit organization that promotes and assists other not-for-profit programs providing lodging and supportive services in a caring environment for families receiving medical care away from home. The Association provides services and technical assistance to established and developing Hospital Hospitality Houses. Membership is available to hospitals, groups, and individuals interested in developing a program in their area, as well as to organizations supporting the goals of the Association. Membership offers participation in an annual national conference designed for networking and education; a national referral directory listing Hospital Hospitality Houses and services; consultation services to newly developing programs; a resource center and clearinghouse to aid HHH programs, staff, and boards; and a newsletter and other publications.

President: Gerry Beck
Executive Director: Robert N. Gray
Year Established: N/A
Organization Members: 135

Publishes the following materials:
hhh ~ *Brochure*
1995 Annual Conference ~ *Newsletter*

1824 NATIONAL ASSOCIATION OF PROTECTION AND ADVOCACY SYSTEMS (NAPAS)

900 Second Street NE
Suite 211
Washington, DC 20002 202-408-9514
Fax: 202-408-9520
TDD: 202-408-9521
E-mail: HN4537@handsnet.org
http://www.protectionandadvocacy.com

The National Association of Protection and Advocacy Systems (NAPAS) is a national voluntary not-for-profit membership organization for the federally mandated nationwide network of disability rights agencies, protection and advocacy systems (P&As), and client assistance programs (CAPs). Established in 1977, NAPAS facilitates coordination of its members; represents the needs of members to federal agencies and Congress; and provides technical assistance and training to member agencies that enhance their effectiveness on the state and local level. NAPAS offers many services including monitoring the activities of legislative, executive, and judicial branches of the federal government as they relate to individuals with disabilities; providing information exchange through telephone, surface mail, and computer link-up; providing fax board and e-mail communications; representing the P&A and CAP network on national coalitions, boards, task forces, etc.; and offering discounted group rates for subscriptions to Clearinghouse Law Review and other publications related to disability law. In addition, NAPAS maintains and operates the Advocacy Training and Technical Assistance Center (ATTAC), a centralized repository of training and technical assistance resources. Although NAPAS provides a variety of membership services, the development of training programs and the provision of technical assistance to meet the needs of its members remain priority activities for NAPAS. The National Association of Protection and Advocacy Systems provides educational materials including brochures and holds an annual conference.

President: Lois Simpson
Executive Director: Curtis L. Decker
Year Established: 1977
Organization Chapters: 55

Publishes the following materials:
P & A Systems ~ *Brochure*
ATTAC Update ~ *Newsletter*
NAPAS Publications ~ *Publication List*
State Protection and Advocacy Agencies ~ *Agency List*
NAPAS Annual Report ~ *Report*
Annual Report of the P & A System (1996-1997) ~ *Booklet*
National Association of Protection and Advocacy Systems (NAPAS) ~ *Brochure*
The Advocacy Training and Technical Assistance Center ~ *Brochure*

1825 NATIONAL ASSOCIATION OF THE DEAF (NAD)

814 Thayer Avenue
Suite 250
Silver Spring, MD 20910-4500 301-587-1788
Fax: 301-587-1791
TDD: 301-587-1789
E-mail: NADHQ@juno.com
http://www.nad.org

The National Association of the Deaf (NAD) is a national, not-for-profit federation dedicated to ensuring that Americans with deafness or hearing impairment have proper access in education, employment, health care, and telecommunications. Established in 1880, NAD, which consists of 51 state affiliates including the District of Columbia, has over 22,000 individual members including individuals with deafness or hearing impairment; parents, children, or other family members of affected individuals; health care professionals and service providers; and other professionals. NAD provides a variety of programs and services including American Sign Language (ASL) and Deaf Studies Teacher Certification; interpreter assessment and certification; biennial conventions and regional conferences; a Junior NAD Chapter Network; and a captioned films and videos project (funded by the US Department of Education). NAD also engages in public policy efforts and educational rights; offers public information and outreach; advocates for expanded telecommunications accessibility; and promotes greater awareness and understanding of deaf culture, community, and language. The National Association of the Deaf offers its "NAD Bookstore Catalog," which lists a variety of educational materials, and has a regular newsletter entitled "The Broadcaster."

President: Benjamin J. Soukup (1995 to Present)
Executive Director: Nancy J. Bloch
Organization Language: American Sign Language.
Year Established: 1880
Organization Chapters: 51
Organization Members: 22,000

Publishes the following materials:
The National Association of the Deaf ~ *Brochure*
Bookstore Catalog 1997 ~ *Pamphlet*

Concerned with the following diseases or disorders:
Neurofibromatosis Type 2 (NF-2); Norrie Syndrome; Waardenburg Syndrome

1826 NATIONAL ASSOCIATION OF THE PHYSICALLY HANDICAPPED, INC. (NAPH)

NAPH Business Office
Bethesda Scarlet Oaks
440 Lafayette Avenue
#GA4
Cincinnati, OH 45220-1073 513-961-8040

The National Association of the Physically Handicapped, Inc. (NAPH) is a non-profit organization dedicated to the advancement of the social, economic, and physical welfare of the physically handicapped. Established in 1958, NAPH's objectives are to promote public awareness of the needs of handicapped people and to push for government and legislation to meet those needs. Presently, its goals include the adjustment of buildings for handicapped people (e.g., wider doorways and proper ramps for wheelchairs, etc.); equal education and employment opportunities for the handicapped; and, in collaboration with government agencies, civic groups, and other organizations, the implementation of programs to benefit the handicapped. Consisting of 650 members and 14 chapters, the organization produces educational materials including a brochure entitled "The National Association of the Physically Handicapped, Inc.," a periodic newsletter, and a booklet entitled "What is the Purpose of NAPH." Program activities include physical fitness sessions, sports, and other activity programs; government and legislative concerns; and networking.

President: Clarence O. Averill (1989 to Present)
Year Established: 1958
Organization Chapters: 14
Organization Members: 650

Publishes the following materials:
National Association of the Physically Handicapped, Inc. ~ *Letter*
The National Association of the Physically Handicapped, Inc. ~ *Mission Statement*

The National Assocaition of the Physically Handicapped, Inc. ~ *Brochure*
An Introduction to the National Association of the Physically Handicapped ~ *Mission Statement*
What is the Purpose of NAPH? ~ *Fact Sheet*

1827 NATIONAL ATAXIA FOUNDATION (NAF)

2600 Fernbrook Lane
Suite 119
Minneapolis, MN 55447 612-553-0020
Fax: 612-553-0167
E-mail: naf@mr.net
http://www.ataxia.org/

The National Ataxia Foundation is a national not-for-profit organization that seeks to identify people with hereditary ataxia and to improve the physical and emotional well-being of affected individuals and their families. Hereditary ataxia is a group of progressive, chronic neurological disorders that affect coordination. Established in 1957, the National Ataxia Foundation encourages and supports research efforts into identifying the causes and mechanisms of the hereditary ataxias, improving diagnosis, and developing treatment models; locates families affected by ataxia or at risk for ataxia in order to offer information and education; identifies needs and services for purposes of referral; creates and makes available educational programs for ataxia families, health care professionals, and the general public; and increases public awareness of hereditary ataxia. In addition, the National Ataxia Foundation provides informational materials, counseling, referrals, and avenues to support groups and is responsive to the needs of its membership by achieving an acceptable balance among the funding of the various programs of education/awareness, patient services, research, administration, and fund-raising. The organization produces informational materials including brochures on hereditary ataxia, financial planning, and health insurance issues. The VHS video tape entitled "Together... There is Hope" and a newsletter entitled "Generations" are also distributed by the National Ataxia Foundation. There are currently 45 affiliated chapters and support groups of the National Ataxia Foundation is the United States and Canada.

President: DeNiece Roach (1987-Present)
Executive Director: Donna Gruetzmacher
Year Established: 1957
Organization Chapters: 47

Publishes the following materials:
Hereditary Ataxia ~ *Brochure*
Hereditary Ataxia (HA) The Facts ~ *Factsheet*
Financial Planning ~ *Factsheet*
Health Care Coverage for Ataxia Patients ~ *Factsheet*
Generations ~ *Newsletter*

Concerned with the following diseases or disorders:
Aniridia Cerebellar Ataxia Mental Deficiency; Ataxia Telangiectasia; Ataxia, Friedreich's; Ataxia, Hereditary; Ataxia, Marie's; Kennedy Disease; Marinesco Sjogren Syndrome; Olivopontocerebellar Atrophy

1828 NATIONAL BONE MARROW TRANSPLANT LINK (NATIONAL BMT LINK)

29209 Northwestern Highway #624
Southfield, MI 48034 248-932-8483
800-546-5268
Fax: 248-932-8483
http://comnet.org/nbmtlink

The National Bone Marrow Transplant Link is a not-for-profit voluntary organization dedicated to improving the quality of life of those undergoing bone marrow transplantation (BMT) and to promote public understanding of BMT through programs of education and research. Established in 1992, its primary goal was to assist individuals involved in the bone marrow transplantation process. However, the National BMT Link also educates the public about bone marrow transplantation; works as an advocate for national recognition of BMT as an effective, insurable procedure; supports the continuation of BMT research; and serves as a clearinghouse for information about transplants, transplant centers, donor centers, and bone marrow collection sites. In addition, the organization acts as a resource center of up-to-date medical and scientific reports on BMT and offers a networking service, which is a person-to-person connection that puts potential patients in touch with experienced and accessible peers. The National BMT Link is funded through private, foundation, and corporate donations.

President: Myra Jacobs (Director)
Organization Language: Spanish (written).
Year Established: 1992

Publishes the following materials:
NBMT LINK ~ *Newsletter*
Bone Marrow Transplant Resource Guide. Friends Helping Friends ~ *Booklet*

National Bone Marrow Transplant Link A Second Chance at Life is Our First Priority ~ *Brochure*

Concerned with the following diseases or disorders:
Hyper IgM Syndrome; Wiskott Aldrich Syndrome

1829 NATIONAL BRAIN TUMOR FOUNDATION (NBTF)

785 Market Street
Suite 1600
San Francisco, CA 94103 415-284-0208
800-934-2873
Fax: 415-284-0209
E-mail: nbtf@braintumor.org
http://www.braintumor.org

The National Brain Tumor Foundation is a national not-for-profit voluntary organization that serves as a comprehensive center for information regarding resources and support services for people whose lives are affected by brain tumor disease. Established in 1981, the National Brain Tumor Foundation also provides financial support for investigational studies into the causes, prevention, and treatments of brain tumors. To these ends, the National Brain Tumor Foundation has funded basic and applied laboratory research and clinical trials of new treatments at major institutions in the United States. The organization has also supported research into quality of life issues that regularly confront people with brain tumors. A comprehensive guide is available for affected individuals and their families who want to learn more about brain tumors. The National Brain Tumor Foundation also produces a variety of educational materials including a newsletter entitled "Search." Affected individuals and family members may also receive referrals to a network of support groups throughout the United States.

President: Sharon Lamb
Executive Director: Janis C. Brewer
Year Established: 1981

Publishes the following materials:
National Brain Tumor Foundation Order Form ~ *Order Form*
Research - Resources - Recovery ~ *Fact Sheet*
Coping With a Diagnosis of a Brain Tumor ~ *Fact Card*
Support Groups for Brain Tumor Patients & Families in North America ~ *Booklet*
SEARCH ~ *Newsletter*
Brain Tumors - A Guide ~ *Booklet*

Concerned with the following diseases or disorders:
Astrocytoma, Benign; Astrocytoma, Malignant; Brain Tumors, General; Glioblastoma Multiforme; Medulloblastoma; Meningioma

1830 NATIONAL BURN VICTIM FOUNDATION (NBVF)

246A Madisonville Road
P.O. Box 409
Basking Ridge, NJ 07920 908-953-9091
800-803-5789
Fax: 908-953-9099
E-mail: nbvf@intac.com
http://www.nbvf.org

The National Burn Victim Foundation (NBVF) is a national not-for-profit organization dedicated to providing advocacy services to burn victims and their families free of charge. Established in 1973, the Foundation is committed to assisting in the development of burn centers and rehabilitation programs for burn victims; assisting in medical research to improve the treatment of burns, reduce time spent in the hospital, and reduce associated costs; participating in the development of personnel training programs in burn care; and developing a burn prevention program for the general public. The NBVF also has developed the "Forensic Burn Unit (FBU)" to investigate and forensically reconstruct how burn injuries have occurred for child protective services cases, medical personnel, law enforcement agencies, etc. In addition, the Foundation has developed a disaster response system; serves as a national resource for burn related information and referrals; and offers professional seminars on several topics including returning to school after burns, burn awareness, disaster support services, and post traumatic stress disorders. The NBVF's educational materials include a variety of brochures and pamphlets including "Guard Your Child Against Burns," "Child Abuse ... Think Again," and "Our Hopes, Our Mission."

President: Professor Harry J. Gaynor (1973 to Present)
Executive Director: Gary S. Stocco
Year Established: 1973

Publishes the following materials:
Guard Your Child Against Burns ~ *Brochure*
National Burn Victim Foundation. Future solutions now... ~ *Brochure*
National Burn Victim Foundation. Man's Environment ~ *Brochure*

1831 NATIONAL CENTER FOR LEARNING DISABILITIES (NCLD)

381 Park Avenue South
#1420
New York, NY 10016 212-545-7510
Fax: 212-545-9665
http://www.ncld.org

The National Center for Learning Disabilities is a national voluntary not-for-profit organization dedicated to improving the lives of millions of Americans affected by learning disabilities. Established in 1977, the Center works toward several goals: supporting and funding research; educating teaching professionals so that they are better equipped to assist individuals with learning disabilities; advocating on behalf of individuals with learning disabilities; and raising public awareness and understanding. In addition, the Center disseminates information to the public, medical professionals, and individuals with learning disabilities. Local and regional referrals are also provided by the organization. The Center for Learning Disabilities produces a wide variety of educational and support materials including brochures, pamphlets, videotapes, a newsletter, and reports.

Executive Director: Shirley C. Cramer
Year Established: 1977
Organization Members: 2,000

Publishes the following materials:
Learning Disabilities - A National Responsibility ~ *Report*

Concerned with the following diseases or disorders:
Attention Deficit Hyperactivity Disorder; Dyslexia; Triplo X Syndrome

1832 NATIONAL CENTER FOR YOUTH WITH DISABILITIES (NCYD)

Institute for Health & Disability
University of Minnesota
Box 721
420 Delaware Street South East
Minneapolis, MN 55455-0392 612-626-2825
Fax: 612-626-2134
TDD: 612-624-3939
E-mail: instihd@tc.umn.edu
http://www.peds.umn.edu/Centers/ihd

The National Center for Youth with Disabilities (NCYD) is located in the University of Minnesota's Adolescent Health Program. Established in 1985, the National Center for Youth with Disabilities is an information, policy, and resource center focusing on adolescents with chronic illness and disabilities and the issues that surround their transition to adult life. The Center's mission is to raise awareness of the needs of adolescents with chronic illness and disabilities and expand the knowledgebase and level of involvement of professionals who provide services to youth. In addition, the Center promotes programs and strategies that enhance the ability of adolescents and young adults to grow, develop, work, and participate in community life to their fullest capacity. Educational materials produced and distributed by the Center include a newsletter, a series of annotated bibliographies, and special reports.

Executive Director: Nancy A. Okinow, MSW
Year Established: 1985

Publishes the following materials:
National Center for Youth with Disabilites ~ *Fact Sheet*
National Center for Youth with Disabilities Publications List ~ *Publications List/Order Form*

1833 NATIONAL CENTER OF CHROMOSOME INVERSIONS

1029 Johnson Street
Des Moines, IA 50315 515-287-6798
Fax: 515-287-6798

The National Center for Chromosome Inversions is a non-profit voluntary health organization that helps support basic medical research on chromosomal inversions and functions as a point of connection for parents of affected children. Chromosome inversions are a rare defect in which two or more portions of a chromosome break off, become separated, and rejoin the chromosome in the wrong order. Established in 1992, the National Center for Chromosome Inversions plans to develop a variety of educational materials including brochures, newsletters, and videos.

President: Jacqueline Barker (1995-Present)
Executive Director: Jacqueline Barker
Year Established: 1993
Organization Chapters: 1
Organization Members: 30

Publishes the following materials:
Articles of Incorporation ~ *Incorporation Documents*

Concerned with the following diseases or disorders:
Cat Eye Syndrome

1834 NATIONAL COALITION FOR CANCER SURVIVORSHIP (NCCS)

1010 Wayne Avenue
Suite 505
Silver Spring, MD 20910 301-650-8868
Fax: 301-565-9670
access.digex.net/~mkragen/cansearch.htm

The National Coalition for Cancer Survivorship (NCCS) is a national non-profit consumer group dedicated to representing the interests of all people with all types of cancer in order to maximize their potential for living the best quality of life possible following a diagnosis of cancer. Established in 1986, the Coalition is comprised of independent institutes and 2,300 members, organizations, individuals, and families affected by cancer. The goals of NCCS are to identify and address the needs of long-term cancer survivors and to advocate for appropriate change in health care delivery and policy to maximize survivors' access to optimal treatment and support. To this end, NCCS facilitates communication among people involved with cancer survivorship; promotes peer support; serves as an information clearinghouse; advocates for the interests of cancer survivors; and promotes research on cancer survivorship. Publications include the group's newsletter "NCCS Networker" and informational brochures such as "Working It Out: Your Employment Rights As A Cancer Survivor" and "Teamwork...The Cancer Patient's Guide to Talking with Your Doctor."

President: Elizabeth Johns Clark, Ph.D. (1995 to Present)
Executive Director: Ellen Stovall
Year Established: 1986
Organization Chapters: 7
Organization Members: 2300

Publishes the following materials:
You Have The Right To Be Hopeful ~ *Brochure*
"From the time of discovery and for the balance of life, an individual diagnosed with cancer is a survivor." ~ *Brochure*
NCCS Networker ~ *Newsletter*
National Coalition For Cancer Survivorship Publications List and Order Form ~ *Order Form*
NCCS Vision, Mission and Goals ~ *Mission Statement*
Working It Out: Your Employment Rights As a Cancer Survivor ~ *Booklett*
Teamwork. The Cancer Patient's Guide To Talking With Your Doctor ~ *Booklet*
What Cancer Survivors Need to Know About Health Insurance ~ *Booklet*

1835 NATIONAL COUNCIL AGAINST HEALTH FRAUD, INC.

Room 204C
Evans Hall
Loma Linda University
P.O. Box 1276
Loma Linda, CA 92354-1276 909-824-4690
Fax: 909-824-4838
E-mail: wjarvis@ccmaail.11u.edu
http://www.ncahf.org

The National Council Against Health Fraud, Inc. (NCAHF) is a voluntary nonprofit organization dedicated to investigating and evaluating claims made for controversial health practices, products, and services; providing a center for communication for individuals and organizations concerned about the negative impact of health misinformation, fraud, and quackery; and educating consumers, professionals, business people, legislators, law enforcement personnel, organizations, and agencies about health misinformation, fraud, and quackery. The organization also works to develop a constituency of concerned citizens who will support sound consumer protection laws and oppose legislation and policies that undermine consumer protection; stimulate, encourage, and aid in legal actions against consumer protection law violators; and provide a resource for the media that will articulate the position of consumer protection and science on controversial health issues. NCAHF was established in 1984 when consumer health education specialists became alarmed over the proliferation of health misinformation, fraud, and quackery within society and the perceived failure of established social institutions to cope with these problems. Employing the voluntary health agency concept, it organized concerned citizens and experts within academia, health care, public health, law, and related fields to actively combat these social problems. Consisting of 1,100 members and 10 chapters, NCAHF produces educational materials including a newsletter, reports, and referrals. In addition, NCAHF encourages networking, advocates in regard to government legislation, and supports research. NCAHF maintains a web site on the Internet at [http://www.ncahf.org].

President: William Jarvis, Ph.D.
Year Established: 1984
Organization Chapters: 10
Organization Members: 1,100

Publishes the following materials:
National Council Against Helath Fraud ~ *Fact Sheet*

1836 NATIONAL COUNCIL ON PATIENT INFORMATION AND EDUCATION (NCPIE)

666 Eleventh Street, NW
Suite 810
Washington, DC 20001 202-347-6711
Fax: 202-638-0773

The National Council on Patient Information and Education (NCPIE) is a not-for-profit coalition of organizations dedicated to improving communication between health care professionals, patients, and consumers about prescription medicines. Established in 1982 and consisting of approximately 300 members, NCPIE works toward its goal to encourage patients to work with their health care providers and to follow their medication therapy safely and effectively. NCPIE members are national and international organizations representing physician, pharmacy, nursing, and other health care professional groups; pharmaceutical research and manufacturing companies; managed care organizations; and the Food and Drug Administration (FDA). The objectives of the organization are to increase consumer awareness of the right to know and the need to know about medicines, the availability of useful medicine information, and how to obtain it; to increase patient awareness of the benefit of communicating with health professionals about prescription therapy and to appropriately use prescribed medicines; to increase health professionals' communication of useful prescription medicine information to patients, both orally and in supportive written form; and to assist in the development of more useful prescription medicine information in keeping with the federal Healthy People public health goals for the years 2000 and 2006. NCPIE's materials include pamphlets, a series of brochures, a quarterly newsletter entitled "The NCPIE News," and the annual "Talk About Prescriptions Month Planning Guide."

Executive Director: William Ray Bullman
Organization Language: Spanish (written).
Year Established: 1982
Organization Members: 300

Publishes the following materials:
National Council on Patient Information and Education ~ *Brochure*
Prescription Medicines and You. A Consumer Guide (Spanish) ~ *Brochure*
Prescription Medicines and You ~ *Brochure*
The Active Consumer. Getting the most from your medicines ~ *Brochure*
Get The Answers ~ *Brochure*
Medicines: What Every Woman Should Know ~ *Brochure*
A Parent's Guide For Medicine Use by Children ~ *Brochure*
Medicine: Before you take it, talk about it ~ *Brochure*
Alcohol and Medicines: Ask Before You Mix ~ *Brochure*
Talk About Prescriptions. Planning Guide ~ *Leaflet*

1837 NATIONAL COUNCIL ON RADIATION PROTECTION AND MEASUREMENTS (NCRP)

7910 Woodmont Avenue
Suite 800
Bethesda, MD 20814-3095 301-657-2562
Fax: 301-907-8768
E-mail: ncrp@ncrp.com
http://www.ncrp.com

The National Council on Radiation Protection and Measures (NCRP) is a not-for-profit, voluntary corporation chartered by Congress in 1964. The organization is dedicated to collecting, analyzing, and disseminating information and recommendations about protection against radiation and radiation measurements, quantities and units, particularly those concerned with radiation protection. The organization also strives to provide a means by which organizations concerned with the scientific and related aspects of radiation protection and of radiation quantities may cooperate for effective utilization of their combined resources and to stimulate the work of such organizations. The NCRP works to develop basic concepts about radiation quantities, units and measurements, about the application of these concepts, and about radiation protection. The organization cooperates with the International Commission on Radiological Protection, the International Commission on Radiation Units and Measurements, and other national and international organizations, government and private, concerned with radiation quantities, units and measurements and with radiation protection. The Council is the successor to the National Committee on Radiation Protection and Measurements that was formed in 1929. The Council members are from public and private universities, medical centers, national and private laboratories, and industry. The Council produces specific scientific reports.

President: Charles Meinhold
Year Established: 1964
Organization Members: Non-Membership

Publishes the following materials:
The NCRP ~ *Mission Statement*

Concerned with the following diseases or disorders:
Radiation Syndromes

1838 NATIONAL DYSAUTONOMIA RESEARCH FOUNDATION (NDRF)

P.O. Box 211153
Eagan, MN 55121-2553 715-594-3140
Fax: 715-594-3140
E-mail: ndrf@ndrf.org
http://www.ndrf.org

The National Dysautonomia Research Foundation (NDRF) is a national not-for-profit voluntary organization dedicated to providing information and support to individuals affected by dysfunction of the autonomic nervous system (dysautonomia). The autonomic nervous system controls involuntary (automatic or reflex) activities of the organs, blood vessels, glands, and a variety of tissues in the body. The autonomic nervous system is divided into two parts: the sympathetic nervous system, which, in general, heightens activity in the body (e.g., accelerating the heart beat and breathing rate) and the parasympathetic nervous system, which, in general, lessens activity in the body (e.g., decreasing the heart rate). Many disorders may be associated with dysautonomia including Shy-Drager Syndrome (Multiple System Atrophy), Postural Orthostatic Tachycardia Syndrome (POTS), Familial Dysautonomia, and Neurocardiogenic Syncope. The NDRF strives to provide contacts to additional organizations that may be of assistance to individuals with dysautonomia; advocate on behalf of affected individuals in support of ongoing research efforts to determine the causes of and treatments for dysautonomia; supply news organizations with timely and accurate information on dysautonomia; and raise funds for the purpose of ongoing medical and scientific research concerning dysautonomia. The Foundation provides a variety of educational materials including a regular newsletter that contains information on ongoing efforts to find cures and treatments for those affected by any of the various forms of dysautonomia. In addition, the Foundation maintains a web site at [http://www.ndrf.org] that provides general information on autonomic dysfunction as well as specific information on the various forms of dysautonomia; references to physicians and medical facilities that specialize in the research and treatment of dysautonomia; a Frequently Asked Questions (FAQ) and answers area; and more.

President: Daniel Smith
Executive Director: Lynn B. Eldred (Contact Person)
Year Established: 1997

Publishes the following materials:
NDRF ~ *Mission Statement*

Concerned with the following diseases or disorders:
Chagas Disease; Hypotension, Orthostatic; Mitral Valve Prolapse Syndrome; Shy Drager Syndrome

1839 NATIONAL EASTER SEAL SOCIETY, INC.

230 W. Monroe St.
Suite 1800
Chicago, IL 60606-4802
312-726-6200
800-221-6827
Fax: 312-726-1494
TDD: 312-726-4258
E-mail: nessinfo@seals.com
http://www.seals.com

The National Easter Seal Society, Inc. is a voluntary nonprofit service organization established in 1919 to serve the needs of children and adults with disabilities and to help them achieve independence. Easter Seals currently consists of a nationwide network of 105 affiliate societies that operates approximately 400 centers throughout the United States and Puerto Rico. The Society provides rehabilitation services; technological assistance; and disability prevention, advocacy and public education programs. Among its programs and services are the provision of physical, occupational, and speech therapy for children and adults; screening programs to identify vision, speech, and hearing problems, scoliosis, and other disabling conditions; and daycare programs for children with disabilities and their non-disabled peers that foster early acceptance of persons with disabilities. In addition, Easter Seals operates parent resource centers with adaptive toys and play therapy programs for young children; offers educational evaluation services; offers job evaluation, training, and placement for people with disabilities; provides loans of such equipment as braces, crutches, wheelchairs, and hearing aids; provides medical treatment and prosthetic care; and offers head trauma programs for children and adults. The National Easter Seal Society maintains a web site at [http://www.seals.com].

President: James E. Williams, Jr. (CEO)
Executive Director: Don E. Jackson (Chief Operations Officer)
Year Established: 1919
Organization Chapters: 225

Concerned with the following diseases or disorders:
Cerebral Palsy; Spina Bifida

1840 NATIONAL EATING DISORDERS ORGANIZATION (NEDO)

6655 South Yale Avenue
Tulsa, OK 74136
918-481-4044
Fax: 918-481-4076
http://www.laureate.com

The National Eating Disorders Organization (NEDO) is an international nonprofit self-help organization dedicated to increasing understanding and contributing toward the prevention of all forms of eating disorders and obesity. Eating disorders are extreme expressions of a range of weight and food issues experienced by both males and females. These include self-starvation and excessive weight loss (anorexia nervosa), a secretive cycle of binge eating followed by purging (bulimia nervosa), and compulsive overeating. NEDO was established in 1977 and was originally known as the National Anorexic Society. NEDO's mission is to provide support, education, and treatment to individuals with eating disorders based on an approach that takes into consideration biological, social, psychological, and familial factors. The organization produces educational materials including an information packet, audio tapes, an international treatment resource directory, a quarterly newsletter, and a video tape entitled "Skin Deep." In addition, NEDO provides information and guidance to those interested in developing local support groups. The National Eating Disorders Organization maintains a web site on the Internet at [http://www.laureate.com].

Executive Director: Barbara Fleming, L.S.W. (Coordinator)
Year Established: 1977
Organization Members: 550

Publishes the following materials:
Introduction To the National Eating Disorders Organization ~ *Mission Statement*
Eating Disorders Warning Signs ~ *Fact Sheet*

Concerned with the following diseases or disorders:
Anorexia Nervosa; Bulimia

1841 NATIONAL EYE CARE PROJECT (NECP)

P.O. Box 429098
San Francisco, CA 94142-9098
800-222-3937
Fax: 415-561-8567
E-mail: tjuring@aao.org
http://www.eyenet.org

The National Eye Care Project, which was established in 1986, is a not-for-profit organization dedicated to providing medical and surgical eye care to the financially disadvantaged elderly who cannot afford care. The program is designed so that volunteer ophthalmologists provide eye care at no out-of-pocket cost to the individual, regardless of insurance coverage (or lack thereof). In order to qualify for this program, the patient must be at least 65 years of age, have citizenship or legal residency in the United States, and must demonstrate a need for financial aid, and must have no access to an ophthalmologist or an alternative method of receiving care (e.g., HMO, Veteran's Hospital). The purpose of the NECP is to provide a unique program that enables senior citizens to receive the proper eye care treatment that they need, as well as encourage the public to recognize the need for more affordable medical care in the United States, particularly in the elderly community. Program activities include patient advocacy, patient and general education, brochures and pamphlets, and referrals.

President: B. Thomas Hutchinson, Chair
Year Established: 1986

Publishes the following materials:
National Eye Care Project ~ *Mission Statement*
National eye Care Project. The Foundation of the American Academy of Ophthalmology ~ *Pamphlet*
Glaucoma: What you don't know can hurt you ~ *Fact Sheet*
Cataract: A cause of poor vision ~ *Fact Sheet*
Diabetes: It can harm your sight ~ *Fact Sheet*
Macular Degeneration: When you can't see the center ~ *Fact Sheet*

1842 NATIONAL EYE RESEARCH FOUNDATION (NERF)

910 Skokie Boulevard
Suite 207A
Northbrook, IL 60062
847-564-4652
800-621-2258
Fax: 847-564-0807
E-mail: nerf1955@aol.com
http://www.eyemac.com/nerf

The National Eye Research Foundation (NERF) is a nonprofit, international organization dedicated to improving eye care for the public and meeting the professional needs of eye care practitioners. The Foundation sponsors eye research projects on contact lens applications and eye care problems. Established in 1955, NERF is committed to professional enrichment through special study sections in such fields as orthokeratology, primary eye care, pediatrics, and through continuing education programs. The Foundation provides eye care information for the public and professionals. Consisting of 300 members, the organization produces educational materials including pamphlets entitled "National Eye Research Foundation, Pioneers in Contact

Lenses Eye and Health Care Research Since 1955," "Visual Color Fields, The Diagnostic Eye Test for Early Warning Health Screening," and "Corrective Vision Care." Program activities include education and referrals. NERF can be reached at its e-mail address at [nerf1955@aol.com.] or its web site at [www.eyemac.com/nerf].

President: Andrew K. Kim (1996 to Present)
Executive Director: Dr. Newton K. Wesley (Chairperson/Founder)
Year Established: 1955
Organization Members: 300

Publishes the following materials:
History of NERF ~ *Mission Statement*
Open Your Eyes. The Big Picture: Myopia Control ~ *Fact Sheet*
Myopia: Can We Prevent It? ~ *Reprint*
Weighing the Options? ~ *Reprint*
Do You Know What Your Cornea Looks Like? ~ *Reprint*
National Eye Research Foundation ~ *Brochure*
Visual Color Fields. The diagnostic eye test for early warning health screening ~ *Brochure*
The NERF Wellness Center. Employee Benefits Program ~ *Brochure*
Corrective Vision Care ~ *Brochure*
Professional Ortho-keratology ~ *Brochure*
Dealing with Myopia. Causes. Symptoms. Treatments. "Your Eyes Can Get Better" ~ *Brochure*
Ortho-K. Nearsightedness (Myopoia. Astigmatism and Orthokeratology ~ *Brochure*

Concerned with the following diseases or disorders:
Aniridia Cerebellar Ataxia Mental Deficiency; Apraxia, Ocular Motor, Cogan Type; Keratomalacia; Retinopathy, Arteriosclerotic; Retinopathy, Hypertensive; WAGR Syndrome

1843 NATIONAL FAMILY CAREGIVERS ASSOCIATION (NFCA)

9621 East Bexhill Drive
Kensington, MD 20895-3104 301-942-6430
800-896-3650
Fax: 301-942-2302
E-mail: info@nfcacares.org
http://www.nfcacares.org

The National Family Caregivers Association is a not-for-profit membership organization dedicated to improving the quality of life for family caregivers. Established in 1992, the organization provides services in research, information and education, support and validation, respite care, and advocacy. Consisting of 1,200 members, the organization produces educational materials including a newsletter entitled "Take Care," an article entitled "America's Family Caregivers: An Invisible Multi-Billion Dollar Industry at Risk," and several informational brochures and pamphlets. Other materials disseminated by the NFCA include reports, a journal, and audiovisual aids. Programs offered by NFCA include lobbying efforts, networking, and maintenance of a World Wide Web site on the Internet at [http://www.nfcacares.org].

President: Suzanne Geffen Mintz (1992 to Present)
Executive Director: Diane Walden
Year Established: 1992
Organization Members: 1,200

Publishes the following materials:
Improving the Lives of America's Family Caregivers ~ *Brochure*
In Sickness and in Health ~ *Reprint*
What is Caregiving ~ *Fact Sheet*
NFCA Publications, Speaking Engagements, Testimony and Media Appearances - 1994 and 95 ~ *Publication List*
National Family Caregivers Week. "Family Caregiving counts!" ~ *Pamphlet*
No "Happily Ever After" ~ *News Release*

1844 NATIONAL FATHERS' NETWORK (NFN)

Kindering Center
16120 NE Eighth Street
Bellevue, WA 98008-3937 425-747-4004
Fax: 425-747-1069
E-mail: jmay@fathersnetwork.org
http://www.fathersnetwork.org

The National Fathers' Network (NFN) is a national voluntary not-for-profit organization dedicated to advocating and providing resources and support to fathers and families of children with chronic illness, developmental disabilities, and special health care needs. Established in 1986 and funded by a grant from the Maternal and Child Health Bureau, the National Fathers' Network currently consists of over 5,000 members and more than 80 chapters. The NFN provides a variety of programs and services including developing national and statewide databases with information concerning fathers from diverse ethnic, racial, and geographic backgrounds; offering father support and mentoring programs; developing curriculum (monographs and videos) designed to enhance the involvement of fathers in the home and service provision (i.e., health care settings, schools); offering technical assistance to organizations and agencies to ensure that their services are increasingly "father friendly"; and sponsoring local and regional conferences. In addition, the National Father's Network offers a variety of educational materials including monographs; a "how to" manual for developing effective and successful programs for men; videos; and discussion and resource guides. The Network also regularly publishes articles in national magazines and journals, has a monthly column in "Exceptional Parent" Magazine called "Fathers' Voices," and publishes a regular newsletter entitled "DADS Newsletter: Dads Advocating for Dads." In addition, the NFN maintains a web site on the Internet at [http://www.fathersnetwork.org/].

President: James May (1986 to Present)
Organization Language: Spanish (written).
Year Established: 1986
Organization Chapters: 83
Organization Members: 5,000

Publishes the following materials:
DADS Newsletter ~ *Newsletter*
National Fathers' Network ~ *Reprint*

1845 NATIONAL FEDERATION OF THE BLIND (NFB)

1800 Johnson Street
Baltimore, MD 21230
410-659-9314
800-638-7518
Fax: 410-685-5653
E-mail: nfb@access.digex.net
http://www.nfb.org

The National Federation of the Blind is a national, voluntary not-for-profit organization dedicated to providing information and support to individuals who are blind, their families, and professionals; ensuring complete integration of affected individuals into society; and acting as a vehicle for collective self-expression of the blind. Established in 1940, the organization, which has over 50,000 members, has more than 600 affiliates throughout the United States. The Federation engages in patient and family advocacy; provides job opportunities in cooperation with the Department of Labor; offers referrals and scholarships; and assists in the development and evaluation of technology for blind individuals. The Federation provides appropriate medical and support referrals; promotes and supports research; and provides a variety of aids and devices for affected individuals. The Federation also offers a wide range of educational and support materials for affected families and professionals. These include a monthly publication entitled "The Braille Monitor"; quarterly publications, such as "Future Reflections" for parents and educators and "Voice of the Diabetic"; brochures; and audio tapes.

President: Marc Maurer (1986-Present)
Year Established: 1940
Organization Chapters: 600
Organization Members: 50,000

Concerned with the following diseases or disorders:
Cataract Dental Syndrome; Choroideremia; Coats' Disease; Leber's Optic Atrophy; Lenz Microphthalmia Syndrome; Norrie Syndrome; Retinitis Pigmentosa; Septo Optic Dysplasia; Usher's Syndrome; Waardenburg Syndrome

1846 NATIONAL FOUNDATION FOR DEPRESSIVE ILLNESS, INC. (NAFDI)

P.O. Box 2257
New York, NY 10116-2257
800-248-4344
http://www.depression.org

The National Foundation for Depressive Illness, Inc. (NAFDI) is a national not-for-profit organization dedicated to informing the public, primary health care providers, other health care professionals, and corporations about depression and manic depression and providing information about correct diagnosis, treatment, and the availability of qualified doctors and support groups. There are various forms of depression. Major depression may be characterized by a period of depressed mood associated with a lack of pleasure or interest in the individual's usual activities. Associated symptoms may include fatigue, disturbances in appetite and/or sleeping patterns, difficulty with concentration, and/or other abnormalities. Manic depression may be characterized by cycles of varying intensity between degrees of depression and mania. Manic episodes may be characterized by an elevated or irritable mood accompanied by decreased need for sleep, distractibility, talkativeness, hyperactivity or agitation, and/or reckless behavior. NAFDI was established in 1983 to correct myths and misconceptions that may often surround mental illness and help reverse the negative effects depression and manic depression may have on affected individuals, family members, and society. NAFDI's services include maintaining 12 "800" help lines; mailing out thousands of information packets every month; maintaining current listings of physicians and support groups by state; engaging in public service announcement campaigns; holding symposia including participants from Congress, other public officials, leading business figures, and the press to increase awareness; providing speakers and materials for workshops, symposia, and seminars in the mental health community; and engaging in patient advocacy and lobbying efforts to ensure the proper awareness, diagnosis, and treatment of these disorders. Educational materials include brochures, pamphlets, article reprints, and a regular newsletter. NAFDI also has a web site at [http://www.depression.org].

President: Donald F. Klein (1983 to Present)
Executive Director: Peter Ross
Year Established: 1983
Organization Members: Non-Membership

Publishes the following materials:
Now We Can Successfully Treat The Illness Called Depression ~ *Leaflet*
Depression is a Disease; but few get treatment ~ *Reprint*
51 Tips On Coping With Mental Illness In The Family ~ *Fact Sheet*
Manic Depression ~ *Fact Sheet*
Personal Health ~ *Reprint*
Depression in the Old Can Be Deadly, But the Symptoms Are Often Missed ~ *Reprint*
Bouncing Back ~ *Reprint*
Man-To-Man ~ *Reprint*
Personal Health ~ *Reprint*
Suicide Myths Cloud Efforts To Save Children ~ *Reprint*
Depression. The Growing Role of Drug Therapies ~ *Reprint*
The Stigma of Mental Illness ~ *Reprint*
As Fellow Traveler of Other Illness, Depression Often Goes in Disguise ~ *Reprint*
One Answer for Manic Depression ~ *Reprint*
Is That Child Bad Or Depressed? ~ *Reprint*
NAFDI Purpose and Activities ~ *Mission Statement*
National Foundation for Depressive Illness, Inc. ~ *Bibliography*

Concerned with the following diseases or disorders:
Dysthymia; Manic Depression, Bipolar

1847 NATIONAL FOUNDATION FOR FACIAL RECONSTRUCTION (NFFR)

317 East 34th St.
#901
New York, NY 10016 212-263-6656
800-422-3223
Fax: 212-263-7534

The National Foundation for Facial Reconstruction is a not-for-profit research organization dedicated to helping people affected by craniofacial disorders lead productive and fulfilling lives. Established in 1951, the National Foundation for Facial Reconstruction, through its support of the Institute of Reconstructive Plastic Surgery at New York University Medical Center, provides assistance to those affected by craniofacial conditions. The Foundation's broad programs include sponsorship of medical research; professional training; social, psychological, and financial assistance; and programs of public education. Educational materials produced and distributed by the Foundation include a variety of informative brochures.

Executive Director: Calliope Ligelis
Organization Language: Spanish.
Year Established: 1951
Organization Members: 4,000

Concerned with the following diseases or disorders:
Apert Syndrome; Branchio Oculo Facial Syndrome; Craniometaphyseal Dysplasia; Fraser Syndrome; Goodman Syndrome; Marshall Syndrome; Maxillonasal Dysplasia, Binder Type; Oral Facial Digital Syndrome; Oto Palato Digital Syndrome Type I and II; Pallister W Syndrome; Sakati Syndrome; Summitt Syndrome; Velocardiofacial Syndrome

1848 NATIONAL FOUNDATION FOR JEWISH GENETIC DISEASES (NFJGD)

250 Park Avenue
Suite 1000
New York, NY 10017 212-371-1030

The National Foundation for Jewish Genetic Diseases is a not-for-profit voluntary health and research organization devoted to supporting medical research and informing the public and medical communities about the seven most common Jewish genetic diseases. These diseases include Gaucher Disease, Dystonia, Familial Dysautonomia, Tay-Sach's Disease, Bloom Syndrome, Niemann-Pick Disease, and Mucolipidosis IV. The National Foundation for Jewish Genetic Diseases aims to advance progress toward the cure and/or prevention of these disorders. The major efforts of the Foundation are directed to help physicians and researchers understand the nature of these rare genetic diseases so that newer and better means of diagnosis, management, treatment, and prevention can be developed. Informational fact sheets on each of these diseases are produced by the Foundation and describe the specific nature of the genetic defect, diagnostic tests, and available disease management and treatments. The National Foundation for Jewish Genetic Diseases also supports research and training programs through endowed scholarship programs and direct funding to academic and medical research centers.

President: George Crohn Jr. (1975-Present)
Executive Director: Doris Shaw Gluck
Year Established: 1975

Publishes the following materials:
What You Should Know About... Jewish Genetic Diseases ~ *Pamphlet*

Concerned with the following diseases or disorders:
Bloom Syndrome; Dubin Johnson Syndrome; Dystonia, Torsion; Leukodystrophy, Canavan's; Tay Sachs Disease

1849 NATIONAL FOUNDATION FOR VITILIGO AND PIGMENT DISORDERS

9032 South Woemandy Lane
Centerville, OH 45458 937-885-5739

The National Foundation for Vitiligo and Pigment Disorders is a voluntary not-for-profit organization dedicated to educating affected individuals, family members, health care professionals, and the public about vitiligo and pigment disorders. Vitiligo is an acquired dermatological condition characterized by areas of decreased pigmentation of the skin. The lesions are usually sharply demarcated with increased coloring on the borders. Established in 1986, the National Foundation for Vitiligo and Pigment Disorders provides support to affected individuals and their families; raises funds for research; engages in patient advocacy; and provides appropriate referrals to physicians and researchers. The Foundation also provides educational and support information through its directory and various educational materials published by its parent organization, the National Vitiligo Foundation.

President: Ms. Sandy Wenner
Executive Director: Sandy Wenner
Year Established: 1986

Concerned with the following diseases or disorders:
Schmidt Syndrome; Vitiligo

1850 NATIONAL GAUCHER FOUNDATION, INC. (NGF)

11140 Rockville Pike
Suite 350
Rockville, MD 20852-3106 301-816-1515
800-925-8885
Fax: 301-816-1516
E-mail: ngf@gaucherdisease.org
http://www.gaucherdisease.org

The National Gaucher Foundation is a not-for-profit organization that supports medical research into causes of Gaucher Disease. Gaucher Disease is a rare metabolic disorder characterized by the accumulation of a fatty substance, a lipid called glucocerebrosidase. The most common symptoms of Gaucher Disease are enlargement of the liver and spleen, anemia, reduced platelets (resulting in easy bruising and long clotting times), bone infarctions often leading to damage to the shoulder or hip joints, and a generalized demineralization of the bones (osteoporosis). The weakening of the bones can then lead to spontaneous fractures. The course of the disease is quite variable, ranging from no overt symptoms to skeletal problems, liver or spleen damage, bleeding, or other problems. Founded in 1984, the National Gaucher Foundation encourages scientific investigation into developing treatments for Gaucher Disease. The organization hopes that this research will ultimately lead to a cure for the disease. In addition to funding vital research, the National Gaucher Foundation offers an extensive range of services to people with Gaucher Disease and their families. These services include financial assistance and patient and physician education programs. The Foundation also publishes a quarterly newsletter.

President: Dr. Robin Ely Berman
Executive Director: Rhonda P. Buyers
Year Established: 1984
Organization Chapters: 5
Organization Members: 1,000

Concerned with the following diseases or disorders:
Gaucher Disease

1851 NATIONAL HEAD INJURY FOUNDATION, INC. (AND FAMILY HELPLINE) (NHIF)

1776 Massachusetts Avenue NW
Suite 100
Washington, D.C. 20036 202-296-6443
800-444-6443
Fax: 202-296-8850
http://www.biausa.org

Established in 1980, the National Head Injury Foundation, Inc. (NHIF) is a voluntary not-for-profit organization dedicated to promoting advocacy for people who have survived traumatic brain injury (TBI); securing and developing community based services for survivors of TBI and their families; supporting research that will enhance the lives of affected people; and promoting the prevention of brain injuries through public awareness, education, and legislation. The National Head Injury Foundation has a nationwide network of more than 800 support groups; provides direct financial assistance to people with a brain injury and their families; hosts nationwide conferences and symposia for physicians, rehabilitation specialists, trial lawyers, pharmaceutical representatives, and other professionals; and promotes a multifaceted public awareness campaign. The Foundation also spearheads a network of information exchange through its toll-free Family Helpline; Defense and Veterans Head Injury Program; advisory groups (e.g., the Survivor and Family Councils); and the Brain Injury Resource Center, an interactive computer-based multimedia system. The Foundation also offers a national directory of head injury services; a quarterly magazine, "TBI Challenge!"; regular newsletters; and an extensive library that includes TBI research indexes, TBI professional series, books, videos, audiotapes, brochures, information packets, training materials, article reprints, and posters.

President: George A. Zitnay, PhD (1990-Present)
Executive Director: Fred Krause (Chief Operating Officer)
Year Established: 1980
Organization Chapters: 200
Organization Members: 15,000

Publishes the following materials:
National Head Injury Foundation - Mission Statement ~ *Mission Statement*
National Head Injury Foundation ~ *Fact Sheet*
Catalouge of Educational Materials 1994 Edition ~ *Catalog*

Concerned with the following diseases or disorders:
Agnosia, Primary Visual

1852 NATIONAL HEADACHE FOUNDATION (NHF)

428 West Saint James Place # 2
Chicago, IL 60614-2750 773-388-6399
800-843-2256
Fax: 773-525-7357
http://www.headaches.org

Established in 1970, the National Headache Foundation is a not-for-profit organization dedicated to serving as an information resource to affected individuals, their families, and the physicians who treat them. The organization is also committed to promoting research into the causes of and treatments for headaches as well as increasing awareness among the public concerning the seriousness of headaches and the need for understanding and continuity of care for affected individuals. The National Headache Foundation funds ongoing medical research; sponsors public and professional education seminars across the country; and has a nationwide network of local support groups. In addition, the Foundation, which functions as a clearinghouse of information on headaches, provides a regular newsletter, brochures, and audio and video tapes. Some materials are available in Spanish.

President: Robert S. Kunkel, M.D.
Executive Director: Suzanne E. Simons
Year Established: 1970
Organization Members: 15,000

Publishes the following materials:
NHF Educational Materials ~ *Order Form*
National Headache Foundation ~ *Fact Sheet*

Concerned with the following diseases or disorders:
Cyclic Vomiting Syndrome; Headache, Cluster; Tolosa Hunt Syndrome

1853 NATIONAL HEALTHY MOTHERS, HEALTHY BABIES (NHMHB)

409 12th Street SW
Washington, D.C. 20024 202-863-2458
Fax: 202-554-4346
None.

National Healthy Mothers, Healthy Babies is a not-for-profit, self-help, service organization dedicated to promoting public awareness and education concerning perinatal health issues, particularly preventive health habits for pregnant women and their families. Established in 1990, this national coalition has over 100 members, representing national voluntary organizations, health professional organizations, and the Federal Government. This service group is organized into several working issue committees: adolescent pregnancy, breast feeding promotion, genetics, immunization, injury/violence prevention, oral health, and substance abuse. National Healthy Mothers, Healthy Babies assists the development of state and local Healthy Mothers, Healthy Babies Coalitions. The organization provides technical assistance and resource materials; develops networks for sharing information among groups concerned about improving the health of mothers and babies; and conducts quarterly membership meetings. It promotes maternal and infant health educational campaigns and conducts biennial national conferences for health care professionals and administrators. Healthy Mothers, Healthy Babies also distributes public and professional educational materials including a quarterly newsletter, brochures, audiovisual aids, posters, and resource lists of additional publications.

President: Stephanie Harrison
Executive Director: Anita Boles
Year Established: 1990
Organization Members: 104

1854 NATIONAL HEART ASSIST AND TRANSPLANT FUND, INC. (NHATF)

6 Bryn Mawr Avenue
P.O. Box 258
Bryn Mawr, PA 19010 610-527-5056
800-642-8399
Fax: 610-527-5210
E-mail: txfund:@libertynet.org
http://www.libertynet.org/~txfund

Established in 1983 by a group of medical professionals, the National Heart Assist and Transplant Fund (NHATF) is a not-for-profit service organization dedicated to assisting heart, heart/lung, and lung transplant patients and their families with the social and financial problems that develop as a result of their disorders. The Fund also promotes education through organ donor drives, awareness seminars, and lectures. It provides local support groups with information and materials; advocates on behalf of all people affected by heart/lung transplant diseases; raises money for medical grants and patients' ongoing expenses; and gives fund-raising advice to transplant candidates. Members of the organization's Board of Directors receive no compensation, and the Fund's staff is composed of professionals and volunteers working with a limited budget. The National Heart Assist and Transplant Fund produces and disseminates a wide variety of educational and support materials. These materials include an informational brochure, an organ donation brochure, a regular newsletter, audio-visual aids, bumper stickers, patient application packets, and a corporate matching gift list.

President: Jacob Kolff, M.D. (1983-Present)
Executive Director: Patricia M. Kolff
Year Established: 1983

1855 NATIONAL HOME OF YOUR OWN ALLIANCE (NHOYOA)

7 Leavitt Lane
Suite 101
Institute on Disability
Durham, NH 03824-3522 603-862-0550
Fax: 603-862-0555
E-mail: mcaulk@hopper.unh.edu
http://iod.unh.edu

The National Home of Your Own Alliance (NHOYOA), a not-for-profit organization, was established in 1993 as a national information and technical assistance center on home ownership and control to help individuals with developmental disabilities overcome potential barriers to home ownership. Founded by the U.S. Administration on Developmental Disabilities through a cooperative agreement with the Institute on Disability at the University of New Hampshire, the Alliance is dedicated to creating an infrastructure of exemplary practices and public and private sector partnerships that will link the home mortgage and social service industries to better serve people with disabilities. Focused on broad systems change and local efforts to create opportunities for individuals, the Alliance is addressing the need for local, state, and national systems change through three primary activities: intensive technical assistance in selected states, leadership of people with disabilities in all aspects of the Alliance, and information and referral on person-owned/controlled housing and support. Specifically, the Alliance is working to provide technical assistance and training in selected states to achieve systems change at the state and local level; include individuals and families in technical assistance and systems change efforts; analyze national and state policies that impact the availability of housing and support; implement strategies to overcome identified policy barriers; establish a national information and referral system to respond to requests for assistance in dealing with barriers that prevent people from controlling their housing and supports; and disseminate information about effective strategies for creating person-controlled housing and support. The Alliance has a variety of materials including brochures, pamphlets, reports, videos, training materials, information packets, and a regular newsletter. The NHOYOA also has a web site on the Internet at [http://iod.unh.edu].

Executive Director: Jay Klein
Year Established: 1993
Organization Members: Non-Membership

Publishes the following materials:
Home of Your Own ~ *Newsletter*
A Home of My Own. Institute on Disability ~ *Video Tape*
Home Of Your Own ~ *Newsletter*
"I Can Do What I Want When I Want" ~ *Brochure*
National Home of Your Own Alliance ~ *Brochure*
Publications List ~ *Bibliography*

1856 NATIONAL HOSPICE ORGANIZATION (NHO)

1901 North Moore Street
Suite 901
Arlington, VA 22209 703-243-5900
800-658-8898
Fax: 703-525-5762
E-mail: drsnho@cais.com
http://www.nho.org

The National Hospice Organization (NHO) is a national nonprofit membership organization dedicated to promoting and maintaining quality care for terminally ill individuals and their families and making hospice an integral part of the U.S. health care system. Hospice is a comprehensive, medically directed, team-oriented program of care that seeks to treat and comfort terminally ill patients and their families in a home or home-like setting. Established in 1978, the NHO is committed to educating about and advocating for the fundamental philosophy and principles of hospice care to meet the unique needs of each terminally ill person and his or her family. Consisting of approximately 2,200 hospices and 5,000 individual professional members, the NHO engages in patient advocacy and lobbying, promotes research, engages in patient and professional education, and provides referrals. The NHO offers a variety of materials including pamphlets, brochures, educational booklets, a resource directory listing hospices throughout the United States by city and state, a journal, and a regular newsletter. The National Hospice Organization also has a web site on the Internet at [http://www.nho.org] that provides a searchable online directory of hospices in the United States, links to other hospice sites on the web, links to discussion groups, conference information for hospice professionals, and more.

President: John J. Mahoney
Organization Language: Spanish (written/spoken).
Year Established: 1978
Organization Chapters: 3,000
Organization Members: 7,200

Publishes the following materials:
The 1997/98 Guide to the Nation's Hospices ~ *Book*
"You matter to the last moment of your life..." ~ *Leaflet*
National Hospice Organization (Spanish) ~ *Brochure*
About Hospice ~ *Booklet*
Helping Your Child Grieve ~ *Booklet*
About Infection Control in the Home ~ *Booklet*
About Universal Precautions (Spanish) ~ *Booklet*
Hospice Under Medicare ~ *Booklet*
About Caring For Patients With Active TB ~ *Booklet*
Advance Medical Directives. Something to think about ~ *Booklet*
Hospice Volunteers. Making each day count! ~ *Booklet*
About Caring For People With Aids ~ *Booklet*
About Wound Care At Home ~ *Booklet*
Helping Confused Patients ~ *Booklet*
Caring For Someone With Alzheimer's Disease ~ *Booklet*
About Dying ~ *Booklet*
Going Through Bereavement. When a loved one dies ~ *Booklet*
Grief. Living with loss ~ *Booklet*
About DNR Orders. Do not resuscitate orders ~ *Booklet*
About Pain Management ~ *Booklet*
What Everyone should know about Aids ~ *Booklet*
About Caregiving ~ *Booklet*

Concerned with the following diseases or disorders:
Creutzfeldt Jakob Disease

1857 NATIONAL HYDROCEPHALUS FOUNDATION

22427 South River Road
Joliet, IL 60436 815-467-6548
E-mail: hydrobrat@aol.com

The National Hydrocephalus Foundation is a national not-for-profit voluntary organization dedicated to providing information and support to families of individuals affected by Hydrocephalus. Hydrocephalus is an abnormal accumulation of cerebrospinal fluid, causing a build-up of pressure inside the head. Established in 1979, the Foundation is also committed to funding and promoting medical research on Hydrocephalus and enabling affected families to exchange information, resources, and support. The National Hydrocephalus Foundation, in cooperation with the Hydrocephalus Research Foundation, provides a quarterly, 20-page publication and gives access to the networking database. The quarterly publication includes medical and technical articles, human interest stories, and updates on resources, clinical trials, special education services, and more. The News & Notes database connects affected families with one another and with researchers and provides access to a variety of articles on

Hydrocephalus. The National Hydrocephalus Foundation also provides additional materials, including video tapes and survey results concerning affected individuals and family members.

President: James A. Mazzetti
Executive Director: Debbi Fields (Contact Person)
Year Established: 1979
Organization Members: 350

Publishes the following materials:
National Hydrocephalus Foundation ~ *Brochure*
Dear National Hydrocephalus Foundation Members ~ *Form Letter*

Concerned with the following diseases or disorders:
Acrocallosal Syndrome, Schinzel Type; Agenesis of Corpus Callosum; Craniosynostosis, Primary; Dandy Walker Malformation; Diencephalic Syndrome; Encephalocele; Hydranencephaly; Hydrocephalus; MASA Syndrome; Walker Warburg Syndrome

1858 NATIONAL HYPOGLYCEMIA ASSOCIATION (NHA)

P.O. Box 120
Ridgewood, NJ 07451 201-670-1189

The National Hypoglycemia Assocation was founded in 1982 as a support group, information resource, and educator about hypoglycemia. NHA also runs support groups, conducts research, advocates on behalf of affected individuals, produces audio-visual aids, publishes a newsletter, and offers a referral service.

President: Lenore L. Cohen
Year Established: 1982

Concerned with the following diseases or disorders:
Hypoglycemia

1859 NATIONAL INFERTILITY NETWORK EXCHANGE (NINE)

P.O. Box 204
East Meadow, NY 11554 516-794-5772
Fax: 516-794-0008
E-mail: NINE204@aol.com

The National Infertility Network Exchange (NINE) is a national not-for-profit organization dedicated to helping men, women, and couples affected by infertility. Established in 1988, NINE provides information and support concerning infertility, family planning and decisionmaking, medical options, and legal options such as adoption. The Exchange's programs and services include a "Talkline" information and support service; support groups; networking opportunities that enable affected individuals to exchange information, assistance, and resources; and patient advocacy services. NINE also promotes research, conducts monthly educational meetings, offers a referral service, maintains a reference library, and provides several educational materials including brochures, booklets, audiotapes, and a regular newsletter.

President: Ilene Stargot (1988 to Present)
Organization Language: Spanish (written).
Year Established: 1988
Organization Members: 300

Publishes the following materials:
National Infertility Network Exchange ~ *Brochure*
News From Nine ~ *Newsletter*
Monthly Nine Meetings ~ *Audio Casette List*
News From NINE ~ *Newsletter Spring 1997*

1860 NATIONAL INFORMATION CENTER FOR CHILDREN AND YOUTH WITH DISABILITIES (NICHCY)

P.O. Box 1492
Washington, D.C. 20009 202-884-8200
800-695-0285
Fax: 202-884-8441
TDD: 800-695-0285
E-mail: nichcy@aed.org
http://www.nichcy.org

The National Information Center for Children and Youth with Disabilities is an information clearinghouse that provides free information on disabilities and disability-related issues. Children and youth (aged birth to 22) are a special focus of the Information Center. Founded in 1982, the National Information Center for Children and Youth with Disabilities provides personal responses to questions on disability issues including early intervention, special education, individualized education programs, and family, legal and adult transitional issues. Referrals are made to other agencies including national, state, and regional groups, professional associations, information centers, and parent and advocacy groups. The National Information Center for Children and Youth with Disabilities provides up-to-date information on disabilities by searching the Center's databases and library. Free publications include resource sheets, fact sheets, briefing papers, parent guides, and bibliographies.

Executive Director: Suzanne Ripley
Organization Language: Spanish.
Year Established: 1982

Publishes the following materials:
NICHCY ~ *Mission Statement*
Publications List 1995 ~ *Publications List*

Concerned with the following diseases or disorders:
Penta X Syndrome; Triplo X Syndrome

1861 **NATIONAL INFORMATION CENTER ON DEAFNESS (NICD)**
Gallaudet University
800 Florida Avenue, NE
Washington, D.C. 20002 202-651-5051
Fax: 202-651-5054
TDD: 202-651-5052
E-mail: nicd@gallux.gallaudet.edu
http://www.gallaudet.edu/~nicd

Established in 1980, the National Information Center on Deafness (NICD) is a not-for-profit organization located on the Gallaudet University campus in Washington, DC. The Center functions as a centralized source of current information on topics dealing with deafness and hearing loss. The Center responds to questions from individuals who are deaf or hard of hearing, their families, professionals who work with affected individuals and families, and the general public. The Center collects, develops, and disseminates information concerning hearing impairment; maintains contacts with a multitude of resources and experts on the University campus and across the United States; and makes referrals to other organizations and agencies. The National Information Center on Deafness produces and distributes a wide variety of brochures and pamphlets. These include information on deafness for children and their teachers, career and employment information, and details on assistive devices and hearing aids.

Executive Director: Loraine DiPietro
Year Established: 1980

Publishes the following materials:
Genetics and Deafness ~ *Fact Sheet*
Publications from the National Information Center on Deafness ~ *Publication List*
A Provider Of Information That Can Make A Difference ~ *Pamphlet*

Concerned with the following diseases or disorders:
Alstrom Syndrome; Bjornstad Syndrome; Carbohydrate deficient Glycoprotein Syndrome Type I; Jansen Type Metaphyseal Chondrodysplasia; Norrie Syndrome; Usher's Syndrome; Waardenburg Syndrome; Wildervanck Syndrome

1862 **NATIONAL INSTITUTE FOR REHABILITATION ENGINEERING (NIRE)**
Box T
Hewitt, NC 07421 973-853-6585
800-736-2216
E-mail: nire@theoffice.net

The National Institute for Rehabilitation Engineering (NIRE) is a voluntary organization dedicated to providing custom-made devices, training, and onsite services for severely handicapped individuals. Established in 1967, the Institute is an onsite technology training organization and research and development facility. Its staff designs custom-made devices for handicapped persons who are trial-fitted, trained, counseled, and evaluated in the field. Such devices include special field-expander glasses for monocular vision, loss of one half the field vision in both eyes (hemianopsia), and tunnel vision; low vision cataract glasses; night vision aids; and macular degeneration glasses. Conventional vision, hearing, and other services are provided for persons otherwise handicapped. In addition, electronic speech aids are available, and aids for the totally deaf and special visual aids for deaf people with impaired vision are also provided by the Institute. The organization supplies specifically designed mobility aids for individuals with cerebral palsy, paralysis, or paralysis of all four limbs (quadriplegia). The Institute also provides self-care aids, communication aids, and occupational aids. In addition, NIRE provides computers and specially modified computer programs with educational and employment applications for handicapped individuals; provides driver assessment and/or training for persons with a wide range of disabilities; offers technical assistance to handicapped persons trying to set up their own businesses; and coordinates outreach programs that provide most of these services and aids in clients' own local areas such as schools, clinics, homes, and places of employment. The Institute supports the Swedish and Norwegian languages in both spoken and written form, and the French, Spanish, German, and Italian languages in written form only.

President: Reverend Tom Schwanda (1987 to Present)
Executive Director: Donald Selwyn
Organization Language: Swedish (written/spoken). Norwegian (written/spoken). French (written). Spanish (written). German (written). Italian (written).
Year Established: 1967
Organization Members: Non-Membership

Publishes the following materials:
National Institute for Rehabilitation Engineering ~ *Mission Statement*

1863 NATIONAL KIDNEY FOUNDATION (NKF)

30 East 33rd Street
New York, NY 10016 212-889-2210
800-622-9010
Fax: 212-689-9261
http://www.kidney.org

Established in 1950, the National Kidney Foundation is a voluntary not-for-profit organization dedicated to preventing kidney and urinary tract diseases, improving the health and well-being of individuals and families affected by these diseases, and increasing the availability of organs for transplantation. The Foundation is committed to gaining adequate support for research and research training; fostering continuing education of health care professionals; expanding and developing patient services and community resources; increasing public awareness of kidney diseases; monitoring health policy development; and increasing fund-raising for new programs and research. In addition, the Foundation supports and promotes medical research into the causes, prevention, and treatment of kidney diseases. A wide variety of educational materials is produced and distributed by the Foundation. These materials are listed in a booklet entitled Public and Professional Education Materials.

President: Garabed Eknoyan, M.D.
Executive Director: John Davis
Organization Language: Spanish.
Year Established: 1950
Organization Chapters: 51

Concerned with the following diseases or disorders:
Alport Syndrome; Arginino Succinic Aciduria; Bartter's Syndrome; Blue Diaper Syndrome; Branchio Oto Renal Syndrome; Carbamyl Phosphate Synthetase Deficiency; Carcinoma, Renal Cell; Citrullinemia; Cystinuria; Drash Syndrome; Fraser Syndrome; Galloway Mowat Syndrome; Goldenhar Syndrome (Oculo Auriculo Vertebral Spectrum); Goodpasture Syndrome; Hematuria, Benign, Familial; Hemolytic Uremic Syndrome; Hepatic Fibrosis, Congenital; IGA Nephropathy; Loken Senior Syndrome; MURCS Association; Medullary Cystic Disease; Medullary Sponge Kidney; Mullerian Aplasia; Myeloma, Multiple; N-Acetyl Glutamate Synthetase Deficiency; Nail Patella Syndrome; Ochoa Syndrome; Ornithine Transcarbamylase Deficiency; Polycystic Kidney Diseases; Purpura, Henoch Schonlein; Renal Agenesis, Bilateral; Renal Glycosuria; Retroperitoneal Fibrosis; WAGR Syndrome; Wegener's Granulomatosis; Wilms' Tumor

1864 NATIONAL LEAD INFORMATION CENTER (NLIC)

1025 Connecticut Avenue, NW
Suite 1200
Washington, DC 20036 202-293-2270
800-424-5323
Fax: 202-659-1192
TDD: 202-293-0113
E-mail: leadctr@nsc.org
http://www.nsc.org/ehc/lead.htm

The National Lead Information Center (NLIC) is a national not-for-profit environmental health organization dedicated to bringing the public, health, housing, and environmental communities together to combat childhood lead poisoning. A major cause of childhood lead poisoning is known to be old deteriorating lead-based paint (and the dust and contaminated soil that come from it) in 57 million residences in the United States. Established in 1992, NLIC is committed to providing accurate, timely information on lead poisoning prevention. The Center disseminates several informational pamphlets and brochures including "Questions Parents Ask About Lead Poisoning," "Home Repairs and Renovations: What You Should Know About Lead-Based Paint," and "Testing Your Home For Lead." NLIC also operates a web site on the Internet that can be reached at [http://www.nsc.org/ehc/lead.htm]. Resources available on the web site include general information on lead-based paints and lead poisoning prevention; information on the federal real estate notification and disclosure rules; state and local contacts for additional information on lead; links to other related web sites in both English and Spanish; and bibliographic citations for information on lead in soil, dust, and water. Also available on the web site is NLIC's quarterly newsletter "LeadInform."

President: Jerry Scannell
Executive Director: Bud Ward
Organization Language: Spanish (written/spoken).
Year Established: 1992
Organization Members: Non-Membership

Publishes the following materials:
NLIC List of Clearinghouse Materials ~ *Pamphlet*
EPA Lead Poisoning and your Children ~ *Brochure*
National Center for Lead-Safe Housing ~ *Mission Statement*
Questions Parents Ask About Lead Poisoning ~ *Fact Sheet*
Home Repairs and Renovations: What you should know about lead-based paint ~ *Fact Sheet*
EPA. HUD ~ *Fact Sheet*
Testing your home for lead ~ *Fact Sheet*
NLIC on the World Wide Web ~ *Fact Sheet*
State Contacts for Additional Information on Lead ~ *Leaflet*

Concerned with the following diseases or disorders:
Heavy Metal Poisoning

1865 NATIONAL LIPID DISEASES FOUNDATION

1201 Corbin Street
Elizabeth, NJ 07201 908-527-8000
800-527-8005
Fax: 908-527-8004

Established in 1965, the National Lipid Diseases Foundation is a voluntary not-for-profit organization dedicated to raising research funds for lipid storage diseases. Lipid storage diseases are a group of rare inherited metabolic disorders characterized by an abnormal accumulation of lipids (fatty or fatty-like substances) in different tissues of the body. Symptoms may vary greatly and depend on the affected organ system(s). The Foundation's funds currently go to Columbia Presbyterian Hospital to purchase research equipment and to Massachusetts General Hospital to support clinical research on Gaucher's Disease. The National Lipid Diseases Foundation provides referrals to those who are interested in receiving genetic counseling and/or educational materials concerning lipid storage diseases.

President: Harriet Klein
Executive Director: Joy Avidan
Year Established: 1965

Concerned with the following diseases or disorders:
Broad Beta Disease; Fabry Disease; I Cell Disease; Leukodystrophy, Metachromatic; Niemann Pick Disease; Schindler Disease

1866 NATIONAL LYMPHATIC AND VENOUS DISEASES FOUNDATION, INC. (NLVF)

255 Commandants Way
Chelsea, MA 02150 617-889-2103
800-301-2103
Fax: 617-887-1089

The National Lymphatic and Venous Foundation, Inc. is a not-for-profit organization dedicated to helping individuals affected by chronic lymphedema and venous diseases. Established in 1978, the Foundation has a nationwide membership. The National Lymphatic and Venous Foundation, Inc. provides appropriate referrals, including those to support groups; engages in patient advocacy; promotes legislation beneficial to affected individuals; and supports and promotes research. The Foundation also offers educational and support information to affected individuals, family members, and health care professionals through its database, regular newsletter, brochures, and audio-visual aids.

President: Mary F. Bellini (1987-Present)
Executive Director: Ellen Fox (Co-Founder)
Year Established: 1978
Organization Chapters: 6
Organization Members: 250

Concerned with the following diseases or disorders:
Cystic Hygroma; Lymphangioma, Cavernous; Lymphedema, Hereditary; Waldmann Disease

1867 NATIONAL LYMPHEDEMA NETWORK (NLN)

2211 Post Street
Suite 404
San Francisco, CA 94115-3427 415-921-1306
800-541-3259
Fax: 415-921-4284
E-mail: lymphnet@hooked.net
http://www.hooked.net/~lymphnet

The National Lymphedema Network (NLN) is a not-for-profit organization dedicated to providing education and support to affected individuals and health care professionals by disseminating information on the prevention and management of primary and secondary lymphedema. Established in 1988, the National Lymphedema Network provides a toll-free information hotline that offers 24-hour recorded information. NLN also offers emotional support and education as well as referrals to health care professionals, treatment centers, and local support groups. The Network is dedicated to supporting research into the causes of and possible alternative treatments for lymphedema; offering national educational conferences; and providing training workshops for health care professionals who are interested in organizing lymphedema treatment centers. NLN's long-term goal is to aid in the implementation of standardized quality treatment for lymphedema affected individuals nationwide. NLN provides a variety of educational materials to affected individuals, health care professionals, and the public. These materials include a quarterly newsletter, article reprints, brochures, and a Resource Guide that provides a listing of health care professionals and lymphedema treatment centers. The Network also maintains an informational database on lymphedema.

President: Saskia R.J. Thiadens, RN (1988-Present)
Executive Director: Saskia R. J. Thiadens
Organization Language: Dutch. German.
Year Established: 1988
Organization Chapters: 1
Organization Members: 2,500

Publishes the following materials:
Information About the NLN ~ *Factsheet*
Lymphedema Education Support Referral ~ *Brochure*
National Lymphedema Network Newsletter ~ *Newsletter*
Lymphedema Questionnaire ~ *Questionnaire*

Concerned with the following diseases or disorders:
Lymphedema, Hereditary

1868 NATIONAL MPS (MUCOPOLYSACCHARIDOSES/MUCOLIPIDOSES) SOCIETY, INC.

17 Kraemer Street
Hicksville, NY 11801 516-931-6338
Fax: 516-822-2041
E-mail: cohenZEE@aol.com
INATTIC1@aol.com
http://members.aol.com/mpssociety/index.html

The National MPS Society is a not-for-profit organization dedicated to acting as a support group for families affected by mucopolysaccharidoses (MPS) and other related disorders; increasing professional and public awareness; and raising funds to further research into such disorders. Mucopolysaccharidoses, mucolipidoses (ML), and other related disorders are rare inherited diseases in which the body is deficient in certain enzymes. As a result, progressive damage occurs as complex sugars and/or fats accumulate in various tissues of the body. Established in 1974, the National MPS Society promotes patient advocacy, provides referrals to genetic counseling and other services, and has established regional contact families to assist new families and conduct local support meetings. The National MPS Society produces a variety of educational and support materials including a membership directory, books, reports, brochures, videos of conferences, and a quarterly newsletter entitled "Courage." The Society also has a series of booklets on MPS and ML disorders that are designed to be daily living guides for families as well as tools for professionals who work with affected individuals. Support to families of children and young adults with mucopolysaccharide and related diseases.

President: Marie Capobianco (1978-Present)
Executive Director: Marie Capobianco
Year Established: 1974
Organization Chapters: 9
Organization Members: 800

Concerned with the following diseases or disorders:
Aspartylglycosaminuria; Fucosidosis; Hunter Syndrome; Hurler Syndrome; I Cell Disease; Mannosidosis; Maroteaux Lamy Syndrome; Morquio Syndrome; Mucopolysaccharidosis; Pseudo Hurler Polydystrophy; Sanfilippo Syndrome; Sialidosis; Sly Syndrome

1869 NATIONAL MARROW DONOR PROGRAM (NMDP)

3433 Broadway NE
Suite 500
Minneapolis, MN 55413 612-627-5800
800-526-7809
Fax: 612-627-5899
http://www.marrow.org

The National Marrow Donor Program (NMDP) is a not-for-profit organization dedicated to establishing, maintaining, and improving a system that provides transplants of bone marrow and other hematopoietic cells from volunteer, unrelated donors for individuals with leukemia and other life-threatening blood diseases. Established in 1988, NMDP maintains a registry of 2,795,616 volunteer marrow donors; its network consists of 101 donor centers, 114 collection centers, 107 transplant centers, and 12 recruitment centers. There is a special need for volunteer marrow donors from the African American, Asian/Pacific Islander, Hispanic, and American Indian/Alaskan Native communities. To address this need, NMDP is currently conducting four specially targeted national recruitment campaigns to increase Registry representation of minority volunteers. NMDP maintains a database on unrelated transplant outcomes for research, as well as an office of patient advocacy to assist affected individuals and their families regarding medical and financial concerns. Organizational materials include "Global Hope," "The Search Newsletter," and "The Marrow Messenger." NMDP maintains a web site at [http://www.marrow.org].

Executive Director: Craig W.S. Howe, M.D. (Chief Executive Officer)
Organization Language: Spanish (written/spoken).
Year Established: 1986
Organization Members: 322

Publishes the following materials:
Share Life ~ *Leaflet*
The Marrow Messenger ~ *Newsletter 1996*
The Search ~ *Newsletter Winter/Spring 1996*
The National Marrow Donor Program ~ *Mission Statement*
National Marrow Donor Program. Global Hope ~ *Fact Sheet*

1870 NATIONAL MENTAL HEALTH ASSOCIATION

1021 Prince Street
Alexandria, VA 22314-2971 703-684-7722
800-969-6642
Fax: 703-684-5968
TDD: 800-433-5959
E-mail: nmhainfo@aol.com
http://www.nmha.org

Established in 1909, the National Mental Health Association (NMHA) is a not-for-profit voluntary organization that addresses the mental health needs of individuals throughout the United States. The Association, which has over 300 affiliates in 35 states, has a network of volunteers across the country that work to meet the mental health needs of their communities. Activities include support groups, community outreach and education, information and referral programs, patient advocacy, and a wide array of other services. Nationally, the Association works with the media to keep the public informed about mental health and mental illness and with the Federal government to promote research and services for people with mental health problems. The Association also works with other major organizations to ensure that the nation's mental health needs are understood and addressed. Services include fact sheet and pamphlet distribution; buddy and companion programs; client services and case management; education and training programs; referral services; and social and recreational programs, workshops, and seminars. Educational materials distributed by the Association include quarterly newsletters entitled "Prevention Update" and "The Bell."

President: Michael Faenza
Executive Director: Rob Gabriel
Year Established: 1909
Organization Chapters: 300

Concerned with the following diseases or disorders:
Anorexia Nervosa; Antisocial Personality Disorder; Attention Deficit Hyperactivity Disorder; Autism; Bulimia; Conversion Disorder; Depersonalization Disorder; Dysthymia; Fetal Alcohol Syndrome; Kleine Levin Syndrome; Manic Depression, Bipolar; Mutism, Selective; Neurasthenia; Neuroleptic Malignant Syndrome; Obsessive Compulsive Disorder; Organic Mood Syndrome; Organic Personality Syndrome; Panic Anxiety Syndrome; Pica; Tardive Dyskinesia; Trichotillomania; XYY Syndrome

1871 NATIONAL MENTAL HEALTH CONSUMER SELF-HELP CLEARINGHOUSE (NMHCSHC)

1211 Chestnut Street
Philadelphia, PA 19107-4103 215-751-1810
800-553-4539
Fax: 215-636-6310
E-mail: thekey@delphi.com
http://www.kibertynet.org/~mha/cl_house.htm
l

The National Mental Health Consumer Self-Help Clearinghouse is a self-help, service, and advocacy organization that was established in 1985. The Clearinghouse handles thousands of inquiries annually from people who are concerned with mental health issues. Health care consumers, affected individuals, family members, professionals, and other interested people request information and technical assistance on locating local groups and becoming involved in the self-help movement. The Clearinghouse also provides on-site consultations to individuals and groups interested in mental health self-help group development. In addition, the Clearinghouse sponsors conferences and training events and has developed a wide variety of printed pamphlets and manuals on mental illness. A national quarterly newsletter entitled "The Key" provides assistance to affected individuals, their families, and physicians.

President: Joe Rogers
Executive Director: Marie D. Verna
Organization Language: Spanish.
Year Established: 1985
Organization Members: 8

Concerned with the following diseases or disorders:
Anorexia Nervosa; Antisocial Personality Disorder; Attention Deficit Hyperactivity Disorder; Autism; Bulimia; Conversion Disorder; Depersonalization Disorder; Dysthymia; Fetal Alcohol Syndrome; Kleine

Levin Syndrome; Manic Depression, Bipolar; Mutism, Selective; Neurasthenia; Neuroleptic Malignant Syndrome; Organic Mood Syndrome; Panic Anxiety Syndrome; Pica; Trichotillomania; XYY Syndrome

1872 NATIONAL ORGANIZATION FOR ALBINISM AND HYPOPIGMENTATION (NOAH)

1530 Locust Street
#29
Philadelphia, PA 19102 215-545-2322
800-473-2310
Fax: 609-858-4337
E-mail: noah@albinism.org
http://www.albinism.org

The National Organization for Albinism and Hypopigmentation (NOAH) is a national voluntary not-for-profit organization for people with albinism, their families, and professionals who work with them. Established in 1982, NOAH provides a network of local chapters and contact persons; offers information, support, and appropriate referrals; and promotes public and professional education. The organization also provides networking for those with special interests related to albinism and promotes and supports research and funding that will improve diagnosis and management of albinism and hypopigmentation. Through participating in the Albinism World Alliance, NOAH networks with support groups for people with albinism in other countries and promotes development of albinism support groups throughout the world. NOAH also sponsors workshops, conferences, and outreach programs and offers a variety of educational materials including a regular newsletter, information bulletins, brochures, and information packets for libraries.

President: Charla McMillan (1996-Present)
Organization Language: Spanish.
Year Established: 1982
Organization Chapters: 22
Organization Members: 1,000

Publishes the following materials:
Albinism ~ *Brochure*
Chapters ~ *Address List*
NOAH News ~ *Newsletter*
Social and Emotional Aspects of Albinism ~ *Brochure*
Assisting Students with Albinism ~ *Brochure*
What is Albinism? ~ *Brochure*
Resources for Persons with Albinism ~ *Brochure*
African Americans and Albinism ~ *Brochure*
Ocular Albinism ~ *Brochure*
Hermansky-Pudlak Syndrome ~ *Brochure*
Low Vision Aids ~ *Brochure*
Sun Protection ~ *Brochure*

Concerned with the following diseases or disorders:
Albinism; Chediak Higashi Syndrome; Waardenburg Syndrome

1873 NATIONAL ORGANIZATION FOR RARE DISORDERS, INC. (NORD)

P.O. Box 8923
New Fairfield, CT 06812-8923 203-746-6518
800-999-6673
Fax: 203-746-6481
TDD: 203-746-6927
E-mail: orphan@nord-rdb.com
http://www.nord-rdb.com/~orphan

The National Organization for Rare Disorders, Inc. (NORD) is a not-for-profit federation of voluntary health organizations dedicated to helping people with rare orphan diseases and assisting the organizations that serve them. Established in 1983, NORD, which played a pivotal role in the passage of the Orphan Drug Act, is committed to the identification, treatment, and cure of rare disorders through programs of education, advocacy, research, and service. NORD's primary goal is to educate the public as well as the medical community by serving as an international clearinghouse of information on rare "orphan" diseases (i.e., disorders that affect fewer than 200,000 people in the United States). Through its Rare Disease Database (RDB) NORD provides reports in understandable, layperson's terminology on more than 1,100 rare disorders. The organization also provides articles on thousands of additional rare disorders in response to inquiries from affected individuals, family members, medical professionals, researchers, educators, social workers, librarians, and the general public. NORD is also committed to increasing funding for clinical research for rare disorders. It works to fulfill this goal by funding "seed" grants for the investigation of new treatments for rare disorders, advocating for increased government research funds, and referring affected individuals to clinical trials and genetic investigations. In addition, the National Organization for Rare Disorders links thousands of families with others who have the same disorders through its Networking Program; gives referrals to additional organizations, clearinghouses, registries, and support groups that can benefit families with rare disorders; offers Medication Assistance Programs that provide certain prescription pharmaceuticals to needy patients who cannot afford to purchase them; and, through its Patient Services Department, advises affected individuals and family members who need assistance in accessing benefits and services in their local communities. The National Organization for Rare Disorders also sponsors an annual Patient/Family Conference to create opportunities for networking, support, information exchange, and medical community interface. The organization also conducts an annual conference for support group leaders and publishes a regular newsletter entitled "Orphan Disease Update." In addition to maintaining the reports within its Rare Disease Database, NORD also compiles the medical textbook "Physicians' Guide to Rare Diseases."

President: Abbey S. Meyers, Ph.D. (Honorary)
Year Established: 1983
Organization Chapters: 5
Organization Members: 103,000

Publishes the following materials:
Literature Order Form ~ *Order Form*
NORD Resource Guide (Third Edition) ~ *Book*
Orphan Disease Update ~ *Newsletter*
Physicians' Guide to Rare Diseases (Second Edition) ~ *Book*
Physician's Guide to NORD Services ~ *Brochure*
National Organization for Rare Disorders, Inc. ~ *Brochure*
Patient/Family Networking Program ~ *Form*
1,100 Disease Reports on Rare Disorders ~ *Report*
NORD Online Database Subscription Service ~ *Brochure*
1998 NORD 15th Anniversary Commemorative Calendar ~ *Calendar*
Patient/Family Conference ~ *Brochure*
Patient/Family Conference Tapes ~ *Audio Tapes*
Journal of Rare Diseases ~ *Journal*
Membership Application ~ *Form*

Concerned with the following diseases or disorders:
Birth Defects; Cardiovascular Diseases; Chromosomal Disorders; Connective Tissue Disorders; Dermatologic Disorders; Dysmorphic Syndromes; Endocrine Disorders; Environmental/Toxic Disorders; Gastrointestinal Disorders; Genetic Diseases; Genitourinary Disorders; Hematologic Disorders; Immunologic Disorders; Inborn Errors of Metabolism; Infectious Diseases; Mitochondrial Disorders; Neurologic Disorders; Oncologic Disorders; Ophthalmologic Disorders; Psychiatric Disorders; Renal Disorders; Respiratory Diseases

1874 NATIONAL ORGANIZATION OF SOCIAL SECURITY CLAIMANTS' REPRESENTATIVES (NOSSCR)

6 Prospect Street
Suite 2A
Midland Park, NJ 07424 201-444-1415
800-431-2804
Fax: 204-444-1823
E-mail: nosscr@worldnet.att.net
http://www.nosscr.org

The National Organization of Social Security Claimants' Representatives (NOSSCR) is a nonprofit professional advocacy organization dedicated to promoting a better understanding of Social Security law and procedure through research, discussion, and courses of study and encouraging a high standard of representation for all individuals seeking benefits through the Social Security Administration. Established in 1979, NOSSCR has more than 3,000 members including attorneys, non-attorney representatives, and others who work in the field of Social Security Disability Law. NOSSCR provides several services to help Social Security and SSI claimants' representatives ensure the highest legal representation for their clients. Social services include sponsoring two annual national continuing legal education conferences; providing a research clearinghouse for practitioners, including briefs, case citations, memoranda of law, questionnaires, etc.; providing assistance with complex research problems; monitoring class actions of national and statewide scope; and publishing a monthly newsletter entitled the "Social Security Forum," which follows current developments at the Social Security Administration, in the federal courts, in legal practice, and in federal legislation. NOSSCR also has a web site on the Internet at [http://www.nosscr.org].

President: Shelley Davidson (1996 to Present)
Executive Director: Nancy G. Shor
Organization Language: Spanish (written).
Year Established: 1979
Organization Members: 3,100

Publishes the following materials:
NOSSCR ~ *Mission Statement*
Social Security Disability and SSI Claims. Your Need For Representation (Spanish) ~ *Brochure*
Social Security Disability and SSI Claims. Your Need For Representation ~ *Brochure*
Research Materials ~ *List*
NOSSCR Social Security Forum ~ *Newsletter August 1996*

1875 **NATIONAL ORGANIZATION ON DISABILITY (NOD)**

910 16th Street NW
Suite 600
Washington, DC 20006 202-293-5960
Fax: 202-293-7999
TDD: 202-293-5968
E-mail: ability@nod.org
http://www.nod.org

The National Organization on Disability (NOD) is a not-for-profit organization dedicated to promoting the full and equal participation of America's 49 million men, women, and children with disabilities in all aspects of life. NOD was founded in 1982 at the conclusion of the United Nations International Year of Disabled Persons. NOD is the only national disability network organization concerned with all disabilities, all age groups, and all disability issues. NOD believes real change takes place in the communities where America's 49 million men, women, and children with disabilities go about their lives. People with disabilities want to and can participate in and contribute to the life of their community; full participation of people with disabilities can best be achieved by fostering partnerships of individuals with and without disabilities. Closing the significant gap in the levels of participation between persons with and without disabilities is good for America and for all its citizens. Consisting of 4,500 members and 250 chapters, NOD produces educational materials including fact sheets, brochures, a directory, and various booklets including "From Barriers To Bridges" and "Loving Justice." Program activities include the Community Partnership Program, a nationwide network of towns, cities, and counties that promote the replication of effective local disability programs; the National Organization Partnership Program, which assists 35 national non-disability associations in promoting disability action programs among their local affiliates; the CEO Council, which promotes expanded employment of people with disabilities through recognition of corporate leaders and their companies; the Religion and Disability program, which helps congregations of all faiths become more accessible and welcoming to people with disabilities; the Start On Success (S.O.S) student internship program, which provides paid internships to high school students with disabilities to give them first time work experience and to increase their chances for future self-sufficiency; the Attitude Surveying Program, which provides reliable disability data on attitudes and stereotypes so that public acceptance will be more readily achieved; and the World Committee on Disability, NOD's international arm, which promotes commitment and action by international organizations and leaders of nations in furtherance of the United Nations World Programme Of Action Concerning Disabled Persons.

President: Alan A. Reich
Organization Language: Spanish (spoken).
Year Established: 1982
Organization Chapters: 250
Organization Members: 4,500

Publishes the following materials:
A Ramp is Not Enough. Art the gifts of people with disabilities welcomed in your congregation and community? ~ *Brochure*
NOD Fact Sheet ~ *Mission Statement*
Community Partnership Program ~ *Fact Sheet*
National Organization Partnership Program ~ *Leaflet*

1876 **NATIONAL PARENT NETWORK ON DISABILITIES (NPND)**

1200 G Street North West
Suite 800
Washington, DC 20005 202-434-8686
Fax: 202-638-0509
TDD: 202-434-8686
E-mail: npnd@cs.com
http://www.npnd.org

The National Parent Network on Disabilities is a voluntary not-for-profit coalition of parent organizations, specific disability organizations, professionals who work with persons with disabilities, and concerned friends. It was established in 1988 to provide a presence and a national voice for parents of children, youth, and adults with special needs. The National Parent Network on Disabilities provides up-to-date reporting on governmental policy and planning; provides a strong advocacy voice to communicate the needs of its members; and maintains a system of sharing experiences that can be used to develop effective policy recommendations. It shares its resources and information in order to promote and support parents' abilities to influence policy issues concerning the needs of people with disabilities and their families. In addition, the Network provides appropriate referrals and offers a variety of educational and support materials including brochures, reports, and a regular newsletter.

President: Joanne Butts (1994-Present)
Executive Director: Patricia McGill Smith
Year Established: 1988
Organization Members: 525

NPPSIS News (Spring 1997) ~ *Newsletter*
Tips for Networking ~ *Fact Sheet*
NPPSIS Facts ~ *Fact Sheet*
The goals of NPPSIS ~ *Mission Statement*
Fact Sheet ~ *Fact Sheet*

1877 NATIONAL PARENT TO PARENT SUPPORT AND INFORMATION SYSTEM, INC. (NPPSIS)

P.O. Box 907
Blue Ridge, GA 30513 706-632-8822
800-651-1151
Fax: 706-632-8830
TDD: 706-632-8822
E-mail: judd103w@wonder.em.cdc.gov
http://www.NPPSIS.org

The National Parent To Parent Support and Information System, Inc. (NPPSIS) is a not-for-profit organization dedicated to strengthening, supporting, and empowering families by establishing one to one parent to parent contacts. NPPSIS enhances the ability of parents to access services and resources for children with special needs by providing information and resources to parents, professionals, and other health related disability organizations. Established in 1994, NPPSIS nationally links families whose children have rare disorders or special health care needs; provides parents with local, state, and national information, resources, and referrals to appropriate services; supports and empowers families to participate in parent programs and disability organizations; and provides information to professionals on national parent support and disability issues. Educational materials consist of a quarterly newsletter entitled "NPPSIS News" and a fact sheet containing managed care information.

President: Kathleen Judd
Organization Language: Spanish (written).
Year Established: 1994
Organization Members: Non-Membership

Publishes the following materials:
National Parent to Parent Support and Information System, Inc. ~ *Mission Statement*
Family Information ~ *Application*
Family Resource Sheet on Managed Care ~ *Factsheet*
Matches Matches Matches ~ *News Release*
Homeschool Resources ~ *Resource List*
Resources for Starting a Parent to Parent Program ~ *Resource List*
Outline of Listening Skills ~ *Outline*
Parent Information ~ *Networking Form*
Dear Parent, November 27, 1995 ~ *Letter*
Directory Resource Form ~ *Resource Form*
Grantee Information ~ *Information Sheet*
National Parent to Parent Support & Information System, Inc. ~ *Brochure*

1878 NATIONAL PATIENT AIR TRANSPORT HELPLINE (NPATH)

P.O. Box 1940
Manassas, VA 20108-0804 703-361-1191
800-296-1217
Fax: 703-361-1792
E-mail: npath@aol.com
http://www.mercymedical.org

The National Patient Air Transport Helpline (NPATH) is operated by Mercy Medical Airlift (MMA) and Children's Transport for Life (CTL), and all organizations dedicated to facilitating charitable medical transportation on a national level. MMA and CTL fund and operate NPATH on behalf of the Air Care Alliance (ACA) and the entire national charitable air medical transport systems. Founded in 1984, NPATH provides services for those who must find a way to travel considerable distances for specialized evaluation, diagnosis, treatment, rehabilitation, and/or recovery necessitated by illness or accidents. The organization also gives information to health care professionals who must find the most cost-effective way to move affected individuals and their family members long distances as well as volunteer pilots who wish to serve with one of the volunteer pilot agencies that are part of the ACA. A 24 hour "helpline" is available so that individuals can access available resources. Referrals are based on an evaluation of the patient's medical condition, type of transport required, and departure/destination locations. This service is staffed by people who take the time to explain all known appropriate options.

President: Dr. Pierpont Buck (1994 to Present).
Executive Director: Edward R. Beyer
Year Established: 1984
Organization Members: Non-Membership

Publishes the following materials:
N-P-A-T-H ~ *Referral List*
National Patient Air Transport Helpline ~ *Brochure*

1879 NATIONAL PERINATAL ASSOCIATION (NPA)

3500 East Fletcher Avenue
Suite 209
Tampa, FL 33613 813-971-1008
Fax: 813-971-9306
E-mail: npaonline@aol.com

The National Perinatal Association (NPA) is a voluntary organization dedicated to perinatal health issues from preconception through infancy within a multicultural perspective. Established in 1976, NPA fosters optimal perinatal care by promoting education, supporting research, influencing national priorities, and encouraging collaboration among all concerned constituencies, including health care providers and consumers. Consisting of 1,111 members and approximately 45 chapters, NPA produces educational materials including a self-titled brochure, a journal flyer, the bimonthly "Journal of Perinatology," audiotapes, and various bulletins. The NPA holds an annual clinical conference and exhibition; works to construct a national framework for advocacy; strives to increase multidisciplinary involvement and understanding; conducts educational seminars; offers speakers from varied disciplines; and holds an annual fund-raiser.

President: Maureen Greer (1997 to Present)
Executive Director: Julie Leachman
Year Established: 1976
Organization Chapters: 45
Organization Members: 1,111

Publishes the following materials:
National Perinatal Association ~ *Brochure*
Bulletin ~ *Newsletter*
Network ~ *Pamphlet*

1880 NATIONAL PERINATAL INFORMATION CENTER (NPIC)

One State Street
Suite 102
Providence, RI 02908 401-274-0650
Fax: 401-455-0377
http://www.npic.org

The National Perinatal Information Center is a not-for-profit organization dedicated to serving the perinatal medical community through providing information, performing research, and conducting educational programs. Established in 1985, the NPIC strives to develop a solid research program for maternal and child health; to enhance the present state of perinatal health care and increase the awareness of its importance to the medical community; and to provide information, education, and, when necessary, consultations on perinatal health care. Educational materials include a newsletter entitiled "NPIC Newsletter" and brochures. Program services include a directory, reports, networking, and lobbying efforts.

President: David E. Gagnon
Year Established: 1985

Publishes the following materials:
National Perinatal Information Center ~ *Brochure*
NPIC Newsletter (December 1996) ~ *Newsletter*
NPIC Newsletter (March 1997) ~ *Newsletter*

1881 NATIONAL PLATELET ASSOCIATION (NPA)

2807 Fifth Avenue
Baltimore, MD 21234-3009 410-668-9346
E-mail: ebunker@platelet.org
http://www.platelet.org

The National Platelet Association (NPA) is a grassroots voluntary organization dedicated to increasing public awareness about the need for a large and diverse pool of platelet donors. Platelets are a component of the blood that aid in the clotting process. Platelets donated by human volunteers are used in the treatment of cancers, aplastic anemia, leukemia, and other medical conditions. Established in 1996 and consisting of 20 members, the Association, along with a group of platelet donors, recruitment professionals, patient advocates, and representatives from various non-profit organizations, joined together to promote "National Platelet Awareness Week." This is a strategy for increasing public awareness about the need for a larger and more diverse pool of platelet donors.

President: Edward B. Bunker, M.P.H. (May 1996 to Present)
Year Established: 1996
Organization Members: 20

Publishes the following materials:
National Platelet Donation Awareness Week ~ *Pamphlet*
National Platelet Association. Volunteers Helping Patients Who Need Platelets ~ *Pamphlet*

1882 NATIONAL REGISTRY FOR ICHTHYOSIS AND RELATED DISORDERS

University of Washington
Dermatology Department, Box 356524
1959 N.E. Pacific
Seattle, WA 98195-6524 206-616-3179
800-595-1265
Fax: 206-616-4302
E-mail: fleck@u.washington.edu or
geoff@u.washington.edu

The mission of the National Registry for Ichthyosis and Related Disorders is to identify individuals and families in the United States with the Ichthyoses and related disorders and to encourage them to participate in the registry. The Ichthyoses are a group of rare, inherited disorders characterized by abnormally dry, scaly, thickened skin due to abnormalities in the production of the protein keratin. The goal of the Registry is to obtain data for study by skin biologists, pharmacologists, and other scientists in order to promote research into the diagnosis and treatment of these disorders. Interested individuals will be asked to complete a "Patient Enrollment Form"; their physicians will need to complete the "Physician's Form." The Registry is supported by the National Institutes of Health, The Society of Investigative Dermatology, and the Foundation for Ichthyosis and Related Skin Types (FIRST). Individuals with Ichthyosis Vulgaris are not included in this registry.

President: Geoffrey W. Hamil, R.N. (1995 to present) (Coordinator)
Executive Director: Philip Gleckman, M.D. (Principal Investigator)
Year Established: 1994

Publishes the following materials:
National Registry for Ichthyosis and Related Disorders ~ *Patient Enrollment Form*
National Registry for Ichthyosis and Related Disorders ~ *Patient Enrollment Form*

Concerned with the following diseases or disorders:
Cardio Facio Cutaneous Syndrome; Erythrokeratodermia with Ataxia; Ichthyosis; Ichthyosis Congenita; Ichthyosis Hystrix, Curth Macklin Type; Ichthyosis Vulgaris; Ichthyosis, Erythrokeratodermia Progressiva Symmetrica; Ichthyosis, Harlequin Type; Ichthyosis, Keratosis Follicularis Spinulosa Decalvans; Ichthyosis, Lamellar Recessive; Ichthyosis, Netherton Syndrome; Ichthyosis, Tay Syndrome; Ichthyosis, X-Linked; Refsum Syndrome

1883 NATIONAL REHABILITATION ASSOCIATION (NRA)

633 South Washington Street
Alexandria, VA 22314 703-836-0850
Fax: 703-836-0848
TDD: 703-836-0849
http/www.allware.com/rehab/

The National Rehabilitation Association (NRA) is a national not-for-profit professional organization dedicated to advocating, supporting, and enhancing the lives of individuals with disabilities and their families. Established in 1925, the Association is the oldest and largest advocacy organization for individuals with disabilities. The NRA disseminates up-to-date information, conducts educational seminars, and provides opportunities through knowledge and diversity for professionals in the field of rehabilitation. The National Rehabilitation Association has approximately 11,000 members and 69 chapters across the country. It produces educational materials such as the "The Journal of Rehabilitation" and "Contemporary Rehab." In addition, the Association sponsors an annual training conference with exhibits displaying the latest in rehabilitation technologies, gives out annual awards to individuals and organizations who make major contributions in the field of rehabilitation, and provides access to a nationwide employment network.

President: Brian Fitzgibbons
Executive Director: Michelle Vaughn (Acting Executive Director)
Year Established: 1925
Organization Chapters: 69
Organization Members: 11,000

Publishes the following materials:
National Rehabilitation Association - Seventy Years ~ *Brochure*
National Rehabilitation Association ~ *Brochure*
Contemporary Rehab ~ *Newsletter*
The Journal of Rehabilitation ~ *Booklet*

1884 NATIONAL REHABILITATION INFORMATION CENTER (NARIC)

8455 Colesville Road
Suite 935
Silver Spring, MD 20190-3319 301-588-9284
800-346-2742
Fax: 301-587-1967
TDD: 301-495-5626
E-mail: naric@capaccess.org
http://www.naric.com/naric

Funded by the National Institute on Disability and Rehabilitation Research (NIDRR), the National Rehabilitation Information Center (NARIC) was established in 1977 as a national disability and rehabilitation library and information center that collects and disseminates the results of NIDRR-funded research projects. The collection, which now has more than 50,000 documents on all aspects of disability and rehabilitation, includes commercially published books, journal articles, and audiovisual aids. NARIC also has several databases available that provide abstracts on NARIC's entire library collection; list national disability-related organizations and directories; describe journals and newsletters related to disability or rehabilitation; and contain information on current and past NIDRR-funded projects. NARIC's professionally trained Information Specialists will provide customized searches of its various databases (sometimes for a small fee). NARIC also provides resource guides on various topics and a variety of resources and directories.

Executive Director: Mark X. Odum
Organization Language: American Sign Language.
Year Established: 1977

Publishes the following materials:
NARIC Quarterly ~ *Newsletter*
New Publications Address Consumer and Practitioner Needs ~ *Information Directory*
NARIC Publications List & Order Form ~ *Order Form*
1994 Calendar of Events in Disability, Rehabilitation, and Assistive Technology ~ *List of Events*
REHABDATA ~ *Brochure*
NARIC ~ *Brochure*
The Able Inform ~ *Brochure*
ABLEDATA Serving the Nation ~ *Brochure*
ABLEDATA on CD-ROM ~ *Brochure*

Concerned with the following diseases or disorders:
Phocomelia Syndrome

1885 NATIONAL RESOURCE CENTER ON HOMELESSNESS AND MENTAL ILLNESS (NRCHMI)

Policy Research Associates, Inc.
262 Delaware Avenue
Delmar, NY 12054 518-439-7415
800-444-7415
Fax: 518-439-7612
E-mail: nrc@prainc.com
http://www.prainc.com/nrc

The National Resource Center on Homelessness and Mental Illness (NRCHMI) is the only national technical assistance center specifically focused on the needs of people who are homeless and have serious mental illness. Established in 1988, the NRCHMI, which receives federal funding from the Center for Mental Health Services (CMHS), Bethesda, Maryland, provides on-site technical assistance to CMHS grantees on system integration, mental health treatment, and housing for people who are homeless; telephone consultation to other providers, researchers, and policy makers; targeted workshops and training institutes; and papers on emerging topics. NRCHMI's materials include a free periodic bulletin entitled "Access," a resource list entitled "National Organizations Concerned with Mental Health, Housing, and Homelessness," a series of annotated bibliographies on topics related to homelessness and serious mental illness, and an extensive database of published and unpublished materials to assist researchers and others. The NRCHMI also has a web site on the Internet at [http://www.prainc.com/nrc].

President: Henry J. Steadman, Ph.D. (Director)
Executive Director: Deborah Dennis, M.A.
Year Established: 1988
Organization Members: 5,500

Publishes the following materials:
The National Resource Center on Homelessness and Mental Illness ~ *Brochure*
Access ~ *Newsletter*
National Resource Center on Homelessness and Mental Illness ~ *Fact Sheet*
NRC Publications ~ *Fact Sheet*
Homeless Programs Branch ~ *Fact Sheet*

1886 NATIONAL RESPITE LOCATOR SERVICE

800 Eastowne Drive
Suite 105
Chapel Hill, NC 27514-2204 919-490-5577
800-773-5433
Fax: 919-490-4905
E-mail: HN4735@connectinc.com
http://www.chtop.com/locator.htm

The National Respite Locator Service is a national not-for-profit organization dedicated to assisting parents, caregivers and professionals find temporary relief "respite" services in their state and local area. Established in 1994, the National Respite Locator Service provides care for children with disabilities, chronic or terminal illnesses, and to children at risk of abuse and neglect. The National Respite Locator Service provides appropriate referrals for further assistance and has a leaflet describing the organization.

Executive Director: Linda Baker
Year Established: 1994

Publishes the following materials:
The National Respite Locator Sevice ~ *Mission Statement*

1887 NATIONAL RESPITE NETWORK

800 Eastowne Drive
Suite 105
Chapel Hill, NC 27514-2204 919-490-5577
800-473-1727
Fax: 919-490-4905
E-mail: HN4735@connectinc.com
http://www.chtop.com/nrn.htm

The National Respite Network (NRN) is a national not-for-profit organization dedicated to keeping families together by promoting the development of respite options nationwide. For caregivers in stressful situations, respite provides temporary relief from the ongoing responsibilities of caring for loved ones in the home. Established in 1994, the NRN is committed to providing information, training, and referral services to families, caregivers, agencies, and other organizations seeking respite options; offering information, training, and consultation to programs and agencies interested in initiating or expanding respite options for caregivers; providing information regarding public policy initiatives in areas of respite, caregiver, and family support services; increasing public awareness regarding the needs of families and caregivers; and promoting the expansion of respite services through research, evaluation, and other initiatives. The NRN has two major divisions. It offers nationwide training, consultation, and technical assistance through The ARCH National Resource Center for Respite and Crisis Care Services. ARCH's professional staff offers training and technical assistance to state and local agencies to assist their efforts in developing and maintaining effective respite programs. NRN also has a national policy division, which includes The National Respite Coalition, an advocacy organization for parents, health care professionals, and others that provides information and teaching tools to respite advocates throughout the country. NRN also offers a National Respite Locator Service for providers and families at (800) 7 RELIEF, engages in lobbying efforts, and offers a variety of educational materials for parents, caregivers, service providers, advocates, and others. Such materials include a regular newsletter, a directory of national resource organizations, fact sheets, a lending library catalog, public awareness packets, training guides, National Respite Locator Service insert and rolodex card, and more. The NRN also has a web site on the Internet at [http://www.chtop.com/nrn.htm].

Executive Director: Linda Baker
Year Established: 1994
Organization Members: 375

Publishes the following materials:
ARCH Product List ~ *Resource List*
Strengthening Familes and Caregivers Through Respite Services ~ *Mission Statement*
Respite for Children with Disabilities ~ *Factsheet*
Siblings of Children with Special Health and Developmental Needs ~ *Factsheet*
Nurturing Our Children, Building a Future ~ *Annual Report*
Say "Hello" to Relief ~ *Insert*
Access to Respite Care and Help ~ *Brochure*
National Respite Network ~ *Mission Statement*

1888 NATIONAL SELF-HELP CLEARINGHOUSE

25 West 43rd Street
Suite 620
New York, NY 10036 212-354-8525
Fax: 212-642-1956
http://www.selfhelpweb.org

The National Self-Help Clearinghouse is a self-help organization dedicated to facilitating access to self-help groups and increasing the awareness of the importance of mutual support. Established in 1978, the clearinghouse conducts training for self-help group leaders and professionals about self-help and ways to work with mutual aid groups; carries out research activities; and maintains a database of information and referrals to self-help groups. Educational materials include training materials and a periodic newsletter entitled "The Self-Help Reporter." The Clearinghouse maintains a World Wide Web site at [http://www.selfhelp.org].

President: Frank Riessman (Director)
Year Established: 1978
Organization Members: Non-Membership

Publishes the following materials:
The Self-Help Reporter ~ *Newsletter*
National Self-Help Clearinghouse ~ *Brochure*

1889 NATIONAL SHARED HOUSING RESOURCE CENTER (NSHRC)

321 East 25th Street
Baltimore, MD 21218 410-235-4454
Fax: 410-235-4454

The National Shared Housing Resource Center (NSHRC) is a nonprofit volunteer organization dedicated to promoting shared living as an affordable and secure housing option. The National Shared Housing Resource Center's goal is to return the national office to its status as a true resource center for shared housing consumers and the general public. Established in 1981, the NSHRC focuses on linking consumers to existing programs and linking programs to each other through volunteer regional coordinators. Consisting of 300 members, the organization produces educational materials including conference opportunities for its membership, information about shared housing for the general public, and a quarterly newsletter. Services include public advocacy on issues that affect shared housing and referrals.

President: Marjorie Marlin and Helen Head
Year Established: 1981
Organization Members: 300

Publishes the following materials:
National Shared Housing Resource Center ~ *Mission Statement*
Shared Housing News ~ *Newsletter*

1890 NATIONAL SLEEP FOUNDATION (NSF)

729 15th Street, NW
4th Floor
Washington, D.C. 20005 202-347-3471
Fax: 202-347-3472
E-mail: natsleep@erols.com
http://www.sleepfoundation.org

The National Sleep Foundation (NSF) is a not-for-profit organization dedicated to improving the quality of life for those who are affected by sleep disorders (e.g., Sleep Apnea, Narcolepsy, Restless Legs Syndrome, and Periodic Limb Movement Disorder) and preventing accidents related to sleep deprivation or sleep disorders. Established in 1991, the National Sleep Foundation increases public awareness of sleep disorders through all forms of media; encourages the development of patient services, community resources, and support groups for affected individuals; and creates partnerships with business and government to extend its educational reach. The National Sleep Foundation also provides referrals to regional sleep disorder centers; conducts symposia for physicians across the United States; and provides research grants and fellowships. The Foundation offers a variety of educational and supportive information through its database, brochures and pamphlets designed for physicians and the general public, a regular newsletter for physicians entitled "Sleep Medicine Alert," and "NSF Connection," a newsletter for the public.

President: Lorraine L. Wearley, Ph.D.
Executive Director: Reid Blank
Year Established: 1990
Organization Members: 600

Publishes the following materials:
The Nature of Sleep and Its Disorders ~ *Pamphlet*
Drive Alert Arrive Alive ~ *Brochure*
Wake Up ~ *Pamphlet*
Understanding Narcolepsy ~ *Pamphlet*
When You Can't Sleep ABCs of ZZZs ~ *Pamphlet*
National Sleep Foundation ~ *Brochure*
The NSF Connection ~ *Newsletter*
Sleep Medicine Review ~ *Newsletter for Physicians*

Concerned with the following diseases or disorders:
Kleine Levin Syndrome

1891 NATIONAL SPINAL CORD INJURY ASSOCIATION (NSCIA)

8300 Colesville Road
Suite 551
Silver Spring, MD 20910 301-588-6959
800-962-9629
Fax: 301-588-9414
E-mail: NSCIA2@aol.com
http://www.spinalcord.org

The National Spinal Cord Injury Association is a not-for-profit, voluntary organization dedicated to enabling people with spinal cord injury (SCI) to make choices and take actions to achieve their highest level of independence and personal fulfillment. Spinal cord injury results from trauma to or disease of the spinal cord. The primary result of SCI is paralysis. Established in 1948 as a response to the medical and social problems that result from injury to the spinal cord, NSCIA has 12,000 members with 55 chapters and support groups. Members are encouraged to help with peer-to-peer counseling, disability rights, and general advocacy. The National Spinal Cord Injury Association has an Early Intervention Project that provides comprehensive vocational and rehabilitative services immediately after spinal cord injury; an Employment Opportunity Program that serves persons with a wide range of disabilities who are seeking comprehensive employment services; and "teleconferences" and "videoconferences" for SCI professionals and consumers. Educational materials include a quarterly magazine entitled "SCI Life," fact sheets pertaining to various aspects of Spinal Cord injuries, and audiotape lectures. NSCIA maintains a web site at [http://www.spinalcordorg],and e-mail at [NSCIA2@AOL.com].

President: Mark X. Odum (1995 to Present)
Executive Director: Thomas H. Countee, Jr., Esq.
Year Established: 1948
Organization Chapters: 33
Organization Members: 6,000

Publishes the following materials:
National Spinal Cord Injury Asssociation In Brief ~ *Mission Statement*
Thomas Hilaire Countee, Jr ~ *Resume*
Every day more than thirty people become paralyzed ~ *Brochure*
Common Questions About Spinal Cord Injury. Factsheet 1 ~ *Pamphlet*

Spinal Cord Injury Statistical Information. Factsheet 2 ~ *Pamphlet*
Sexuality After Spinal Cord Injury. Factsheet 3 ~ *Pamphlet*
Choosing A Spinal Cord Injury Rehab Program. Factsheet 4 ~ *Pamphlet*
What's New in Cure and Treatment Research? Factsheet 5 ~ *Pamphlet*
The Importance of Basic Science in Research. Factsheet 6 ~ *Pamphlet*
Tendon Transfer Surgery to Restore Hand Function in Persons with Quadriplegia. Factsheet 7 ~ *Pamphlet*
SCI Awareness: The Importance of Language and Images. Factsheet 8 ~ *Pamphlet*
Functional Electrical Stimulation, Clinical Applications. Factsheet 9 ~ *Pamphlet*
Male Reproductive Function After Spinal Cord Injury. Factsheet 10 ~ *Pamphlet*
What is a Physiatrist? Factsheet 11 ~ *Fact Sheet*
Medical Facilities and Resources for Ventilator Users. Factsheet 12 ~ *Pamphlet*
Reading Resources. Factsheet 13 ~ *Pamphlet*
Resources for Pediatric Spinal Cord Injury. Factgsheet 14 ~ *Pamphlet*
Travel After Spinal Cord Injury. Factsheet 15 ~ *Pamphlet*
What is Autonomic Dysreflexia? Factsheet 17 ~ *Pamphlet*
Starting a support group or a discussion group. Factsheet 18 ~ *Pamphlet*

Concerned with the following diseases or disorders:
Arachnoiditis; Syringobulbia

1892 NATIONAL SPINAL CORD INJURY HOTLINE

2200 Kernan Drive
Baltimore, MD 21207 410-448-6623
800-526-3456
Fax: 410-448-6627
E-mail: SCIHOTLINE@aol.com
http://users.aol.com/scihotline

Established in 1984, the National Spinal Cord Injury Hotline, a not-for-profit organization, is a toll-free information and referral service that is available to individuals who have sustained a traumatic spinal cord injury. The staff is composed of medical professionals and health administrators. The Hotline facilitates the callers' search for support and resources by referring them to others who have personal experience or to professionals with expertise in spinal cord injuries. Referrals to a wide variety of resources include rehabilitation facilities and other spinal cord injury organizations. The Hotline works with people with spinal cord injuries and their families to find answers to questions ranging from therapeutic programs to house modifications, from medical equipment to sports and recreation.

Executive Director: Cindy Miller
Year Established: 1984

Publishes the following materials:
National Spinal Cord Injury Hotline ~ *Factsheet*

Concerned with the following diseases or disorders:
Arachnoiditis; Stenosis, Spinal; Syringobulbia; Syringomyelia

1893 NATIONAL TAY-SACHS AND ALLIED DISEASES ASSOCIATION, INC. (NTSAD)

2001 Beacon Street
Suite 204
Brookline, MA 02146-4227 617-277-4463
800-906-8723
Fax: 617-277-0134
E-mail: NTSAD-Boston@worldnet.att.net
mcrcr2.med.nyu.edu/~murphp01/taysachs.htm

The National Tay-Sachs and Allied Diseases Association, Inc. (NTSAD) is a voluntary not-for-profit health organization dedicated to the prevention and eradication of Tay-Sachs and 40 related genetic disorders. Established in 1956, the Association has expanded to encompass active chapters in major metropolitan areas, a Scientific Advisory Committee, and a Parent Peer Support Group that extends worldwide. Through the guidance and expertise of its Scientific Advisory Committee, the Association promotes Tay-Sachs carrier screening, sponsors a Tay-Sachs Laboratory Quality Control Program, and publishes a current listing of participating labs. It approves candidates for research fellowships and maintains a repository of specialized knowledge for affected individuals, family members, health care professionals, and others who seek a greater understanding of lysosomal storage diseases. The Association also conducts an annual conference and provides support, referral, and advocacy services from its national office and affiliate chapters. In addition, the National Tay-Sachs and Allied Diseases Association offers a variety of educational and support materials. These materials include a directory of families, a directory of Tay-Sachs Test Centers, regular newsletters, fact sheets, brochures, videos, and a child care manual. The Association also provides a lending library and a traveling educational display.

President: Yvonne Sacks (1993-Present)
Executive Director: Debbi Gutter, MSW
Year Established: 1956
Organization Chapters: 7
Organization Members: 2,000

Publishes the following materials:
Tay-Sachs Is ~ *Brochure*
Tay-Sachs Is (Ukranian) ~ *Brochure*
There is only one child in the world and the child's name is ALL Children ~ *Brochure*
Breakthrough ~ *Newsletter*
Adult Onset Tay-Sachs Disease ~ *Bibliography*
Parent Peer Group Lending Library Booklet ~ *Fact Sheet*
Late Onset Tay-Sachs Disease ~ *Fact Sheet*
Tay-Sachs - The Dreaded Inheritance ~ *Reprint*
The NTSAD Family ~ *Brochure*
What Every Family Should Know ~ *Booklet*
The Home Care Book ~ *Booklet*
Prevent A Tragedy 1995 Test Center Directory ~ *Booklet*

Concerned with the following diseases or disorders:
Acanthocytosis; Batten Disease; Fabry Disease; Fucosidosis; Kufs Disease; Leukodystrophy; Leukodystrophy, Canavan's; Leukodystrophy, Metachromatic; Multiple Sulfatase Deficiency; Niemann Pick Disease; Sandhoff Disease; Santavuori Disease; Schindler Disease; Tangier Disease; Tay Sachs Disease

1894 NATIONAL UREA CYCLE DISORDERS FOUNDATION (NUCDF)

P.O. Box 32
Sayreville, NJ 08872
800-386-8233
E-mail: lemons@interserv.com
http://www.execpc.com/~fenders/nucdf.html

The National Urea Cycle Disorders Foundation is a voluntary not-for-profit organization dedicated to providing information and guidance to families affected by urea cycle disorders; educating health care professionals concerning the diagnosis and treatment of these disorders; and increasing public awareness. Urea cycle disorders are rare genetic disorders in which an enzyme deficiency causes an excessive accumulation of ammonia in the blood. Established in 1989, the National Urea Cycle Disorders Foundation is also committed to promoting and supporting medical research; networking families to promote the exchange of mutual support, information, and resources; and educating legislators on the needs of affected families. In addition, the Foundation provides appropriate referrals; engages in patient, professional, and community education; and offers educational and supportive information through its national database, directory, biannual newsletter, brochures, and pamphlets. The Foundation's goals include creating a national network of families who together can stimulate medical research activities and eventually find a cure for urea cycle disorders.

President: Chip Bagnal
Executive Director: Cynthia Le Mons
Year Established: 1989
Organization Members: 410

Publishes the following materials:
National Urea Cycle Foundation ~ *Brochure*
National Urea Cycle Disorders Foundation Membership Directory ~ *Directory*
Urea Cycle Disorders ~ *Pamphlet*

Concerned with the following diseases or disorders:
Arginase Deficiency; Arginino Succinic Aciduria; Carbamyl Phosphate Synthetase Deficiency; Citrullinemia; Glutaricaciduria I; Glutaricaciduria II; N-Acetyl Glutamate Synthetase Deficiency; Ornithine Transcarbamylase Deficiency

1895 NATIONAL VASCULAR MALFORMATIONS FOUNDATION, INC. (NVMF)

8320 Nightingale
Dearborn Heights, MI 48127 313-274-1243
Fax: 313-274-1243

The National Vascular Malformations Foundation, Inc. is a voluntary not-for-profit organization established to help anyone affected by vascular malformations. Vascular malformations are tumors or flat lesions consisting of abnormally sized blood vessels; such abnormal growths may occur anywhere in the body. The Foundation is committed to promoting and supporting biomedical research in all aspects of such disorders; providing information concerning the latest medical findings; and sponsoring national and international meetings among the medical professions for the exchange of information concerning progress in this field. The Foundation is also committed to giving financial assistance to affected individuals who cannot afford the necessary treatment; developing a National Vascular Malformations Center; and providing educational funds for doctoral and postdoctoral studies for specialization in the study and treatment of vascular malformations. The National Vascular Malformations Foundation also engages in patient advocacy; provides appropriate referrals; and offers educational and supportive materials including brochures and information packets.

President: Mary P. Burris (1990-Present)
Year Established: N/A
Organization Members: 400

Publishes the following materials:
The National Vascular Malformations Foundation, Inc. ~ *Brochure*
Finding the Answers Together by Caring and Sharing ~ *Brochure*

Concerned with the following diseases or disorders:
Arteriovenous Malformation; Cavernous Hemangioma; Vascular Malformations of the Brain

1896 NATIONAL VULVODYNIA ASSOCIATION (NVA)

P.O. Box 4491
Silver Spring, MD 20914-4491 301-299-0775
Fax: 301-299-3999
E-mail: matenva@graphcom.com
http://www.nva.org

The National Vulvodynia Association is a non-profit organization created in 1994 to improve the lives of individuals affected by vulvodynia, a group of chronic vulvar pain disorders. The National Vulvodynia Association seeks to educate affected women about vulvodynia to enable them to make informed choices about their treatment; encourage affected individuals to develop self-help strategies to deal with the physical and emotional aspects of these disorders; provide a support network for interested members; involve and educate family members to promote a supportive family environment; and coordinate a centralized source of information on suspected causes, current treatments, and ongoing research for healthcare professionals and affected individuals. The National Vulvodynia Association works cooperatively with other health organizations to improve understanding of vulvodynia and promote public attention to these disorders. Educational materials produced by the organization include a brochure and newsletter.

President: Phyllis Mate (1996 to Present)
Executive Director: Phyllis Mate (1996 to Present)
Year Established: 1994
Organization Members: 1,700

Publishes the following materials:
National Vulvodynia Association ~ *Brochure*
NVA News ~ *Newsletter*
National Association Established to Aid Victims of Debilitating Gynecological Disorder ~ *Facts Sheets*

Concerned with the following diseases or disorders:
Lichen Sclerosus; Vulvovaginitis

1897 NATIONAL WOMEN'S HEALTH NETWORK (NWHN)

514 10th Street NW
Suite 400
Washington, D.C. 20004 202-628-7814
Fax: 202-347-1168

The National Women's Health Network is a national not-for-profit voluntary health organization that functions as an advocate for health issues that affect women. The Network also functions as a clearinghouse for information on women's health issues and lifetime wellness. The Women's Health Information Service distributes brochures on topics such as Breast and Ovarian Cancer, Fibrocystic Disease, Interstitial Cystitis, Pelvic Inflammatory Disease, Vulvodynia, Urinary Tract Infections, and Toxic Shock Syndrome. The Network also distributes a regular newsletter.

Executive Director: Cynthia Pearson
Year Established: 1976
Organization Members: 12,000

Concerned with the following diseases or disorders:
Ahumada Del Castillo Syndrome; Amenorrhea, Primary; Asherman's Syndrome; Endometriosis; Forbes Albright Syndrome; Lichen Sclerosus; Stein Levanthal Syndrome

1898 NATIONAL WOMEN'S HEALTH RESOURCE CENTER (NWHRC)

5255 Loughboro Road, NW
Washington, D.C. 20016 202-537-4015
Fax: 301-320-3762
E-mail: nwhrc02@erols.com
http://www.healthywomen.org

The National Women's Health Resource Center is a national voluntary not-for-profit organization committed to providing information that enables women and their health care providers to make informed health decisions. Established in 1988, the Center, which is a subsidiary of the Columbia Hospital for Women Foundation, has a membership that consists of individual consumers, health professionals, and organizations. The Center uses its Information Database to provide current information in response to consumer inquiries. It collaborates with national corporations to develop women's health campaigns and disseminate information across the country and uses its National Referral Database to refer callers to women's health care providers in all regions of the United States. The Center also conducts conferences and work site programs, sponsors special events, serves as a women's health information resource for the media and members of Congress, and authors the Women's Book of Health (published by William Morrow). The National Women's Health Resource Center's goals include establishing and coordinating a clinical research program with major women's health providers in the United States.

Executive Director: Amy Niles
Year Established: 1988
Organization Members: 2,000

Publishes the following materials:
National Women's Health Report ~ *Report*
National Women's Health Resource Center ~ *Factsheet*

Concerned with the following diseases or disorders:
Ahumada Del Castillo Syndrome; Forbes Albright Syndrome; Lichen Sclerosus

1899 NEW DIRECTIONS FOR PEOPLE WITH DISABILITIES, INC.

5276 Hollister Avenue
Suite 207
Santa Barbara, CA 93111 805-967-2841
Fax: 805-964-7344
E-mail: mogan@silcom.com

New Directions for People with Disabilities, Inc., a not-for-profit organization established in 1985, is dedicated to providing local, national, and international travel and foreign exchange programs for people with disabilities. The purpose of the programs is to promote the understanding, acceptance, and appreciation of people with disabilities as important and contributing members of our society as well as to promote a sense of accomplishment, belonging, and self-worth for participants by providing a wide range of challenging activities. Such activities include skiing, river rafting, biking tours, and hot air ballooning. The Tour Guides/Chaperones are special educational instructors, recreation therapists, residential counselors, nurses, nurses' aides, vocational and independent living skill counselors, and other professional staff who have been trained to work with people with disabilities. Each year, New Directions serves over 350 children, adults, and seniors who have developmental, emotional, and physical disabilities such as cerebral palsy, Down Syndrome, autism, schizophrenia, blindness, hearing impairment, and mental retardation. Participants live in state hospitals, board and care homes, residential treatment centers, and nursing homes. Most have not previously had a vacation, and many have not been away from their facilities or treatment centers for 10 or more years. New Directions annually sponsors trips in the United States and abroad to locations including Hawaii, Washington D.C., New York City, Las Vegas, Disneyland, the Grand Canyon, Australia, Ireland, Japan, and Mexico.

Executive Director: Dee Duncan
Organization Language: Spanish (spoken). American Sign Language. Braille.
Year Established: 1985
Organization Members: Non-Membership

Publishes the following materials:
New Directions Fact Sheet ~ *Factsheet*
New Directions ~ *Newsletter*

1900 NEW YORK COALITION FOR ALTERNATIVES TO PESTICIDES, INC. (NYCAP)

353 Hamilton Street
Albany, NY 12210-1709 518-426-8246
Fax: 518-426-3052
E-mail: nycap@crisny.org

The New York Coalition for Alternatives to Pesticides, Inc. (NYCAP) is a voluntary not-for-profit organization dedicated to reducing hazardous chemical pesticide use through outreach and education. Established in 1989, NYCAP actively promotes the use of safer alternatives to chemical pesticides, the development of environmentally sound public policy, and the empowerment of all people seeking to improve environmental health. Consisting of 1,500 members, the Coalition produces educational materials including a brochure entitled "NYCAP, New York Coalition for Alternatives to Pesticides," reports, booklets, fact sheets, books, videos, and a directory. In addition, the organization supports government legislation, promotes education, provides referrals, works to create a partnership for healthy schools, serves as an information clearinghouse, and provides integrated pest management training.

President: Robert Ross (1996 to Present)
Executive Director: James Moore
Year Established: 1989
Organization Members: 1,500

Publishes the following materials:
NYCAP ~ *Brochure*
Solutions ~ *Newsletter*

1901 **NORTH AMERICAN CHRONIC PAIN ASSOCIATION OF CANADA (NACPAC)**

150 Central Park Drive
Unit 105
Brampton
Ontario, L6T 2T9
Canada
905-793-5230
800-616-7246
Fax: 905-793-8781
E-mail: nacpac@sympatico.ca
http://www3.sympatico.ca/nacpac

The North American Chronic Pain Association of Canada (NACPAC) is a nonprofit self-help organization dedicated to providing assistance and hope to individuals with chronic pain. NACPAC defines chronic pain as any frequent or continuous pain that has lasted more than a few months. This includes, but is not limited to, lower back pain, fibromyalgia, arthritis, headaches and migraines, and neck and shoulder pain. NACPAC was established in 1986 and currently consists of approximately 1,000 members. NACPAC brings together affected individuals through mutual support groups operating throughout Canada. Where no group exists, NACPAC provides materials and guidance on how to establish a support group. Members are encouraged by their peers to share ways of coping with chronic pain and to live full, productive lives. Group leaders are individuals who have themselves learned to function well despite their pain. NACPAC also provides education about pain related problems through a series of brochures, pamphlets, and a quarterly newsletter entitled "NACPAC Track." In addition, speakers, videotapes, and books are available to assist members to learn about their pain problems in layperson's language. NACPAC also provides referrals to other organizations and maintains a web site at [http://www3.sympatico.ca/nacpac].

President: Alan Gaudet (1997 to present).
Executive Director: Debbie Deschenes
Year Established: 1986
Organization Chapters: 40
Organization Members: 1,000

1902 **OKADA, LTD. (OKADA)**

W5634 Stearns Road
P.O. Box 650
Fontana, WI 53125
414-275-5226
Fax: 414-275-0127
TDD: 414-275-5226
E-mail: okada@elknet.net
http://www.elknet.net/okada

Okada, Ltd. is a not-for-profit organization dedicated to promoting human independence and personal enrichment of individuals by utilizing the unique qualities of specially trained dogs. Established in 1986, Okada has established its reputation and credibility as a provider of hearing dogs, companion dogs, and seizure dogs and recently has begun research and development on "Alzheimer Dogs." Seizure dogs live at home with persons coping with life-threatening seizure disorders. The dogs are trained to identify the onset of their partners' seizures, activate a special mechanical device designed to call for help through the telephone line, and stay close to their partners until help arrives. Alzheimer's Dogs are trained to help control wandering episodes of individuals with Alzheimer's Syndrome. The majority of dogs trained come from animal shelters. The name "Okada" is American Indian for "asking for a place." These once abandoned animals are carefully trained by Okada to enhance human life, to guide, and to give and/or maintain independence. The dogs have "their place" and enable persons with disabilities to become independent and take "their place" in life. Okada, Ltd. is a voting member of Assistance Dogs International (ADI), a coalition of assistance dog providers formed to promote standards of excellence, facilitate communication between providers, and educate the public. Affiliation with ADI demonstrates that Okada has met the minimum standards for training assistance dogs. Okada's founder was named to the ADI Board of Directors at its International Congress in 1990, for a three year term. Okada, Ltd. maintains a web site on the Internet at [http://www.elknet.net/okada].

President: Pat Putnam
Organization Language: American Sign Language.
Year Established: 1986
Organization Members: Non-Membership

Publishes the following materials:
Discover Okada ~ *Brochure*
Okada Specialty Dogs ~ *Brochure*
Woman's Best Friend ~ *Reprint*
Specialty Dogs ~ *Reprint*

Canine Companions Provide Special Services for Special ~ *Reprint*
Woman's Best Friend - Janesville Gazette ~ *Reprint*
Wisconsin - The Milwaukee Journal Magazine ~ *Reprint*
Canines Lend an Ear ~ *Reprint*
Gallaudet's Student's Hearing Guide Dog ~ *Reprint*
Animals and Physically Challenged Adults ~ *Reprint*
Betting on a Friendship ~ *Reprint*
Dogs Train for New Careers in Human Service ~ *Reprint*
The Mystery Dog ~ *Reprint*
Gandi Fell Victim to Steel-Jawed Leg-Hold Trap ~ *Reprint*
Her Dogs Become Ears for the Deaf ~ *Reprint*
Old Dogs Lerning There are New Tricks ~ *Reprint*
Hearing Aids ~ *Reprint*
Molly - A Greyhound witha Mission ~ *Reprint*
Niles Canine Foster Parent Becomews Dog's Best Friend ~ *Reprint*
It's Puppy Love ~ *Reprint*
Alert - Years Best Hearing Dog Has Talents Exceeding Her Training ~ *Reprint*
Discover OKADA Specialty Guide dogs ~ *Brochure*

1903 OLEY FOUNDATION

214 Hun Memorial A-23
Albany Medical Center
Albany, NY 12208-3478 518-262-5079
800-776-6539
Fax: 518-262-5528
http://www.wizvax.net/oleyfdn

The Oley Foundation is a national non-profit organization dedicated to providing educational and emotional support, outreach activities, and clinical outcome information for individuals who depend on home intravenous (parenteral) and tube (enteral) nutrition, their families, professionals, and others. Individuals who depend on such nutrition include those who cannot receive enough nutrients from the food they eat because of severe gastrointestinal disorders that may impair their swallowing or intestinal absorption. Founded in 1983, the Foundation publishes a bimonthly newsletter entitled "LifelineLetter" that includes articles contributed by individuals who depend on home nutrition for their survival, their families and caregivers, clinicians, researchers, and homecare services. The Foundation facilitates a national network of regional volunteers who provide emotional support and outreach at the local level. Comprised of individuals who are themselves users of home nutrition and their family members, the network offers services ranging from telephone support and hospital visitation to lectures and self-help get-togethers. The Oley Foundation also sponsors two conferences each year that bring together home nutrition users with experts in the field. Educational materials produced by the Oley Foundation include brochures, audio-visual aids, and information about travel, swimming, and other topics.

President: Donald Young (1995 to Present)
Year Established: 1983
Organization Members: 4,500

Publishes the following materials:
The Oley Foundation. For Home Parenteral and Enteral Nutrition ~ *Brochure*
Lifeline Letter ~ *Newsletter*
North American Home Parenteral and Enteral Nutrition Patient Registry. Annual Report With Outcome Profiles ~ *Booklet*
If You Depend Upon Home-Infused Nutritional Support. ~ *Fact Sheet*
The Oley Foundation. For those people whose daily survival depends on the technology of home-infused nutrition sup ~ *Brochure*
The Oley Foundation ~ *Brochure*

1904 ONCOLINK: THE UNIVERSITY OF PENNSYLVANIA CANCER CENTER RESOURCE

E-mail: editors@oncolink.upenn.edu
http://cancer.med.upenn.edu/

OncoLink is a multimedia oncology information resource on the World Wide Web on the Internet. OncoLink's mission "is consistent with that of the University of Pennsylvania Medical Center and the University of Pennsylvania Cancer Center, which have sanctioned the site's use and development. OncoLink is accessible worldwide to anyone with Internet access, and there is no charge for its use. Oncolink has been established with the following objectives: (1) dissemination of information relevant to the field of oncology; (2) education of health care personnel; (3) education of affected individuals, families, and other interested parties; and (4) rapid collection of information pertinent to the specialty. OncoLink's home page includes the following headings: Disease Oriented Headings (i.e., specific types of cancer); Medical Specialty Oriented Menus (i.e., medical specialities that deal with cancer, chemotherapy information, etc.); Psychosocial Support and Personal Experiences; Cancer Causes, Screening, and Prevention; Clinical Trials; Global Resources for Cancer Information; Cancer FAQs (frequently asked questions); Medical Supportive Care for the Cancer Patient; Conferences and Meetings; and Financial Issues for Cancer Patients.

Concerned with the following diseases or disorders:
Cancer, Breast; Cancer, Colon; Cancer, Lung; Cancer, Prostate; Cancers, Skin, General; Carcinoma, Renal Cell; Carcinoma, Squamous Cell; Nevoid Basal Cell Carcinoma Syndrome; Tongue Carcinoma

1905 ORGAN TRANSPLANT FUND, INC. (OTF)

1102 Brookfield
Suite 202
Memphis, TN 38119 901-684-1697
800-489-3863
Fax: 901-684-1128
E-mail: otfnatl@aol.com
http://www.otf.org

The Organ Transplant Fund, Inc. (OTF) is a national not-for-profit organization dedicated to helping individuals who are in need of organ or bone marrow transplants through financial assistance, advocacy, and emotional support. The Organ Transplant Fund was established in 1983 in Memphis, TN as the Liver Organ Transplant Fund to assist an individual in the local area who was in critical need of a liver transplant, but unable to afford the procedure. The small group of volunteers who founded OTF went to work to raise philanthropic contributions to pay for the transplant and related expenses. Hearing of the success of this first effort, other candidates for liver and other types of transplants turned to the new organization for assistance in raising the funds needed to help pay for their transplants. What began as a local limited endeavor evolved into an organization that is helping hundreds of organ and tissue transplant candidates and recipients nationwide. OTF provides candidates with fund-raising training and advice that can enable a patient campaign to raise up to $250,000 for the cost of a transplant and related expenses. The assistance provided by OTF ranges from helping to organize the volunteer fund-raising efforts, to counseling on the use of various fund-raising techniques and approaches, to acknowledging the charitable donations to the campaigns. In assisting with the patient campaigns, OTF also helps with publicity, negotiates bills, and processes payments to hospitals, physicians, pharmacies, and other providers of transplant-related services. Another OTF program is the "Celebration of Life" Campaigns that focus on the ongoing financial needs to transplant recipients, whose transplant-related expenses (e.g., life-sustaining immunosuppressant medication costs) pose continuing monetary obstacles. "Celebration of Life" Campaigns are created as mini- models of the patient campaigns and are implemented on a long-term basis, through the sustained efforts of transplant recipients and their volunteers. Additionally, emergency funds and short-terms assistance are available to assist with airfare, lodging, insurance premiums, home health care, and other transplant services and/or equipment. The Organ Transplant Fund also publishes "Reaching Out To Help," a quarterly newsletter and maintains a site on the World Wide Web at [http://www.otf.org].

President: Len Edwards
Executive Director: Gary L. McMahan
Year Established: 1983
Organization Members: Non-Membership

Publishes the following materials:
The Fund News ~ *Newsletter*
Only the Good Die Young ~ *Brochure*
Organ Transplant Fund, Inc. ~ *Mission Statement*
What is Organ Transplant Fund Inc.? ~ *Services List*
Reaching Out to Help ~ *Information Packet*
OTF ~ *Brochure*
"Reaching Out To Help". (1st Quarter 1997) ~ *Newsletter*
"Reaching Out To Help" (2nd Quarter 1997) ~ *Newsletter*

1906 ORGANIC ACIDEMIA ASSOCIATION (OAA)

14600 41st Avenue North
Plymouth, MN 55446 612-559-1797
Fax: 612-694-0017
E-mail: OAANews@aol.com
just4u.com/oaa/ or http://www.oaanews.org

The Organic Acidemia Association is a voluntary not-for-profit self-help organization dedicated to providing information and support to families of children with inborn errors of metabolism. Established in the early 1980s, the Organic Acidemia Association provides information to affected families and health care professionals across the country and internationally. The Association publishes the Organic Acidemia Association Newsletter three times yearly, which includes updates, editorials, and letters from and for affected families.

President: Kathi Stagni
Executive Director: Carol Barton (Vice President)
Year Established: 1980
Organization Members: 500

Publishes the following materials:
Organic Acidemia Association Newsletter ~ *Newsletter*

Concerned with the following diseases or disorders:
Acidemia, Isovaleric; Acidemia, Methylmalonic; Acidemia, Propionic; Carnitine Deficiency Syndromes;

Glutaricaciduria I; Glutaricaciduria II; Long Chain Acyl CoA Dehydrogenase Deficiency (LCAD); Medium Chain Acyl CoA Dehydrogenase Deficiency; Muscular Dystrophy, Landouzy Dejerine; Non-Ketotic Hyperglycinemia; Pyruvate Dehydrogenase Deficiency; Short Chain Acyl CoA Dehydrogenase Deficiency (SCAD)

1907 OSTEOPOROSIS AND RELATED BONE DISEASES NATIONAL RESOURCE CENTER (ORBD/NRC)

1150 17th Street NW
Suite 500
Washington, DC 20036-4603 202-223-0344
800-624-2663
Fax: 202-223-2237
TDD: 202-466-4315
E-mail: orbdnrc@nof.org
http://www.osteo.org

Osteoporosis and Related Bone Diseases National Resource Center (ORBD-NRC) is dedicated to expanding awareness and enhancing knowledge and understanding of the prevention, early detection, and treatment of these diseases, as well as strategies for coping with them. Osteoporosis is a disease characterized by low bone mass and structural deterioration on bone tissue, leading to bone fragility and an increased susceptibility to fractures of the hip, spine, and wrist. Founded in 1994, ORBD-NRC provides affected individuals, families, health-care professionals and families with an important link to resources and information on metabolic bone diseases. The Center collects information on materials, programs, and support services on metabolic bone diseases and disseminates this information widely through publications (e.g., "Fast Facts on Primary Hyperparathyriodism," "Hypophosphatasia," and "Myeloma Bone Disease"), online services, professional and patient meetings and general media outreach. In addition, its extensive database provides individuals with answers to their questions or refers them to sources of additional information. The Resource Center is supported by the National Institute of Arthritis and Musculoskeletal and Skin Disease, National Institutes of Health.

Executive Director: Janet Meleney (Contact Person)
Organization Language: Spanish (written).
Year Established: 1994

Publishes the following materials:
Professional Information Packets ~ *Order Form*
Fast Facts on Osteoporosis ~ *Fact Sheet*
Fast Facts on Osteogenesis Imperfecta ~ *Fact Sheet*
Fast Facts on Fibrous Dysplasia ~ *Fact Sheet*
Fast Facts on Paget's Disease of Bone ~ *Fact Sheet*
Fast Facts on Primary Hyperparathyroidism ~ *Fact Sheet*
Hypophosphatasia ~ *Fact Sheet*
Myeloma Bone Disease ~ *Fact Sheet*
Hearing Loss and Bone Disorders ~ *Fact Sheet*
Latino Women and Osteoporosis ~ *Fact Sheet*
Osteoporosis in Men ~ *Fact Sheet*
Osteoporosis and Asian American Wormen ~ *Fact Sheet*
Rodding Surgery in Children with Osteogenesis Imperfecta ~ *Fact Sheet*
Osteoporosis. A Woman's Guide ~ *Pamphlet*
Bone Basics For Men of All Ages ~ *Pamphlet*
Strategies for Safer Living. Fall Prevention for Older Adults ~ *Pamphlet*
1996 and 2015 Osteoporosis Prevalence Figures. State-by-State Report ~ *Booklet*
Osteopetrosis. Annotated Bibliography (December 1996) ~ *Pamphlet*
Calcium. Annotated Bibliography (March 1997) ~ *Pamphlet*

Concerned with the following diseases or disorders:
Osteopetrosis; Paget's Disease; Singleton Merten Syndrome

1908 OXALOSIS AND HYPEROXALURIA FOUNDATION (OHF)

5727 Westcliffe Drive
St. Louis, MO 63129 314-846-3645
Fax: 314-846-6779
E-mail: info@ohf.org
http://www.ohf.org/

The Oxalosis and Hyperoxaluria Foundation is a national voluntary organization established to inform the public, especially affected individuals, families, physicians, and medical professionals about hyperoxaluria and related conditions such as oxalosis and calcium-oxalate kidney stones. The Foundation endeavors to provide a support network to those affected by hyperoxaluria. Founded in 1989, the group supports and encourages research studies to find a cure for hyperoxaluria. The organization publishes educational materials including a summer camp list, reprints of medical journal articles, a patient resource list, and brochures entitled "Understanding Oxalosis" and "Hyperoxaluria and Low Oxalate Diet List." The organization also supports a toll-free telebraille number ([800] 833-6385).

President: Tim Berra (1997 to Present).
Executive Director: Tammy Murphy
Year Established: 1989
Organization Members: 441

Publishes the following materials:
Understanding Hyperoxaluria and Oxalosis ~ *Brochure*

Concerned with the following diseases or disorders:
Hyperoxaluria, Primary (Type I)

1909 **PHP—PARENTS HELPING PARENTS, INC.**

3041 Olcott Street
Santa Clara, CA 95054-3222 408-727-5775
Fax: 408-727-0182
E-mail: info@php.com
http://www.php.com

PHP—Parents Helping Parents, Inc. is a multifaceted, comprehensive not-for-profit parent directed family resource center dedicated to assisting children with any type of special need (mental, physical, emotional, or learning disability). The organization was founded in 1976 as a parent support group, but now parent support is only one of numerous services offered by this organization. The mission of the Center is to help children with special needs receive love, hope, respect, and services needed to achieve their full potential by strengthening their families and the professionals who serve them. This mission is attained through well-informed, supportive, assertive, and caring families; knowledgeable professionals who are well-trained and sensitive to ongoing social, financial, emotional, and educational needs of families with children who have special needs; and family-centered care that is coordinated and based in the community. The Center has developed and implemented numerous programs including bulletin board services, workshops for physicians, a special needs library, networking, and peer counseling training. Parents Helping Parents produces a variety of educational and support materials including information packets, brochures, a database, audio-visual aids, and a quarterly newsletter.

Executive Director: Mary Ellen Peterson
Organization Language: Spanish. French. Catonese. Vietnamese.
Year Established: 1976
Organization Chapters: 20

1910 **PAGET FOUNDATION FOR PAGET'S DISEASE OF BONE AND RELATED DISORDERS**

120 Wall Street
#1602
New York, NY 10005 212-509-5335
800-237-2438
Fax: 212-509-8492
E-mail: pagetfdn@aol.com
http://www.healthanswers.com/paget

The Paget Foundation for Paget's Disease of Bone and Related Disorders is a voluntary health agency devoted to serving people affected by Paget's Disease of Bone and to assisting the professionals in the medical community who treat this disorder. Established in 1978, the Paget Foundation continues to provide affected individuals and their families with up-to-date information about Paget's Disease; refers individuals diagnosed with Paget's Disease to physicians who specialize in treating this disorder; and enhances public awareness of Paget's Disease of Bone and related disorders. The Foundation also provides ongoing professional education to the medical community and promotes ongoing medical research into the causes, prevention, and treatment of Paget's Disease. The Foundation produces educational and support materials including brochures, pamphlets, audiovisual aids, a newsletter entitled "Update," and a guide for people affected by Paget's Disease.

President: Frederick R. Singer, M.D. (1989-Present)
Executive Director: Charlene Waldman
Year Established: 1978
Organization Members: Non-membership.

Publishes the following materials:
Questions & Answers About Primary Hyperparathyroidism ~ *Brochure*
Questions & Answers about Paget's Disease of the Bone ~ *Brochure*
A Patient's Guide to Paget's Disease of Bone ~ *Booklet*
Update - The Newsletter of the Paget Foundation ~ *Newsletter*

Concerned with the following diseases or disorders:
Dysplasia, Fibrous; McCune Albright Syndrome; Osteopetrosis; Paget's Disease

1911 **PARALYZED VETERANS OF AMERICA**

801 18th Street NW
Washington, DC 20006 202-872-1400
800-424-8200
http://www.pva.org

The Paralyzed Veterans of America (PVA) is a voluntary not-for-profit organization dedicated to serving the needs of its members — all of whom have catastrophic paralysis caused by spinal cord injury or disease. Established in 1946, PVA has been in the forefront of improving health care, rehabilitation, and access to society for paralyzed veterans and all citizens with a disability. As part of its mission, PVA's Research and Education Program has funded a wide range of educational materials and videotapes for people with disabilities, their families, the general public, and professionals in the field of spinal cord dysfunction. The materials include a booklet entitled "An Introduction to Spinal Cord Injury - Understanding the Changes," a pamphlet entitled "Resource Connection," and brochures. PVA consists of 16,000 members and 54 chapters and also has 59 service offices nationwide that serve the needs of all veterans seeking Department of Veteran Affairs claims and benefits. PVA's national advocacy program focuses on obtaining full Civil Rights for those with a disability. In addition, the organization funds the National Spinal Cord Hotline (800-526-3456). PVA maintains a web site on the Internet at [http://www.pva.org].

President: Kenneth Huber
Executive Director: Gordon Mansfield
Organization Language: Spanish (written).
Year Established: 1946
Organization Chapters: 54
Organization Members: 16,000

Publishes the following materials:
Resource Connection. Paralyzed Veterans of America
Research and Education Program ~ *Bibliography*
An Introduction to Spinal Cord Injury ~ *Booklet*

1912 PARENT CARE, INC.

9041 Colgate Street
Indianapolis, IN 46268-1210 800-808-2224
Fax: 317-872-0795
E-mail: acch@clark.net
http://www.acch.org

Parent Care, Inc. is a national not-for-profit organization established in 1982 by parents and professionals familiar with the needs of newborns and families who have experienced stays in neonatal intensive care units (NICU). The mission of Parent Care is to improve the neonatal intensive care experiences and the futures of babies, families, and caregivers through a partnership of parents and professionals. Parent Care addresses its mission by advocating family-centered care and uniting families and health care providers in the provision of services of NICU babies and their families. Parent Care also seeks to educate the general public about the need for family-centered services and support the development of family or professional partnerships. It provides social, emotional, and informational support for families and caregivers involved in neonatal intensive care. Parent Care is governed by a volunteer Board of Directors composed of parents and professionals from across the United States and is funded by membership dues, corporate sponsors, educational grants, donations, and product sales. Parent Care produces many educational and support materials including brochures, guidebooks, a quarterly newsletter entitled "News Brief," and books for parents, professionals, and siblings of babies requiring special care after birth.

President: Frank Andrews (1995-Present)
Executive Director: Sarah Killion
Year Established: 1982
Organization Members: 500

1913 PARENT PALS (A GIFTED AND SPECIAL EDUCATION WEB SITE ON THE INTERNET FOR PARENTS)

E-mail: superpal@parentpals.com
http://www.parentpals.com

Parent Pals, a Gifted and Special Education Web site on the Internet, provides a variety of information and services for parents of children who are gifted or who have certain disabilities including Attention Deficit Disorder, autism, hearing impairment, emotional disturbances, learning disabilities, mental retardation, mobility impairment, speech and language impairment, stuttering, visual impairment, traumatic brain injury, and/or other health impairments. Parent Pals provides newsletters from therapists, teachers, and psychiatrists; general information on such topics as special education services, early intervention services, and individualized education programs (IEPs); a dictionary of terms used in special education; and an index of definitions concerning certain disorders. The site also provides specific educational and therapy games to enhance children's learning and language skills. These teaching ideas are organized by four levels, ranging from level 1 with preschool tasks to level 4 for gifted students. Parent Pals also provides weekly tips for parents of gifted children or children with certain disabilities. In addition, the site offers dynamic links to additional web sites in several different categories including "education links," "therapy links," "special education legislation links," and "medical links." Parent Pals is located at [http://www.parentpals.com].

President: Leslie Kirchoff M.A. C.C.C. (Founder)

1914 PARENT TO PARENT OF NEW ZEALAND

P.O. Box 234
Waikato Mail Center
Hamilton,
New Zealand 647-834-1108
Fax: 647-834-1108
E-mail: 100353.2754@compuserve.com
www.nzhealth.co.nz/everybody/parent.htm

The Parent to Parent of New Zealand is a non-profit organization dedicated to providing support to parents who have children with special needs. Support is provided voluntarily by trained support parents who have a child with the same or similar needs. Formed in 1983, the group has built up a support network that is now nationwide. The organization is affiliated with similar groups around the world and maintains close links with other organizations and professionals who work in related fields. Parent to Parent provides contact with a Support Parent, community seminars, workshops, family camps, and a resource library on different conditions. In addition to resource materials, a newsletter entitled "Parent to Parent" is available. Consisting of 14 chapters and more than 400 members, the organization also offers support groups, and patient networking.

President: Linda Davies (1996 to Present)
Executive Director: Shirley Wass
Year Established: 1983
Organization Chapters: 14
Organization Members: 400

Publishes the following materials:
Who Are Parent To Parent? ~ *Brochure*
Disabilities, Special Needs, Health Impairments, Rare Syndromes ~ *Pamphlet*
Parent to Parent National Newsletter ~ *Newsletter*

1915 PEDIATRIC CROHN'S & COLITIS ASSOCIATION, INC. (PCCA)

P.O. Box 188
Newton, MA 02168 617-489-5854
Fax: 617-489-5854

The Pediatric Crohn's and Colitis Association, Inc. (PCCA) is an international not-for-profit service organization dedicated to providing information and emotional support to families of children with inflammatory bowel disease (IBD) to help ensure that affected children reach their potential in today's society. Crohn's Disease and Ulcerative Colitis, collectively known as Inflammatory Bowel Disease, are chronic digestive diseases of unknown cause. While Crohn's Disease may affect any part of the gastrointestinal tract and often results in swelling, soreness, and inflammation of layers of the large and/or small intestinal wall, Ulcerative Colitis affects only the colon (large intestine), causing inflammation of the inner lining and resulting in diarrhea, often mixed with blood, cramping abdominal pain, and other symptoms. The Association was founded in 1988 by a group of parents with children affected by IBD to address the broad range of issues faced by the pediatric population with these disorders. Currently consisting of over 1,200 members, PCCA is dedicated to promoting pediatric research; providing educational, emotional, social, academic, and psychological support; and addressing the role of family dynamics in dealing with a chronic illness. The organization's services include a parent hotline; support groups; patient advocacy; networking services; and medical, educational, and psychological symposia. The organization also provides a variety of educational materials including brochures, pamphlets, an information packet, and a regular newsletter.

President: Mary Jayne Suchy (1995 to Present)
Executive Director: Harriet Kahn
Year Established: 1988
Organization Members: 1,200

Publishes the following materials:
The ABC;S of Pediatric Inflammatory Bowel Disease ~ *Brochure*
Pediatric Crohn's & Colitis Association, Inc. ~ *Brochure*
Crohn's Disease, Ulcerative Colitis and School ~ *Leaflet*
Pediatric Crohn's & Colitis Association Newsletter ~ *Newsletter*

Concerned with the following diseases or disorders:
Colitis, Collagenous; Colitis, Ulcerative; Crohn's Disease

1916 PEN PAL SUPPORT GROUP FOR CHRONIC DIZZINESS AND BALANCE DISORDERS

307 2nd Street
P.O. Box 305
Elliott, IA 51532 712-767-2325

The Pen Pal Support Group for Chronic Dizziness and Balance Disorders is a not-for-profit organization dedicated to bringing people together who have problems coping with their disability or with family and friends who do not understand. Established in 1987, the Pen Pal Support Group consists of 70 members. The organization provides a pen pal contact list.

President: Sharen Artlip
Year Established: 1987
Organization Members: 70

1917 PERSPECTIVES NETWORK, INC. (TPN, INC.)

P.O. Box 1859
Cumming, GA 30028-1859 770-844-6898
800-685-6302
Fax: 770-844-6898
E-mail: dktaylor@tbi.org
http://www.tbi.org

The Perspectives Network, Inc. (TPN) is a nonprofit organization dedicated to identifying and encouraging individual potential by providing various forums and opportunities wherein affected individuals, family members and friends, professionals and community members are encouraged to discuss issues relating to treatment, recovery, and reentry as well as creating positive changes following traumatic and acquired brain injury. TPN was established in 1990 by Dena K. Taylor, a brain injury survivor herself. The Perspectives Network provides information and education, but perhaps most importantly, it provides hope to those who survived a brain injury and to those who care for them. Educational materials include a quarterly magazine with an international circulation written by survivors, family members, and professionals; fact brochures; and a lending library and file archives containing books, videos, and topical articles. Program activities include peer communication networks for survivors, spouses, offspring, parents, and siblings; brain injury awareness workshops; support groups; and education. TPN can be reached at its e-mail address at [dktaylor@tbi.org] or its website at [http://www.tbi.org].

President: Dena K. Taylor (1990 to Present)
Organization Language: Spanish (written).
Year Established: 1990
Organization Members: Non-Membership

Publishes the following materials:
From Bump on the Head to Coma: We are all Interlinked ~ *Brochure*
The Perspectives Network ~ *Brochure*
Brain Injury. Prevention is worth a pound of cure but sometimes it happens anyway! ~ *Brochure*
Brain Injury Empathy and Awareness ~ *Brochure*

1918 PILOT PARENT PROGRAM

2818 San Gabriel
Austin, TX 78705 512-476-7044
Fax: 512-476-9054
http://www.main.org/arc/

The Pilot Parent Program provides support and information for families of children with disabilities, chronic illnesses, or other special needs. There are no fees for services and the only eligibility requirement is that families want to participate. The program distributes resource information about funding sources, child care and respite, local support groups, community services, local conferences, and specific disabilities and syndromes. A special program called Kristen's Fund was established as a limited source of funding to assist parents of children with special needs who find themselves unable to pay for essential resources. The Program also operates a parent matching program for those with children who have similar special needs. Other services include weekly educational and support groups, used equipment exchange, and a lending resource library. The ARC of the Capital Area is the parent group of the Pilot Parent Program.

Executive Director: Susan Eason
Organization Language: Spanish.
Year Established: 1980
Organization Members: 1,000

1919 PITUITARY TUMOR NETWORK ASSOCIATION (PTNA)

16350 Ventura Boulevard
Suite 231
Encino, CA 91436 805-499-2262
Fax: 805-499-1523
E-mail: ptna@pituitary.com
http://www.pituitary.com

The Pituitary Tumor Network Association (PTNA) is a support organization dedicated to promoting, supporting, and, where possible, funding research on pituitary tumors in a sustained effort to find a cure for these illnesses. Established in 1992 by four pituitary patients undergoing experimental treatment, the Association is now the world's largest pituitary support network. Its members include affected individuals, physicians, and pharmaceutical companies. The Association disseminates information to affected families, the medical community, and the public concerning early detection, symptoms, treatments, and resources available to pituitary patients. The Pituitary Tumor Network Association publishes a regular newsletter and a comprehensive resource guide. The guide, entitled "The Pituitary Patient Resource Guide," assists affected individuals to locate a variety of medical, surgical, insurance, occupational, lifestyle, and health maintenance services. It also helps primary-care physicians and other medical personnel to determine where to call for advice and consultation, where to send patients for specialized treatment and surgery, and what other medical specialties should be involved in treatment.

President: Robert Knutsen (Chairman)
Year Established: 1992
Organization Members: 5,000

Publishes the following materials:
Dedicated to improving the quality of life and well-being for all patients ~ *Brochure*
Network ~ *Newsletter*
The Pituitary Tumor Network Association ~ *Fact Sheet*
Why I Joined the PTNA ~ *Fact Sheet*
Brief Biography of Robert Knutzen ~ *Fact Sheet*
The Pituitary Patient Resource Guide ~ *Book*
The Pituitary Patient Resource Guide ~ *Book*

Concerned with the following diseases or disorders:
Brain Tumors, General; Diabetes Insipidus

1920 PREGNANCY AND INFANT LOSS SUPPORT, INC. (SHARE)

National SHARE Office
St. Joseph Health Center
300 First capitol Drive
St. Charles, MO 63301 314-947-6164
800-821-6819
Fax: 314-947-7486
http://www.NationalSHAREOffice.com

Pregnancy and Infant Loss Support, Inc. (SHARE) is a not-for-profit, self-help organization whose purpose is to serve those who are touched by the death of a baby through miscarriage, stillbirth, or newborn death. Established in 1977, SHARE's primary purpose is to provide support toward the positive resolution of grief experienced at the time of and/or following the death of an infant. The secondary purpose is to provide information, education, and resources on the needs and rights of bereaved parents and siblings. Currently, SHARE has 115 groups with a total of 1,400 members. Educational materials include informational brochures, bereavement resources, and an information packet. The packet includes a video catalog, bibliography, and the organization's self-titled newsletter which is published six times per year.

Executive Director: Catherine A. Lammert, R.N.
Organization Language: Spanish (written/spoken).
Year Established: 1977
Organization Members: 1,400

Publishes the following materials:
SHARE. Bereavement Resources ~ *Brochure*
SHARE ~ *Brochure*
SHARE. Pregnancy and Infant Loss Support, Inc. ~ *Pamphlet*

1921 PRESCRIPTION PARENTS (FOR PARENTS OF CHILDREN WITH CLEFT LIP AND PALATE)

22 Ingersoll Road
Wellesley, MA 02181 617-965-2946
E-mail: seltzer@samizdat.com
http://www.samizdat.com/pp1.html

Prescription Parents is a not-for-profit voluntary health organization dedicated to providing information and support to parents of children born with cleft lip and cleft palate. Established in the mid-1970s, Prescription Parents conducts parent support groups and a newborn program; provides referrals to genetic counseling and other services; holds informational meetings for members; and conducts social events for affected families. Prescription Parents also promotes patient advocacy and legislation beneficial to affected individuals and families. The organization offers a variety of educational and support materials through its directory, regular newsletter, booklets, brochures, and videotapes. Its informational materials highlight important issues concerning parents of affected children. These issues include various procedures in cleft lip and cleft palate rehabilitation, caring for an affected newborn, hearing and behavior in affected children, and matters of importance to affected adolescents.

President: Barb Sectzer
Year Established: 1975
Organization Members: 200

Concerned with the following diseases or disorders:
Catel Manzke Syndrome; Cerebrocostomandibular Syndrome; Oral Facial Digital Syndrome; Pierre Robin Syndrome

1922 PREVENT BLINDNESS AMERICA

500 East Remington Road
Schaumberg, IL 60173 708-843-2020
800-331-2020
Fax: 847-843-8458
E-mail: info@preventblindness.org
http://www.preventblindness.org

Prevent Blindness America is a nonprofit voluntary organization dedicated to fighting blindness and saving sight. Established in 1908, Prevent Blindness America and its nationwide network of affiliates, divisions, and chapters serve millions of people each year through public and professional education, community and patient service programs, and research. Consisting of 35,000 volunteers and 43 chapters, the organization produces educational materials including brochures entitled "Age-Related Macular Degeneration," "Signs of Possible Eye Trouble in Adults," and "Your Child's Sight." The organization also produces videos, posters, and brochures in Spanish, Portuguese, and Chinese. Program activities include support groups, patient advocacy, referrals, and a toll-free help line.

President: Richard T. Hellner (Chief Executive Officer)
Executive Director: Kent D. Stuckey (Chairman)
Organization Language: Spanish (written). Portuguese (written). Chinese (written).
Year Established: 1908
Organization Chapters: 43
Organization Members: Non-Membership

Publishes the following materials:
Prevent Blindness America. Organizational Materials List ~ *List*
Publications and Video Catalog ~ *Catalog*

Concerned with the following diseases or disorders:
Bardet Biedl Syndrome; Chandler's Syndrome; Cogan Reese Syndrome; Essential Iris Atrophy; Keratomalacia; Laurence Moon Syndrome

1923 PROSTATE POINTERS

E-mail: gary@rattler.cameron.edu
http://rattler.cameron.edu/prostate/

Prostate Pointers is a Web site on the Internet dedicated to providing the online community with a full spectrum of information available about prostate cancer and other problems of the prostate. The site provides information concerning several subjects related to prostate cancer or other prostate problems. It also contains a series of dynamic links to: support groups for affected individuals and family members; online "e-mailing" lists (listservs) concerning prostate cancer or other prostate problems; FAQs (Frequently Asked Questions); specific medical journal articles of interest; clinical trial information; web sites of peer-reviewed medical journals; physicians' web pages; prostate cancer centers; foundations; sources of financial assistance; web sites of medical libraries; additional web sites concerning prostate cancer and other prostate health problems; and more.

1924 PULL-THRU NETWORK

4 Woody Lane
Westport, CT 06880 203-221-7530
Fax: 203-221-9212
E-mail: PullthruNW@aol.com
members.aol.com/pullthrunw/Pullthru.html

The Pull-thru Network, a chapter of the United Ostomy Association, is a not-for-profit self-help organization dedicated to providing mutual support to families of children born with anorectal malformations. The Network provides information and support to families whose children have or will have a pull-thru type surgery to correct an anorectal malformation. The Network is also dedicated to providing information and support to families with a child who is incontinent and/or has a permanent or temporary ostomy. Established in 1988, the Network offers appropriate referrals, conducts support group meetings, gives phone support, provides a national networking service for its members, and offers a pen pal service. In addition, the organization provides a variety of educational and support materials, including pamphlets and a quarterly newsletter entitled "The Pull-thru Network News" that features articles with tips on dealing with diaper rash, personal stories, current events, and new techniques that may benefit affected children.

President: Karen and Scott Brownlow
Year Established: 1991
Organization Chapters: 1
Organization Members: 450

Concerned with the following diseases or disorders:
Hirschsprung's Disease; Imperforate Anus; Johanson Blizzard Syndrome

1925 PURINE RESEARCH SOCIETY

5424 Beech Avenue
Bethesda, MD 20814-1730 301-530-0354
Fax: 301-564-9597
E-mail: purine@erols.com
http://www2.dgsys.com/~purine/

The Purine Research Society (formerly known as Purine 24) is a national nonprofit charitable organization dedicated to funding research and treatments for purine-related metabolic diseases. Errors in the metabolism of purines (compounds commonly found in food) can lead to a variety of disorders. Established in 1986 by parents of children with purine autism (autistic children who excrete too much uric acid in their urine), the Society serves people with purine metabolic disorders and their families, health care professionals, and the general public. The Society has contributed a significant amount of money to fund M.D./Ph.D. researchers to find out why their children with autism were excreting excess uric acid, the end product of purines. The Purine Research Society provides appropriate referrals to affected individuals and offers educational pamphlets and brochures.

Executive Director: Mrs. Tahma Metz
Year Established: 1986
Organization Members: 25

Concerned with the following diseases or disorders:
Lesch Nyhan Syndrome

1926 RAISING OUR CHILDREN'S KIDS (ROCKING, INC.)

241 Pokagon St.
P.O. Box 96
Niles, MI 49120

Raising Our Children's Kids: An Intergenerational Network of Grandparenting, Inc. (ROCKING, Inc.) is a network of support groups for grandparents raising their grandchildren. As a non-membership organization, ROCKING, Inc. instead creates community-support groups and helps grandparents locate their community's resources to ease household, financial, physical, or emotional difficulties and enable them to keep their family unit intact. ROCKING, Inc. publishes brochures, offers a referral service, and provides a directory of all of their support groups, along with information and guidance on how to start your own group. ROCKING, Inc. is a nonprofit organization, and although it is not mandatory, postage fee payment is appreciated.

President: Mary A. Fron, R.N.
Year Established: 1992

Publishes the following materials:
Raising our Children's Kids ~ *Mission Statement*
Empowerment of Grandparents ~ *Pamphlet*
Are You Raising Your Grandchild? ~ *Pamphlet*
What is This Thing Called Kinship Care? ~ *Pamphlet*
Ideas and Considerations for Starting a Self-Help Support Group for Grandparents as Caregivers ~ *Information Sheet*

1927 RARE CHROMOSOME DISORDER SUPPORT GROUP OF AUSTRALASIA

66 Albion Street
Surry Hills
New South Wales, 2010
Australia

The Rare Chromosome Disorder Support Group of Australasia is a voluntary self-help organization dedicated to serving families and children affected by rare chromosome abnormalities. The Group's aims are to act as a family support group; promote awareness of chromosome abnormalities; hold meetings where families and relevant specialists can meet; link families whose children have similar clinical problems; and raise funds to support the group. Established in 1994, the Group also conducts seminars for families and professionals and holds an annual picnic day. The Group produces educational information through its database, pamphlets, and a regular newsletter.

President: Marlene Brightwell (1994 to Present)
Year Established: 1994
Organization Members: Non-Membership

1928 RARE DISEASE INFORMATION CENTER (ITALY)

Istituto di Ricerche Farmacologiche Mario Negri
Via G.B. Camozzi 3
24020, Ranica
Bergamo,
Italy 003935516516
Fax: 003935514503
http://irfmn.mnegri.it

The Istituto di Ricerche Farmacologiche Mario Negri (Clinical Research Center for Rare Disease) in Ranica, Italy is a not-for-profit foundation established in 1963. The Center operates on three levels: the Clinical Research Center, the Information Center for Rare Diseases; and the European School for Rare Diseases. The Clinical Research Center is a fully equipped hospital devoted entirely to clinical research. The aim is to develop research projects with special emphasis on rare diseases and innovative diagnostic and therapeutic procedures. The Information Center for Rare Diseases is a service to the public that provides up-to-date information on rare disorders with emphasis on causes, genetics, prevention, and investigational treatments of these disorders. The goal of the center is to create a computerized Rare Disease Database containing updated information on rare disorders and a directory of specialized physicians and clinical research centers in Europe that are familiar with a variety of rare diseases. The European School for Rare Diseases functions as a forum for cultural activities aimed at specialists and health professionals. Workshops and conferences are scheduled throughout the year. Clinical training includes short "basic" courses, intensive courses, and clinical research studies.

President: Prof. Silvio Garattini
Executive Director: Giuseppe Remuzzi, M.D.
Organization Language: Italian.
Year Established: 1992
Organization Members: raredisgcyberg.it

Publishes the following materials:
Mario Negri Institute for Pharmacological Research ~ *Pamphlet*

1929 RECOVERY, INC.

802 North Dearborn Street
Chicago, IL 60610 312-337-5661
Fax: 312-337-5756
E-mail: spot@recovery-inc.com
http://www.recovery-inc.com

Recovery, Inc. is a nonprofit self-help organization for people with anxiety and nervous disorders and panic attacks. Based on the Recovery Method developed by the late Dr. Abraham Low, Recovery, Inc. provides support, encouragement, and training to help individuals cope with their fears and overcome any possible relapses. Since it was founded in 1939, Recovery has grown to become an international support system for people, with over 800 chapters throughout the world. Recovery also publishes a newsletter, directory, and numerous brochures; produces audio-visual aids; and is frequently highlighted in medical and community publications. A limited number of materials are available in Spanish and French. Members must be at least 18 years old, but guests (i.e., spouses, family) are welcome at meetings. The meetings are free of charge, but donations are appreciated.

President: Lauretta Lucien (1997 to 1998)
Executive Director: Shirley Sachs
Organization Language: Spanish (written). French (written).
Year Established: 1939
Organization Chapters: 800

Publishes the following materials:
Recovery 1997 Directory of Group Meeting Information ~ *Pamphlet*
Self-Help for Nervous Symptoms and Fears ~ *Brochure*
Rx: Recovery, Inc. ~ *Brochure*
Recovery, Inc. What it is and How it Developed ~ *Booklet*
Recovery, Inc., as an Adjunct to Treatment in an Era of Managed Care ~ *Reprint*
Community Psychiatrist ~ *Reprint*
No Hopeless Cases ~ *Reprint*
Interview with Mark Hansen, M.D. Department of Psychiatry, Mayo Clinic, Rochester, Minnesota ~ *Reprint*
Finding Strength To Will Yourself Back In Control ~ *Reprint*
Self-Help Group With A Method Fights Mental Ills ~ *Reprint*
Help for anxiety sufferers ~ *Reprint*
Hospital and Community Psychiatry ~ *Reprinted*
A Method of Will Training ~ *Reprint*
Self-help and the Chicago Connection ~ *Reprint*
Self-help keeps mental health wounds healed ~ *Reprint*
"Partners in Wellness—Self-Help Groups and Professionals" ~ *Reprint*
Help yourself by helping your employee ~ *Reprint*
Recovery Inc. helps build strong minds ~ *Reprint*
A Complement to Clinical Practice ~ *Reprint*
Self-help group key to recovery ~ *Reprint*
Chicago Tribune. Ann Landers ~ *Reprint*
Don't panic: You're not alone and there's help ~ *Reprint*

Concerned with the following diseases or disorders:
Chiari Frommel Syndrome; Stein Levanthal Syndrome

1930 REHABILITATION RESEARCH AND TRAINING CENTER ON AGING WITH MENTAL RETARDATION (RRTC ON AGING WITH MENTAL RETA)

Institute on Disability and Human Development
University of Illinois at Chicago
1640 West Roosevelt Road
Chicago, IL 60608-6904 312-413-1520
800-996-8845
Fax: 312-996-6942
TDD: 312-413-0453
E-mail: gailpynd@uic.edu
http://www.uic.edu/orgs/rrtcamr/index.html

The Rehabilitation Research and Training Center (RRTC) on Aging with Mental Retardation is a not-for-profit research organization dedicated to promoting independence, productivity, community inclusion, and full citizenship of older adults with mental retardation through a coordinated program of research, training, technical assistance, and dissemination activities. Established in 1988 and funded by the U.S. Department of Education, Office of Special Education and Rehabilitative Services, RRTC's current research projects address six priority areas: increasing empowerment and self-advocacy; understanding how age related changes affect medical and psychosocial well-being; developing service models to meet the needs of families from diverse cultures; coping with changing capabilities through in-home interventions and assistive technology; supporting individuals through life transitions including the loss of significant others; and expanding retirement, financial, health, and independent living options. The RRTC is a national resource for researchers, planners, providers, self-advocates, families, and students in the field of aging with mental retardation. The RRTC's Clearinghouse on Aging and Developmental Disabilities has a computerized database containing over 2,000 reprints, bibliographies, manuals, and monographs on topics addressing issues of aging with mental retardation. The RRTC also disseminates RRTC research reports, training materials, and other educational materials and publishes a biannual newsletter entitled "A/DDVANTAGE," concerning aging and developmental disabilities.

Executive Director: Tamar Heller, Ph.D.
Year Established: 1988

Publishes the following materials:
RRTC Institute on Disability and Human Development.
College of Associated Health Professions ~ *Brochure*
Clearinghouse on Aging and Developmental Disabilities Publications List ~ *Pamphlet*
Older Adults with Mental Retardation and their Aging Family Caregivers ~ *Fact Sheet*
Getting Involved in Research and Training Projects: A Guide for Persons with Disabilities ~ *Booklet*
Aging with Mental Retardation ~ *Leaflet*
Addvantage ~ *Newsletter*

1931 RESEARCH TRUST FOR METABOLIC DISEASES IN CHILDREN (RTMDC)

Golden Gates Lodge
Weston Road,
Crewe, CW2 SXN
United Kingdom. 01270250221
Fax: 01270250244

The Research Trust for Metabolic Diseases in Children (RTMDC) is an international voluntary health agency located in the United Kingdom. Established in 1981, the Trust is dedicated to furthering medical research into the nature of metabolic diseases in children; encouraging the ongoing investigations of the prenatal diagnosis of these diseases; providing information, counseling, and financial support to caregivers; and providing information to health care professionals. In addition, the organization is dedicated to assisting in the care of affected children in hospitals, homes, or institutions and educating the public about metabolic diseases. The Research Trust for Metabolic Diseases networks parents of affected children for mutual benefit and support. The Trust also provides a regular newsletter, brochures, videos, and other educational materials.

President: Peter Greene, OBE (1985-Present)
Executive Director: Helen Carter
Organization Language: French. German.
Year Established: 1981
Organization Chapters: 23
Organization Members: 3,000

Publishes the following materials:
Some Questions and Answers ~ *Brochure*
HELP ~ *Brochure*
RTMDC 14th Annual Conference ~ *Pamphlet*
RTMDC Video Library ~ *Video List*
To Help Children with Metabolic Diseases ~ *Brochure*
RTMDC NEWS ~ *Newsletter*

Concerned with the following diseases or disorders:
5 Oxoprolinuria; Acanthocytosis; Acidemia, Isovaleric; Acidemia, Methylmalonic; Acidemia, Propionic; Acrodermatitis Enteropathica; Adrenal Hyperplasia, Congenital (General); Adrenoleukodystrophy; Alkaptonuria; Andersen Disease; Arginase Deficiency; Arginino Succinic Aciduria; Aspartylglycosaminuria; Batten Disease; Blue Diaper Syndrome; Carbamyl Phosphate Synthetase Deficiency; Carbohydrate deficient Glycoprotein Syndrome Type I; Carboxylase Deficiency, Multiple; Carnitine Deficiency Syndromes; Carnitine Palmitoyltransferase Deficiency; Carnosinemia; Citrullinemia; Cockayne Syndrome; Crigler Najjar Syndrome Type I; Cystinosis; Cytochrome C Oxidase Deficiency; Erythropoietic Protoporphyria (EPP); Fabry Disease; Farber's Disease; Forbes Disease; Fructosuria; Galactosemia; Ganglioside Sialidase Deficiency; Glucose-6-Phosphate Dehydrogenase Deficiency; Glutaricaciduria I; Glutaricaciduria II; Glycogen Storage Disease VIII; Hallervorden Spatz Disease; Hartnup Disease; Hers Disease; Histidinemia; Homocystinuria; Hunter Syndrome; Hurler Syndrome; Hutchinson Gilford Progeria Syndrome; Hyperchylomicronemia; Hyperoxaluria, Primary (Type I); Hyperprolinemia Type I; Hyperprolinemia Type II; Hypokalemia; Hypophosphatasia; I Cell Disease; Leigh's Disease; Leprechaunism; Lesch Nyhan Syndrome; Leukodystrophy, Krabbe's; Lipodystrophy; Long Chain Acyl CoA Dehydrogenase Deficiency (LCAD); MELAS Syndrome; MERRF Syndrome; Mannosidosis; Maple Syrup Urine Disease; Maroteaux Lamy Syndrome; McArdle Disease; Medium Chain Acyl CoA Dehydrogenase Deficiency; Morquio Syndrome; Multiple Sulfatase Deficiency; N-Acetyl Glutamate Synthetase Deficiency; Niemann Pick Disease; Non-Ketotic Hyperglycinemia; Ornithine Transcarbamylase Deficiency; Osteopetrosis; PEPCK Deficiency, Mitochondrial; Pelizaeus Merzbacher Brain Sclerosis; Phosphoglycerate Kinase Deficiency; Pompe Disease; Porphyria Cutanea Tarda; Porphyria, ALA-D; Porphyria, Acute Intermittent; Porphyria, Congenital Erythropoietic; Porphyria, Hereditary Coproporphyria; Porphyria, Variegate; Pseudo Hurler Polydystrophy; Pyruvate Carboxylase Deficiency; Pyruvate

Dehydrogenase Deficiency; Refsum Syndrome; Renal Glycosuria; Sanfilippo Syndrome; Schindler Disease; Short Chain Acyl CoA Dehydrogenase Deficiency (SCAD); Sialidosis; Sly Syndrome; Sucrose Isomaltose Malabsorption, Congenital; Tarui Disease; Tay Sachs Disease; Tetrahydrobiopterin Deficiency; Trimethylaminuria; Tyrosinemia, Hereditary; Valinemia; Von Gierke Disease

1932 ROCKY MOUNTAIN RESOURCE & TRAINING INSTITUTE (RMRTI)

6355 Ward Road
#310
Arvada, CO 80004 303-420-2942
Fax: 303-420-8675
TDD: 303-420-2942

The Rocky Mountain Resource & Training Institute (RMRTI) is a not-for-profit, state government (CO) organization that serves people with disabilities and provides training to the agencies that assist them. Established in 1989, the Institute is dedicated to facilitating disabled individuals' transition from school to adult life; providing information and resources concerning assistive technology, devices, and services; promoting and ensuring compliance with the federal Americans with Disabilties Act(ADA) and other legislation promoting the rights and inclusion of people with disabilites; and promoting supported employment, positive behavior support strategies, total quality improvement, strategic planning, and organizational development.

Executive Director: Judith Emery
Year Established: 1989
Organization Members: 15

1933 RONALD MCDONALD HOUSE CHARITIES

One Kroc Drive
Oak Brook, IL 60521 630-623-7048
Fax: 630-623-7488
http://www.mcdonald.com

Ronald McDonald House Charities' goal is to lift "kids to a better tomorrow." It supports more than 170 Ronald McDonald Houses and makes grants to other not-for-profit organizations that help children in neighborhoods worldwide. Its cornerstone program is "Ronald McDonald Houses," which serve as homes away from home for families who must travel far outside their own communities to seek medical treatment for a child. Ronald McDonald Houses are located near hospitals that provide specialized care for children. Parents and family members receive a room of their own with beds, kitchen and laundry facilities, and toys for the kids. Houses are designed to encourage interaction among guests to help them cope during such a difficult time. Such services are offered for a small contribution; if that is not possible, no one is turned away. Since its inception in 1974, more than 2 million families have been served in approximately 13 countries. The Charities also provide grants to other children's organizations and support major, national initiatives, such as health care and medical research, education and the arts, and civic and social services.

Year Established: 1974

1934 ROSWELL PARK FAMILY CANCER REGISTRY (RPCI)

Elm & Carlton Streets
Buffalo, NY 14263 716-845-5815
800-685-6825
Fax: 716-845-8980
E-mail:
mrodriguez@sc3101.med.buffalo.edu

Roswell Park Family Cancer Registry is a research organization dedicated to registering families at risk of developing cancers. The Registry seeks to educate affected individuals and family members in the areas of prevention, early detection, and treatment of cancer, as well as risk assessment of such family members. Established in 1992, this research program is designed to obtain detailed medical and family history information from people who, because of their family history or other risk factors, may have an increased potential of developing cancer. To this end, the Registry takes blood and other tissue samples. This material is provided to research scientists studying cancer genes. The affected individuals or families are thus provided with updated information on genetics, genetic cancers, and testing. The Registry produces educational materials including a pamphlet entitled "Hereditary Non-polyposis Colorectal Cancer." The organization supports such program activities as genetic counseling, patient and general education, and research.

Executive Director: Miguel A. Rodriguez-Bigas, M.D. (Director)
Organization Language: Spanish (spoken).
Year Established: 1992
Organization Members: Non-Membership

Publishes the following materials:
Hereditary Non-Polyposis Colorectal Cancer ~ *Brochure*

Concerned with the following diseases or disorders:
Polyposis, Familial

1935 ROYAL SOCIETY FOR MENTALLY HANDICAPPED CHILDREN & ADULTS (MENCAP)

Mencap National Center
123 Golden Lane
London, EC1Y 0RT
United Kingdom

The Royal Society for Mentally Handicapped Children and Adults (MENCAP) is a non-profit organization exclusively concerned with learning disabled people of all degrees, their families, and caregivers. Since 1946, the Society has dedicated itself to providing support, opportunity, and advice to individuals with learning disabilities and their families, and today, MENCAP is the largest national organization of its type. Through its divisional and district offices, its federation of Gateway Clubs, and its associations with the International League of Societies for Mentally Handicapped Children and Adults and other national consortia, MENCAP offers a wide range of programs and services. These services include residential homes, training facilities and employment opportunities, support groups, networking, and public awareness campaigns. MENCAP also conducts research, publishes reports and a newsletter, produces audio-visual aids, and maintains a database of information. MENCAP only serves the United Kingdom, not including Scotland.

President: The Lord Rix, CBE DL
Executive Director: Fred Heddell
Year Established: 1946
Organization Members: 47,000

Publishes the following materials:
MENCAP Publications List ~ *Publications List*
Mencap's Work & Services ~ *Brochure*

1936 SCHEPENS EYE RESEARCH INSTITUTE

20 Staniford Street
Boston, MA 02114-2500 617-742-3140
Fax: 617-523-3463
E-mail: geninfo@vision.eri.harvard.edu

The Schepens Eye Research Institute, a not-for-profit organization, is a prominent center for research on the eye, vision, and blinding diseases. Established in 1950 and an affiliate of the Department of Ophthalmology at Harvard Medical School, the Schepens Eye Research Institute is dedicated to research that improves the understanding, management, and prevention of eye diseases and visual deficiencies; fosters collaboration among its faculty members; trains young scientists and clinicians from around the world; promotes communication with scientists in allied fields; and is a leader in the worldwide dispersion of basic scientific knowledge of vision. The Schepens Eye Research Institute's research program focuses on eye studies and the search for causes of disease in several core areas, including retinal and macular diseases (macular degeneration and diabetic retinopathy), corneal and ocular surface diseases (dry eye syndrome and corneal infection and injury), anterior segment diseases (glaucoma), ocular immunology (ocular cancer, inflammation, viral infections), transplantation (retinal and corneal transplants), and low vision aids and diagnostic technologies. The Schepens Eye Research Institute provides a variety of materials including brochures, reports and a magazine.

President: Richard Godfrey
Executive Director: J. Wayne Streilein, M.D.
Year Established: 1950
Organization Members: 170

Publishes the following materials:
The Schepens Eye Research Institute ~ *Annual Report*
The Schepens Eye Research Institute ~ *Annual Report*
Sundial ~ *Newsletter*

Concerned with the following diseases or disorders:
Chalazion; Chandler's Syndrome; Duane Syndrome; Eales Disease; Retinopathy, Arteriosclerotic; Retinopathy, Hypertensive

1937 SECOND WIND LUNG TRANSPLANT ASSOCIATION, INC.

9030 West Lakeview Court
Crystal River, FL 34428 352-563-0135
888-222-2690
Fax: 352-563-0728
E-mail: secondwind@xtalwind.net
http://www.arthouse.com/secondwind

Second Wind Lung Transplant Association, Inc. is a not-for-profit organization dedicated to improving the quality of life for lung transplant recipients, lung surgery candidates, people with related pulmonary concerns, and their families. The Association provides support, advocacy, education, information, and guidance through a spirit of service, "adding years to their lives and life to their years." Established in 1995 by a group of lung transplant recipients, candidates, and their families, Second Wind has quarterly support group meetings to provide educational programs (e.g., on nutrition, effects of medications and exercise, physical therapy) for both lung transplant candidates and recipients; to share experiences; and to enjoy social activities. Second Wind also is developing a directory of candidates and lung transplant recipients to provide networking opportunities; is establishing a mentor program to offer fellowship to affected individuals and families during the transplant experience; and is planning to establish low-cost Lung Transplant Housing near transplant hospitals for use by candidate and recipient transplant affected individuals and their support person. In addition, the organization provides educational programs; seeks to increase Organ Donor Awareness; and provides a quarterly newsletter entitled "AirWays" to their members. The Second Wind Lung Transplant Association also has a web site on the Internet that provides information to individuals who seekinformation on lung transplantation. The site also provides linkage to information on certain specific pulmonary disorders; describes Second Wind's mentoring program; and provides information concerning financing lung transplantation. Such information includes listings of organizations that may provide advocacy, assistance with fund-raising, financial grants, and/or medication or pharmaceutical payment assistance grants or programs.

President: Tom and Judy Wright, Co-President (1996 to Present)
Year Established: 1995
Organization Chapters: 3
Organization Members: 500

Publishes the following materials:
Second Wind Lung Transplant Association, Inc. "Support Through Service" ~ *Brochure*
Lung Transplant Association, Inc. ~ *Fact Pamphlet*
Second Wind Lung Transplant Association, Inc. ~ *Fact Pamphlet*

Concerned with the following diseases or disorders:
Lymphangioleiomyomatosis

1938 SELF HELP FOR HARD OF HEARING PEOPLE, INC. (SHHH)

7910 Woodmont Avenue
Suite 1200
Bethesda, MD 20814 301-657-2248
Fax: 301-913-9413
TDD: 301-657-2249
E-mail: 71162.634@compuserve.com
http://www.shhh.org

Self-Help for Hard of Hearing People, Inc. (SHHH) is an international non-profit self-help organization dedicated to the well-being of people of all ages and communication skills who do not hear well. The aims of SHHH are to educate affected individuals, their families, hearing health care providers, educators, industry, and government about hearing loss and those options available to help deal with hearing loss. Established in 1979 and consisting of 240 chapters, SHHH provides information on several aspects of hearing loss, from technological and medical advances to coping and parenting strategies. The organization also advocates for improved communication access for people with hearing loss in the workplace, hotels, schools, court systems, medical, and entertainment facilities. SHHH also encourages and supports research to improve hearing aids, assistive listening devices, and other technology needs of people with hearing loss, as well as research into understanding the causes of hearing loss and for development of new treatments. Self-Help for Hard of Hearing People, Inc. provides support in setting up local support groups and publishes "Hearing Loss," a bi-monthly magazine. Discounted publications and resource materials covering all aspects of hearing loss such as causes, coping strategies and technological devices are also available. SHHH maintains a site on the World Wide Web at [http://www.shhh.org].

President: Marcia Dugan (Present to 1998)
Executive Director: Donna L. Sorkin
Year Established: 1979
Organization Chapters: 240
Organization Members: 12,000

Publishes the following materials:
Hearing Loss: You can do something about it! ~ *Brochure*
Self Help for Hard of Hearing People, Inc. (1997 Publications Catalog) ~ *Catalog*

1939 **SEXUALITY INFORMATION AND EDUCATION COUNCIL OF THE U.S. (SIECUS)**
130 West 42nd Street
Suite 350
New York, NY 10010 212-819-9770
Fax: 212-819-9776
E-mail: siecus@siecus.org
http://www.siecus.org

The Sexuality Information and Education Council of the U.S. (SIECUS) is a nonprofit organization dedicated to developing, collecting, and disseminating information; promoting comprehensive education about sexuality; and advocating the rights of individuals to make responsible sexual choices. Established in 1964, SIECUS has many different programs including "Guidelines for Comprehensive Sexuality Education," which is used in kindergarten through twelfth grade. The guidelines were developed by the National Guidelines Task Force comprised of 20 leading health, education, and sexuality experts, and was initially convened in response to findings from a SIECUS study of programs for school sexuality and HIV/AIDS education. Another program is the "Condom Availability Program." This includes a fact sheet that provides information about the human immunodeficiency virus (HIV) and young people; their need for protection against infection from HIV and other sexually transmitted diseases (STDs) and unwanted pregnancy; and information about condoms and their use in comprehensive sexuality and HIV/AIDS education programs. Educational materials include a booklet entitled "How to Talk to Your Children About AIDS," a pamphlet entitled "SIECUS Publications Catalog," and a bimonthly journal entitled the "SIECUS Report." The organization provides appropriate referrals, encourages lobbying efforts, and supports education. SIECUS maintains the Mary S. Calderone Library; the library has more than 5,000 books, 2,000 journals and newsletters, and 500 sexuality and AIDS curricula. The library also has a computerized database with more than 10,000 citations.

President: Debra Hafner, M.P.H. (1988 to Present)
Organization Language: Spanish (written/spoken).
Year Established: 1964

Publishes the following materials:
SIECUS Publications 1995 ~ *Catalog*
SIECUS Annotated Bibliography of Available Print and Audiovisual Materials ~ *Bibliography*
Mary S. Calderone Library ~ *Information Sheet*
SIECUS Sexuality information and education council of the United States ~ *MIssion Statement*

Concerned with the following diseases or disorders:
AIDS (Acquired Immune Deficiency Syndrome); Bowenoid Papulosis; Condyloma; Fitz Hugh Curtis Syndrome; Proctitis; Reiter's Syndrome; Syphilis, Acquired

1940 **SHORT STATURE FOUNDATION (SSF)**
4521 Campus Drive
#310
Irvine, CA 92715 714-559-7131
800-243-9273
Fax: 714-258-1933

The Short Stature Foundation is a not-for-profit organization founded in 1984 to provide services to people with dwarfism or short stature. The Foundation serves as an advocate for people of short stature and seeks to enhance the positive well-being and independence of people with short stature or various forms of dwarfism. The organization encourages patient and professional education and supplies referrals to local physicians and support systems. In addition, the Foundation maintains a toll-free number that offers touch-tone services leading to a variety of resources.

President: Tina Schafnitz
Executive Director: Tina Schafnitz
Year Established: 1984

Concerned with the following diseases or disorders:
Achondrogenesis; Achondroplasia; Acrodysostosis; Acromesomelic Dysplasia; Acromicric Dysplasia; Arthrogryposis Multiplex Congenita; Camptomelic Syndrome; Conradi Hunermann Syndrome; Costello Syndrome; Diastrophic Dysplasia; Dyschondrosteosis; Ear, Patella, Short Stature Syndrome; Fairbank Disease; Floating-Harbor Syndrome; Froelich's Syndrome; Growth Delay, Constitutional; Growth Hormone Deficiency; Hypochondroplasia; Jansen Type Metaphyseal Chondrodysplasia; Johanson Blizzard Syndrome; Juberg Marsidi Syndrome; Kenny Caffe Syndrome; Kniest Syndrome; LEOPARD Syndrome; Laron Dwarfism; Leri Pleonosteosis; McKusick Type Metaphyseal Chondrodysplasia; Megalocornea Mental Retardation Syndrome; Mulibrey Nanism Syndrome (Perheentupa Syndrome); Myhre Syndrome; Robinow Syndrome; Rothmund Thomson Syndrome; Russell Silver Syndrome (RSS); SHORT Syndrome; Seckel Syndrome; Septo Optic Dysplasia; Spondyloepiphyseal Dysplasia Tarda; Spondyloepiphyseal Dysplasia, Congenital; Three M Syndrome; Weismann Netter Stuhl Syndrome

1941 SIBLING INFORMATION NETWORK

A.J. Pappanikou Center
62 Washington Street
Middletown, CT 06457-2844 860-344-7500
Fax: 860-344-7595
TDD: 860-344-7590

The Sibling Information Network is a national not-for-profit organization that was founded in 1981. The Network was established to assist individuals interested in the unique needs and concerns of families of persons with disabilities. In addition, it functions as a clearinghouse for information relating to brothers and sisters who have a sibling with a disability. Educational materials produced by the Network include a newsletter entitled "Sibling Information Network Newsletter," a listing of sibling groups and programs, an extensive bibliography of articles relating to sibling issues, and booklets entitled "Issues Relating to Developmental Disabilities: A Bibliography for Families" and "Children's Literature for Sisters and Brothers of Children with Special Needs." Guidelines for starting sibling programs and a list of videotape resources are also available from the Network.

President: Lisa Glidden
Year Established: 1981
Organization Members: 2,000

1942 SIBLING SUPPORT PROJECT

Children's Hospital and Medical Center
P.O. Box 5371
CL-09
Seattle, WA 98105-0371 206-368-4911
Fax: 206-368-4816
E-mail: dmeyer@chmc.org
http://www.chmc.org/departmt/sibsupp

The Sibling Support Project (SSP) is an organization dedicated to creating statewide systems of peer support and education programs for brothers and sisters of children with special needs throughout the United States. Established in 1990, SSP provides training, demonstrations, and technical assistance on creating programs specifically for brothers and sisters; works to increase the awareness of sibling issues and concerns through presentations to family members and service providers; and disseminates educational materials. Such materials include brochures and a newsletter entitled "The NASP Newsletter." The SSP has a Sibshop model that details the goals of the organization: to provide brothers and sisters of children with special needs an opportunity to meet other siblings in a relaxed, recreational setting; to provide brothers and sisters with an opportunity to discuss common concerns with other siblings; to provide brothers and sisters with an opportunity to learn how others handle situations commonly experienced by siblings of children with special needs; to provide brothers and sisters with an opportunity to learn more about the implications of their siblings' special needs; and to provide parents and service providers with opportunities to learn more about common concerns of brothers and sisters. The organization maintains a World Wide Web site at [http://www.chmc.org/departmt/sibsupp].

Executive Director: Donald J. Meyer
Year Established: 1990
Organization Chapters: 150

Publishes the following materials:
The Sibling Support Project. Resources for Parents and Service Providers ~ *Resource List*
The Sibling Support Project. A brief Description of the Sibshop Model ~ *Mission Statement*
NASP ~ *Neswletter*
The Sibling Support Project. Creating Opportunities for Brothers and Sisters of Children with Special Health and D ~ *Fact Sheet*
Announcing SibKids and SibNet! ~ *Fact Sheet*
Uncommon Fathers. Reflections on Raising a Child with a Disability ~ *Order Form*

1943 SIBLINGS FOR SIGNIFICANT CHANGE (SSC)

United Charities Building
East 22nd Street
Room 710
New York, NY 10010 212-420-0776
800-841-8251
Fax: 212-677-0696
E-mail: gerri@ix.netcom.com

Established in 1981, Siblings for Significant Change is a voluntary not-for-profit organization created by sisters of disabled individuals. The organization was founded on the belief that siblings as well as parents deserved support and guidance. Members of the organization include siblings of individuals with physical, emotional, and/or sensory impairments, cancer, or AIDS. Many members are preparing to assume the role of full-time caregiver to their siblings. Siblings for Significant Change provides advocacy training to siblings of disabled individuals. It offers counseling for siblings in need of support; engages in crisis intervention when required by families; and provides legal assistance to help siblings with matters of disability law and guardianship. In addition, the group promotes legislation that is beneficial to individuals with disabilities and their families; engages in professional education; works to educate the general public through informational multi-media programs; and provides appropriate referrals. The organization also conducts workshops and conferences for siblings; holds regular monthly meetings; conducts informal gatherings for families; and distributes a wide variety of educational and support materials. These include regular newsletters, article reprints, personal stories written by siblings, brochures, and audio-visual aids.

Executive Director: Gerry Zatlow
Year Established: 1981
Organization Chapters: 2
Organization Members: 75

Publishes the following materials:
Who are we? Siblings, What do we want? Significant Change ~ *Brochure*
The Sibling Perspective ~ *Report*

1944 SKIN CANCER FOUNDATION

245 Fifth Avenue
Suite 1403
New York, NY 10016 212-725-5176
800-754-6490
Fax: 212-725-5751
E-mail: info@skincancer.org

The Skin Cancer Foundation is a not-for-profit international educational health organization dedicated to providing information on detection and prevention of and support to individuals with skin cancer. The Foundation seeks to educate the public about the different forms of skin cancer and promotes and supports ongoing medical research into the causes and treatment of these diseases. Established in 1977, the Skin Cancer Foundation has a growing membership of over 130 leading physicians. The Foundation provides support for medical research and training; functions as a major resource center for the media; and works to educate the public. Programs include screening clinics, health fairs, and corporate and community wellness programs. Educational materials produced by the organization include a wide variety of brochures, posters, books, newsletters, and audio-visual materials.

President: Perry Robins (1977-Present)
Executive Director: Mitzl Moulds
Organization Language: Spanish (written). German (written). French (written).
Year Established: 1977
Organization Members: 1,000

Publishes the following materials:
The Skin Cancer Foundation Journal ~ *Journal*
Simple Guidelines To Help Protect You From The Damaging Rays Of The Sun ~ *Fact Sheet*
Skin Cancer Facts & Figures - 1993 ~ *Fact Sheet*
The Skin Cancer Foundation Seal of Recommendation ~ *Product List*
Sun & Skin News ~ *Newsletter*
The Melanoma Letter ~ *Newsletter*
Sun Fitness For All Ages ~ *Pamphlet*
Types and descriptions of Skin Cancers ~ *Pamphlet*
What You Need To Know About Skin Cancer ~ *Pamphlet*
Dysplastic nevi and malignant malanoma ~ *Pamphlet*
The ABCD's of Moles & Melanoma ~ *Pamphlet*
It's never too early to stop skin cancer... ~ *Pamphlet*
Skin Cancer: If You Can Spot It, You Can Stop It. ~ *Brochure*
Simple Steps To Sun Safety ~ *Pamphlet*
Sunproofing Your Baby ~ *Brochure*
Squamous Cell Carcinoma ~ *Brochure*
For Every Child Under the Sun ~ *Brochure*
Basal Cell Carcinoma - The Most Common Cancer ~ *Brochure*
The Many Faces Of Malignant Melanoma ~ *Brochure*

Concerned with the following diseases or disorders:
Bowen's Disease; Cancers, Skin, General; Carcinoma, Squamous Cell; De Santis Cacchione Syndrome; Dysplastic Nevus Syndrome; Melanoma, Malignant; Mycosis Fungoides; Nevoid Basal Cell Carcinoma Syndrome; Paget's Disease of the Breast; Xeroderma Pigmentosum

1945 SMELL AND TASTE CENTER

Smell and Taste Center
University of Pennsylvania 5 Ravdin Building
3400 Spruce Street
Philadelphia, PA 19104 215-662-6580
Fax: 215-349-5266

The Smell and Taste Center at the University of Pennsylvania was established in 1980 as the result of funding received from the National Institute of Neurological Disorders and Stroke, the Hoffman Fund, and other sources. It is the first clinical research center in the United States devoted to the senses of taste and smell and has achieved world-wide prominence for its research and clinical activities. In addition, the Center has plans to expand its facilities, clinical service, research programs, and staff. The Center is focused on three primary goals: to provide clinical evaluation, treatment, and counseling for patients ex affected individuals experiencing taste and smell disorders; to provide the facilities and an intellectual focus for research in both basic and applied aspects of chemoreception; and to provide training for students and doctoral level scientists and other interested medical personnel in both basic and applied aspects of chemoreception science. Foreign language translators are available from other departments at the University to speak with callers in most languages.

Executive Director: Richard L. Doty, Ph.D
Organization Language: Italian. Spanish. French. German.
Year Established: 1980
Organization Members: 20

Concerned with the following diseases or disorders:
Macroglossia; Tongue, Fissured; Tongue, Geographic; Tongue, Hairy

1946 SMITH-MAGENIS SYNDROME CONTACT GROUP (SMS CONTACT GROUP.)

1 Poppyfields
Chester-le-Street
Durham, DH2 2NA
United Kingdom 191-388-8868
E-mail: blue.J@bigfoot.com

Located in the United Kingdom, the Smith-Magenis Syndrome Contact Group is an international self-help organization dedicated to providing information and support to individuals with Smith-Magenis Syndrome and their families. Smith-Magenis Syndrome is an extremely rare congenital disorder in which chromosomal material is absent from a certain portion of the short arm (p) of chromosome 17 (interstitial deletion 17p11.2) due to a spontaneous (de novo) genetic change early in embryonic development. Affected individuals may have a variety of associated symptoms and physical abnormalities including characteristic malformations of the head and facial area; abnormalities of the fingers and hands; speech delays and an unusually deep, hoarse voice; hearing loss; and/or moderate to severe mental retardation. In addition, many affected children may demonstrate self-destructive behavior. Established in 1992, the Smith-Magenis Syndrome Contact Group is committed to disseminating information concerning Smith-Magenis Syndrome to affected families and health care professionals; promoting awareness of the disorder in the United Kingdom; and providing networking opportunities to affected families to enable them to exchange information, support, and resources. The Contact Group also promotes research; engages in patient, professional, and general education; and provides a variety of materials including pamphlets, brochures, and a regular newsletter.

President: Julie Jowitt (1992 to Present).
Year Established: 1992
Organization Members: 45

Concerned with the following diseases or disorders:
Smith Magenis Syndrome

1947 SOCIETY FOR MUSCULAR DYSTROPHY INFORMATION INTERNATIONAL (SMDI INTERNATIONAL)

P.O. Box 479
Bridgewater
Nova Scotia, B4V 2X6
Canada 902-685-3961
Fax: 902-685-3962
E-mail: smdi@auracom.com

The Society for Muscular Dystrophy Information International (SMDI) is a not-for-profit registered Canadian charity dedicated to assisting people in helping themselves by reducing the national and international isolation of individuals and organizations concerned with neuromuscular disorders/disabilities (e.g., muscular dystrophy and over 50 allied disorders). In general, "neuromuscular disorder" is a term used to describe a group of over 50 diseases affecting the body's motor neurons (nerves and muscles). Symptoms may include varying degrees of progressive muscle weakness and loss of muscle mass (wasting). SMDI was established in 1983 to provide a non-technical information link for individuals with neuromuscular disorders and for organizations around the world; to link people with other people and organizations concerned with their disorder; to share information to assist people in helping themselves; and to create increased public awareness of this group of disorders. The Society publishes two quarterly newsletters entitled "S.M.D.I. International Newsletter," a publication for those concerned with muscular dystrophy or the allied disorders and "Access - Able Information," a quarterly disability information resource publication. In addition to educational materials, brochures and referrals are available. SMDI provides a toll-free hotline for affected individuals and their families for support.

President: James Dobson (1983 to Present)
Executive Director: Linda Dobson
Year Established: 1983

Publishes the following materials:
SMDI International ~ *Mission Statement*
Access-able Information. Helping People Help Themselves (Spring 1977) ~ *Resource Publication*
Society for Muscular Dystrophy Information International (Spring 1997) ~ *Newsletter*
Society for Muscular Dystrophy Information (Summer 1997) ~ *Newsletter*
SMDI International ~ *Mission Statement*
Access-Able Information. Helping People Help Themselves (Summer 1997) ~ *Resource Publication*

Concerned with the following diseases or disorders:
Muscular Dystrophy, Becker; Muscular Dystrophy, Duchenne; Muscular Dystrophy, Emery Dreifuss; Muscular Dystrophy, Fukuyama Type; Muscular Dystrophy, Landouzy Dejerine; Muscular Dystrophy, Limb Girdle; Muscular Dystrophy, Oculo-Gastrointestinal

1948 SOCIETY FOR PROGRESSIVE SUPRANUCLEAR PALSY (SPSP)

Johns Hopkins Outpatient Center
Suite 5065
601 N. Caroline Street
Baltimore, MD 21287 410-955-2954
800-457-4777
Fax: 410-614-9260
E-mail: epkatz@erols.com
spsp@erols.com
http://www.psp.org

The Society for Progressive Supranuclear Palsy is a not-for-profit voluntary service organization dedicated to providing information to families, health care professionals, and others interested in or affected by Progressive Supranuclear Palsy (PSP). In addition, the Society is an advocate for affected individuals and acts as a self-help organization for people with this disorder. Established in late 1990, the Society supports and promotes research into the causes, treatment, and potential cure for Progressive Supranuclear Palsy. The Society has a medical advisory board of neurologists from the United States, England, France, and Italy. The organization publishes a quarterly newsletter entitled the "PSP Advocate." The publication reports findings in the area of PSP and includes editorials, updates, and comprehensive strategies for managing the disorder. In addition, the organization holds symposia and regional lectures, provides referral cards, brochures, and videotapes.

President: Joanne Armstrong (1992-Present)
Executive Director: Ellen Pam Katz
Year Established: 1990
Organization Members: 2,800

Publishes the following materials:
Personality Changes in PSP ~ *Brochure*
Advocacy and Support ~ *Brochure*
PSP Some Answers ~ *Brochure*
PSP Advocate ~ *Newsletter*

Concerned with the following diseases or disorders:
Progressive Supranuclear Palsy

1949 SPINA BIFIDA AND HYDROCEPHALUS ASSOCIATION OF CANADA (SBHAC)

220-388 Donald Street
Winnipeg
Manitoba, R3B 2J4
Canada 204-925-3650
800-565-9488
Fax: 204-925-3654
E-mail: spinab@mts.net
http://www.sbhac.ca

The Spina Bifida and Hydrocephalus Association of Canada (SBHAC) is a not-for-profit support organization dedicated to improving the quality of life of individuals with spina bifida and/or hydrocephalus and their families through awareness, education, and research. Spina bifida is a neural tube defect occurring early during fetal development, in which part of one or more of the bones of the spine (vertebrae) fail to develop completely, leaving a portion of the spinal cord exposed and resulting in damage to exposed nerve tissue. Hydrocephalus is a condition in which there is abnormal accumulation of cerebrospinal fluid in the skull, causing increased pressure on the brain. Established in 1981, the SBHAC currently has approximately 2,400 members in 11 chapters throughout Canada. The Association provides a variety of programs and services including and 800 Help Line, support networking, educational workshops and seminars, and annual educational conference, research grants, scholarship programs for students with spina bifida and/or hydrocephalus, and public awareness programs. The Association also offers a variety of educational guides and materials for schools, professionals, parents, and the general public including fact sheets; articles; a lending library of materials including books, guides, handbooks, and videos; and a regular newsletter entitled "Podium." SBHAC also maintains a web site on the Internet [http://www.sbhac.ca].

President: Colleen Talbot (1996 to Present)
Executive Director: Andrea Salmon
Organization Language: French (written/spoken). Spanish (written).
Year Established: 1981
Organization Chapters: 11
Organization Members: 2,400

Publishes the following materials:
A Bright Future (English/French) ~ *Book Mark*
Folic Acid. What every woman should know before becoming pregnant ~ *Brochure*
Folic Acid. What every woman should know before becoming pregnant (French) ~ *Brochure*
Folic Acid. What every woman should know before becoming pregnant (Japanese) ~ *Brochure*
Spina Bifida and Hydrocephalus (English/French) ~ *Brochure*
Latex in the hospital environment ~ *Fact Sheet*
Catalogue of Library Articles for People with Spina Bifida and/or Hydrocephalus, Their Families and Their Friends ~ *Catalogue*

Concerned with the following diseases or disorders:
Fetal Valproate Syndrome; Spina Bifida; Tethered Spinal Cord Syndrome

1950 SPINAL CORD SOCIETY (SCS)

Wendell Road
Fergus Falls, MN 56537 218-739-5252
Fax: 218-739-5262
http://users.aol.com/scsweb

The Spinal Cord Society is a not-for-profit organization whose members include individuals with spinal cord injuries, their families and friends, and scientists and physicians who are dedicated to finding a cure for spinal cord paralysis through improved treatment and research. Established in 1978, the Society is a grassroots organization linked by over 200 chapters and more than 4,000 members throughout the United States and around the world. The Society raises funds for medical research, promotes citizen advocacy, and provides appropriate referrals to treatment and support. The Spinal Cord Society has been instrumental in establishing civilian research conferences and cure research/treatment centers for spinal cord injury. Other projects include pioneering computerized walking technology (functional electronic stimulation) for such injuries; artificial bone substitutes; autologous cell transplants (transplants to the spinal cord of cells cultured from the patient's own body); and regeneration research. The Spinal Cord Society also publishes a monthly newsletter.

President: Dr. Charles E. Carson
Year Established: 1978
Organization Chapters: 200
Organization Members: 4,000

Concerned with the following diseases or disorders:
Arachnoiditis; Myelitis

1951 SPOTLIGHT 6

2617 Ted Toad Road
Rising Sun, MD 21911 410-658-6264

Spotlight 6 is a not-for-profit self-help organization dedicated to gathering and sharing information on abnormalities of chromosome 6 in children. Established in 1993, this parent-run organization provides support and information to affected families, caregivers, and concerned health care professionals. Spotlight 6 publishes a newsletter for members that includes medical journal abstracts, article reprints, research updates, and more.

President: Ted Wiggins
Executive Director: Valeria Wiggins
Year Established: N/A

Concerned with the following diseases or disorders:
Chromosome 6 Ring; Chromosome 6, Partial Trisomy 6q

1952 STARLIGHT CHILDREN'S FOUNDATION

International Headquarters
12424 Wilshire Boulevard
Suite 1050
Los Angeles, CA 90025 310-207-5558
800-274-7827
Fax: 310-207-2554
http://www.starlight.org

The Starlight Children's Foundation is a not-for-profit organization dedicated to granting the wishes of seriously ill children and their families. Established in 1983 by Emma Samms and film executive Peter Samuelson, the Starlight Children's Foundation brightens the lives of seriously ill children from ages four to 18 years. Nearly 46,000 children benefit each month from Starlight programs including wish granting, Starlight Fun Centers, and Starlight Rooms. The types of wishes granted include trips (e.g., Disneyland), tangible items (e.g., computer, bikes, toys), event/experiences (e.g., Laker Girl, space camp), and celebrity meetings. The Fun Center Program provides hospitalized kids all over the world with mobile entertainment units that are rolled into action into a child's hospital room. These units contain a color television, VCR, and video games. Starlight Rooms are state of the art pediatric play rooms that enable hospitalized children an escape from their sterile hospital room environments. In addition, the Foundation provides hospital parties for seriously ill children. The Starlight Children's Foundation consists of 13 chapters across the United States and in the United Kingdom, Australia, and Canada. Starlight produces educational materials including fact sheets, brochures, a booklet entitled "Starlight Foundation," and a newsletter entitled "The Shining Star." The organization supports fund-raising activities, provides administrative support, and maintains a database. The Starlight Children's Foundation also maintains a web site on the Internet at [http://www.starlight.org].

Executive Director: Katherine Culpepper
Organization Language: Spanish (written/spoken).
Year Established: 1983
Organization Chapters: 13
Organization Members: Non-Membership

Publishes the following materials:
Starlight Fact Sheet ~ *Fact Sheet*
Starlight Foundation International. 1995-1996 Annual Report ~ *Leaflet*
The Shining Star ~ *Newsletter*
Starlight Children's Foundation ~ *Leaflet*

1953 SUDDEN ARRHYTHMIA DEATH SYNDROMES FOUNDATION (SADS)

P.O. Box
58767
549 Arapee Drive Suite 207
Salt Lake City, UT 84158 801-582-1934
800-786-7723
Fax: 801-582-1941

The Sudden Arrhythmia Death Syndromes (SADS) Foundation is a national not-for-profit organization that was established in 1991. The mission of the Foundation is to save the lives of children and young adults who are genetically predisposed to sudden death due to abnormal rhythym or rate of the heart beat (cardiac arrhythmias). The Foundation seeks to educate health care providers and the public about Sudden Arrhythmia Death Syndromes to promote early diagnosis and treatment. The Foundation encourages and funds ongoing medical research into Long QT Syndrome and other genetic cardiovascular diseases that predispose young people to sudden death. SADS serves as a physician referral resource center and provides advice to physicians who care for people with Long QT Syndrome. In addition, the Foundation is interested in the identification of individuals and families at risk for these diseases and to assisting families and friends affected by Long QT Syndrome. Educational materials distributed by the organization include reprints of medical articles and an informational brochure on Long QT Syndrome.

President: G. Michael Vincet, M.D. (1992-Present)
Executive Director: Charlene Holmstrom
Year Established: 1991

1954 SUPERKIDS, INC. (NEWSLETTER FOR FAMILIES AND FRIENDS OF CHILDREN WITH LIMB DIFFERENCES)

60 Clyde Street
Newton, MA 02160

Superkids is a newsletter for families and friends of children with limb differences. It is published twice a year and is free to interested families and professionals. The newsletter offers timely information and support to those affected by limb differences.

President: Peggy McLoughlin
Executive Director: Peter McLoughlin
Year Established: 1981
Organization Members: 3,000

Publishes the following materials:
Superkids ~ *Newsletter*

Concerned with the following diseases or disorders:
Adams Oliver Syndrome; Clubfoot; Cornelia de Lange Syndrome; Dysplasia, Epiphysealis Hemimelica; Holt Oram Syndrome; Phocomelia Syndrome; Schinzel Syndrome

1955 SUPPORT ORGANIZATION FOR TRISOMY 13/18 AND RELATED DISORDERS, UK (S.O.F.T. UK)

Tudor Lodge
Redwood
Ross-on-Wye
Herefordshire, HR9 5UD
United Kingdom 198-956-7480

Support Organisation for Trisomy 13/18 and Related Disorders is an international UK-based organization that serves families affected by Trisomy 13/18, related disorders, and rare conditions for whom no other organisation exists. SOFT provides support, assistance, and information for families in many different situations and stages of diagnosement, caregiving, and for some, grief. SOFT offers informational packets, booklets, a "link list"networking service, a newsletter, support groups, patient education, advocacy, a journal, a database, and a variety of audio-visual aids. SOFT serves the UK, the USA (in conjunction with SOFT USA), Scandinavia, Europe, New Zealand, and Australia; and through member resources, SOFT supports the English, Italian, French, German, Danish, and Swedish languages.

President: Jenny Robbins
Organization Language: Italian. French. German. Danish.
Year Established: 1990
Organization Chapters: 9
Organization Members: 1,000

Concerned with the following diseases or disorders:
Chromosome 9, Trisomy 9P (Multiple Variants); Trisomy 13 Syndrome; Trisomy 18 Syndrome

1956 SUPPORT ORGANIZATION FOR TRISOMY 18, 13, AND RELATED DISORDERS (SOFT)

2982 S. Union Street
Rochester, NY 14624-1926 716-594-4621
800-716-7638
Fax: 716-594-4621

The Support Organization for Trisomy 18, 13, and Related Disorders (SOFT) is a voluntary not-for-profit network consisting of affected families and professionals who are involved in the care of individuals with Trisomy 18, Trisomy 13, and other related disorders (e.g., other chromosomal abnormalities involving the duplication of genetic material). Established in 1979, SOFT was created to provide affected families and professionals with the additional information and support they often need when confronted with a diagnosis of Trisomy 18, 13, or related chromosomal disorders. The Organization enables parents to share information and support; promotes education of health care professionals; provides appropriate referrals to affected families; holds local chapter gatherings for interested members; and conducts an annual international conference with seminars and cost-free consultations with doctors and other professionals. Educational material distributed by the Organization include a quarterly national newsletter containing letters from affected families and articles by a variety of professionals, booklets and brochures, and audio visual aids. A computer database is also maintained by SOFT.

President: Barbara Van Herrewegle
Year Established: 1979
Organization Chapters: 50
Organization Members: 2,000

Publishes the following materials:
Support Organization for Trisomy 18, 13, and Related Disorders ~ *Brochure*
Trisomy 13 Facts ~ *Brochure*
Trisomy 18 Facts ~ *Brochure*
The Soft Touch ~ *Booklet*
Guidebook Order Form ~ *Order Form*
Common Problems of Babies with Trisomy 18 or 13 ~ *Pamphlet*
Background: The Need for S.O.F.T. ~ *Pamphlet*
Available S.O.F.T. Materials ~ *Factsheet*
Trisomy in Review ~ *Pamphlet*
Your Baby - Facts for Families ~ *Booklet*
Prenatal Diagnosis ~ *Booklet*
Your Baby - Facts for Families ~ *Booklet*
SOFT ~ *Pamphlet*
SOFT Newsletter No. 16 ~ *Newsletter*

Concerned with the following diseases or disorders:
Chromosome 10, Distal Trisomy 10q; Chromosome 11, Partial Trisomy 11q; Chromosome 14, Trisomy Mosaic; Chromosome 15, Distal Trisomy 15q; Chromosome 18, Monosomy 18p; Chromosome 18, Tetrasomy 18p; Chromosome 22, Trisomy Mosaic; Chromosome 3, Trisomy 3q2; Chromosome 4, Partial Trisomy Distal 4q; Chromosome 4, Trisomy 4p; Chromosome 5, Trisomy 5p; Chromosome 6, Partial Trisomy 6q; Chromosome 7, Monosomy 7p2; Chromosome 9, Tetrasomy 9p; Chromosome 9, Trisomy 9P (Multiple Variants); Chromosome 9, Trisomy Mosaic; Penta X Syndrome; Trisomy; Trisomy 13 Syndrome; Trisomy 18 Syndrome

1957 SUPPORT FOR PEOPLE WITH ORAL AND HEAD AND NECK CANCER, INC. (SPOHNC)

P.O. Box 53
Locust Valley, NY 11560-0053 516-759-5333
Fax: 516-671-7637
E-mail: spohnc@ix.netcom.com
http://www.cybermedical.com/spohnc/

Support for People with Oral and Head and Neck Cancer (SPOHNC) is a patient-directed not-for-profit organization dedicated to addressing the broad emotional, physical, and humanistic needs of oral and head and neck cancer patients. Founded in 1991, the organization produces educational materials including "News from SPOHNC," a newsletter that is published quarterly. SPOHNC facilitates small group meetings, networking and one-to-one support. It also has educational programs for affected individuals and families and provides referrals to additional resources. SPOHNC encourages and promotes increased scientific clinical research and development in the improvement of quality of life for individuals affected by oral and head and neck cancer.

President: Nancy E. Leupold (1991 to Present)
Year Established: 1991
Organization Chapters: 1
Organization Members: 300

Publishes the following materials:
SPOHNC ~ *Mission Statement*
News From SPOHNC (February 1997) ~ *Newsletter*
Products to Help Improve the Quality of Life for People with Oral and Head and Neck Cancer ~ *Leaflet*
News From SPOHNC (March 1997) ~ *Newsletter*
News From SPOHNC (April 1997) ~ *Newsletter*
News From SPOHNC (Summer 1997) ~ *Newsletter*

1958 THRESHOLD (FOR UNCONTROLLED SEIZURE DISORDERS)
PO Box 7002
Hackettstown, NJ 07840 732-974-1144
E-mail: fscnj@aol.com
http://www.efnj.com

THRESHOLD, sponsored by the Epilepsy Foundation of New Jersey, is a newsletter dedicated to providing information and support to parents of children with Intractable Seizure Disorder (uncontrolled seizure disorders). Established in 1988, THRESHOLD is published and distributed to more than 1,000 affected families and concerned health care professionals across the United States and throughout the world. The newsletter provides information on uncontrolled seizure disorders as well as parent-to-parent support information.

President: Cheryl Cooper-Kinney
Executive Director: Eric Joice
Year Established: 1988
Organization Members: 1,000

Concerned with the following diseases or disorders:
Alpers Disease; Cardio Facio Cutaneous Syndrome; Lennox Gastaut Syndrome; Perisylvian Syndrome, Congenital Bilateral; West Syndrome

1959 TAKING ACTION AGAINST LANGUAGE DISORDERS FOR KIDS, INC. (TALK)
22980 Donna Lane
Bend, OR 97701 541-389-0004
Fax: 541-389-0004
E-mail: TALK@Hwy97.net

Taking Action Against Language Disorders for Kids, Inc. (TALK) is a service organization dedicated to educating the medical and educational communities and the public on the importance of early recognition of speech and language disorders in children. Established in 1992, the organization promotes the exchange of current information on speech and language disorders or impairments and other topics such as parental issues, research, behavior modification approaches, and speech/language and occupational therapy techniques. This is accomplished through an established nationwide network that is available to the public and educational and medical communities. The organization also offers parental support to affected families, providing such families with resources, articles, and other materials. It is hoped that this support will enable parents to become advocates for their children to help ensure their rights under the law. The organization also offers support to the siblings of affected children through informational literature and other resources. TALK also exchanges current information and resources with organizations and agencies locally, nationally, and worldwide and makes a library of relevant materials available to the public and medical and educational communities. In addition, the organization provides a directory and a regular newsletter.

President: Linda Newland (1992-Present)
Executive Director: Linda Newland
Year Established: 1992
Organization Chapters: 1
Organization Members: 350

Publishes the following materials:
T.A.L.K. ~ *Newsletter*
Dear Bobbie: ~ *Letter*

Concerned with the following diseases or disorders:
Acidemia, Methylmalonic

1960 TELECOMMUNICATIONS FOR THE DEAF, INC. (TDI)
8630 Fenton Street
Suite 604
Silver Spring, MD 20910-3803 301-589-3786
Fax: 301-589-3797
TDD: 301-589-3006
E-mail: tdiexdir@aol.com

Telecommunications for the Deaf, Inc. (TDI) is a non-profit advocacy organization dedicated to promoting full visual access to information and telecommunications through consumer education and involvement; technical assistance and consulting; application of existing and emerging technologies; networking and collaboration; uniformity of standards; and national policy development and advocacy. The or. The organization serves people who are deaf, hear of hearing, deaf/blind, and/or speech impaired. TDI's main objectives are promoting text telephone compatibility with existing communication devices; increasing toll-free services for TTY users; improving emergency access; and improving communications between TTY and other telephone users through comprehensive telecommunications relay services training. Telecommunications for the Deaf, Inc. also develops, implements, and evaluates new strategies for improving the quality and availability of visual telecommunications; encourages progress in key technologies such as television captioning; creates improved specifications and standards for equipment, telecommunications relay, and emergency services; educates the public about and supports legislation to improve telecommunications services; and builds coalitions of consumers and service providers to meet the needs of the deaf, heard of hearing, and speech-impaired. In addition, TDI provides training to industry groups and service providers who need assistance in service implementation. TDI provides a comprehensive overview of deafness and deaf culture; explains the influence of American Sign Language on TTY communication; trains personnel in telecommunications relay and emergency services; and conducts needs assessment studies, manages focus groups, and designs surveys to guide service-improvement projects. TDI comprises 9,000 members and three chapters. The organization's e-mail address is [tdiexdir@aol.com].

President: Roy Miller
Executive Director: Claude Stout
Organization Language: American Sign Language.
Year Established: 1968
Organization Chapters: 3
Organization Members: 9,000

Publishes the following materials:
Promoting Telecommunication - Access For All ~ *Brochure*
GA-SK Newsletter ~ *Newsletter*
When a Life is on the Line, Will Your TTY Call be Understood? ~ *Brochure*
Emergency Access Self Evaluation ~ *Order Form*
TDI Products Order Form ~ *Order Form*
Is Your Organization listed in the National Directory of TTY Numbers ~ *Directory Listing Application*
Is Your Name Listed in the "Blue Book"? ~ *Directory Listing Application*
Telecommunications for the Deaf, Inc. Promoting telecommunication access for all ~ *Brochure*

1961 THE ARC (A NATIONAL ORGANIZATION ON MENTAL RETARDATION)

500 East Border Street
Suite 300
Arlington, TX 76010 817-261-6003
800-433-5255
Fax: 817-277-3491
TDD: 817-277-0553
E-mail: thearc@metronet.com
http://thearc.org/welcome.html

The Arc is the largest organization in the United States that is solely devoted to improving the lives of all children and adults with mental retardation. The organization offers support to families affected by mental retardation and fosters research and educational programs on the prevention of mental retardation. The Arc is committed to securing opportunities for all people with mental retardation. To this end, the organization emphasizes personal opportunities for choice in education, housing, employment, and entertainment. The Arc is further committed to reducing the incidence and limiting the consequences of mental retardation through research, advocacy, and mutual support. The Arc provides leadership in the field of mental retardation and develops necessary human and financial resources to attain its goals. In addition, the Arc provides a wide variety of educational materials for parents, teachers, health care professionals, and others, including a regular newsletter, handbooks, instruction packets, reports, booklets, audio-visual aids, posters, and brochures. Many materials are available in Spanish.

President: Quincy Abbot (1996-Present)
Executive Director: Alan Aberson
Year Established: 1950
Organization Chapters: 1,100
Organization Members: 140,000

Publishes the following materials:
Publications Catalog ~ *Catalog*
Q&A Introduction to The Arc ~ *Fact Sheet*
Q&A Inroduction to Mental Retardation ~ *Fact Sheet*

Concerned with the following diseases or disorders:
5 Oxoprolinuria; AIDS Dysmorphic Syndrome; Acidemia, Isovaleric; Acidemia, Methylmalonic; Acidemia, Propionic; Adrenoleukodystrophy; Agenesis of Corpus Callosum; Aicardi Syndrome; Alagille Syndrome; Alexander's Disease; Anemia, Pernicious; Angelman Syndrome; Aniridia; Apert Syndrome; Arginase Deficiency; Beckwith Wiedemann Syndrome; Carnosinemia; Chromosome 18, Tetrasomy 18p; Chromosome 3, Trisomy 3q2; Chromosome 8, Monosomy 8p2; Chromosome 9, Partial Monosomy 9p;

Chromosome 9, Tetrasomy 9p; Coffin Lowry Syndrome; Coffin Siris Syndrome; Conradi Hunermann Syndrome; Cornelia de Lange Syndrome; Cri du Chat Syndrome; Crouzon Disease; DiGeorge Syndrome; Down Syndrome; Dubowitz Syndrome; Ectodermal Dysplasias; Encephalitis, Rasmussen's; Fetal Alcohol Syndrome; Froelich's Syndrome; Ganglioside Sialidase Deficiency; Gaucher Disease; Glutaricaciduria I; Goldenhar Syndrome (Oculo Auriculo Vertebral Spectrum); Hallermann Streiff Syndrome; Hallervorden Spatz Disease; Hartnup Disease; Homocystinuria; Hunter Syndrome; Hurler Syndrome; Hydranencephaly; Hydrocephalus; I Cell Disease; Ichthyosis, Sjogren Larsson Syndrome; Joubert Syndrome; KBG Syndrome; Kufs Disease; Larsen Syndrome; Laurence Moon Syndrome; Leigh's Disease; Leprechaunism; Lesch Nyhan Syndrome; Leukodystrophy, Krabbe's; Lipodystrophy; Lowe's Syndrome; Mannosidosis; Maple Syrup Urine Disease; Meningitis; Moebius Syndrome; Non-Ketotic Hyperglycinemia; Noonan Syndrome; Norrie Syndrome; Oral Facial Digital Syndrome; Pallister Killian Mosaic Syndrome; Paraplegia, Hereditary Spastic; Phenylketonuria; Pseudo Hurler Polydystrophy; Pyruvate Dehydrogenase Deficiency; Retrolental Fibroplasia; Rett Syndrome; Rubella, Congenital; Rubinstein Taybi Syndrome; Russell Silver Syndrome (RSS); Saethre Chotzen Syndrome; Sanfilippo Syndrome; Schindler Disease; Seckel Syndrome; Septo Optic Dysplasia; Sialidosis; Sly Syndrome; Smith Lemli Opitz Syndrome; Sotos Syndrome; Sturge Weber Syndrome; Tetrahydrobiopterin Deficiency; Toxoplasmosis; Trisomy; Trisomy 13 Syndrome; Trisomy 18 Syndrome; Tuberous Sclerosis; Tyrosinemia, Hereditary; Wiedemann Rautenstrauch Syndrome; Williams Syndrome; Wilms' Tumor; Xeroderma Pigmentosum; Zellweger Syndrome

1962 THINK FIRST FOUNDATION (TFF)

22 South Washington Street
Park Ridge, IL 60068 — 847-692-2740
800-844-6556
Fax: 847-692-2394
E-mail: thinkfirst@aans.org
http://www.thinkfirst.org

The Think First Foundation (TFF) is a not-for-profit voluntary organization dedicated to preventing brain and spinal cord injuries through education of individuals, community leaders, and creators of public policy. Established in 1986, TFF was founded by the American Association of Neurological Surgeons and the Congress of Neurological Surgeons. Consisting of more than 200 chapters, TFF produces educational materials including a catalog entitled "1997 Catalog, Think First," the "Think First Fact Sheet," and brochures. The Foundation conducts high school presentations, develops local programs engaging in public policy initiatives, supports public and community awareness projects, and has the "Think First For Kids" program which is implemented in elementary schools by local teachers. TFF includes more than 200 active local programs throughout the United States, Chile, Canada, Mexico, and Brazil. Each program includes a sponsoring licensed physician and program coordinator who participate in the Think First high school program. More than five million students have attended Think First program presentations. TFF maintains a web site on the Internet at [http://www.thinkfirst.org].

President: Thomas G. Saul, M.D. (Chairperson) (1996 to Present)
Executive Director: Frederick Grubbe (CEO)
Organization Language: Spanish (written).
Year Established: 1986
Organization Chapters: 200
Organization Members: Non-Membership

Publishes the following materials:
Think First Fact Sheet ~ *Mission Statement*
Think First ~ *Fact Sheet*
Good follows bad ~ *Reprint*
Think First for kids curriculum summary ~ *Fact Sheet*
Street Smart. Relaxin at the play ground! ~ *Comic*
Street Smart. Time to make a splash! ~ *Comic*
Prevention ~ *Newsletter*
Think First Foundation. 1995 Annual Report ~ *Booklet*

1963 THYROID FOUNDATION OF AMERICA, INC. (TFA)

Ruth Sleeper Hall
RSL 350
40 Parkman Street
Boston, MA 02114-2698 — 617-726-8500
800-832-8321
Fax: 617-726-4136

The Thyroid Foundation of America, Inc. (TFA) was established in 1986 as a national not-for-for profit organization dedicated to providing support and information to affected individuals and health care professionals on all types of thyroid diseases. Thyroid diseases are a group of disorders of the thyroid gland typically involving overactivity of the thyroid (hyperthyroidism) or underactivity of the thyroid (hypothyroidism). TFA currently consists of 12 chapters and interest groups and approximately 4,500 members. The goals of the Foundation include increasing public awareness of thyroid diseases; lending moral support to affected individuals and their families; and raising and distributing funds for thyroid research. TFA produces a variety of educational materials including a quarterly newsletter entitled "The Bridge," brochures, and reprints of medical articles.

President: Lawrence C. Wood, M.D. (1985-Present)
Organization Language: Spanish.
Year Established: 1985
Organization Chapters: 12
Organization Members: 4,500

Publishes the following materials:
Thyroid Topics Childhood Head and Neck Irradiation ~ *Brochure*
Thyroid Topics Postpartum Thyroiditis ~ *Brochure*
Thyroid Topics Thyroid Disease in the Elderly ~ *Brochure*
Thyroid Topics Cancer Of The Thyroid Papillary and Follicular Thyroid Cancer ~ *Brochure*
Thyroid Topics Graves' Disease Hyperthryoidism Caused by Diffuse Toxic Goiter ~ *Brochure*
Thyroid Topics Hyperthyroidism ~ *Brochure*
Thyroid Topics Hypothyroidism ~ *Brochure*
Thyroid Topics Thyroid Hormone Treatment ~ *Brochure*
The Thyroid Foundation of America, Inc. ~ *Factsheet*
Thyroid Foundation of America Bibliography ~ *Factsheet*
The Thyroid Foundation of America Publications List ~ *Factsheet*
Brochure and Book Order Form ~ *Order Form*

Concerned with the following diseases or disorders:
Graves' Disease; Hashimoto's Syndrome; Hypoparathyroidism; Hypothyroidism; Schmidt Syndrome; Sheehan Syndrome

1964 THYROID FOUNDATION OF CANADA

1040 Gardiners Road
Suite C
Kingston, M3H 1H1
Canada 613-634-3426
800-267-8822
Fax: 613-634-3483
E-mail: thyroid@ican.net
http://www.home.ican.net/~thyroid/Canada.html

The Thyroid Foundation of Canada (TFC) was founded in 1980 as a not-for-profit organization in response to the needs of affected individuals and their families for more information and support on all forms of thyroid diseases. Thyroid diseases are a group of disorders of the thyroid gland typically involving overactivity of the thyroid (hyperthyroidism) or underactivity of the thyroid (hypothyroidism). TFC has 22 chapters and 4,200 members. The aims of the Foundation are to increase public interest in and awareness of thyroid diseases; lend moral support to individuals and families affected by thyroid disease; and to assist in fundraising for thyroid disease research. TFC publishes a quarterly newsletter entitled "Thyrobulletin" and other patient-directed educational material. In addition, it conducts public education meetings with medical experts, and raises funds for thyroid disease research. TFC maintains a web site at [http://www.home.ican.net/~thyroid/Canada.html]; its e-mail address is [thyroid2ican.net].

President: Arliss Beardmore (1997-2000)
Executive Director: Katherine Keen
Organization Language: French (written/spoken).
Year Established: 1980
Organization Chapters: 22
Organization Members: 4,200

Publishes the following materials:
Thyroid Disease is real. Know The Facts (French) ~ *Brochure*
Thyroid Disease is real. Know The Facts ~ *Brochure*
The Thyroid Gland. A General Introduction ~ *Brochure*
To Confirm the Clinical Diagnosis ~ *Brochure*
Hypothyroidism ~ *Brochure*
Thyroid Nodules ~ *Brochure*
Throiditis ~ *Brochure*
Graves' Hyperthyroidism (Thryotoxicosis) ~ *Brochure*
Graves' Eye Disease (Ophthalmopathy) ~ *Brochure*
Thyroid Disease, Pregnancy and Fertility ~ *Brochure*
Thyroid Disease in Childhood ~ *Brochure*
Thyroid Disease in Late Life ~ *Brochure*
Surgical Treatment of Thyroid Disease ~ *Brochure*
Thyroid Cancer ~ *Brochure*
THYRObulletin ~ *Newsletter Spring 1997*

Concerned with the following diseases or disorders:
Graves' Disease; Hashimoto's Syndrome; Hypoparathyroidism

1965 TRANSWEB: ALL ABOUT TRANSPLANTATION AND DONATION

Trans Web
The Norther Brewery Bldg.
1327 Jones Drive, Suite 105
Ann Arbor, MI 48105 313-998-7314
Fax: 313-998-6710
E-mail: transweb@umich.edu
http://www.transweb.org

TransWeb is an online resource on the World Wide Web dedicated to providing information concerning organ transplantation and donation. Its goals include providing a resource for transplant patients and families world wide with information specifically dealing with transplant issues and problems; providing an index of sources for transplant related information available through the Internet and otherwise; and providing information about organ donation and transplantation to the general public in order to improve organ and tissue procurement efforts world wide. TransWeb's home page includes the following headings: News; Focus on Transplant Patients; Information for Medical Professionals; Organ and Tissue Donation: Issues and Answers; Transplantation Resources on the Internet; and Library and Index.

1966 TRANSPLANT RECIPIENTS INTERNATIONAL ORGANIZATION, INC. (TRIO)

1000 16th Street NW
Suite 602
Washington, DC 20036-5705 202-293-0980
800-874-6386
Fax: 202-293-0973
E-mail: trio@primenet.com
http://www.primenet.com/~trio

Transplant Recipients International Organization, Inc. (TRIO) is a nonprofit organization dedicated to improving the quality of life of transplant candidates, recipients, and their families. Through the TRIO Headquarters and a network of chapters, TRIO serves its members by promoting organ and tissue donation; providing support to transplant candidates; providing current information on developments in organ and tissue donation; and making known to federal, state, and local government bodies the concerns and needs that affect the welfare of transplant candidates, recipients, their families, and donor family members. The Organization hopes to effectively communicate its views to the general public on issues in the field of transplantation and organ and tissue donation. Established in 1987 and consisting of 4,000 members, TRIO provides numerous educational materials including brochures and a fact sheet. In addition, TRIO works closely with the United Network of Organ Sharing (UNOS) to manage the Organ Procurement Transplant Network and the Scientific Registry.

President: Bruce Weir
Executive Director: Lisa Kory, R.N., B.S.N., C.P.T.C.
Year Established: 1987
Organization Chapters: 80
Organization Members: 4,000

Publishes the following materials:
TRIO ~ *Membership Application*
Transplant Recipients International Organization, Inc. ~ *Mission Statement*
TRIO Fact Sheet ~ *Factsheet*

1967 TRAVELIN' TALK NETWORK

130 Hillcrest Drive
Suite 102
Clarksville, TN 37043-3534 615-552-6670
Fax: 615-552-1182
E-mail: trvlntlk@aol.com

The Travelin' Talk Network is a self-help organization dedicated to helping travelers with disabilities. Established in 1988, Travelin' Talk is a network of people willing to answer their telephones and share their knowledge of their hometowns with travelers with disabilities who are visiting or passing through specific areas in the United States and throughout the world. The organization consists of 1,200 members and two chapters. Educational materials include a quarterly newsletter to update members on the network's progress, introduce the numerous resources available to travelers, share travel tips, and share stories about the many ways members are helping travelers with disabilities; a brochure entitled "The Travelin' Talk Network" and a directory entitled "The Travelin' Talk Directory."

President: Rick Crowder
Year Established: 1988
Organization Chapters: 2
Organization Members: 1,200

Publishes the following materials:
Travelin' Talk Network ~ *Brochure*

1968 TRIPLET CONNECTION

8900 Thornton Road
Suite 25
P.O. Box 99571
Stockton, CA 95209 209-474-0885
Fax: 209-474-2233
E-mail: triplets@inreach.com
http://www.inreach.com/triplets

The Triplet Connection is a not-for-profit organization dedicated to providing support and information to families who have or, particularly, who are expecting triplets, quadruplets, or quintuplets. Established in 1983, the organization provides information regarding the prevention of preterm birth in larger multiple gestations, and helps expectant parents know exactly what they can do in order to enhance the best possible outcomes to their pregnancies. Consisting of 12,000 members, the organization produces educational materials including a quarterly self-titled newsletter, a packet of information for expectant parents, and various reports. The organization coordinates support and networking opportunities for families of multiple births; maintains a database of medical information regarding larger multiple pregnancies and their outcomes; has an advisory board comprised of physicians who are in charge of research; and provides resources to help families who have lost one or more of their children. The Triplet Connection is a vital "lifeline" to expectant parents, a source of encouragement to parents of larger multiple births, and a thorough resource for health care professionals.

President: Janet Bleyl (1983 to Present)
Year Established: 1983
Organization Members: 12, 000

Publishes the following materials:
The Triplet Connection ~ *Mission Statement*
A Network of Caring and Sharing for Multiple Birth Families ~ *Brochure*
Seeing is Believing ~ *Photo Galley*
The Triplet Connection, Volume 12, Number 1 ~ *Newsletter*

1969 TWIN HOPE (TWIN-TWIN TRANSFUSION SYNDROME)

2592 West 14th Street
Cleveland, OH 44113 216-228-8887
E-mail: twinhope@mail.ohio.net
http://www.twinhope.com

Twin Hope is an international not-for-profit organization dedicated to providing information and support to parents of children with Twin-Twin Transfusion Syndrome and other related disorders that may affect twins (including Cerebral Palsy and Conjoined Twinning). During the development of identical twins, there are often blood vessels in the fetuses' shared placenta that connect their blood circulations (placental anastomoses). In cases of Twin-Twin Transfusion Syndrome, the blood begins to flow unevenly, with one fetal twin receiving too much blood (recipient) and one receiving too little (donor). The recipient twin may experience heart failure due to continual strain on its heart and blood vessels. The donor twin, on the other hand, may experience life-threatening anemia due to its inadequate supply of blood. In some cases, both twins may receive an inadequate supply of oxygen during pregnancy or due to early delivery; as a result, brain damage may occur, potentially causing Cerebral Palsy. Twin Hope is committed to promoting awareness of TTTS and other related disorders among the medical community and the general public; engaging in patient advocacy; and promoting research. Established in 1994, Twin Hope also provides networking services for affected families, has a registry, conducts presentations, and offers a variety of educational materials. Such materials include a biannual newsletter entitled "TwinLines," a Family Support Guide, brochures, articles, multiple birth loss information, a Medical Professional Resource Manual, and other publications.

President: Jill MacNiven (1994 to Present).
Year Established: 1994
Organization Chapters: 2
Organization Members: 500

Publishes the following materials:
Twin Lines ~ *Newsletter*
Pioneering procedure saves twins ~ *Reprint*
Twin Hope, Inc. ~ *Brochure*
Twin Hope Support Group ~ *Brochure*
Twin To Twin Transfusion Syndrome Network, Inc. Family Support Guide ~ *Booklet*

Concerned with the following diseases or disorders:
Twin-Twin Transfusion Syndrome

1970 TWIN TO TWIN TRANSFUSION SYNDROME FOUNDATION

National Office
411 Longbeach Parkway
Bay Village, OH 44140 216-899-8887
Fax: 440-366-6148
E-mail: tttsfound@aol.com
http://www.tttsfoundation.com

The Twin to Twin Transfusion Syndrome Foundation is a national voluntary not-for-profit organization dedicated to providing educational, emotional, and financial support to families, caregivers, and medical professionals before, during, and after pregnancies diagnosed with Twin to Twin Transfusion Syndrome (TTTS). Twin to Twin Transfusion Syndrome is a rare disorder that affects identical twins during pregnancy when blood passes unequally from one fetus to the other through connecting blood vessels in their shared placenta. Established in 1992, the Twin to Twin Transfusion Syndrome Foundation is dedicated to educating families, health care professionals, and the general public about TTTS and the latest available treatments. The Foundation seeks to inform the public about other complications of high-risk, multiple pregnancies and endeavors to save affected babies and improve their future health and care. The organization provides financial assistance to further medical research into TTTS and related complications and works with medical experts in the field of placental research to develop a protocol for analyzing placental tissue. The group is working to develop and maintain a national registry of all TTTS pregnancies. The Twin to Twin Transfusion Syndrome Foundation promotes patient and family advocacy; offers financial assistance through corporate sponsors to affected families who require treatment; and provides a referral network. In addition, The Twin to Twin Transfusion Syndrome Foundation offers a variety of educational and support materials, including a regular newsletter, directory, reports, journals, brochures, educational packets, and videos.

President: Mary Slaman-Forsythe (1992-Present)
Executive Director: Linda DeAngelis
Year Established: 1992
Organization Chapters: 12
Organization Members: 3,000

Publishes the following materials:
The Twin to Twin Transfusion Syndrome Foundation ~ *Brochure*
A Diagnosis Has Been Made... ~ *Pamphlet*
Compassionate Deliveries ~ *Pamphlet*
Patient Profile ~ *Brochure*

Concerned with the following diseases or disorders:
Twin-Twin Transfusion Syndrome

1971 UNIQUE - RARE CHROMOSOME DISORDER SUPPORT GROUP (UNIQUE)

160 Locket Road
Harrow Weald
Middlesex, HA3 7NZ
United Kingdom 0181 863 3557
Fax: 0181 863 3557

UNIQUE - The Rare Chromosome Disorder Support Group is a not-for-profit voluntary organization dedicated to promoting awareness of chromosome abnormalities. The organization was originally known as the Trisomy 9 Support Group, which was founded in 1984 and served as a source of mutual support and self-help to families of children suffering from this rare group of chromosomal conditions. In 1989, with the support of In Touch Trust and Contact A Family, the group expanded to include families whose children have any chromosomal abnormality. In 1993 the group was granted charity status and the new logo "UNIQUE" was adopted. UNIQUE's mission is to provide support and information to families of children with similar clinical problems although the children may have different chromosomal abnormalities. Consisting of 1,000 members, UNIQUE acts as a family support group; produces a newsletter three times each year; promotes awareness of chromosome abnormalities; links families whose children have similar clinical problems; raises funds to support the group and produce informational literature. The organization also helps to make hospitals, doctors, health professionals, and genetic clinics aware of the group so that they may have early contact with new families; helps to research and coordinate the centralization of information; arranges for families to assist in research into these disorders; and holds an annual conference where families and medical specialists can meet.

President: Edna Knight (1980 to Present)
Year Established: 1989
Organization Members: 1,000

Publishes the following materials:
Unique ~ *Mission Statement*
Unique - Rare Chromosome Disorder Support Group ~ *Flyer*
UNIQUE Support Group for the families of children born with Rare Chromosome Abnormalities ~ *Brochure*

Concerned with the following diseases or disorders:
Chromosome 10, Distal Trisomy 10q; Chromosome 10, Monosomy 10p; Chromosome 11, Partial Monosomy 11q; Chromosome 11, Partial Trisomy 11q; Chromosome 13, Partial Monosomy 13q; Chromosome 14 Ring; Chromosome 14, Trisomy Mosaic; Chromosome 15 Ring; Chromosome 15, Distal Trisomy 15q; Chromosome 18, Ring; Chromosome 18, Tetrasomy 18p; Chromosome 18q- Syndrome; Chromosome 21 Ring; Chromosome 22 Ring; Chromosome 22, Trisomy Mosaic; Chromosome 3, Monosomy 3p2; Chromosome 3, Trisomy 3q2; Chromosome 4 Ring; Chromosome 4, Monosomy 4q; Chromosome 4, Partial Trisomy Distal 4q; Chromosome 4, Trisomy 4p; Chromosome 6 Ring; Chromosome 6, Partial Trisomy 6q; Chromosome 7, Monosomy 7p2; Chromosome 8, Monosomy 8p2; Chromosome 9 Ring; Chromosome 9, Partial Monosomy 9p; Chromosome 9, Tetrasomy 9p; Chromosome 9, Trisomy 9P (Multiple Variants); Chromosome 9, Trisomy Mosaic; Triplo X Syndrome; Triploid Syndrome; Trisomy 13 Syndrome; Trisomy 18 Syndrome; XYY Syndrome

1972 US TOO INTERNATIONAL, INC., PROSTATE CANCER SURVIVOR SUPPORT GROUPS

930 North York Road
Suite 50
Hinsdale, IL 60521-2993 630-323-1002
800-808-7866
Fax: 630-323-1003
E-mail: ustoo@ustoo.com
http://www.ustoo.com

US TOO International, Inc., an international voluntary not-for-profit self-help organization, is dedicated to helping survivors of prostate cancer and Benign Prostatic Hypertrophy (BPH) and their families lead healthy and productive lives, physically, mentally, and spiritually, by offering fellowship, shared counseling, and discussions pertaining to current medical options and a positive mental outlook. Prostate cancer is characterized by malignant cell development arising in the prostate gland. Symptoms may include increased frequency of urination, poor flow of urine, and difficulties beginning urination due to enlargement of the prostate. Benign Prostatic Hypertrophy (BPH), meaning enlargement of the prostate gland, refers to a benign, noninflammatory condition common in men over the age of 50 years. BPH is, however, a progressive condition that may cause increased frequency of urination, pain during urination, and urinary tract infections. US TOO was established in 1990 by five men, each of whom had been diagnosed and treated for prostate cancer and were interested in discussing their common situations and concerns with others. US TOO consists of approximately 550 support groups throughout the United States and other countries including Canada that each function as independent chapters and, together, form a network under the aegis of the parent group, US TOO International, Inc. Each chapter holds regular meetings for prostate cancer survivors and their families. At such meetings, members of the medical profession speak on some phase of diagnosis, stages, treatment options, or other related topics. Participants have the opportunity to discuss individual experiences that may be of interest to the group and receive various sources of information on prostate cancer and BPH. These shared experiences may be beneficial in understanding the disease, communicating with physicians, and making informed decisions. US TOO provides a variety of educational materials including brochures, pamphlets, monthly "Hot Sheets" containing information on clinical trials and current issues, and a regular newsletter entitled "US TOO Prostate Cancer Communicator." US TOO International also has a web site on the Internet at [http://www.us-too.com].

President: Henry A. Porterfield (Chairman/CEO)
Organization Language: Spanish (written).
Year Established: 1990
Organization Chapters: 550
Organization Members: Non-Membership

Publishes the following materials:
Us Too International, Inc. ~ *Mission Statement*
Hormonal Therapy for Prostate Cancer ~ *Brochure*
Learning to Cope Through Knowledge and Hope ~ *Leaflet*
Prostate Cancer Hot Sheet ~ *Newsletter*
Communicator ~ *Newsletter*

Concerned with the following diseases or disorders:
Cancer, Prostate

1973 UNITED LEUKODYSTROPHY FOUNDATION

2304 Highland Drive
Sycamore, IL 60178
815-895-3211
800-728-5483
Fax: 815-895-2432
E-mail: ulf@ceet.niu.edu
http://www.ulf.org/

The United Leukodystrophy Foundation (ULF) is a voluntary not-for-profit organization dedicated to helping children and adults with leukodystrophy and assisting the family members, caregivers, and professionals who serve them. Leukodystrophy is a group of rare, progressive diseases that affect the white matter of the brain. Established in 1982, the United Leukodystrophy Foundation is committed to the identification, treatment, and cure of all leukodystrophies through programs of education, advocacy, research, and service. The Foundation also provides appropriate referrals, including to support groups; promotes professional and patient education; and offers a variety of educational and support materials. These include a regular newsletter, brochures, and audiovisual aids.

President: Paula Brazeal (1984-Present)
Executive Director: Ron Brazeal
Year Established: 1982
Organization Members: 3,500

Publishes the following materials:
The Facts About Leukodystrophy ~ *Brochure*
ULF Resource Materials Order Form ~ *Resource Listing*
ULF News ~ *Newsletter*

Concerned with the following diseases or disorders:
Adrenoleukodystrophy; Alexander's Disease; Balo Disease; Carbohydrate deficient Glycoprotein Syndrome Type I; Leukodystrophy; Leukodystrophy, Canavan's; Leukodystrophy, Krabbe's; Leukodystrophy, Metachromatic; Pelizaeus Merzbacher Brain Sclerosis; Refsum Syndrome; Seitelberger Disease (Infantile Neuroaxonal Dystrophy); Wiedemann Rautenstrauch Syndrome; Zellweger Syndrome

1974 **UNITED LIVER ASSOCIATION (ULA)**

11646 West Pico Boulevard
Los Angeles, CA 90064-2987 310-445-4204
Fax: 310-575-3871

The United Liver Association is a not-for-profit organization dedicated to providing support services to individuals with liver disease, family members, and caregivers. The Association seeks to increase awareness and understanding of liver diseases in the medical and lay communities and promote ongoing medical research into the causes, management, and potential cure of these disorders. Established in 1985, the United Liver Association has a telephone hot line under the direction of liver specialists and other trained professionals; and holds group support sessions for affected individuals and families. It offers psychologist-led sessions and conducts educational seminars for patients, families, and health care professionals. The Association also gives appropriate referrals; provides limited direct assistance for out-of-area liver transplant patients and families, based on financial need; engages in patient, family, and community education; and promotes patient and family advocacy. The United Liver Association also provides a variety of educational materials, including a regular newsletter and a brochure.

President: Gloria Moret
Executive Director: Francine Pierce Jackson
Year Established: 1985
Organization Chapters: 4

Publishes the following materials:
United Liver Association (ULA) ~ *Factsheet*
Through Patient Support, Research, and Education. Reversing Years of Neglect ~ *Brochure*
Report Spring 1994 ~ *Newsletter*

Concerned with the following diseases or disorders:
Alagille Syndrome; Antithrombin III Deficiency; Banti's Syndrome; Biliary Atresia, Extrahepatic; Budd Chiari Syndrome; Caroli Disease; Cholangitis, Primary Sclerosing; Cholestasis; Cirrhosis, Primary Biliary; Crigler Najjar Syndrome Type I; Dubin Johnson Syndrome; Fascioliasis; Gilbert Syndrome; Hepatitis B; Hepatitis, Neonatal; Hepatitis, Non-A, Non-B (Hepatitis C); Kernicterus; Polycystic Liver Disease; Vitamin E Deficiency; Wilson's Disease

1975 **UNITED MITOCHONDRIAL DISEASE FOUNDATION**

P.O. Box 1151
Monroeville, PA 15146-1151 412-856-1297
Fax: 412-856-1297
E-mail: 74743.2705@compuserve.com
http://biochemgen.ucsd.edu/umdf

The United Mitochondrial Disease Foundation is a voluntary not-for-profit self-help organization dedicated to providing education and support to individuals diagnosed with Cytochrome C Oxidase (COX) deficiency or other mitochondrial disorders, their families, and medical professionals. Established in 1993, the United Mitochondrial Disease Foundation networks families affected by these disorders, enabling them to engage in information-sharing and support. In addition, the Foundation networks with research professionals and alerts affected individuals and family members to upcoming clinical studies and their required protocols. The United Mitochondrial Disease Foundation provides educational and support materials to affected individuals, family members, and medical professionals through its computer database, directory, pamphlets, and regular newsletter. The Education and Support Exchange (the research division of the COX Foundation) can be reached at P.O. Box 1151 Monroeville, PA 15146-1151.

Executive Director: Joyce Vaught
Year Established: 1993
Organization Members: 175

Concerned with the following diseases or disorders:
Alpers Disease; Carnitine Deficiency Syndromes; Cytochrome C Oxidase Deficiency; Kearns Sayre Syndrome (KSS); Leber's Optic Atrophy; Leigh's Disease; Long Chain Acyl CoA Dehydrogenase Deficiency (LCAD); MELAS Syndrome; MERRF Syndrome; Medium Chain Acyl CoA Dehydrogenase Deficiency; PEPCK Deficiency, Mitochondrial; Pyruvate Carboxylase Deficiency; Pyruvate Dehydrogenase Deficiency; Short Chain Acyl CoA Dehydrogenase Deficiency (SCAD); Wolfram Syndrome

1976 **UNITED OSTOMY ASSOCIATION, INC. (UOA)**

19772 MacArthur Boulevard
Suite 200
Irvine, CA 92612-2405 714-660-8624
800-826-0826
Fax: 714-660-9262
E-mail: uoa@deltanet.com
http://www.uoa.org

Established in 1960, the United Ostomy Association, Inc. is a national not-for-profit organization dedicated to offering support and information to parents of children who have had ostomy surgery. The Association, which has approximately 40,000 members and 600 chapters nationwide, offers networking programs, distributes educational materials, provides referrals to other resources, and conducts a yearly national conference. The Association also operates a camp for children between the ages of 12 and 17 who have had ostomy surgery or have bowel or bladder concerns. The United Ostomy Association produces educational materials including a quarterly newsletter, a national newsletter on issues related to children who have had ostomy surgery, and activity books for affected children.

President: Helen DuBois
Executive Director: Darlene Smith
Year Established: 1955
Organization Chapters: 525
Organization Members: 35,000

Concerned with the following diseases or disorders:
Colitis, Ulcerative; Crohn's Disease; Gardner Syndrome; Hirschsprung's Disease; Imperforate Anus; Intestinal Pseudoobstruction; Muscular Dystrophy, Oculo-Gastrointestinal; Polyposis, Familial

1977 UNITED STATES SOCIETY FOR AUGMENTATIVE AND ALTERNATIVE COMMUNICATION (USSAAC)

P.O. Box 5271
Evanston, IL 60204-5271 847-869-2122
Fax: 847-869-2161
E-mail: ussaac@northshore.net

The United States Society for Augmentative and Alternative Communication (USSAAC) is a not-for-profit voluntary organization dedicated to enhancing the communication effectiveness of persons who can benefit from augmentative and alternative communication (AAC) and to supporting the purposes of the International Society for Augmentative and Alternative Communication through individual, local, state, regional, and national efforts. USSAAC's specific purposes are to assist individuals with AAC needs in the pursuit of their right to communicate, allowing full participation in society; to promote public awareness of communication disability and AAC options; to influence public policy and legislation at national and state levels; to disseminate legislative, regulatory, and funding information; to facilitate the development, expansion, and refinement of quality service delivery programs and systems; to promote the development of and to support existing local, state, and regional AAC groups and activities; and to develop alliances and cooperate with organizations that serve the interests of persons with AAC needs. Established in 1989 and consisting of 600 members, the organization produces educational materials including a newsletter entitled "Speak-Up." The organization also promotes education and provides referrals.

Executive Director: James Neils
Year Established: 1989
Organization Members: 600

Publishes the following materials:
USSAAC ~ *Mission Statement*

1978 VAINCRE LES MALADIES LYSOSOMALES (ASSOCIATION VML)

9 Place du 19 Mars 1962,
Evry Cedex, 91035
France 33160917500
Fax: 33169369350
E-mail: VML@provnet.fr
http://www.provnet.fr/VML/

Vaincre Les Maladies Lysosomales is a voluntary not-for-profit organization in France dedicated to providing information and support to individuals with lysosomal disorders and their families; improving the quality of life of affected individuals; and promoting and supporting research for these disorders (e.g., Pompe Disease, the Lipidoses, Mucolipidoses, Mucopolysaccharidoses, and Glycoproteinoses). Established in 1990, Vaincre Les Maladies Lysosomales provides referrals to appropriate support groups; promotes public awareness campaigns; and offers informational conferences and weekend retreats for affected individuals, families, and health care professionals. Vaincre Les Maladies Lysosomales also offers a variety of educational materials to affected individuals, family members, and health care professionals including regular newsletters, brochures, books, and videos.

President: Daniel Walschaerts (1990-Present)
Organization Language: French.
Year Established: 1990
Organization Members: 1,200

Concerned with the following diseases or disorders:
Carbohydrate deficient Glycoprotein Syndrome Type I; Cystinosis; Farber's Disease; Fucosidosis; Gaucher Disease; Hunter Syndrome; Hurler Syndrome; I Cell Disease; Mannosidosis; Maroteaux Lamy Syndrome; McArdle Disease; Morquio Syndrome; Mucopolysaccharidosis; Multiple Sulfatase Deficiency; Non-Ketotic Hyperglycinemia; Pompe Disease; Pseudo Hurler Polydystrophy; Sanfilippo Syndrome; Santavuori Disease; Schindler Disease; Sialidosis; Sly Syndrome; Tarui Disease

1979 VESTIBULAR DISORDERS ASSOCIATION (VEDA)

P.O. Box 4467
Portland, OR 97208-4467 503-229-7705
800-837-8428
Fax: 503-229-8064
E-mail: veda@teleport.com
http://www.teleport.com/~veda

The Vestibular Disorders Association is a national not-for-profit organization dedicated to providing informational services and support to people with dizziness, balance disorders, and related hearing problems. Established in 1983, the Association provides educational materials about vestibular disorders and related topics, supports a network for people with dizziness and balance disorders, engages in public and professional education, and supports research and clinical activities that may improve the quality of life for people affected by vestibular disorders. The Association's quarterly newsletter "On the Level" provides current information about medical diagnosis, treatment, and research as well as tips on diet, exercise, safety, stress, and other issues that are important to people with vestibular disorders.

President: Janet Lunde
Executive Director: Jerry Underwood, PhD
Year Established: 1983
Organization Members: 5,000

Publishes the following materials:
Vestibular Disorders Association ~ *Brochure*
Printed Materials Order Form ~ *Order Form*
Videotape Rental Form ~ *Rental Form*
Order Form for Patient-Education Materials ~ *Order Form*

Concerned with the following diseases or disorders:
Meniere Disease; Nystagmus, Benign Paroxysmal Positional; Tinnitus

1980 VETERANS FAMILY HEALTH SERVICES, INC. (VFHS, INC.)

P.O. Box 2465
Darien, CT 06820 203-656-0003
800-521-0198
Fax: 203-656-1957
E-mail: VFHSInc@aol.com

Veterans Family Health Services, Inc. (VFHS) is a nonprofit organization dedicated to providing case management social services and limited medical assistance to Vietnam and Gulf War veterans and their families. VFHS exists to address the special needs of these veterans and their families. VFHS's programs combine family-guided case management and advocacy assistance while building social and community support. Established in 1978, VFHS administers a national hotline for veterans and their families who have inquiries or who need assistance; maintains a special fund providing limited emergency economic assistance and relief for veteran families in crisis; and creates partnerships with other agencies that make it possible to secure services and equipment at reduced rates or at no cost for families in need. VFHS's educational materials include brochures.

President: Frank McCarthy (1978 to Present)
Executive Director: James Sparrow
Year Established: 1978
Organization Members: Non-Membership

Publishes the following materials:
Veterans Family Health Services, Inc. Two Decades of Service to Veterans and Their Families ~ *Pamphlet*
Vietnam Veterans Agent Orange Victims, Inc. ~ *Fact Sheet*

1981 VISION FOUNDATION, INC.

818 Mt. Auburn Street
Watertown, MA 02172 617-926-4232
800-852-3029
Fax: 617-926-1412

Vision Foundation, Inc. is a not-for-profit self-help organization dedicated to providing practical and emotional support to individuals affected by visual impairment. The Vision Foundation was founded in 1970 by people who were losing their sight but were not legally blind. At that time, all agencies serving people who were blind or visually impaired required legal blindness for service eligibility. The founders wanted to prepare themselves for blindness by sharing information and providing emotional support. The Vision Foundation remains committed to these two ideals, but has grown to offer support groups, a referral center, a "buddy" telephone system, programs for seniors, and educational materials for affected individuals, medical professionals, and other interested groups or individuals. Such materials include a resource list and a bimonthly newsletter entitled "Vision Resource Update." The Foundation also has a computer database that is accessible by print, large print, and speech. The Vision Foundation supports several languages including English, Spanish, Creole, and Russian. The toll-free number is operational is Massachusetts only.

President: Caper Barkus (1994-Present)
Executive Director: Barbara R. Kibler
Organization Language: Spanish. Creole. Russian.
Year Established: 1970
Organization Chapters: 33
Organization Members: 300

Publishes the following materials:
Vision Resource List - 15th Edition ~ *Resource List*

Concerned with the following diseases or disorders:
Aniridia; Aniridia Cerebellar Ataxia Mental Deficiency; Bardet Biedl Syndrome; Cataracts; Choroideremia; Choroiditis, Serpiginous; Eales Disease; Epitheliopathy, Acute Posterior Multifocal Placoid Pigment; Keratoconus; Keratomalacia; Laurence Moon Syndrome; Leber's Optic Atrophy; Lenz Microphthalmia Syndrome; Macular Degeneration; Macular Degeneration, Polymorphic; Megalocornea Mental Retardation Syndrome; Norrie Syndrome; Papillitis; Posterior Uveitis; Retinopathy, Diabetic; Retinoschisis; Rieger Syndrome; Smith Magenis Syndrome; Treacher Collins Syndrome; WAGR Syndrome; Wolfram Syndrome

1982 VISION WORLD WIDE, INC.

5707 Brockton Drive
#302
Indianapolis, IN 46220-5481 317-254-1332
800-431-1739
Fax: 317-251-6588
E-mail: visionww@aol.com
www.netdirect.net/vision-enhancement/

Vision World Wide, Inc. is an international nonprofit organization dedicated to helping address the needs of individuals who are visually impaired. Special emphasis is given to the aging population. Established in 1995, Vision World Wide accomplishes its mission through operating an information and referral toll-free telephone number, disseminating fact sheets and brochures, and working closely with rehabilitation agency administrators, counselors, educators, researchers, and radio information services with the aim of providing a variety of services and assistance to affected individuals. The organization's materials are available in large print, on audiocassette, and on PC and Macintosh computer disks. All materials are furnished at no cost or at a substantially reduced price. The organization also provides individuals with the opportunity to network with medical professionals including optometrists, ophthalmologists, hospitals, and low vision centers. The organization publishes a quarterly magazine entitled "Vision Enhancement" and maintains a web site at [http://www.netdirect.net/vision-enhancement/].

President: Patricia L. Price (1977 to Present)
Year Established: 1995
Organization Members: Non-Membership

Publishes the following materials:
Vision World Wide, Inc. ~ *Mission Statement*
Vision Enhancement. A Quarterly Publication Providing Information and Resources for Persons with Vision Loss ~ *Booklet*

Concerned with the following diseases or disorders:
Cataract Dental Syndrome; Macular Degeneration; Retinitis Pigmentosa

1983 VOICE OF THE RETARDED (VOR)

5005 Newport Drive
Suite 108
Rolling Meadows, IL 60008 847-253-6020
Fax: 847-253-6054
E-mail: vor@compuserve.com

Voice of the Retarded (VOR) is a national not-for-profit voluntary organization that was founded in 1983. The organization provides information, support, and advocacy services to individuals and family members affected by mental retardation and seeks to keep public officials, legislators, and the public informed about issues that affect people with mental retardation. VOR supports alternatives in residential living and rehabilitation systems that serve the individual needs of affected individuals and their families. The organization's activities include testimony before federal, state, and local governmental officials on issues of importance to people with mental retardation; advocacy on behalf of groups and individuals in residential, community, or home settings; and cooperation and interaction with other parent organizations that share the same concerns as VOR. The Voice of the Retarded has members in all 50 states including parents, families, providers, professionals, friends, and affiliated groups. VOR's educational materials include brochures and a quarterly newsletter.

President: Polly Spare (1992-Present)
Executive Director: Tamie Hopp
Year Established: 1983

Publishes the following materials:
Voice of the Retarded ~ *Brochure*
VOR Newsletter ~ *Newsletter*

1984 WE MOVE

Mt. Sinai Medical Center
One Gustave L. Levy Place Box 1052
New York, NY 10029 212-241-8567
800-437-6682
Fax: 212-987-7363
E-mail: wemove@smtplink.mssm.edu.
http://www.wemove.org

WE MOVE is an international educational program endorsed by the Movement Disorder Society. It is dedicated to promoting awareness of neurological movement disorders for the purpose of early diagnosis, appropriate treatment, and patient support. The primary focus of the program is to educate the health care community about movement disorders. To that end, the organization sponsors education programs and produces teaching materials designed for medical professionals including neurologists, family practitioners, physical therapists, speech pathologists, and other health care workers. WE MOVE serves as a communication link between physicians, affected individuals, and support groups around the world. The program also publishes the "International Guide to Patient Support Organizations" and a brochure entitled "Educator's Resource Materials." In addition, the organization maintains a web site at [http://www.mssm.edu/neurology/html/we move.html].

President: NA
Executive Director: Judith Blazer, M.S.
Year Established: 1991

Publishes the following materials:
International Guide to Patient Support Organizations ~ *Directory*
WE MOVE ~ *Brochure*

Concerned with the following diseases or disorders:
Allan Herndon Syndrome; Ataxia Telangiectasia; Ataxia, Friedreich's; Ataxia, Hereditary; Ataxia, Marie's; Blepharospasm, Benign Essential; Cerebral Palsy; Chorea, Sydenham's; Corticobasal Degeneration; Dysphonia, Chronic Spasmodic; Dystonia, Torsion; Epilepsy, Myoclonic Progressive Familial; Huntington's Disease; Locked In Syndrome; MASA Syndrome; Meige Syndrome; Myelitis; Myoclonus, General; Myotonia Congenita; Olivopontocerebellar Atrophy; Paramyotonia Congenita; Parkinson's Disease; Progressive Supranuclear Palsy; Restless Legs Syndrome; Shy Drager Syndrome; Spasmodic Torticollis; Subacute Sclerosing Panencephalitis; Tardive Dyskinesia; Tourette Syndrome; Wilson's Disease

1985 WHEELCHAIR ACCESS, INC.

P.O. Box 12
Glenmoore, PA 19343 610-942-3266
Fax: 610-942-0282
E-mail: wanews@chesco.com
http://www.inet-usa.com/wca/

Wheelchair Access, Inc. is a voluntary organization dedicated to providing comprehensive information to individuals with disabilities concerning wheelchair accessible homes for sale or for rent, vans, wheelchairs, and any other equipment they may require. Established in 1994, the organization also produces a variety of educational materials including a regular newsletter. Wheelchair Access maintains a web site at [http://www.inet-usa.com/wca/].

President: Frank Gomez (1994 to Present)
Year Established: 1994
Organization Members: Non-Membership

Publishes the following materials:
W.A. & News ~ *Newsletter*

1986 WIDE SMILES (WS)

P.O. Box 5153
Stockton, CA 95205-0153 209-942-2812
Fax: 209-464-1494
E-mail: widesmiles@aol.com
http://www.widesmiles.org

Wide Smiles is a not-for-profit organization dedicated to providing support, information, and networking services to families dealing with the challenges associated with clefting. Incomplete closure of the roof of the mouth (cleft palate) and/or the presence of an abnormal groove in the upper lip (cleft lip) are considered among the most common facial birth defects. Approximately one child in 700 is born with a cleft. Wide Smiles offers networking services to affected family members; provides referrals to physicians and clinics that specialize in clefting; has a cleft lip and cleft palate research registry; offers a variety of educational materials on all aspects of clefting; provides supportive materials; and has a regular magazine entitled "Wide Smiles Quarterly." Wide Smiles also has a web site on the Internet that offers several online networking opportunities including an e-mail discussion list (listserv), regular chats, and an area called "Cleft Links" that provides over 400 articles and answers to questions in several categories that concern all aspects of clefting. Such topic categories include "New Parents," "Feeding Issues," "Terms Defined," "For All Parents," "Speech," "Ears and Hearing," "Insurance," "Uplifting Thoughts," "Clefts and Syndromes," "Resources and References," and more. The Wide Smiles web site also provides a Frequently Asked Questions (FAQ) and answers area, offers parents the opportunity to register themselves and/or their children in the Cleft Lip and Palate Registry, provides a guide to physicians and clinics in the United States and Canada (that is organized by state and province), and offers several additional services. The Wide Smiles web site is located at [http://www.widesmiles.org/].

President: Joanne Green (Director) (1991 to Present)
Year Established: 1991
Organization Members: 1,600

Publishes the following materials:
Wide Smiles...We're an Information Network for families of children born with cleft ~ *Brochure*
Partners In Care ~ *Booklet*
Wide Smiles (Fall 1996) ~ *News Booklet*
Wide Smiles...We're an Informaion Network for families of children born with cleft ~ *Brochure*

Concerned with the following diseases or disorders:
Catel Manzke Syndrome; Cerebrocostomandibular Syndrome; Chromosome 4, Monosomy Distal 4Q; Cleft Palate and Cleft Lip; Orocraniodigital Syndrome; Pierre Robin Syndrome; Popliteal Pterygium Syndrome

1987 WORLD HEALTH ORGANIZATION (WHO) REGIONAL OFFICE FOR THE AMERICAS (AMRO)

Pan American Health Organization (PAHO)
525 23rd Street NW
Washington, DC 20037 202-974-3000
Fax: 202-974-3663
E-mail: postmaster@paho.org
http://www.who.ch/

The World Health Organization is an international organization with headquarters in Geneva, Switzerland and regional offices across the world including the Regional Office for the Americas (AMRO)/ Pan American Health Organization (PAHO) in Washington, D.C. The objective of WHO is the attainment by all peoples of the highest possible level of health. Health, as defined in the WHO Constitution, is a state of complete physical, mental, and social well-being and not merely the absence of disease or infirmity. In support of its main objective, the Organization has a wide range of functions including acting as the directing and coordinating authority on international health work; assisting Governments, upon request, in strengthening health services; furnishing appropriate technical assistance and, in emergencies, necessary aid, upon the request or acceptance of Governments; and stimulating and advancing work on the prevention and control of epidemic, endemic, and other diseases. WHO is also committed to promoting, in cooperation with other specialized agencies where necessary, the improvement of nutrition, housing, sanitation, recreation, economic, or working conditions and other aspects of environmental hygiene; promoting and coordinating biomedical and health services research; and promoting improved standards of teaching and training in the health, medical, and related professions. The World Health Organization also establishes and stimulates the establishment of international standards for biological, pharmaceutical, and similar products and standardizes diagnostic procedures; fosters activities in the field of mental health, particularly those activities affecting the harmony of human relations; proposes conventions, agreements, and regulations and makes recommendations about international nomenclature of diseases, causes of death, and public health practices; and develops, establishes, and promotes international standards concerning foods and biological, pharmaceutical, and similar substances. WHO maintains a web site at [http://www.who.ch/].

Concerned with the following diseases or disorders:
Acanthocheilonemiasis; Babesiosis; Balantidiasis; Bartonellosis; Bejel; Blastomycosis; Brucellosis; Bubonic Plague; Candidiasis; Chagas Disease; Chikungunya; Cholera; Colorado Tick Fever; Congenital Varicella Syndrome; Cowpox; Creutzfeldt Jakob Disease; Cryptococcosis; Cysticercosis; Dengue Fever; Dracunculosis; Encephalitis, Japanese; Filariasis; Giardiasis; Hantavirus Pulmonary Syndrome; Hemolytic Uremic Syndrome; Human Granulocytic Ehrlichiosis (HGE); Human Monocytic Ehrlichiosis (HME); Legionnaire's Disease; Leptospirosis; Malaria; Meningitis; Meningitis, Bacterial; Meningitis, Meningococcal; Paracoccidioidomycosis; Pertussis; Pinta; Q Fever; Rabies; Rheumatic Fever; Sennetsu Fever; Simian B Virus Infection; Toxic Shock Syndrome; Toxocariasis; Typhoid; Varicella Zoster; Weil Syndrome; Wolf Hirschhorn Syndrome; Yaws; Yellow Fever

1988 **WORLD LIFE FOUNDATION (WLF)**

P.O. Box 571
Bedford, TX 76095
800-289-5433
800-289-5433
Fax: 817-285-0216

The World Life Foundation is a voluntary not-for-profit domestic and international information network dedicated to supporting research, medical, and scientific projects into the nature of rare metabolic disorders. Established in 1992, the Foundation believes that information networking among physicians, researchers, affected individuals, and their families is critical to progress in improving clinical care and the understanding of rare metabolic diseases. The Foundation disseminates information to affected individuals and/or family members; assists in fulfilling affected families' ground/air transportation needs to treatment centers; and publishes a regular newsletter.

President: Louis F. Baum
Executive Director: Vicki Baum (Vice President)
Year Established: 1992

Publishes the following materials:
World Life Foundation: In Support Of ~ *Report*

Concerned with the following diseases or disorders:
Rocky Mountain Spotted Fever

1989 **WORLDWIDE CONGRESS ON PAIN**

c/o Dannemiller Memorial Educational Foundation
12500 Network Blvd.
Suite 101
San Antonio, TX 78249-3302
http://www.pain.com

The Worldwide Congress on Pain is a web site on the Internet sponsored by the Dannemiller Memorial Educational Foundation. The Foundation, which was founded in 1984 in memory of Francis Joseph Dannemiller, M.D., Chairman and Director of the Anesthesiology Residency Training Program at Wilford Hall USAF Medical Center, San Antonio, Texas, designed the Worldwide Congress on Pain web site to provide both consumers and health care professionals with current information on pain and pain management. The web site provides access to a searchable "Virtual Library" of journal articles, case studies, and abstracts on pain and pain management from hundreds of professional medical publications; listings of and dynamic linkage to pain societies and associations, international societies and associations, general health resources, and more; and listings of medical journals and newsletters concerning pain and pain management. The Worldwide Congress on Pain's web site also provides online users with the ability to locate pain management specialists and pain clinics by state; has an "Ask the Doctor" column that enables online users to submit questions to a network of practicing pain management physicians; has a weekly column called "Straight from the Top," which is written by an individual who shares her secrets for dealing with chronic pain; and provides an area entitled "Support Groups and Stories." The Worldwide Congress on Pain web site is located at [http://www.pain.com].

Concerned with the following diseases or disorders:
Reflex Sympathetic Dystrophy Syndrome (RSDS)

1990 **YOUNG AT HEART**

P.O. Box 366
Mattydale, NY 13211
315-454-2059
800-377-9044
Fax: 315-453-5777
E-mail: tracy@mail.dec.com
http://www.dreamscape.com/young@heart

Young At Heart is a nonprofit organization dedicated to providing information and emotional support to individuals with heart conditions including pre-operative and post-operative heart surgery patients. Established in 1991, Young at Heart is also committed to assisting professional organizations and physicians who provide services to heart patients. The organization's services include visiting and encouraging individuals anticipating or recovering from heart surgery; assisting established rehabilitation programs for cardiac patients; and providing support and services to families of individuals recovering from cardiovascular conditions. The organization produces educational materials including a monthly newsletter entitled "HEART TALK" AND BOOKS.

Executive Director: Bargara Tracy (Founder)
Year Established: 1991
Organization Members: 350

Publishes the following materials:
HeartMates. A guide for the spouse and family of the heart patient ~ *Book*
Young at Heart. A Support Group for Cardiac Patients and their Families ~ *Brochure*
Young at Heart ~ *Mission Statement*
Heart Talk ~ *Newsletter July 1997*

1991 ZAIN HANSEN MPS FOUNDATION (ZHMPS FD)
1200 Fernwood Drive
Arcata, CA 95521 707-822-5421
800-767-3121

The Zain Hansen MPS Foundation is a national nonprofit organization that provides information to families and professionals who work with children with mucopolysaccharidosis (MPS) and mucolipidosis (ML). MPS is a rare group of genetic degenerative disorders that are caused by a lack of a specific enzyme in various tissues of the body. This enzyme abnormality affects the way the body deals with carbohydrates and results in the accumulation of unwanted susbstances (mucopolysaccharidoses) in the tissues. Mucolipidoses involve a similar process that results in the abnormal accumulation of a fatty substance (lipids) in various tissues of the body. Established in 1987, the Foundation provides educational materials and referrals to resources that may benefit affected children and families. Individual fund-raising support is made available on a case-by-case basis.

President: Marshall Hansen (1995 to Present)
Year Established: 1987
Organization Chapters: 3
Organization Members: Non-Membership

Publishes the following materials:
Glossary of Acronyms ~ *Pamphlet*
No. Coast Resource Guide for Parents and Caregivers of Medically Fragile, Chronically Ill or Terminally Ill Infants ~ *Leaflet*

1992 **ABLEDATA**
8455 Colesville Road
Suite 935
Silver Spring, MD 20910-3319 301-588-9284
800-227-0216
Fax: 301-587-1967
TDD: 301-495-5626

1993 **AGENCY FOR HEALTH CARE POLICY AND RESEARCH PUBLICATIONS CLEARINGHOUSE**
P.O. Box 8547
Silver Spings, MD 20907-8547 410-381-3150
800-358-9295

1994 **CDC NATIONAL AIDS CLEARINGHOUSE (CDC NAC)**
P.O. Box 6003
Rockville, MD 20849-6003 800-458-5231
800-458-5231
Fax: 301-738-6616

The CDC (Centers for Disease Control and Prevention) National AIDS Clearinghouse is the nation's reference, referral, and distribution service for HIV/AIDS-related information. A government service organization founded in 1987, the CDC National AIDS Clearinghouse (CDC NAC) has served a diverse network of people in local, state, and national settings and has designed its services to facilitate sharing of information and resources on education and prevention programs, research findings, and trends among clearinghouse users. The CDC NAC offers a variety of informational publications including brochures, posters, videotapes, and reports. In addition, the CDC NAC offers many specialized services including an electronic bulletin board (NAC on-line); referral and networking services; access to databases; publications distribution Resource Centers in Rockville, MD and Atlanta, GA; the Business and Labor Resource Service; the AIDS Clinical Trials Information Service; the HIV/AIDS Treatment Information Service; and an International Access phone number. Many of the CDC NAC's publications are available in Spanish. Postage and handling payment is required for bulk orders of materials.

Executive Director: Ruthann Bates
Organization Language: Spanish.
Year Established: 1987

Publishes the following materials:
Information to Help Prevent the Spread of HIV ~ *Brochure*

1995 **CENTERS FOR DISEASE CONTROL AND PREVENTION (CDC)**
1600 Clifton Road NE
Atlanta, GA 30333 404-639-3534
800-342-2437
http://www.cdc.gov/

Concerned with the following diseases or disorders:
AIDS (Acquired Immune Deficiency Syndrome); AIDS Dysmorphic Syndrome; Acanthocheilonemiasis; Agammaglobulinemias, Primary; Arthritis, Infectious; Aspergillosis; Babesiosis; Balantidiasis; Bartonellosis; Bejel; Berylliosis; Blastomycosis; Botulism; Bowenoid Papulosis; Brucellosis; Bubonic Plague; Candidiasis; Cat Scratch Disease; Chagas Disease; Chikungunya; Chlamydia; Cholera; Chorea, Sydenham's; Chronic Fatigue Syndrome; Ciguatera Fish Poisoning; Colorado Tick Fever; Condyloma; Cowpox; Cryptococcosis; Cysticercosis; Cytomegalovirus Infection; Dengue Fever; Dracunculosis; Elephantiasis; Encephalitis, Herpetic; Encephalitis, Japanese; Encephalitis, Rasmussen's; Encephalomyelitis, Myalgic; Endocarditis, Infective; Endomyocardial Fibrosis; Enterobiasis; Eosinophilia Myalgia; Eosinophilic Fasciitis; Fascioliasis; Filariasis; Fitz Hugh Curtis Syndrome; Gianotti Crosti Syndrome; Giardiasis; Hand Foot Mouth Syndrome; Hantavirus Pulmonary Syndrome; Hepatitis B; Hepatitis, Non-A, Non-B (Hepatitis C); Herpes Zoster; Herpes, Neonatal; Kawasaki Syndrome; Legionnaire's Disease; Leprosy; Leptospirosis; Listeriosis; Lyme Disease; Malaria; Measles; Meningitis; Meningitis, Bacterial; Meningitis, Meningococcal; Meningitis, Tuberculous; Meningococcemia; Mumps; Nocardiosis; Opportunistic Infections; Paracoccidioidomycosis; Pertussis; Pica; Pinta; Pneumonia, Eosinophilic; Post Polio Syndrome; Psittacosis; Q Fever; Rabies; Reiter's Syndrome; Reye Syndrome; Rheumatic Fever; Rocky Mountain Spotted F ever; Roseola Infantum; Rubella; Simian B Virus Infection; Streptococcus, Group B; Syphilis, Acquired; TORCH Syndrome; Toxic Shock Syndrome; Toxocariasis; Toxoplasmosis; Tropical Sprue; Tuberculosis; Typhoid; Varicella Zoster; Weil Syndrome; Whipple's Disease; Yaws; Yellow Fever

1996 **DIVISION OF BIRTH DEFECTS AND DEVELOPMENTAL DISABILITIES**

4740 Buford
Highway
NE
Mailstop F-34
Atlanta, GA 30341-3724 770-488-7150
Fax: 770-488-7156

Concerned with the following diseases or disorders:
Botulism; Brucellosis; Heavy Metal Poisoning; Listeriosis

1997 **ERIC CLEARINGHOUSE ON DISABILITIES AND GIFTED EDUCATION**

1920 Association Drive
Reston, VA 20191 703-264-9474
800-328-0272
Fax: 703-264-9494
TDD: 703-264-9449
E-mail: ericec@cec.sped.org
http://www.cec.sped.org/ericec.htm

ERIC Clearinghouse on Disabilities and Gifted Education is a federal government organization that provides information on special and gifted education. Founded in 1966, the Clearinghouse provides referrals, offers patient networking services, and provides information on current research programs. The organization focuses its efforts on prevention, identification, assessment, intervention, and enrichment both in special settings and within mainstream communities. The Clearinghouse offers a variety of materials including brochures and Spanish language materials.

Organization Language: Spanish (written).
Year Established: 1966

Publishes the following materials:
ERIC ~ *Flyer*
CEF Leads the Way in Special Education ~ *Pamphlet*
Eric Clearinghouse on Disabilities and Gifted Education ~ *Brochure*
1997 CEC Spring Resources Catalog ~ *Catalog*

1998 **FOOD AND DRUG ADMINISTRATION (FDA) OFFICE OF INQUIRY & CONSUMER INFORMATION**

Office of Inquiry and Consumer Information
5600 Fisher Lane
Room 12-A-40
Rockville, MD 20857 301-827-4420
http://www.fda.gov/fdahomepage.html

1999 **FOOD AND DRUG ADMINISTRATION (FDA) OFFICE OF ORPHAN PRODUCT DEVELOPMENT**

5600 Fishers Lane
HF-35
Room 8-73
Rockville, MD 20857 301-827-3666
800-300-7469

President: Marlene Haffner, M.D.

2000 **GENOME DATABASE AND ONLINE MENDELIAN INHERITANCE IN MAN (OMIM)**

Lay Gottesman
Applied Research Laboratory
Johns Hopkins University School of Medicine
2024 East Monument Street
Baltimore, MD 21205-2100 410-955-7058
http://www.ncbi.nlm.nih.gov/Omim/

2001 **HIV/AIDS TREATMENT INFORMATION SERVICE (ATIS)**

P.O. Box 6303
Rockville, MD 20849-6303 301-519-0459
800-448-0440
Fax: 301-738-6616
TDD: 800-243-7012
E-mail: atis@cdcnac.org
http://www.hivatis.org

The HIV/AIDS Treatment Information Service (ATIS) is a coordinated Public Health Service project sponsored by seven Public Health Service agencies: the Centers for Disease Control and Prevention (CDC), Agency for Health Care Policy and Research, Health Resources and Services Administration, Indian Health Service, National Institute of Allergy and Infectious Diseases, National Library of Medicine, and Substance Abuse and Mental Health Services Administration. Human Immunodeficiency Virus (HIV) is the cause of Acquired Immunodeficiency Syndrome (AIDS) and AIDS-related complex. HIV may be transmitted through sexual contact or exposure to contaminated blood or other body fluids. AIDS, an acquired deficiency of cell-mediated immunity, has a prolonged incubation period, followed by a progressive, debilitating course. Initial symptoms may include night sweats, fatigue, periodic fever, chills, lack of appetite, weight loss, diarrhea, and depression. As the disease progresses, affected individuals have an abnormal susceptibility to certain recurring infections and certain forms of cancer. Initiated in 1994, ATIS is a free telephone reference service for affected individuals, family members, friends, and health care professionals that provides information about federally approved treatment guidelines for HIV and AIDS. ATIS is staffed by bilingual (English and Spanish) health information specialists who answer questions on HIV treatment options using HSTAT, the National Libraryof Medicine database of HIV/AIDS treatment information, as well as other Federal resources. ATIS health information service specialists may also provide copies of federally approved HIV/AIDS treatment guidelines and refer callers to an extensive network of Federal information services and national and community-based organizations for treatment-related information. ATIS also has a web site on the Internet that provides direct access to HSTAT free of charge as well as dynamic linkage to additional sources of information on the web (such as the AIDS Clinical Trials Information Service web site). The ATIS web site is located at [http://www.hivatis.org].

Executive Director: Cynthia Cadden
Organization Language: Spanish (written/spoken).
Year Established: 1994
Organization Members: Non-Membership

Publishes the following materials:
Questions about treatment for HIV disease? (spanish) ~ *Mission Statement*
Questions about treatment for HIV disease? ~ *Mission Statement*

Concerned with the following diseases or disorders:
AIDS (Acquired Immune Deficiency Syndrome)

2002 HOUSING AND URBAN DEVELOPMENT

P.O. Box 6091
Rockville, MD 20849 301-251-5154
800-245-2691
Fax: 301-251-5767
TDD: 800-483-2209
E-mail: huduser@aspensys.com

2003 INDIAN HEALTH SERVICE

5300 Homestead Road NE
Alberquerque, NM 87110 505-837-4245
Fax: 505-837-4257

2004 INDOOR AIR QUALITY INFORMATION CLEARINGHOUSE (IAQ INFO)

P.O. Box 37133
Washington, DC 20013-7133 202-484-1307
800-483-4318
Fax: 202-484-1510

President: Susan Dolgin
Executive Director: Nina S. Faye
Organization Language: AT&T Language Line.
Year Established: N/A

2005 NIH CONSENSUS DEVELOPMENT PROGRAM

Office of Medical Applications of Research
Federal Building, RM 618
7550 Wisconsin Avenue MSC 9120
Bethesda, MD 20892-9120
E-mail: consensus@nih.gov
http://odp.od.nih.gov/consensus/

The National Institutes of Health's (NIH's) Consensus Development Program, established in 1977, is the premier health technology assessment and transfer program in American medicine. Under this program, the Office of Medical Applications of Research at NIH organizes major conferences that produce consensus statements and technology assessment statements on controversial issues in medicine important to health care providers, patients, and the general public. Consensus and Technology Assessment Statements are independent reports of the panels in question and are not policy statements of the NIH nor the Federal Government. The NIH Consensus Development Program has a web site on the Internet at [http://odp.od.nih.gov/consensus/] that provides full text of all NIH Consensus Statements and Technology Assessment Statements, information on upcoming conferences, recent news releases summarizing conference results, a Frequently Asked Questions (FAQ) and answers area, a search engine to help online users locate particular Consensus

Statements and Technology Assessment Statements, dynamic linkage to other NIH sites that provide valuable information and services, and more. Inquiries about the NIH Consensus Development Program should be addressed to the Office of Medical Applications of Research at the mailing address above. In addition to being available on the web, full text printed copies of consensus statements and technology assessment statements that are still medically currentare also available free of charge from: NIH Consensus Program Information Service, P.O. Box 2577, Kensigton, MD 20891, fax (301) 816-2494, phone (800) 644-6627.

Year Established: 1977

2006 NIH/DEVELOPMENTAL ENDOCRINOLOGY BRANCH

Bldg 10, Room 10N262
10 Center Drive
Bethesda, MD 20892 301-496-4686
Fax: 301-402-0574

Concerned with the following diseases or disorders:
Endomyocardial Fibrosis; POEMS Syndrome

2007 NIH/HEMATOLOGY BRANCH, NATIONAL HEART, LUNG AND BLOOD INSTITUTE (NHLBI)

301-402-0764
Fax: 301-402-3088
E-mail: zamaniwe@gwgate.nhlbi.nih.gov
www.nhlbi.nih.gov/nhlbi/seekpat/hematol.htm

The Hematology Branch at the National Institutes of Health (NIH) National Heart, Lung and Blood Institute (NHLBI) conducts clinical research studies on a number of hematologic diseases including aplastic anemia, myelodysplasia, chronic autoimmune thrombocytopenic purpura, multiple myeloma, and T-large granular lymphocytic leukemia. The Hematology Branch also has a strong interest in evaluating individuals with fanconi's anemia, paroxysmal nocturnal hemoglobinuria, and post-hepatitis aplastic anemia for possible novel therapies. For individuals to be admitted to the NIH Clinical Center, they must be referred by a physician and meet specific protocol requirements. There is no charge for medical care at the Clinical Center since patients are participating in research studies. In most instances, patients are expected to pay the costs of their travel and local lodging. Patients may contact Wanda Zamani by e-mail at [zamaniwe@gwgate.nhlbi.nih.gov], phone (301) 402-0764, or fax (301) 402-3088 for more information. Physicians may call Dr. Neal Young, Chief of the Hematology Branch or Dr. John Barrett, Chief of the Bone Marrow Transplant Unit by phone (301) 496-5093 or fax (301) 496-8396 for further information.

President: Dr. Neal Young, Chief

Concerned with the following diseases or disorders:
Anemia, Aplastic; Anemia, Fanconi's; Hemoglobinuria, Paroxysmal Nocturnal; Myeloma, Multiple; Purpura, Idiopathic Thrombocytopenic

2008 NIH/INSTITUTE ON ALCOHOL ABUSE AND ALCOHOLISM

6000 Executive Blvd Ste 400
Bethesda, MD 20892-7003 301-443-3885
Fax: 301-443-7043

Concerned with the following diseases or disorders:
Fetal Alcohol Syndrome

2009 NIH/NATIONAL ARTHRITIS AND MUSCULOSKELETAL AND SKIN DISEASES INFORMATION CLEARINGHOUSE

One AMS Circle
Bethesda, MD 20892-3675 301-495-4484
Fax: 301-587-4352
TDD: 301-565-2966

Concerned with the following diseases or disorders:
Achondroplasia; Acne Rosacea; Acromegaly; Adams Oliver Syndrome; Alkaptonuria; Alopecia Areata; Amyloidosis; Ankylosing Spondylitis; Aplasia Cutis Congenita; Arthritis, Juvenile; Arthritis, Psoriatic; Arthrogryposis Multiplex Congenita; Behcet's Syndrome; Blue Rubber Bleb Nevus; Bowen's Disease; Bullous Pemphigoid; Coffin Lowry Syndrome; Conradi Hunermann Syndrome; Cutis Laxa; Darier Disease; De Santis Cacchione Syndrome; Dermatitis, Contact; Duhring Disease; Dupuytren's Contracture; Dysplasia, Epiphysealis Hemimelica; Dystrophy, Asphyxiating Thoracic; Engelmann Disease; Epidermal Nevus Syndrome; Epidermolysis Bullosa; Epidermolytic Hyperkeratosis; Erythrokeratodermia with Ataxia; Farber's Disease; Felty Syndrome; Fibrodysplasia Ossificans Progressiva (FOP); Focal Dermal Hypoplasia; Forestier's Disease; Freeman Sheldon Syndrome; Gianotti Crosti Syndrome; Gordon Syndrome; Granuloma annulare; Grover's Disease; Holt Oram Syndrome; Hyperostosis Frontalis Interna;

Hypophosphatasia; Ichthyosis; Ichthyosis Vulgaris; Ichthyosis, Erythrokeratodermia Progressiva Symmetrica; Ichthyosis, Erythrokeratodermia Variabilis; Ichthyosis, Erythrokeratolysis Hiemalis; Ichthyosis, Keratosis Follicularis Spinulosa Decalvans; Ichthyosis, Lamellar Recessive; Ichthyosis, Netherton Syndrome; Ichthyosis, Sjogren Larsson Syndrome; Ichthyosis, Tay Syndrome; Kearns Sayre Syndrome (KSS); Keratitis Ichthyosis Deafness Syndrome; Keratosis, Seborrheic; Kienbock Disease; Klippel Feil Syndrome; LADD Syndrome; Larsen Syndrome; Leiner Disease; Lupus; Lyelles Syndrome; Lyme Disease; Maffucci Syndrome; Marfan Syndrome; Marinesco Sjogren Syndrome; Mastocytosis; McCune Albright Syndrome; Myositis, Inclusion Body; Myotonia Congenita; Oculo Dento Digital Dysplasia; Osgood Schlatter's Disease; Osteopetrosis; Paget's Disease; Panniculitis, Idiopathic Nodular; Paramyotonia Congenita; Parsonage Turner Syndrome; Peeling Skin Syndrome; Pemphigoid, Benign Mucosal; Pemphigus; Poland Syndrome; Polychondritis; Proteus Syndrome; Prune Belly Syndrome; Psoriasis; Pyoderma Gangrenosum; Rapp Hodgkins Syndrome; Reflex Sympathetic Dystrophy Syndrome (RSDS); Reiter's Syndrome; Rothmund Thomson Syndrome; Scleroderma; Sjogren Syndrome; Split Hand Deformity; Sweet Syndrome; Tarsal Tunnel Syndrome; Tietze Syndrome; Xeroderma Pigmentosum; Yellow Nail Syndrome

2010 NIH/NATIONAL CANCER INSTITUTE

Office of Cancer Communications
Building 31 Rm 10A16
9000 Rockville Pike
Bethesda, MD 20892 301-496-5583
800-422-6237
http://www.nci.nih.gov/

Concerned with the following diseases or disorders:
Alopecia Areata; Beckwith Wiedemann Syndrome; Brain Tumors, General; Bullous Pemphigoid; Cancer, Breast; Cancer, Prostate; Cancers, Skin, General; Candidiasis; Chromosome 13, Partial Monosomy 13q; Epidermolysis Bullosa; Hodgkin's Disease; Pemphigus; Pseudomyxoma Peritonei

2011 NIH/NATIONAL CENTER FOR HUMAN GENOME RESEARCH (ELSI) ETHICAL LEGAL AND SOCIAL IMPLICATIONS BRANCH

Building 38A Rm 617
38 Library Dr MSC 6050
Bethesda, MD 20892-6050 301-402-4997
Fax: 301-402-1950
E-mail: ThomsonE@ODDER.NCHGR.NIH.GOV

2012 NIH/NATIONAL DIABETES INFORMATION CLEARINGHOUSE

1 Information Way
Bethesda, MD 20892-3560 301-654-3327
800-891-5388
Fax: 301-907-8906

Concerned with the following diseases or disorders:
Diabetes Insipidus; Diabetes, Insulin Dependent; Wolfram Syndrome

2013 NIH/NATIONAL DIGESTIVE DISEASES INFORMATION CLEARINGHOUSE

2 Information Way
Bethesda, MD 20892-3570 301-654-3810
800-891-5389
Fax: 301-907-8906

Concerned with the following diseases or disorders:
APECED Syndrome; Achalasia; Acidemia, Isovaleric; Acidemia, Methylmalonic; Acidemia, Propionic; Acrodermatitis Enteropathica; Addison's Disease; Alagille Syndrome; Arginase Deficiency; Arginino Succinic Aciduria; Banti's Syndrome; Barrett Esophagus; Blue Diaper Syndrome; Budd Chiari Syndrome; Carbamyl Phosphate Synthetase Deficiency; Carboxylase Deficiency, Multiple; Caroli Disease; Celiac Sprue; Cholangitis, Primary Sclerosing; Cholecystitis; Cirrhosis, Primary Biliary; Citrullinemia; Colitis, Collagenous; Colitis, Ulcerative; Crohn's Disease; Cronkhite Canada Disease; Cushing Syndrome; Cystic Fibrosis; Degos Disease; Diverticulitis; Diverticulosis; Dubin Johnson Syndrome; Edema, Idiopathic; Erythropoietic Protoporphyria (EPP); Forbes Disease; Fructose Intolerance, Hereditary; Galactosemia; Ganglioside Sialidase Deficiency; Gastritis, Giant Hypertrophic; Gastroesophageal Reflux; Gilbert Syndrome; Graves' Disease; Hashimoto's Syndrome; Hepatitis, Neonatal; Hirschsprung's Disease; Homocystinuria; Hurler Syndrome; Hyperchylomicronemia; Hyperoxaluria, Primary (Type I); Hypoglycemia; Hypoparathyroidism; Hypothyroidism; I Cell Disease; Imperforate Anus; Irritable Bowel Syndrome; Jejunal Atresia; Korsakoff's Syndrome; Lipodystrophy; Mannosidosis; Maple Syrup Urine Disease; Maroteaux Lamy Syndrome; McArdle Disease; Mediterranean Fever, Familial; Mesenteritis, Retractile; Morquio Syndrome; N-Acetyl Glutamate Synthetase Deficiency; Non-Ketotic Hyperglycinemia; Ornithine Transcarbamylase Deficiency; PEPCK Deficiency, Mitochondrial; Pancreatic Islet Cell Tumor; Peutz Jeghers Syndrome; Polyposis, Familial; Porphyria; Porphyria Cutanea Tarda; Porphyria, ALA-D; Porphyria, Acute Intermittent; Porphyria,

Congenital Erythropoietic; Porphyria, Hereditary Coproporphyria; Porphyria, Variegate; Proctitis; Prune Belly Syndrome; Pseudo Hurler Polydystrophy; Pseudohypoparathyroidism; Renal Glycosuria; Retroperitoneal Fibrosis; Rickets, Hypophosphatemic; Rickets, Vitamin D Deficiency; Sanfilippo Syndrome; Schmidt Syndrome; Sheehan Syndrome; Shwachman Syndrome; Sialidosis; Sly Syndrome; Sucrose Isomaltose Malabsorption, Congenital; Tarui Disease; Tropical Sprue; Vitamin B12 Deficiency; Vitamin E Deficiency; Waldmann Disease; Whipple's Disease

2014 **NIH/NATIONAL EYE INSTITUTE**

Building 31 Rm 6A32
31 Center Dr MSC 2510
Bethesda, MD 20892-2510 301-496-5248
Fax: 301-402-1065
E-mail: 2020@b31.nei.nih.gov
http://www.nei.nih.gov/

Concerned with the following diseases or disorders:
Ablepharon Macrostomia Syndrome; Adie Syndrome; Alstrom Syndrome; Aniridia; Aniridia Cerebellar Ataxia Mental Deficiency; Apraxia, Ocular Motor, Cogan Type; Behcet's Syndrome; Brown Syndrome; Cataract Dental Syndrome; Cataracts; Chalazion; Chandler's Syndrome; Choroideremia; Choroiditis, Serpiginous; Chromosome 13, Partial Monosomy 13q; Coats' Disease; Cogan Reese Syndrome; Cone Dystrophy; Congenital Varicella Syndrome; Conjunctivitis, Ligneous; Conradi Hunermann Syndrome; Corneal Dystrophy; Cytomegalovirus Infection; Devic Disease; Duane Syndrome; Eales Disease; Epitheliopathy, Acute Posterior Multifocal Placoid Pigment; Essential Iris Atrophy; Goldenhar Syndrome (Oculo Auriculo Vertebral Spectrum); Horner's Syndrome; Juberg Marsidi Syndrome; Kearns Sayre Syndrome (KSS); Keratitis Ichthyosis Deafness Syndrome; Keratoconjunctivitis, Vernal; Keratoconus; Keratomalacia; Leber's Congenital Amaurosis; Leber's Optic Atrophy; Lenz Microphthalmia Syndrome; Loken Senior Syndrome; Macular Degeneration; Macular Degeneration, Polymorphic; Marcus Gunn Phenomenon; Marshall Syndrome; Megalocornea Mental Retardation Syndrome; Mulibrey Nanism Syndrome (Perheentupa Syndrome); Mulvihill Smith Syndrome; Norrie Syndrome; Oculocerebral Syndrome with Hypopigmentation; Papillitis; Pars Planitis; Posterior Uveitis; Pseudoxanthoma Elasticum (PXE); Retinitis Pigmentosa; Retinoblastoma; Retinopathy, Arteriosclerotic; Retinopathy, Diabetic; Retinopathy, Hypertensive; Retinoschisis; Retrolental Fibroplasia; Rieger Syndrome; Rothmund Thomson Syndrome; SHORT Syndrome; Santavuori Disease; Schwartz Jampel Syndrome; Seitelberger Disease (Infantile Neuroaxonal Dystrophy); Stevens Johnson Syndrome; Stickler Syndrome; Toxocariasis; Usher's Syndrome; Vogt Koyanagi Harada Syndrome; Von Hippel Lindau Disease; WAGR Syndrome; Waardenburg Syndrome; Weill Marchesani Syndrome; Wildervanck Syndrome; Wolfram Syndrome; Wyburn Mason Syndrome; X-linked Juvenile Retinoschisis

2015 **NIH/NATIONAL HEART, LUNG AND BLOOD INSTITUTE**

31 Center Drive MSC 2480
Building 31A Rm 4A16
Bethesda, MD 20892-2480 301-594-1348
Fax: 301-480-4907
http://www.nhlbi.nih.gov/nhlbi/nhlbi.htm

Concerned with the following diseases or disorders:
Aase Syndrome; Alveolitis, Fibrosing; Anemia, Aplastic; Anemia, Blackfan Diamond; Anemia, Fanconi's; Anemia, Hereditary Nonspherocytic Hemolytic; Anemia, Hereditary Spherocytic Hemolytic; Anemia, Megaloblastic; Anemia, Pernicious; Angioedema, Hereditary; Antithrombin III Deficiency; Cor Triatriatum; Dilatation of the Pulmonary Artery, Idiopathic; Endocardial Fibroelastosis (EFE); Factor XIII Deficiency; Heart Block, Congenital; Hemangioma Thrombocytopenia Syndrome; Hemorrhagic Telangiectasia, Hereditary; Hypoplastic Left Heart Syndrome; Lymphedema, Hereditary; Maffucci Syndrome; Perniosis; Polycythemia Vera; Pure Red Cell Aplasia, Acquired; Pyruvate Kinase Deficiency; Thalassemia Minor; Vitamin B12 Deficiency; Waldenstrom Macroglobulinemia

2016 **NIH/NATIONAL HEART, LUNG AND BLOOD INSTITUTE INFORMATION CENTER**

P.O. Box 30105
Bethesda, MD 20824-0105 301-251-1222
Fax: 301-251-1223
E-mail: nhlbiic@dgsys.com

Concerned with the following diseases or disorders:
Afibrinogenemia, Congenital; Agranulocytosis, Acquired; Alpha-1-Antitrypsin Deficiency; Anemia, Hemolytic, Acquired Autoimmune; Anemia, Hemolytic, Cold Antibody; Anemia, Sideroblastic; Antiphospholipid Syndrome; Arteritis, Giant Cell; Arteritis, Takayasu; Atrial Septal Defects; Atrioventricular Septal Defect; Bernard Soulier Syndrome; Broad Beta Disease; Bronchopulmonary Dysplasia (BPD); Buerger's Disease; Cardio Auditory Syndrome; Castleman's Disease; Cat Eye Syndrome; Catel Manzke Syndrome; Cavernous Hemangioma; Cerebrocostomandibular Syndrome; Chromosome 10, Distal Trisomy 10q; Chromosome 11, Partial Monosomy 11q; Churg Strauss Syndrome; Conn Syndrome; Cryoglobulinemia, Essential Mixed; Dextrocardia with Situs Inversus; Dyskeratosis Congenita; Eisenmenger Syndrome; Emphysema, Congenital Lobar; Endocarditis, Infective; Factor IX Deficiency; Goldenhar Syndrome (Oculo Auriculo

Vertebral Spectrum); Goodman Syndrome; Graft versus Host Disease; Hageman Factor Deficiency; Hallervorden Spatz Disease; Hemophilia; Hiccups, Chronic; Histiocytosis X; Holt Oram Syndrome; Hyper IgM Syndrome; Hypercholesterolemia; Hyperlipoproteinemia Type IV; LEOPARD Syndrome; Lymphangioleiomyomatosis; May Hegglin Anomaly; McKusick Type Metaphyseal Chondrodysplasia; Mitral Valve Prolapse Syndrome; Myelofibrosis, Idiopathic; Myopathy, Desmin Storage; Neutropenia, Chronic; Neutropenia, Cyclic; Pneumonia, Interstitial; Pseudoxanthoma Elasticum (PXE); Pulmonary Alveolar Proteinosis; Pulmonary Hypertension,Primary; Pulmonary Hypertension, Secondary; Purpura, Henoch Schonlein; Purpura, Idiopathic Thrombocytopenic; Purpura, Thrombotic Thrombocytopenic; Raynaud's Disease and Phenomenon; Recurrent Respiratory Papillomatosis; Respiratory Distress Syndrome, Adult; Respiratory Distress Syndrome, Infant; Rh Disease; Romano Ward Syndrome; Shwachman Syndrome; Sickle Cell Disease; Singleton Merten Syndrome; Sneddon Syndrome; Tetralogy of Fallot; Thalassemia Major; Thrombasthenia of Glanzmann and Naegeli; Thrombocythemia, Essential; Thrombocytopenia Absent Radius Syndrome; Thrombocytopenia, Essential; Truncus Arteriosus, Persistent; Vasculitis; Vasculitis, Cutaneous Necrotizing; Ventricular Septal Defects; Von Willebrand Disease; Wegener's Granulomatosis; Wiskott Aldrich Syndrome; Wolff Parkinson White Syndrome; Wolfram Syndrome; Yellow Nail Syndrome; Yunis Varon Syndrome

2017 NIH/NATIONAL HUMAN GENOME RESEARCH INSTITUTE

9000 Rockville Pike
Building 31, Rm 4B09
Bethesda, MD 20892 301-402-0911
http://www.nhgri.nih.gov/

2018 NIH/NATIONAL INFORMATION CLEARINGHOUSE FOR INFANTS WITH DISABILITIES

University of South Carolina
Benson Building
Columbia, SC 29208
800-922-9234

2019 NIH/NATIONAL INSTITUTE OF ALLERGY AND INFECTIOUS DISEASES

9000 Rockville Pike
Building 31A
Bethesda, MD 20892 301-496-5717
Fax: 301-402-0120
http://www.niaid.nih.gov/

Concerned with the following diseases or disorders:
AIDS (Acquired Immune Deficiency Syndrome); AIDS Dysmorphic Syndrome; Acanthocheilonemiasis; Agammaglobulinemias, Primary; Alveolitis, Extrinsic Allergic; Anaphylaxis; Babesiosis; Balantidiasis; Bartonellosis; Bejel; Berylliosis; Blastomycosis; Botulism; Bubonic Plague; Candidiasis; Chagas Disease; Chediak Higashi Syndrome; Chikungunya; Cholera; Chronic Fatigue Syndrome; Colorado Tick Fever; Cowpox; Cryptococcosis; Cysticercosis; Cytomegalovirus Infection; Dengue Fever; Dracunculosis; Elephantiasis; Encephalitis, Herpetic; Encephalitis, Japanese; Encephalomyelitis, Myalgic; Enterobiasis; Fascioliasis; Filariasis; Gianotti Crosti Syndrome; Giardiasis; Granulomatous Disease, Chronic; Hand Foot Mouth Syndrome; Hepatitis B; Hepatitis, Non-A, Non-B (Hepatitis C); Herpes Zoster; Herpes, Neonatal; Hidradenitis Suppurativa; Ichthyosis Hystrix, Curth Macklin Type; Ichthyosis, CHILD Syndrome; Ichthyosis, Chanarin Dorfman Syndrome; Ichthyosis, Harlequin Type; Kawasaki Syndrome; Keratoconjunctivitis, Vernal; Kikuchi's Disease; Legionnaire's Disease; Leprosy; Leptospirosis; Listeriosis; Lymphadenopathy, Angioimmunoblastic with Dysproteinemia; Malaria; Measles; Meningitis; Meningitis, Meningococcal; Myelitis; Nezelof's Syndrome; Nocardiosis; Opportunistic Infections; Panniculitis, Idiopathic Nodular; Paracoccidioidomycosis; Pertussis; Pinta; Pneumonia, Eosinophilic; Polyarteritis Nodosa; Posterior Uveitis; Psittacosis; Purpura, Henoch Schonlein; Q Fever; Rheumatic Fever; Rocky Mountain Spotted Fever; Roseola Infantum; Rubella; Sarcoidosis; Severe Combined Immunodeficiency; Simian B Virus Infection; Stevens Johnson Syndrome; Subacute Sclerosing Panencephalitis; TORCH Syndrome; Toxic Shock Syndrome; Toxocariasis; Toxoplasmosis; Tuberculosis; Typhoid; Urticaria Pigmentosa; Urticaria, Cholinergic; Urticaria, Cold; Urticaria, Papular; Urticaria, Physical; Varicella Zoster; Vulvovaginitis; Weil Syndrome; Wiskott Aldrich Syndrome; X-Linked Lymphoproliferative Syndrome; Yaws; Yellow Fever

2020 NIH/NATIONAL INSTITUTE OF ARTHRITIS AND MUSCULOSKELETAL AND SKIN DISEASES

9000 Rockville Pike
Bethesda, MD 20892 301-496-8188
Fax: 301-587-4352
http://www.nih.gov/niams/

Concerned with the following diseases or disorders:
Ablepharon Macrostomia Syndrome; Acanthosis Nigricans; Arthritis, Infectious; Bjornstad Syndrome; Chondrocalcinosis, Familial Articular; Cochin Jewish Disorder; DOOR Syndrome; Dermatitis, Atopic;

Dermatomyositis; Diastrophic Dysplasia; Dysplasia, Fibrous; Dystrophy, Myotonic; Ear, Patella, Short Stature Syndrome; Ehlers Danlos Syndrome; Eosinophilia Myalgia; Erb's Palsy; Erythema Multiforme; Erythromelalgia; Fibromyalgia; Gorham's Disease; Hajdu Cheney Syndrome; Hay Well's Syndrome; Hermansky Pudlak Syndrome; Hidradenitis Suppurativa; Hyperhidrosis, Primary; Hypochondroplasia; Hypomelanosis of ITO; Ichthyosis, X-Linked; Incontinentia Pigmenti; Kohler Disease; Laband Syndrome; Legg Calve Perthes Disease; Leri Pleonosteosis; Lichen Planus; Lichen Sclerosus; Lymphocytic Infiltrate of Jessner; Maxillonasal Dysplasia, Binder Type; Mediterranean Fever, Familial; Mixed Connective Tissue Disease (MCTD); Myopathy, Scapuloperoneal; Ollier Disease; Osteogenesis Imperfecta; Pityriasis Rubra Pilaris; Polymyalgia Rheumatica; Pseudoxanthoma Elasticum (PXE); Rubinstein Taybi Syndrome; Russell Silver Syndrome (RSS); Sarcoidosis; Schinzel Syndrome; Setleis Syndrome; Singleton Merten Syndrome; Stenosis, Spinal; Stevens Johnson Syndrome; Tricho Dento Osseous Syndrome; Trichorhinophalangeal Syndrome Type I; Trichorhinophalangeal Syndrome Type II; Trichorhinophalangeal Syndrome Type III; Vitiligo; Wieacker Syndrome

2021 NIH/NATIONAL INSTITUTE OF CHILD HEALTH & HUMAN DEVELOPMENT (PREG & PERINAT)
Pregnancy and Perinatology Branch
6100 Executive Blvd Rm 4B03
Bethesda, MD 20892-7510 301-496-5575

Concerned with the following diseases or disorders:
Aspartylglycosaminuria; Carnitine Palmitoyltransferase Deficiency; Galloway Mowat Syndrome; McKusick Type Metaphyseal Chondrodysplasia; Myhre Syndrome; Spondyloepiphyseal Dysplasia, Congenital

2022 NIH/NATIONAL INSTITUTE OF CHILD HEALTH AND HUMAN DEVELOPMENT
9000 Rockville Pike
Building 31 Rm 2A32
MSC 2425
Bethesda, MD 20892 301-496-5133
Fax: 301-496-7101
http://www.nih.gov/nichd/

Concerned with the following diseases or disorders:
Aarskog Syndrome; Aase Syndrome; Acrodysostosis; Adrenal Hyperplasia, Congenital (General); Ahumada Del Castillo Syndrome; Albinism; Amenorrhea, Primary; Amniotic Bands; Anencephaly; Angelman Syndrome; Antley Bixler Syndrome; Apert Syndrome; Apnea, Infantile; Beckwith Wiedemann Syndrome; Bloom Syndrome; CHARGE Syndrome; Carnosinemia; Carpenter Syndrome; Cayler Syndrome; Cerebral Palsy; Cerebrocostomandibular Syndrome; Chiari Frommel Syndrome; Chromosome 10, Monosomy 10p; Chromosome 11, Partial Monosomy 11q; Chromosome 18, Monosomy 18p; Chromosome 18, Tetrasomy 18p; Chromosome 3, Trisomy 3q2; Chromosome 7, Monosomy 7p2; Chromosome 8, Monosomy 8p2; Chromosome 9, Partial Monosomy 9p; Chromosome 9, Trisomy Mosaic; Clubfoot; Cockayne Syndrome; Coffin Siris Syndrome; Cornelia de Lange Syndrome; Cri du Chat Syndrome; Crouzon Disease; Dextrocardia with Situs Inversus; DiGeorge Syndrome; Down Syndrome; Dubowitz Syndrome; Dysplasia, Epiphysealis Hemimelica; Dystrophy, Asphyxiating Thoracic; Endomyocardial Fibrosis; Fairbank Disease; Forbes Albright Syndrome; Goldenhar Syndrome (Oculo Auriculo Vertebral Spectrum); Gottron's Syndrome; Greig Cephalopolysyndactyly Syndrome; Hallermann Streiff Syndrome; Hermaphroditism, True; Holt Oram Syndrome; Hutchinson Gilford Progeria Syndrome; Ichthyosis Congenita; Jarcho Levin Syndrome; KBG Syndrome; Kenny Caffe Syndrome; Kernicterus; Klinefelter Syndrome; Klippel Feil Syndrome; LEOPARD Syndrome; Larsen Syndrome; Laurence Moon Syndrome; Lowe's Syndrome; Meckel Syndrome; Melnick Needles Syndrome; Noonan Syndrome; Pallister Killian Mosaic Syndrome; Pfeiffer Syndrome; Phocomelia Syndrome; Pierre Robin Syndrome; Polymyositis; Prader Willi Syndrome; Precocious Puberty; Rh Disease; Roberts Syndrome; Robinow Syndrome; Rubella, Congenital; Rubinstein Taybi Syndrome; Saethre Chotzen Syndrome; Seckel Syndrome; Sirenomelia Sequence; Smith Lemli Opitz Syndrome; Sotos Syndrome; Spondyloepiphyseal Dysplasia Tarda; Stein Levanthal Syndrome; Tay Sachs Disease; Telecanthus with Associated Abnormalities; Tethered Spinal Cord Syndrome; Tooth and Nail Syndrome; Treacher Collins Syndrome; Trichorhinophalangeal Syndrome Type I; Triploid Syndrome; Trisomy 13 Syndrome; Trisomy 18 Syndrome; Turner Syndrome; VACTERL Association; Wiedemann Rautenstrauch Syndrome; Williams Syndrome; Wolf Hirschhorn Syndrome

2023 NIH/NATIONAL INSTITUTE OF DENTAL RESEARCH
31 Center Dr MSC 2290
Building 31 Rm 2C35
Bethesda, MD 20892-2290 301-496-4261
Fax: 301-496-9988
http://www.nidr.nih.gov/

Concerned with the following diseases or disorders:
Cataract Dental Syndrome; Cochin Jewish Disorder; Gorlin Chaudhry Moss Syndrome; Johanson Blizzard Syndrome; Laband Syndrome; Papillon Lefevre Syndrome; Rothmund Thomson Syndrome; Tooth and Nail Syndrome

2024 **NIH/NATIONAL INSTITUTE OF DIABETES, DIGESTIVE & KIDNEY DISEASES**

Endocrine Diseases Metabolic Diseases Branch
Building 31 Rm 9A04
31 Center Dr
Bethesda, MD 20892 301-496-3583
Fax: 301-496-7422

Concerned with the following diseases or disorders:
Aspartylglycosaminuria; Carnitine Palmitoyltransferase Deficiency; Cytochrome C Oxidase Deficiency; Fructosuria; Hers Disease; Histidinemia; Hyperprolinemia Type I; Hyperprolinemia Type II; Hypoglycemia; Medium Chain Acyl CoA Dehydrogenase Deficiency; Phosphoglycerate Kinase Deficiency; Pyruvate Carboxylase Deficiency; Short Chain Acyl CoA Dehydrogenase Deficiency (SCAD); Valinemia; Von Gierke Disease

2025 **NIH/NATIONAL INSTITUTE OF DIABETES, DIGESTIVE AND KIDNEY DISEASES**

Building 31 Rm 9A04
31 Center Dr
Bethesda, MD 20892-2560 301-496-3583
Fax: 301-496-7422

Concerned with the following diseases or disorders:
ACTH Deficiency; Acanthocytosis; Achard Thiers Syndrome; Andersen Disease; Bartter's Syndrome; Biliary Atresia, Extrahepatic; Branchio Oto Renal Syndrome; Burning Mouth Syndrome; Carnitine Deficiency Syndromes; Cholestasis; Conn Syndrome; Dercum Disease; Gardner Syndrome; Gastritis, Chronic, Erosive; Glucose-6-Phosphate Dehydrogenase Deficiency; Glycogen Storage Disease VIII; Hartnup Disease; Hemochromatosis, Hereditary; Hemolytic Uremic Syndrome; Hunter Syndrome; Hypokalemia; Intestinal Pseudoobstruction; Kernicterus; Lactose Intolerance; Leprechaunism; Madelung's Disease; Microvillus Inclusion Disease; Mucopolysaccharidosis; Pica; Polycystic Liver Disease; Pompe Disease; Renal Agenesis, Bilateral; Tyrosinemia, Hereditary; Zollinger Ellison Syndrome

2026 **NIH/NATIONAL INSTITUTE OF ENVIRONMENTAL HEALTH SCIENCES**

Public Affairs Office
P.O. Box 12233
Resrch Triangle Prk, NC 27709 919-541-3345
Fax: 919-541-4395

2027 **NIH/NATIONAL INSTITUTE OF ENVIRONMENTAL HEALTH SCIENCES CLEARINGHOUSE**

EnviroHealth
2605 Meridian Parkway Ste 115
Durham, NC 27713 919-361-9408
800-643-4794

Concerned with the following diseases or disorders:
Alveolitis, Extrinsic Allergic; Berylliosis; Formaldehyde Poisoning; Heavy Metal Poisoning; Mountain Sickness, Acute

2028 **NIH/NATIONAL INSTITUTE OF GENERAL MEDICAL SCIENCES**

45 Center Dr MSC 6200
Bethesda, MD 20892-6200 301-496-7301
Fax: 301-402-0224

Concerned with the following diseases or disorders:
Malignant Hyperthermia; Pseudocholinesterase Deficiency

2029 **NIH/NATIONAL INSTITUTE OF MENTAL HEALTH**

5600 Fishers Lane
Rockville, MD 20857-8030 301-443-4513
http://www.nimh.nih.gov/

Concerned with the following diseases or disorders:
Anorexia Nervosa; Antisocial Personality Disorder; Attention Deficit Hyperactivity Disorder; Autism; Bulimia; Conversion Disorder; Depersonalization Disorder; Dysthymia; Fetal Alcohol Syndrome; Kleine Levin Syndrome; Manic Depression, Bipolar; Mutism, Selective; Neurasthenia; Neuroleptic Malignant Syndrome; Obsessive Compulsive Disorder; Organic Mood Syndrome; Panic Anxiety Syndrome; Pica; Tardive Dyskinesia; Trichotillomania; XYY Syndrome

2030 **NIH/NATIONAL INSTITUTE OF MENTAL HEALTH (DEPRESSION HOTLINE)**

800-421-4211

Concerned with the following diseases or disorders:
Dysthymia; Manic Depression, Bipolar

2031 NIH/NATIONAL INSTITUTE OF NEUROLOGICAL DISORDERS AND STROKE

31 Center Dr MSC 2540
Building 31 Rm 8A16
Bethesda, MD 20892 301-496-5751
800-352-9424
Fax: 301-402-2186
http://www.ninds.nih.gov/

Concerned with the following diseases or disorders:
Adrenoleukodystrophy; Agenesis of Corpus Callosum; Aicardi Syndrome; Alexander's Disease; Alzheimer's Disease; Amyotrophic Lateral Sclerosis; Apnea, Infantile; Apnea, Sleep; Arachnoiditis; Arnold Chiari Syndrome; Arteriovenous Malformation; Astrocytoma, Malignant; Ataxia Telangiectasia; Ataxia, Friedreich's; Ataxia, Marie's; Autism; Balo Disease; Batten Disease; Bell's Palsy; Benign Essential Tremor; Blepharospasm, Benign Essential; Carpal Tunnel Syndrome; Central Core Disease; Central Hypoventilation Syndrome, Congenital; Cerebral Palsy; Charcot Marie Tooth Disease; Coffin Lowry Syndrome; Creutzfeldt Jakob Disease; Cryptococcosis; Dandy Walker Malformation; Dejerine Sottas Disease; Dysautonomia, Familial; Dyslexia; Dystonia, Torsion; Dystrophy, Myotonic; Encephalitis, Herpetic; Encephalitis, Rasmussen's; Epilepsy; Fabry Disease; Frey's Syndrome; Froelich's Syndrome; Gaucher Disease; Guillain Barre Syndrome; Huntington's Disease; Hydranencephaly; Hydrocephalus; Hypotonia, Benign Congenital; Joseph's Disease; Joubert Syndrome; Jumping Frenchmen of Maine; Kufs Disease; Landau Kleffner Syndrome; Laurence Moon Syndrome; Leigh's Disease; Leukodystrophy, Canavan's; Leukodystrophy, Krabbe's; Leukodystrophy, Metachromatic; Meige Syndrome; Muscular Dystrophy, Duchenne; Myasthenia Gravis; Myoclonus, General; Myopathy, Congenital, Batten Turner Type; Myotonia Congenita; Narcolepsy; Nemaline Myopathy; Neurofibromatosis Type 1 (NF-1); Neuropathy, Peripheral; Niemann Pick Disease; Nystagmus, Benign Paroxysmal Positional; Paraplegia, Hereditary Spastic; Parkinson's Disease; Pelizaeus Merzbacher Brain Sclerosis; Phenylketonuria; Progressive Supranuclear Palsy; Pyruvate Dehydrogenase Deficiency; Refsum Syndrome; Rett Syndrome; Reye Syndrome; Sandhoff Disease; Schindler Disease; Seitelberger Disease (Infantile Neuroaxonal Dystrophy); Shy Drager Syndrome; Spasmodic Torticollis; Spina Bifida; Stiff Man Syndrome; Sturge Weber Syndrome; Sudden Infant Death Syndrome; Syringobulbia; TORCH Syndrome; Tangier Disease; Tay Sachs Disease; Tetrahydrobiopterin Deficiency; Tolosa Hunt Syndrome; Tourette Syndrome; Trigeminal Neuralgia (Tic Douloureux); Tuberous Sclerosis; Werdnig Hoffman Disease; Wiedemann Rautenstrauch Syndrome; Wilson's Disease; Zellweger Syndrome

2032 NIH/NATIONAL INSTITUTE ON AGING

PO Box 8057
Gaithersburg, MD 20892-8057 301-496-1752
800-222-2225

Concerned with the following diseases or disorders:
Alzheimer's Disease; Binswanger's Disease; Cerebellar Degeneration, Subacute; Fragile X Syndrome; Hyperthermia; Pick's Disease; Werner Syndrome

2033 NIH/NATIONAL INSTITUTE ON DEAFNESS AND OTHER COMMUNICATION DISORDERS (BALANCE)

National Temporal Bone Hearing
and Balance Pathology Resource Registry
243 Charles Street
Boston, MA 02114-3096 617-573-3711
800-822-1327
Fax: 617-573-3838
TDD: 617-573-3888

Concerned with the following diseases or disorders:
Acoustic Neuroma; Alstrom Syndrome; Dysphonia, Chronic Spasmodic; Kluver Bucy Syndrome; Landau Kleffner Syndrome; Meniere Disease; Neurofibromatosis Type 2 (NF-2); Patulous Eustachian Tube; Tinnitus; Usher's Syndrome

2034 NIH/NATIONAL INSTITUTE ON DEAFNESS AND OTHER COMMUNICATION DISORDERS INFORMATION CLEARINGHOUSE

1 Communication Avenue
Bethesda, MD 20892-3456 301-907-8830
800-241-1044
Fax: 301-907-8830
TDD: 800-241-1105
E-mail: NIDCD@AERIE.COM
http://www.nih.gov/nidcd/

Concerned with the following diseases or disorders:
Allan Herndon Syndrome; Autism; Bjornstad Syndrome; Cerebrocostomandibular Syndrome; Chromosome 11, Partial Monosomy 11q; Cornelia de Lange Syndrome; Ear, Patella, Short Stature Syndrome; Fountain Syndrome; Jansen Type Metaphyseal Chondrodysplasia; Juberg Marsidi Syndrome; MASA Syndrome; Treacher Collins Syndrome; Trichorhinophalangeal Syndrome Type II

2035 **NIH/NATIONAL INSTITUTE ON DRUG ABUSE**
5600 Fischer Lane
Rockville, MD 20857 301-443-1124
800-729-6686

2036 **NIH/NATIONAL INSTITUTES OF HEALTH, MAIN OFFICE**
9000 Rockville Pike
Bldg 10
Bethesda, MD 20892 301-496-4000

2037 **NIH/NATIONAL KIDNEY AND UROLOGIC DISEASES INFORMATION CLEARINGHOUSE**
3 Information Way
Bethesda, MD 20892-3580 301-651-4415
800-891-5390
Fax: 301-907-8906

Concerned with the following diseases or disorders:
Alport Syndrome; Carcinoma, Renal Cell; Chromosome 10, Distal Trisomy 10q; Cystinosis; Exstrophy of the Bladder; Galloway Mowat Syndrome; Goodpasture Syndrome; Hematuria, Benign, Familial; Hepatic Fibrosis, Congenital; Hepatorenal Syndrome; IGA Nephropathy; Interstitial Cystitis; Loken Senior Syndrome; MURCS Association; Medullary Cystic Disease; Medullary Sponge Kidney; Mullerian Aplasia; Nail Patella Syndrome; Ochoa Syndrome; Peyronie Disease; Polycystic Kidney Diseases; Prostatitis

2038 **NIH/NATIONAL ORAL HEALTH INFORMATION CLEARINGHOUSE**
1 NOHIC Way
Bethesda, MD 20892-3500 301-402-7364
Fax: 301-907-8830
TDD: 301-656-7581
E-mail: nidr@aerie.com
http://www.aerie.com/nohicweb/

Concerned with the following diseases or disorders:
Ameloblastoma; Amelogenesis Imperfecta; Anodontia; Burning Mouth Syndrome; Cleft Palate and Cleft Lip; Dentin Dysplasia, Coronal; Dentin Dysplasia, Radicular; Dentinogenesis Imperfecta Type III; Ectodermal Dysplasias; Focal Dermal Hypoplasia; Macroglossia; Mikulicz Syndrome; Oculo Dento Digital Dysplasia; Oral Facial Digital Syndrome; Parry Romberg Syndrome; Sialadenitis; Sjogren Syndrome; Sutton's Disease II; Temporomandibular Joint Dysfunction (TMJ); Tongue, Fissured; Tongue, Geographic; Tongue, Hairy; Tooth and Nail Syndrome; Tricho Dento Osseous Syndrome; Trigeminal Neuralgia (Tic Douloureux); Velocardiofacial Syndrome; Waardenburg Syndrome

2039 **NIH/NATIONAL SOCIETY FOR CHILDREN AND ADULTS WITH AUTISM**
1234 Massachusetts Ave.
Suite 1017
Washington, DC 20005

Concerned with the following diseases or disorders:
Autism

2040 **NIH/OFFICE OF ALTERNATIVE MEDICINE**
9000 Rockville Pike MSC 2182
Building 31 Rm 5B38
Bethesda, MD 20892 301-402-4741
800-531-1794

2041 **NIH/OFFICE OF RARE DISEASES**
Steve Groft, Pharm.D.
31 Center Drive, MSC 2082
Room 1B03
Bethesda, MD 20892-2082 301-402-4336
Fax: 301-402-0420
E-mail: sg18b@nih.gov
http://rarediseases.info.nih.gov/ord/

The Office of Rare Diseases was established in 1993 within the Office of the Director (OD), National Institutes of Health (NIH), to respond to the reporting requirements on the Orphan Drug Act; to implement the recommendations of the National Commission on Orphan Diseases; and to respond to requests for information on rare diseases. The Office of Rare Diseases develops and maintains a centralized database on rare disease clinical research supported by the NIH; stimulates rare disease research by supporting scientific workshops and symposia to identify such research opportunities; responds to requests for information on highly technical matters and matters of public policy relative to rare diseases and orphan products; provides information to the Office of the Director, NIH, on matters relating to rare diseases and orphan products; coordinates and serves as a liaison with Federal and non-Federal national and international organizations concerned with rare disease research and orphan products development; and prepares the NIH Director's annual report to Congress on rare disease and condition research activities sponsored by NIH. The Office of Rare Diseases also provides a web site on the Internet to help meet the need for up-to-date, accurate information frequently requested by patients and their family members or caregivers, health care providers, and research investigators. The site provides information on rare diseases and conditions; ongoing or planned research including clinical trials; and support services provided by voluntary health organizations. This site provides links to disease-specific information; to searchable databases that provide information on clinical studies; and to other government and non-government home pages and other voluntary health organizations that provide information and support services.

Year Established: 1993

2042 NIH/OFFICE OF RECOMBINANT DNA ACTIVITIES

Building 31
Room 4B11
Bethesda, MD 20892

2043 NIH/OFFICE OF RESEARCH ON WOMEN'S HEALTH (ORWH)

9000 Rockville Pike
Building 1, Rm 201
Bethesda, MD 20892 301-402-1770
Fax: 301-402-1798
http://ohrm.od.nih.gov/orwh/index.html

The NIH/Office of Research on Women's Health (ORWH) serves as a focal point for women's health research at the National Institutes of Health (NIH) in setting and monitoring policy, promoting and directing research, and enhancing scientific career development. Established in 1990 within the Office of the Director of the NIH, ORWH works in partnership with the NIH Institutes, Centers, and Divisions (ICDs) to ensure that women's health research becomes an integral part of the scientific fabric at NIH and throughout the scientific community. ORWH has a threefold mandate: to strengthen and enhance research related to diseases, disorders, and conditions that affect women and to ensure that research conducted and supported by the NIH adequately addresses issues regarding women's health; to ensure that women are adequately represented in biomedical and behavioral research studies supported by NIH; and to develop opportunities and support for recruitment, retention, reentry, and advancement of women in biomedical careers. Using its threefold mandate as a basis for action, ORWH is focusing its efforts in the major following areas: Implementation of a Research Agenda for Women's Health in collaboration with the NIH (ICDs); Recruitment and Retention of Women in Clinical Studies; Implementation of a Tracking System and Other Activities to Monitor the Inclusion of Women in NIH-Supported Biomedical and Behavioral Research; Recruitment, Retention, Reentry, and Advancement of Women in Biomedical Careers; and Policy Development Activities including Legal and Ethical Issues Associated with Inclusion of Women in Clinical Studies, Women's Health Curriculum in Medical Academic and Clinical Training, and Collaboration on the "NIH Women's Health Initiative," a prevention study to examine the major causes of death, disability, and frailty in postmenopausal women of all races and socioeconomic strata. The ORWH has a web site on the Internet at [http://ohrm.od.nih.gov/orwh/index.html].

Year Established: 1990

Concerned with the following diseases or disorders:
Cancer, Breast

2044 NIH/PATIENT REFERRAL SERVICES UNIT

Warren Grant Magnuson Clinical Center
Patient Referral and Recruitment Center
Quarters 15 D-2
Bethesda, MD 20892 301-496-4891
800-411-1222
E-mail: prrc@cc.nih.gov
http://www.cc.nih.gov/

Executive Director: Elaine Robinovitz

Concerned with the following diseases or disorders:
Ataxia Telangiectasia; Brain Tumors, General; Carcinoma, Renal Cell; Fibromatosis, Congenital Generalized; Gardner Syndrome; Glioblastoma Multiforme; Leukemia, Chronic Lymphocytic;

Leukemia, Hairy Cell; Leukodystrophy, Canavan's; Leukodystrophy, Krabbe's; Lynch Syndromes; Maffucci Syndrome; Medulloblastoma; Meningioma; Myeloma, Multiple; Panniculitis, Idiopathic Nodular; Peutz Jeghers Syndrome; Polyposis, Familial; Von Hippel Lindau Disease; Waldenstrom Macroglobulinemia; Williams Syndrome

2045 NATIONAL CANCER INSTITUTE PHYSICIAN DATA QUERY (PDQ) CANCER INFORMATION SERVICE
9000 Rockville Pike
Bethesda, MD 20892
800-422-6237
http://cancernet.nci.nih.gov/trials

2046 NATIONAL CENTER FOR HEALTH STATISTICS
6525 Belcrest Road
Hyattsville, MD 20782 301-436-8500
Fax: 301-436-3796
E-mail: nhicinfo@health.org

2047 NATIONAL CLEARINGHOUSE FOR ALCOHOL AND DRUG INFORMATION (NCADI)
11426 Rockville Pike
Suite 200
Rockville, MD 20852-3007 301-468-2600
800-729-6686
Fax: 301-468-6433
TDD: 800-487-4889
E-mail: info@health.org
http://www.health.org

Executive Director: John Noble
Organization Language: Spanish (written/spoken).
Year Established: 1987
Organization Members: Non-Membership

Publishes the following materials:
Life is a journey. Help your child choose wisely ~ *Brochure*
How Not To Get High, Get Stupid, Get Aids. A Guide To Partying ~ *Brochure*
Drugs and Alcohol in the Work Place (Spanish) ~ *Brochure*
Tips For Teens About Smoking ~ *Brochure*
Tips For Teens About Inhalants ~ *Brochure*
Tips For Teens About Crack and Cocaine ~ *Brochure*
Tips For Teens About Alcohol ~ *Brochure*
Tipis For Teens About Aids ~ *Brochure*
How getting High Can Get You Aids ~ *Brochure*
How to Cut Down on Your Drinking ~ *Brochure*
Healthy Women/Healthy Lifestyles: What you need to know about alcohol and illicit drugs ~ *Leaflet*
Your Body. Your Life. Your Choice. Choose Wisely. ~ *Brochure*
Tips For Teens About Steroids ~ *Brochure*
Moving forward with your life! ~ *Leaflet*
Say "NO"! Stay Smart! Don't Start! (Spanish) ~ *Brochure*
Publications Catalog ~ *Catalog*

2048 NATIONAL CLEARINGHOUSE FOR PRIMARY CARE INFORMATION
2070 Chain Bridge Road
Suite 450
Vienna, VA 22182 703-821-8955
Fax: 703-821-2098

2049 NATIONAL CLEARINGHOUSE ON FAMILY SUPPORT AND CHILDREN'S MENTAL HEALTH
P.O. Box 751
Portland, OR 97207-0751 503-725-4040
800-628-1696
Fax: 503-725-4180
TDD: 503-725-4165

2050 NATIONAL CLEARINGHOUSE ON POSTSECONDARY EDUCATION FOR INDIVIDUALS WITH DISABILITIES (HEATH)
1 Dupont Circle NW
Suite 800
Washington, DC 20036-1193 202-939-9320
800-544-3284
Fax: 202-833-4760
E-mail: heath@ace.nche.edu

2051 NATIONAL COUNCIL ON DISABILITY
1331 F Street
NW
Suite 1050
Washington, DC 20004-1107 202-272-2004
Fax: 202-205-2022
TDD: 202-272-2074

2052 **NATIONAL INSTITUTE FOR OCCUPATIONAL SAFETY AND HEALTH (NIOSH)**

Washington Office (Headquarters)
200 Independence Avenue, SW
Washington, DC 20201
800-356-4674
E-mail: pubstaft@cdc.gov
http://www.cdc.gov/niosh/homepage.html

The National Institute for Occupational Safety and Health (NIOSH) is a federal agency established by the Occupational Safety and Health Act of 1970. NIOSH, a part of the Centers for Disease Control and Prevention (CDC) and the Department of Health and Human Services, is a research agency responsible for identifying the causes of work-related diseases and injuries and the potential hazards of new work technologies and practices. With this information, NIOSH determines new and effective ways to protect workers from chemicals, machinery, and hazardous working conditions. The Institute's responsibilities include investigating potentially hazardous working conditions as requested by employers or employees; evaluating hazards in the workplace; creating and disseminating methods for preventing disease, injury, and disability; and conducting research and providing scientifically valid recommendations for protecting workers. NIOSH has a web site on the Internet that provides information on NIOSH activities in all states within the United States; NIOSH database information; a searchable NIOSH directory; NIOSH publications; "What's New at NIOSH," which enables online users to read full-text press releases (listed by month and year) on topics ranging from preventing work-related latex allergies to surveillance reports on work-related lung disease; a compendium of occupational and environmental questionnaires; information concerning ergonomics; dynamic linkage to additional, helpful sources of information on the Web; and more.

President: Linda Rosenstock, M.D., M.P.H. (Director)
Executive Director: William Halperin, M.D., M.P.H. (Deputy Director)
Year Established: 1970

2053 **NATIONAL LIBRARY SERVICE FOR THE BLIND AND PHYSICALLY HANDICAPPED**

Library of Congress
1291 Taylor Street
NW
Washington, DC 20542 202-707-5100
Fax: 202-707-0712
TDD: 202-707-0744

2054 **NATIONAL MATERNAL AND CHILD HEALTH CLEARINGHOUSE (NMCHC)**

2070 Chain Bridge Road
Suite 450
Vienna, VA 22181-2536 703-356-1964
Fax: 703-821-2098
E-mail: nmchc@circsol.com
http://www.circsol.com/mch

The National Maternal and Child Health Clearinghouse distributes informational materials developed by the Federal Maternal and Child Health Bureau (MCHB) or its grantees. MCHB is an agency within the Health Resources and Services Administration (HRSA), U.S. Department of Health and Human Services (DHHS). The Clearinghouse also provides referrals to other organizations that offer information and support to affected mothers and children. The Clearinghouse responds to requests for information from health care professionals, program planners, educators, researchers, policy makers, and the general public. Most of the educational materials distributed by the Clearinghouse are written for professionals; however, it also distributes materials written for the public. Subject areas include adolescent health, perinatal and infant health, breastfeeding and nutrition, children with special health needs, emergency medical services for children, violence and injury prevention, and other topics that comprise the broad area of maternal and child health.

Executive Director: Linda Cramer
Organization Language: Spanish.
Year Established: 1981

Publishes the following materials:

Maternal and Child Health 1994 Publications Catalog ~ *Catalog*
Equals in This Partnership ~ *Booklet*
Understanding DNA Testing ~ *Booklet*
Starting Point... ~ *Book*
Technology-Dependent Children: Hospital vs. Home Care ~ *Book*
Project SPOON: Special Program of Oral Nutrition for

Children with Special Needs ~ *Book*
Family/Professional Collaboration ~ *Book*
Dear Colleague: ~ *Survey Results*
EPSDT A Guide For Educational Programs ~ *Program Guide*
Thalassemia Among Asians - Vietnamese ~ *Brochure*
Thalassemia Among Asians - Korean ~ *Brochure*
Thalassemia Among Asians - English ~ *Brochure*
Thalassemia Among Asians - Laotian ~ *Brochure*
Newborn Screening For Sickle Cell Disease: Issues And Implications ~ *Book*
A Parents' Handbook for Sickle Cell Disease Part I ~ *Book*
Problem Oriented Management of Sickle Syndromes ~ *Book*
Pediatric Home Care ~ *Book*
A Reader's Guide for Parents of Children With Mental, Physical, or Emotional Disabilities ~ *Book*
Koneksyon Familial ~ *Brochure*
Thalassemia Among Asians - Tagalog ~ *Brochure*
Reaching Out to Culturally Diverse Hemophilia Populations ~ *Book*
Nutrition Services for Children with Special Health Needs ~ *Book*

Concerned with the following diseases or disorders:
Congenital Varicella Syndrome

2055 NATIONAL NEUROLOGICAL RESEARCH SPECIMEN BANK (NNRSB OR BRAIN BANK)
West Los Angeles VA Medical Center
11301 Wilshire Boulevard
Building 212
Room 16
Los Angeles, CA 90073 310-268-3536
Fax: 310-268-4768
E-mail: wourtel@ucla.edu.

President: W.W. Tourtellotte, M.D., Ph.D. (Director)
Executive Director: Iris P. Rosario, R.N., M.A. (Assistant Director)
Year Established: 1961
Organization Members: 2,000

Publishes the following materials:
Human Neuro-Specimen Banking ~ *Mission Statement*
Gift of Hope ~ *Donor Packet*
Human Neurospecimen Bank for Epilepsy ~ *Brochure*
National Neurological Research Specimen Bank. "A Gift of Hope" ~ *Brochure*
Multiple Sclerosis Human Neurospecimen Bank ~ *Brochure*
National Neurological Research Specimen Bank ~ *Brochure*

2056 OFFICE OF FAIR HOUSING AND EQUAL OPPORTUNITY
Department of Housing and Urban Development
820 1st Street
NE
Suite 420
Washington, DC 20002 202-275-0848
Fax: 202-275-0779
TDD: 202-275-0772

2057 OFFICE OF MINORITY HEALTH RESOURCE CENTER
P.O. Box 37337
Washington, DC 20013-7337
800-444-6472
Fax: 301-589-0884
TDD: 301-589-0951

2058 OFFICE OF SPECIAL EDUCATION AND REHABILITATIVE SERVICES (OSERS)
United States Department of Education
Switzer Building
330 C Street
SW
Washington, DC 20202 202-272-2004
Fax: 202-205-9252
TDD: 202-205-8241

2059 PRESIDENT'S COMMITTEE ON EMPLOYMENT OF PEOPLE WITH DISABILITIES
1331 F Street, NW
3rd Floor
Washington, DC 20004 202-376-6200
Fax: 202-376-6219
TDD: 202-376-6205

2060 PRESIDENT'S COMMITTEE ON MENTAL RETARDATION
Wilbur J. Cohen Building
Room 5325
330 Independence Avenue
SW
Washington, DC 20201 202-619-0634
Fax: 202-205-9519

2061 SKIN DISEASE RESEARCH CORE CENTERS OF THE NATIONAL INSTITUTE OF ARTHRITIS
Emory University School of Medicine
S. Wright Caughman, M.D.
Department of Dermatology
1639 Pierce Drive, Room 5001 WMB
Atlanta, GA 30322 404-727-5872

Concerned with the following diseases or disorders:
Bullous Pemphigoid; De Santis Cacchione Syndrome; Hyperhidrosis, Primary; Lichen Planus; Mucha Habermann Disease; Sweet Syndrome

2062 SOCIAL SECURITY ADMINISTRATION
6401 Security Boulevard
Baltimore, MD 21235 410-965-7700
800-772-1213
Fax: 410-965-0695
TDD: 800-325-0778

2063 U.S DEPT. OF HHS/ADMINISTRATION ON DEVELOPMENTAL DISABILITIES
United States Department of Health and Human Services
HHH Building Room 329D
200 Independence Avenue
SW
Washington, DC 20201 202-690-6590
Fax: 202-690-6904
TDD: 202-690-6415

2064 U.S. DEPARTMENT OF THE INTERIOR
National Park Service
P.O. Box 37127
Washington, DC 20013-7127 202-208-4747
Fax: 202-219-0910

2065 U.S. RESOURCE CENTER ON SUBSTANCE ABUSE
1819 L Street
NW
Suite 300
Washington, DC 20036 202-628-8080
Fax: 202-628-3812
TDD: 202-638-5862

Name and Keyword Index

Name and Keyword Index

A

Name and Keyword Index

Name and Keyword Index

Name and Keyword Index

Name and Keyword Index

B

Name and Keyword Index

C

Name and Keyword Index

Name and Keyword Index

Name and Keyword Index

Name and Keyword Index

D

Name and Keyword Index

E

Name and Keyword Index

F

Name and Keyword Index

G

Name and Keyword Index

H

Name and Keyword Index

I

Name and Keyword Index

J

K

Name and Keyword Index

L

M

Name and Keyword Index

Name and Keyword Index

Name and Keyword Index

O

Name and Keyword Index

Q

R

S

Name and Keyword Index

T

Name and Keyword Index

Name and Keyword Index

U

V

W

X

Y

Z